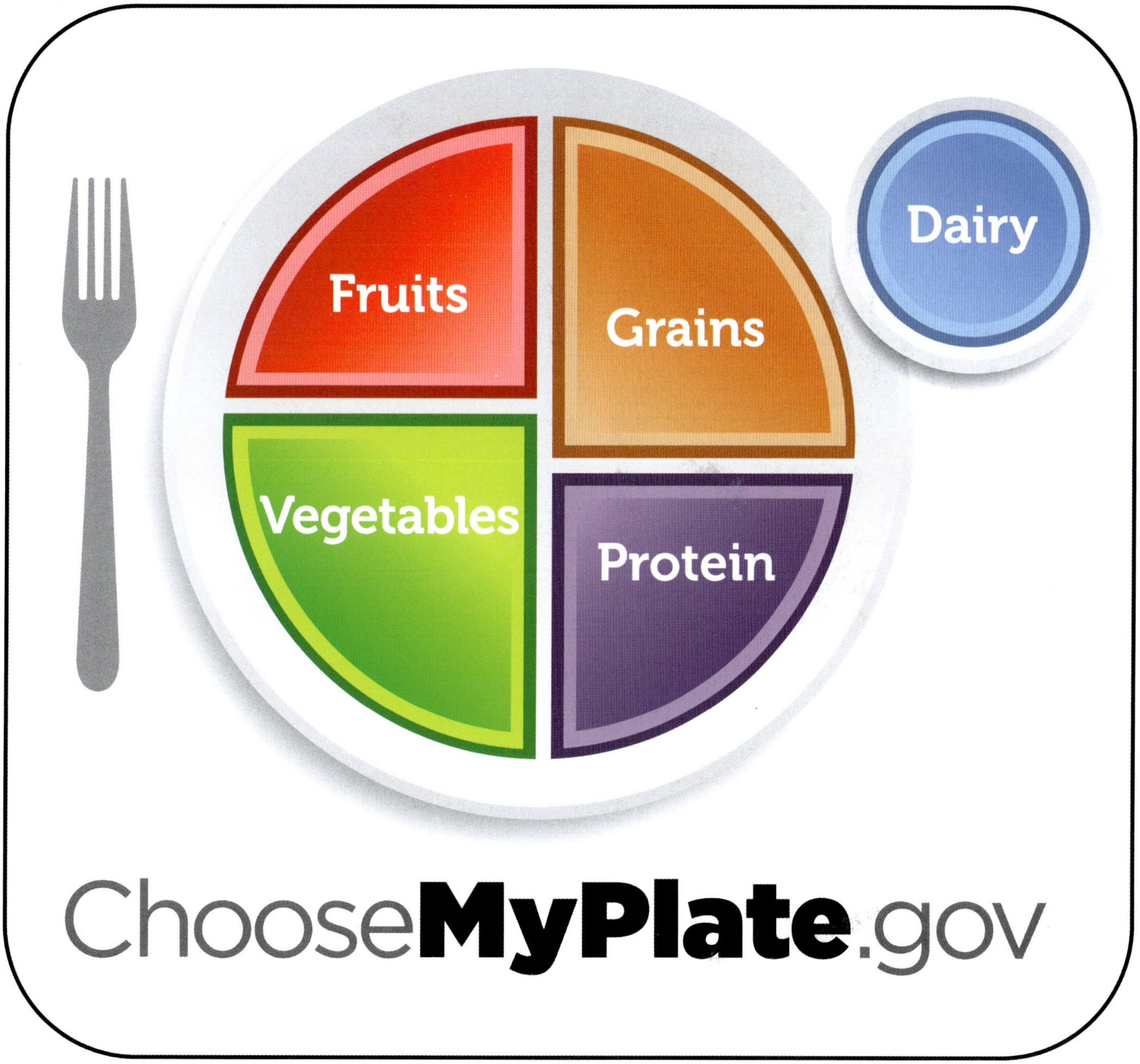
Fruits
Grains
Dairy
Vegetables
Protein
ChooseMyPlate.gov

Criteria and Dietary Reference Intake Values: FOR ENERGY BY ACTIVE INDIVIDUALS BY LIFE STAGE GROUP[a]

Life Stage Group	Criterion	ACTIVE PAL EER[b] (kcal/d) Male	ACTIVE PAL EER[b] (kcal/d) Female
0 through 6 mo	Energy expenditure plus energy deposition	570	520 (3 mo)
7 through 12 mo	Energy expenditure plus energy deposition	743	676 (9 mo)
1 through 2 y	Energy expenditure plus energy deposition	1,046	992 (24 mo)
3 through 8 y	Energy expenditure plus energy deposition	1,742	1,642 (6 y)
9 through 13 y	Energy expenditure plus energy deposition	2,279	2,071 (11 y)
14 through 18 y	Energy expenditure plus energy deposition	3,152	2,368 (16 y)
>18 y	Energy expenditure	3,067[c]	2,403[c] (19 y)
Pregnancy			
14 through 18 y	Adolescent female EER plus change in Total Energy Expenditure (TEE) plus pregnancy energy deposition		
1st trimester			2,368 (16 y)
2nd trimester			2,708 (16 y)
3rd trimester			2,820 (16 y)
19 through 50 y	Adult female EER plus change in TEE plus pregnancy energy deposition		
1st trimester			2,403[c] (19 y)
2nd trimester			2,743[c] (19 y)
3rd trimester			2,855[c] (19 y)
Lactation			
14 through 18 y	Adolescent female EER plus milk energy output minus weight loss		
1st 6 mo			2,698 (16 y)
2nd 6 mo			2,768 (16 y)
19 through 50 y	Adult female EER plus milk energy output minus weight loss		
1st 6 mo			2,733[c] (19 y)
2nd 6 mo			2,803[c] (19 y)

Reproduced with permission from Energy Calculations for Active Individuals by Life Stage Group. In *Dietary Reference Intakes for Water, Potassium, Sodium, Chloride, and Sulfate*, National Academy of Sciences. Washington, DC: National Academies Press, 2005.

[a]For healthy active Americans and Canadians. Based on the cited age, an active physical activity level, and the reference heights and weights cited in Table 1.1. Individualized EERs can be determined by using the equations in Chapter 5.

[b]PAL = Physical Activity Level, EER = Estimated Energy Requirement. The intake that meets the average energy expenditure of individuals at the reference height, weight, and age (see Table 1.1).

[c]Subtract 10 kcal/d for males and 7 kcal/d for females for each year of age above 19 years.

Dietary Reference Intakes (DRIs): DIETARY ALLOWANCES AND ADEQUATE INTAKES, TOTAL WATER, AND MACRONUTRIENTS (Food and Nutrition Board, National Academy of Medicine)

Life Stage Group	Total Water (L/d)	PROTEIN		CARBOHYDRATE		FIBER		FAT		*n*-6 POLYUNSATURATED FATTY ACIDS (α-linoleic acid)		*n*-3 POLYUNSATURATED FATTY ACIDS (α-linoleic acid)	
		RDA/AI g/day[a]	AMDR[b]	RDA/AI g/day	AMDR[b]	RDA/AI g/day	AMDR[b]	RDA/AI g/day	AMDR[b]	RDA/AI g/day	AMDR[b]	RDA/AI g/day	AMDR[d]
Infants													
0–6 mo	0.7*	9.1	ND[c]	60	ND	ND	ND	31		4.4*	ND	0.5*	ND
7–12 mo	0.8*	**11.0**	ND	95	ND	ND	ND	30		4.6*	ND	0.5*	ND
Children													
1–3 y	1.3*	**13**	5–20	**130**	45–65	19*	ND	ND	30–40	7*	5–10	0.7*	0.6–1.2
4–8 y	1.7*	**19**	10–30	**130**	45–65	25*	ND	ND	25–35	10*	5–10	0.9*	0.6–1.2
Males													
9–13 y	2.4*	**34**	10–30	**130**	45–65	31*	ND	ND	25–35	12*	5–10	1.2*	0.6–1.2
14–18 y	3.3*	**52**	10–30	**130**	45–65	38*	ND	ND	25–35	16*	5–10	1.6*	0.6–1.2
19–30 y	3.7*	**56**	10–35	**130**	45–65	38*	ND	ND	20–35	17*	5–10	1.6*	0.6–1.2
31–50 y	3.7*	**56**	10–35	**130**	45–65	38*	ND	ND	20–35	17*	5–10	1.6*	0.6–1.2
51–70 y	3.7*	**56**	10–35	**130**	45–65	30*	ND	ND	20–35	14*	5–10	1.6*	0.6–1.2
>70 y	3.7*	**56**	10–35	**130**	45–65	30*	ND	ND	20–35	14*	5–10	1.6*	0.6–1.2
Females													
9–13 y	2.1*	**34**	10–30	**130**	45–65	26*	ND	ND	25–35	10*	5–10	1.0*	0.6–1.2
14–18 y	2.3*	**46**	10–30	**130**	45–65	26*	ND	ND	25–35	11*	5–10	1.1*	0.6–1.2
19–30 y	3.7*	**46**	10–35	**130**	45–65	25*	ND	ND	20–35	12*	5–10	1.1*	0.6–1.2
31–50 y	3.7*	**46**	10–35	**130**	45–65	25*	ND	ND	20–35	12*	5–10	1.1*	0.6–1.2
51–70 y	3.7*	**46**	10–35	**130**	45–65	21*	ND	ND	20–35	11*	5–10	1.1*	0.6–1.2
>70 y	3.7*	**46**	10–35	**130**	45–65	21*	ND	ND	20–35	11*	5–10	1.1*	0.6–1.2
Pregnant													
≤18 y	3.0*	**71**	10–35	**175**	45–65	28*	ND	ND	20–35	13*	5–10	1.4*	0.6–1.2
19–30 y	3.0*	**71**	10–35	**175**	45–65	28*	ND	ND	20–35	13*	5–10	1.4*	0.6–1.2
31–50 y	3.0*	**71**	10–35	**175**	45–65	28*	ND	ND	20–35	13*	5–10	1.4*	0.6–1.2
Lactating													
≤18 y	3.8*	**71**	10–35	**210**	45–65	29*	ND	ND	20–35	13*	5–10	1.3*	0.6–1.2
19–30 y	3.8*	**71**	10–35	**210**	45–65	29*	ND	ND	20–35	13*	5–10	1.3*	0.6–1.2
31–50 y	3.8*	**71**	10–35	**210**	45–65	29*	ND	ND	20–35	13*	5–10	1.3*	0.6–1.2

Dietary cholesterol, *trans* fatty acids, saturated fatty acids: As low as possible while consuming a nutritionally adequate diet.

Added sugars: Limit to no more than 25% of total energy.[e]

Dietary Reference Intakes for Energy, Carbohydrate, Fiber, Fat, Fatty Acids, Cholesterol, Protein, and Amino Acids. Washington, DC: The National Academies Press, 2002.

Note: This table represents Recommended Dietary Allowances (RDAs) in **bold type** and *Adequate Intakes (AIs) in ordinary type. RDAs and AIs may both be used as goals for individual intake. RDAs are set to meet the needs of almost all (97%–98%) individuals in a group. For healthy breastfed infants, the AI is the mean intake. The AI for other life-stage and gender groups is believed to cover the needs of all individuals in the group, but lack of data prevents being able to specify with confidence the percentage of individuals covered by this intake.

[a]Based on 1.5 g/kg/day for infants, 1.1 g/kg/day for 1–3 y; 0.95 g/kg/day for 4–13 y, 0.85 g/kg/day for 14–18 y, 0.8 g/kg/day for adults, and 1.1 g/kg/day for pregnant (using prepregnancy weight) and lactating women.

[b]Acceptable Macronutrient Distribution Range (AMDR) is the range of intake for a particular energy source that is associated with reduced risk of chronic disease while providing intakes of essential nutrients. If an individual has consumed in excess of the AMDR, there is a potential of increasing the risk of chronic diseases and insufficient intakes of essential nutrients.

[c]ND 5 Not determinable due to lack of data of adverse effects in this age group and concern with regard to lack of ability to handle excess amounts. Source of intake should be from food only to prevent high levels of intake.

[d]Approximately 10% of the total can come from longer-chain, *n*-3 fatty acids.

Dietary Reference Intakes (DRIs): RECOMMENDED DIETARY ALLOWANCES AND ADEQUATE INTAKES, VITAMINS (Food and Nutrition Board, National Academy of Medicine)

Life Stage Group	Vitamin A (μg/d)[a]	Vitamin C (mg/d)	Vitamin D (μg/d)[b,c]	Vitamin E (mg/d)[d]	Vitamin K (μg/d)	Thiamin (mg/d)	Riboflavin (mg/d)	Niacin (mg/d)[e]	Vitamin B_6 (mg/d)	Folate (μg/d)[f]	Vitamin B_{12} (μg/d)	Pantothenic Acid (mg/d)	Biotin (μg/d)	Choline (mg/d)[g]
Infants														
0–6 mo	400*	40*	13	4*	2.0*	0.2*	0.3*	2*	0.1*	65*	0.4*	1.7*	5*	125*
7–12 mo	500*	50*	**15**	5*	2.5*	0.3*	0.4*	4*	0.3*	80*	0.5*	1.8*	6*	150*
Children														
1–3 y	**300**	**15**	**15**	**6**	30*	**0.5**	**0.5**	**6**	**0.5**	**150**	**0.9**	2*	8*	200*
4–8 y	**400**	**25**	**15**	**7**	55*	**0.6**	**0.6**	**8**	**0.6**	**200**	**1.2**	3*	12*	250*
Males														
9–13 y	**600**	**45**	**15**	**11**	60*	**0.9**	**0.9**	**12**	**1.0**	**300**	**1.8**	4*	20*	375*
14–18 y	**900**	**75**	**15**	**15**	75*	**1.2**	**1.3**	**16**	**1.3**	**400**	**2.4**	5*	25*	550*
19–30 y	**900**	**90**	**15**	**15**	120*	**1.2**	**1.3**	**16**	**1.3**	**400**	**2.4**	5*	30*	550*
31–50 y	**900**	**90**	**15**	**15**	120*	**1.2**	**1.3**	**16**	**1.3**	**400**	**2.4**	5*	30*	550*
51–70 y	**900**	**90**	**15**	**15**	120*	**1.2**	**1.3**	**16**	**1.7**	**400**	**2.4**[h]	5*	30*	550*
>70 y	**900**	**90**	**20**	**15**	120*	**1.2**	**1.3**	**16**	**1.7**	**400**	**2.4**[h]	5*	30*	550*
Females														
9–13 y	**600**	**45**	**15**	**11**	60*	**0.9**	**0.9**	**12**	**1.0**	**300**	**1.8**	4*	20*	375*
14–18 y	**700**	**65**	**15**	**15**	75*	**1.0**	**1.0**	**14**	**1.2**	**400**[i]	**2.4**	5*	25*	400*
19–30 y	**700**	**75**	**15**	**15**	90*	**1.1**	**1.1**	**14**	**1.3**	**400**[i]	**2.4**	5*	30*	425*
31–50 y	**700**	**75**	**15**	**15**	90*	**1.1**	**1.1**	**14**	**1.3**	**400**[i]	**2.4**	5*	30*	425*
51–70 y	**700**	**75**	**15**	**15**	90*	**1.1**	**1.1**	**14**	**1.5**	**400**	**2.4**[h]	5*	30*	425*
>70 y	**700**	**75**	**20**	**15**	90*	**1.1**	**1.1**	**14**	**1.5**	**400**	**2.4**[h]	5*	30*	425*
Pregnancy														
14–18 y	**750**	**80**	**15**	**15**	75*	**1.4**	**1.4**	**18**	**1.9**	**600**[j]	**2.6**	6*	30*	450*
19–30 y	**770**	**85**	**15**	**15**	90*	**1.4**	**1.4**	**18**	**1.9**	**600**[j]	**2.6**	6*	30*	450*
31–50 y	**770**	**85**	**15**	**15**	90*	**1.4**	**1.4**	**18**	**1.9**	**600**[j]	**2.6**	6*	30*	450*
Lactation														
14–18 y	**1,200**	**115**	**15**	**19**	75*	**1.4**	**1.6**	**17**	**2.0**	**500**	**2.8**	7*	35*	550*
19–30 y	**1,300**	**120**	**15**	**19**	90*	**1.4**	**1.6**	**17**	**2.0**	**500**	**2.8**	7*	35*	550*
31–50 y	**1,300**	**120**	**15**	**19**	90*	**1.4**	**1.6**	**17**	**2.0**	**500**	**2.8**	7*	35*	550*

SOURCES: *Dietary Reference Intakes for Calcium, Phosphorus, Magnesium, Vitamin D, and Fluoride* (1997); *Dietary Reference Intakes for Thiamin, Riboflavin, Niacin, Vitamin B_6, Folate, Vitamin B_{12}, Pantothenic Acid, Biotin, and Choline* (1998); *Dietary Reference Intakes for Vitamin C, Vitamin E, Selenium, and Carotenoids* (2000); Dietary Reference Intakes for Vitamin A, *Vitamin K, Arsenic, Boron, Chromium, Copper, Iodine, Iron, Manganese, Molybdenum, Nickel, Silicon, Vanadium, and Zinc* (2001); *Dietary Reference Intakes for Water, Potassium, Sodium, Chloride, and Sulfate* (2005); and *Dietary Reference Intakes for Calcium and Vitamin D* (2011). These reports may be accessed via www.nap.edu.

NOTE: This table (taken from the DRI reports; see www.nap.edu) presents Recommended Dietary Allowances (RDAs) in **bold type** and Adequate Intakes (AIs) in ordinary type followed by an asterisk (*). An RDA is the average daily dietary intake level; sufficient to meet the nutrient requirements of nearly all (97%–98%) healthy individuals in a group. It is calculated from an Estimated Average Requirement (EAR). If sufficient scientific evidence is not available to establish an EAR for calculating an RDA, an AI is usually developed. For healthy breastfed infants, an AI is the mean intake. The AI for other life-stage and gender groups is believed to cover the needs of all healthy individuals in the groups, but lack of data or uncertainty in the data prevent being able to specify with confidence the percentage of individuals covered by this intake.

[a]As retinol activity equivalents (RAEs). 1 RAE = 1 μg retinol, 12 μg β-carotene, 24 μg β-carotene, or 24 μg β-cryptoxanthin. The RAE for dietary provitamin A carotenoids is twofold greater than retinol equivalents (RE), whereas the RAE for preformed vitamin A is the same as RE.

[b]As cholecalciferol. 1 μg cholecalciferol = 40 IU vitamin D.

[c]Under the assumption of minimal sunlight.

[d]As α-tocopherol. α-Tocopherol includes *RRR*-α-tocopherol, the only form of α-tocopherol that occurs naturally in foods, and the *2R*-stereoisomeric forms of α-tocopherol (*RRR*-, *RSR*-, *RRS*-, and *RSS*-α-tocopherol) that occur in fortified foods and supplements. It does not include the *2S*-stereoisomeric forms of α-tocopherol (*SRR*-, *SSR*-, *SRS*-, and *SSS*-α-tocopherol), also found in fortified foods and supplements.

[e]As niacin equivalents (NE). 1 mg of niacin = 60 mg of tryptophan; 0–6 months = preformed niacin (not NE).

[f]As dietary folate equivalents (DFE). 1 DFE = 1 μg food folate = 0.6 μg of folic acid from fortified food or as a supplement consumed with food = 0.5 μg of a supplement taken on an empty stomach.

[g]Although AIs have been set for choline, there are few data to assess whether a dietary supply of choline is needed at all stages of the life cycle, and it may be that the choline requirement can be met by endogenous synthesis at some of these stages.

[h]Because 10% to 30% of older people may malabsorb food-bound B_{12}, it is advisable for those older than 50 years to meet their RDA mainly by consuming foods fortified with B_{12} or a supplement containing B_{12}.

[i]In view of evidence linking folate intake with neural tube defects in the fetus, it is recommended that all women capable of becoming pregnant consume 400 μg from supplements or fortified foods in addition to intake of food folate from a varied diet.

[j]It is assumed that women will continue consuming 400 μg from supplements or fortified food until their pregnancy is confirmed and they enter prenatal care, which ordinarily occurs after the end of the periconceptional period—the critical time for formation of the neural tube.

Dietary Reference Intakes (DRIs): RECOMMENDED DIETARY ALLOWANCES AND ADEQUATE INTAKES, ELEMENTS (Food and Nutrition Board, National Academy of Medicine)

Life-Stage Group	Calcium (mg/d)	Chromium (μg/d)	Copper (μg/d)	Fluoride (mg/d)	Iodine (μg/d)	Iron (mg/d)	Magnesium (mg/d)
Infants							
0–6 mo	200*	0.2*	200*	0.01*	110*	0.27*	30*
7–12 mo	260*	5.5*	220*	0.5*	130*	**11**	75*
Children							
1–3 y	**700***	11*	**340**	0.7*	**90**	**7**	**80**
4–8 y	**1000***	15*	**440**	1*	**90**	**10**	**130**
Males							
9–13 y	**1,300***	25*	**700**	2*	**120**	**8**	**240**
14–18 y	**1,300***	35*	**890**	3*	**150**	**11**	**410**
19–30 y	**1,000***	35*	**900**	4*	**150**	**8**	**400**
31–50 y	**1,000***	35*	**900**	4*	**150**	**8**	**420**
51–70 y	**1,200***	30*	**900**	4*	**150**	**8**	**420**
>70 y	**1,200***	30*	**900**	4*	**150**	**8**	**420**
Females							
9–13 y	**1,300***	21*	**700**	2*	**120**	**8**	**240**
14–18 y	**1,300***	24*	**890**	3*	**150**	**15**	**360**
19–30 y	**1,000***	25*	**900**	3*	**150**	**18**	**310**
31–50 y	**1,000***	25*	**900**	3*	**150**	**18**	**320**
51–70 y	**1,200***	20*	**900**	3*	**150**	**8**	**320**
>70 y	**1,200***	20*	**900**	3*	**150**	**8**	**320**
Pregnancy							
≤18 y	**1,300***	29*	**1,000**	3*	**220**	**27**	**400**
19–30 y	**1,000***	30*	**1,000**	3*	**220**	**27**	**350**
31–50 y	**1,000***	30*	**1,000**	3*	**220**	**27**	**360**
Lactation							
≤18 y	**1,300***	11*	**1,300**	3*	**290**	**10**	**360**
19–30 y	**1,000***	15*	**1,300**	3*	**290**	**9**	**310**
31–50 y	**1,000***	45*	**1,300**	3*	**290**	**9**	**320**

SOURCES: *Dietary Reference Intakes for Calcium, Phosphorus, Magnesium, Vitamin D, and Fluoride* (1997); *Dietary Reference Intakes for Thiamin, Riboflavin, Niacin, Vitamin B_6, Folate, Vitamin B_{12}, Pantothenic Acid, Biotin, and Choline* (1998); *Dietary Reference Intakes for Vitamin C, Vitamin E, Selenium, and Carotenoids* (2000); *Dietary Reference Intakes for Vitamin A, Vitamin K, Arsenic, Boron, Chromium, Copper, Iodine, Iron, Manganese, Molybdenum, Nickel, Silicon, Vanadium, and Zinc* (2001); *Dietary Reference Intakes for Water, Potassium, Sodium, Chloride, and Sulfate* (2005); and *Dietary Reference Intakes for Calcium and Vitamin D* (2011). These reports may be accessed via www.nap.edu.

Dietary Reference Intakes (DRIs): ESTIMATED AVERAGE REQUIREMENTS (Food and Nutrition Board, National Academy of Medicine)

Life Stage-Group	Calcium (mg/d)	CHO (g/kg/d)	Protein (g/d)	Vitamin A (μg/d)[a]	Vitamin C (mg/d)	Vitamin D (μg/d)	Vitamin E (mg/d)[b]	Thiamin (mg/d)	Riboflavin (mg/d)	Niacin (mg/d)[c]	Vitamin B_6 (mg/d)	Folate (μg/d)[d]	Vitamin B_{12} (μg/d)	Copper (μg/d)	Iodine (μg/d)	Iron (mg/d)	Magnesium (mg/d)	Molybdenum (μg/d)	Phosphorus (mg/d)	Selenium (μg/d)	Zinc (mg/d)
Infants																					
0–6 mo																					
7–12 mo			1.0													6.9					2.5
Children																					
1–3 y	500	100	0.87	210	13	10	5	0.4	0.4	5	0.4	120	0.7	260	65	3.0	65	13	380	17	2.5
4–8 y	800	100	0.76	275	22	10	6	0.5	0.5	6	0.5	160	1.0	340	65	4.1	110	17	405	23	4.0
Males																					
9–13 y	1,100	100	0.76	445	39	10	9	0.7	0.8	9	0.8	250	1.5	540	73	5.9	200	26	1,055	35	7.0
14–18 y	1,100	100	0.73	630	63	10	12	1.0	1.1	12	1.1	330	2.0	685	95	7.7	340	33	1,055	45	8.5
19–30 y	800	100	0.66	625	75	10	12	1.0	1.1	12	1.1	320	2.0	700	95	6	330	34	580	45	9.4
31–50 y	800	100	0.66	625	75	10	12	1.0	1.1	12	1.1	320	2.0	700	95	6	350	34	580	45	9.4
51–70 y	800	100	0.66	625	75	10	12	1.0	1.1	12	1.4	320	2.0	700	95	6	350	34	580	45	9.4
>70 y	1,000	100	0.66	625	75	10	12	1.0	1.1	12	1.4	320	2.0	700	95	6	350	34	580	45	9.4
Females																					
9–13 y	1,100	100	0.76	420	39	10	9	0.7	0.8	9	0.8	250	1.5	540	73	5.7	200	26	1,055	35	7.0
14–18 y	1,100	100	0.71	485	56	10	12	0.9	0.9	11	1.0	330	2.0	685	95	7.9	300	33	1,055	45	7.3
19–30 y	800	100	0.66	500	60	10	12	0.9	0.9	11	1.1	320	2.0	700	95	8.1	255	34	580	45	6.8
31–50 y	800	100	0.66	500	60	10	12	0.9	0.9	11	1.1	320	2.0	700	95	8.1	265	34	580	45	6.8
51–70 y	1,000	100	0.66	500	60	10	12	0.9	0.9	11	1.3	320	2.0	700	95	5	265	34	580	45	6.8
>70 y	1,000	100	0.66	500	60	10	12	0.9	0.9	11	1.3	320	2.0	700	95	5	265	34	580	45	6.8
Pregnancy																					
14–18 y	1,000	135	0.88	530	66	10	12	1.2	1.2	14	1.6	520	2.2	785	160	23	335	40	1,055	49	10.5
19–30 y	800	135	0.88	550	70	10	12	1.2	1.2	14	1.6	520	2.2	800	160	22	290	40	580	49	9.5
31–50 y	800	135	0.88	550	70	10	12	1.2	1.2	14	1.6	520	2.2	800	160	22	300	40	580	49	9.5
Lactation																					
14–18 y	1,000	160	1.05	885	96	10	16	1.2	1.3	13	1.7	450	2.4	985	209	7	300	35	1,055	59	10.9
19–30 y	800	160	1.05	900	100	10	16	1.2	1.3	13	1.7	450	2.4	1,000	209	6.5	255	36	580	59	10.4
31–50 y	800	160	1.05	900	100	10	16	1.2	1.3	13	1.7	450	2.4	1,000	209	6.5	265	36	580	59	10.44

SOURCES: *Dietary Reference Intakes for Calcium, Phosphorus, Magnesium, Vitamin D, and Fluoride* (1997); *Dietary Reference Intakes for Thiamin, Riboflavin, Niacin, Vitamin B_6, Folate, Vitamin B_{12}, Pantothenic Acid, Biotin, and Choline* (1998); *Dietary Reference Intakes for Vitamin C, Vitamin E, Selenium, and Carotenoids* (2000); *Dietary Reference Intakes for Vitamin A, Vitamin K, Arsenic, Boron, Chromium, Copper, Iodine, Iron, Manganese, Molybdenum, Nickel, Silicon, Vanadium, and Zinc* (2001); *Dietary Reference Intakes for Energy, Carbohydrate, Fiber, Fat, Fatty Acids, Cholesterol, Protein, and Amino Acids* (2002/2005); and *Dietary Reference Intakes for Calcium and Vitamin D* (2011). These reports may be accessed via www.nap.edu.

Note: An Estimated Average Requirement (EAR) is the average daily nutrient intake level estimated to meet the requirements of the healthy individuals in a group. EARs have not been established for vitamin K, pantothenic acid, biotin, choline, chromium, fluoride, manganese, or other nutrients not yet evaluated via the DRI process.

[a]As retinol activity equivalents (RAEs). 1 RAE = 1 μg retinol, 12 μg β-carotene, 24 μg α-carotene, or 24 μg β-cryptoxanthin. The RAE for dietary provitamin A carotenoids is two-fold greater than retinol equivalents (RE), whereas the RAE for preformed vitamin A is the same as RE.

[b]As α-tocopherol. α-Tocopherol includes *RRR*-α-tocopherol, the only form of α-tocopherol that occurs naturally in foods, and the *2R*-stereoisomeric forms of α-tocopherol (*RRR-*, *RSR-*, *RPS-*, and *RSS*-α-tocopherol) that occur in fortified foods and supplements. It does not include the *2S*-stereoisomeric forms of α-tocopherol (*SRR-*, *SSR-*, *SRS-*, and *SSS*-α-tocopherol), also found in fortified foods and supplements.

[c]As niacin equivalents (NE). 1 mg of niacin = 60 mg of tryptophan.

[d]As dietary folate equivalents (DFE). 1 DFE = 1 μg food folate = 0.6 μg of folic acid from fortified food or as a supplement consumed with food = 0.5 μg of a supplement taken on an empty stomach.

Dietary Reference Intakes (DRIs): TOLERABLE UPPER INTAKE LEVELS, VITAMINS (Food and Nutrition Board, National Academy of Medicine)

Life-Stage Group	Vitamin A (μg/d)[a]	Vitamin C (mg/d)	Vitamin D (μg/d)	Vitamin E (mg/d)[b,c]	Vitamin K	Thiamin	Riboflavin	Niacin (mg/d)[c]	Vitamin B_6 (mg/d)	Folate (μg/d)[c]	Vitamin B_{12}	Pantothenic Acid	Biotin	Choline (g/d)	Carotenoids[d]
Infants															
0–6 mo	600	ND[e]	25	ND	ND	ND	ND	ND	ND	ND	ND	ND	ND	ND	ND
7–12 mo	600	ND	38	ND	ND	ND	ND	ND	ND	ND	ND	ND	ND	ND	ND
Children															
1–3 y	600	400	63	200	ND	ND	ND	10	30	300	ND	ND	ND	1.0	ND
4–8 y	900	650	75	300	ND	ND	ND	15	40	400	ND	ND	ND	1.0	ND
Males															
9–13 y	1,700	1,200	100	600	ND	ND	ND	20	60	600	ND	ND	ND	2.0	ND
14–18 y	2,800	1,800	100	800	ND	ND	ND	30	80	800	ND	ND	ND	3.0	ND
19–30 y	3,000	2,000	100	1,000	ND	ND	ND	35	100	1,000	ND	ND	ND	3.5	ND
31–50 y	3,000	2,000	100	1,000	ND	ND	ND	35	100	1,000	ND	ND	ND	3.5	ND
51–70 y	3,000	2,000	100	1,000	ND	ND	ND	35	100	1,000	ND	ND	ND	3.5	ND
>70 y	3,000	2,000	100	1,000	ND	ND	ND	35	100	1,000	ND	ND	ND	3.5	ND
Females															
9–13 y	1,700	1,200	100	600	ND	ND	ND	20	60	600	ND	ND	ND	2.0	ND
14–18 y	2,800	1,800	100	800	ND	ND	ND	30	80	800	ND	ND	ND	3.0	ND
19–30 y	3,000	2,000	100	1,000	ND	ND	ND	35	100	1,000	ND	ND	ND	3.5	ND
31–50 y	3,000	2,000	100	1,000	ND	ND	ND	35	100	1,000	ND	ND	ND	3.5	ND
51–70 y	3,000	2,000	100	1,000	ND	ND	ND	35	100	1,000	ND	ND	ND	3.5	ND
>70 y	3,000	2,000	100	1,000	ND	ND	ND	35	100	1,000	ND	ND	ND	3.5	ND
Pregnancy															
14–18 y	2,800	1,800	100	800	ND	ND	ND	30	80	800	ND	ND	ND	3.0	ND
19–30 y	3,000	2,000	100	1,000	ND	ND	ND	35	100	1,000	ND	ND	ND	3.5	ND
31–50 y	3,000	2,000	100	1,000	ND	ND	ND	35	100	1,000	ND	ND	ND	3.5	ND
Lactation															
14–18 y	2,800	1,800	100	800	ND	ND	ND	30	80	800	ND	ND	ND	3.0	ND
19–30 y	3,000	2,000	100	1,000	ND	ND	ND	35	100	1,000	ND	ND	ND	3.5	ND
31–50 y	3,000	2,000	100	1,000	ND	ND	ND	35	100	1,000	ND	ND	ND	3.5	ND

SOURCES: *Dietary Reference Intakes for Calcium, Phosphorus, Magnesium, Vitamin D, and Fluoride* (1997); *Dietary Reference Intakes for Thiamin, Riboflavin, Niacin, Vitamin B_6, Folate, Vitamin B_{12}, Pantothenic Acid, Biotin, and Choline* (1998); *Dietary Reference Intakes for Vitamin C, Vitamin E, Selenium, and Carotenoids* (2000); *Dietary Reference Intakes for Vitamin A, Vitamin K, Arsenic, Boron, Chromium, Copper, Iodine, Iron, Manganese, Molybdenum, Nickel, Silicon, Vanadium, and Zinc* (2001); and *Dietary Reference Intakes for Calcium and Vitamin D* (2011). These reports may be accessed via www.nap.edu.

Note: A Tolerable Upper Intake Level (UL) is the highest level of daily nutrient intake that is likely to pose no risk of adverse health effects to almost all individuals in the general population. Unless otherwise specified, the UL represents total intake from food, water, and supplements. Due to a lack of suitable data, ULs could not be established for vitamin K, thiamin, riboflavin, vitamin B_{12}, pantothenic acid, biotin, and carotenoids. In the absence of a UL, extra caution may be warranted in consuming levels above recommended intakes. Members of the general population should be advised not to routinely exceed the UL. The UL is not meant to apply to individuals who are treated with the nutrient under medical supervision or to individuals with predisposing conditions that modify their sensitivity to the nutrient.

[a]As preformed vitamin A only.

[b]As α-tocopherol; applies to any form of supplemental α-tocopherol.

[c]The ULs for vitamin E, niacin, and folate apply to synthetic forms obtained from supplements, fortified foods, or a combination of the two.

[d]β-Carotene supplements are advised only to serve as a provitamin A source for individuals at risk of vitamin A deficiency.

[e]ND = Not determinable due to lack of data of adverse effects in this age group and concern with regard to lack of ability to handle excess amounts. Source of intake should be from food only to prevent high levels of intake.

Dietary Reference Intakes (DRIs): TOLERABLE UPPER INTAKE LEVELS, ELEMENTS (Food and Nutrition Board, National Academy of Medicine)

Life-Stage Group	Arsenic[a]	Boron (mg/d)	Calcium (mg/d)	Chromium	Copper (μg/d)	Fluoride (mg/d)	Iodine (μg/d)	Iron (mg/d)	Magnesium (mg/d)[b]	Manganese (mg/d)	Molybdenum (μg/d)	Nickel (mg/d)	Phosphorus (g/d)	Selenium (μg/d)	Silicon[c]	Vanadium (mg/d)[d]	Zinc (mg/d)	Sodium (g/d)	Chloride (g/d)
Infants																			
0–6 mo	ND[e]	ND	1,000	ND	ND	0.7	ND	40	ND	ND	ND	ND	ND	45	ND	ND	4	ND	ND
7–12 mo	ND	ND	1,500	ND	ND	0.9	ND	40	ND	ND	ND	ND	ND	60	ND	ND	5	ND	ND
Children																			
1–3 y	ND	3	2,500	ND	1,000	1.3	200	40	65	2	300	0.2	3.0	90	ND	ND	7	1.5	2.3
4–8 y	ND	6	2,500	ND	3,000	2.2	300	40	110	3	600	0.3	3.0	150	ND	ND	12	1.9	2.9
Males																			
9–13 y	ND	11	3,000	ND	5,000	10	600	40	350	6	1,100	0.6	4.0	280	ND	ND	23	2.2	3.4
14–18 y	ND	17	3,000	ND	8,000	10	900	45	350	9	1,700	1.0	4.0	400	ND	ND	34	2.3	3.6
19–30 y	ND	20	2,500	ND	10,000	10	1,100	45	350	11	2,000	1.0	4.0	400	ND	1.8	40	2.3	3.6
31–50 y	ND	20	2,500	ND	10,000	10	1,100	45	350	11	2,000	1.0	4.0	400	ND	1.8	40	2.3	3.6
51–70 y	ND	20	2,000	ND	10,000	10	1,100	45	350	11	2,000	1.0	4.0	400	ND	1.8	40	2.3	3.6
>70 y	ND	20	2,000	ND	10,000	10	1,100	45	350	11	2,000	1.0	3.0	400	ND	1.8	40	2.3	3.6
Females																			
9–13 y	ND	11	3,000	ND	5,000	10	600	40	350	6	1,100	0.6	4.0	280	ND	ND	23	2.2	3.4
14–18 y	ND	17	3,000	ND	8,000	10	900	45	350	9	1,700	1.0	4.0	400	ND	ND	34	2.3	3.6
19–30 y	ND	20	2,500	ND	10,000	10	1,100	45	350	11	2,000	1.0	4.0	400	ND	1.8	40	2.3	3.6
31–50 y	ND	20	2,500	ND	10,000	10	1,100	45	350	11	2,000	1.0	4.0	400	ND	1.8	40	2.3	3.6
51–70 y	ND	20	2,000	ND	10,000	10	1,100	45	350	11	2,000	1.0	4.0	400	ND	1.8	40	2.3	3.6
>70 y	ND	20	2,000	ND	10,000	10	1,100	45	350	11	2,000	1.0	3.0	400	ND	1.8	40	2.3	3.6
Pregnancy																			
14–18 y	ND	17	3,000	ND	8,000	10	900	45	350	9	1,700	1.0	3.5	400	ND	ND	34	2.3	3.6
19–30 y	ND	20	2,500	ND	10,000	10	1,100	45	350	11	2,000	1.0	3.5	400	ND	ND	40	2.3	3.6
31–50 y	ND	20	2,500	ND	10,000	10	1,100	45	350	11	2,000	1.0	3.5	400	ND	ND	40	2.3	3.6
Lactation																			
14–18 y	ND	17	3,000	ND	8,000	10	900	45	350	9	1,700	1.0	4.0	400	ND	ND	34	2.3	3.6
19–30 y	ND	20	2,500	ND	10,000	10	1,100	45	350	11	2,000	1.0	4.0	400	ND	ND	40	2.3	3.6
31–50 y	ND	20	2,500	ND	10,000	10	1,100	45	350	11	2,000	1.0	4	400	ND	ND	40	2.3	3.6

Note: A Tolerable Upper Intake Level (UL) is the highest level of daily nutrient intake that is likely to pose no risk of adverse health effects to almost all individuals in the general population. Unless otherwise specified, the UL represents total intake from food, water, and supplements. Due to a lack of suitable data, ULs could not be established for vitamin K, thiamin, riboflavin, vitamin B_{12}, pantothenic acid, biotin, and carotenoids. In the absence of a UL, extra caution may be warranted in consuming levels above recommended intakes. Members of the general population should be advised not to routinely exceed the UL. The UL is not meant to apply to individuals who are treated with the nutrient under medical supervision or to individuals with predisposing conditions that modify their sensitivity to the nutrient.

[a]Although the UL was not determined for arsenic, there is no justification for adding arsenic to food or supplements.

[b]The ULs for magnesium represent intake from a pharmacologic agent only and do not include intake from food and water.

[c]Although silicon has not been shown to cause adverse effects in humans, there is no justification for adding silicon to supplements.

[d]Although vanadium in food has not been shown to cause adverse effects in humans, there is no justification for adding vanadium to food and vanadium supplements should be used with caution. The UL is based on adverse effects in laboratory animals; this data could be used to set a UL for adults but not children and adolescents.

[e]ND = Not determinable due to lack of data of adverse effects in this age group and concern with regard to lack of ability to handle excess amounts. Source of intake should be from food only to prevent high levels of intake.

SOURCES: *Dietary Reference Intakes for Calcium, Phosphorus, Magnesium, Vitamin D, and Fluoride* (1997); *Dietary Reference Intakes for Thiamin, Riboflavin, Niacin, Vitamin B6, Folate, Vitamin B12, Pantothenic Acid, Biotin, and Choline* (1998); *Dietary Reference Intakes for Vitamin C, Vitamin E, Selenium, and Carotenoids* (2000); *Dietary Reference Intakes for Vitamin A, Vitamin K, Arsenic, Boron, Chromium, Copper, Iodine, Iron, Manganese, Molybdenum, Nickel, Silicon, Vanadium, and Zinc* (2001); *Dietary Reference Intakes for Water, Potassium, Sodium, Chloride, and Sulfate* (2005); and *Dietary Reference Intakes for Calcium and Vitamin D* (2011). These reports may be accessed via www.nap.edu.

Body Mass Index Table

	NORMAL						OVERWEIGHT					OBESE										EXTREME OBESITY														
BMI	19	20	21	22	23	24	25	26	27	28	29	30	31	32	33	34	35	36	37	38	39	40	41	42	43	44	45	46	47	48	49	50	51	52	53	54
Height (inches)																Body Weight (pounds)																				
58	91	96	100	105	110	115	119	124	129	134	138	143	148	153	158	162	167	172	177	181	186	191	196	201	205	210	215	220	224	229	234	239	244	248	253	258
59	94	99	104	109	114	119	124	128	133	138	143	148	153	158	163	168	173	178	183	188	193	198	203	208	212	217	222	227	232	237	242	247	252	257	262	267
60	97	102	107	112	118	123	128	133	138	143	148	153	158	163	168	174	179	184	189	194	199	204	209	215	220	225	230	235	240	245	250	255	261	266	271	276
61	100	106	111	116	122	127	132	137	143	148	153	158	164	169	174	180	185	190	195	201	206	211	217	222	227	232	238	243	248	254	259	264	269	275	280	285
62	104	109	115	120	126	131	136	142	147	153	158	164	169	175	180	186	191	196	202	207	213	218	224	229	235	240	246	251	256	262	267	273	278	284	289	295
63	107	113	118	124	130	135	141	146	152	158	163	169	175	180	186	191	197	203	208	214	220	225	231	237	242	248	254	259	265	270	278	282	287	293	299	304
64	110	116	122	128	134	140	145	151	157	163	169	174	180	186	192	197	204	209	215	221	227	232	238	244	250	256	262	267	273	279	285	291	296	302	308	314
65	114	120	126	132	138	144	150	156	162	168	174	180	186	192	198	204	210	216	222	228	234	240	246	252	258	264	270	276	282	288	294	300	306	312	318	324
66	118	124	130	136	142	148	155	161	167	173	179	186	192	198	204	210	216	223	229	235	241	247	253	260	266	272	278	284	291	297	303	309	315	322	328	334
67	121	127	134	140	146	153	159	166	172	178	185	191	198	204	211	217	223	230	236	242	249	255	261	268	274	280	287	293	299	306	312	319	325	331	338	344
68	125	131	138	144	151	158	164	171	177	184	190	197	203	210	216	223	230	236	243	249	256	262	269	276	282	289	295	302	308	315	322	328	335	341	348	354
69	128	135	142	149	155	162	169	176	182	189	196	203	209	216	223	230	236	243	250	257	263	270	277	284	291	297	304	311	318	324	331	338	345	351	358	365
70	132	139	146	153	160	167	174	181	188	195	202	209	216	222	229	236	243	250	257	264	271	278	285	292	299	306	313	320	327	334	341	348	355	362	369	376
71	136	143	150	157	165	172	179	186	193	200	208	215	222	229	236	243	250	257	265	272	279	286	293	301	308	315	322	329	338	343	351	358	365	372	379	386
72	140	147	154	162	169	177	184	191	199	206	213	221	228	235	242	250	258	265	272	279	287	294	302	309	316	324	331	338	346	353	361	368	375	383	390	397
73	144	151	159	166	174	182	189	197	204	212	219	227	235	242	250	257	265	272	280	288	295	302	310	318	325	333	340	348	355	363	371	378	386	393	401	408
74	148	155	163	171	179	186	194	202	210	218	225	233	241	249	256	264	272	280	287	295	303	311	319	326	334	342	350	358	365	373	381	389	396	404	412	420
75	152	160	168	176	184	192	200	208	216	224	232	240	248	256	264	272	279	287	295	303	311	319	327	335	343	351	359	367	375	383	391	399	407	415	423	431
76	156	164	172	180	189	197	205	213	221	230	238	246	254	263	271	279	287	295	304	312	320	328	336	344	353	361	369	377	385	394	402	410	418	426	435	443

SOURCE: Adapted from Clinical Guidelines on the Identification, Evaluation, and Treatment of Overweight and Obesity in Adults: The Evidence Report. Bethesda, MD: National Heart, Lung, and Blood Institute, 1998.

The Dental Hygienist's Guide to Nutritional Care

5th edition

Cynthia A. Stegeman, RDH, EdD, RDN, LD, CDE

Ohio Delegate to the Academy of Nutrition and Dietetics
National Board Dental Hygiene Examination Test Construction Committee
Commission on Dental Competency Assessments Consultant
Professor and Chairperson, Dental Hygiene Program
University of Cincinnati, Blue Ash
Cincinnati, Ohio

Judi Ratliff Davis, MS, RDN

Former Quality Assurance Nutrition Consultant
Women, Infants and Children (WIC) Program
Texas Department of State Health Services
Austin, Texas

ELSEVIER

ELSEVIER

3251 Riverport Lane
St. Louis, Missouri 63043

THE DENTAL HYGIENIST'S GUIDE TO NUTRITIONAL CARE, FIFTH EDITION ISBN: 978-0-323-497275

Library of Congress Cataloging-in-Publication Data

Names: Stegeman, Cynthia A., author. | Davis, Judi Ratliff, author.
Title: The dental hygienist's guide to nutritional care / Cynthia A. Stegeman, RDH, EdD, RDN, LD, CDE, Ohio Delegate to the Academy of Nutrition and Dietetics, Associate Professor, Dental Hygiene Program, University of Cincinnati, Cincinnati, Ohio, Judi Ratliff Davis, MS, RDN, Former Quality Assurance Nutrition Consultant, Women, Infants and Children (WIC) Program, Texas Department of State Health Services, Austin, Texas.
Description: Fifth edition. | St. Louis, Missouri : Elsevier, Inc., [2019] | Includes bibliographical references and index.
Identifiers: LCCN 2017059590| ISBN 9780323497275 (pbk. : alk. paper) | ISBN 9780323569460 (ebook)
Subjects: LCSH: Nutrition and dental health. | Dental hygienists.
Classification: LCC RK60.7 .S74 2019 | DDC 617.6/01–dc23 LC record available at https://lccn.loc.gov/2017059590

Content Strategist: Kristin R. Wilhelm
Senior Content Development Manager: Ellen M. Wurm-Cutter
Senior Content Development Specialist: Rebecca M. Leenhouts
Publishing Services Manager: Deepthi Unni
Project Manager: Radhika Sivalingam
Designer: Brian Salisbury

Printed in China

Last digit is the print number: 9 8 7 6 5

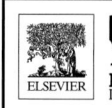

This fifth edition is dedicated to all of the dental hygiene students, faculty, and practitioners throughout the world who read and apply information from this text. Your curiosity and desire to gain evidence-based and applicable information regarding the role of nutrition in oral health continues to guide the content.

Cyndee and Judi

and

To my husband, son, family, and dental hygiene and dietetic colleagues for their encouragement, support, visions, and humor.

Cyndee

and

To my friends and family, especially my five granddaughters: Riley, Avery, Ellie, Maggie, and Callie, and my newest addition, at last, a grandson, Falcon.

Judi

Preface

The *fifth* edition of this nutrition textbook for dental professionals!!! Why is nutrition information always changing? Concisely, nutrition is a relatively new science. It has long been recognized that certain food factors are important to health: in the early 1800s, all English ships carried lime juice, with a portion given to each sailor daily. However, isolation and discovery of the exact elements in foods and the role they play in maintaining health and preventing disease is more complicated. The B vitamins were only discovered as late as the twentieth century. Scientists continue to research the nutrient content of foods, the specific physiologic uses of vitamins and minerals, and the quantity resulting in beneficial or harmful effects. Advances in technology continue to guide us in the functions and interactions of nutrients. After discovering vitamins and determining which minerals and elements are essential to health, even more food components have been discovered, such as antioxidants and polyphenols, leading to shifting directions and policies. Expect further changes as research delves into the effects of the microbiome and nutrigenomics in maintaining optimal health and preventing chronic diseases. The science of nutrition is further complicated by such factors as personal food habits and nutrient interactions. You will realize in studying this subject that nutrition is a dynamic field relevant to both you and your patients.

The study of nutrition is a rewarding topic for dental hygiene students and practitioners, not only as it relates to patient education but also for how it can affect the dental hygienist's own health. ***The Dental Hygienist's Guide to Nutritional Care*** is designed to show both dental hygiene students and practicing dental professionals how to apply sound nutrition principles when assessing, diagnosing, planning, implementing, and evaluating the total care of patients, as well as to help them contribute to the nutritional well-being of patients. The Academy of Nutrition and Dietetics, American Dental Hygienists' Association, and American Dental Association each recognize nutrition as an integral component of oral health. The dental professional should be able to assess the oral cavity in relation to the patient's nutrition, dietary habits, and overall health status. A holistic approach to dietary management of a disease by all members of the health care team is especially appropriate to coordinate managed health care.

Since the subject of nutrition is a hot topic in today's world, the consumer is challenged to comprehend and apply the overwhelming amount of nutritional information that can be confusing and conflicting. As the health source that patients may see most often, dental professionals should be able to knowledgeably and authoritatively discuss nutritional practices with their patients or provide appropriate referrals as needed.

New to This Edition

This expertly revised edition provides the most recent developments in the field and new and improved resources for instructors, including:

- The latest federal nutrition standards, including the *2020 Dietary Guidelines for Americans* and *MyPlate*
- Updated art program, featuring modern illustrations, more clinical photos, and food-source photos within micronutrient chapters
- Content on interdisciplinary practice and the Food Safety Modernization Act (FSMA), plus expanded coverage of older adults, vitamin D, and nutrigenomics
- Information on the role of biochemistry in dental hygiene and nutrition
- TEACH Lesson Plans, PowerPoints, Answer Keys, and Student Handouts provided for the instructor
- An expanded and improved Test Bank with cognitive leveling based on Bloom's Taxonomy and mapping to the National Board Dental Hygiene Examination (NBDHE) blueprint

Organization

Part I, Orientation to Basic Nutrition, deals with basic principles of nutrition. A basic understanding of fundamental nutrition facts enables the dental hygienist to make wise judgments about eating habits, educate patients about needed dietary changes, and evaluate the flood of new information available. Nutrient deficiencies and excesses are addressed in sections entitled *Hyper-States* and *Hypo-States,* terms that are more congruent with real-life occurrences. Chapters addressing vitamins and minerals are arranged to cover the specific nutrients involved in oral calcified structures or oral soft tissues. The chapter entitled *Concepts in Biochemistry* introduces a basic understanding of biochemistry, the foundation for understanding and applying principles of nutrition. This chapter serves as a valuable resource throughout the textbook.

Part II, Considerations of Clinical Nutrition, addresses problems specifically involved in the application of basic nutrition principles through the lifespan within ethnic groups and socioeconomically deprived individuals. Because of the ever-changing, diverse population in the United States, food pyramids or food guides from eight different cultural groups are provided within the chapters or on the back cover. This helps dental hygienists recognize that food choices different from their own eating patterns may be nutritionally healthy. By approaching any necessary modifications with sensitivity and respect, patients are more likely to make suggested changes. Alterations in nutritional requirements and eating patterns affected by various stages of life—specifically for females, infants and children, and older adults—are discussed.

Part III, Nutritional Aspects of Oral Health, looks at factors involved in oral problems and the nutritional treatment of these problems. In these chapters, *Dental Considerations* and *Nutritional Directions* boxes provide specific information to consider during an assessment and educational dialogue by the dental professional, including (1) *physical* status and *dietary* habits; (2) *interventions*, or factors that need to be considered when caring for the patient; and (3) *evaluations* concerning the patient's ability or motivation to make changes based on what has been learned during the appointment. A nutritional assessment is a basic procedure in dental management for the nutritional well-being of all patients. This involves performing a medical and dental assessment, evaluating dietary intake/history, and educating patients about healthful changes in food choices. Many conditions or their outcome are improved by encouraging patients to eat a wide variety of foods and beverages in appropriate portion sizes or to make minor changes in food choices to improve their health.

A variety of features throughout the text help to enhance the learning experience:

- **Student Learning Outcomes:** A list of outcomes accompanies each chapter to provide a guide to the important information to acquire from the chapter.
- **Key Terms:** Definitions of unfamiliar terms for each chapter in **bold** and **blue** letters within the text; also compiled in the **Glossary** for easy reference.
- **Test Your NQ** (nutrition quotient): True-false pretests to stimulate interest in the reading assignment; answers conveniently located in the back of the book.
- **Dental Considerations:** Practical information affecting the patient's care or nutritional status.
- **Nutritional Directions:** Information to teach the patient to improve oral health and overall health status; stimulating discussions with the patient using the educational information for improvement of oral health, food choices, and/or overall health status.
- **Health Applications:** Current "hot topics" in nutrition, including the ways to obtain an adequate balance of nutrients by a vegetarian; understanding the difficulty in diagnosing persons with gluten sensitivity or intolerance, and adhering to a gluten-free diet; causes and treatment of obesity; and appropriate use of vitamin and mineral supplements.
- **Case Application:** Potential patient situations describing a clinical situation and providing the five-step care plan to help "pull it all together."
- **Student Readiness:** Questions at the end of each chapter for students to determine their comprehension of the subject.
- **Case Studies:** Practical case studies for students to test their ability to make sound judgments when faced with real-life patient scenarios.

About Evolve

The Evolve website offers a variety of additional learning tools that greatly enhance the text for both students and instructors.

For the Student

Evolve Student Resources offers the following:

- **Practice Quizzes.** Each chapter contains approximately 400 National Board Dental Hygiene Examination-style questions with instant-feedback answers, rationales, and page number references for remediation.
- **Illustrated Case Studies.** Written scenarios with accompanying photographs, and follow-up questions present situations observed frequently. These case studies serve as an excellent review source for the National Board Dental Hygiene Examination.
- **Nutritrac Nutrition Analysis Version 5.0:** An online tool allows users to analyze specifics of food intake and energy expenditure, manage weight loss and gain goals, and analyze nutrition and weight status.
- **Food Pyramids and Guides from Around the World.** Food pyramids and guides from a variety of countries are provided, including Mexico, Puerto Rico, the Philippines, Korea, China, Canada, Great Britain, Germany, Australia, Portugal, and Sweden. Also included are the Native American Food Pyramid, Mediterranean Diet Pyramid, DASH Eating Plan, Healthy Vegetarian Eating Patterns, My Vegan Plate, and MyPlate for Older Adults (©Tufts University).
- **Food Diary and Food Analysis Forms.** Printable versions of forms needed to complete the Personal Assessment Project as well as printable versions for Carbohydrate Intake Analysis and Menu Planning Record.
- **MNA Mini Nutritional Assessment.** A validated nutrition screening tool that can be used to asses for malnutrition in patients 65 years and older.

For the Instructor

Evolve Instructor Resources offers the following:

- **Testbank.** An extensive test bank makes the creation of quizzes and exams easier.
- **TEACH Instructor Resources.**
  - **Lesson Plans** organize chapter content into 50-minute class times and map to educational standards and chapter learning objectives.
  - **PowerPoints** provide lecture presentations with talking points for discussion, all mapped to chapter learning objectives.
  - **Student Handouts** are PDFs of the lecture presentations for easy posting and sharing with students.
- **Image Collection.** An image collection with the illustrations from the textbook is provided for ease of incorporating a photo or drawing into a lecture or quiz.
- **Personal Assessment Project.** A classroom learning activity is provided for students to objectively assess their own personal dietary patterns, practice the process of recording and analyzing food intake for its nutritive and cariogenic value, and use nutritional and dental knowledge to contribute to better general and oral health for self and patients.

Note From the Authors

With a better understanding of the importance of food choices, the members of a multidisciplinary health care team can complement each other's work and provide optimal care for the patient. Even though specific amounts of nutrients are mentioned, the intent of this text is not for prescriptive use. Instead, its purpose is to provide dental hygiene students and practicing dental professionals with a relative idea of the amounts of various nutrients needed so that viable food sources can be recommended.

Dr. Cynthia Stegeman
Judi Ratliff Davis

Acknowledgments

Because of the diversity of subjects presented in a general nutrition textbook, a compilation of the work of many people, whether direct or indirect, is necessary to present current and evidence-based information that is relevant to dental professionals. Whether the aid was in the area of a research study or verbal or written communications, each person's help and support is truly appreciated.

Our sincere thanks to Barbara Altshuler, Assistant Professor Emeritus, Caruth School of Dental Hygiene, Baylor College of Dentistry, who "birthed" this nutrition textbook for dental hygienists and took this baby to W. B. Saunders to develop a resource for dental hygienists to assess the nutritional status of their patients. While your "early retirement" is a true loss to the dental hygiene profession, we hope you are enjoying your family time. It takes a team of experts to complete a textbook. We would like to acknowledge the hard work of Dr. Scott Tremain, Associate Professor in the Department of Chemistry at the University of Cincinnati Blue Ash, for creating a practical and usable chapter in biochemistry. Condensing complex information into one chapter is quite a feat. Another valuable contributor to the textbook is Dr. Amy Sullivan, RDH, at the University of Mississippi Medical Center. She worked diligently to improve Chapters 18 to 21. In addition to her knowledge in dental issues, her excellent photos provide an important supplement to the text. We also thank her dental hygiene students for their participation in the photos to demonstrate various education concepts. Special thanks to the dental hygiene faculty, staff, and students at the University of Cincinnati Blue Ash for their encouragement, expertise, and provision of research. Their consistent support and praise make the monumental task of updating a nutrition textbook easier and rewarding.

A special thanks to the librarians at the Texas Department of State Health Services, Carolyn Medina and David McLellan, who were superb at locating scientific references for "dramatic findings" publicized by the press. In addition to those listed, there are countless other friends and relatives to whom we wish to express our gratitude for their encouragement and support. Objective critiques from reviewers are invaluable to a good publication. We appreciate the insight, perspective, words of encouragement, and valuable ideas of the following reviewers:

Wanda Cloet, RDH, MS, Central Community College, Hastings, Nebraska; Nanette Feil-Megill, BSc, DDS, RRDH, CAE, Canadian National Institute of Health, Ottawa, Ontario, Canada; Deborah L. Johnson, RDH-EPP, MS, Eastern Washington University, Spokane, Washington; Jodi Olmsted, RDH, PhD, School of Health Care Professions, University of Wisconsin, Stevens Point, Wisconsin; Nancy Shearer, RDH, BS, MEd, Cape Cod Community College, West Barnstable, Massachusetts; Julie Stage-Rosenberg, RDH, MPH, Truckee Meadows Community College, Reno, Nevada.

In addition, we appreciate the editing "eagle eye" of Professor Luke Burroughs, RDH, MPH, an assistant professor in the dental hygiene program at the University of Cincinnati Blue Ash.

We also wish to thank the many staff members at Elsevier who worked so tirelessly in the various phases of planning and producing this book. We are especially grateful to Kristin Wilhelm, Director, Private Sector Education Content, and Becky Leenhouts, Senior Content Development Specialist, for their helpful ideas and for seeing us through this project.

About the Authors

Cynthia A. Stegeman, RDH, EdD, RDN, LD, CDE, FAND is the Chairperson and Professor in the Dental Hygiene Program at the University of Cincinnati Blue Ash. She has taught Nutrition and Health Education for over 30 years. Dr. Stegeman has been a dental hygienist for over 35 years and a long-time member of the American Dental Hygienists' Association and the Academy of Nutrition and Dietetics. She is currently the Ohio delegate to the Academy of Nutrition and Dietetics, a member of the National Board Dental Hygiene Examination test construction committee, a consultant in the evaluation process of licensure of candidates for the dental hygiene profession for the Commission on Dental Competency Assessments, and a Certified Diabetes Educator. In addition, she speaks to numerous community and professional groups nationally and internationally, and has published over 80 articles on nutrition, dentistry, and diabetes. Dr. Stegeman received an Associate of Applied Science in Dental Hygiene from the University of Cincinnati, Bachelor of Science in Public Health Dentistry from Indiana University Purdue University at Indianapolis, Master of Education in Nutrition from the University of Cincinnati, dietetic internship from The Christ Hospital in Cincinnati, and Doctorate of Education in Instructional Design and Technology from the University of Cincinnati.

Judi Ratliff Davis, MS, RDN has been working in the field of nutrition and dietetics for 50 years. She worked for the Texas Department of State Health Services as a Quality Assurance Nutrition Consultant for the Women, Infants and Children (WIC) program for over 10 years. Despite retirement in Austin, Texas, she continues to be very active, serving as a volunteer in community service and church organizations locally—Lake Travis Crisis Ministries (local food bank), Healthcare Volunteer Associates Clinic, Lake Travis Mobile Meals, and Austin Disaster Relief Network–helping to ensure unmet nutritional needs of the less fortunate, both physically and economically. She also enjoys volunteering for the Texas Performing Arts at the University of Texas. An active member of the Academy of Nutrition and Dietetics for 50 years, she has held numerous offices and served on many committees in the Fort Worth Dietetic Association and the Austin Dietetic Association. She has had a variety of experiences in the field of nutrition, including teaching, clinical dietitian, and consultant. She taught various nutrition courses to dental hygiene, nursing, and child development students as well as food service courses at Tarrant County College in Fort Worth, Texas. Her roles as a clinical dietitian and Certified Nutrition Support Specialist include Home-Based Community Support (HCS), Tarrant County Mental Health Mental Retardation; Rehabilitation Hospital of North Texas, Arlington, Texas; Fort Worth State School, Fort Worth, Texas; Rex Hospital, Raleigh, North Carolina; and Baptist Memorial Hospital, San Antonio, Texas. As a nutrition consultant, she worked in long-term care facilities and mental health facilities in western Virginia, San Antonio, and the Dallas–Fort Worth area, and for the Greenhouse, a health spa in Arlington, Texas. She also coauthored the nursing textbook *Applied Nutrition and Diet Therapy for Nurses* and has written several chapters for nursing references and textbooks. She received her Bachelor of Science degree in Foods and Nutrition from the University of Texas, Austin; Master of Science degree in Nutrition from Texas Woman's University, Denton; and completed a dietetic internship at Indiana University Medical Center, Indianapolis.

Contents

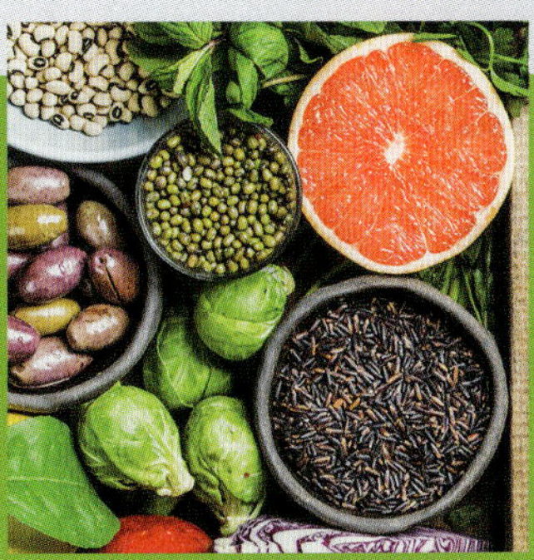

1 Overview of Healthy Eating Habits

STUDENT LEARNING OUTCOMES

Upon completion of this chapter, the student will be able to achieve the following student learning outcomes:

1. Discuss why dental hygenists, registered dietitians, and nutritionists need to be competent in assessing and providing basic nutritional education to patients.
2. List and describe the general physiologic functions of the six nutrient classifications of foods. Also, describe factors that influence patients' food habits.
3. Discuss government concerns with nutrition, as well as the purpose and objectives of *Healthy People 2020*.
4. Discuss Dietary Reference Intakes (DRIs).
5. Describe the purpose of the *2015-2020 Dietary Guidelines for Americans*, and determine the number of food equivalents needed from each food group and subgroup based on the Healthy U.S.-Style Eating Pattern for various calorie levels.
6. Describe healthy eating patterns, and discuss the importance of vegetables, fruits, dairy, protein foods, and oils.
7. Discuss nutrients to limit, as well as other dietary components such as alcohol and caffeine.
8. Describe how physical activity and physical fitness are important factors for an individual's overall health, and how healthful choices should be supported by all systems.
9. Assess the dietary intake of a patient using the *MyPlate* system. Also, discuss other food guides and how they compare to the *MyPlate* system.
10. Master how to read a nutritional label.

KEY TERMS

Acceptable macronutrient distribution ranges (AMDRs)
Adequate Intake (AI)
Bariatric surgery
Body mass index (BMI)
Calorie (cal)
c-eq
Daily Value (DV)
Dietary Reference Intakes (DRIs)
Energy
Enrichment
Estimated Average Requirement (EAR)
Estimated Energy Requirement (EER)
Fortification
Ghrelin
Health claim
Healthy U.S.-Style Eating Pattern (U.S.-Pattern)
Hydrogenation
Hypertension
Kilocalorie (kcal)
Low nutrient density
Macronutrients
Micronutrients
Nutrient content claims
Nutrient-dense
Nutrients
Nutrition
Nutrition and Dietetic Technician, Registered (DTR)
Nutrition Facts label
Nutritionist
Obesity
Overweight
oz-eq
Physical activity
Physical fitness
Phytochemicals
Precursor
Qualified health claims
Recommended Dietary Allowances (RDAs)
Registered dietitian (RD)/registered dietitian nutritionist (RDN)
Satiety
Tolerable Upper Intake Level (UL)
***Trans* fatty acids**
Unqualified health claims
Whole grains

TEST YOUR NQ

1. **T/F** Milk is a perfect food for everyone.
2. **T/F** According to the *Dietary Guidelines for Americans*, consumption of all sugars should be reduced.
3. **T/F** Water is the most important nutrient.
4. **T/F** Dietary Reference Intakes (DRIs) are required daily intakes essential for all patients to be healthy.
5. **T/F** Good nutrition is possible regardless of a patient's cultural habits.
6. **T/F** Based on *MyPlate*, two to four servings daily are needed from the fruit and vegetable group.
7. **T/F** The *Dietary Guidelines for Americans* were written for healthy people to help reduce their risk of developing chronic diseases.
8. **T/F** Sugar is the leading cause of chronic health problems.
9. **T/F** The goal of the *MyPlate Food Guidance System* is to convey the importance of variety, moderation, and proportion.
10. **T/F** The only nutrients that provide energy are carbohydrates, fats, and vitamins.

The dental hygiene profession continues to grow and rapidly move into the forefront of health care. To function as valuable members of today's health care team, the dental hygienist must be knowledgeable in various aspects of health care. Because of the lifelong, synergistic, bidirectional relationship between oral health and nutritional status, dental hygienists and registered dietitians and nutritionists need to be competent in assessing and providing basic education to patients and provide referrals to each other to effect comprehensive patient care.

All registered dietitians and some nutritionists are considered experts in the field of food and nutrition, but their training prepares them for slightly different specialties. A **nutritionist** may have a 4-year degree in foods and nutrition and usually works in a public health setting assisting people in the community, such as pregnant women or older individuals, with diet-related health issues. In many states, a nutritionist is legally defined and is licensed or certified. Nutritionists work in local or state health departments and in the extension service of a land-grant university. A **registered dietitian (RD)** or **registered dietitian nutritionist (RDN)** has completed a minimum of a bachelor's degree in foods and nutrition with training in normal and clinical nutrition, food science, food service management, research, and medical nutrition therapy. The credential RDN is granted by the Commission on Dietetic Registration for the Academy of Nutrition and Dietetics for those who have passed a national registration examination and who maintain updated knowledge of the field through continuing education. RDNs working in hospitals, long-term care facilities, health care providers' offices, and pharmaceutical companies may be more involved with medical nutrition therapy or specialized diets. RDNs may also work in settings dealing principally with basic nutrition, such as in schools, community and research settings, wellness and fitness centers, public health and community programs, educational institutions, and health and wellness preventive programs. The addition of the term *nutritionist* helps identify the type of work performed. Actually, all registered dietitians are nutritionists, but not all nutritionists are registered dietitians.

A **Nutrition and Dietetic Technician, Registered (NDTR)** has completed a 2-year degree program in a dietetic technician program or has a 4-year degree from an approved program (approved by the Accreditation Council for Education in Nutrition and Dietetics). An NDTR, like the RDN, must pass a national registration examination and receive continuing education. The DTR normally works under the supervision of an RDN in such practice areas as hospitals, clinics, and nursing homes, but they may also work independently to provide general nutrition education to healthy populations.

Dental professionals typically see patients on a more regular basis than other health care professionals; this allows observation of many physical signs, particularly oral signs, of a nutrient deficiency or medical condition that affects nutritional status before it is diagnosed. Recognition of abnormal conditions and early referral to an appropriate health care professional can lead to positive health outcomes for patients. Assessment of dietary information obtained from a patient can also uncover habits detrimental to oral health readily addressed in the dental office. Additionally, compromised oral health may affect food choices. For example, patients with missing dentition or ill-fitting dentures may avoid foods that are hard to chew and reduce the quality and variety of their diets.

Finally, dental hygienists can follow up on goals established by patients to evaluate their understanding and compliance. Overall, the dental hygienist is committed to prevention of oral disease as well as the promotion of health and wellness. All health care professionals must work together to enhance patient care. This textbook provides the dental professional with the nutrition information that can realistically be applied to and practiced with patients in the dental setting.

Basic Nutrition

Nutrition is the process by which living things use food to obtain nutrients for energy, growth and development, and maintenance. **Energy** is the ability or power to do work. **Nutrients** are biochemical substances that can be supplied only in adequate amounts from an outside source, normally from food. One aspect of nutrition is the integration of physiologic and biochemical reactions within the body: (a) digesting food to make nutrients available, (b) absorbing and delivering nutrients to the cells where they are used, and (c) eliminating waste products.

Nutrition is a relatively new science and still an evolving discipline. People want science to be definitive; they become confused and concerned when scientific research challenges what they assume to be factual. In nutrition, something that is considered to be true today may be disrupted by future research refuting established beliefs. In many cases, the media exacerbate this situation by reporting new research and recommendations as soon as they are released. These findings may not necessarily be reproduced in further research. Often, it is difficult to separate a medical certainty from what is merely solid scientific conjecture. The pace of research has quickened; this text is based on current, well-established, and evidence-based nutrition advice. Everyone in the health care field must continue to stay abreast of ongoing research to knowledgeably respond to questions from patients.

Americans are interested in food and health issues and are concerned about their diet, their physical activity, and substances in foods they eat, but most Americans find it easier to do their own taxes than to choose an adequate balanced diet. This may be related to the fact that nutrition information is ever changing.

Psychological and social factors that enter into frequent decisions concerning food choices are also important aspects of nutrition. Freedom of choice and variety in consumption are important components of an individual's personal and social life. Tastes, budget, environment, and cultural attitudes influence food choices. Systemic and environmental effects of nutrients, which are determined by these food choices, affect dental health.

Physiologic Functions of Nutrients

Physiologically, foods eaten are used for energy, tissue building, maintenance and replacement, and obtaining or producing numerous regulatory substances. Nutrients obtained from foods are the following: (1) water, (2) proteins, (3) carbohydrates, (4) fats, (5) minerals, and (6) vitamins. Other naturally occurring substances in various foods, such as **phytochemicals** (plant chemicals) also promote health.

Of these nutrients, only proteins, carbohydrates, and fats provide energy. Alcohol also provides calories but limited or no nutrients. The potential energy value of foods within the body is expressed in terms of the kilocalorie, more frequently referred to as the **calorie**. A **kilocalorie (kcal)** is a measure of heat equivalent to 1000 calories.

Nutrients work together and interact in complex metabolic reactions. Proteins, carbohydrates, and fats provide energy the body needs for metabolic processes. However, the body cannot use energy from these caloric-containing components of food without adequate amounts of vitamins and minerals. Vitamins and minerals, along with protein and water, are essential for the body to build and maintain body tissues and to regulate essential body processes.

Basic Concepts of Nutrition

Foods differ in the amount of nutrients they furnish. Any individual food can be compatible with good nutrition but should be evaluated in the context of the patient's physiologic needs, the food's nutrient content, and other food choices. The premise of nutritional care is that, in any cultural or environmental circumstance or for any personal taste or preference, good nutrition is possible. The total diet or overall pattern of food intake is the most important focus of healthful eating.

Increasing the variety of healthful foods consumed reduces the probability of developing isolated nutrient deficiencies, nutrient excesses, and toxicities resulting from nonnutritive components or contaminants in any particular food. A dietary change to eliminate or increase intake of one specific food component or nutrient usually alters the intake of other nutrients. For instance, because red meats are an excellent source of iron and zinc, decreasing cholesterol intake by limiting these meats can reduce dietary iron and zinc intake.

Essential nutrients are needed throughout life on a regular basis; only the amounts of nutrients require change. The patient's consumption of foods and beverages, stage of growth and development, sex, body size, weight, physical activity, and state of health influence nutrient requirements.

Some nutrients can be converted by the body to meet physiologic needs. Nonessential nutrients can be used by the body but either are not required or can be synthesized from dietary precursors. **Precursors** are substances from which an active substance is formed. An example is carotene, found in fruits and vegetables, which the liver can convert into an active form of vitamin A.

Water is the most important nutrient. After water, nutrients of highest priority are those providing energy, which must be obtained from foods or supplied from physiologic stores. The human body has adaptive mechanisms that allow toleration of modest ranges in nutrient intakes. For instance, the metabolic rate usually decreases as a result of decreased caloric intake.

DENTAL CONSIDERATIONS

- Because nutrients work interdependently, a lack or excess of one can interfere with or prevent use of another. Asking the patient to record food and beverage intake for the past 24 to 72 hours allows assessment of nutrient intake.
- Evaluation of the patient's intake of food and beverages can help determine whether intake is adequate or excessive.
- Abnormalities in the oral cavity can affect systemic health and nutrition. Additionally, nutritional conditions or their treatments can affect the oral cavity or the feasibility of delivering dental care.

NUTRITIONAL DIRECTIONS

- No single food contains all the essential nutrients in amounts needed for optimal health.
- Nutritional intake can either improve or adversely affect health.

Government Nutrition Concerns

Before 1977, nutritional efforts focused on ensuring that the food supply provided adequate nutrients to prevent deficiency diseases. The U.S. government recognized health and nutritional problems related to food choices in 1977 with the *United States Dietary Goals*, which addressed excessive consumption of some nutrients. In 1988, the Surgeon General issued a report confirming that 5 of the 10 leading causes of death (cardiovascular disease [CVD], certain types of cancer, stroke, diabetes mellitus, and atherosclerosis) were associated with dietary intake. These reports provided comprehensive science-based objectives to improve the health of the U.S. population and to establish national objectives for promoting health and preventing disease.

Healthy People Nutrition Objectives

Healthy People 2000: National Health Promotion and Disease Prevention Objectives, initially introduced in 1990 by the U.S. Department of Health and Human Services (USDHHS), established objectives and goals to measure progress in specific areas. The objectives for *Healthy People* focus on (a) increasing the quality and years of healthy life, (b) eliminating health disparities among racial and ethnic groups, (c) creating social and physical environments that promote good health for everyone, and (d) promoting quality of life and healthful development and behaviors of all age groups. Based on progress toward these objectives by 2010, many of the 10-year national objectives were continued if they had not been met and/or goals were adjusted, and new goals were set for 2020. New topics continue to be added as needed.

Healthy People 2020 (*Healthy People)* identifies emerging public health priorities and aligns them with health promotion strategies driven by the best evidence available. *Healthy People 2020* is organized into 42 topic areas with about 600 measurable objectives to be accomplished by 2020. It targets 22 objectives related to nutrition, physical activity, and weight, and 17 objectives related to oral health.[1]

A midcourse progress report on these objectives indicates that there was little or no detectable change for the prevalence of obesity among adults or children and adolescents or in mean daily intake of vegetables, but goals were met for adults meeting physical activity and muscle-strengthening objectives. The number of children, adolescents, and adults who had an annual dental visit declined. Two oral health objectives showing significant improvement are to increase the percentage of the U.S. population served by community water systems that are optimally fluoridated and the proportion of children who have received dental sealants.[2] Little to no progress has been accomplished in the area of reducing health disparities for minority and low-income groups. Many other objectives showed small improvements.

Other relevant objectives are referenced throughout this text. The *Healthy People* website (https://www.healthypeople.gov/) is updated frequently, providing consumers and health care providers the opportunity to monitor progress.

Nutrient Recommendations: Dietary Reference Intakes

Recommendations for the amounts of required nutrients have undergone significant changes over the years, and the revised sets of nutrient-based reference values are collectively called the **Dietary Reference Intakes (DRIs**; see pp. iii–vi). In 1993, the Food and Nutrition Board of the Institute of Medicine (IOM, now the National Academy of Medicine) undertook this major project, which was completed in 2004. The DRIs, published by the National Academy of Medicine, are established by an expert group of scientists and RDNs from the United States and Canada. These groups of experts base their recommendations on the most current scientific knowledge from different types of studies involving nutrients for healthy populations.

Previous **Recommended Dietary Allowances (RDAs)** focused on amounts of nutrients necessary to prevent deficiency diseases. The current DRIs also attempt to (a) estimate amounts of required nutrients to improve long-term health and well-being by reducing risk of chronic diseases affected by nutrition, for example, heart disease, diabetes, osteoporosis, and cancer; and (b) establish maximum safe levels of tolerance. The four categories of nutrient-based reference values are relevant for various stages of life. The DRIs were intended for planning and assessing diets of healthy Americans and Canadians. The DRIs are inappropriate for malnourished individuals or patients whose requirements are affected by a disease state. Because of emerging evidence involving potential roles of nutrients or other food substances in ameliorating chronic diseases, the National Academies appointed a committee to make recommendations for establishing DRIs for specific nutrients that could ameliorate the risk of chronic diseases. In 2017, *Guiding Principles for Developing Dietary Reference Intakes Based on Chronic Disease* ad hoc committee established guiding principles to support future DRI committees in making decisions about recommending chronic disease DRIs.

Estimated Average Requirement

The **Estimated Average Requirement (EAR)** is the amount of a nutrient that is estimated to meet the needs of half of the healthy individuals in a specific age and gender group. This set of values is useful in assessing nutrient adequacy or planning intakes of population groups, not individuals.

Recommended Dietary Allowance

The new RDA is generally higher than the EAR and provides a sufficient amount of a nutrient to meet the requirements of nearly all healthy individuals (97%–98%). These recommendations provide a generous margin of safety and are intended as a goal for achieving adequate intakes. No health benefits are established for consuming intakes greater than the RDA.

Adequate Intakes

If sufficient scientific evidence was unavailable to determine an EAR or RDA, an **Adequate Intake (AI)** was established based on scientific judgments. An AI, which is derived from mean nutrient intakes by groups of healthy people, is the average amount of a nutrient that seems to maintain a defined nutritional state. An AI is expected to exceed average requirements of virtually all members of a life stage/gender group but is more tentative than an RDA. AI values were established for various life stages for several nutrients, including fluoride, because of uncertainties about the scientific data to determine EAR and RDA values that would reduce the risk of chronic disease.

Tolerable Upper Intake Level

A **Tolerable Upper Intake Level (UL)** is the maximum daily level of nutrient intake that probably would not cause adverse health effects or toxic effects for most individuals in the general population. The potential risk of adverse effects increases as intake exceeds the UL. The term Tolerable Intake was selected to avoid implying that these higher levels would result in beneficial effects. These values are especially helpful because of increased consumption of nutrients in the form of dietary supplements or from enrichment and fortification. This recommendation pertains to habitual daily use and is based on combined intake of food, water, dietary supplements, and fortified foods, with a few exceptions: the UL for magnesium applies only to intake from nonfood sources; ULs for vitamin E, niacin, and folate apply only to fortified foods or supplement sources; and UL for vitamin A applies only to intake of preformed retinol, regardless of the source.

Acceptable Macronutrient Distribution Ranges

Acceptable Macronutrient Distribution Ranges (AMDRs) were established for the macronutrients, fat, carbohydrate, protein, and two polyunsaturated fatty acids, to ensure sufficient intakes of essential nutrients (carbohydrate, protein and fat), while potentially reducing risk of chronic disease. **Macronutrients** are energy-providing nutrients needed in larger amounts than **micronutrients**, for example, vitamins and minerals. The AMDR is a range of intakes for food components that provide calories; these are expressed as a percentage of total energy intake because the intake of each depends on intake of the others or of total energy requirement of the individual. Increasing or decreasing one energy source while consuming a set amount of calories affects intake of the other sources of energy. For instance, if an individual who routinely consumes 2000 cal reduces fat intake, either protein or carbohydrate intake would need to increase to provide 2000 cal. Consuming amounts outside of the ranges increases risk of insufficient intake of essential nutrients. Recommended ranges for carbohydrates, fats, and proteins allow more flexibility in eating patterns for healthy individuals and as well as accomodating individual preferences.

Estimated Energy Requirement

The **Estimated Energy Requirement (EER)** is defined as dietary energy intake that is predicted to maintain energy balance in healthy, normal-weight individuals of a defined age, gender, weight, height, and physical activity level consistent with good health. The EER is similar to the EAR, and no RDA was established because consuming more calories than are needed would result in weight gain. Because energy requirement depends on activity level, four different activity levels are provided.

Summary of Dietary Reference Intakes

Because nutrient requirements are influenced by age and sexual development, the DRIs are listed for 16 groups, separating gender groups after 10 years of age. Separate levels are established for three categories of pregnant and lactating women. Also, two age groups for the older American population are available.

These guidelines apply to average daily intakes. Meeting the recommendations for every nutrient on a daily basis is very difficult and unnecessary. These nutrient goals are intended to be met by consuming a variety of foods whenever possible.

DENTAL CONSIDERATIONS

- Use of DRIs as an assessment guide is for healthy patients only.
- An individual's exact requirement for a specific nutrient is not known for certain.
- The ULs may be used to warn patients that excessive intake of nutrients from nutritional supplements could lead to adverse effects if taken on a regular basis.
- Generally, specific foods or food groups, rather than nutrients, should be discussed with patients.
- If an individual's food consumption is below the RDA for a nutrient over several days, more food choices containing that particular nutrient should be encouraged.

NUTRITIONAL DIRECTIONS

- The DRIs are general guidelines for good health rather than specific requirements.
- Choosing a wide variety of foods will probably result in meeting established nutrient requirements.

Food Guidance System for Americans

Identification of nutrients and knowledge of their physiologic functions are significant developments. However, consumers eat and think in terms of food, not nutrients. Nutrient requirements and information must be interpreted into the "food" language that consumers understand. In 2015, the USDHHS and the U.S. Department of Agriculture (USDA) released the *Dietary Guidelines for Americans 2015–2020 (Dietary Guidelines)*, the eighth edition of the guidelines. These *Dietary Guidelines* are based on scientific knowledge to meet nutrient requirements, promote health, support active lives through physical activity, and reduce risks of chronic disease. The *Dietary Guidelines* are the foundation for *MyPlate* (www.ChooseMyPlate.gov), released in 2011 to help consumers become healthier by making wise food choices.

Another helpful tool is the food label that helps consumers determine what kind and how much food to eat. Nutrition labeling, required for most packaged foods, provides information on certain nutrients. The **Nutrition Facts label** enumerates nutrient content of food for the serving size specified and discloses the number of servings in the package. Knowing how to interpret labels enables consumers to accurately apply *Dietary Guideline* messages that correspond to the nutrients and other information on the label.

2015–2020 Dietary Guidelines for Americans

The objective of the five key guidelines is to help consumers make healthful choices from each of the food groups that, with an awareness of caloric intake, will result in an overall healthful eating pattern (Fig. 1.1). An eating pattern represents all the foods and beverages consumed over time or a customary way of eating. Ideally, it meets nutritional needs without exceeding limitations with regard to saturated fats, added sugars, sodium, and total calories. The long-range goal of the *Dietary Guidelines* is to prevent, or at least decrease, the rate of chronic disease and mortality. Interestingly, a recent study attributed dietary factors as a substantial cause of mortality from heart disease, stroke, and type 2 diabetes.

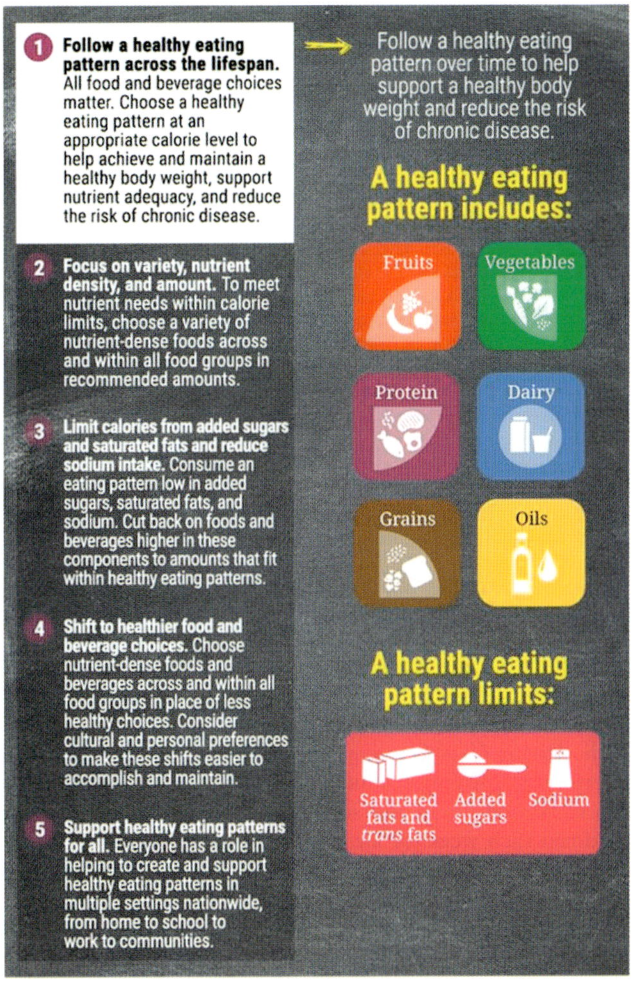
1 Follow a healthy eating pattern across the lifespan. All food and beverage choices matter. Choose a healthy eating pattern at an appropriate calorie level to help achieve and maintain a healthy body weight, support nutrient adequacy, and reduce the risk of chronic disease.
2 Focus on variety, nutrient density, and amount. To meet nutrient needs within calorie limits, choose a variety of nutrient-dense foods across and within all food groups in recommended amounts.
3 Limit calories from added sugars and saturated fats and reduce sodium intake. Consume an eating pattern low in added sugars, saturated fats, and sodium. Cut back on foods and beverages higher in these components to amounts that fit within healthy eating patterns.
4 Shift to healthier food and beverage choices. Choose nutrient-dense foods and beverages across and within all food groups in place of less healthy choices. Consider cultural and personal preferences to make these shifts easier to accomplish and maintain.
5 Support healthy eating patterns for all. Everyone has a role in helping to create and support healthy eating patterns in multiple settings nationwide, from home to school to work to communities.
Follow a healthy eating pattern over time to help support a healthy body weight and reduce the risk of chronic disease.
A healthy eating pattern includes:
Fruits
Vegetables
Protein
Dairy
Grains
Oils
A healthy eating pattern limits:
Saturated fats and trans fats
Added sugars
Sodium

• **Figure 1.1** *2015–2020 Dietary Guidelines for Americans*. (From the U.S. Department of Agriculture and U.S. Department of Health and Human Services: *2015-2020 Dietary Guidelines for Americans*. 8th ed. Washington, DC; U.S. Government Printing Office: December 2015. https://health.gov/dietaryguidelines/2015/.)

TABLE 1.1 Healthy U.S.-Style Eating Pattern: Recommended Amounts of Food From Each Food Group at 12 Calorie Levels

Calorie Level of Pattern[a]	1000	1200	1800	2000	2400	3000
Food Group	**Daily Amount**[b] of Food From Each Group (vegetable and protein foods subgroup amounts are per week)					
Vegetables	**1 c-eq**	**1½ c-eq**	**2½ c-eq**	**2½ c-eq**	**3 c-eq**	**4 c-eq**
Dark-green vegetables (c-eq/wk)	½	1	1½	1½	2	2½
Red and orange vegetables (c-eq/wk)	2½	3	5½	5½	6	7½
Legumes (beans and peas; c-eq/wk)	½	½	1½	1½	2	3
Starchy vegetables (c-eq/wk)	2	3½	5	5	6	8
Other vegetables (c-eq/wk)	1½	2½	4	4	5	7
Fruits	**1 c-eq**	**1 c-eq**	**1½ c-eq**	**2 c-eq**	**2 c-eq**	**2½ c-eq**
Grains	**3 oz-eq**	**4 oz-eq**	**6 oz-eq**	**6 oz-eq**	**8 oz-eq**	**10 oz-eq**
Whole grains[c] (oz-eq/day)	1½	2	3	3	4	5
Refined grains (oz-eq/day)	1½	2	3	3	4	5
Dairy	**2 c-eq**	**2½ c-eq**	**3 c-eq**	**3 c-eq**	**3 c-eq**	**3 c-eq**
Protein Foods	**2 oz-eq**	**3 oz-eq**	**5 oz-eq**	**5½ oz-eq**	**6½ oz-eq**	**7 oz-eq**
Seafood (oz-eq/wk)	3	4	8	8	10	10
Meats, poultry, eggs (oz-eq/wk)	10	14	23	26	31	33
Nuts, seeds, soy products (oz-eq/wk)	2	2	4	5	5	6
Oils	**15 g**	**17g**	**24 g**	**27 g**	**31 g**	**44 g**
Limit on calories for other uses, calories (% of calories)[d]	150 (15%)	100 (8%)	170 (9%)	270 (14%)	350 (15%)	470 (16%)

[a]Food intake patterns at 1000, 1200, and 1400 calories are designed to meet the nutritional needs of 2- to 8-year-old children. Patterns from 1600 to 3200 calories are designed to meet the nutritional needs of children 9 years and older and adults. If a child 4 to 8 years of age needs more calories and, therefore, is following a pattern at 1600 calories or more, that child's recommended amount from the dairy group should be 2.5 cups per day. Children 9 years and older and adults should not use the 1000-, 1200-, or 1400-calorie patterns.
[b]Food group amounts shown in cup-equivalents (c-eq) or ounce-equivalents (oz-eq), as appropriate for each group, based on caloric and nutrient content.
[c]Amounts of whole grains in the Patterns for children are less than the minimum of 3 oz-eq in all Patterns recommended for adults.
[d]All foods are assumed to be in nutrient-dense forms; lean or low-fat; and prepared without added fats, sugars, refined starches, or salt. If all food choices to meet food group recommendations are in nutrient-dense forms, a small number of calories remain within the overall calorie limit of the Pattern (i.e., limit on calories for other uses). The number of these calories depends on the overall calorie limit in the Pattern and the amounts of food from each food group required to meet nutritional goals. Calories from protein, carbohydrates, and total fats should be within the Acceptable Macronutrient Distribution Ranges (AMDRs).
From U.S. Department of Health and Human Services, U.S. Department of Agriculture: *2015–2020 Dietary Guidelines for Americans.* 8th ed. Washington, DC: 2015 (Dec), USDHHS/USDA. https://health.gov/dietaryguidelines/2015/guidelines/appendix-3/.

Intakes of high sodium, low nuts/seeds, highly processed meats, low seafood omega-3 fats, low fruits, and high sugar-sweetened beverages were related to diet-related deaths.[3] All these nutrients/foods are addressed in the *Dietary Guidelines.*

The *Dietary Guidelines* reference the **Healthy U.S.-Style Eating Pattern (U.S.-Pattern)** that indicates the number of food equivalents from each food group and subgroups for 12 caloric levels to be consumed each week for an adequate healthful diet (Table 1.1). Foods providing similar kinds of nutrients are grouped together and, as a rule, foods in one group cannot replace those in another (Table 1.2). This U.S.-Pattern can be adapted easily using various types and proportions of foods that Americans typically consume; however, to provide all the essential nutrients, foods need to be nutrient dense and in appropriate amounts to prevent exceeding calorie limits and other limiting dietary components. **Nutrient-dense** foods provide substantial amounts of vitamins and minerals but relatively few calories. When many **low nutrient-density** foods or beverages (containing high fat, sugar, or alcohol) are chosen, obtaining adequate amounts of essential nutrients without gaining weight is unachievable. The consumption of excessive calories from fats, added sugars, and refined grains reduces intake of nutrient-dense foods and beverages without exceeding caloric requirements.

Portion control is very important to stay within the desired caloric level. Portion size is different than serving size. The amounts from each food group and subgroup change as needed among the different caloric levels to meet nutrient and *Dietary Guidelines* standards and comply with calories and overconsumed dietary components. Fig. 1.2 is a simple tool from the USDHHS that provides relationships consumers can relate to for estimating portion sizes. Within the U.S.-Pattern, serving or portion sizes are depicted as c-eq or oz-eq. Vegetables, fruits, and dairy food groups are represented with **c-eq**, which is the amount of a food or beverage considered equal to 1 cup or one portion. A serving size of many popular foods or beverages differs due to (1) concentration (e.g.,

TABLE 1.2 Principal Nutrient Contributions of Each Food Group

Nutrients	Vegetable	Fruit	Meat	Milk	Grain
Protein			X	X	X
Vitamin A	X	X			
Vitamin D				X[a]	
Vitamin E	X				
Vitamin C	X	X			
Thiamin			X		X[b]
Riboflavin				X	X[b]
Niacin			X		X[b]
Vitamin B_6			X	X	
Folate/folic acid	X	X			X[b]
Vitamin B_{12}			X[c]	X[c]	
Calcium				X	
Phosphorus			X	X	X
Magnesium	X			X	X[d]
Iron			X		X[b]
Zinc			X	X	X
Fiber	X	X			X[d]

[a]If fortified
[b]If enriched
[c]Only animal products
[d]Whole grains

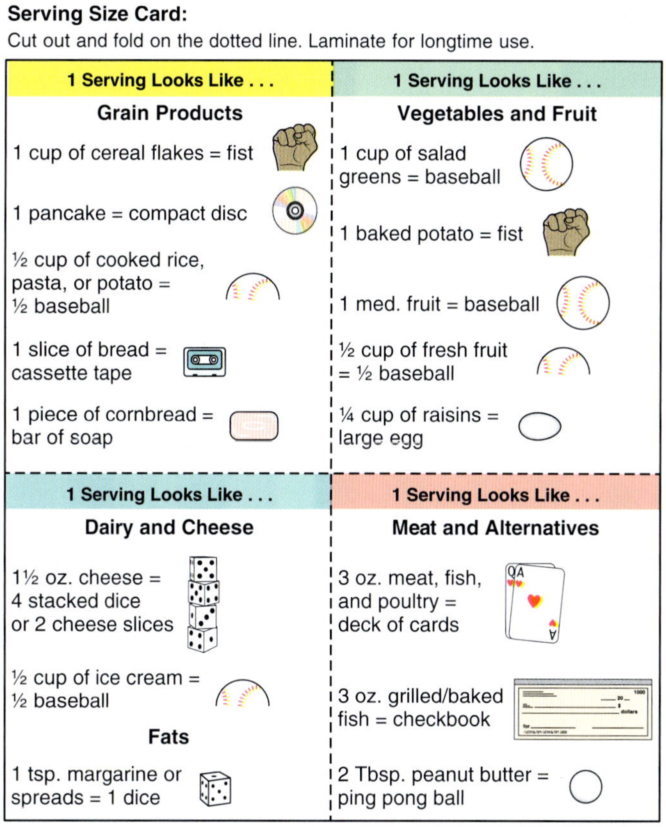
Serving Size Card:
Cut out and fold on the dotted line. Laminate for longtime use.
1 Serving Looks Like . . .
Grain Products
1 cup of cereal flakes = fist
1 pancake = compact disc
½ cup of cooked rice, pasta, or potato = ½ baseball
1 slice of bread = cassette tape
1 piece of cornbread = bar of soap
1 Serving Looks Like . . .
Vegetables and Fruit
1 cup of salad greens = baseball
1 baked potato = fist
1 med. fruit = baseball
½ cup of fresh fruit = ½ baseball
¼ cup of raisins = large egg
1 Serving Looks Like . . .
Dairy and Cheese
1½ oz. cheese = 4 stacked dice or 2 cheese slices
½ cup of ice cream = ½ baseball
Fats
1 tsp. margarine or spreads = 1 dice
1 Serving Looks Like . . .
Meat and Alternatives
3 oz. meat, fish, and poultry = deck of cards
3 oz. grilled/baked fish = checkbook
2 Tbsp. peanut butter = ping pong ball

• **Figure 1.2 Serving size card.** This tool can be used when estimating appropriate serving sizes when choosing/serving foods. (From U.S. Department of Health and Human Services, National Heart, Lung and Blood Institute, Obesity Education Initiative. Serving sizes and portions: and servings: what's the difference? Portion distortion. https://www.nhlbi.nih.gov/health/educational/wecan/downloads/servingcard7.pdf.)

raisins or tomato paste), (2) fresh produce that does not compress into a cup (e.g., salad greens), or (3) foods that are measured in a different form (e.g., meat and cheese). A serving portion of food from the grain or protein groups is equivalent to one ounce (oz-eq). If a food is concentrated or contains minimal amounts of water (e.g., nuts, peanut butter, jerky, cooked beans, rice or pasta), its portion size may be less than a measured ounce (by weight). If it contains a large amount of water (e.g., tofu, cooked beans, cooked rice or pasta), it may be more than a measured ounce (weight).

The U.S.-Patterns meet the RDA for almost all nutrients. Vitamins D and E and potassium are marginal in the U.S.-Patterns for many or all age–sex groups. Intake below the RDA or AI for these nutrients is not considered to be of public health concern.

Other meal patterns endorsed in the 2015–2020 *Dietary Guidelines* include the Dietary Approaches to Stop Hypertension (DASH) diet (see Chapter 12), Mediterranean-Style Eating Pattern (see Evolve website), and Healthy Vegetarian Eating Pattern (see Chapter 5 and Evolve website).

Key Recommendations for Healthy Eating Patterns

A healthful eating pattern includes vegetables, fruits, dairy, protein foods, and oils, as summarized in the Key Recommendations (Box 1.1).

Calorie Balance

Individuals should consume a healthy eating pattern that includes all foods and beverages within an appropriate caloric level to achieve and/or maintain a healthy body weight. The basic element for healthful eating patterns is managing caloric balance, an average equilibrium between calories consumed (food and beverages) and calories expended (metabolic processes and physical activity). For a person to maintain a set weight, energy consumed from foods and beverages must equal calories expended in normal physiologic functions and physical activity. The average intake for Americans age 20 years and over in 2011 to 2012 was 2191 cal per day (1837 cal/day for women and 2567 cal/day for men).[4] Because weight loss is a challenge requiring changes in many behaviors and patterns, avoiding excess pounds is ideal. Even small decreases in caloric intake can help prevent weight gain. A reduction in daily intake of 100 calories to prevent gradual weight gain is much easier than reducing daily intake by 500 calories to lose weight. In general, the best choice for weight loss involves a change in lifestyle, both in diet and physical activity. By frequently monitoring body weight, consumers can determine whether their eating patterns are providing an appropriate amount of calories and thereby adjust food intake and/or activity level. All Americans are encouraged to achieve and/or maintain a healthy body weight:

• BOX 1.1 *2015–2020 Dietary Guidelines for Americans* Executive Summary: Key Recommendations

Consume a healthful eating pattern that accounts for all foods and beverages within an appropriate calorie level.

A Healthy Eating Pattern Includes:*

- A variety of vegetables from all of the subgroups–dark green, red and orange, legumes (beans and peas), starchy, and other
- Fruits, especially whole fruits
- Grains, at least half of which are whole grains
- Fat-free or low-fat dairy, including milk, yogurt, cheese, and/or fortified soy beverages
- A variety of protein foods, including seafood; lean meats and poultry; eggs; legumes (beans and peas); and nuts, seeds, and soy products
- Oils

A Healthy Eating Pattern Limits:

- Saturated fats and *trans* fats, added sugars, and sodium

Key recommendations that are quantitative are provided for several components of the diet that should be limited. These components are of particular public health concern in the United States, and the specified limits can help individuals achieve healthy eating patterns within calorie limits:

- Consume less than 10% of calories per day from added sugars[a]
- Consume less than 10% of calories per day from saturated fats[b]
- Consume less than 2300 milligrams (mg) per day of sodium[c]
- If alcohol is consumed, it should be consumed in moderation—up to one drink per day for women and up to two drinks per day for men—and only by adults of legal drinking age.[d]

**Definitions for each food group and subgroups are provided in subsequent sections of this chapter.*

[a]The recommendation to limit intake of calories from added sugars is a target based on evidence that demonstrates the need to limit added sugars to meet food group and nutrient needs within calorie limits.

[b]The recommendation to limit intake of calories from saturated fats is a target based on evidence that replacing saturated fats with unsaturated fats is associated with reduced risk of cardiovascular disease.

[c]The recommendation to limit intake of sodium is the UL for individuals ages 14 years and older set by the National Academy of Medicine (formerly the Institute of Medicine).

[d]The amount of alcohol and calories in beverages varies and should be accounted for within the limits of healthy eating patterns. There are many circumstances in which individuals should not drink, such as during pregnancy.

From U.S. Department of Health and Human Services, U.S. Department of Agriculture, 2015–2020 Dietary Guidelines for Americans, *8th ed. Washington, DC: USDHHS/USDA, 2015. https://health.gov/dietaryguidelines/2015/guidelines/executive-summary/#key-recs.*

- Children and adolescents are encouraged to maintain calorie balance to support normal growth and development without promoting excess weight gain.
- Women are encouraged to achieve and maintain a healthy weight, and women who are pregnant are encouraged to gain weight within gestational weight gain guidelines (see Chapter 13).
- Adults who are overweight or obese should change both eating habits and physical activity to prevent additional weight gain and/or promote weight loss.
- Older adults (65 years and older) who are overweight or obese are encouraged to prevent additional weight gain. Intentional weight loss is beneficial for patients who have chronic conditions such as CVD or diabetes.

Body weight can be evaluated in relation to a person's height using **body mass index (BMI)** to determine health risks that increase at higher levels of **overweight** (BMI 25.0–29.9) and **obesity** (BMI >30.0). BMI is a preferred method of defining healthy weight because it correlates more closely with actual body fat than height and weight tables. BMI can be determined by using the table on page ix and Table 1.3 to classify body weight category (underweight, normal weight, overweight, or obese). A BMI of less than 25 is generally considered a healthy weight; chronic disease risk increases in most people who have a BMI above 25. BMI reflects overall fat distribution and can be calculated quickly and inexpensively. BMI is not appropriate for pregnant and nursing women, infants and children younger than age 2 years (see special table on the Evolve website for children 2 to 20 years old), or some athletes with a large percentage of muscle.

TABLE 1.3 Body Mass Index and Corresponding Body Weight Categories for Children and Adults

Body Weight Category	Children and Adolescents (Ages 2–19 y; BMI-for-Age Percentile Range)	Adults (BMI)
Underweight	< 5th percentile	< 18.5 kg/m^2
Normal weight	5th percentile to < 85th percentile	18.5–24.9 kg/m^2
Overweight	85th to < 95th percentile	25.0–29.9 kg/m^2
Obese	≥ 95th percentile	≥ 30.0 kg/m^2

From U.S. Department of Health and Human Services, U.S. Department of Agriculture: *2015–2020 Dietary Guidelines for Americans.* 8th ed. 2015 (Dec), USDHHS/USDA. https://health.gov/dietaryguidelines/2015/guidelines/.

BMI reveals little about overall body composition. It is a starting point in assessing an individual's health status and risks that is noninvasive, inexpensive, and quick. Limitations of relying solely on a person's BMI include the following: (1) women tend to have more body fat; (2) BMI can underestimate body fat in an elderly person who has lost lean body mass; (3) ethnic background can impact bone mineral density; and (4) BMI overestimates body fat in individuals who have very high levels of lean body mass. Athletes usually have high BMIs because of their increased muscle mass, not excess fat. On the other hand, a frail or inactive person with a normal-range BMI may have excess body fat and not appear out of shape. Additional muscle tissue aids body functions, but excessive fat interferes with normal metabolism. A healthy weight depends on the amount and location of body fat and other health indicators, such as blood pressure, glucose, and cholesterol and triglyceride levels.

Major ethnic differences exist regarding BMI. For example, Asian Americans or persons from India are at risk of health problems at a lower BMI (18.5–23.9 is a better range) than whites; African Americans can have higher BMIs (28.0) than other populations without developing health problems. Older adults can tolerate slightly more body fat and tend to have a better survival rate with a BMI in the upper range of normal.[5]

All foods and some beverages contain varying amounts of calories based on their nutrient content. Macronutrients include carbohydrates and protein that contribute 4 cal/g; fats, 9 cal/g; and alcohol, which, although not a nutrient, contributes 7 cal/g when consumed. Most foods and beverages contain combinations of macronutrients in varying amounts. There is little evidence that any individual macronutrient has a unique impact on body weight. Caloric intake is the key factor to controlling body weight, not by manipulating the proportions of fat, carbohydrates, and protein but by balancing overall calories with energy expenditure.

A patient's caloric requirements are based on size (height and weight), age, sex, and level of physical activity. Many Americans consume more calories than they need and spend large portions of their days engaged in sedentary behaviors that expend minimal calories. Consequently, many children and adults routinely consume more calories than they expend.

For weight maintenance, caloric requirements typically range from 1600 to 2400 calories daily for adult women and 2000 to 3000 calories for adult men, with variances depending on physical activity. The metabolic rate decreases with age, thus lowering caloric requirements for older adults.

Vegetables

Vegetables are primary sources of the required nutrients dietary fiber, vitamin A (carotenoids), vitamin C, folic acid, and potassium (Table 1.4). Most vegetables are naturally low in fat and are cholesterol free. Because of their high water and fiber content, most vegetables are relatively low in calories. Dark-green vegetables provide calcium, iron, magnesium, and riboflavin. Beans are unusual because they are in both the vegetable and protein groups. Beans contain protein, fiber, calcium, folic acid, and potassium. Choosing dark-green, red, and orange vegetables; legumes (beans and peas); starchy vegetables; and other vegetables several times a week is encouraged to provide the many nutrients contributed by different vegetables.

Despite an abundance of nutritious foods available in the United States, many individuals do not choose the variety of nutrient-dense foods that provide all their nutrient requirements and enable them to remain within their calorie needs.

Vegetable choices include all fresh, frozen, canned, and dried options, cooked or raw, in addition to vegetable juices. Nutrient-dense vegetables are limited in the amount of salt, butter, or creamy sauces added. The U.S.-Pattern for a 2000-calorie diet includes 2½ c-eq of vegetables daily. For each vegetable subgroup, weekly amounts are recommended to ensure variety and meet nutrient needs.

Fruits

All fruits or 100% fruit juices count as part of the fruit group. Fruits are naturally low in fat, sodium, and calories, and do not contain cholesterol. They are also important sources of potassium, dietary fiber, vitamin C, and folate (see Table 1.4). Fresh, frozen, canned, or dried fruits are recommended for their fiber content, but fruit juice should be minimized because it does not contain fiber and excess amounts can contribute extra calories.

Because of their high water content, fruits are more filling than juices, with fewer calories. Fruit juice can be part of a healthful diet, but only the proportion that is 100% fruit juice counts because these products usually contain added sugars. The percentage of juice in a beverage is indicated on the package label. Fruit juices containing added sugars are classified as sugar-sweetened beverages. The recommendation for children 6 months to 6 years old limits 100% fruit juice to 4 to 6 fluid ounces per day (infants under 6 months old should not be given any juice).

At least half of the recommended amount of fruit should be from whole fruits (fresh, canned, frozen, or dried). Fruits that contain a small amount of added sugar can be chosen as long as daily calories from added sugars does not exceed 10% and total caloric intake remains within limits. With canned fruits, those containing the least amount of added sugar should be selected. The recommended amount of fruits in the U.S-Pattern for 2000 cal is 2 c-eq daily (see Table 1.1 for amounts for different caloric levels).

TABLE 1.4 Contributions of Selected Fruits and Vegetables

Fruit/Vegetable	Vitamin A[a,b]	Vitamin C[c,d]	Fiber[e,f]
Acorn squash	#	#	#
Apple with skin			#
Avocado		#	†
Banana		#	#
Bell pepper		†	
Bok choy	†	†	
Broccoli, cooked	†	†	#
Brussels sprouts		†	#
Cabbage		†	#
Cantaloupe	†	†	
Carrot	†	#	#
Cauliflower		†	
Collard greens	†	†	
Grapefruit	#	†	
Iceberg lettuce	#		
Kale	†	†	#
Kiwi		†	#
Kohlrabi		†	#
Mango	†	†	
Orange		†	
Papaya	†	†	
Pear			#
Prune, dried			†
Romaine lettuce	†		
Spinach	†	#	
Strawberry		†	
Sweet potato	†	†	#
Swiss chard	†	†	
Tomato	#	†	

[a]# = Good source: 500–950 IU/100 g
[b]† = Excellent source: ≥ 950 IU/100 g
[c]# = Good source: 6–11.4 mg/100 g
[d]† = Excellent source: ≥ 11.4 mg/100 g
[e]# = Good source: 2.5–4.75 g/100 g
[f]† = Excellent source: ≥ 4.75 g/100 g
Data from U.S. Department of Agriculture, Agricultural Research Service, Nutrient Data Laboratory. *USDA National Nutrient Database for Standard Reference, Release 28.* Version current: September 2015, slightly revised May 2016. Accessed August 8, 2017. https://www.ars.usda.gov/ba/bhnrc/ndl

Grains

Grains are principally carbohydrates or starchy foods and are essential for a healthful diet. The U.S.-Patterns include whole grains and refined grains, but products made with refined grains, especially those high in saturated fats, added sugars, and/or sodium, such as cookies, cakes, and some snack foods are limited. All whole-grain, refined and enriched, or fortified-grain products are included in these two groups, for example, barley, buckwheat, bulgur, corn, millet, rice, rye, oats, sorghum, wheat, and wild rice.

At the 2000-cal level, the U.S.-Pattern indicates a total of 6 oz-eq per day. Most Americans are consuming more than the recommended amount of refined grains, but the Dietary Guidelines Advisory Committee estimates that 95% of Americans do not reach guideline amounts for whole grains.[6]

Whole grains are grains and grain products made from the entire grain seed, usually called the *kernel,* which consists of bran, germ, and endosperm. If the kernel has been cracked, crushed, or flaked, it must retain all components of the original grain kernel (bran, germ, and endosperm) to be called *whole grain.* Whole wheat, oatmeal, brown rice, whole rye, and quinoa are all whole grains. When selecting whole grains, the first or second ingredient listed on the ingredient panel should contain the words *whole grain.* One oz-eq of whole grains has 16 g of whole grains; a food that contains 8 g/oz-eq or more whole grains is at least half whole grains. Product labels usually indicate the grams of whole grain to help consumers identify food choices having a substantial amount of whole grains.

The difficulty in identifying whole grains is a major barrier. Labels such as "100% wheat," "stone-ground," and "multigrain" do not guarantee that the food contains whole grain. Multiple conflicting definitions exist for identifying whole-grain products, causing confusion for consumers. Color is a poor indicator of whole grains because molasses or caramel food coloring may be added. As a result of the *Dietary Guidelines,* food manufacturers have introduced more processed foods with higher whole-grain content.

Most whole grains are a good source of dietary fiber and are needed to meet the daily fiber recommendation. Whole grains differ from a nutritional perspective, with significant variations in levels and effects of the fiber. Whole-grain products contribute more fiber, magnesium, phosphorus, and zinc than do enriched products (Table 1.5). When whole grains are refined, vitamins, minerals, and dietary fiber are lost in the process.

Most refined grains are enriched with some of the nutrients lost in the process, but dietary fiber and some vitamins and minerals are not routinely added back in the enrichment process. **Enrichment** is the process by which iron, thiamin, riboflavin, folic acid, and niacin removed during processing are restored to approximate their original levels. This process is controlled by the U.S. Food and Drug Administration (FDA), which establishes the quantity of nutrients permitted.

Fortification is the process by which nutrients not present in the natural product are added or increased in the original product. Most processed breakfast cereals are fortified to achieve nutrient levels higher than those naturally occurring in the grain. Whole grains are a poor source of folic acid; thus, rather than relying exclusively on whole grains, some cereal products fortified with folic acid should be selected. Products that are enriched with folic acid are especially important for women who are pregnant or capable of becoming pregnant. Serious birth defects may occur during early pregnancy if adequate amounts of folic acid are not consumed. Despite the fact that enriched grains have a positive role in providing some vitamins and minerals, excessive amounts can result in excess calories being consumed. The recommended amount of refined grains is less than 3 oz-eq servings daily; at least one-half of an individual's grain choices should be whole grains.

TABLE 1.5 Comparison of Nutrient Values of Selected Whole-Grain and Enriched Breads (1 slice)

Nutrients	Enriched White	Whole Wheat	Multigrain	Whole Grain	Rye
Protein (g)	3.0	3.98	3.47	4.0	2.72
Total dietary fiber (g)	0.6	1.9	1.9	3.0	1.9
Thiamin (mg)	0.20	0.126	0.73	0.740	0.139
Riboflavin (mg)	0.13	0.053	0.034	0.340	0.107
Niacin (mg)	1.89	1.420	1.051	1.20	1.218
Vitamin B_6 (mg)	0.01	0.069	0.068	0.080	0.024
Total folate (mcg)	72	13	20	Unk	48
Iron (mg)	1.10	0.79	0.65	0.72	0.91
Zinc (mg)	0.21	0.57	0.44	0.60	0.36
Sodium (mg)	120	146	99	150	193
Calcium (mg)	4.0	52.0	27.0	20.0	23.0
Phosphorus (mg)	24.0	68.0	59.0	80.0	40.0
Magnesium (mg)	6.0	24.0	20.0	32.0	13.0

U.S. Department of Agriculture, Agricultural Research Service. 2016. *USDA Food and Nutrient Database for Dietary Studies 2011–2012.* Release 28. https://ndb.nal.usda.gov/ndb/. Accessed March 20, 2017.

Dairy

Healthful eating patterns include fat-free and low-fat (1%) dairy, including milk, yogurt, cheese, and/or fortified soy beverages. Soy beverages fortified with calcium and vitamins A and D are similar to milk in nutrient composition and can replace traditional cow's milk. The U.S.-Pattern recommends 2 c-eq per day for children ages 2 to 3 years, 2½ c-eq for children ages 4 to 8 years, and 3 c-eq per day for adolescents and adults. Children who establish the habit of drinking milk are more likely to drink milk as adults. Most age-sex groups (except children 1–3 years old) fall below the recommended amount.

Milk products provide calcium and potassium and may be a good source of vitamin D. Fortified milk products are important sources of vitamin D. However, many milk substitutes (cheese, yogurt, and ice cream) are not fortified with vitamin D (unless made with fortified milk). Whole milk and many cheeses are high in saturated fat and can have negative health implications. Low-fat or fat-free milk products providing little or no fat should be chosen most often to avoid consuming more calories than needed. These products contain similar amounts of nutrients as the higher-fat options. Fat-free milk and yogurt contain less saturated fat and sodium and more potassium and vitamins A and D than cheese; therefore, decreasing the proportion of cheese-to-milk consumption improves overall nutritional intake. If a consumer does not drink milk, efforts should be made to obtain adequate amounts of calcium, potassium, magnesium, and vitamins A and D from other food sources.

The dairy group does not include high-fat products, such as butter and cream, because they are not high in calcium, riboflavin, and protein. Other milks—such as almond, rice, coconut, and hemp milks—may contain calcium but are not part of the dairy group because overall nutritional content is inferior to dairy milk and fortified soy milk.

The consumption of dairy products can help children and adolescents achieve peak bone mass and reduce the risk of low bone mass and osteoporosis. In terms of oral health, studies indicate that higher dairy product consumption is associated with decreased prevalence and severity of periodontal disease.[7]

Protein Foods

The U.S.-Patterns include a variety of nutrient-dense forms of protein foods, including legumes (beans and peas). The U.S.-Patterns divide protein foods into subgroups, as follows, with recommended amounts of each to encourage nutritional balance and flexibility: seafood; meats, poultry, and eggs; and nuts, seeds, and soy products.

These foods are important sources of protein, B vitamins (niacin, thiamin, riboflavin, and B_6), vitamin E, iron, zinc, and magnesium. A variety of foods from this group is advisable because each food has distinct nutritional advantages (Table 1.6). By varying choices and including fish, nuts, beans, and seeds, the intake of healthful fats, such as monounsaturated fatty acids and polyunsaturated fatty acids, is increased.

Red meats include all forms of beef, pork, lamb, veal, goat, and nonbird game (e.g., venison, bison, elk). Chicken, turkey, duck, geese, guineas, and game birds are classified as poultry. To decrease intake of saturated fats and calories, lean cuts of meat and skinless poultry should be chosen; seafood, nuts, and seeds should replace some of the meat and poultry. Fish, nuts, and seeds contain a healthful type of fat; thus, they should be chosen more often than meat or poultry.

Dry beans and peas, such as kidney beans, pinto beans, lima beans, black-eyed peas, and lentils, are included in this group, as well as in the vegetable group. Dried beans and peas do not contain significant quantities of fat and are excellent sources of plant protein and dietary fiber. They also contribute other nutrients found in meats, poultry, and fish. Whether they are counted as a vegetable or a meat, several cups a week are recommended.

TABLE 1.6 Outstanding Contributions of Various Protein Foods

Protein Food	Nutrient
Lean red meats	Iron B vitamins Zinc
Pork	Thiamin Zinc
Poultry	Potassium Niacin
Liver and egg yolks	Vitamin A Iron Zinc
Dry peas and beans, soybeans, and nuts	Magnesium Fiber Zinc

Seafood includes all edible marine animals from saltwater and freshwater sources, including fish (e.g., salmon, tuna, trout, tilapia) and shellfish (e.g., shrimp, crab, oysters). The adult recommendation for seafood is approximately 20% of total intake of protein foods. Moderate evidence shows that 8 oz-eq or more of seafood per week from a variety of seafood sources provides omega-3 fatty acids associated with prevention of CVD. Pregnant or breastfeeding women should avoid fish high in mercury—such as tilefish, shark, swordfish, and king mackerel—and should limit white tuna to 6 oz-eq per week.

The size portion for nuts or seeds is only ½ ounce rather than 1 ounce because of the high calorie content of these foods; thus, small portions should replace other protein foods (meat or poultry). Nuts and seeds should be unsalted to control sodium intake.

Vegetarians can choose eggs, beans, nuts, nut butters, peas, and soy products to obtain adequate amounts of protein (see Chapter 5).

The U.S.-Pattern recommends 5 to 6½ oz-eq of protein foods, with the specific recommendation of at least 8 oz-eq of seafood per week. Most individuals consume adequate amounts (or more) of protein foods, but leaner types of protein foods need to be chosen more often. Although consuming significantly higher amounts of protein may not be harmful, high-fat meats may be an undesirable source of calories, cholesterol, and/or saturated fatty acids. Protein supplements promoted to increase muscle mass may not contain nutrients important for health and should be used only after consulting a health care provider or an RDN.

Oils

Lipids (oils and fats) are not a food group, but these nutrients are important in a healthful diet. Individuals should be mindful of the type and total amount of fats chosen. Oils are distinctly different from fats because oils, liquids at room temperature, contain a higher percentage of monounsaturated and polyunsaturated fats. Commonly selected oils include canola, corn, olive, peanut, safflower, soybean, and sunflower oils; these are also present in nuts, seeds, seafood, olives, and avocados. Coconut oil, palm kernel, and palm oils are called *oils* because they are derived from tropical plants, but nutritionally they are considered solid fats because they are solid at room temperature due to their high percentages of saturated fatty acids.

The U.S.-Patterns contain some oils, measured in grams (g), but because they are a concentrated source of calories, amounts are limited to within calorie limits and the AMDR (20%–35% of calories) for total fat intake. Fats are classified by the type and percentage of fatty acids they contain. Polyunsaturated fatty acids, monounsaturated fatty acids, saturated fatty acids, and *trans* fatty acids are prevalent in American foods. Polyunsaturated and monounsaturated fats are included in the U.S.-Patterns as long as the amounts are within caloric limitations, but saturated and *trans* fats are addressed in the subsequent discussion in the Nutrients to Limit section. A more detailed explanation of lipids is provided in Chapters 2 and 6.

Highlights of Nutrient-Dense Foods

- Meet recommended intakes with energy needs by adopting balanced dietary habits using the U.S.-Patterns, *MyPlate*, Mediterranean-style pattern (see Fig. 6.7), DASH Eating Plan (see Chapter 12), or Healthy Vegetarian Eating Pattern (see Table 5.5) as a guide for food choices.
- Consume a sufficient amount of fiber-rich fruits and vegetables while staying within energy needs. Per day, 2 c-eq of fruit and 2½ c-eq of vegetables are recommended for a reference 2000-cal intake, with higher or lower amounts depending on the calorie level.
- Choose a variety of fruits and vegetables each day. In particular, select from all five vegetable subgroups (dark green, orange and red, legumes, starchy vegetables, and other vegetables) several times a week.
- Adding more fruits, vegetables, whole grains, and fat-free or low-fat dairy products may have beneficial health effects and provide good sources of nutrients commonly lacking in American diets.
- Consume 3 or more oz-eq per day of whole-grain products, with the rest of the recommended grains coming from enriched products. In general, at least half the grains should come from whole grains.
- Replace most refined-grain food choices with whole-grain foods that are nutrient dense (low in added sugars and fats) to keep total caloric intake within limits.
- Because fruit juices contain little or no fiber, whole fruits (fresh, frozen, canned, or dried) are preferable choices.
- Protein-containing foods are important, but most Americans consume adequate amounts; therefore, for most, an increase is not recommended.
- Keep total fat intake between 20% and 35% of calories, with most fats coming from sources of polyunsaturated and monounsaturated fatty acids, such as fish, nuts, and vegetable oils.
- When selecting and preparing meat, poultry, dry beans, and dairy products, choose lean, low-fat, or fat-free options to decrease intake of saturated fats and calories.

Nutrients to Limit

Total Caloric Intake

The U.S.-Patterns indicate food group and nutrient recommendations for caloric needs, which can only be achieved by choosing foods in a nutrient-dense form (without added sugar and lean and/or very-low-fat dairy and protein foods). To remain within a specific caloric range, only a limited number of calories are available after eating the specified amounts of all the food groups, and this is based on choosing nutrient-dense foods. For example, the amount of additional calories for added sugars or additional fats is only 270 cal for a 2000-cal diet (see Table 1.1). These additional calories can be used for foods that are not nutrient dense (added sugars, additional refined starches, or fats) or to eat more than the recommended amount of nutrient-dense foods. Many foods in the American food supply provide excess calories without contributing wholesome nutrients or meeting food group recommendations and thus exceed the recommended caloric amount to maintain a healthy body weight.

Added Sugars

Naturally occurring sugars found in fruits and milk are not added sugars. Added sugars are listed in Box 1.2. Consumption of foods containing added sugars increases the difficulty of obtaining adequate nutrients without weight gain.

Sugars, whether they are naturally present or added to the food, and grains supply physiologic energy in the form of glucose. The physiologic response of naturally occurring sugars is similar to the response from added sugars, but added sugars supply calories with few or no nutrients. Additionally, the frequency and duration of sugars and refined-grain consumption are important factors in caries risk by increasing exposure to cariogenic substrates.

The recommendation is to limit added sugars to less than 10% of calories per day. At lower caloric levels (below 2000 calories), the amount of calories remaining after meeting food group recommendations, even using nutrient-dense foods, is less than 10% per day of the total caloric goal. The limited amount of added sugars can be used to improve the palatability of nutrient-dense foods as long as calories from added sugars do not exceed 10% per day, total carbohydrate intake remains within the AMDR, and total calorie intake remains within limits.

• BOX 1.2 Sources of Other Sugars

Agave
Barley malt
Beet sugar
Brown sugar
Cane sugar/juice
Coconut palm sugar (or coconut sugar)
Confectioner's sugar
Corn sweetener
Date sugar
Dextrose
Evaporated cane juice
Fructose
Fruit juice concentrate
Fruit sugar
Glucose
High-fructose corn syrup
Honey
Invert sugar
Lactose
Maltose
Molasses
Palm sugar
Raw sugar
Refiner's syrup
Sucrose
Syrups (malt, corn, brown rice, malt, maple, refiner's sorghum)
Trehalose
Turbinado sugar

High-intensity sugars (saccharin, aspartame, acesulfame potassium [Ace-K], and sucralose) can replace added sugars to reduce caloric intake, but their effectiveness in long-term weight management is uncertain. Moderate intake of these high-intensity sugars has been deemed safe for the general population.

Saturated Fats, Trans *Fats, and Cholesterol*

Usually, high fat intake (more than 35% of calories) is associated with a higher intake of saturated fat, *trans* fatty acid and cholesterol, and excess calories. These unnecessary lipid components of food may raise undesirable blood lipids. On the other hand, if fat intake is less than 20% of calories, inadequate intakes of vitamin E and essential fatty acids may lead to unfavorable changes in the good type of blood lipids and triglycerides.

Saturated fatty acids should provide less than 10% of calories and should be replaced with monounsaturated and polyunsaturated fatty acids while keeping total dietary fats within the age-appropriate AMDR. There is no dietary requirement of saturated fats for persons 2 years and older because the human body produces more than enough to meet physiologic and structural requirements. Solid fats usually contain a high percentage of saturated fatty acids. Saturated fats are consumed as food (high-fat meats and dairy products) or as ingredients in mixed dishes (e.g., burgers, pizza, hamburgers, tacos, shortening in a cake, hydrogenated oils in fried foods). These fats, abundant in the American diet, contribute significantly to excess caloric intake and exceeding the 10% per day recommendation.

Trans fatty acid consumption should be as low as possible. Commercially produced solid fats may contain a high percentage of *trans* fatty acids. Partially hydrogenated oils in margarines are synthetic sources of ***trans* fatty acids** produced by a process called **hydrogenation**. This process was implemented by food manufacturers to make products more resistant to spoilage and rancidity. In partial hydrogenation, some of the unsaturated fats are converted to saturated fatty acids, but some of the unsaturated fats are changed to the *trans* configuration associated with increased risk of CVD. These *trans* fatty acids are frequently found in partially hydrogenated oils (some margarines, snack foods, and prepared desserts). Due to heightened consumer awareness and federal regulations, the amount of artificial *trans* fats in processed foods has decreased significantly in recent years.

Naturally occurring *trans* fats produced by ruminant animals are present in small quantities in dairy products and meats. They do not have the same undesirable effects as commercially produced *trans* fats.

Cholesterol is a very important component in the body for physiologic and structural functions, but adequate amounts are naturally produced; making dietary cholesterol unnecessary. Individuals should eat as little dietary cholesterol as possible while consuming a healthy diet. As a general rule, foods high in fats, such as fatty meats and high-fat dairy products, are also high in cholesterol and saturated fats. Because the U.S.-Pattern limits saturated fats, dietary cholesterol is naturally low—100 to 300 mg of cholesterol. Dietary cholesterol is present only in animal foods such as egg yolk, high-fat dairy products, shellfish, meats, and poultry. Eggs and shellfish are high in dietary cholesterol but not in saturated fats.

Sodium

Sodium is an essential nutrient, but the body requires relatively small quantities available from naturally occurring sodium in foods. The natural sodium content of food only accounts for approximately 10% of total intake; discretionary sodium (i.e., salt added at the table or in cooking) provides another 5% to 10% of intake. Manufacturers and food establishments add more than 75% to prepared foods. Because most of the sodium consumed in American diets is from processed foods, the goal should concentrate primarily on reducing sodium added during food processing and on changing food selections to more fresh foods and fewer processed items.

Most Americans consume an average of 3440 mg sodium daily; the recommended intake (per the *Dietary Guidelines*, UL from the National Academy of Medicine, and the American Heart Association) is less than 2300 mg per day for adults and children ages 14 years and older. Decreasing sodium intake is advisable for all, but persons with high blood pressure may benefit by a further reduction to 1500 mg per day.

In general, high sodium intake is associated with **hypertension** (high blood pressure). Hypertension increases an individual's risk of CVD, stroke, congestive heart failure, and kidney disease. The DASH diet is recommended for people with hypertension (see Chapter 12). The *Dietary Guidelines* endorses this diet for all Americans to ensure adequate essential nutrients while reducing undesirable ones.

Caloric intake is associated with sodium intake; the more foods and beverages consumed, the more sodium is consumed. By reducing calorie intake, sodium intake is lowered somewhat. Additionally, sodium intake can be reduced by choosing fewer processed foods (e.g., pizza, burgers, sandwiches, tacos, soups). Manufacturers are endeavoring to reduce sodium content of processed foods.

Highlights of Nutrients to Limit

- Consume a variety of nutrient-dense foods and beverages within and among the basic food groups while limiting foods containing saturated and *trans* fats, cholesterol, added sugars, salt, and alcohol.
- Consume less than 2300 mg of sodium (approximately 1 tsp of salt) per day. Individuals ages 51 years and older; all African Americans; and people with hypertension, diabetes, or chronic kidney disease should further reduce intake to 1500 mg sodium per day.
- Processed meats and poultry are preserved by smoking, curing, salting, and/or the addition of chemical preservatives. Processed meats, such as hot dogs and luncheon meats, contain larger amounts of sodium and saturated fats. However, these products can be accommodated as long as sodium, saturated fats, and total calories are within limits of the U.S.-Pattern.
- To decrease intake of saturated fats, lean cuts of meat and skinless poultry should be chosen. Seafood, nuts, and seeds should replace some of the protein foods, as they are higher in monounsaturated and polyunsaturated fatty acids.
- Read nutrition labels and choose and prepare foods with less sodium.
- Choose fresh or frozen vegetables over canned versions.
- For 2000 cal per day intake, solid fats and added sugars should comprise less than 13% of the calories, or approximately 258 cal.
- Avoid processed foods containing synthetic sources of *trans* fats, such as partially hydrogenated oils.
- Limit consumption of refined grains to three servings daily, especially those containing solid fats, added sugars, and sodium.
- Reduce the incidence of dental caries by practicing good oral hygiene and consuming sugar- and starch-containing foods and beverages less frequently.

Other Dietary Components

Alcohol

Alcohol (also referred to as adult beverages) is not a component of the U.S.-Pattern but as a substance frequently chosen by Americans, contributes to overall caloric intake. There is no nutritional reason for a person to begin consuming alcohol, and many reasons exist for abstinence.

In the past two decades, both the number of people consuming adult beverages and the amount consumed have increased, representing approximately 17% of total caloric intake.[8] Women who are pregnant or anticipate a pregnancy should not consume alcohol.

Alcohol consumption can have beneficial or harmful effects depending on the amount consumed, age, and other characteristics of the person consuming the alcohol and other circumstances. Because alcoholic beverages supply calories with few nutrients, adequate nutrient intake without weight gain is difficult with excessive alcohol consumption.

The U.S.-Pattern categorizes adult beverages as drink-equivalents. One alcoholic beverage contains 14 g (0.6 fl oz) of pure alcohol. One alcoholic drink-equivalent (oz-eq) is defined as 12 fluid oz of regular beer (5% alcohol), 5 fluid oz of wine (12% alcohol), or 1.5 fluid oz of 80 proof distilled spirits (40% alcohol). If alcohol is consumed, it should be in moderation—up to one drink per day for women and limited to two drinks per day for men, and only by adults of legal drinking age. Moderation is not intended as an average over several days, but rather as the amount consumed on any single day.

Caffeine

Caffeine is a desirable dietary component (not an essential nutrient) for many Americans; more than 90% consume caffeine-containing foods and/or beverages. Caffeine functions as a stimulant in the body.

Popular plant sources of naturally occurring caffeine are coffee beans, tea leaves, cocoa beans, and kola nuts, consumed as coffee, tea, and soda. Caffeine is also added to foods and beverages, such as caffeinated soft drinks and energy drinks. Caffeine added to foods and beverages must be included in the ingredient list on the food label.

The amount of caffeine in frequently consumed beverages varies widely (see Box 12.1). Average intake of caffeine ranges from 110 to 260 mg per day, although 400 mg per day is considered the highest safe amount.[6] Women who are pregnant or capable of becoming pregnant, or breastfeeding, should follow the advice of their health care providers regarding caffeine consumption. Further discussion about the health effects of caffeine is provided in Chapter 12.

Highlights of Other Dietary Components

- Moderate coffee consumption (3–5 8-oz cups/day or up to 400 mg/day of caffeine) can be incorporated into healthful eating patterns, but people who do not currently consume caffeine (in various forms) are not encouraged to begin.
- Adults of legal drinking age should consume alcoholic beverages in moderation—up to one drink daily for women and two drinks per day for men.
- Excessive drinking is an important health problem, not limited to college-age individuals.
- Alcoholic beverages should not be consumed by some individuals, including those who cannot limit their alcohol intake; women of childbearing age who may become pregnant; pregnant and lactating women; children and adolescents; or individuals taking prescription or over-the-counter medications that can interact with alcohol, those engaging in activities requiring attention, skill, or coordination (e.g., driving or operating machinery), and those with specific medical conditions (e.g., liver disease, hypertriglyceridemia, and pancreatitis).
- Caution is advised for individuals who choose to mix caffeine and alcohol together or consume them at the same time.

Physical Activity Guidelines

The principal focus of the *Dietary Guidelines* is to ensure that Americans choose foods that promote overall health and well-being. Part of the objective to improve and/or maintain health and prevent chronic disease includes maintaining a healthy weight. Excess weight can contribute to many health problems, including CVD, diabetes, and hypertension. Because of the prevalence of overweight and obesity, the *Dietary Guidelines* frequently mentions the other side of the balance—calorie expenditure, which is a significant factor in attaining a healthy weight.

Physical Activity

Regular physical activity and physical fitness are important factors for an individual's health, sense of well-being, and maintenance of a healthy body weight. **Physical activity** is defined as any body movement produced by skeletal muscles resulting in energy expenditure. Physical activity is not the same as physical fitness. **Physical fitness** is related to the ability to perform physical activity. People with high levels of physical fitness are at lower risk of developing chronic diseases, whereas a sedentary lifestyle increases the risk of weight gain and overweight, obesity, and the development of many chronic diseases. Active individuals have longer life expectancies. Furthermore, physical activity can help manage mild to moderate depression and anxiety.

Different intensities and types of exercise yield distinct benefits. Vigorous activity improves physical fitness more than moderate physical activity and burns more calories per unit of time. Resistance exercise increases muscular strength and endurance and maintains or increases muscle mass. Weight-bearing exercise increases peak bone mass during growth, maintains peak bone mass during adulthood, and reduces the rate of bone loss during aging. It also may reduce the risk of osteoporosis. Also, regular exercise can help prevent falls, common sources of injury, and disability in older adults.

Physical activity may be accomplished in short bouts (10-minute periods) of moderate-intensity activity performed three to six times during the course of a day; the cumulative total is the factor in improving health status and increasing caloric expenditure. The higher a person's physical activity level, the more calories can be consumed without gaining weight. This makes it easier to plan a daily food intake pattern providing recommended nutrient requirements without exceeding caloric requirements.

In addition to physical activity, a high-quality diet without excess calories enhances the health of most Americans. This may include healthful, nutrient-dense foods and beverages that meet nutrient requirements within individual calorie needs. In general, individuals should become more mindful of what they eat and what they do. The *Dietary Guidelines* encourage adherence to the Physical Activity Guidelines for Americans (https://www.health.gov/paguidelines) to help promote health, reduce the risk of chronic disease, and achieve and maintain a healthy body weight.

Highlights of Physical Activity Guidelines

- To prevent gradual weight gain over time, make small decreases in calories from foods and beverages and increase physical activity.
- Engage in regular physical activity and reduce sedentary activities to promote health, psychological well-being, and a healthy body weight.
- For adults to reduce the risk of chronic disease: Engage in at least 30 minutes of moderate-intensity physical activity, beyond usual activity, on most days of the week.
- To help adults manage body weight and prevent gradual unhealthy body weight gain: Engage in approximately 60 minutes of moderate- to vigorous-intensity activity on most days of the week while not exceeding caloric intake requirements.
- For adults to sustain weight loss: Participate in at least 60 to 90 minutes of daily moderate-intensity physical activity while not exceeding caloric intake requirements. (Some people may need to consult a health care provider before participating in this level of activity.)
- For most adults, greater health benefits can be obtained by engaging in physical activity of more vigorous intensity or longer duration. Achieve physical fitness by including cardiovascular conditioning, stretching exercises for flexibility, and resistance exercises or calisthenics for muscle strength and endurance.

DENTAL CONSIDERATIONS

- The *Dietary Guidelines* do not necessarily apply to individuals with conditions that interfere with normal nutrition and require a special diet or for children younger than 2 years of age.
- Nutrient-dense foods provide substantial amounts of vitamins and minerals and relatively few calories. Suggestions for foods to recommend are noted in Table 1.7.
- Fats provide energy and essential fatty acids and are important for absorption of fat-soluble vitamins A, D, E, and K, and carotenoids.
- Processed foods and oils provide approximately 80% of *trans* fats, with the remainder coming from natural sources or animal foods. *Trans* fats from natural sources are not considered detrimental.
- Provide the patient with a definition or example of moderation (e.g., 1 tsp salt per day or 5-oz glass of wine for a woman per day).
- Many patients understand the general concepts of healthful eating, but they lack specific knowledge or motivation to help implement the recommendations. Most questions or misunderstandings are related to servings and food group placement.
- Dental hygienists should be knowledgeable enough to provide foundational information about the food groups, whole grains, types of fats, and physical activity.
- Assess each patient's diet to determine nutrient adequacy or inadequacy. (For example, if a patient eliminates fruits and vegetables, vitamin A and C deficiencies may develop; if milk and other milk products are eliminated, calcium and vitamin D deficiencies may develop.)
- Ensure that patients are aware of the number and size of servings recommended from each food group daily to obtain adequate nutrients.
- Although consumers are aware that they need to make positive dietary and lifestyle changes, putting that advice into practice is challenging and confusing for many (Fig. 1.3).
- A large proportion of Americans, regardless of their weight, are malnourished in terms of vitamin and mineral intake. However, they should not be told to eat less food but rather to choose more nutrient-dense foods.
- Remind patients that a serving size is a measured amount of food or drink (as indicated on a nutrition label) and portion is the amount actually consumed.

NUTRITIONAL DIRECTIONS

- The *Dietary Guidelines* support healthful eating habits to improve health and quality of life, as shown in the sample menu in Fig. 1.4.
- Choosing foods that follow the *Dietary Guidelines* will provide all the nutrients needed for growth and health.
- Make your plate look like a rainbow–consume dark-green, orange, and red vegetables; legumes; fruits; whole grains; and low-fat milk and milk products.
- Choose fewer refined grains, total fats (especially saturated and *trans* fats), added sugars, and calories.
- Read food labels when choosing foods high in fiber or low in fats to determine whether the calories or grams of sugar have increased.
- Limit saturated fat intake to 20 g or less if trying to limit intake to 2000 cal daily.
- Fruits, vegetables, grains, and milk are important sources of many nutrients but should be chosen wisely, within the context of a calorie-controlled diet.
- By reducing frequency and duration of oral exposure to fermentable carbohydrate intake and optimizing oral hygiene practices, such as drinking fluoridated water, brushing, and flossing, dental caries can be minimized.
- A person's preference for salt is not fixed; the desire for salty foods tends to decrease after consuming foods lower in salt for a period of time.
- The recommended dietary fiber intake is 14 g per 1000 cal consumed.
- Within each food group, individual foods can vary widely in the number of calories furnished; therefore, knowledge about serving sizes is important.
- If nutrient-dense foods are selected from each food group in the amounts recommended, a small amount of discretionary calories can be consumed as added fats or sugars, alcohol, or other foods.
- Dairy products are poor sources of iron and vitamin C, but they are good sources of protein, calcium, and riboflavin.
- Caloric consumption can be decreased by substituting low-fat or skim milk for whole milk. The nutrient content is the same for whole milk and low-fat milk, except for the amount of fat and calories. Skim milk (1%) or fat-free milk is recommended for all healthy Americans older than age 2 years.
- Foods in the grains group are economical as well as nutritious; they may be staple items for those in lower socioeconomic groups. However, whole-grain products may be more expensive; thus, encourage patients to increase these food choices as much as possible.
- Elimination or reduction of one or more food groups will reduce the variety of food intake, thereby reducing the number or amount of nutrients consumed.
- Adults watching their weight should choose minimal amounts of servings from all groups and limit portion sizes.

Support Healthy Eating Patterns for All

The final guideline discusses a social-ecological model for understanding individual lifestyle and motivators affecting food choices. To achieve a healthful eating pattern, food must be readily accessible and safe to eat (free from harmful diseases or bacteria). Food access is influenced by many factors, including distance to a store that stocks healthy foods, financial resources, and neighborhood-level resources (e.g., average income of the neighborhood and availability of public transportation). An individual's perception and food preferences are also influenced by race/ethnicity, socioeconomic status, and geographic location (see Chapter 16). The presence of a disability can be a real hindrance to having access to healthful foods.

TABLE 1.7 Frequency of Use of Foods for Implementing the *Dietary Guidelines*

Food Groups	Choose More Often	Choose Less Often	Major Contributions
Fats	Corn, cottonseed, olive, sesame, soybean, safflower, sunflower, peanut, canola oils Mayonnaise or salad dressing (made from olive oils) Avocado Olives	Butter, lard Margarine made from hydrogenated (*trans*) or saturated fats Coconut or palm oil Hydrogenated vegetable shortening Bacon Meat/fat drippings, gravy, sauces	Vitamin A, calories, essential fatty acids
Soups	Lightly salted soups with fat skimmed Cream-style soups (with low-fat milk)	Commercially prepared soups and mixes	Fluid, calories (may contain a variety of vitamins, minerals, and proteins, depending on type)
Sweets and desserts	Desserts that have been sweetened lightly or contain only moderate fat, such as puddings made from skim milk, angel food cake, fruit-based desserts	Desserts high in sugar or fats, candy, pastries, cakes, pies, whole-milk puddings, cookies	Calories (fats, carbohydrates)
Beverages	Water Unsweetened soft drinks Decaffeinated drinks	Sweetened beverages Caffeine-containing beverages Alcoholic beverages	Fluid, calories (unless sugar-free)
Milk and milk products	Low-fat or skim milk Low-fat cheese Low-fat yogurt	Whole-milk Whole-milk cheeses Whole-milk yogurt Ice cream	Calories, calcium, protein, phosphorus, vitamins A and D, riboflavin
Vegetables, including starchy vegetables	Fresh, frozen, or canned; potatoes—baked or boiled Include one dark-green or deep-orange vegetable daily	Deep-fried vegetables, chips Pickled vegetables Highly salted vegetables or juices	Calories, vitamins A and C, dietary fiber, potassium, zinc, cobalt, folic acid
Fruits	Unsweetened fruits or juices Include one citrus fruit/juice or one tomato juice daily	Sweetened fruits or juices Coconut	Calories, dietary fiber, vitamins A and C
Breads, starches, and cereals	Whole-grain breads or cereals Muffins, bagels, tortillas Enriched pasta, rice, grits, or noodles	Snack chips or crackers Sweetened cereals Pancakes, doughnuts, and biscuits	Calories, B-complex vitamins, magnesium, copper, iron, dietary fiber
Meats or substitutes	Lean meats, fish, shellfish, poultry without skin Low-fat cheese (e.g., cottage cheese and part skim mozzarella) Peanut butter Soybeans, tofu Dry beans and peas	Fried or fatty meats/fish Fried poultry or poultry with skin High-fat cheeses (e.g., cheddar and processed cheese) Nuts	Calories, protein, iron, zinc, copper, B-complex vitamins
Miscellaneous	Herbs, spices, flavorings	Salt and salt/spice combinations	Sodium

From Peckenpaugh NJ. *Nutrition Essentials and Diet Therapy.* 11th ed, Philadelphia, PA: W. B. Saunders: 2010.

Healthful choices (both food choices and activity) should be supported by all systems (e.g., governments, education, health care, and transportation), organizations (e.g., public health, community, and advocacy), and businesses and industries (e.g., planning and development, agriculture, food and beverage, retail, entertainment, marketing, and media). All sectors can have an important role in encouraging individuals to make healthful choices. Not only should available food be healthful and affordable but foods must be safe (free of microbes and contaminants) to prevent foodborne illness (see Chapter 16).

MyPlate System

MyPlate is part of a comprehensive communications initiative to promote healthful food choices. The *MyPlate* icon (Fig. 1.5), replaced the well-known *MyPyramid* symbol in 2011. The *MyPlate* food guidance system provides assistance in implementing the recommendations of the *Dietary Guidelines* and the DRIs. *MyPlate* has been well received; nearly two-thirds of Americans recognize the icon.[9]

The *MyPlate* icon is divided into four quadrants; each section is a different color that represents a food type. The quadrants indicate the recommended proportions on a plate for protein, grain, fruit, and vegetables at each meal, the same food groups discussed in the *Dietary Guidelines*. This icon does not indicate specific amounts to eat, however. Portion sizes in relation to items consumer can relate to are shown in Fig. 1.2. The main message of the plate to consumers is: (a) fruits (red section) and vegetables (green section) should fill half the plate; (b) lean protein foods (purple section) should occupy one-fourth of the plate; (c) whole

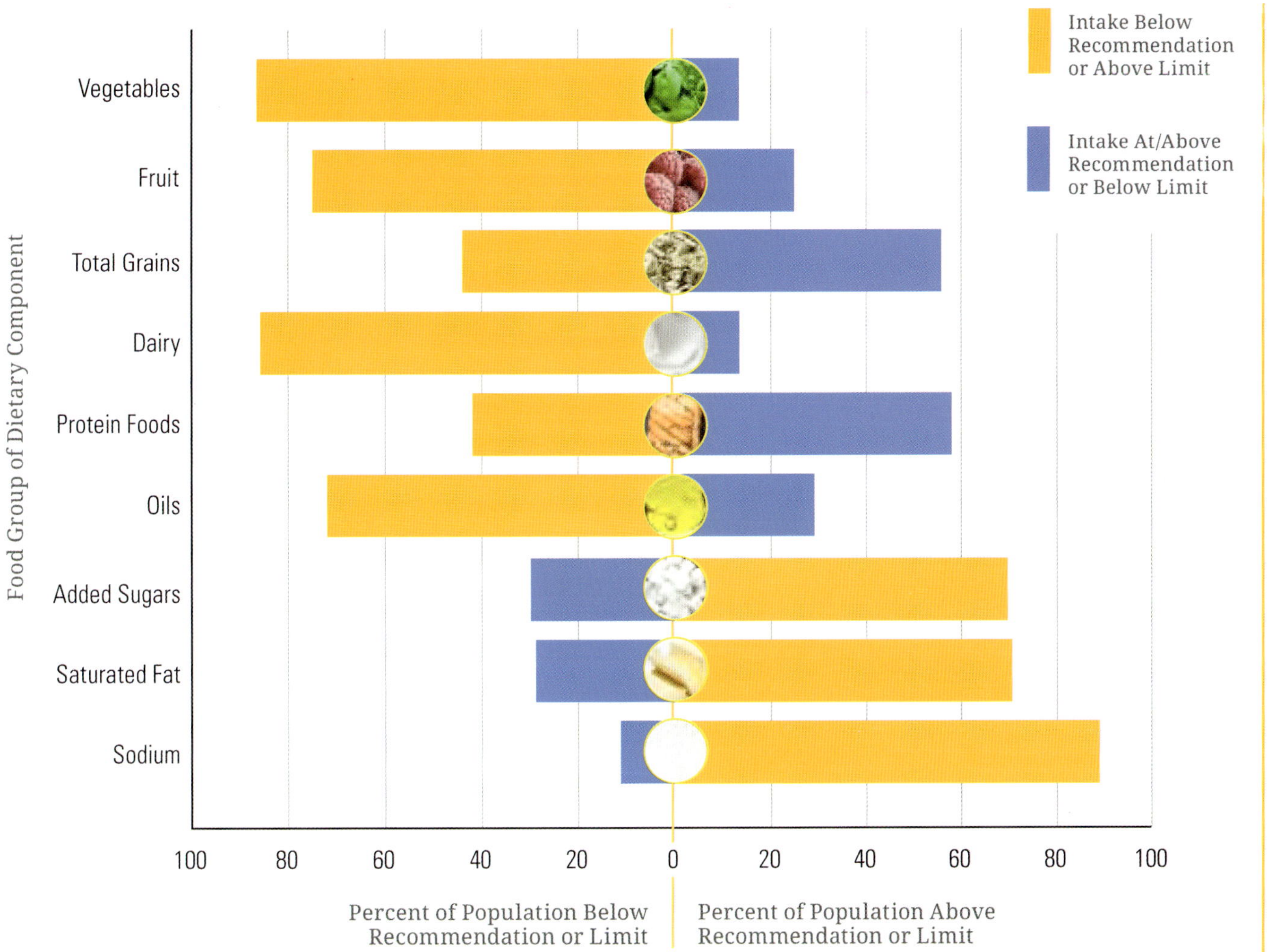

NOTE: The center (0) line is the goal or limit. For most, those represented by the orange sections of the bars, shifting toward the center line will improve their eating pattern.

DATA SOURCES: What We Eat in America, NHANES 2007-2010 for average intakes by age-sex group. Healthy U.S.-Style Food Patterns, which vary based on age, sex, and activity level, for recommended intakes and limits.

The What We Eat in America (WWEIA) Food Categories provide an application to analyze foods and beverages as consumed. Each of the food and beverage items that can be reported in WWEIA, National Health and Nutrition Examination Survey, are placed in one of the mutually exclusive food categories. More information about the WWEIA Food Categories is available at: https://health.gov/dietaryguidelines/2015/guidelines/chapter-2/current-eating-patterns-in-the-united-states/. Accessed October 7, 2017.

• **Figure 1.3** Dietary intakes compared to recommendations. Percent of the U.S. population ages 1 year & older who are below, at, or above each dietary goal or limit.

grains (brown section) should fill about one-fourth of the plate; and (4) dairy products (blue circle) should also be chosen. Fig. 1.6 is a concise synopsis of the *Dietary Guidelines*; it is available online in English and Spanish.

The key tool of this guidance system is the website, *www.chooseMyPlate.gov.* This food guidance system is revolutionary for a number of reasons. The website is an interactive nutrition education tool intended to help consumers apply personalized dietary guidance to achieve a healthful lifestyle through better eating and increased physical activity. This website continues to change through "facelift designs" and expand and update information available.

The *MyPlate* homepage provides quick access to the food groups and their content, website organization for various age groups, social media sharing, access to online tools, and interactive quizzes to test basic nutrition knowledge.[10] Most of the materials (brochures, tip sheets, graphics, and archived material) on the website can be printed or forwarded in English or Spanish.

MyPlate serves as a simple, research-based icon that sends a clear message on proportionality (balance, variety, and moderation) and exemplifies what should be on a plate of healthful foods. The tools, particularly the graphics, are designed to help Americans make food choices adequate to meet nutritional needs. They also

Breakfast

1 ½ c Frosted Mini-Wheat cereal
1 ½ c skim milk
12 oz black coffee

Mid-morning snack

12 oz water
1 oz (22) dry roasted almonds, unsalted
1 medium orange

Lunch

Sandwich with:
- 1 c tuna salad with egg, low-calorie mayonnaise
- ¼ c thin sliced cucumber
- 3 thin slices tomato
- Lettuce leaf
- 2 thin slices 100% wheat bread

6 raw baby carrots
1 medium applesauce cookie
1 c grapes

Mid-afternoon snack

6 oz vanilla yogurt, low fat
12 oz herbal tea with low calorie sweetener

Dinner

3 oz pot roast beef, braised, lean only with ¼ c sauteed mushrooms
1 c white and wild rice blend, cooked with margarine and ¼ c vegetable juice
2 c garden salad with avocado, lettuce, tomato, carrots
- ¼ c shredded low fat Muenster cheese
- 2 tbsp vinaigrette salad dressing

⅛ medium cantaloupe
12 oz tea with low calorie sweetener

Evening snack

3 c low fat microwave popcorn
12 oz water

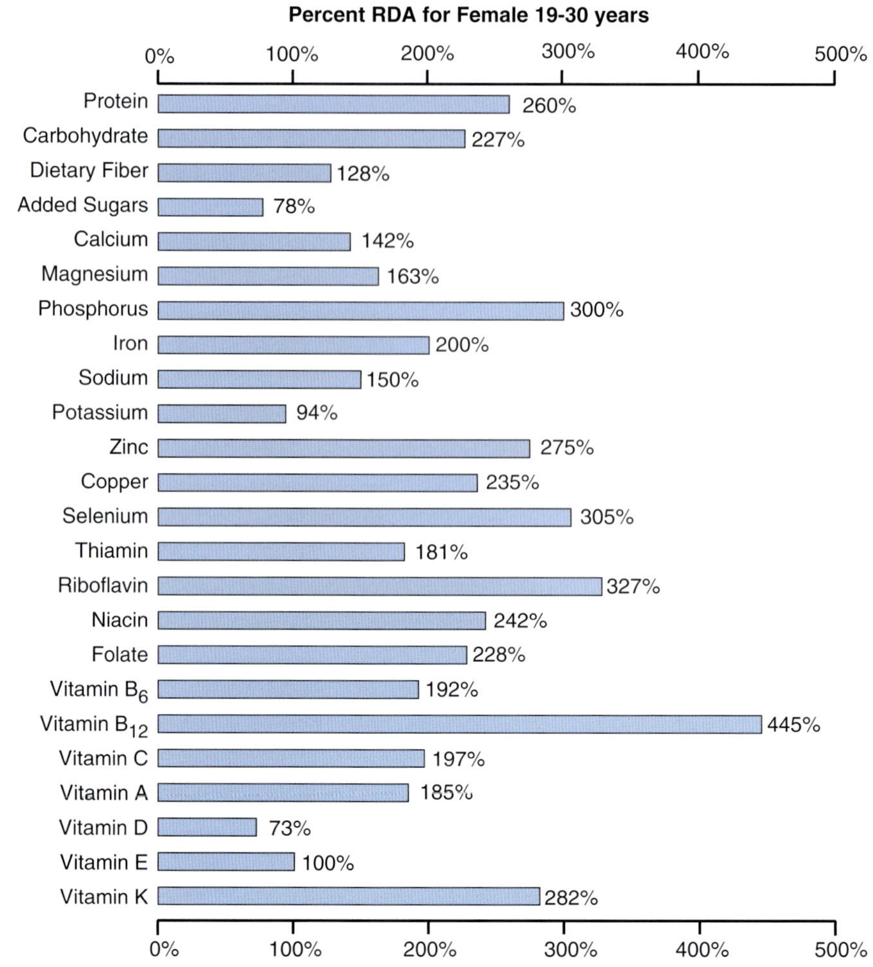

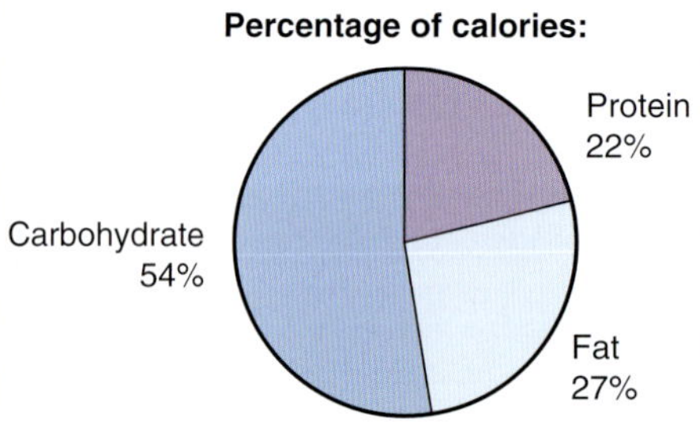

	Target	Eaten	Status
Grains	7 oz	7½ oz	OK
Vegetables	3 cups	3 cups	OK
Fruits	2 cups	2 cups	OK
Dairy	3 cups	2¾ cups	OK
Protein Foods	6 oz	3½ oz	Over

• **Figure 1.4** Sample menu based on the *Dietary Guidelines for Americans* and *MyPlate*.*

Balancing Calories

- Enjoy your food, but eat less.
- Avoid oversized portions.

Foods to Increase

- Make half your plate fruits and vegetables.
- Make at least half your grains whole grains.
- Switch to fat-free or low-fat (1%) milk.

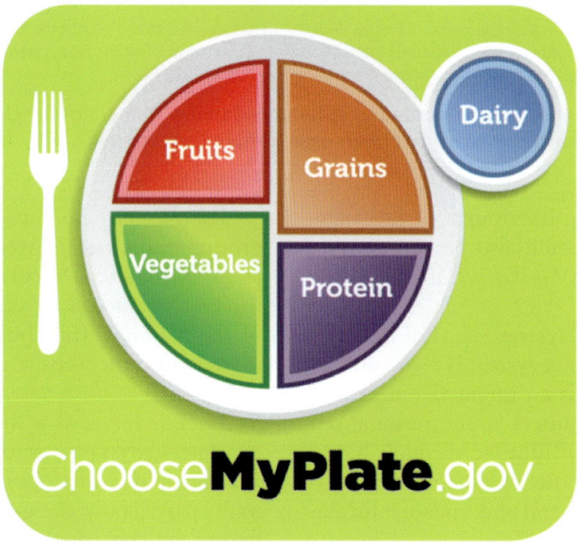

Foods to Reduce

- Compare sodium in foods like soup, bread and frozen meals--and choose the foods with lower numbers.
- Drink water instead of sugary drinks.

• **Figure 1.5** The *MyPlate* icon. (From United Stated Department of Agriculture: ChooseMyPlate.gov, 2011.)

MyPlate, MyWins: Make it yours

Find your healthy eating style. Everything you eat and drink over time matters and can help you be healthier now and in the future.

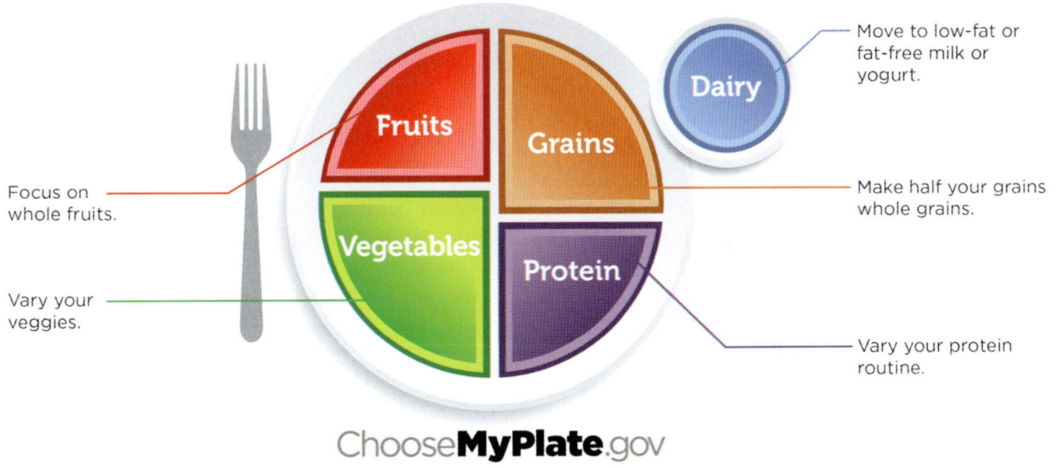
Fruits
Grains
Dairy
Vegetables
Protein
Focus on whole fruits.
Vary your veggies.
Move to low-fat or fat-free milk or yogurt.
Make half your grains whole grains.
Vary your protein routine.
ChooseMyPlate.gov

Limit — **Limit the extras.** Drink and eat beverages and food with less sodium, saturated fat, and added sugars.

MyWins — **Create 'MyWins' that fit your healthy eating style.** Start with small changes that you can enjoy, like having an extra piece of fruit today.

Fruits	Vegetables	Grains	Dairy	Protein
Focus on whole fruits and select 100% fruit juice when choosing juices. Buy fruits that are dried, frozen, canned, or fresh, so that you can always have a supply on hand.	Eat a variety of vegetables and add them to mixed dishes like casseroles, sandwiches, and wraps. Fresh, frozen, and canned count, too. Look for "reduced sodium" or "no-salt-added" on the label.	Choose whole-grain versions of common foods such as bread, pasta, and tortillas. Not sure if it's whole grain? Check the ingredients list for the words "whole" or "whole grain."	Choose low-fat (1%) or fat-free (skim) dairy. Get the same amount of calcium and other nutrients as whole milk, but with less saturated fat and calories. Lactose intolerant? Try lactose-free milk or a fortified soy beverage.	Eat a variety of protein foods such as beans, soy, seafood, lean meats, poultry, and unsalted nuts and seeds. Select seafood twice a week. Choose lean cuts of meat and ground beef that is at least 93% lean.

Daily Food Group Targets — Based on a 2,000 Calorie Plan
Visit SuperTracker.usda.gov for a personalized plan.

2 cups	2½ cups	6 ounces	3 cups	5½ ounces
1 cup counts as:	*1 cup counts as:*	*1 ounce counts as:*	*1 cup counts as:*	*1 ounce counts as:*
1 large banana 1 cup mandarin oranges ½ cup raisins 1 cup 100% grapefruit juice	2 cups raw spinach 1 large bell pepper 1 cup baby carrots 1 cup green peas 1 cup mushrooms	1 slice of bread ½ cup cooked oatmeal 1 small tortilla ½ cup cooked brown rice ½ cup cooked grits	1 cup milk 1 cup yogurt 2 ounces processed cheese	1 ounce tuna fish ¼ cup cooked beans 1 Tbsp peanut butter 1 egg

Water — **Drink water instead of sugary drinks.** Regular soda, energy or sports drinks, and other sweet drinks usually contain a lot of added sugar, which provides more calories than needed.

Activity — **Don't forget physical activity!** Being active can help you prevent disease and manage your weight.
Kids ≥ 60 min/day | Adults ≥ 150 min/week

MyPlate, MyWins
Healthy Eating Solutions for Everyday Life
ChooseMyPlate.gov/MyWins

Center for Nutrition Policy and Promotion
May 2016
CNPP-29
USDA is an equal opportunity provider, employer, and lender.

• **Figure 1.6** *MyPlate* miniposter. Used in conjunction with the *MyPlate* icon (Fig. 1.5), this concisely summarizes the food groups and portions providing 2000 calories. (From U.S. Department of Agriculture, Center for Nutrition Policy and Promotion: *MyPlate* Miniposter (ChooseMyPlate.gov). *MyPlate, MyWins*. Center for Nutrition Policy and Promotion, May 29, 2016. https://choosemyplate-prod.azureedge.net/sites/default/files/printablematerials/mini_poster.pdf. Accessed March 18, 2017.)

promote food choices moderate in energy level (calories) and in food components or nutrients often consumed in excess (fats, added sugars, and sodium). *MyPlate* is intended to be used as food guidance for the general public and not a therapeutic diet for any specific health condition.

The ChooseMyPlate.gov/website (also available in Spanish, choosemyplate.gov/en-espanol.html) provides numerous materials and useful information to help implement the principles of the *Dietary Guidelines* for both consumers and health professionals. The *MyPlate, MyWins* initiative helps consumers find solutions for common problems experienced in trying to provide healthful meals considering time, budget, and cooking skills. Through the *MyPlate, MyWins* video series, the USDA Center for Nutrition Policy and Promotion has added (1) upbeat animated videos to educate consumers about the components of healthful eating and how to make small changes to live a healthier lifestyle, and (2) documentary interviews with testimonial videos of American families.

SuperTracker is an interactive food, physical activity, and weight tracking tool to help implement the *Dietary Guidelines.* A database of over 8000 foods provides information about a specific food (calories, serving size, food group, and nutrient content) to evaluate a consumer's diet. Approximately 600 types of physical activity are available to assist in balancing food intake with activity to help achieve a healthier weight. Continual updates to this part of the *MyPlate* website include recipe analysis and the ability to track intake of added sugars. *What'sCooking* features tips for healthful meal planning, cooking, and grocery shopping with an extensive database of healthy recipes and cookbooks.

Other Food Guides

Not all health care professionals agree that *MyPlate* is the ideal method to promote health and wellness. However, the recommendations in *MyPlate* are remarkably consistent with other population-based recommendations designed to control obesity, diabetes, CVD and stroke, hypertension, cancer, and osteoporosis. Although different guides were derived from different types of nutrition research and for different purposes, they share consistent messages: eat more fruits, vegetables, legumes, and whole grains; eat less added sugar and saturated fat; and emphasize plant oils. Primary differences are in the types of recommended vegetables and protein sources, and the amount of recommended dairy products and total oil/fats. Overall nutrient values are also similar for most nutrients.

The recommendations in *MyPlate* are similar to the guidelines of the DASH eating plan (discussed in Chapter 12), the American Heart Association (discussed in Chapter 6), the American Diabetes Association (discussed in Chapter 7), the National Cholesterol Education Program Expert Panel on Detection, Evaluation and Treatment of High Blood Cholesterol in Adults (Adult Treatment Panel III), and the American Cancer Society. Calculated nutrient intakes associated with following any of these guidelines are generally within the ranges of nutrient recommendations of the *Dietary Guidelines.* Another alternative food guide is the Healthy Eating Plate created by nutrition faculty at the Harvard School of Public Health (see the Evolve website). While their goal is similar to the USDA's *MyPlate,* more specific information is provided, including visual reminders for increasing fluid intake and physical activity.

Canada's Food Guide

Canada has also developed a pictorial food guide to help Canadians choose food wisely (Fig. 1.7). The *Food Guide* rainbow encourages consumers to find their own healthy lifestyle—a pot of gold. The website (https://www.hc-sc.gc.ca/fn-an/food-guide-aliment/order-commander/myguide-monguide/index-eng.php) is interactive, allowing consumers to personalize the food guide, providing recipes, tips for healthful eating and physical activity, and other educational materials.

Other Nations' Guides

Many nations eat very differently than Americans. No one food is essential for good health. People in many countries are healthy (sometimes healthier than Americans) despite eating very different types of foods. This is further discussed in Chapter 16; food guides from other countries are shown on the inside of the back cover.

Nutrition Labeling

Nutrition Facts Label

In a concerted effort by the USDA and FDA to help people make informed decisions about choosing foods to improve their health and well-being, the Nutrition Facts label graphic was designed. It is encouraging that half of all adults read this Nutrition Facts label "always" or "most of the time."[11] Initially introduced approximately 20 years ago, the Nutrition Facts label was revised in 2016 to reflect new recommendations of the *Dietary Guidelines*, changes in the modern American diet, and to improve the graphics to make information clearer to consumers (Fig. 1.8). The Nutrition Facts label enhances nutritional knowledge by focusing attention on information important for addressing current public health problems, such as obesity. The label indicates the nutrients in a food, enabling consumers to compare the nutrient content of various products. The labeling regulation requires that approximately 90% of all foods sold in the United States provide specific information based on the nutrient content, including imported foods.

The USDA's Food Safety and Inspection Service requires packages of ground or chopped meat and poultry and the most popular whole, raw cuts of meat and poultry (such as chicken breast or steak) to have nutritional information either on the package labels or on display for consumers. Currently, these products are labeled with the number of calories and grams of total fat and saturated fat in the product. For foods not packaged, the information must be displayed at the point of purchase (e.g., counter card, sign, or booklet). These nutrition labels differ from the Nutrition Facts label required by the FDA; the USDA's Food Safety and Inspection Service has proposed amending nutrition labeling for meat and poultry products to be more consistent with the FDA Nutrition Facts panel.

The updated design of the Nutrition Facts label requires calories and portion sizes to be in large bold type. Serving sizes more closely reflect the amounts of food Americans currently consume, but this amount may not be consistent with portion sizes. Packages containing between one and two servings (e.g., a 20-oz soft drink) list the calories and other nutrients as one serving because typically the full amount is consumed in one sitting. Individuals sometimes consume certain multi-serving foods in one sitting; these foods (e.g., one pint of ice cream) must indicate both "per serving" and

• BOX 1.3 Daily Values (Updated)

Total fat: 65 g to 78 g
Total carbohydrate: 300 g to 275 g
Dietary fiber: 25 g to 28 g
Sodium: 2400 mg to 2300 mg
Potassium: 3500 mg to 4700 mg
Calcium: 1000 mg to 1300 mg
Vitamin D: 400 IUs (10 μg)

"per package" calorie and nutrition information, displaying this information in a two-column format.

Because research indicates that the type of fat consumed is more important than the amount of fat, only total fat, saturated fat, and *trans* fat amounts are listed. *Trans* fats, while practically absent from processed foods, still appear on the label because ruminant sources, while not harmful, contribute to intake. Dietary fiber and total and added sugars are all itemized under the bolded Total Carbohydrate. Grams and percent daily value (%DV) for dietary fiber and added sugars must be listed. Only specific added fibers can be reflected in the carbohydrate count. Other fibers currently added to foods will be reviewed by the FDA before they can be counted. This may be confusing for consumers during the transition period. Consuming required nutrients and staying within one's calorie limit is difficult when added sugars make up more than 10% of the total calories.

Sodium, dietary fiber, and vitamin D are based on updated daily values, consistent with the National Academy of Medicine recommendations and *Dietary Guidelines* (Box 1.3). The updated footnote better clarifies the %DV and puts calories in the context of the daily diet. Both the actual amount and %DV are revealed for vitamin D, calcium, iron, and potassium. Survey data indicate that Americans do not consume adequate amounts of vitamin D and potassium. Vitamins A and C are no longer required because deficiencies are rare, but this information may be included voluntarily.

Daily Values (%) on the label provide a rough guide indicating whether the food contains a small or large amount of a nutrient for comparison purposes. Foods that provide 20% or more of the DV are considered high in a nutrient. The requirement to label products has resulted in reformulation of many foods to provide healthier products. The 2016 Nutrition Facts label must be implemented by large food manufacturers by January 2020, but smaller companies will have an additional year to comply. Some large food manufacturers have requested additional time for compliance due to a lack of consensus regarding the definition of dietary fiber.

Nutrient Content and Health Claims

Two categories of claims currently can be used on foods in the United States: nutrient content claims and health claims. **Nutrient content claims** identify the nutrients in a product and provide information to assess its relative value. **Health claims** describe a relationship between a food or food component and its ability to reduce risk of a disease or health-related condition. These claims are based on a very high standard of scientific evidence.

Nutrient content claims describe the quantity of a nutrient in a product using words defined by the FDA, such as "free," "low," or "high." Comparative terms—such as "more" or "reduced"—can be used to indicate a difference to a similar food. "Healthy," "lean," or "light" are descriptions of nutrient contents. The food must meet FDA definitions to use these terms. A label cannot include an explicit or implied nutrient content claim unless it uses terms defined by the FDA. Box 1.4 defines some of the established terms and definitions used on food labels.

Only health claims that have been approved and authorized by the FDA can be used on food products and dietary supplements (Box 1.5). To use a health claim, the food must meet specific criteria regarding the amount of that specific nutrient and sometimes other nutrients in the product. Products making a claim are required to use the FDA's exact wording.

Health claims on foods require preapproval from the FDA; these are limited and regulated in an effort to protect consumers from false or misleading claims. **Unqualified health claims** must be supported by qualified experts agreeing that scientific evidence is available determining a relationship between a nutrient and a specific disease. **Qualified health claims** are supported by some evidence, but they lack significant scientific agreement; thus, their claim must be accompanied by a disclaimer as specified by the FDA. Since 2002, when the FDA began allowing companies to petition for qualified health claims, fewer than 20 qualified health claims have been approved. A health claim must use the exact wording specified by the FDA. For instance, the first qualified claim allowed by the FDA was the association between nuts and heart disease; verbiage on the package must read: "Scientific evidence suggests but does not prove 1.5 ounces per day of most nuts such as (insert name of specific nut) as part of a diet low in saturated fat and cholesterol may reduce the risk of heart disease."[12]

Additional Nutrition Labels

Many consumers are confused by the Nutrition Facts panel and prefer information in a quicker and easy-to-read format. Food manufacturers, supermarket chains, trade associations, and health organizations have developed comprehensive mechanisms to provide information about the nutritional quality of foods and beverages either on product packaging or shelf tags in retail setting nutrition labeling systems.

Since 1985, the American Heart Association has tried to make heart-healthy grocery shopping easier with its heart check symbol. A food has to meet certain criteria to qualify for using this symbol. The Whole Grain Council has different stamps indicating two different levels of whole grain in a serving (see Chapter 4). The Produce for Better Health Foundation's More Matters icon, Kraft's Sensible Solutions, and Sara Lee's Nutritional Spotlight are several other programs that have been developed. These food rating programs can help individuals make better food choices, as will the revised Nutrition Facts label. Furthermore, in order to make wise choices, food should be selected within the context of the whole diet.

The FDA is apprehensive about these different labeling programs, fearing they may mislead consumers about the health benefits of the food. Multiple systems may create more confusion, and other systems' criteria may not be stringent enough or consistent with the *Dietary Guidelines*. Another concern is that they may encourage consumers to choose highly processed foods and refined grains rather than fruits, vegetables, and whole grains. The FDA has considered developing a single standardized guidance system for front-of-package labels. Whether all nutrition and health claims from the front of processed food packages will be eliminated is yet to be determined.

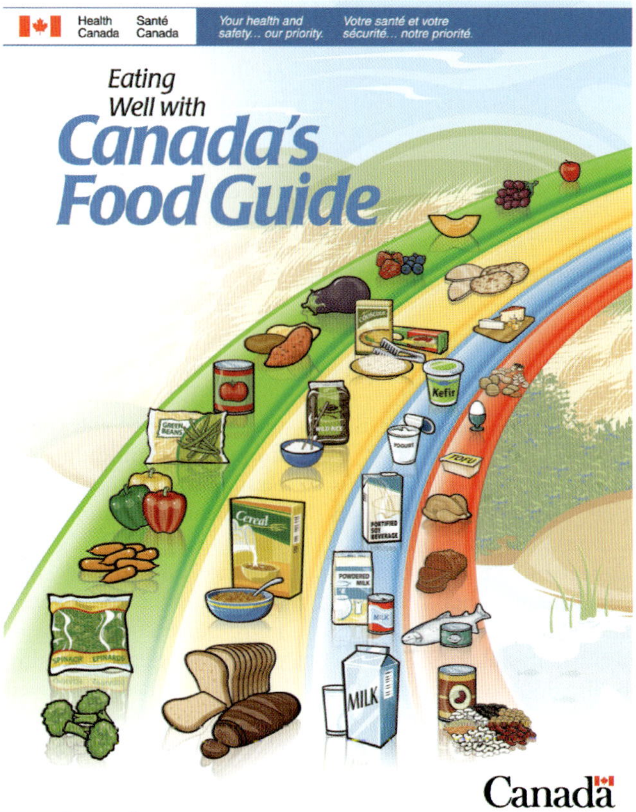

Recommended Number of Food Guide Servings per Day

	Children			Teens		Adults			
Age in Years	2-3	4-8	9-13	14-18		19-50		51+	
Sex	Girls and Boys			Females	Males	Females	Males	Females	Males
Vegetables and Fruit	4	5	6	7	8	7-8	8-10	7	7
Grain Products	3	4	6	6	7	6-7	8	6	7
Milk and Alternatives	2	2	3-4	3-4	3-4	2	2	3	3
Meat and Alternatives	1	1	1-2	2	3	2	3	2	3

What is One Food Guide Serving?
Look at the examples below.

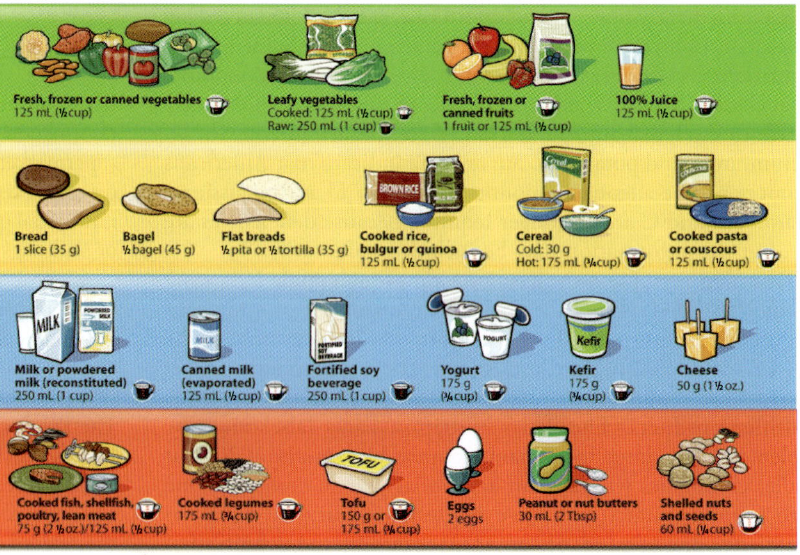
Fresh, frozen or canned vegetables
125 mL (½cup)
Leafy vegetables
Cooked: 125 mL (½cup)
Raw: 250 mL (1 cup)
Fresh, frozen or canned fruits
1 fruit or 125 mL (½cup)
100% Juice
125 mL (½cup)
Bread
1 slice (35 g)
Bagel
½ bagel (45 g)
Flat breads
½ pita or ½ tortilla (35 g)
Cooked rice, bulgur or quinoa
125 mL (½cup)
Cereal
Cold: 30 g
Hot: 175 mL (¾cup)
Cooked pasta or couscous
125 mL (½cup)
Milk or powdered milk (reconstituted)
250 mL (1 cup)
Canned milk (evaporated)
125 mL (½cup)
Fortified soy beverage
250 mL (1 cup)
Yogurt
175 g (¾cup)
Kefir
175 g (¾cup)
Cheese
50 g (1 ½ oz.)
Cooked fish, shellfish, poultry, lean meat
75 g (2 ½ oz.)/125 mL (½cup)
Cooked legumes
175 mL (¾cup)
Tofu
150 g or 175 mL (¾cup)
Eggs
2 eggs
Peanut or nut butters
30 mL (2 Tbsp)
Shelled nuts and seeds
60 mL (¼cup)

The chart above shows how many Food Guide Servings you need from each of the four food groups every day.

Having the amount and type of food recommended and following the tips in *Canada's Food Guide* will help:

- Meet your needs for vitamins, minerals and other nutrients.
- Reduce your risk of obesity, type 2 diabetes, heart disease, certain types of cancer and osteoporosis.
- Contribute to your overall health and vitality.

Oils and Fats

- Include a small amount – 30 to 45 mL (2 to 3 Tbsp) – of unsaturated fat each day. This includes oil used for cooking, salad dressings, margarine and mayonnaise.
- Use vegetable oils such as canola, olive and soybean.
- Choose soft margarines that are low in saturated and trans fats.
- Limit butter, hard margarine, lard and shortening.

A

• **Figure 1.7** Eating well with Canada's food guide. (From *Canada's Guide*. Last modified: May 23, 2012. © Her Majesty the Queen in Right of Canada, represented by the Minister of Health Canada, 2011. This publication may be reproduced without permission. No changes permitted. HC Pub.: 4651 Cat.: H164-38/1-2011E-PDF ISBN: 978-1-100-19255-0. Web site. http://www.hc-sc.gc.ca/fn-an/food-guide-aliment/order-commander/index-eng.php. Accessed March 20, 2017.)

Make each Food Guide Serving count…
wherever you are – at home, at school, at work or when eating out!

- **Eat at least one dark green and one orange vegetable each day.**
  - Go for dark green vegetables such as broccoli, romaine lettuce and spinach.
  - Go for orange vegetables such as carrots, sweet potatoes and winter squash.
- **Choose vegetables and fruit prepared with little or no added fat, sugar or salt.**
  - Enjoy vegetables steamed, baked or stir-fried instead of deep-fried.
- **Have vegetables and fruit more often than juice.**

- **Make at least half of your grain products whole grain each day.**
  - Eat a variety of whole grains such as barley, brown rice, oats, quinoa and wild rice.
  - Enjoy whole grain breads, oatmeal or whole wheat pasta.
- **Choose grain products that are lower in fat, sugar or salt.**
  - Compare the Nutrition Facts table on labels to make wise choices.
  - Enjoy the true taste of grain products. When adding sauces or spreads, use small amounts.

- **Drink skim, 1%, or 2% milk each day.**
  - Have 500 mL (2 cups) of milk every day for adequate vitamin D.
  - Drink fortified soy beverages if you do not drink milk.
- **Select lower fat milk alternatives.**
  - Compare the Nutrition Facts table on yogurts or cheeses to make wise choices.

- **Have meat alternatives such as beans, lentils and tofu often.**
- **Eat at least two Food Guide Servings of fish each week.***
  - Choose fish such as char, herring, mackerel, salmon, sardines and trout.
- **Select lean meat and alternatives prepared with little or no added fat or salt.**
  - Trim the visible fat from meats. Remove the skin on poultry.
  - Use cooking methods such as roasting, baking or poaching that require little or no added fat.
  - If you eat luncheon meats, sausages or prepackaged meats, choose those lower in salt (sodium) and fat.

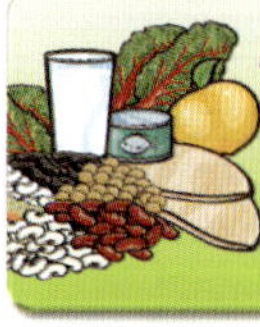

Enjoy a variety of foods from the four food groups.

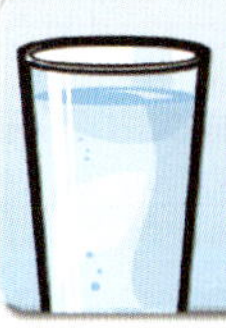

Satisfy your thirst with water!

Drink water regularly. It's a calorie-free way to quench your thirst. Drink more water in hot weather or when you are very active.

* Health Canada provides advice for limiting exposure to mercury from certain types of fish. Refer to www.healthcanada.gc.ca for the latest information.

Advice for different ages and stages…

Children

Following *Canada's Food Guide* helps children grow and thrive.

Young children have small appetites and need calories for growth and development.

- Serve small nutritious meals and snacks each day.
- Do not restrict nutritious foods because of their fat content. Offer a variety of foods from the four food groups.
- Most of all... be a good role model.

Women of childbearing age

All women who could become pregnant and those who are pregnant or breastfeeding need a multivitamin containing **folic acid** every day. Pregnant women need to ensure that their multivitamin also contains **iron**. A health care professional can help you find the multivitamin that's right for you.

Pregnant and breastfeeding women need more calories. Include an extra 2 to 3 Food Guide Servings each day.

Here are two examples:
- Have fruit and yogurt for a snack, or
- Have an extra slice of toast at breakfast and an extra glass of milk at supper.

Men and women over 50

The need for **vitamin D** increases after the age of 50.

In addition to following *Canada's Food Guide*, everyone over the age of 50 should take a daily vitamin D supplement of 10 μg (400 IU).

Eat well and be active today and every day!

The benefits of eating well and being active include:

- Better overall health.
- Lower risk of disease.
- A healthy body weight.
- Feeling and looking better.
- More energy.
- Stronger muscles and bones.

Be active

To be active every day is a step towards better health and a healthy body weight.

Canada's Physical Activity Guide recommends building 30 to 60 minutes of moderate physical activity into daily life for adults and at least 90 minutes a day for children and youth. You don't have to do it all at once. Add it up in periods of at least 10 minutes at a time for adults and five minutes at a time for children and youth.

Start slowly and build up.

Eat well

Another important step towards better health and a healthy body weight is to follow *Canada's Food Guide* by:

- Eating the recommended amount and type of food each day.
- Limiting foods and beverages high in calories, fat, sugar or salt (sodium) such as cakes and pastries, chocolate and candies, cookies and granola bars, doughnuts and muffins, ice cream and frozen desserts, french fries, potato chips, nachos and other salty snacks, alcohol, fruit flavoured drinks, soft drinks, sports and energy drinks, and sweetened hot or cold drinks.

Read the label

- Compare the Nutrition Facts table on food labels to choose products that contain less fat, saturated fat, trans fat, sugar and sodium.
- Keep in mind that the calories and nutrients listed are for the amount of food found at the top of the Nutrition Facts table.

Nutrition Facts
Per 0 mL (0 g)

Amount		% Daily Value
Calories 0		
Fat 0 g		0 %
Saturates 0 g		0 %
+ Trans 0 g		
Cholesterol 0 mg		
Sodium 0 mg		0 %
Carbohydrate 0 g		0 %
Fibre 0 g		0 %
Sugars 0 g		
Protein 0 g		
Vitamin A 0 %	Vitamin C	0 %
Calcium 0 %	Iron	0 %

Limit trans fat

When a Nutrition Facts table is not available, ask for nutrition information to choose foods lower in trans and saturated fats.

Take a step today…

- ✓ Have breakfast every day. It may help control your hunger later in the day.
- ✓ Walk wherever you can – get off the bus early, use the stairs.
- ✓ Benefit from eating vegetables and fruit at all meals and as snacks.
- ✓ Spend less time being inactive such as watching TV or playing computer games.
- ✓ Request nutrition information about menu items when eating out to help you make healthier choices.
- ✓ Enjoy eating with family and friends!
- ✓ Take time to eat and savour every bite!

For more information, interactive tools, or additional copies visit Canada's Food Guide on-line at:
www.healthcanada.gc.ca/foodguide

or contact:
Publications
Health Canada
Ottawa, Ontario K1A 0K9
E-Mail: publications@hc-sc.gc.ca
Tel.: 1-866-225-0709
Fax: (613) 941-5366
TTY: 1-800-267-1245

Également disponible en français sous le titre : Bien manger avec le Guide alimentaire canadien

This publication can be made available on request on diskette, large print, audio-cassette and braille.

How do I count Food Guide Servings in a meal?

Here is an example:

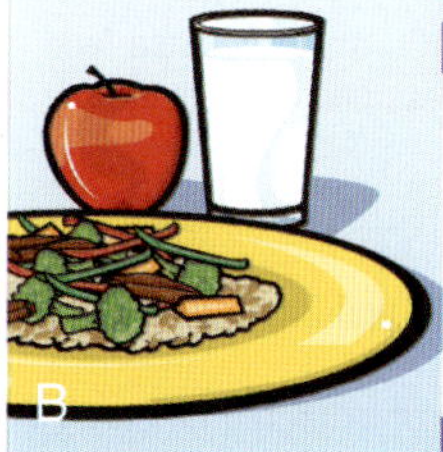

Vegetable and beef stir-fry with rice, a glass of milk and an apple for dessert		
250 mL (1 cup) mixed broccoli, carrot and sweet red pepper	=	2 **Vegetables and Fruit** Food Guide Servings
75 g (2½ oz.) lean beef	=	1 **Meat and Alternatives** Food Guide Serving
250 mL (1 cup) brown rice	=	2 **Grain Products** Food Guide Servings
5 mL (1 tsp) canola oil	=	part of your **Oils and Fats** intake for the day
250 mL (1 cup) 1% milk	=	1 **Milk and Alternatives** Food Guide Serving
1 apple	=	1 **Vegetables and Fruit** Food Guide Serving

B

• **Figure 1.7,** cont'd

The New and Improved Nutrition Facts Label – Key Changes

The U.S. Food and Drug Administration has finalized a new Nutrition Facts label for packaged foods that will make it easier to make informed food choices that support a healthy diet. The updated label has a fresh new design and reflects current scientific information, including the link between diet and chronic diseases.

1. Servings

The number of "servings per container" and the "Serving Size" declaration have increased and are now in larger and/or bolder type. Serving sizes have been updated to reflect what people actually eat and drink today. For example, the serving size for ice cream was previously ½ cup and now is ¾ cup.
There are also new requirements for certain size packages, such as those that are between one and two servings or are larger than a single serving but could be consumed in one or multiple sittings.

2. Calories

"Calories" is now larger and bolder.

3. Fats

"Calories from Fat" has been removed because research shows the type of fat consumed is more important than the amount.

4. Added Sugars

"Added Sugars" in grams and as a percent Daily Value (%DV) is now required on the label. "Added Sugars" include sugars that have been added during the processing or packaging of a food. Scientific data shows that it is difficult to meet nutrient needs while staying within calorie limits if you consume more than 10 percent of your total daily calories from added sugar.

NEW LABEL

Nutrition Facts

8 servings per container
Serving size 2/3 cup (55g)

Amount per serving	
Calories	**230**
	% Daily Value*
Total Fat 8g	**10%**
Saturated Fat 1g	**5%**
Trans Fat 0g	
Cholesterol 0mg	**0%**
Sodium 160mg	**7%**
Total Carbohydrate 37g	**13%**
Dietary Fiber 4g	**14%**
Total Sugars 12g	
Includes 10g Added Sugars	**20%**
Protein 3g	
Vitamin D 2mcg	10%
Calcium 260mg	20%
Iron 8mg	45%
Potassium 235mg	6%

* The % Daily Value (DV) tells you how much a nutrient in a serving of food contributes to a daily diet. 2,000 calories a day is used for general nutrition advice.

Manufacturers will need to use the new label by January 1, 2020, and small businesses will have an additional year to comply. During this transition time, you will see the current Nutrition Facts label or the new label on products.

5. Nutrients

The lists of nutrients that are required or permitted on the label have been updated. Vitamin D and potassium are now required on the label because Americans do not always get the recommended amounts. Vitamins A and C are no longer required since deficiencies of these vitamins are rare today. The actual amount in grams in addition to the %DV must be listed for vitamin D, calcium, iron, and potassium.
The daily values for nutrients have also been updated based on newer scientific evidence. The daily values are reference amounts of nutrients to consume or not to exceed and are used to calculate the %DV.

6. Footnote

The footnote at the bottom of the label has changed to better explain the meaning of %DV. The %DV helps you understand the nutrition information in the context of a total daily diet.

JULY 2016

For more information about the new Nutrition Facts label, visit:
www.fda.gov/Food/GuidanceRegulation/GuidanceDocumentsRegulatoryInformation/LabelingNutrition/ucm385663.htm

• **Figure 1.8** Changes finalized in May 2016 to the Nutrition Facts label for packaged foods to reflect new scientific information. (From Geiger CJ. Deconstructing the updated Food Label for informed consumer choices. Presented at the Food and Nutrition Conference and Exhibition, Academy of Nutrition and Dietetics, Boston, MA. October 2016.)

• BOX 1.4 Definitions of Commonly Used Nutrient Content Claims

Calories

- *Calorie free*: Fewer than 5 calories per RACC (reference amounts customarily consumed)
- *Low calorie*: 40 calories or less per RACC, or per 50 g of the food
- *Reduced or fewer calories*: At least 25% fewer calories per RACC than reference food

Fat

- *Fat free*: Less than 0.5 g of fat per RACC
- *Saturated fat free*: Less than 0.5 g per RACC, and the level of *trans* fatty acids does not exceed 1% of total fat
- *Low fat*: 3 g or less per RACC, or per 50 g of the food
- *Low saturated fat*: 1 g or less per RACC and not more than 15% of calories from saturated fatty acids
- *Reduced or less fat*: At least 25% less per RACC than reference food
- *Reduced or less saturated fat*: At least 25% less per RACC than reference food

Cholesterol

- *Cholesterol free*: Less than 2 mg of cholesterol and 2 g or less of saturated fat per RACC
- *Low cholesterol*: 20 mg or less or 2 g or less of saturated fat per RACC, or per 50 g of the food
- *Reduced or less cholesterol*: At least 25% less and 2 g or less of saturated fat per RACC than reference food

• BOX 1.4 Definitions of Commonly Used Nutrient Content Claims—cont'd

Sodium

- *Sodium-free*: Less than 5 mg per RACC
- *Low sodium*: 140 mg or less per RACC, or per 50 g of the food
- *Very low sodium*: 35 mg or less per RACC, or per 50 g of the food
- *Reduced or less sodium*: At least 25% less per RACC than reference food

Fiber

- *High fiber*: 5 g or more per RACC (foods with high-fiber claims must meet the definition for low fat or the level of total fat must appear next to the high-fiber claim)
- *Good source of fiber*: 2.5–4.9 g per RACC
- *More or added fiber*: At least 2.5 g more per RACC than reference food

Sugar

- *Sugar free*: Less than 0.5 g per RACC
- No added sugar, without added sugar, or no sugar added:
  - No sugars are added during processing or packaging, including ingredients that contain sugars (e.g., fruit juices, applesauce, or dried fruit).
  - Processing does not increase the sugar content to an amount higher than is naturally present in the ingredients (a functionally insignificant increase in sugars is acceptable from processes used for purposes other than increasing sugar content).
  - The food that resembles it and for which it substitutes normally contains added sugars.
  - If it does not meet the requirements for a low- or reduced-calorie food, that product bears a statement that the food is not low calorie or reduced calorie and directs consumers' attention to the nutritional panel for additional information on sugars and calorie content.
- *Reduced sugar*: At least 25% less sugar per RACC than reference food

Healthy*

The regulatory criteria for use of the nutrient content claim "healthy" is being re-evaluated, a lengthy process, but enforcement discretion may be exercised during this period. Products may use the term "healthy" in the product name or as a claim on the label or in the labeling of a food that is useful in creating a diet that is consistent with dietary recommendations. If the product is not low in fat, it should have a fat profile makeup of predominantly mono- and polyunsaturated fats (i.e., sum of monounsaturated fats and polyunsaturated fats are greater than the total saturated fat content of the food). The food must supply at least 10% of the Daily Value per reference amount customarily consumed (RACC) of for at least one of six nutrients: vitamins A and C, calcium, iron, protein, or fiber, or if the food instead contains at least 10% of the DV of potassium or vitamin D. Whichever nutrient is used as the basis for eligibility should be declared in the Nutrition Facts label. From U.S. Food and Drug Administration: *Food labeling guide*. Revised January 2013. https://www.fda.gov/downloads/Food/GuidanceRegulation/UCM265446.pdf

**U.S Department of Health and Human Services, Food and Drug Administration.* Use of the Term "Healthy" in the Labeling of Human Food Products: Guidance for Industry. *Center for Food Safety and Applied Nutrition; College Park, MD, September 2016.* https://www.fda.gov/Food/GuidanceRegulation/GuidanceDocumentsRegulatoryInformation/ucm521690.htm

• BOX 1.5 Health Claims Authorized by the U.S. Food and Drug Administration

- Calcium and reduced risk of osteoporosis; calcium, vitamin D, and reduced risk of osteoporosis
- Sodium and increased risk of hypertension
- Dietary fat and increased risk of cancer
- Saturated fat and cholesterol and increased risk of heart disease
- Fiber-containing grain products, fruits, and vegetables, and reduced risk of cancer
- Fruits, vegetables, and grain products that contain fiber, particularly soluble fiber, and reduced risk of heart disease
- Fruits and vegetables and reduced risk of cancer
- Folate and reduced risk of neural tube defects during pregnancy
- Noncariogenic carbohydrate sweeteners (D-tagatose, sugar alcohols, isomaltulose, sucralose) and reduced risk of dental caries
- Soluble fiber from certain foods (oat products, barley, and soluble fiber from psyllium husk) and reduced risk of coronary heart disease
- Soy protein and reduced risk of coronary heart disease
- Plant sterol/stanol esters and reduced risk of coronary heart disease

The following must meet specific nutrient requirements and use specific wording:

- Whole-grain foods and risk of heart disease and certain cancers
- Whole-grain foods with moderate fat content and risk of heart disease
- Potassium and reduced risk of hypertension and stroke
- Fluoride and decreased risk of dental caries
- Saturated fat, cholesterol, and *trans* fats and reduced risk of heart disease
- Substitution of saturated fat with unsaturated fatty acids and decreased risk of heart disease

DENTAL CONSIDERATIONS

- The dental hygienist must ensure that the appropriate RDIs are used for the patient's age or grouping (e.g., when talking to a pregnant patient, the RDI for pregnancy should be used).
- To prevent confusion, the acronym RDI is not used on labels; however, dental hygienists need to be aware of the basis for the information presented.
- Review a label together with the patient and family. Ask the patient to bring in several labels of commonly used foods in the household for you to discuss.
- Encourage patients to keep portion sizes consistent with activity level.
- On a label, point out the DVs that indicate calories (carbohydrate, fat, and protein), those indicating they should be limited (saturated and *trans* fat, cholesterol, and sodium), and how to determine whether a product contains a small or large amount of a nutrient (see Fig. 1.8).

NUTRITIONAL DIRECTIONS

- Read labels carefully. Ingredients are listed in order of quantity (by weight). Choose products that have less fat or oils or in which fats are listed last.
- Food labels are a useful tool to compare nutrient values of foods and learn valuable sources of nutrients. Fortified foods and supplements should not be purchased in an attempt to meet 100% of the RDIs because this may result in greater nutrient consumption than is needed, especially for young children. Concerns should be addressed to a health care provider or RDN.
- A product labeled "low fat" or "low sodium" may or may not be more healthful than another product. These claims are comparative to a previous product's fat or sodium content, not the whole product. Other nutrients in the product may be modified also, possibly negatively. Read the whole Nutrition Facts label carefully to know if the product is healthful or nutrient dense.
- When looking at the Nutrition Facts label to compare products, consider portion sizes between products because these can vary.
- Products labeled as "dietetic," "sugar-free," or "reduced fat" may not be low in calories; this is dependent on other ingredients in the food.
- Unsweetened juices and milk contain significant amounts of natural sugars.

HEALTH APPLICATION 1

Obesity

The U.S. population is leading the rest of the world in obesity, but this health problem has become a global issue–affecting around 13% of people worldwide. By 2025, one-fifth of adults worldwide will be obese unless effective interventions are adopted. China and the United States now have the most obese people in the world, with the United States having the most severely obese people of any country.[13] Obesity is a threat to the world's future food security and could precipitate a catastrophic epidemic of diabetes. The global cost of obesity is $2 trillion annually, which is nearly as much as the global cost of smoking ($2.1 trillion).[14]

Although the prevalence of obesity has shown signs of leveling off, obesity rates in 2016 were approximately 38% and extremely obese 8% (BMI >40.0).[15] During the past 20 years, groups with the heaviest BMIs have been increasing at the fastest rates.[16] As shown in Fig. 1.9, approximately 6.6% of adults were severely obese (more than 100 pounds over a healthy weight) in 2010, up from 3.9% in 2000. More alarming is the forecast that the prevalence of obesity may reach 51% by 2030.[17] Additionally, the statistics are very discouraging in ethnic groups (i.e., Hispanics, African Americans, Native Americans, and Alaska Natives) because the prevalence of obesity is markedly higher than in white Americans.

The goals of the *Healthy People 2020* nutritional objectives include increasing the proportion of adults who are at a healthy weight to 33.9% compared with the current level of 30.8% in 2005 to 2008 and reducing the proportion of adults who are obese to 30.5% compared with 33.9% who were obese in 2005 to 2008.[18] The Midcourse Review indicated little or no detectable change between 2005 and 2008 (30.8%) and 2009 and 2012 (29.5%) for increasing numbers of adults who are at a healthy weight and an undesirable change in the proportion of adults with obesity (from 33.9% to 35.3%).[19]

Other 2020 goals related to objectives to attain a healthy weight include (1) decreasing the proportion of adults who did not engage in any leisure-time physical activity, (2) increasing the proportion of adults who engaged in aerobic physical activity of light/moderate intensity for 150 minutes or more per week or vigorous intensity for 75 minutes or more per week, and (3) adults who met the physical activity guidelines for both aerobic physical activity and muscle strengthening. Midcourse review showed these objective exceeded their 2020 targets.[20]

According to the State of Obesity 2017, five states exceed 35% rates of obesity, 25 states are at or above 30%, and all states have a more than 20% rate of obesity. U.S. adult obesity rates decreased in one state (Kansas), increased in four (Colorado, Minnesota, Washington, and West Virginia), and remained steady in the rest between 2015 and 2016.[15]

Preventing weight gain or maintaining a healthy weight is a major goal to reduce the burden of illness and its consequent reduction in quality of life and life expectancy. Obesity and overweight in adulthood go hand in hand with preventable chronic diseases. These include hypertension, osteoarthritis, elevated blood cholesterol or triglyceride levels, heart disease, stroke, insulin resistance or type 2 diabetes, gallbladder disease, sleep apnea and respiratory problems, and certain types of cancers. Overweight takes a toll on the joints, especially knees, and overweight people are at increased risk of sleep apnea and asthma. Most of these conditions may have an impact on life expectancy but significantly impact quality of life.

Obesity affects many other aspects of life related to weight stigma or biases and discrimination: education, income, employability, and social position. Obesity also impacts psychological and social factors related to negative attitudes that affect interpersonal interactions.

Because overweight and obesity contribute to other health problems, their economic impact on the health care system is immense. Obesity costs more than $150 billion in health care costs in the U.S. and billions more in lost productivity.[15] A U.S. adult who is "healthy" but obese could eventually cost society anywhere from about $17,000 to just over $36,000.[21] Obesity-related medical costs in general are expected to rise significantly, especially because today's obese children are likely to become tomorrow's obese adults. Reducing obesity could save billions of dollars for the health care industry.

Weight management is very difficult for most individuals. Individuals who maintain a stable lean body shape throughout life have the lowest mortality.[22,23] Obesity and overweight at a young age and substantial weight gain are significantly associated with low physical performance in old age.[24] Because weight loss is so difficult, prevention of weight gain should be strongly emphasized.

In addition to BMI, weight distribution is also a factor in predicting health risk. Excess fat in the abdominal area (the "apple-shaped" body) is characteristic of men, but some women also tend to accumulate more fat around the waist, especially after menopause. Accumulation of fat in the hips or thighs (the "pear-shaped body") is typical of women. Any amount of increased abdominal fat (larger waist size) is a greater risk for heart attacks than body weight because it is associated with an accumulation of fat around the heart, liver, and other internal organs.[25,26] In contrast, lower body obesity has been thought to be relatively benign. However, patients with gluteal adipose tissue of obesity have more difficulty losing weight and maintaining a healthy weight.

A quick way to help determine fat intraabdominal accumulation, thereby determining overall health risks, is waist-to-height ratio (compares the waist measurement to height). A rule of thumb to determine abdominal fat is that the waist measurement should be less than half of the person's height (Fig. 1.10). A high BMI is associated with a high mortality risk, but waist-to-height ratio appears to be a more accurate indicator of mortality risk.[27]

HEALTH APPLICATION 1

Obesity—cont'd

Abdominal obesity increased in the United States through 2008, and a recent study reveals waist circumference increased progressively and significantly from 37.6 inches in 1999 to 2000 to 38.8 inches in 2011 to 2012. At a time when the prevalence of obesity may have plateaued and BMIs have remained relatively stable, waistlines of U.S. adults continue to expand.[28]

Researchers worldwide continue to study which method of measurement is best for different genders and nationalities. Gold standard methods that determine body fat more accurately—such as magnetic resonance imaging (MRI), dual-energy x-ray absorptiometry (DEXA) scans, and bioelectrical impedance scales—are significantly more expensive and require specialized equipment.

Obesity is the result of consistent caloric overconsumption in excess of energy expenditure. The average daily energy intake increased almost 7% for men and approximately 22% for women between 1971 and 2010. American men consume an average of 2600 cal, and women consume approximately 1850 cal.[29] This increased intake reflects a consumption level that is conducive for weight gain in inactive individuals.

Genetic influence is a significant factor contributing to obesity. Body weight is affected by genes, metabolism, hormones, food choices, behavior, environment, culture, and socioeconomic status. Although genetics and the environment may increase the risk of weight gain, environmental factors may overrule genetic risks.[30] The foods and portion sizes an individual consumes significantly affect body weight.

The United States has cultivated an environment with an abundance of foods containing hidden fats and sugars that can promote obesity. Many factors in the American culture have made food more accessible, including fast food restaurants, prepackaged food, and soft drinks. Fast foods account for 11.3% of total daily calories.[31] Portion sizes have also increased, and more people are eating at home less often. When people eat out, they tend to consume more calories—many restaurant meals average almost 1500 calories.[32] Contrary to popular belief, pizza, burgers, chicken, and french fries from restaurants and fast food establishments account for less energy than breads, grain-based desserts, pasta, and soft drinks from stores.[33]

In some cases, understanding physiologic benefits of weight loss can be motivating for patients. Weight loss is highly desirable in individuals with certain risk factors and advisable for others. A 10% weight loss is associated with a decrease in serum glucose, cholesterol, systolic blood pressure, and uric acid. Other physical symptoms that can be expected to improve with weight loss include shortness of breath, easy fatigability, fluid retention, gastric disorders, headaches, energy level, sexual interest, joint pains, muscle cramps, elevated pulse rate, sleeping disorders, urinary infection, and varicose veins.

Treatment of obesity has a high level of noncompliance and failure. Any caloric restriction triggers several biologic adaptations designed to prevent starvation. These adaptations may undermine the long-term effectiveness of lifestyle modification in most individuals who are overweight, particularly in an environment that promotes gluttony.[34] One of the reasons for regaining weight after struggling to lose it relates to appetite. People who successfully lose weight experience a surge in appetite–the body prompts a proportional increase in appetite to eat about 100 calories daily per kilogram of lost weight more than usual. The effect of appetite is three times stronger than the slowed metabolism.[35]

The incidence of obesity needs to be approached on four levels: (1) individuals need to be accountable for their food choices; (2) families must assume responsibility for foods available to their children, with parents acting as role models for healthful diet and exercise habits; (3) communities should provide opportunities for exercise (parks, sidewalks, sports programs) and schools should provide healthful food choices; and (4) more research is needed in this area to discover optimal, effective ways of weight management.

Any treatment for weight loss should always be a serious undertaking with a high level of motivation and long-term commitment. Such an approach increases the likelihood both of successful weight loss and maintaining a healthy weight. To lose weight involves a lifelong commitment to change one's lifestyle—regular exercise, wise food choices, and behavior modifications. Weight loss should be motivated by internal rather than external reasons ("I am doing this for myself," rather than "I will lose weight for my son's wedding").

One pound of fat equals 3500 cal. Losing weight can be accomplished by eating fewer calories, increasing activity, or a combination of both. A 0.5- to 2-lb per week weight loss is recommended to lose body fat while minimizing muscle loss. To accomplish this goal, food intake must be 500 cal less than needed per day, which results in loss of 1 lb per week. An additional energy expenditure of 500 cal per day is recommended to lose an additional pound of weight. When weight loss is achieved slowly, it is usually more effective and is maintained for a longer period. A realistic goal regarding the rate and amount of weight loss must be established for each individual trying to lose weight. A 3% to 5% weight loss that is maintained may produce clinically relevant health improvement.[36]

Numerous strategies have been implemented to treat overweight and obesity. No one treatment is best for everyone; each modality varies in effectiveness, risk, and cost. Drugs, medical devices, and surgical procedures currently being used for weight loss are beyond the scope of this text.

Millions of obese individuals have chosen **bariatric surgery** (surgical procedure on the stomach or small intestine for weight reduction), which usually results in greater, sustained weight loss than conventional methods in addition to diabetes remission, reduced incidence of cardiovascular events and hypertension, and a longer life.[37–39] This drastic but effective measure has many drawbacks and side effects, including limited absorption of many nutrients, pulmonary embolism, and some postoperative deaths.

Popular weight-reduction diets devised for weight loss are abundant (see the Evolve website). Although many different plans "guarantee" weight loss, no guaranteed easy cure exists for maintaining a healthy weight. A weight reduction diet needs to be followed for an extended time; it must be appealing, flexible, and affordable for the individual trying to lose weight. It can be balanced in terms of nutrients, yet hypocaloric. Reducing caloric intake to less than 1200 cal for women and 1400 cal for men is not recommended because adequate amounts of nutrients are not provided.

Popular diets vary in their nutritional adequacy and consistency with guidelines for risk reduction. The low-carbohydrate, high-protein diet has come into a favorable light as a result of numerous studies indicating that low-carbohydrate, high-protein diets are more effective in promoting weight loss and reducing blood lipid levels. A dietary regimen that stresses high-protein foods but eliminates sugar and most carbohydrates may be more successful at helping people lose weight because high-protein foods provide greater **satiety** (feeling of fullness). Higher-protein diets appear to have small to moderate improvements in weight loss, BMI, waist circumference, lean body mass, and a slightly negative effect on body fat storage.[40–42] Proteins may suppress **ghrelin** (an appetite-stimulating hormone) production better than carbohydrates and lipids. Diets that are considered high fat may cause undesirable cholesterol levels to increase, but weight loss as a result of inadequate calorie intake itself usually improves blood lipid levels regardless of the macronutrient composition. Reviews about various popular diets are available from the Academy of Nutrition and Dietetics at http://www.eatright.org/resources/media/trends-and-reviews/bookreviews.

Different diets work for different people; all components of energy balance—including energy intake from carbohydrates, protein, and fat, and expenditure—interact with one another to impact body weight. A change to

Continued

HEALTH APPLICATION 1

Obesity—cont'd

any one aspect will correspond to profound changes in the other side of the equation. Unreasonable expectations and unrealistic predictions are frequently made about weight-loss benefits of exercise and dietary interventions.

A diet that totally eliminates one category (fat or carbohydrate) or a specific group of foods (fruits or meats) is not advisable. The best diets are easy to follow, nutritious, safe, and effective for weight loss and prevent chronic health conditions associated with obesity.

Indispensable to any weight-loss program is a preplanned food allotment with specified times for eating throughout the day to lessen feelings of deprivation and to eliminate excessive food intake. The total amount of food should be divided into at least three feedings. Eating only once or twice a day is associated with consuming more calories, impulsive snacking, and increased adipose tissue and serum cholesterol. Some "free" foods or beverages (foods containing less than 20 cal per serving) may be available for snack periods, but regular mealtimes are important. A diet that requires the least amount of change in usual dietary patterns has better long-term success. A 1200- to 1500-cal diet is relatively safe; when accompanied by an exercise program, the rate of weight loss is augmented, and muscle mass is maintained.

A weight-reduction diet should satisfy the following criteria: (a) meets all nutrient needs except energy, (b) suits tastes and habits, (c) minimizes hunger and fatigue, (d) is accessible and socially acceptable, (e) encourages a change in eating pattern, and (f) favors improvement in overall health. Box 1.6 provides some questions to help determine the validity of a weight-reduction diet. Common reasons indicated for discontinuing a weight-loss regimen: (a) trouble controlling food choices, (b) difficulty motivating oneself to eat appropriately, and (c) using food as a reward.

Treatment of obesity is improved when increased energy expenditure occurs along with decreased caloric intake. Exercise alone has a modest effect on weight loss. Exercise positively affects energy metabolism, whereas decreased energy intake and loss of muscle mass will result in a lower metabolic rate. Initiation of an exercise regimen may lead to weight gain in the form of muscle mass, but the health benefits are significant, including improved cardiovascular fitness, improved plasma lipoprotein profile, improved carbohydrate metabolism, increased energy expenditure, and enhanced psychological well-being.

Comprehensive lifestyle interventions—including diet, physical activity, and behavior therapy provided by a skilled professional team of RDNs, exercise specialists, and behaviorists—have shown the highest success rate.[43] Behavior modification for weight control refers to getting in touch with the reality of foods being consumed and in what quantity, and when and why eating occurs (mindful eating). One of the most important components of an effective weight control program is learning new ways of dealing with old habits. Comprehensive behavior-modification programs include diet and exercise programs individually tailored for patients. A team approach—including a health care provider, a psychologist, an RDN, and family members—is effective in helping the individual make necessary long-lasting changes in food choices and lifestyle behaviors. A food diary for recording amounts and types of food eaten, emotional status, and environmental factors helps provide new insights to devise strategies for dealing with eating habits.

Although behavior-modification approaches to weight control are helpful, maintaining weight loss remains a major problem. Studies indicate that programs need to be approximately 20 to 24 weeks long and more comprehensive, including relapse prevention training and use of social support systems.

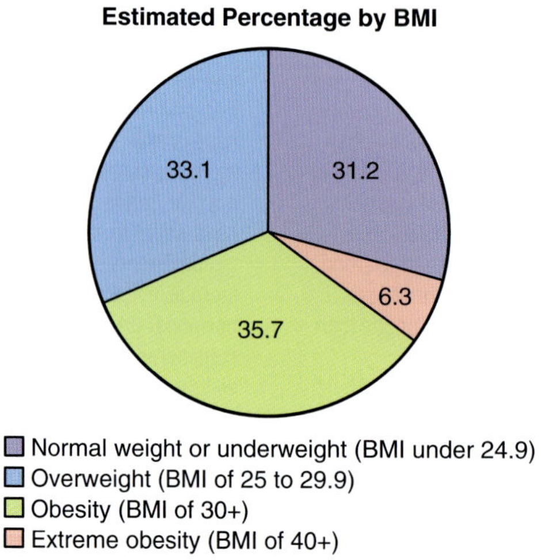

• **Figure 1.9** Overweight and obesity among adults age 20 and older, United States, 2009–2010. (Source: National Health and Nutrition Examination Survey, 2009–2010. https://www.niddk.nih.gov/health-information/health-statistics/Pages/overweight-obesity-statistics.aspx. Accessed March 20, 2017.)

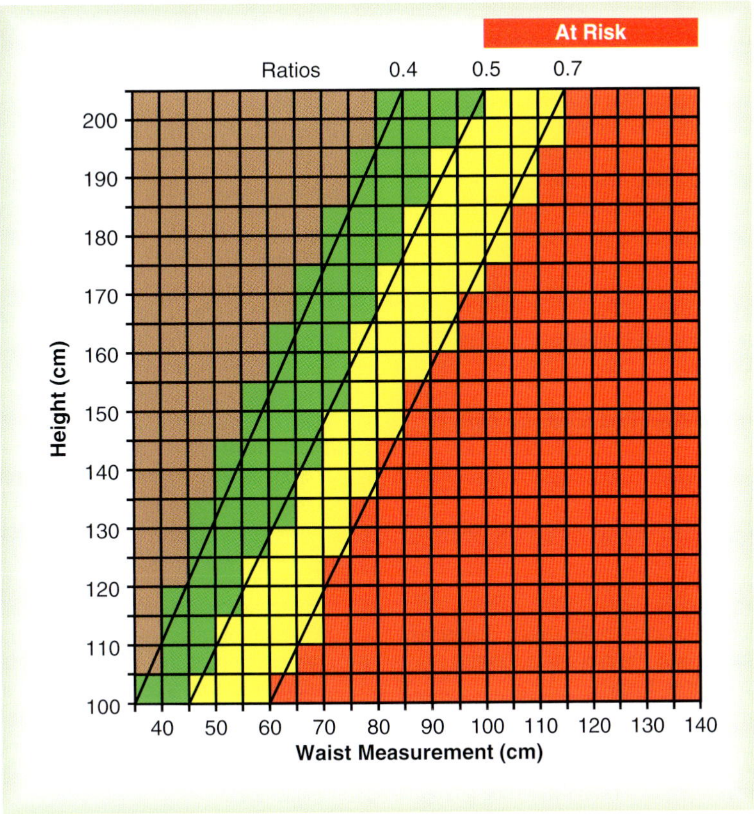

Waist-To-Height Ratio less than 0.5 - Low Risk Level. The boundary at a ratio of 0.4 represents low risks for 'normal' body shape (green) and potentially slight risks from being underweight for height (brown).

Waist-To-Height Ratio above 0.5 - Moderate to High Risk Level. The boundary at a ratio of 0.6 represents moderate risks (yellow) and high risks (red).

• **Figure 1.10** Waist circumference-to-height ratio chart. (Courtesy of Dr. John Anderson.)

• BOX 1.6 Evaluating Weight Loss Diets or Programs

The program should evaluate the individual's body mass index and whether the weight is principally from increased fat stores or increased muscle mass and possible contributing factors.

The cost of the program should be realistic and reasonable.

The program should be adaptable for various lifestyles and something an individual can continue indefinitely.

Tips for Evaluating Safety and Effectiveness of Reduction Diets

1. Stay current with scientific research. Nutrition is a relatively new science, and new developments are still evolving to increase our knowledge base.
2. Evaluate diet trends and claims for effects on overall health.
3. Compare recommendations with known nutrition science and recommendations, such as *MyPlate* and *Dietary Guidelines for Americans*.
4. Calculate nutritional requirements of the individual considering the diet and determine what nutrients would be lacking.
5. Evaluate diets using the following principles:
   - What is the weight loss recommendation?
   - What is the success rate of the program?
   - What is the basis for advertisements and endorsements?
   - Has any scientific research been done to evaluate the safety and effectiveness of the diet?
   - What is the cost of the program? Are special foods or nutrient supplements required and what do they cost? Are there other additional fees?
   - Is the program medically supervised?
   - Are any major food groups excluded?
   - Are the foods appealing to the individual? Does the program allow occasional consumption of favorite foods?
   - Is it permissible to eat in restaurants and other people's homes at least occasionally?
   - Are certain foods avoided because they cause specific problems?
   - Are certain foods used to "cure"?
   - Are dramatic statements made that contradict well-established nutrition principles or reputable scientific organizations?
   - Are exercise and behavior modification included?
   - Can an individual live on the program for a lifetime?
   - Is there a maintenance plan?
   - Does it promote good food habits?

CASE APPLICATION FOR THE DENTAL HYGIENIST

A young healthy mother who has a 3-year-old son at home comes to the dental office for a 6-month recare appointment. She expresses concern about foods she should be eating and feeding her husband and son to improve and maintain their overall health for optimal growth and development of the child. She has learned a little about the food groups, the *Dietary Guidelines*, and nutrition labels from the press but does not know how to implement them.

Nutritional Assessment

- Willingness to seek nutritional information
- Desire for increased control of nutritional health habits
- Knowledge of community resources
- Cultural or religious influences
- Knowledge regarding the *Dietary Guidelines*, food labels, and *MyPlate*
- Definition of optimal nutrition

Nutritional Diagnosis

Health-seeking behaviors related to lack of knowledge concerning optimal nutrition and current standards.

Nutritional Goals

The patient verbalizes correct information concerning the *Dietary Guidelines* and food labels and can name the food groups, the number of servings needed, and portion sizes from each group of *MyPlate*.

Nutritional Implementation

Intervention: Ask the patient to write down everything she ate yesterday from the time she got up yesterday until this morning when she got up.

Rationale: This will help you tailor the information you provide to the patient's needs.

Intervention: Encourage variety of food intake, using *MyPlate*. Review the number of servings needed and serving size.

Rationale: The total balance of food intake matters; the best balance incorporates variety to promote optimal nutrition. Providing the minimal number of servings prevents nutritional deficiencies in healthy individuals.

Intervention: (a) Suggest that the mother and her husband have their blood lipid profiles checked if not recently done; (b) emphasize a decreased intake of saturated and *trans* fats by trimming excess fat and eating smaller servings of meat (about the size of a fist or a deck of cards).

Rationale: Decreasing saturated and *trans* fats helps reduce the risk of heart disease. By decreasing these two types of fats, total fat and cholesterol should be within acceptable AMDRs.

Intervention: (a) Stress the importance of eating vegetables, fruits, and grains, and (b) explain that complex carbohydrates are not fattening.

Rationale: Dietary fiber is important for healthy bowel functioning and can reduce symptoms of chronic constipation, diverticular disease, and hemorrhoids, and decrease the risk of developing obesity, cancer, and diabetes.

Intervention: (a) Explain how to read labels for sugar. The names of most sugars end in "-ose." (b) Emphasize moderation of sugar intake. (c) Explain that "dietetic" and "sugar-free" do not mean that the product is low in calories. (d) Explain the relationship between sugar and tooth decay and emphasize the importance of proper oral hygiene after sugar consumption.

Rationale: Refined sugar contains calories and no other nutrients but is acceptable when used in items that contain appreciable amounts of other nutrients (e.g., a pudding would provide more nutrients than a gelatin dessert or carbonated beverage).

Intervention: (a) Stress using sodium and salt in moderation; (b) emphasize that "no salt added" does not mean that the product is low in sodium.

Rationale: Good habits that do not foster a high level of salt preference are recommended to prevent development of high blood pressure.

Intervention: Emphasize that any alcohol intake should be in moderation (one drink a day for women and two drinks a day for men), if at all.

Rationale: Alcohol is high in calories and contains few, if any, nutrients.

Intervention: (a) Review an entire label with the mother to help her understand how to interpret it. (b) Determine a serving size. (c) Explain the types of carbohydrates. (d) Determine the percentage of fat in a product by multiplying the grams of fat by 9, and compare this number with the total calories; if the amount is more than 30%, do not consume that product every day. (e) Emphasize that "no cholesterol" does not indicate that the product contains no saturated or *trans* fat. (f) Point out the sodium level, and if it is greater than 400 mg, encourage its use in moderation.

Rationale: Knowledge increases compliance and allows informed choices regarding food choice.

Intervention: Refer the patient to county extension agencies or to a registered dietitian.

Rationale: These agencies and nutritional professionals provide practical guidelines via newsletters, workshops, and written materials for healthy patients wanting to improve health.

Evaluation

To determine effectiveness of care, the patient reads labels and chooses the best buy for the nutrient content. The patient states the basic guidelines for nutrition; the hygienist explains to her that serving sizes for her son are different than the standard serving size (available on the *ChooseMyPlate* website). Additionally, the patient should be able to plan a menu using recommended foods and to state how to obtain and use community information/support. The patient should be able to indicate how changes in food choices would not only improve overall health, but also maintain health of the oral cavity and ensure optimal growth of her son with minimal or no problems in the oral cavity.

Student Readiness

1. A patient asks you the difference between food and nutrition. What would you say?
2. Locate an advertisement in a popular magazine or newspaper for a weight-reduction product or program and list the merits of the product or program stated in the ad. Then, list information about the product or program that might have been omitted or should be questioned. Evaluate the product or program using information from Box 1.6.
3. Discuss popular weight-reduction diets (see the Evolve website) and how they may have adverse effects.
4. Distinguish between nutrient recommendations and requirements.
5. Keep a record of all the foods you eat for 24 hours. Was your intake adequate as evaluated by *MyPlate?* In what areas did you do well? Where can you improve? Provide specific recommendations for making changes.
6. Collect nutrition labels for three similar products. Compare the nutrient values to determine which is a better source of nutrients. Which is a better buy for the amount of nutrients it contains?
7. List the *Dietary Guidelines*. In which areas do you do well? In which areas would you like to improve your choices? Do you believe you have enough information to make knowledgeable changes?
8. Discuss the pros and cons of allowing nutritional claims on products.

9. If a food label indicates that one serving of the product has 23 g of carbohydrate and 15 g of sugar with 140 cal (total), how many teaspoons of sugar does the product contain? What percentage of carbohydrate does this product contain?

References

1. CDC/National Center for Health Statistics. Healthy People 2020. Last reviewed November 6, 2015. https://www.cdc.gov/nchs/healthy_people/hp2020.htm. Accessed March 21, 2017.
2. National Center for Health Statistics. Chapter IV: Leading health indicators. Healthy People 2020 Midcourse Review. Hyattsville, MD: U.S. Department of Health and Human Services; 2016. https://www.healthypeople.gov/2020/data-search/midcourse-review. Accessed March 21, 2017.
3. Micha R, Peñalvo JL, Cudhea F, et al. Association between dietary factors and mortality from heart disease, stroke, and Type 2 Diabetes in the United States. *JAMA*. 2017;317(9):912–924.
4. U.S. Department of Agriculture. Agricultural Research Service. Energy Intakes: Percentages of Energy from Protein, Carbohydrate, Fat, and Alcohol By Gender and Age–What We Eat in America. NHANES 2011-2012. https://www.ars.usda.gov/ARSUserFiles/80400530/pdf/1314/Table_5_EIN_GEN_13.pdf. Accessed March 21, 2017.
5. Kam K. Why your BMI doesn't tell the whole story. Reviewed September 20, 2014. WebMD, LLC. http://www.webmd.com/diet/features/bmi-drawbacks-and-other-measurements#1. Accessed March 21, 2017.
6. U.S. Department of Health and Human Services, U.S. Department of Agriculture. 2015-2020 Dietary Guidelines for Americans. 8th ed. Washington, DC: USDHHS/USDA; 2015. https://health.gov/dietaryguidelines/2015/. Accessed March 21, 2017.
7. Adegboye AR, Boucher BJ, Kongstad J, et al. Calcium, vitamin D, casein and whey protein intakes and periodontitis among Danish adults. *Public Health Nutr*. 2016;19(3):503–510.
8. Butler L, Poti JM, Popkin BM. Trends in energy intake from alcoholic beverages amont US adults by sociodemographic characteristics, 1989-2012. *J Acad Nutr Diet*. 2016;116:1087–1100.
9. Tagtow A, Raghavan R. Assessing the reach of MyPlate using National Health and Nutrition Examination Survey Data. *J Acad Nutr Diet*. 2017;117(2):181–183.
10. Herring D, Chang S, Bard S. Five years of MyPlate–Looking back and what's ahead. *J Acad Nutr Diet*. 2016;116(7):1069–1071.
11. U.S. Food and Drug Administration (FDA). Constituent Updates: FDA releases 2014 Health and Diet Survey Findings. May 6, 2016. https://www.fda.gov/food/newsevents/constituentupdates/ucm499141.htm. Accessed March 14, 2017.
12. U.S. Food & Drug Administration (FDA). Qualified health claims: Letter of enforcement discretion–nuts and coronary heart disease. July 14, 2003. https://www.fda.gov/food/ingredientspackaginglabeling/labelingnutrition/ucm072926.htm. Accessed March 14, 2017.
13. NCD Risk Factor Collaboration. Trends in adult body-mass index in 200 countries from 1975 to 2014: a pooled analysis of 1698 population-based measurement studies with 19.2 million participants. *Lancet*. 2016;387(10026):1377–1396.
14. Dobbs R, Sawers C, Thompson F, et al. How the world could better fight obesity. McKinsey Global Institute. November 2014. http://www.mckinsey.com/industries/healthcare-systems-and-services/our-insights/how-the-world-could-better-fight-obesity. Accessed March 19, 2017.
15. Segal LM, Rayburn J, Beck SE. The State of Obesity: Better Policies for a Healthier America; 2017. Washington DC: Robert Wood Johnson Foundation. August, 2017. www.healthyAmericans.org. Accessed October 7, 2017.
16. Sturm R. People who are severely overweight remain fastest increasing group of obese Americans. RAND Health, October 1, 2012. http://www.rand.org/news/press/2012/10/01/index1.html. Accessed March 21, 2017.
17. Finkelstein EA, Khavjou OA, Thompson H, et al. Obesity and severe obesity forecasts through 2030. *Am J Prev Med*. 2012;42(6):563–570.
18. CDC/National Center for Health Statistics. Healthy People 2020. 2020 Topics & Objectives. Nutrition and weight status. Hyattsville, MD, 2016. https://www.healthypeople.gov/2020/topics-objectives/topic/nutrition-and-weight-status. Accessed March 21, 2017.
19. CDC/National Center for Health Statistics. Ch. 29: Nutrition and weight Status. Healthy People 2020 Midcourse Review. Hyattsville, MD. 2016. https://www.cdc.gov/nchs/healthy_people/hp2020/hp2020_midcourse_review.htm. Accessed March 21, 2017.
20. CDC/National Center for Health Statistics. Chapter 33: Physical Activity. Healthy People 2020 Midcourse Review. Hyattsville, MD. 2016. https://www.cdc.gov/nchs/healthy_people/hp2020/hp2020_midcourse_review.htm. Accessed March 21, 2017.
21. Fallah-Fini S, Adam A, Cheskin LJ, et al. The additional costs and health effects of a patient having overweight or obesity: a computational model. *Obesity (Silver Spring)*. 2017;25(10):1809–1815.
22. CDC/Centers for Disease Control and Prevention, Data & Statistics. Adult obesity facts. Last reviewed September 1, 2016. https://www.cdc.gov/obesity/data/adult.html. Accessed August 7, 2017.
23. Yu E, Ley SH, Manson JE, et al. Weight history and all-cause and cause-specific mortality in three prospective cohort studies. *Ann Intern Med*. 2017;166(9):613–620.
24. Vu THT, Carnethon MR, Lui K, et al. Obesity status in younger age, 39-year weight change and physical performance in older age: The Chicago Health Aging Study (CHAS). Epidemiology and Prevention/Lifestyle and Cardiometabolic Health 2017 Scientific Sessions. March 7, 2017; Portland, OR.
25. Song M, Hu FB, Wu K, et al. Trajectory of body shape in early and middle life and all cause and cause specific mortality: results from two prospective US cohort studies. *BMJ*. 2016;353:i2195.
26. Egeland GM, Igland J, Vollset SE, et al. High population attributable fractions of myocardial infarction associated with waist-hip ratio. *Obesity (Silver Spring)*. 2016;24(5):1162–1169.
27. Dhana K, Kavousi M, Ikram MA, et al. Body shape index in comparison with other anthropometric measures in prediction of total and cause-specific mortality. *J Epidemiol Community Health*. 2016;70(1):90–96.
28. Ford ES, Maynard LM, Li C. Trends in mean waist circumference and abdominal obesity among US adults, 1999-2012. *JAMA*. 2014;312(11):1151–1153.
29. U.S. Department of Agriculture. Agricultural Research Service. Energy Intakes: Percentages of Energy from Protein, Carbohydrate, Fat, and Alcohol By Gender and Age–What We Eat in America. NHANES 2011-2012. https://www.ars.usda.gov/ARSUserFiles/80400530/pdf/1314/Table_5_EIN_GEN_13.pdf. Accessed August 7, 2017.
30. Walter S, Mejía-Guevara I, Estrada K, et al. Association of a genetic risk score with body mass index across different birth cohorts. *JAMA*. 2016;316(1):63–69.
31. Fryar CD, Ervin RB. Caloric intake from fast food among adults: United States, 2007-2010. NCHS Data Brief No. 114. February 2013. https://www.cdc.gov/nchs/data/databriefs/db114.htm. Accessed March 21, 2017.
32. Urban LE, Weber JL, Heyman MB, et al. Energy contents of frequently ordered restaurant meals and comparison with human energy requirements and U.S. Department of Agriculture database information: a multisite randomized study. *J Acad Nutr Diet*. 2016;116(4):590–598.
33. Drewnowski A, Rehm CD. Energy intakes of US children and adults by food purchase location and by specific food source. *Nutr J*. 2013;12:59.
34. Ochner CN, Tsai AG, Kushner RF, et al. Treating obesity seriously: when recommendations for lifestyle change confront biological adaptations. *Lancet Diabetes Endocrinol*. 2015;3(4):232–234.
35. Polidori D, Sanghvi A, Seeley RJ, et al. How strongly does appetite counter weight loss? Quantification of the feedback control of human energy intake. *Obesity (Silver Spring)*. 2016;24(11):2289–2295.

36. Raynor HA, Champagne CM. Position of the Academy of Nutrition and Dietetics: Interventions for the treatment of overweight and obesity in Adults. *J Acad Nutr Diet*. 2016;116(1):129–147.
37. Bays HE, Jones PH, Jacobson TA, et al. Lipids and bariatric procedures part 1 of 2: Scientific statement from the National Lipid Association, American Society for Metabolic and Bariatric Surgery, and Obesity Medicine Association: EXECUTIVE SUMMARY. *J Clin Lipidol*. 2016;10(1):15–32.
38. National Institute of Diabetes and Digestive and Kidney Diseases (NIDDK). Research Updates: Understanding the health benefits and risks of bariatric surgery. https://www.niddk.nih.gov/news/research-updates/Pages/understanding-the-health-benefits-and-risks-of-bariatric-surgery.aspx. Accessed March 21, 2017.
39. National Institute of Diabetes and Digestive and Kidney Diseases (NIDDK). NIH Research Matters: Weight loss in adults 3 years after bariatric surgery. https://www.nih.gov/news-events/nih-research-matters/weight-loss-adults-3-years-after-bariatric-surgery. Accessed March 21, 2017.
40. Longland TM, Oikawa SY, Mitchell CJ, et al. High compared with lower dietary protein during an energy deficit combined with intense exercise promotes greater lean mass gain and fat mass loss: a randomized trial. *Am J Clin Nutr*. 2016;103(3):738–746.
41. Phillips SM. The impact of protein quality on the promotion of resistance exercise-induced changes in muscle mass. *Nutr Metab (Lond)*. 2016;13:64.
42. Rodriguez NR, Miller SL. Effective translation of current dietary guidance: understanding and communicating the concepts of minimal and optimal levels of dietary protein. *Am J Clin Nutr*. 2015;101(6):1353S–1358S.
43. Millen BE, Wolongevicz DM, Nonas CA, et al. 2013 American Heart Association/American College of Cardiology/The Obesity Society Guidelines for the management of overweight and obesity in adults: implications and new opportunities for Registered Dietitian Nutritionists. *J Acad Nutr Diet*. 2014;114(11):1730–1735.

EVOLVE RESOURCES

Please visit http://evolve.elsevier.com/Stegeman/nutritional for additional practice and study support tools.

2

Concepts in Biochemistry

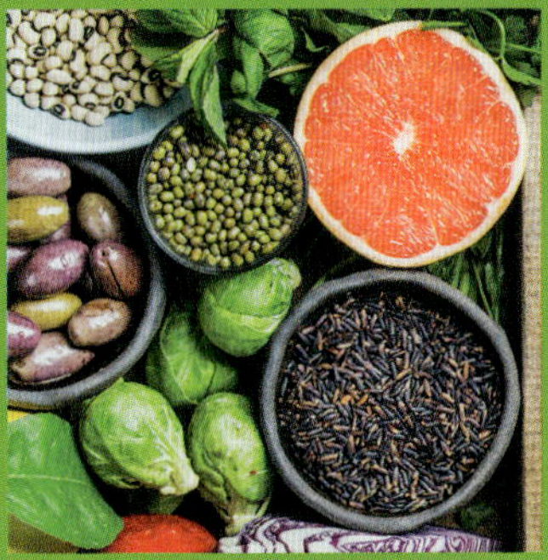

SCOTT M. TREMAIN, PHD

STUDENT LEARNING OUTCOMES

Upon completion of this chapter, the student will be able to achieve the following outcomes:

1. Explain the role of biochemistry in dental hygiene and nutrition.
2. Discuss the fundamentals of biochemistry, including assigning biomolecules according to functional group.
3. Discuss concepts related to principle biomolecules in nutrition:
   - Compare and contrast the structure, function, and properties of the four major classes of biomolecules (carbohydrates, proteins, nucleic acids, and lipids).
   - Outline the structure, function, and properties of monosaccharides, disaccharides, and polysaccharides.
   - Outline the structure, function, and properties of amino acids and proteins.
   - Compare and contrast the roles of enzymes, coenzymes, and vitamins in nutrition.
   - Outline the structure, function, and property of nucleotides and nucleic acids.
   - Outline the structure, function, and property of fatty acids, triglycerides, and steroids.
4. Summarize metabolism, as well as differentiate catabolism from anabolism. In addition, explain connections between metabolic pathways in carbohydrate, protein, and lipid metabolism.

KEY TERMS

Active site
Adenosine 5′-triphosphate (ATP)
Adipose tissue
Aerobic
Amino acids
Amphiphilic
Amylase
Anabolism
Anhydrous
Antioxidants
Bioactive
Bioinformation
Biomolecule
Carbohydrates
Catabolism
Chemical bonds
Cholesterol
***cis* isomer**
Coenzymes
Condensation reaction
Covalent bond
Disaccharide
Disease
Enzymes
Epigenetics
Epinephrine
Essential amino acids (EAAs) or indispensable amino acids
Fatty acids (FAs)
Functional group
Gene
Genome
Genomics
Glucagon
Glycogen
Glucogenic amino acids
Gluconeogenesis
Glycolysis
Glycosidic bond
Hormone
Hydrocarbon
Hydrogenation reaction
Hydrolysis reaction
Hydrophilic
Hydrophobic
Hydroxyapatite
Insulin
Ionic bond
Ketogenic amino acids
Ketone bodies
Linoleic acid
Lipase
Lipids
Lipoproteins
Melting point
Metabolism
Mitochondria
Molecule
Monomer
Monosaccharide
Monounsaturated fatty acid (MUFA)
Nonessential amino acids (NEAAs) or dispensable amino acids
Nucleic acids
Nucleotides
Nutrigenomics or nutritional genomics
Oils
Oxidation
Oxidation-reduction reactions
Oxidative phosphorylation
Peptide bond
Photosynthesis
Polymer
Polypeptide
Polysaccharide
Polyunsaturated fatty acid (PUFA)
Precursor
Protease
Proteins
Redox coenzymes
Reduction
Respiration
Side chain (R group)
Saturated fatty acids
Substrate
Sugar alcohol
***trans* isomer**
Tricarboxylic acid cycle (TCA cycle)
Triglyceride (TG)
Unsaturated fatty acids
Vitamins

TEST YOUR NQ

1. **T/F** A condensation reaction breaks a larger molecule into two smaller molecules.
2. **T/F** Nucleotides are the building blocks of proteins.
3. **T/F** Hydrophilic molecules dissolve readily in water.
4. **T/F** Sucrose is a disaccharide containing glucose and galactose.
5. **T/F** A substrate binds the enzyme active site and is converted into product.
6. **T/F** When the hydrogen atoms are on opposite sides of the double bond, the structure is a *trans* isomer.
7. **T/F** An unsaturated fatty acid with 16 carbons has a lower melting temperature than a saturated fatty acid with 16 carbons.
8. **T/F** Catabolism involves the reduction of carbohydrates into carbon dioxide and water.
9. **T/F** Insulin activates glycogen degradation to regulate carbohydrate and lipid metabolism.
10. **T/F** Humans lack the enzymes to synthesize essential (indispensable) amino acids; thus, they must be obtained from foods.

It is essential for dental professionals to have a basic understanding of biochemistry because it is the foundation for understanding and applying the concepts of nutrition. An overview of the biochemical concepts relevant to nutrition will serve as a useful resource as the learner goes through this textbook. A comprehensive review of chemistry and biochemistry concepts can be found online at Evolve.

What is Biochemistry?

Biochemistry is the study of life at the molecular level. The three major areas of biochemistry are structure, metabolism, and bioinformation. Structure describes the three-dimensional arrangement of atoms in a **molecule**, the smallest particle of a substance that retains all the properties of the substance. Important for life, the structure of a biomolecule determines its function. A **biomolecule** is any molecule that is produced by a living cell or organism, which would include carbohydrates, proteins, nucleic acids, and lipids, as well as other organic compounds found in living organisms. In contrast, a nutrient is a substance required by the body that must be supplied by an outside source, which is usually food. **Metabolism** involves the production and use of energy. In metabolism, energy can be extracted from dietary carbohydrates, proteins, and lipids and used to create the biomolecules required for life. This highly regulated system ensures that energy is not wasted. **Bioinformation** involves the transfer of biological information from deoxyribonucleic acid (DNA) to ribonucleic acid (RNA) to protein. The blueprint for life is stored in DNA, and the resulting proteins carry out all the processes required for life.

Fundamentals of Biochemistry

Atoms in a compound are held together by two types of **chemical bonds**. An **ionic bond** forms between a positively charged metal ion and a negatively charged nonmetal ion. **Hydroxyapatite** in tooth enamel is composed of ionic bonds between calcium ions (Ca^{2+}), phosphate ions (PO_4^{3-}), and hydroxide ions (OH^-). A **covalent bond** forms when electrons are equally shared between two nonmetals. Nitrous oxide, commonly known as laughing gas, is a molecule containing covalent bonds between nitrogen (N) and oxygen (O) atoms. Ultimately, the biomolecules responsible for life are based on the nonmetal carbon (C) because of carbon's ability to form stable covalent bonds to itself and many other atoms, forming long chains and rings. More than 25 different elements—such as hydrogen (H), sulfur (S), and phosphorus (P)—are found in biomolecules, providing for great variety in chemical structure, properties, and reactivity in biological systems. One way to organize this variety in chemical structure is the classification of molecules into functional groups. A **functional group** is a group of atoms that gives a family of molecules its characteristic chemical and physical properties. Molecules that have related functional groups have similar properties. Fig. 2.1 defines and exemplifies a few functional groups found in biochemistry.

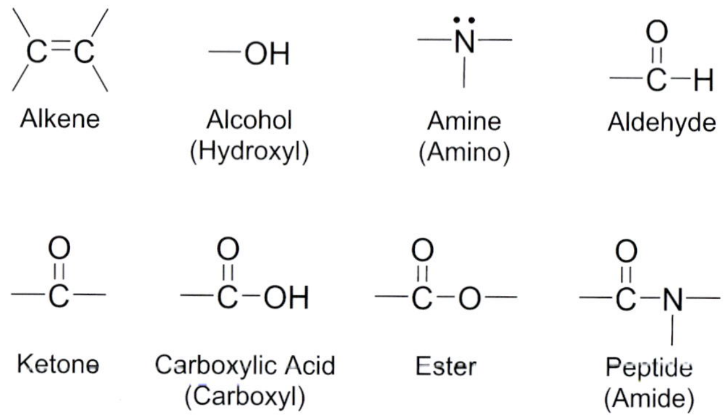

• **Figure 2.1** Common functional groups in biochemistry.

Functional groups can be converted into other functional groups via chemical reactions, such as oxidation–reduction, condensation, and hydrolysis. **Oxidation–reduction reactions** are important in metabolism as biomolecules are degraded or synthesized. **Oxidation** can be defined as a loss of electrons, an increase in charge, a gain of O atoms, or a loss of H atoms. **Reduction** can be defined as a gain of electrons, a decrease in charge, a loss of O atoms, or a gain of H atoms. In metabolism, energy is extracted from glucose ($C_6H_{12}O_6$) by completely oxidizing it to carbon dioxide (CO_2). Condensation and hydrolysis reactions are important in digestion and metabolism. In general, a **condensation reaction** creates a new molecule by forming a bond between two smaller molecules, while a **hydrolysis reaction** breaks a larger molecule into two smaller molecules. When carbohydrates, proteins, and lipids are digested, these biomolecules are hydrolyzed into smaller building blocks for absorption in the digestive system.

Principle Biomolecules in Nutrition

As shown in Table 2.1, the four major classes of biomolecules are carbohydrates, proteins, nucleic acids, and lipids. These biomolecules are characterized by the type of polymer and monomer they contain and by their general function. A **polymer** is a large molecule containing numerous repeating units called monomers. A **monomer** is the smallest repeating unit present in a polymer.

TABLE 2.1 The Four Major Classes of Biomolecules

Polymer	Monomer	Function
Carbohydrates (polysaccharides)	Monosaccharides	Energy source, energy storage form, and structure
Proteins	Amino acids	Structure and biocatalysts (enzymes)
Nucleic acids	Nucleotides	Genetic bioinformation transfer and energy
Lipids	fatty acids	Energy source, energy storage form, and biological membranes

$$6\,CO_2 + 6\,H_2O + \mathit{Energy} \underset{\text{degradation}}{\overset{\text{photosynthesis}}{\rightleftharpoons}} C_6H_{12}O_6 + 6\,O_2$$

• **Figure 2.2** The carbon cycle. Plants utilize photosynthesis (use solar energy) to produce glucose ($C_6H_{12}O_6$) and oxygen (from *left* to *right*), while animals utilize respiration to degrade glucose ($C_6H_{12}O_6$) for energy (from *right* to *left*).

Carbohydrate Structure and Function

The biological function of carbohydrates involves energy metabolism and storage. As shown in Fig. 2.2, plants use photosynthesis to make oxygen (O_2) and glucose ($C_6H_{12}O_6$), the carbohydrate from which animals acquire the energy required for life. Via the process of respiration, animals degrade glucose ($C_6H_{12}O_6$) into CO_2 and water (H_2O), and plants use these products for photosynthesis.

Carbohydrates are classified as monosaccharides, disaccharides, and polysaccharides, depending on the number of sugar monomers present (one, two, or many). Monosaccharides are composed of a single monomeric unit with the molecular formula $C_n(H_2O)_n$, where n is 3 to 8. Fig. 2.3 shows the linear structures of the most common monosaccharides. Monosaccharides undergo oxidation–reduction reactions. When a monosaccharide is reduced, the aldehyde functional group changes to a sugar alcohol (e.g., sorbitol).

In aqueous solution, linear monosaccharides spontaneously form cyclic structures. When two monosaccharides combine, a disaccharide is formed. This involves the formation of a glycosidic bond. As shown in Fig. 2.4, two glucose monomers can combine via a condensation reaction to form maltose. Maltose is a disaccharide that results from the degradation of starch and is used in brewing alcoholic beverages. When glucose and fructose combine, the disaccharide sucrose is formed (Fig. 2.5). This disaccharide is table sugar and one of the sweetest carbohydrates. When the two monosaccharides galactose and glucose combine, the disaccharide lactose is formed (see Fig. 2.5). This disaccharide is found in milk and dairy products.

Many monosaccharides combine to form a polysaccharide. As shown in Table 2.2, polysaccharides can be characterized by the monosaccharide monomer present and overall function. One of the most important dietary polysaccharides is starch, the storage form of energy in plants. Starch is composed of two different polysaccharides (α-amylose and amylopectin). Fig. 2.6 shows the linear structure of the polysaccharide α-amylose.

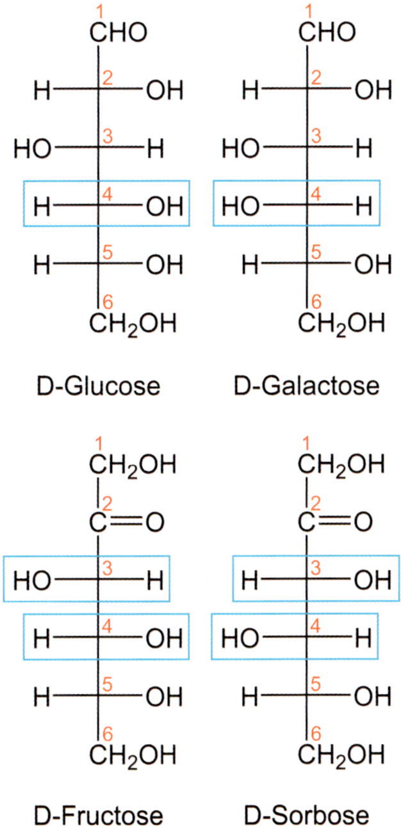

• **Figure 2.3** The linear structures of common monosaccharides. Monosaccharides are classified as aldoses and ketoses. Aldoses contain an aldehyde functional group, while ketoses contain a ketone functional group. D-Glucose ($C_6H_{12}O_6$) is an aldohexose because it contains an aldehyde (represented by CHO at carbon 1) and six carbons. D-Fructose ($C_6H_{12}O_6$) is a ketohexose because it contains a ketone (at carbon 2) and six carbons.

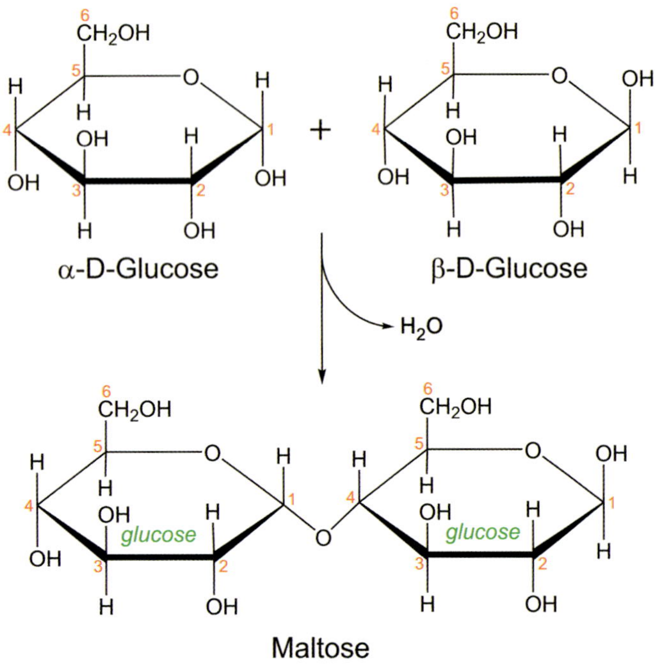

• **Figure 2.4** Formation of the disaccharide maltose from two glucose molecules. Water (H_2O) is released as a product in this condensation reaction.

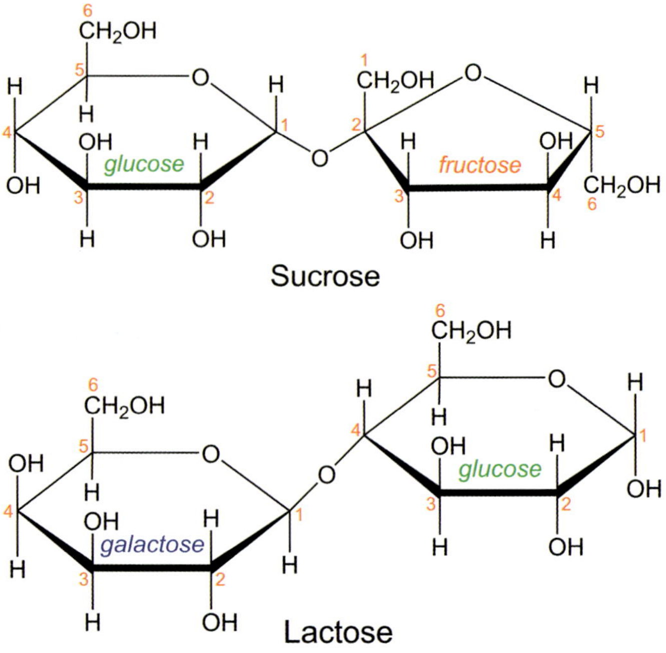

• **Figure 2.5** The structures of the disaccharides sucrose and lactose.

TABLE 2.2 Summary of Common Polysaccharides

Name	Monomer	Biological Function
Amylose (in starch)	Glucose	Nutrient storage (plants)
Amylopectin (in starch)	Glucose	Nutrient storage (plants)
Glycogen	Glucose	Nutrient storage (animals)
Dextran	Glucose	Nutrient storage (yeast and bacteria)
Inulin	Fructose	Nutrient storage (plants)
Cellulose	Glucose	Structure in plants
Pectin	Galacturonic acid	Structural rigidity in plants and gelling agent in yogurt and jelly
Lignin	Coniferyl alcohol	Structural rigidity in plant cell walls

Fig. 2.7 shows the branched structure of the polysaccharide amylopectin. Important for the storage of energy in animals, **glycogen** also is a branched polysaccharide containing glucose monomers. The highly branched structure of glycogen allows its rapid degradation into glucose when energy is needed.

Protein Structure and Function

In an organism, **proteins** are essential for almost every physiologic function, such as providing structure, helping muscles contract, transporting and storing substances, catalyzing reactions, regulating metabolism, and supporting the immune system. Proteins are composed of building blocks or monomer units called **amino acids**. As shown in Fig. 2.8, the general structure of an amino acid consists of an amino group ($–NH_3^+$), a carboxyl group ($–COO^-$), and a **side chain (R group)** that varies from one amino acid to another. The classification of the 20 common amino acids is based on the structure of their side chain. Amino acids polymerize to form long chains called **polypeptides** linked by strong covalent **peptide bonds**. Proteins can consist of as few as 50 to as many as millions of amino acid monomers in one or more polypeptides arranged in a biologically functional way. As shown in Fig. 2.9, a protein will become biologically active when it folds into its distinct compact three-dimensional structure.

Enzymes Catalyze Biochemical Reactions

Enzymes catalyze all biochemical reactions. Enzymes begin the process of digesting dietary proteins (**proteases**), carbohydrates (**amylases**), and lipids (**lipases**). They also execute all the metabolic reactions involving the degradation and biosynthesis of the biomolecules required for life.

As shown in Fig. 2.10, enzymes catalyze reactions by specifically binding a **substrate** and converting it into a product. This chemical transformation takes place in a region of the enzyme called the **active site**. Many enzymes need additional help to complete a specific biochemical reaction. **Coenzymes** are nonprotein organic substances that assist enzymes and are regenerated at the end of a reaction. Many vitamins are converted into these important biologically active coenzymes.

Vitamins or "vital amines" are essential nutrients required in the diet because they cannot be synthesized by the organism itself. Many water-soluble vitamins are **precursors** of coenzymes. As shown in Table 2.3, water-soluble vitamins from foods may need to be converted into a biologically active form (a coenzyme)

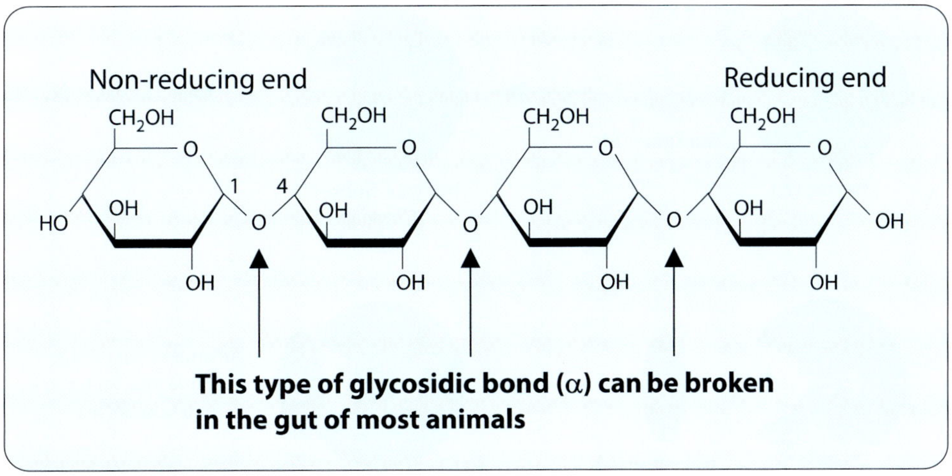

• **Figure 2.6** The linear structure of the polysaccharide α-amylose, a component of starch containing glycosidic linkages that are easily digested. (Reproduced with permission from Batmanian L, Worral S, Ridge J. *Biochemistry for Health Professionals*. Sydney: Elsevier Australia; 2011.)

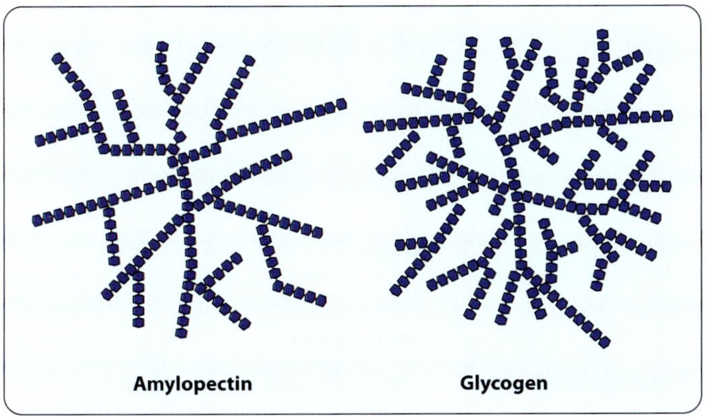

• **Figure 2.7** The branched structures of the polysaccharides amylopectin and glycogen. Amylopectin is a component of starch (the storage form of energy in plants) containing glucose monomers. Glycogen is the storage form of energy in animals containing glucose monomers. (Reproduced with permission from Batmanian L, Worral S, Ridge J. *Biochemistry for Health Professionals*. Sydney: Elsevier Australia; 2011.)

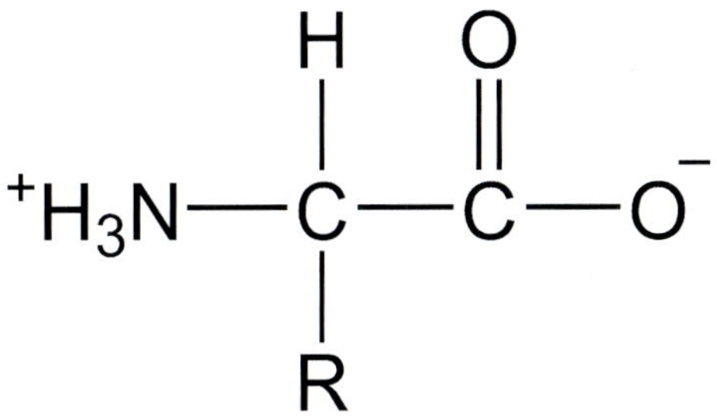

• **Figure 2.8** Structure of an amino acid. At neutral pH, the amino group ($-NH_3^+$) is positively charged, while the carboxyl group ($-COO^-$) is negatively charged.

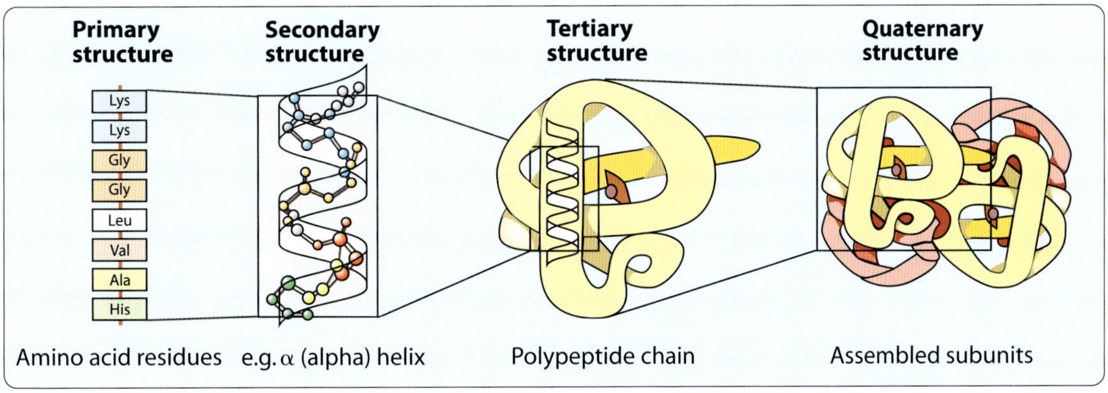

• **Figure 2.9** The four levels of protein structure. The primary (1°) structure is the sequence of amino acids in a protein; it holds the information necessary to form the secondary (2°) structure. The secondary structure is characterized by localized regions of repeating ordered structure that leads to the formation of the compact, biologically active tertiary (3°) structure. The tertiary structure describes the positions of all atoms in the protein or the overall three-dimensional, compactly folded, biologically active structure. The association and organization of two or more protein subunits is the quaternary (4°) structure. (Reproduced with permission from Batmanian L, Worral S, Ridge J. *Biochemistry for Health Professionals*. Sydney: Elsevier Australia; 2011.)

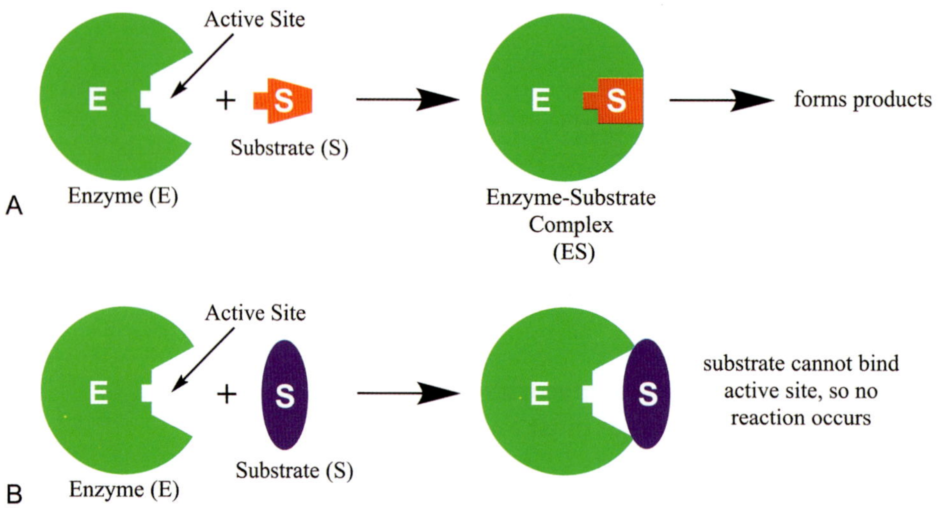

• **Figure 2.10** Enzyme active sites bind substrate and help convert it into product. When substrate binds the active site, an intermediate enzyme–substrate (ES) complex forms and provides the greatest possibility for the reaction to occur and form products. A substrate that neither fits nor induces a fit in the active site cannot undergo reaction by the enzyme. In **A**, both the substrate (S) and the active site of the enzyme (E) are flexible and adjust their shape for optimum binding between the active site and the substrate. In **B**, the substrate (S) does not fit the enzyme (E) active site; thus, a reaction will not occur and product will not form.

TABLE 2.3 Common Vitamins and Coenzymes

Vitamin Type	Coenzyme	Function
Water-Soluble		
Thiamin (vitamin B_1)	Thiamin pyrophosphate (TPP)	Decarboxylation
Riboflavin (vitamin B_2)	Flavin adenine dinucleotide (FAD) and flavin mononucleotide (FMN)	Redox coenzymes (electron transfer)
Niacin (vitamin B_3)	Nicotinamide adenine dinucleotide (NAD^+); nicotinamide adenine dinucleotide phosphate ($NADP^+$)	Redox coenzymes (electron transfer)
Pantothenic acid (vitamin B_5)	Coenzyme A (CoA)	Acetyl group transfer
Pyridoxine (vitamin B_6)	Pyridoxal phosphate (PLP)	Transamination
Cobalamin (vitamin B_{12})	Methylcobalamin	Methyl group transfer
Ascorbic acid (vitamin C)	Ascorbic acid (vitamin C)	Collagen biosynthesis; healing of wounds
Biotin	Biocytin	Carboxylation
Folic Acid	Tetrahydrofolate (THF)	Methyl group transfer
Lipid-Soluble—Biologically Active Form		
Vitamin A	Retinal	Formation of visual pigments
Vitamin D	1,25-Dihydroxycholecalciferol	Absorption of calcium and phosphate, bone development
Vitamin E	α-Tocopherol	Antioxidant; prevents oxidation of vitamin A and unsaturated fatty acids
Vitamin K	Phylloquinone (vitamin K_1) and menaquinone (vitamin K_2)	Synthesis of prothrombin for blood clotting

before binding an enzyme active site. Lipid-soluble or fat-soluble vitamins accumulate in fat deposits and cell membranes in the body. Lipid-soluble vitamins obtained from dietary sources are not involved as coenzymes, but they are converted into a biologically active form.

Nucleic Acid Structure and Function

The biological functions of **nucleic acids** such as DNA and RNA are to store and transfer genetic information. The genetic information in an organism, the **genome**, contains all the information needed for the complete development of a living organism. The

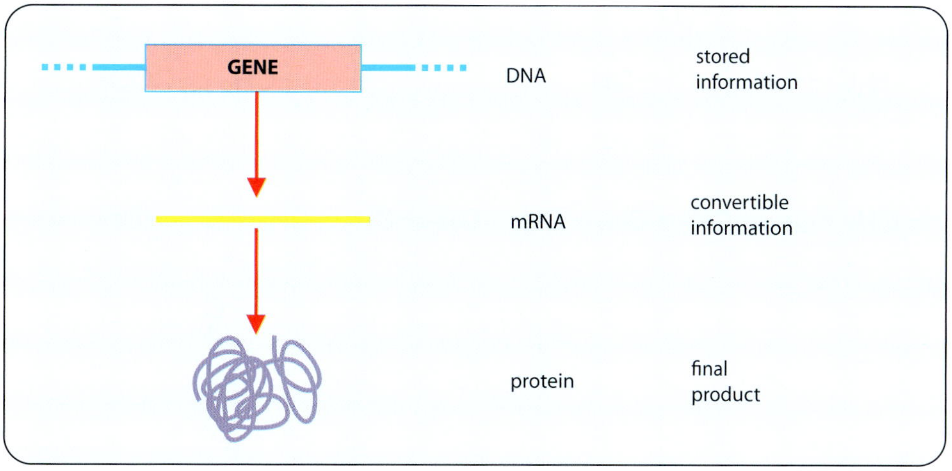

• **Figure 2.11** The central dogma of bioinformation transfer. DNA is composed of genes that are transcribed into messenger RNA (mRNA) and translated into protein. (Reproduced with permission from Batmanian L, Worral S, Ridge J. *Biochemistry for Health Professionals*. Sydney: Elsevier Australia; 2011.)

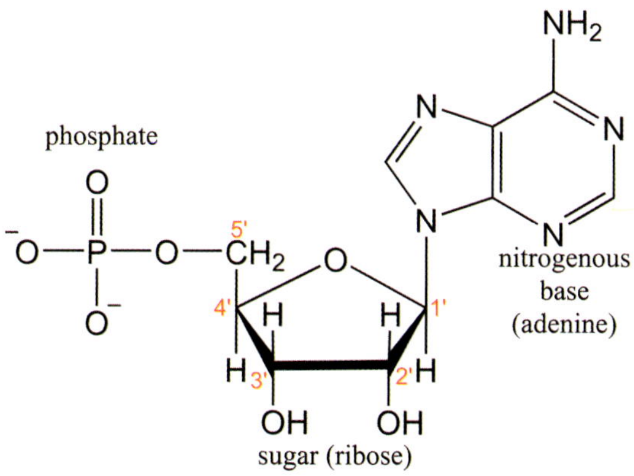

• **Figure 2.12** The structure of the nucleotide adenosine 5′-monophosphate (AMP). AMP consists of the sugar ribose, the nitrogenous base adenine, and a phosphate group.

central dogma shown in Fig. 2.11 describes bioinformation transfer within cells (DNA→RNA→Protein). Messenger RNA carries the message from DNA to the ribosome, the site of protein synthesis. The ribosome is composed of protein and ribosomal RNA. Transfer RNA carries an amino acid to the ribosome for incorporation into the growing polypeptide chain.

Nucleic acids are composed of building blocks called **nucleotides**. As shown in Fig. 2.12, the general structure of a nucleotide consists of sugar attached to a nitrogenous base and phosphate. The sugar is ribose in RNA or deoxyribose in DNA.

Nutrigenomics is an emerging field that studies the interaction of nutrition and the genome. Some **bioactive** molecules found in food can influence how DNA encodes proteins, leading to changes in one's health and wellness. Eventually, personalized diets based on a patient's genetic makeup may help prevent or treat disease (see Health Application 2).

Lipid Structure and Function

Lipids have many different structures and biological functions. They are involved in energy metabolism and storage, serve as structural components of biological membranes, provide insulation and protection, act as **hormones** that regulate the body's major systems, serve as vitamins, and act as detergents in digestion. In contrast to **hydrophilic** ("water-loving") biomolecules, lipids are **hydrophobic** ("water-fearing") compounds that do not readily combine with water.

Fatty acids (FAs) are a structural component present in more complex lipids. FAs are **amphiphilic** ("loving at both ends"), possessing a hydrophilic carboxyl group "head" and hydrophobic **hydrocarbon** chain "tail" containing only carbon and hydrogen atoms. The structure of an FA (e.g., lauric acid which has 12 carbon atoms) can be represented in a number of different ways, but the most common is the skeletal (line) structure, as shown in Fig. 2.13.

FAs can be classified according to the presence or absence of C=C (double) bonds. **Saturated fatty acids**—such as lauric acid, shown in Fig. 2.13—contain only C–C (single) bonds, while **unsaturated fatty acids** are alkenes that contain one or more C=C bonds. As shown in Fig. 2.14, **monounsaturated fatty acids (MUFAs)** such as oleic acid contain just one C=C bond, while **polyunsaturated fatty acids (PUFAs)** such as **linoleic acid** contain more than one C=C bond.

FAs have common names and systematic names, but they also utilize an abbreviated symbol notation that depends on the total number of carbons and C=C bonds present. Table 2.4 summarizes the number of carbon atoms, common name, abbreviated symbol notation, and typical lipid source for many common FAs. In contrast to the delta (Δ) numbering system, the omega (ω) numbering system indicates the position of a C=C bond by numbering the carbon chain from the methyl ($-CH_3$) end. Fig. 2.15 shows how the omega (ω) numbering system is used in the PUFAs linolenic acid and linoleic acid.

In MUFAs and PUFAs, the C=C bond can either be a *cis* isomer or *trans* isomer. As shown in Fig. 2.16, the **cis isomer** of oleic acid has the H atoms on the same side of the C=C bond, so there exists a significant bend, or "kink," in the long hydrocarbon tail. In the **trans isomer** of oleic acid, the H atoms are on opposite sides of the C=C bond and the long hydrocarbon tail remains straight and extended. *Cis* isomers predominate in nature.

The characteristics, properties, and reactivity of an FA can be understood in terms of its structure. One of these properties is

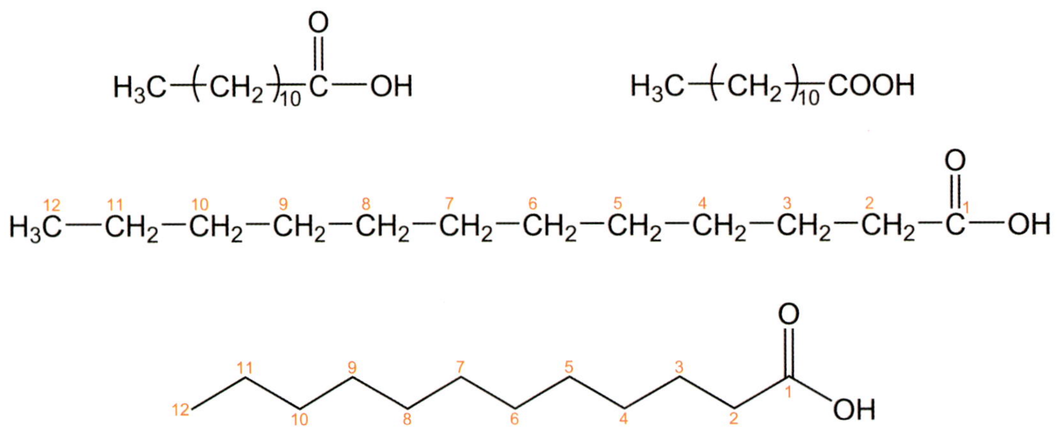

• **Figure 2.13** Four different structural representations of the fatty acid lauric acid. The skeletal (line) structure at the bottom is the most efficient way of representing the numerous carbon atoms in the long hydrocarbon chain.

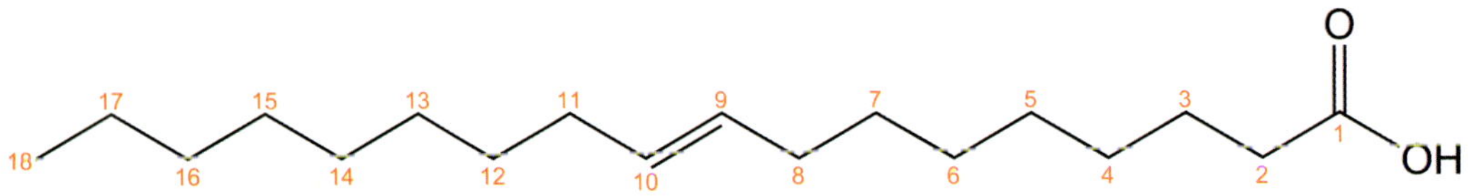

Oleic Acid

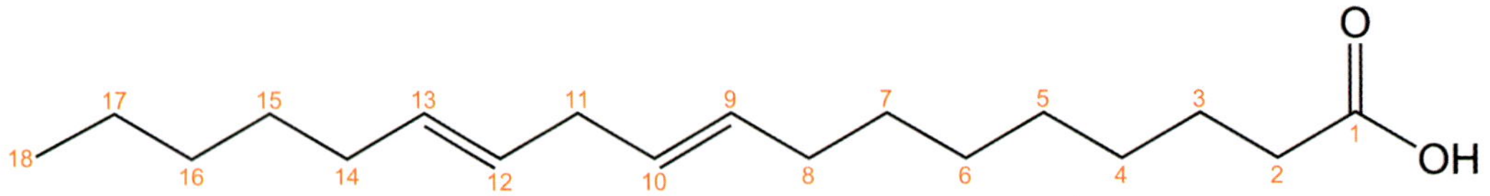

Linoleic Acid

• **Figure 2.14** Structure of unsaturated fatty acids. Oleic acid is a monounsaturated fatty acid (MUFA) with a C=C bond at carbon 9, while linoleic acid is a polyunsaturated fatty acid (PUFA) with C=C bonds at carbon 9 and carbon 12. For oleic acid, the abbreviated symbol notation is $(18:1)^{\Delta 9}$ for which the first number corresponds to the total number of carbons (18), the second number corresponds to the total number of C=C bonds (1) and the superscript corresponds to the delta (Δ) locations of the C=C bonds between carbons 9 and 10 in the long carbon chain numbered starting from the carboxyl (–COOH) end. For linoleic acid, the abbreviated symbol notation is $(18:2)^{\Delta 9,12}$.

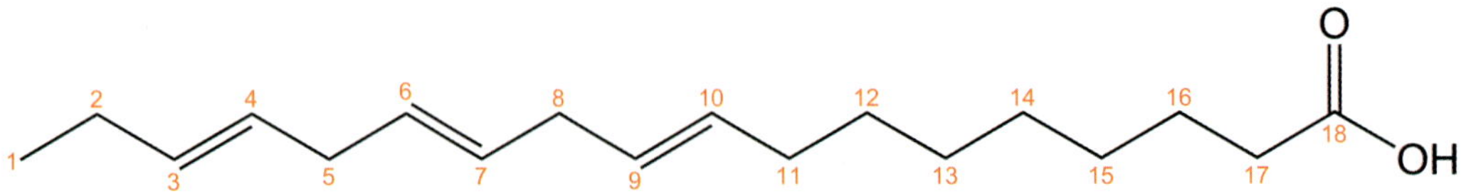

Linolenic Acid (ω-3 Fatty Acid)

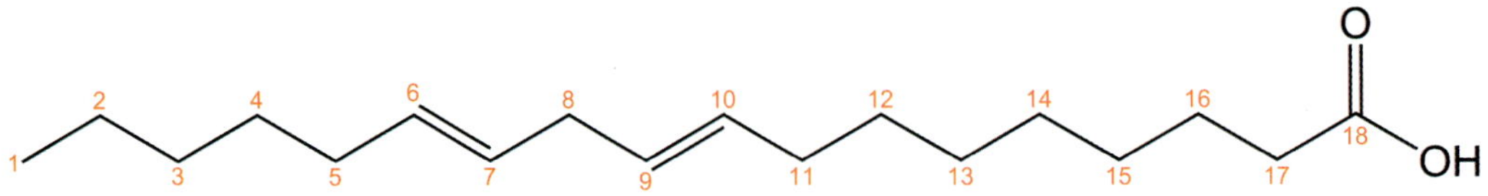

Linoleic Acid (ω-6 Fatty Acid)

• **Figure 2.15** The omega (ω) numbering system for fatty acids. Linolenic acid is an ω-3 polyunsaturated fatty acid, while linoleic acid is an ω-6 polyunsaturated fatty acid.

TABLE 2.4 **Summary of Common Fatty Acids**

Number of Carbon Atoms	Common Name	Abbreviated Symbol Notation	Typical Lipid Source
4	Butyric acid	(4:0)	Butterfat
8	Caprylic acid	(8:0)	Coconut oil
12	Lauric acid	(12:0)	Coconut oil, palm kernel oil
14	Myristic acid	(14:0)	Butterfat, coconut oil
16	Palmitic acid	(16:0)	Palm oil, animal fat
16	Palmitoleic acid	$(16{:}1)^{\Delta 9}$	Some fish oils, beef fat
18	Stearic acid	(18:0)	Cocoa butter, animal fat
18	Oleic acid	$(18{:}1)^{\Delta 9}$	Olive oil, canola oil
18	Linoleic acid	$(18{:}2)^{\Delta 9,12}$	Most vegetable oils; safflower, corn, soybean
18	Linolenic acid	$(18{:}3)^{\Delta 9,12,15}$	Soybean oil, canola oil, walnuts, wheat germ oil
20	Arachidic acid	(20:0)	Peanut oil
20	Arachidonic acid	$(20{:}4)^{\Delta 5,8,11,14}$	Lard, meats
20	Eicosapentaenoic acid (EPA)	$(20{:}5)^{\Delta 5,8,11,14,17}$	Fish oils, shellfish
22	Docosahexaenoic acid (DHA)	$(22{:}6)^{\Delta 4,7,10,13,16,19}$	Fish oils, shellfish

Adapted from Mahan LK, Escott-Stump S, Raymond JL. *Krause's Food and The Nutrition Care Process.* 13th ed. St. Louis: Elsevier/Saunders; 2012.

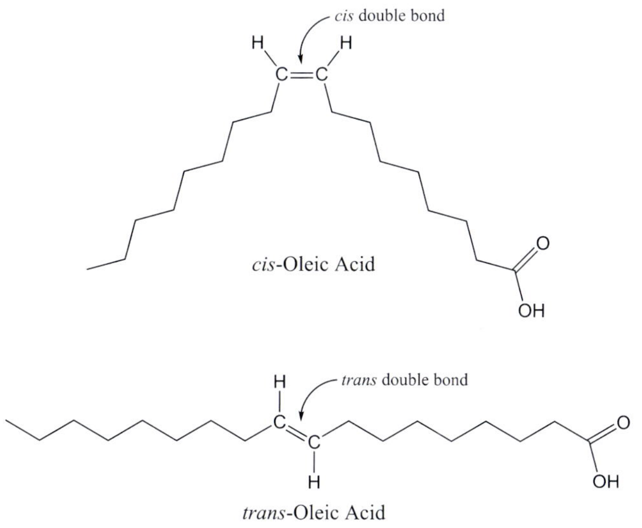

• **Figure 2.16** Structure of *cis-trans* isomers in monounsaturated fatty acids (MUFAs). Oleic acid is an MUFA with a C=C bond at carbon 9.

the **melting point**, the temperature at which a substance changes from a solid to a liquid, or melts. As the number of carbon atoms increases, the melting point of the FA increases because of stronger attractive forces. Moreover, the melting points of saturated FA are higher than unsaturated FAs. Saturated FAs exhibit stronger attractive forces as a result of the compact, tight packing of their long extended hydrocarbon tails, thus they are solids at room temperature. As shown in Fig. 2.16, unsaturated FAs have "kinks" at the *cis* C=C bonds that prevent compact packing, resulting in weaker attractive forces and lower melting points, thus they are liquids (**oils**) at room temperature.

Triglycerides (TGs), also referred to as triacylglycerols, are the storage forms of FAs and considered the metabolic fuel for cells stored in **adipose tissue** or fat. As shown in Fig. 2.17, a TG consists of a 3-carbon glycerol backbone with three FAs attached. The alcohol functional groups of the glycerol backbone react with the carboxylic acid functional groups of three FAs to form the three ester functional groups of a TG. The properties of a TG mirror those of the FAs present. A TG that is solid at room temperature is called a fat, whereas a TG that is liquid at room temperature is called an oil. TGs that are predominantly composed of saturated FAs are solid fats at room temperature, whereas those that are predominantly composed of unsaturated FAs are liquid oils at room temperature.

In TGs, unsaturated FAs that have C=C bonds can be the site of many different types of chemical reactions. A **hydrogenation reaction**, shown in Fig. 2.18, involves the addition of a hydrogen molecule (H_2) to a C=C bond to form a saturated FA with C–C bonds. By controlling the amount of H_2 gas added, it is possible to control how many C=C bonds are converted into C–C bonds, thereby controlling the melting point of the resultant product. Partial hydrogenation of a liquid vegetable oil can be used to create soft semisolid fat products, such as spreadable tub margarines and solid shortening. Partial hydrogenation of vegetable oil results in a small amount of the *cis* C=C bonds being converted into unwanted *trans* C=C bonds. Another common, but unwanted, reaction involving C=C bonds is oxidation. Oxidation of unsaturated fats leads to rancidity; thus, **antioxidants**—such as vitamins C and E, butylated hydroxyanisole, and butylated hydroxytoluene—are added to vegetable oils.

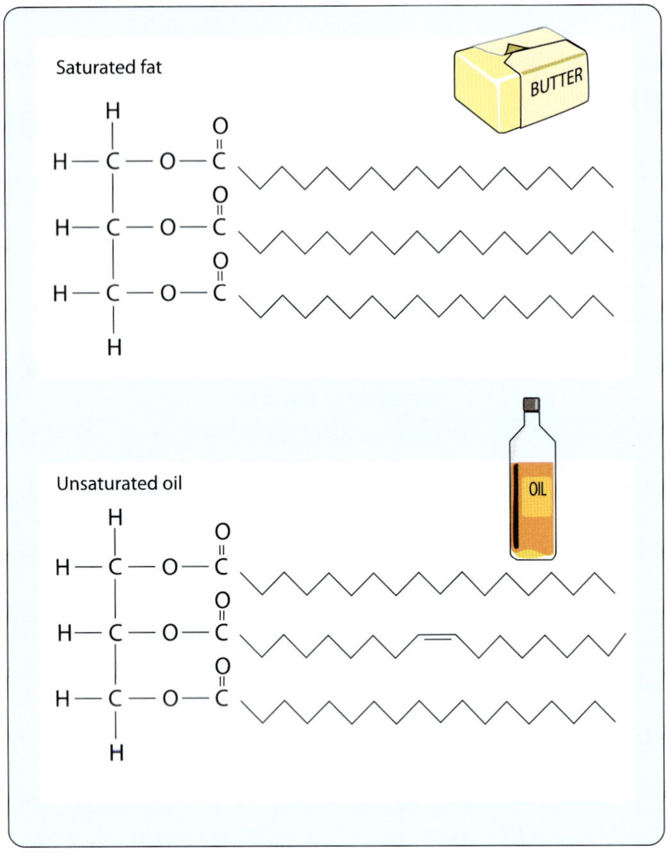

Another class of lipids includes steroids. Steroids are a family of lipids containing a hydrophobic nucleus of four rings fused together. As shown in Fig. 2.19, cholesterol is the most abundant steroid and is an important stabilizing component of biological membranes. Cholesterol is also the precursor of steroid hormones (progesterone, estradiol, and testosterone), bile acids, and lipid-soluble vitamin D.

Lipids must be transported through the bloodstream to be stored, to be used for energy or to make hormones. However, lipids do not readily dissolve in blood. Therefore, they are transported via water-soluble complexes called lipoproteins. As shown in Fig. 2.20, lipoproteins are spherical particles with a hydrophilic surface and a hydrophobic interior that can transport TGs, FAs, and cholesterol in the bloodstream (see Ch. 6 for further discussion).

• **Figure 2.17** Comparison of TGs containing saturated fatty acids (FAs) and unsaturated FAs. The solid fat found in butter is predominantly composed of triglycerides (TGs) containing saturated FAs. The extended hydrocarbon tails of the saturated FAs pack together better, leading to stronger attractive forces. The liquid oil found in vegetable oils is predominantly composed of TGs containing unsaturated FAs. The "kinked" hydrocarbon tails of the unsaturated FAs do not pack well, leading to weaker attractive forces. (Reproduced with permission from Batmanian L, Worral S, Ridge J. *Biochemistry for Health Professionals*. Sydney: Elsevier Australia; 2011.)

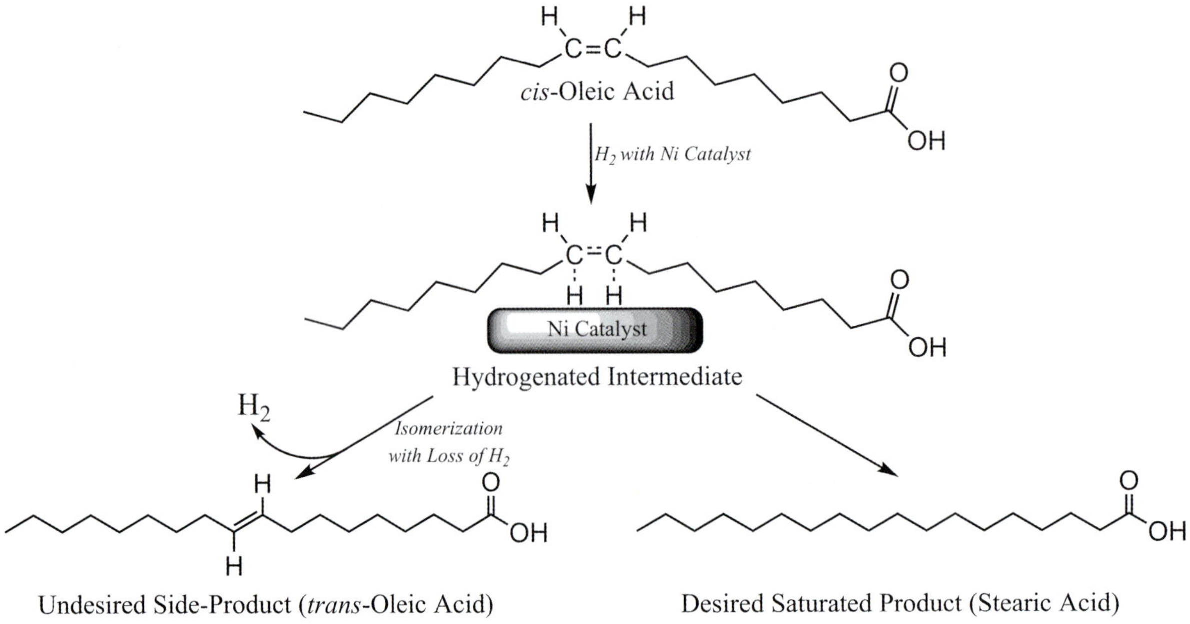

• **Figure 2.18** Hydrogenation of unsaturated fatty acids (FAs) to form saturated FAs. In these hydrogenation reactions, a nickel (Ni) catalyst speeds up the reaction by providing a location for the H atoms to more easily react with the C=C bond. In the hydrogenation process, a slight possibility exists for the two H atoms to react with themselves and not the C=C bond. If this occurs, an undesired *trans* C=C bond results.

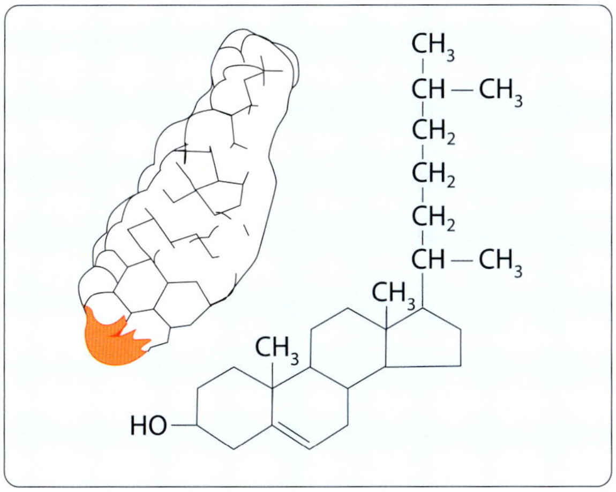

• **Figure 2.19** Structure of cholesterol. Cholesterol consists of a hydrophobic fused ring structure with a single hydrophilic alcohol (–OH) at one end (indicated in red in the globular structure of cholesterol). (Reproduced with permission from Batmanian L, Worral S, Ridge J. *Biochemistry for Health Professionals*. Sydney: Elsevier Australia; 2011.)

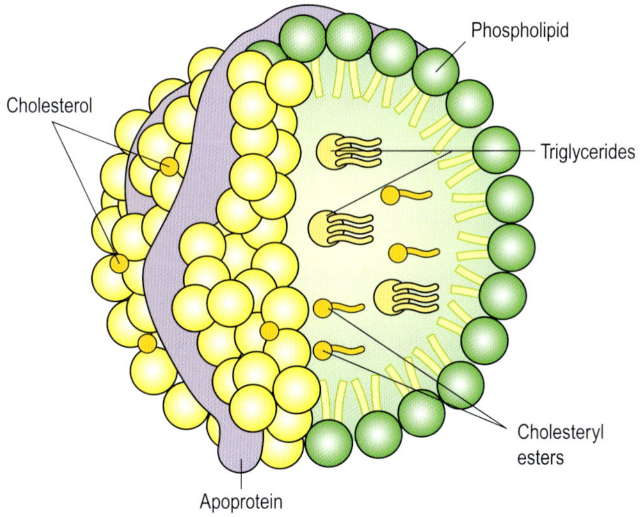

• **Figure 2.20** Structure of a lipoprotein. The hydrophilic surface is composed of protein and membrane phospholipids (or glycerophospholipids) while the hydrophobic core is composed of TGs and cholesterol esters. (From Baynes J, Dominiczak M. *Medical Biochemistry*. 3rd ed. St. Louis, MO: Mosby; 2009.)

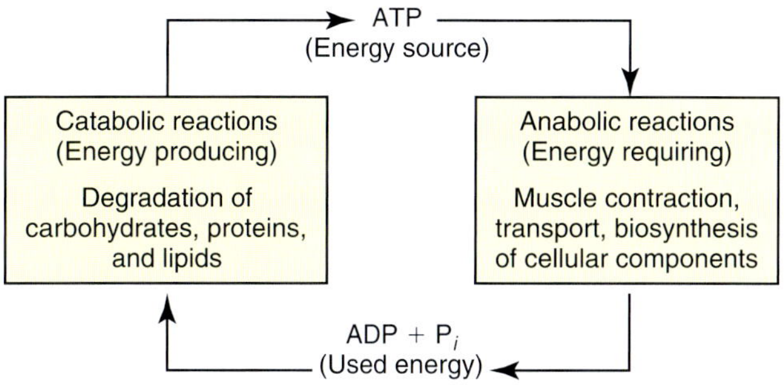

• **Figure 2.21** Energy flow in catabolism and anabolism. Energy is captured in catabolism to synthesize ATP from adenosine diphosphate (ADP) and phosphate (P_i). Energy for this process is extracted from the catabolism of carbohydrates, lipids, and proteins. ATP is used as an energy source in anabolism by being hydrolyzed to ADP and P_i. Muscle contraction, transport, and the biosynthesis of cellular components require energy in the form of ATP.

Summary of Metabolism

Metabolism is how cells acquire, transform, store, and use energy. It is the sum total of all chemical reactions (organized into pathways) in an organism. It also includes the coordination, regulation, and energy requirements of those reactions. The three characteristics of **catabolism** are the production of energy, the degradation of more complex molecules into smaller molecules, and the oxidation of metabolites. In contrast, the three characteristics of **anabolism** are the requirement of energy input, the biosynthesis of more complex biomolecules from simple precursors, and the reduction of metabolites. Fig. 2.21 summarizes the flow of energy in the form of **adenosine 5′-triphosphate (ATP)** within catabolism and anabolism.

Fig. 2.22 summarizes the complex processes involved in catabolism of proteins, carbohydrates, and lipids. Initially, proteins, carbohydrates, and lipids obtained in the diet are hydrolyzed into their simpler building blocks. Dietary protein is broken down into amino acids, dietary carbohydrates into monosaccharides such as glucose, and dietary lipids into glycerol and FAs. Next, amino acids, glucose, and FAs are converted into a common intermediate called acetyl-CoA. Acetyl-CoA then enters the **tricarboxylic acid cycle (TCA cycle)**, the central metabolic pathway also known as the citric acid cycle or Krebs cycle, and is oxidized to CO_2. As nutrients are oxidized in catabolism, electrons are released from the metabolic pathways of glycolysis and the TCA cycle. **Redox coenzymes** capture and transfer these electrons, leading to the conversion of O_2 into H_2O and the synthesis of ATP in the metabolic process called **oxidative phosphorylation**. Two of the redox coenzymes essential for this reaction are derived from the vitamins niacin and riboflavin. Ultimately, the end products of catabolism are CO_2, H_2O, and ammonia (NH_3).

Carbohydrate Metabolism

A major source of energy for the body comes from the degradation of carbohydrates. Complete **aerobic** oxidation of glucose ($C_6H_{12}O_6$) produces CO_2, H_2O, and energy captured as ATP.

$$C_6H_{12}O_6 + 6\ O_2 \rightarrow 6\ CO_2 + 6\ H_2O + 36\ ATP$$

As shown in Fig. 2.22, the digestion of dietary carbohydrates begins in the mouth as amylase enzymes hydrolyze polysaccharides into monosaccharides. These monosaccharides enter the bloodstream and are transported to the tissues that need energy. Glucose oxidation begins with **glycolysis**, entering the TCA cycle with CO_2 being produced. As glucose is oxidized, electrons are transferred by redox coenzymes to the **mitochondria**, the power source of the cell. In oxidative phosphorylation, these electrons ultimately reduce O_2 into H_2O, and the energy is used to synthesize ATP.

Excessive amounts of dietary glucose are stored as the polysaccharide glycogen in muscles and the liver. Later, when blood glucose levels decrease and the body needs energy again, glycogen is converted back into glucose. When glycogen is depleted, **gluconeogenesis** in the liver can convert pyruvate (and other simple

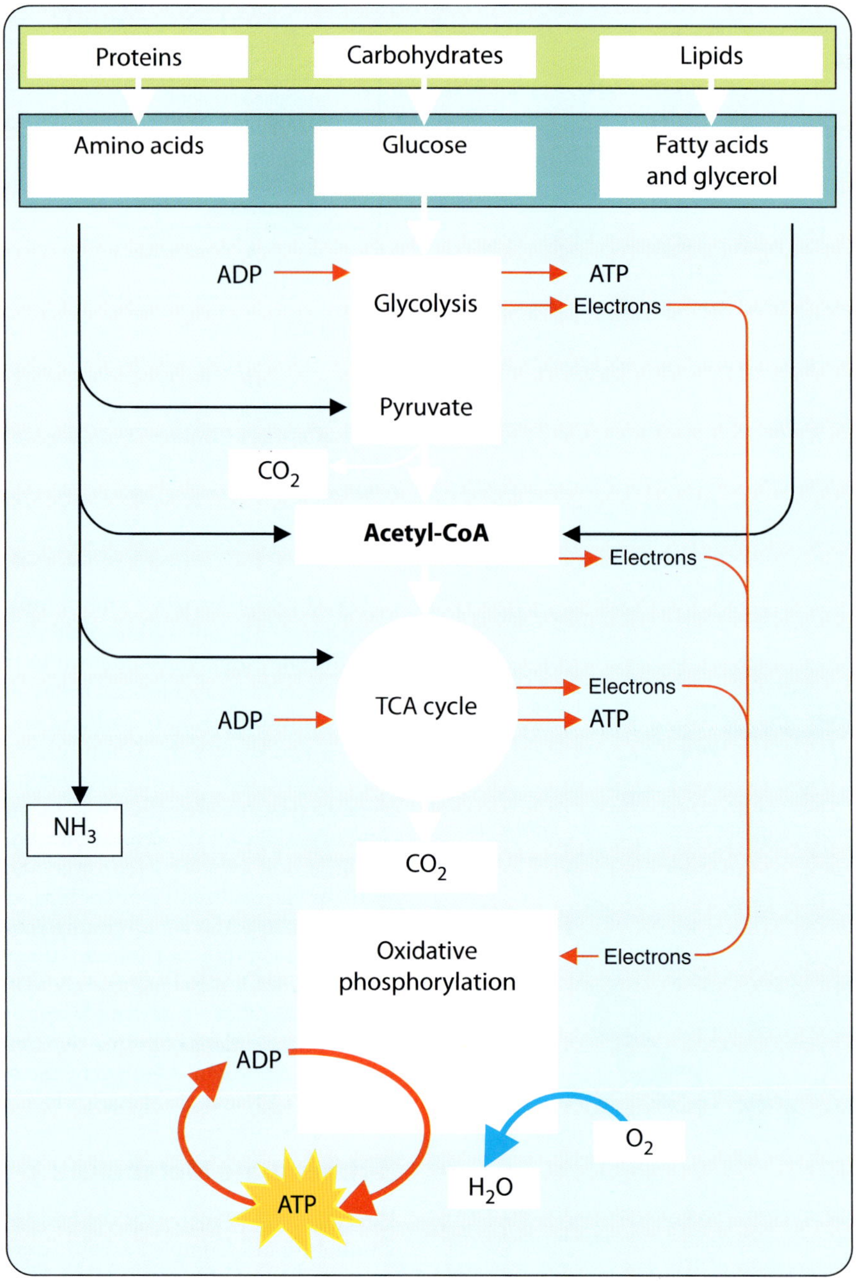

• **Figure 2.22** Summary of catabolism. Proteins, carbohydrates, and lipids are broken down into CO_2, H_2O, and NH_3 with the production of energy. The flow of C, H, O, and N atoms through catabolism are shown in white arrows and black arrows. The flow of energy as ATP and the flow of electrons as redox coenzymes are shown in red arrows. (Adapted from Batmanian L, Worral S, Ridge J. *Biochemistry for Health Professionals*. Sydney: Elsevier Australia; 2011.)

noncarbohydrate precursors like lactate and amino acids) into glucose for energy.

Three hormones regulate carbohydrate metabolism to maintain constant blood glucose levels (Table 2.5). **Insulin** is a signal of the "fed" state and is secreted when blood glucose levels are high. It activates glycolysis and glycogen biosynthesis-metabolic pathways that lower blood glucose levels. **Glucagon** is a signal of the "starved" state and is secreted when blood glucose levels are low. It activates gluconeogenesis and glycogen degradation-metabolic pathways that raise blood glucose levels. **Epinephrine**, the "fight-or-flight" hormone secreted for immediate energy needs, activates glycogen degradation for energy.

Protein Metabolism

The major role of dietary protein is to provide amino acids for the synthesis of new proteins for the body. Amino acids are also a source of N for the synthesis of many biomolecules, such as hormones, heme, and nitrogenous bases. Even though carbohydrates and lipids are the preferred sources of energy, proteins can be an

TABLE 2.5 Hormonal Regulation of Metabolism

Hormone	Increased or Stimulated	Decreased or Inhibited
Insulin	Entry of glucose into cells Glycolysis Glycogen biosynthesis Triglyceride biosynthesis	Gluconeogenesis Triglyceride hydrolysis Glycogen degradation Blood glucose levels
Glucagon	Glycogen degradation (liver) Gluconeogenesis (liver) Blood glucose levels	Glycogen biosynthesis Glycolysis (liver)
Epinephrine	Glycogen degradation (muscle) Glycolysis (muscle) Triglyceride hydrolysis Blood glucose levels	Glycogen biosynthesis

TABLE 2.6 Essential (Indispensable) and Nonessential (Dispensable) Amino Acids

Essential (Indispensable)	Nonessential (Dispensable)
Arginine[a]	Alanine
Histidine[a]	Asparagine
Isoleucine	Aspartic acid
Leucine	Cysteine
Lysine	Glutamic acid
Methionine	Glutamine
Phenylalanine	Glycine
Threonine	Proline
Tryptophan	Serine
Valine	Tyrosine[b]

[a]Arginine and histidine are essential (indispensable) in babies and young children but not adults.
[b]Tyrosine is synthesized from phenylalanine.

energy source of last resort under conditions of fasting and starvation.

As shown in Fig. 2.22, the digestion of proteins begins when enzymes such as proteases hydrolyze proteins into amino acids. When amino acid levels exceed requirements, the amino group is removed, releasing free NH_3. Because high levels of NH_3 are toxic, mammals use the urea cycle to convert excess NH_3 into urea for excretion. Amino acids are further degraded, entering the TCA cycle with CO_2 being produced. The degradation of amino acids for energy can be classified as either ketogenic or glucogenic. **Ketogenic amino acids** degrade into acetyl-CoA and are converted into **ketone bodies**, soluble forms of lipids that can be used as fuel for the body. **Glucogenic amino acids** degrade into pyruvate and other TCA cycle intermediates and can be converted into glucose as a fuel for the body.

When amino acids are synthesized, they utilize common precursors found in metabolic pathways such as glycolysis and the TCA cycle. Unfortunately, humans cannot synthesize all 20 common amino acids because they lack the necessary enzymes; therefore, these **essential amino acids (EAAs) or indispensable amino acids** must be obtained in the diet. The body uses enzymes to synthesize **nonessential amino acids (NEAAs) or dispensable amino acids**. Table 2.6 lists the EAAs and NEAAs.

Lipid Metabolism

Another major source of energy for the body comes from the catabolism of lipids. Because of their structure, lipids can be oxidized to produce more energy than carbohydrates or proteins. Lipids are also **anhydrous** ("without water"); therefore, the energy per gram of lipids (9 kcal/g) is greater than that of carbohydrates (4 kcal/g). Lipids can be stored in adipose tissue in unlimited amounts.

As shown in Fig. 2.22, the digestion of dietary lipids begins when enzymes such as lipase hydrolyze TGs into free FAs and glycerol. FAs are degraded two carbons at a time, producing acetyl-CoA, which enters the TCA cycle and produces CO_2. In the degradation of FAs, electrons are captured by redox coenzymes. Subsequently, ATP is synthesized in the mitochondria via oxidative phosphorylation.

Excess dietary lipids are stored as TGs in adipose tissue. When blood glucose levels are low and glycogen stores are depleted, the utilization of TGs stored in adipose tissue is activated. As shown in Table 2.5, the hormone epinephrine activates TG hydrolysis, yielding free FAs and glycerol for energy.

Under conditions of fasting, starvation, untreated diabetes, and very low-carbohydrate diets, excessive degradation of FAs produces too much acetyl-CoA. Excessive levels of acetyl-CoA and low levels of carbohydrates result in a bottleneck at the TCA cycle. Not all the acetyl-CoA can be degraded; thus, it is converted into ketone bodies and transported via the bloodstream to tissues that need energy, particularly the heart and brain, when blood glucose levels are low.

Student Readiness

1. Explain how the three major areas of biochemistry (structure, metabolism, and bioinformation) are different.
2. For each of the following functional groups, find an example in the textbook of a biomolecule containing that functional group: alkene, alcohol, amine, aldehyde, ketone, carboxylic acid, ester, and peptide (amide).
3. Compare and contrast the functions of carbohydrates, proteins, nucleic acids, and lipids.
4. Differentiate between monosaccharides, disaccharides, and polysaccharides. Give an example of each.
5. Compare and contrast the structure and function of lactose and sucrose.
6. What is the difference between starch and glycogen?
7. What is the difference between enzymes and coenzymes?
8. Explain the structural reason why lipids do not readily dissolve in water.

9. What are the differences between a saturated fatty acid and an unsaturated fatty acid in terms of structure and properties?
10. In your own words, explain the central dogma of bioinformation transfer (DNA→RNA→Protein).
11. Contrast catabolism and anabolism.
12. Draw your own diagram illustrating how proteins, carbohydrates, and lipids are degraded to make energy in metabolism. Indicate on your diagram where ATP is produced. What are the three end products of catabolism containing C, H, O, or N?
13. Compare and contrast the hormones insulin, glucagon, and epinephrine.

HEALTH APPLICATION 2

Nutrigenomics

The word *genome* refers to the entire DNA sequence of an organism. A **gene** is a region of this DNA sequence that contains instructions to produce a specific protein required for life. Human bodies have about 22,000 genes that produce proteins.[1] Mutation of a gene produces an abnormal protein, which can disrupt normal physiologic processes and elicit a **disease**. Virtually every disease has some basis in the individual's genes.

Genomics is the scientific discipline of mapping, sequencing, and analyzing the genome. The Human Genome Project determined the complete DNA sequence of a reference human genome from multiple anonymous people.[2,3] Over the last 15 years, genomics research has lowered the cost to sequence an individual's genome to less than $1000,[4] tailored the drug treatment of a specific cancer based on the genome of the tumor,[5] and developed gene editing techniques that repair mutations in DNA.[6] This information could result in eliminating many diseases in the future.

The emergence of personalized medicine results from slight genetic variations among individuals. Single nucleotide polymorphisms, frequently called SNPs (pronounced "snips"), are the most common type of genetic variation.[7] Each SNP represents a difference in a single nucleotide and basically is an error, or typo, in DNA when it is copied and then passed on from parents to offspring. Most SNPs have no effect on health or development. However, a SNP within a gene can disrupt the function of a protein, increasing the risk of developing disease. Researchers have identified SNPs related to many diseases, such as diabetes, cardiovascular disease (CVD), Parkinson disease, and Crohn disease.[8]

By integrating and applying genomics technology into nutrition research, current studies are focusing on prevention and control of chronic diseases. The scientific study of how foods or their components interact with genes, and how individual genetic variations affect responses to nutrients (and other naturally-occurring compounds), is referred to as **nutrigenomics** or **nutritional genomics**. With further research, nutrigenomics will eventually be able to characterize genetic susceptibility to diet-related chronic diseases and predict molecular responses to nutritional interventions.[8]

Genes have a powerful influence over a person's health but are not the only determinant over destiny because nutrition, emotions, age, lifestyle, and environmental factors also influence health. The scientific study of how these factors regulate gene activity without changing the underlying DNA sequence is referred to as **epigenetics**. Epigenetic changes that switch genes on or off are required for normal development and health; however, they can also be responsible for disease.[9] These factors further complicate research by adding innumerable variables. Of the more than 25,000 bioactive (nonnutrient) food components, many have been identified as epigenetic factors. For example, a tea polyphenol reactivates epigenetically silenced genes in cancer cells.[10] Despite recent advances, there are still many unanswered questions about their modes of interaction and duration of activity.[11]

A nutritionally-related birth defect has almost been cut in half by implementation of a dietary measure.[12] Folate is an example of a nutrient extensively studied because of its impact on DNA synthesis in the human genome. Epigenetic changes and SNPs that affect folate-dependent enzymes increase the risk for developmental conditions, such as neural tube defects.[13] Folate fortification in the food supply was targeted at a distinct group—women of childbearing age who are at genetic risk for having an infant with a neural tube defect—to prevent this birth defect. This public health measure has been successful in lowering the rate of neural tube defects. This is just one example of how a nutritional intervention might be individualized based on knowledge of nutrigenomics.

Nutritional genomics has tremendous potential to not only change the future of personal nutrition recommendations, but also dietary guidelines for the population. Health promotion advice as promoted in the *Dietary Guidelines* is based on population-based data; for example, what is statistically likely to occur with respect to risk factors and disease outcomes.[14] On the other hand, nutrigenomics research focuses on modifying this advice based on an individual's genetics.[15]

The current knowledge base for nutrigenomics is in its infancy. Nutrigenomics will someday provide the basis for personalized dietary recommendations based on the individual's genetic makeup. Chronic disease may be preventable, or delayed, by prescribing a personalized regimen of a specific nutrient based on an analysis of a person's genes. Furthermore, those individuals who are identified as having a higher disease risk through genetic testing may be more motivated to follow dietetic recommendations.[15]

Cutting edge research is exciting and encouraging, but nutrigenomics is not ready for clinical implementation. In its most recent position paper, the Academy of Nutrition and Dietetics states that practical application of nutritional genomics for complex chronic disease is an emerging science and that use of nutrigenetic testing to provide dietary advice is not ready for routine dietetics practice. Most chronic diseases, such as cardiovascular disease, diabetes, and cancer, are multigenetic and multifactorial. Therefore, genetic mutations are only partially predictive of disease. Registered dietitian nutritionists (RDN) who don't have advanced genetic education may not be able to understand, interpret, and communicate complex test results in which the actual risk of developing disease may not be known.[16] Many RDNs are specializing in this field of Integrative and Functional Medical Nutrition Therapy (IFMNT) to earn a certificate to become a Functional Medicine Nutritionist (FMN).

As genetic analysis rapidly develops and becomes more cost effective, potential problems will result in exploitation of the basic hypotheses. Many scientific research studies are essential when determining whether a hypothesis is true, and many of these studies will need to be long-term. A single study claiming to show a specific effect is not considered evidence-based research, ready for implementation in a clinical setting. Unscrupulous individuals will use cutting edge research to make clinical claims that are years or decades premature by basing their work on knowledge that currently does not exist.[17] Currently, clinical claims regarding genomics and nutrition or health conditions are premature and misleading by pretending to be knowledgeable where evidence-based studies do not exist.

Already, websites are claiming to treat autism, multiple sclerosis, Parkinson disease, and other conditions using "nutrigenomics." There is currently no evidence for any nutritional treatment to prevent or cure any of these diseases, and especially not based on genetic types. Nutrigenomics is an exciting legitimate field of research, but it is an area subject to dangerous quackery.

References

1. Pertea M, Salzberg SL. Between a chicken and a grape: estimating the number of human genes. *Genome Biol.* 2010;11(5):206.
2. Lander ES, Linton LM, Birren B, et al. Initial sequencing and analysis of the human genome. *Nature.* 2001;409(6822):860–921.
3. Collins FS, Morgan M, Patrinos A. The Human Genome Project: lessons from large-scale biology. *Science.* 2003;300(5617):286–290.
4. Goodwin S, McPherson JD, McCombie WR. Coming of age: ten years of next-generation sequencing technologies. *Nat Rev Genet.* 2016;17(6):333–351.
5. Zehir A, Benayed R, Shah RH, et al. Mutational landscape of metastatic cancer revealed from prospective clinical sequencing of 10,000 patients. *Nat Med.* 2017;23(6):703–713.
6. Doudna JA, Charpentier E. The new frontier of genome engineering with CRISPR-Cas9. *Science.* 2014;346(6213):1258096.
7. What are single nucleotide polymorphisms (SNPs)?—Genetics Home Reference. U.S. National Library of Medicine. https://ghr.nlm.nih.gov/primer/genomicresearch/snp. Accessed August 24, 2017.
8. Ferguson LR, Caterina RD, Görman U, et al. Guide and position of the International Society of Nutrigenetics/Nutrigenomics on personalised nutrition: Part 1—Fields of precision nutrition. *J Nutrigenet Nutrigenomics.* 2016;9(1):12–27.
9. Simmons D. Epigenetic influence and disease. https://www.nature.com/scitable/topicpage/epigenetic-influences-and-disease-895. Accessed August 24, 2017.
10. Malcomson FC, Mathers JC. Nutrition, epigenetics and health through life. *Nutr Bull.* 2017;42(3):254–265.
11. Yaktine AL, Pool R. *Nutrigenomics and Beyond: Informing the Future: Workshop Summary.* Washington, DC: National Academies Press; 2007.
12. Blom HJ, Shaw GM, Heijer MD, et al. Neural tube defects and folate: case far from closed. *Nat Rev Neurosci.* 2006;7(9):724–731.
13. Liew S-C, Gupta ED. Methylenetetrahydrofolate reductase (MTHFR) C677T polymorphism: epidemiology, metabolism and the associated diseases. *Eur J Med Genet.* 2015;58(1):1–10.
14. U.S. Department of Health and Human Services and U.S. Department of Agriculture. *2015-2020 Dietary Guidelines for Americans.* 8th ed. December 2015. https://health.gov/dietaryguidelines/2015/guidelines/. Accessed August 24, 2017.
15. Kohlmeier M, Caterina RD, Ferguson LR, et al. Guide and position of the International Society of Nutrigenetics/Nutrigenomics on personalized nutrition: Part 2—Ethics, challenges and endeavors of precision nutrition. *J Nutrigenet Nutrigenomics.* 2016;9(1):28–46.
16. Camp KM, Trujillo E. Position of the Academy of Nutrition and Dietetics: Nutritional genomics. *J Acad Nutr Diet.* 2014;114(2):299–312.
17. Novella S. Nutrigenomics—not ready for prime time. Science-based Medicine. Posted January 2, 2013. http://www.sciencebasedmedicine.org/index.php/nutrigenomics-not-ready-for-prime-time/. Accessed August 24, 2017.

EVOLVE RESOURCES

Please visit http://evolve.elsevier.com/Stegeman/nutritional for additional practice and study support tools.

3 The Alimentary Canal: Digestion and Absorption

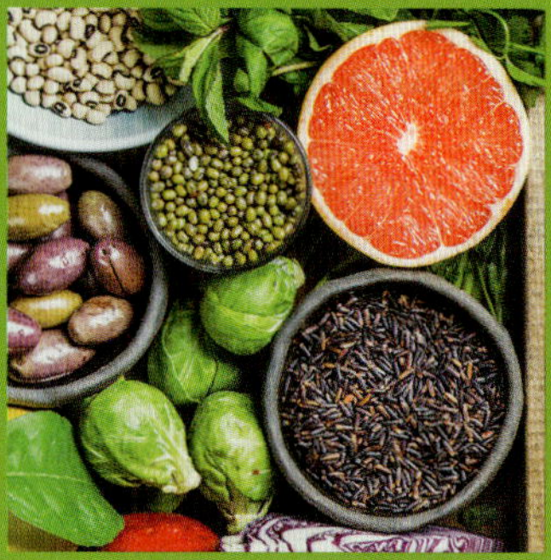

STUDENT LEARNING OUTCOMES

Upon completion of this chapter, the student will be able to achieve the following student learning outcomes:

1. Discuss the physiology of the gastrointestinal tract, including the two basic types of actions on food.
2. Discuss the following related to the oral cavity:
   - Identify oral factors that influence food intake.
   - Explain to patients why saliva flow is important for oral health and overall well-being.
   - Describe the role that teeth play in digestion.
3. Discuss the following related to the esophagus and gastric digestion:
   - Describe how the esophagus works.
   - Discuss gastric digestion, as well as list the two major enzymes found in gastric juice.
4. Discuss the following related to the small intestine:
   - Recognize the nutrients requiring digestion and the absorbable products.
   - Explain the process of osmosis.
   - Discuss with patients how digestion and absorption may affect nutritional status and oral health.
5. Discuss the following related to the large intestine:
   - Describe the function of the large intestine.
   - Discuss the side effects of undigested residue.
   - Define the purpose of microflora.
   - Explain the role of gastrointestinal motility in digestion and absorption.
   - State the purpose of peristalsis.

KEY TERMS

Accessory organs
Active transport
Alimentary canal
Alveolar process
Anorexia
Anosmia
Autoimmune disorder
Bile
Bolus
Cancellous bone
Celiac disease
Chyme
Constipation
Demineralization
Dysgeusia
Emulsification
Gluten
Gustatory
Hypergeusia
Hypogeusia
Iatrogenic
Large intestine
Lower esophageal sphincter
Lymphatic system
Mastication
Masticatory efficiency
Microbiome
Microflora
Microvilli
Nonceliac gluten sensitivity
Olfactory nerves
Osmosis
Pancreatic enzymes
Papillae
Passive diffusion
Pathogenic
Peristalsis
Phantom taste
Portal circulation
Prebiotics
Probiotics
Proteolytic enzymes
Remineralize
Residue
Small intestinal bacterial overgrowth (SIBO)
Small intestine
Sphincter muscles
Symbiotics
Systemic condition
Taste buds
Trabecular bone
Umami
Valves
Wheat allergy
Xerostomia

TEST YOUR NQ

1. **T/F** The alimentary tract is approximately 30 feet long.
2. **T/F** Gurgling sounds in the abdomen are caused by hydrolysis.
3. **T/F** Most absorption occurs in the stomach.
4. **T/F** Fat-soluble nutrients always enter the portal circulation.
5. **T/F** Taste disorders are often the result of problems in smell rather than taste.
6. **T/F** Door-like mechanisms between parts of the intestine are called accessory organs.
7. **T/F** The digestive process begins in the oral cavity.
8. **T/F** Villi are located in the large intestine.
9. **T/F** Missing, decayed, or poorly restored teeth can affect food intake.
10. **T/F** Saliva aids in oral clearance of food.

Foods are composed of large chemical molecules that cannot be used unless they are broken down to an absorbable form. The digestive system is designed to (a) ingest foods; (b) digest or divide complex molecules into simple, soluble materials that can be absorbed; and (c) eliminate unused residues. Only energy-providing macronutrients (carbohydrate, protein, and fat) must be digested for absorption. Most vitamins, minerals, alcohol, and water can be absorbed as eaten.

The gastrointestinal tract can also deliver complex chemical substances, such as oral medications. Medications frequently affect or can be affected by foods, modifying absorption, metabolism, or excretion of either the food or the drug. They may also affect nutritional status by altering taste or salivary flow; these conditions influence the amount and types of foods consumed. The dental hygienist's knowledge of gastrointestinal processes can be an asset in working with patients whose nutritional status and oral health are affected by disturbances in the gastrointestinal tract.

Physiology of the Gastrointestinal Tract

The digestive system includes the alimentary canal and several accessory organs (Fig. 3.1). The alimentary canal is a tubular structure approximately 30 feet long (five times the height of an average man). The **alimentary canal**, extending from the mouth to the anus, comprises all the body parts through which food passes. It includes the oral cavity, pharynx, esophagus, stomach, small intestine, and large intestine. The **small intestine** is comprised of the duodenum, jejunum, and ileum; the **large intestine** includes the cecum, colon, and rectum. **Accessory organs**—the salivary glands, liver, gallbladder, and pancreas—provide secretions essential for digestion and absorption. Digestion involves two basic types of action on food: (1) mechanical and (2) chemical. Mechanical actions include chewing and peristalsis, which break up and mix foods, permitting better blending of foodstuffs with digestive secretions. Chemical actions involve salivary enzymes and digestive juices, reducing foodstuffs to absorbable molecules.

Chemical Action

As discussed in Chapter 2, hydrolysis reactions occur in the digestive tract for nutrients in food to be utilized. The following are basic hydrolysis reactions in food digestion:

$$\text{Protein} + H_2O \rightarrow \text{amino acids}$$

$$\text{Fat} + H_2O \rightarrow \text{fatty acids} + \text{glycerol}$$

$$\text{Carbohydrate} + H_2O \rightarrow \text{monosaccharides}$$

Enzymes produced in the gastrointestinal tract allow these reactions to proceed (Table 3.1).

Mechanical Action

The wall of the gastrointestinal tract is similar from the esophagus to the rectum (Fig. 3.2A). A layer of muscles encircles the tube, allowing the diameter of the tube to expand and contract. Food particles are separated and mixed by the churning action. Outer fibers of the muscular coat (longitudinal muscle) run lengthwise and are responsible for **peristalsis**, involuntary rhythmic waves of contraction traveling the length of the alimentary tract.

Doorlike mechanisms between the digestive segments, called **valves** or **sphincter muscles**, are designed to (a) retain food in each segment until completion of the mechanical actions and digestive juices, (b) allow measured amounts of food to pass into the next segment, and (c) prevent food from "backing up" into the preceding area. Regulation of these valves is complex, involving muscular function and different pressures on each side of the valve.

DENTAL CONSIDERATIONS

- Gurgling sounds, caused by air and fluid in the normal abdomen, indicate peristalsis is occurring.
- If the alimentary tract is not functioning properly and digestion and/or absorption are affected, nutrients may not be absorbed even when ample amounts are consumed. The patient may be prone to nutrient deficiencies, poor healing, or fecal impactions.
- Loss of motility in the stomach and small intestine, observed occasionally in diabetes mellitus, results in impaired gastric and intestinal emptying. This allows excessive growth of bacteria, which may injure the surface of the intestine, cause diarrhea, and interfere with nutrient absorption. Patients who are immobile (because of injury, trauma, or debilitating illness) or patients with uncontrolled diabetes are more prone to these disorders.
- Food–drug interactions have the potential to cause nutritional problems or erratic drug responses. Knowledge of common drugs (including over-the-counter medications, herbals, and supplements) and understanding how they interact with food is important. For example, consuming milk or milk products while taking tetracycline decreases the amount of tetracycline and calcium absorbed.

NUTRITIONAL DIRECTIONS

- Taking over-the-counter enzyme tablets may not be beneficial because enzymes are digested before they can be absorbed. Prescription pancreatic enzymes have a special enteric coating preventing the enzyme from exposure to gastric juices. Lactase, a nonprescription enzyme, is effective for lactose-intolerant individuals because it is either added to or taken with lactose-containing foods, allowing conversion of lactose into two monosaccharides before gastric juices can affect the enzyme (see *Health Application 4: Lactose Intolerance* in Chapter 4).
- Patients reporting gastrointestinal problems should be assessed for adequate nutrient intake using *MyPlate* or the *Dietary Guidelines*. If intake is inadequate, the patient should be referred to the patient's primary care provider or a registered dietitian nutritionist (RDN).

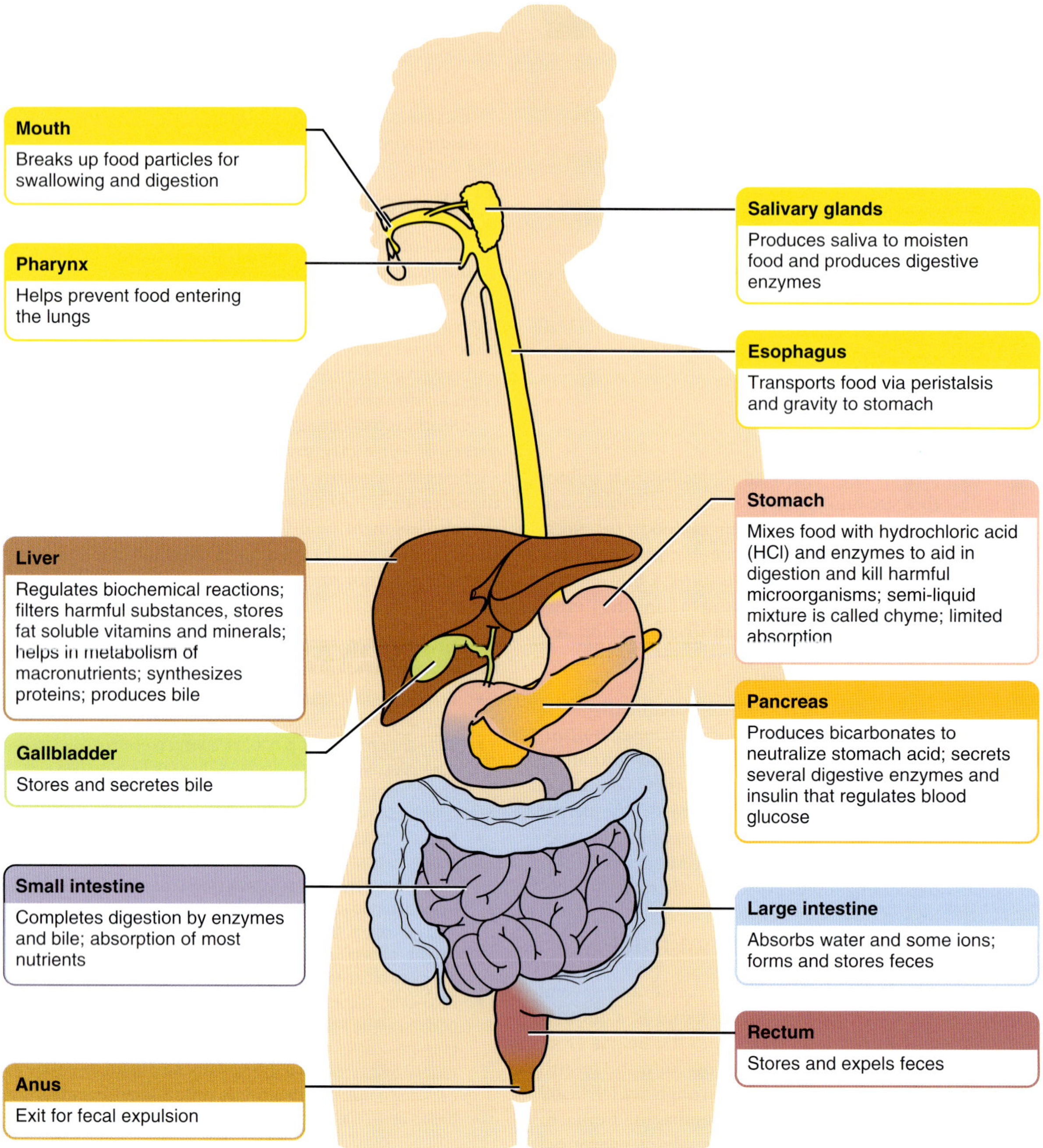
Mouth
Breaks up food particles for swallowing and digestion
Pharynx
Helps prevent food entering the lungs
Liver
Regulates biochemical reactions; filters harmful substances, stores fat soluble vitamins and minerals; helps in metabolism of macronutrients; synthesizes proteins; produces bile
Gallbladder
Stores and secretes bile
Small intestine
Completes digestion by enzymes and bile; absorption of most nutrients
Anus
Exit for fecal expulsion
Salivary glands
Produces saliva to moisten food and produces digestive enzymes
Esophagus
Transports food via peristalsis and gravity to stomach
Stomach
Mixes food with hydrochloric acid (HCl) and enzymes to aid in digestion and kill harmful microorganisms; semi-liquid mixture is called chyme; limited absorption
Pancreas
Produces bicarbonates to neutralize stomach acid; secrets several digestive enzymes and insulin that regulates blood glucose
Large intestine
Absorbs water and some ions; forms and stores feces
Rectum
Stores and expels feces

• **Figure 3.1** Summary of digestive organ functions. *HCl,* hydrochloric acid.

Oral Cavity

Taste and Smell

Generally, food choices are influenced by three sensory perceptions: sight, smell, and taste. **Gustatory** (taste) sensations evoke pronounced feelings of pleasure or aversion; in the United States, taste is the primary determinant of food choices. The presentation of food, its color and aroma, may be the basis for acceptance or rejection. Food flavors are derived from characteristics of substances ingested, including taste, aroma, texture, temperature, and irritating properties. Approximately 75% of flavor is derived from odors. Taste and smell are essential for maintaining sufficient intake to meet physiologic needs.

The mouth, or oral cavity, plays an important role in the digestive system. It is the "port of entry" where receptors for sense of taste, or **taste buds**, are located. A taste bud consists of approximately 50 to 150 cells embedded in the surrounding epithelium, termed **papillae** (Fig. 3.3). Taste papillae appear on the tongue as little red dots, or raised bumps, most numerous on the dorsal epithelium. However, they are also located throughout the mouth—on the palate, epiglottis, and even in the proximal esophagus. These cells replace themselves continually, but they can be affected by disease, drugs, nutritional status, radiation, and age. Despite the well-recognized tongue map (Fig. 3.3) with sections cordoned off for different taste receptors, the receptors that capture these tastes are actually distributed all over the tongue. Different parts of the

TABLE 3.1 Digestive Functions of Saliva

Saliva Component	Classification	Function
Mucous (mucin)	Glycoprotein	Lubricates food for easier passage and protects the lining of the gastrointestinal tract
Ptyalin (salivary amylase)	Enzyme	Initiates hydrolysis of complex carbohydrates to simple sugars
Salivary lipase	Enzyme	Initiates hydrolysis of lipids
Lysozyme (antibody)	Enzyme	Breaks down cell walls of some ingested bacteria

tongue, soft palate, and throat have a lower threshold for perceiving specific tastes but these differences are rather minute. As food is chewed, gustatory receptors come into contact with chemicals dissolved in saliva.

Nerve cells carry messages to the brain, which interprets flavors as sweet, sour, salty, bitter, or **umami** (flavorful, pleasant taste). Umami is detected in foods containing L-glutamine present in amino acids and proteins (specifically soy sauce, meat extracts, aging cheese, bacon, and monosodium glutamate). These five basic tastes reflect specific constituents of food. Genetically related differences affect food preferences, influencing what foods are ingested. Many taste buds degenerate in older adults, causing a decrease in taste sensitivity.

Food stimulates taste buds, and aromas stimulate **olfactory nerves**, receptors for smell. In contrast to the five basic tastes, an almost unlimited number of unique odors can be detected. No tactile sensation indicates the origin of odor sensations. Food-related aromas may be confused with taste sensations, and taste disorders often result from problems in smell rather than taste. Increasing age affects a patient's ability to smell food more than a patient's taste acuity, frequently expressed by the statement, "food just doesn't taste good." Exactly how and why taste preferences shift remains unclear, but preferences are known to change significantly with aging.

Loss of smell, or **anosmia**, results in limited capacity to detect flavor of food and beverages. Ability to smell food being prepared and eaten influences food selection. Smell is also a protective mechanism; odors are used to help determine whether foods are harmful or spoiled. Upper respiratory infections, nasal or sinus problems, neurologic disorders, endocrine abnormalities, aging, or head trauma may cause anosmia. A common cold often impairs a person's sense of smell, causing loss of appetite and limiting the ability to "taste" and enjoy food. The rate of the continuous renewal process undergone by olfactory receptor cells is depressed in malnutrition and by some antibiotics. Some of these disorders are self-limited; however, chemosensory losses from chemotherapy, upper respiratory infection, and aging may be irreversible.

Dysgeusia is persistent, abnormal distortion of taste, including sweet, sour, bitter, salty, or metallic tastes. Dysgeusia without identifiable taste stimuli is called **phantom taste**. Dysgeusia may be caused by a previous viral upper respiratory infection, head trauma, a neurologic or psychiatric disorder, a **systemic condition** (a disease or disorder that affects the whole body), **xerostomia** (dry mouth from inadequate salivary secretion), a severe nutritional deficiency, an invasive dental procedure resulting in nerve damage, an oral bacterial or fungal infection, or burning mouth syndrome, or it may have an iatrogenic causation. **Iatrogenic** refers to an adverse condition resulting from medical treatment, for example, medications, irradiation, and surgery. These conditions may also cause **hypogeusia** or loss of taste, and **hypergeusia** or heightened taste acuity. Mouth breathing may also cause dysgeusia. The dental hygienist is frequently the first health care provider to detect a patient's taste disorder. Hyperkeratinization of the epithelium causing blockage of taste buds and affecting dietary intake may be observed during an oral examination.

Gustatory and olfactory disorders, whether caused by disease or drugs, are not mere inconveniences or neurotic symptoms. They affect food choices and dietary habits. **Anorexia**, lack or loss of appetite resulting in the inability to eat, may occur when medications cause loss of taste acuity. Taste stimulants affect salivary and pancreatic secretions, gastric contractions, and intestinal motility. Therefore, gustatory disorders can also affect digestion.

Because gustatory and olfactory disorders can result in deterioration of a patient's general condition or nutritional status, these abnormalities must always be considered in dental and nutritional care. Potentially adverse compensatory habits may develop (e.g., decreased sweet or salty perceptions may result in excessive usage of sweets or salts). These compensatory habits may be potentially harmful, especially for patients with diabetes or hypertension. Also, additional sugar can increase the risk of weight gain and dental caries. Persistent taste distortions can lead to inadequate caloric intake, resulting in unintentional weight loss or malnutrition.

Saliva

Adequate saliva flow is essential for oral health, which includes maintenance of soft tissues in the oral cavity and taste buds. Saliva, secreted by salivary glands, is essential in taste sensations, functioning to (a) lubricate oral tissues for chewing, swallowing, and digestion; (b) remove debris and microorganisms; (c) provide antibacterial action; (d) neutralize, dilute, and buffer bacterial acids; (e) **remineralize** (restoration or renewal of calcium, phosphates, and other minerals to areas damaged by incipient caries, abrasion, or erosion); (f) prevent plaque accumulation; (g) facilitate taste; and (h) promote ease of speech. An average of 1 to 2 mL/min of this complex fluid helps maintain integrity of teeth against physical, chemical, and microbial insults.

Saliva is supersaturated with calcium phosphates that allow demineralized areas of hydroxyapatite in enamel to be remineralized. **Demineralization** occurs when calcium, phosphate, and other minerals are lost from tooth enamel, causing the enamel to dissolve. This occurs because acids produced by fermentable carbohydrates combine with acidogenic bacteria (see Chapter 18); it is not caused by insufficient calcium. Genetic variations of saliva, especially amylase, affect food preferences and intake by influencing oral sensory properties of food.

Acidic, sour, bitter, and umami tastes stimulate salivary flow. Saliva production is also stimulated by consumption of tasty foods and gum chewing. An increase in oral clearance rate decreases risk of caries formation (see Chapter 18). Saliva moistens food particles to more easily manipulate and prepare them for swallowing.

Some chemical action or hydrolysis of nutrients begins in the mouth. Table 3.1 shows the functions of different constituents in saliva. Because food is normally in the mouth briefly, ptyalin, or salivary amylase, initiates starch digestion. If a carbohydrate food,

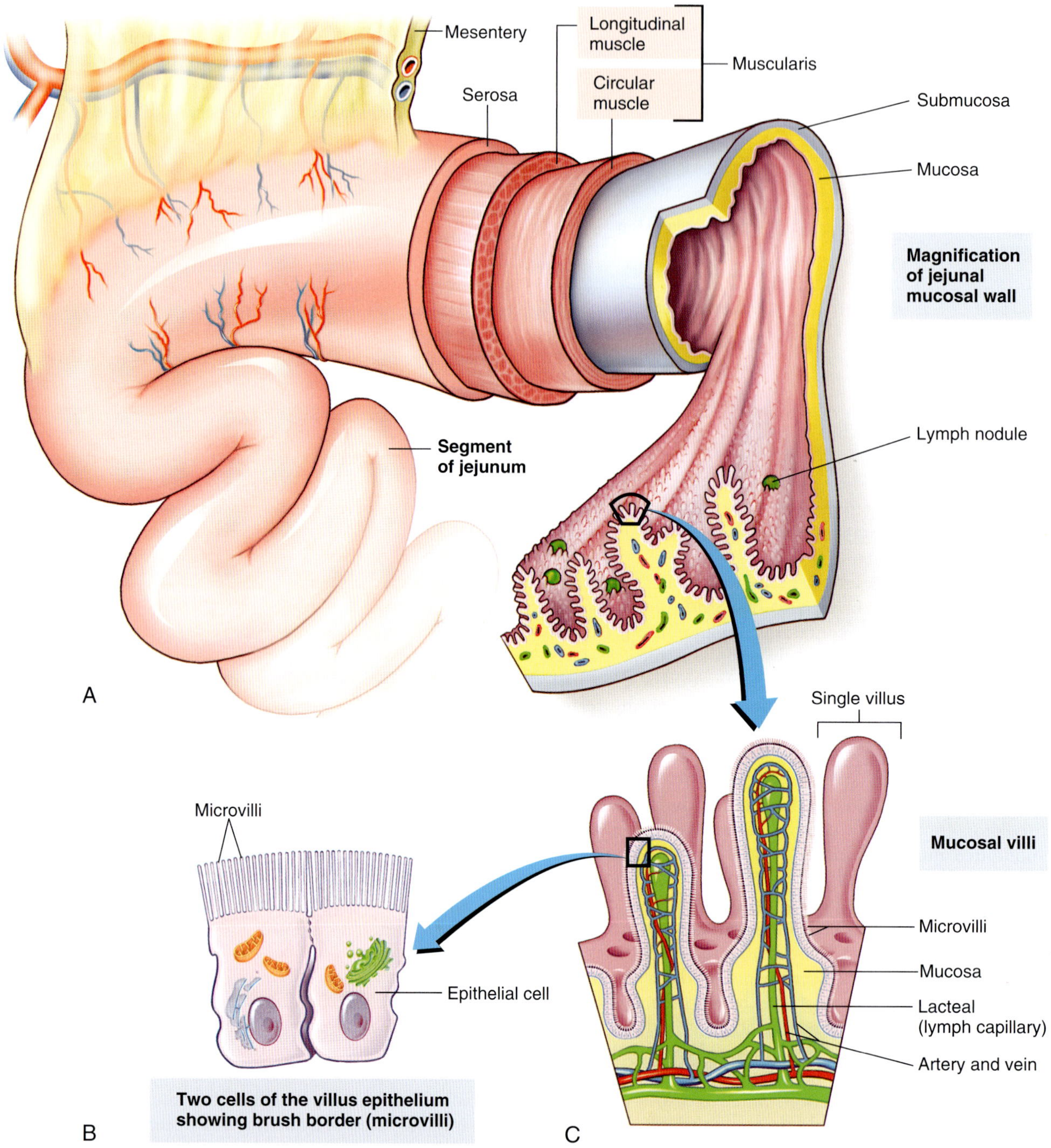

• **Figure 3.2** Wall of the small intestine. (A) Layers composing the intestinal wall. (B) The villi covering the mucosa that absorb nutrients. (C) Further enlargement shows the brush border or microvilli enzymes that are available to hydrolyze nutrients further for absorption. (Reproduced with permission from Standring S. *Gray's Anatomy: The Anatomical Basis of Clinical Practice*, 40th ed. London: Churchill Livingstone; 2009.)

such as a cracker, is chewed and held in the mouth for a few seconds, it will begin to taste sweet, indicating hydrolysis of starch to dextrin and maltose.

Dry mouth from inadequate salivary flow, also called xerostomia, leads to diminished gustatory function (see Chapter 20 for additional details). Xerostomia may result in frequent oral ulcerations, increased sensitivity of the tongue to spices and flavors, and increased risk of dental caries. Many drugs, including diuretics, cause xerostomia. Diuretics, prescribed to help the body eliminate fluids, also cause a decrease in salivary flow. Increasing fluid intake to 8 to 10 cups daily is important to compensate for these losses.

Teeth

Teeth play a major role in digestion by crushing and grinding food into smaller pieces, a process known as **mastication**. In contrast to

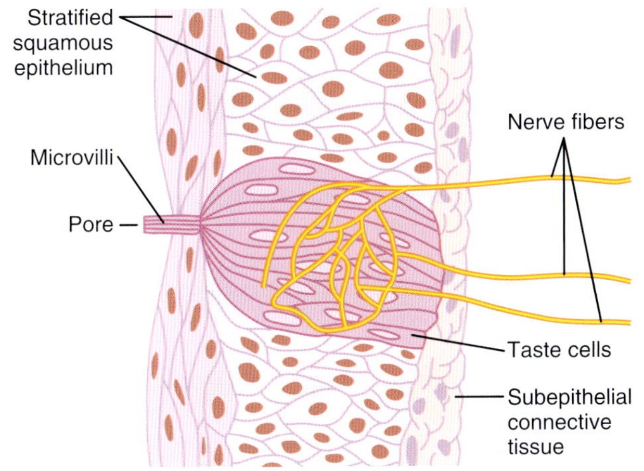

• **Figure 3.3** Taste bud. (Reproduced with permission from Hall JE, Guyton AC. *Guyton and Hall Textbook of Medical Physiology.* Philadelphia, PA: Elsevier; 2016:686.)

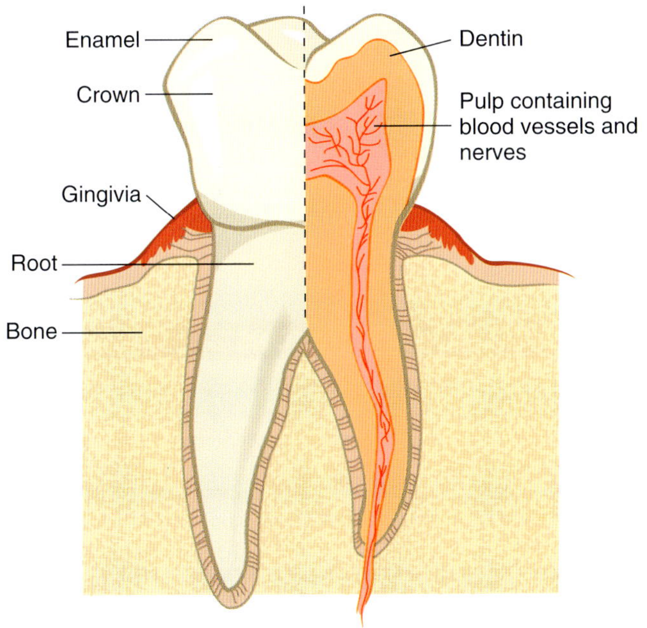

• **Figure 3.4** Diagram of a tooth.

bone, neither tooth enamel nor dentin can be repaired or replaced in significant amounts by natural processes. Only small amounts of enamel and dentin are repaired or replaced through enamel remineralization and through secondary dentin deposition around the pulp chamber of the tooth (Fig. 3.4). Mineral deposition and resorption affect the bone that supports the dentition. This supporting bone, known as alveolar bone, is primarily **trabecular bone** (bony spikes forming a meshwork of spaces) and **cancellous bone** (bone within the spaces created by the network of trabecular bone, which appears spongy and contains bone marrow in small hollows). Negative calcium balance increases susceptibility to resorption and bone loss in the **alveolar process** (comprised of the maxillary and mandibular crest and serves as the bony investment for teeth). The maxilla and mandible to some extent depend on the presence of teeth and occlusal forces associated with chewing to prevent calcium resorption. Chewing firm foods helps maintain proper balance between alveolar bone resorption and new bone formation. Teeth and supporting bone structures are affected by adequate nutrient intake, digestive function, and hormonal balance.

Mastication reduces food particle size. Inability to masticate food adequately may result in larger chunks of food being swallowed. These larger pieces increase potential for obstruction in the airway. Food asphyxiation, which may result in death, may occur in individuals with defective, incomplete, or poorly fitting dentures. Loss of even one permanent molar may decrease **masticatory efficiency** or how well a patient prepares food for swallowing. Even after patients become fully adjusted to well-fitted dentures, masticatory efficiency is less than with their natural teeth.

Digestion of food is facilitated by increasing its surface area. Whether or not particle size affects digestibility is uncertain. However, when elderly patients have digestive problems, masticatory efficiency is usually a factor. Frequently, when masticatory efficiency declines, people either choose foods that require less chewing or use techniques to soften foods, for example, stewing meats, steaming vegetables, or dunking cookies or toast in fluids. In many circumstances, hypersensitive, poorly restored, decayed, abscessed, or periodontally involved teeth affect food choices and limit the variety of foods chosen.

Esophagus

The swallowing reflex moves a **bolus**, or the swallowed mass of food, into the esophagus and is transported to the stomach by peristalsis and gravity. The esophagus is a continuous tube approximately 10 inches (25–30 cm) long connecting the pharynx with the stomach. It penetrates the diaphragm through an opening called the esophageal hiatus. The **lower esophageal sphincter (LES)** comprises a group of very strong circular muscle fibers located just above the stomach. The lower esophageal sphincter relaxes to permit food into the stomach but contracts tightly to prevent regurgitation, or "backwashing," of stomach contents.

DENTAL CONSIDERATIONS

- Assess nutritional status of patients with gustatory or olfactory disorders for changes in dietary habits and appetite that may lead to a dietary deficiency, increased use of spices (especially salt and sugar), food textures, and development of food cravings or dislikes.
- Taste sensations adapt rapidly to dietary changes.
- Patients commonly complain about "taste" or "flavor" of food when olfactory as well as gustatory sensations are impaired.
- Saliva flow helps flush **pathogenic** (harmful) bacteria; enzymes are bactericidal, destroying oral bacteria, including some that cause dental caries. Without salivation, oral tissues may become ulcerated and infected, allowing caries to become rampant.
- Assess patients for possible dietary deficiencies (niacin, vitamins A and B_{12}, zinc, copper, nickel) because these can be related to gustatory abnormalities.
- Loss of umami taste sensation affects quality of life and causes weight loss and health problems, particularly in the older adult.
- Zinc depletion may decrease taste acuity but is not the reason for all cases of hypogeusia. Currently, no tests can accurately assess marginal zinc status in humans.
- Xerostomia may compound nutritional intake problems related to taste loss and make chewing and swallowing more difficult.
- Edentulous patients or patients with ill-fitting dentures should be monitored because quality and quantity of food intake may be compromised.

DENTAL CONSIDERATIONS—cont'd

- Dentures may cause alterations in taste, either caused by altered masticatory efficiency or by the appliance covering the palatal taste buds. Patients with complete dentures exhibit poorer taste and texture tolerance compared to patients with partial dentures or compromised natural dentition.
- Postmenopausal women with low dental bone mass may have decreased levels of total bone mass. If an older woman's (or a man's) mandibular bone density is low, as indicated on radiograph, refer the patient to a health care provider.
- Although food intake often decreases when patients initially receive a set of dentures, after an initial adjustment period, food intake usually increases with improved ability to chew.
- Carefully evaluate anecdotal reports or studies involving limited numbers of patients to support a beneficial effect of vitamins or minerals on dysgeusia.
- Refer patients with persistent gustatory, masticatory, or swallowing difficulties to a health care provider or RDN to determine types of foods needed to obtain adequate nutrients.

NUTRITIONAL DIRECTIONS

- Natural teeth are more efficient for chewing and biting than any prosthesis.
- Tooth loss is not inevitable; most people can maintain their natural dentition throughout life with consistent, preventive dental measures.
- For xerostomia, increase fluid intake with meals to facilitate oral clearance. Nutrient-dense foods in a liquid or semiliquid form are beneficial.
- No proven intervention enhances diminished taste acuity or ameliorates dysgeusia. Encourage experimentation with texture, spiciness, and temperature. Enhance visual presentation of food and serve in a calm, relaxing environment.
- To improve nutrient intake when mastication is less efficient, special cooking techniques (e.g., stewing meats), chewing longer, and choosing soft foods are preferable to pureeing foods. For example, cream-style corn can replace corn on the cob, and stewed apples can replace raw apples.
- Particularly for new denture wearers, herbs and spices and contrasting food flavor combinations (e.g., sweet and sour) can enhance taste perception.
- New denture wearers may slow the rate of alveolar resorption by taking calcium and vitamin D supplements. Refer the patient to a health care provider or RDN for a nutritional assessment.

Gastric Digestion

A bolus entering the stomach is mixed with gastric secretions by peristaltic contractions, producing **chyme**, a semifluid material produced by gastric juices on ingested food. Gastric secretions include mucus, hydrochloric acid, enzymes, and a component called intrinsic factor (Table 3.2).

The low pH of stomach contents (approximately 1.5–3.0) is beneficial for several reasons: (1) kills or inhibits growth of most food bacteria, (2) denatures proteins and facilitates hydrolysis to amino acids, (3) activates gastric enzymes, (4) hydrolyzes some carbohydrates, and (5) increases solubility and absorption of calcium and iron.

Two major enzymes are found in gastric juice: pepsin and lipase. Pepsin is capable of hydrolyzing large protein molecules to smaller fragments. Gastric lipase is involved in digestion of short- and medium-chain triglycerides (e.g., type of fat in butterfat). Mucus forms an alkaline coating in the stomach to protect it against digestion by pepsin. Intrinsic factor, secreted in the stomach, is essential for absorption of vitamin B_{12} in the small intestine.

Normal gastric secretion is regulated by nerves and hormonal stimuli. Visual, olfactory, and gustatory senses stimulate gastric secretions. Fear, sadness, pain, and depression are generally accompanied by decreased secretions; anger, stress, and hostility may increase secretions.

An adult stomach functions as a reservoir to hold an average meal for 3 to 4 hours. The stomach empties at different rates depending on the size of the stomach and composition of the chyme. The rate of passage through the stomach (fastest to slowest) is liquids, carbohydrates, proteins, and fats. When a mixture of foods is presented, this pattern is not as well defined. The smaller the stomach capacity, the more rapidly the stomach empties. (This is exemplified in infants, who must be fed frequently until the stomach size expands.) Fats remain in the stomach longer, providing greater satiety than proteins or carbohydrates. Small amounts of chyme are released from the stomach through the pyloric sphincter to allow for adequate digestion and absorption in the small intestine.

Very little absorption occurs in the stomach because few foods are completely hydrolyzed to nutrients the body can use at this stage. Nutrients can be absorbed from the stomach: water, alcohol, and a few water-soluble substances (e.g., amino acids and glucose).

DENTAL CONSIDERATIONS

- Dietary constituents that increase hydrochloric acid and pepsin secretions are proteins, calcium, caffeine, coffee, and alcohol; patients with ulcers or certain gastrointestinal tract disorders may need to limit or omit these.
- Because gravity facilitates movement of food down the esophagus, patients who are in a supine position may have some difficulty swallowing and may reflux gastric contents, especially after eating. Aspiration of acid reflux into the lungs is possible. To prevent an emergency situation, place the patient in a semisupine position for treatment. If possible, schedule the appointment 3 hours after a meal to minimize reflux.

NUTRITIONAL DIRECTIONS

- Vomiting is one of the body's methods of eliminating toxins from contaminated foods.
- Vomiting can be stimulated by rapid changes in body motion or by drugs.
- Heartburn is a result of regurgitation (reflux) of the stomach contents into the esophagus. Acidic gastric secretions produce discomfort or pain, which may be relieved if the patient remains in an upright position after eating.
- Eating in a calm, relaxing atmosphere helps reduce gastric secretions.
- Over an extended period, chronic problems with vomiting or reflux can result in sensitive teeth and varying degrees of tooth erosion, especially on lingual and occlusal surfaces.

TABLE 3.2 Digestive Process and Physiologic Utilization of Energy-Producing Nutrients

Site	Enzymes	Carbohydrate	Protein	Fat
Nutrient Digestion				
Mouth	Salivary amylase	Starch→maltose	No action	
	Lingual lipase			Triglycerides–diglyceride + free fatty acids
Stomach	Gastric pepsin		Proteins→peptides→amino acids	
	Gastric lipase			Emulsified fats→fatty acids + glycerol
Small intestine	Pancreatic enzyme	Starch→dextrin Dextrin→maltose		
	Pancreatic trypsin, chymotrypsin, carboxypeptidase, ribonuclease and deoxyribonuclease		Protein→polypeptides Ribonucleic acids (RNA) and deoxyribonucleic acids (DNA)→mononucleotides	
	Pancreatic enzyme and intestinal lipase			Emulsified fats—fatty acids + glycerol
	Sucrase, lactase, maltase	Sucrose→glucose + fructose Maltose→glucose + glucose Lactose→glucose + galactose		
	Intestinal aminopeptidase and dipeptidase		Polypeptides→amino acids	
	Nucleotidase		Nucleic acids→nucleotides	
	Nucleosidase and phosphorylase		Nucleosides→purines, pyrimidines and pentose phosphate	
Nutrients Absorption From Small Intestine				
		Glucose, fructose, and galactose absorbed	Amino acids, mononucleotides, dipeptides, and tripeptides absorbed	Fatty acids + glycerol absorbed
Nutrient Utilization				
		Glucose oxidized for energy—CO_2 + H_2O	Amino acids build and repair tissue	Fatty acids + glycerol→new fat
		Unused stored as liver glycogen or changed and stored as body fat	Unused—nitrogen removed, forming urea and carbon, hydrogen, oxygen→glucose	Unused stored as body fat; some fat + phosphorus→phospholipids

Small Intestine

Most of the energy-providing nutrients are completely hydrolyzed and absorbed within the small intestine. Most vitamins and minerals are also absorbed in the small intestine. The small intestine is specially designed to perform these tasks with juices secreted by the accessory organs and its complex luminal wall (see Table 3.2). The small intestine is approximately 15 feet long, and foods are retained there for 3 to 10 hours.

Digestion

Throughout the walls of the small intestine are villi, fingerlike projections rising out of the mucosa into the intestinal lumen (see Figs. 3.2B and 3.2C). These villi increase the surface area of the alimentary tract to approximately 3000 square feet. Each villus is also covered with a layer of epithelial cells containing microvilli, which collectively form the brush border cells. **Microvilli** are minute hairlike folds located on the villi, which greatly increase the intestinal absorptive surface area. The pH change and motility in the small intestine inhibit bacterial growth.

Acidic chyme entering the intestine stimulates hormones to release pancreatic juices into the duodenum. Cholecystokinin, a hormone released in response to the presence of fat in chyme, stimulates the gallbladder to contract and release bile. **Bile**, produced and secreted by the liver, is stored in the gallbladder. The action of bile salts allows insoluble molecules to be divided into smaller particles, a process called **emulsification**. This process allows greater exposure of fats to intestinal and pancreatic lipases. Peristalsis also facilitates mixing and emulsification by bile.

Pancreatic enzymes enter the duodenum through the pancreatic duct and function best in neutralized chyme. Pancreatic enzymes hydrolyze carbohydrates, proteins, and fats. **Proteolytic enzymes**, which hydrolyze proteins, are produced and stored in the pancreas in an inactive form.

Specific digestive enzymes lining the brush border of the microvilli are responsible for completing hydrolysis of carbohydrates, proteins, and fats. Not everything in foods can be completely digested (e.g., the human body lacks enzymes that can digest cellulose, a carbohydrate found in plants). Other factors affecting digestion and absorption are as important to nutritional status as adequate intake: (a) amount of the nutrient consumed; (b) physiologic need; (c) condition of the digestive tract (amount of secretions, motility, and absorptive surface); (d) level of circulating hormones; (e) presence of other nutrients or drugs ingested at the same time enhancing or interfering with absorption; and (f) presence of adequate amounts of digestive enzymes.

Absorption of Nutrients

Only after absorption of the nutrient into the intestinal mucosa is it considered to be "in" the body. Generally, absorption of nutrients occurs by passive diffusion or active transport mechanisms. **Passive diffusion** is the passage of a permeable substance from a more concentrated solution to an area of lower concentration. **Active transport** occurs when absorption is from a region of lower concentration to one of a higher concentration; this mechanism requires a carrier and cellular energy. Approximately 80% to 90% of fluid intake is absorbed in the small intestine by osmosis. **Osmosis** is the passage of a liquid, such as water, through a semipermeable membrane to equalize osmotic pressure exerted by ions in solutions (Fig. 3.5). Water moves freely in both directions across the intestinal mucosa. Absorbable nutrients pass through the microvilli. Water-soluble nutrients enter the portal vein and fat-soluble ones enter through the lymphatic system.

Absorption Into Portal Circulation

Most nutrients (monosaccharides, amino acids, glycerol, water-soluble vitamins, minerals, and short- and medium-chain fatty acids) are absorbed through the mucosa of the small intestine into the **portal circulation** (absorption of nutrients from the gastrointestinal tract and spleen into the bloodstream to the liver via the portal vein). Metabolism of the nutrients then is initiated by the liver.

Absorption of Fat-Soluble Nutrients

The absorption process for long-chain fatty acids is complex because the molecules are large and insoluble. Long-chain fatty acids are broken apart to allow passage through the intestinal wall into the lymphatic system. The **lymphatic system** is comprised of lymph (plasmalike tissue fluid), the lymph nodes, and lymph vessels that are not connected to the blood system. Nutrients are carried through the thoracic duct and flow into the venous blood via the left subclavian vein. Absorption of the four fat-soluble vitamins—A, D, E, and K—is not as complex. Bile salts and lipases increase their water solubility enabling absoprtion of these vitamins along with other fats in the lymphatic system.

DENTAL CONSIDERATIONS

- An enzymatic deficiency in the gastrointestinal tract results in some nutrients not being digested, thus preventing their absorption. The most prevalent enzyme deficiency is lactase deficiency, which is discussed in Chapter 4, *Health Application 4: Lactose Intolerance*.
- Unless preventive care is taken, patients with large portions of the gastrointestinal tract removed, as in bariatric surgery, may develop a nutritional deficiency because digestive secretions or absorptive areas are removed (see Fig. 3.1; Table 3.2).
- If motility is increased, as in diarrhea, nutrients are not exposed to digestive secretions and absorptive surfaces long enough for maximum absorption. Severe or prolonged diarrhea may result in numerous deficiencies, the most rapid being a fluid deficit or dehydration.

NUTRITIONAL DIRECTIONS

- The digestive process may be affected by how well food is broken apart by the teeth.
- Dietary fat should not be eliminated entirely because it increases satiety and transports fat-soluble vitamins in the body.
- Routine use of mineral oil as a laxative is not advisable because it reduces absorption of fat-soluble vitamins.

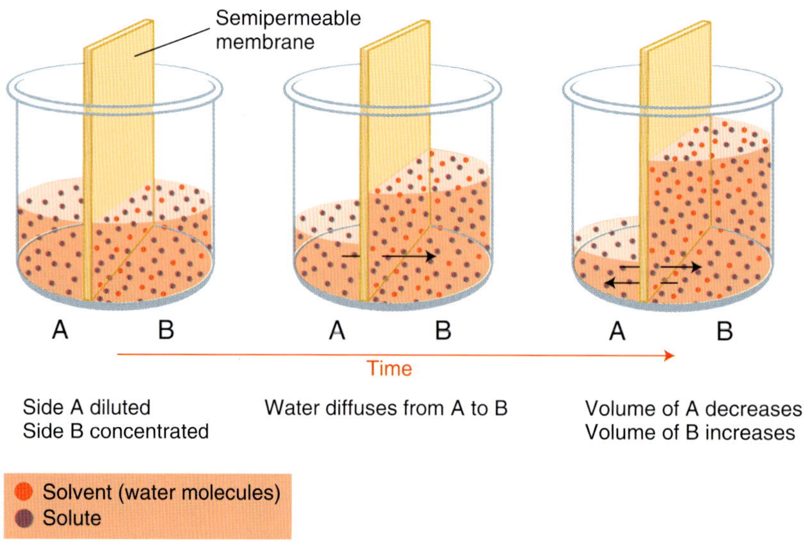

• **Figure 3.5** Osmotic pressure.

Large Intestine

Small amounts of chyme remaining in the ileum are released through the ileocecal valve into the cecum. Only about 5% of ingested foods and digestive secretions continue to the large intestine. For most adults, it takes 16 to 24 hours for foodstuffs to travel the full length of the gut.

Functions

The large intestine, so named because of its large diameter, has little or no digestive function. Its main functions are to reabsorb water and electrolytes (mainly sodium and potassium) and to form and store the residue (feces) until defecation. **Residue** in the intestinal tract is the total amount of fecal solids, including undigested or unabsorbed food, metabolic (bile pigments) and bacterial products. Chyme entering the large intestine with 500 to 1000 mL of water is excreted as feces containing only 100 to 200 mL fluid. Essentially, all absorption occurs in the proximal half of the colon.

The inner lining of the large intestine is smooth, lacking the numerous villi found in the small intestine. Its only important secretion is mucus, which protects the intestinal wall, aids in holding particles of fecal matter together, and helps to control the pH in the large intestine.

Undigested Residues

Fiber, obtained from fruits, vegetables, and whole-grain products, results in increased residue and has a water-holding capacity, contributing to bulkier feces. Dietary fiber is not digestible and works as a laxative. Foods may contain other substances that increase fecal output. One example is prune juice, which yields no residue on chemical digestion but is classified as a high-residue food because inherent chemicals indirectly increase stool volume. Residue has a beneficial side effect of stimulating peristalsis, resulting in improved muscle tone.

Microflora

The body hosts 10 times more microbial cells than "human" cells, including bacterial, fungal, protozoal and other single-cell microorganisms, all of which constitute the **microbiome**. These vast numbers of microbial cells reside throughout the body, in the gut, muscles, nerves, skin, eyes, and nasal passages. The trillions of harmless microrganisms that thrive in the intestines are called **microflora**. These friendly bacteria are present in dozens of different strains. What defines an optimal microbiome has not been identified, but microflora are essential for good health. Individuals have a microbiome as diverse and unique as fingerprints. The microbiome is influenced by many factors (Fig. 3.6).

Types of food and medications ingested influence the type, activity, and relative numbers of bacteria. The composition of intestinal microflora is rapidly affected by food patterns, responding within 3 to 4 hours of dietary alterations. A diet rich in high-fiber foods—such as vegetables, fruits, legumes, and whole grains—is most beneficial to health-promoting gut microbes. The most common bacteria found in the gut belong to groups called *Lactobacillus* and *Bifidobacterium.*

Microflora have several important roles: (a) breaking down substances (fiber and other complex carbohydrates) that human enzymes are unable to digest; (b) synthesizing vitamins needed (vitamins K and B_{12}, biotin, thiamin, and riboflavin); (c) boosting the immune system to improve protection against infection; and (d) inhibiting pathogenic bacteria. Gut microbiota cause fermentation of nondigestible carbohydrates, yielding gases and short-chain fatty acids. These short-chain fatty acids create an inhospitable environment for pathogenic bacteria. Fecal odor is a result of compounds produced by these bacteria.

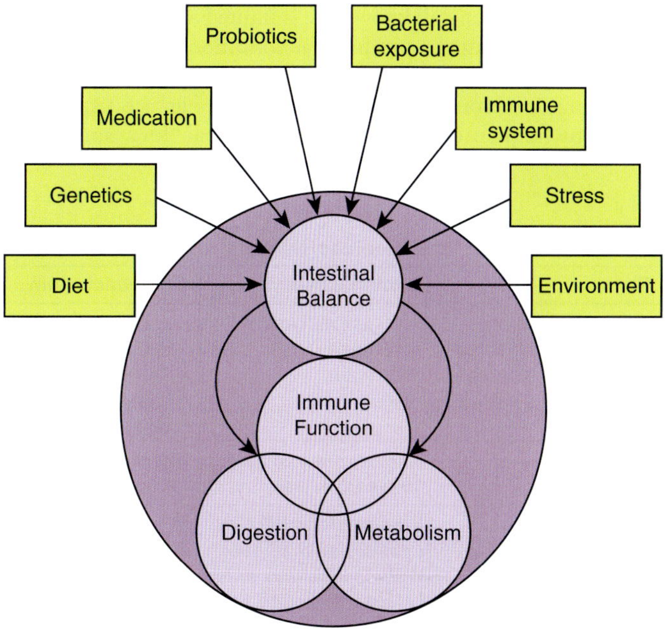

• **Figure 3.6 Digestive balance.** The bacteria environment in the digestive tract is commonly referred to as the intestinal microbiome or the gut microbiota. The "good" bacteria help keep the digestive tract at the right acidity, break down food into more digestible forms, and keep bad bacteria from taking over. Harmful bacteria cause diarrhea and hurt the immune system. The body tries to keep all of the bacteria in balance to maintain good health. These bacterial dynamics have far-reaching effects, including affecting energy metabolism. The biodiversity balance can be influenced by genetics, diet, antibiotic use, surgery, and many other factors. (Reproduced with permission from Del-ImmuneV®. Your digestive balance. https://www.delimmune.com/your-digestive-balance/. Accessed November 30, 2016.)

An imbalance of intestinal flora can impact overall health and may affect mood, anxiety, memory, and concentration. Gastrointestinal microbiota are an integral part of the human genetic landscape helping to shape metabolism and energy balance by influencing energy utilization throughout life.[1,2]

Probiotics are living microorganisms (usually bacteria) that confer a health benefit on the host when present in adequate amounts. While probiotics are essential, they are not classified as nutrients. The term *probiotics* is as general as the term *vitamins.* Currently, scientists do not know exactly how probiotics work. Microflora must be identified and demonstrated to have a beneficial effect in controlled studies to be called probiotics. Each probiotic strain is unique, and the properties and effects of each strain must be assessed individually. A bacterium's name has three parts: the genus (e.g., *Lactobacillus*), species (e.g., *acidophilus*), and strain (such as LA-5; Fig. 3.7). Strains can differ in what they do even within the same species. Sound research studies support only a small number of probiotic strains because of difficulty in identifying the function of each strain. While results indicate positive results for probiotics in general, knowledge is limited about which strains are needed, how much, and in what conditions.

Studies published in the scientific literature support probiotics improving numerous conditions, as listed in Fig. 3.8. Antibiotic treatment frequently disturbs gastrointestinal flora, sometimes resulting in *Clostridium difficile*–associated diarrhea; probiotic treatment is effective in reducing this diarrhea. Limited studies report that certain probiotics can help prevent allergies, decrease *Helicobacter pylori* colonization (a cause of ulcers) in the stomach, prevent recurrence of some inflammatory bowel conditions, and help in controlling oral yeast infections. *Lactobacillus acidophilus* and *Bifidobacterium bifidus*, found in some yogurts and other fermented dairy products, may help prevent pathogenic bacteria from proliferating and becoming toxic. Probiotics have physiologic functions affecting food intake and appetite, but trials regarding weight management are currently limited in sample size and lack long-term follow-up.

Probiotics are considered food or dietary supplements in the United States. Probiotics are found in fermented dairy products, such as kefir, yogurt, and cheeses. New products have been introduced with probiotics added to bread, orange juice, infant formula, cereal, cookies, and even chewing gum. Probiotics are also available from nonanimal sources: coconut milk, yogurt, sauerkraut, pickled or fermented vegetables or fruit (pickles, kimchi), kombucha tea, water, kefir, sourdough bread, and fermented soy products. Commercially available probiotics can be found in various forms, including capsules, tablets, and powders. These products are generally safe with few side effects, relatively inexpensive, and readily available. There is no established recommended intake, but supplements generally contain 10 billion to 20 billion active cultures per dose. Unfortunately, the beneficial effects of probiotic intake or supplements are short-lived, only transiently enriching the microflora.[3]

Consumers are understandably confused about probiotics. The U.S. Food and Drug Administration (FDA) has not established a definition for probiotics. The World Health Organization has

Probiotics: Food Sources, Habitats, and Species

Genus	Lactobacillus	Bifidobacterium
Food sources *Cannot be subjected to pasteurization or high heat, as these will kill the bacteria	• Yogurt with active cultures • Tempeh • Miso	• Yogurt with active cultures • Kefir • Buttermilk • Sauerkraut
Habitat	Urinary tract, GI tract, female genitalia	Mouth, GI tract, female genitalia
Common species/strains	*L. acidophilus W37, L. brevis W63, L. casei W56, L. salivarius W24, L. lactis (W19 and W58)*	*B. bifidum W23, B. lactis W52*

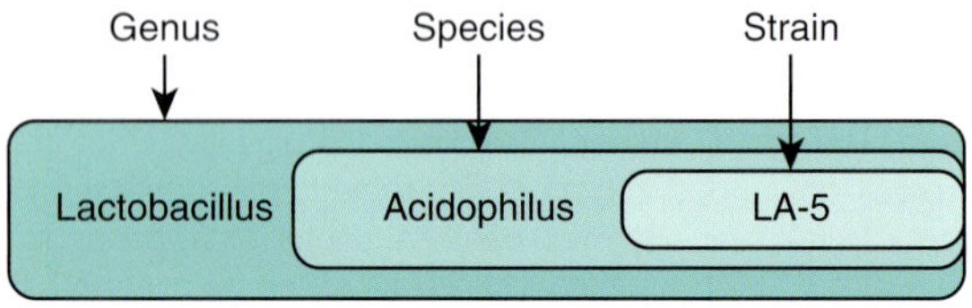

• **Figure 3.7** Probiotics: food sources, habitats, and species. (Courtesy of Rothschild J. Trust your gut: the effect of prebiotics and probiotics on gut microbiome. Webinar presented by Academy of Nutrition and Dietetics, September 10, 2015.)

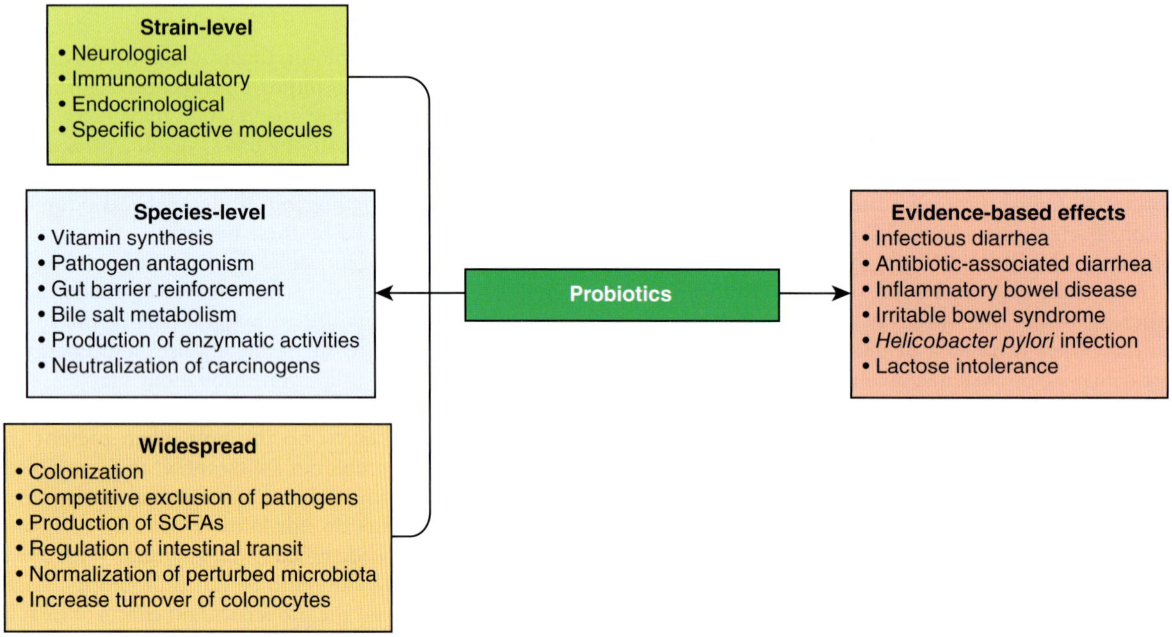

• **Figure 3.8** Beneficial effects attributed to probiotics. (Reproduced with permission from Sánchez B, Delgado S, Aitor Blanco-Míguez A, et al. Probiotics, gut microbiota, and their influence on host health and disease. *Mol Nutr Food Res.* 2017;61(1):1–15; Hill C, Guarner F, Reid G, Gibson GR, et al., Expert consensus document: The International Scientific Association for Probiotics and Prebiotics consensus statement on the scope and appropriate use of the term probiotic. *Nat Rev Gastroenterol Hepatol.* 2014;11:506–514.)

defined probiotics as "live microorganisms which when administered in adequate amounts confer a health benefit on the host."[4] The U.S. government does not test the quality of probiotics or require companies to scientifically demonstrate health benefits before labeling the product as containing beneficial probiotics. Health claims have not been approved by the FDA and the European Food Safety Authority. They are not scrutinized as closely as medications and are not required to meet standards for effectiveness. With lax labeling regulations, it is difficult to know which products have proven health benefits and whether they contain what the label indicates.

Some probiotic products on the market do not meet established minimum criteria. Products do not usually disclose the levels or strain designations of added bacteria; thus, consumers have no assurance as to whether the product has been shown to be efficacious for specific effects. Quality issues include (a) viability of organisms, (b) presence of harmful organisms, (c) protection of organisms from stomach acid, and (d) ability of a pill to properly break apart to release its ingredients.[5] Pasteurization can kill the bacteria. Guidelines for increasing microflora and purchasing probiotics are found in Box 3.1.

Probiotics are an important way to produce specific host benefits through different mechanisms, among which changes in the intestinal microbiota is noteworthy. However, taking probiotics as an "insurance" for preventive protection may lead to adverse side effects. Probiotic users who have impaired gastric and intestinal emptying or take medications that affect gastrointestinal motility have developed **small intestinal bacterial overgrowth (SIBO**; excessive amount of bacteria in the gastrointestinal tract causing nausea, vomiting, bloating, flatulence, and diarrhea). Research is expanding reliable knowledge and understanding of the health benefits of probiotics. Scientific research must continue to be interpreted cautiously. Unfortunately, many products may claim health benefits that have not been validated.

Two oral probiotics have been shown to improve oral health by reducing cariogenic and periodontal pathogen levels.[6–8] Commercially available BLIS K12 and M18 (two types of *S. salivarius)* products contain antibacterial entities that may offer preventative and remedial solutions to attack the root of gingivitis and periodontal disease. Patented probiotic strain BLIS K12 has been approved for an oral-health claim in Canada to promote oral health.

Prebiotics are nondigestible food ingredients (complex carbohydrates) with beneficial effects on the host by selectively providing fuel, stimulating growth or activity, or both, of beneficial colonic microorganisms present in the gastrointestinal tract. Fiber, particularly fermentable fiber, is crucial for good health. Prebiotics are specialized compounds that influence specific bacteria, their fermentation end products, and possible health effects on the host. Prebiotics increase mineral absorption (especially calcium and magnesium) from the foods containing them. Inulin and some sugars and sugar alcohols found in whole grains, onions, bananas, garlic, honey, leeks, and artichokes are natural sources of prebiotics.

Simply put, prebiotics are food for probiotics. Probiotics together with prebiotics that support their growth are called **symbiotics** because they cooperatively promote probiotic benefits more efficiently. The benefits associated with probiotics are strain specific and benefits of prebiotics are substance specific.

• BOX 3.1 Guidelines for Increasing Microflora

- A plant-rich diet (vegetables, fruits, and legumes), high in dietary fiber appears to be beneficial by providing prebiotics for fuel for intestinal bacteria.
- Fermented foods (yogurt, kefir, sauerkraut, kimchi, tempeh) may affect microflora by influencing bacteria already present.
- The *Lactobacillus* bacteria should be "lactofermented" or naturally fermented and raw or unpasteurized since pasteurization kills beneficial bacteria.
- Purchase supplements only from reputable companies; they should contain the United States Pharmacopeia (USP) or the National Formulary (NF) symbol on their packaging.
- Natural food sources of the prebiotic inulin (garlic, leeks, artichokes, asparagus) may help suppress pathogenic bacteria while promoting beneficial bacterial growth.
- Limit processed foods, sugar, and *trans* fats. Diets containing large amounts of highly processed foods may allow pathogenic bacteria to thrive while diminishing the numbers of good bacteria and enhance growth of proinflammatory microbiota.
- Look for words such as "active cultures" or "live cultures" on a food labeled as providing probiotics.
- During and after antibiotic treatments, consume a high-quality probiotic supplement (containing several different strains of *Lactobacillus* and *Bifidobacterium* species, that is, *L. acidophilus, L. reuteri, B. longum, and B.bifidum)* to help recolonize the digestive tract and manage antibiotic-induced diarrhea. (Take probiotic supplements at least 2 hours before or after taking antibiotics.)
- To be effective, microorganisms in a probiotic supplement should be designed to survive the harsh stomach acid.
- Probiotics are generally safe for healthy people, but caution should be used with older patients, those with reduced immunity, children, and pregnant and lactating women.

Peristalsis

The purpose of peristalsis in the large intestine is to force feces into the rectum. These large waves occur only two to three times daily.

Constipation is a common problem for many people. The National Institute of Diabetes and Digestive and Kidney Diseases of the National Institutes of Health defines **constipation** as having a bowel movement fewer than three times per week with hard, dry, small, and difficult-to-pass stools.

DENTAL CONSIDERATIONS

- Bowel habits, stress, exercise, and nutritional intake (especially the amount of fiber and fluid intake) affect gastrointestinal transit rate. Transit time affects the amount of harmful degradation products produced.
- Lengthy retention of feces in the large intestine allows more reabsorption of water, causing feces to become hard and dry and leading to constipation.
- Many patients may have symptoms of a chronic digestive problem, such as heartburn, abdominal pain, constipation, diarrhea, and gastroesophageal reflux disease. Some of these problems can be addressed with dietary or lifestyle changes. Refer these patients to an RDN.
- Prebiotics pass intact into the large intestine, where they stimulate growth and activity of healthy bacteria; in contrast, probiotics influence the types of bacteria present.
- Specific probiotic strains have different biologic activities and provide a variety of health benefits.
- For most patients, microbes in probiotics are beneficial but should be consumed in moderation. However, patients who have a poor immune response should consult a health care provider or RDN before using probiotics.
- Probiotics may be beneficial to treat traveler's diarrhea and can be used to prevent and treat urinary tract infections, irritable bowel disease, and other conditions.
- Antibiotic therapy normally kills bacteria in the colon and inhibits bacterial production of vitamins. Patients on long-term antibiotic therapy may develop deficiencies of vitamins K and B_{12} and biotin.

NUTRITIONAL DIRECTIONS

- Constipation can be treated by increasing fluid intake or by gradually increasing nondigestible food components (fiber) in the diet, or both.
- Activity also affects gastrointestinal mobility. Active individuals who routinely choose high-fiber foods and drink adequate amounts of liquids are less likely to become constipated than sedentary people.
- The frequency of bowel movements varies from after each meal to once every 2 days.
- Probiotics as a dietary supplement may be healthful in providing large amounts of beneficial bacteria if the products are responsibly formulated and stored properly.
- The presence of higher levels of bifidobacteria in the intestines of breastfed infants may be a reason why they are generally healthier than formula-fed infants.

HEALTH APPLICATION 3

Gluten-Related Disorders

In 2012, in response to the prevalence of individuals embracing a gluten-free diet, international experts recognized that gluten reactions are not limited to celiac disease. Three conditions related to the ingestion of gluten are now recognized: (a) an autoimmune genetically predisposed disorder (celiac disease); (b) allergic reactions (wheat allergy), and (c) immune-mediated disorder (nonceliac gluten sensitivity). Although these three conditions are treated with similar diets, they are not the same condition. **Gluten** is a structural protein that is stretchy and viscous, a component of wheat, rye, barley, and triticale (cross-bred hybrid of wheat and rye). Gluten-containing grains are not new, being introduced into the human diet approximately 10,000 years ago.

Celiac disease is an **autoimmune disorder** (condition that causes the body to form antibodies to one's own tissues) caused by a permanent sensitivity to gluten in genetically-susceptible individuals. If the condition is not diagnosed and treated, microvilli in the small intestine are damaged, ultimately impairing absorption of nutrients. Microvilli normally allow nutrients to be absorbed from the small intestine into the bloodstream. **Wheat allergy** is another adverse immunologic reaction specific to wheat proteins. **Nonceliac gluten sensitivity (NCGS)** is characterized by intestinal and other symptoms related to ingesting gluten-containing foods but without celiac disease or wheat allergy. The overall clinical picture is generally less severe and the small intestine is not impaired. Symptoms may appear within hours or days following gluten consumption.

The genes for celiac disease are present in about 30% to 40% of the general population but only a small percentage of carriers develop celiac disease.[9] Diagnosis of celiac disease begins with a blood test for specific antibodies. If this test is positive, the standard for diagnosis is a biopsy from the small intestine, unless the person is following a gluten-free diet. If the individual has been following a gluten-free diet prior to a biopsy, the lining of the small intestine may not show damage, making a definitive diagnosis difficult. The U.S. Preventive Services Task Force determined the effectiveness of screening for celiac disease in asymptomatic individuals is scarce so routine screening is not recommended.[10]

Testing for wheat allergy includes a skin prick test for wheat. NCGS is diagnosed after celiac disease has been ruled out, followed by the skin prick test to determine wheat allergy. The diagnosis protocol for NCGS is based on a link between gluten ingestion and appearance of symptoms. After evaluating the response to a gluten-free diet, gluten is reintroduced and response assessed. NCGS can be unpleasant, but it is not harmful to long-term health; the overall clinical picture is less severe for those without concurrent autoimmune disease.

Symptoms of NCGS include abdominal pain, eczema, headache, foggy mind, fatigue, diarrhea, depression, anemia, numbness in the extremities, and joint pain. For people who suspect they have NCGS, a diagnosis to rule out celiac disease is preeminent before initiating a gluten-free diet to obtain a valid diagnosis. A gluten-free diet should be the last resort when NCGS is suspected. After celiac disease and wheat allergy have been eliminated, the individual should try a gluten-free diet for at least a week, but no longer than a month, to determine if symptoms are alleviated.

Celiac disease is more common in countries predominantly populated by people of European origin, affecting approximately 1.76 million Americans. Less than 10% of the cases have been diagnosed. Between 2009 and 2014, diagnoses of Americans with celiac disease remained stable.[11] More Americans may have gluten sensitivity than celiac disease.

Fatigue is a major symptom for most individuals with celiac disease. Other common signs and symptoms of the disease include diarrhea, abdominal pain, bloating, lactose intolerance, headaches, joint pain, skin rashes, depression, and short stature. A blistering rash, known as dermatitis

HEALTH APPLICATION 3

Gluten-Related Disorders—cont'd

herpetiformis, may be seen in patients with asymptomatic celiac disease. Without treatment, poor absorption of iron, folate, calcium, vitamin D, and other nutrients may result in anemia and osteoporosis. Other long-term serious health complications are neurologic conditions, malignancies, and lymphoid neoplasms. On the other hand, patients' health is not uniformly improved by intervention.[12]

In the oral cavity, enamel defects and recurrent aphthous stomatitis are the most common symptoms. Antibodies generated against gluten can react with a major protein enamel, causing enamel defects in developing teeth. Eruption of teeth in children with celiac disease is delayed. These oral manifestations may be the only presenting features.[13,14] Squamous cell carcinoma of the mouth, oropharynx, and esophagus is a serious long-term oral complication. People with celiac disease must permanently exclude gluten to avoid long-term adverse consequences of this lifelong chronic condition. The only course of treatment is a strict gluten-free diet. While elimination of the offending substance was thought to promote healing and repair of the gastrointestinal tract, despite maintaining a gluten-free diet for 1 year, mucosal recovery did not occur in all the children with celiac disease.[15]

Many Americans who suffer from irritable bowel syndrome are probably sensitive to gluten and may benefit from a gluten-free diet. Patients with wheat allergy may also benefit from a gluten-free diet, but strict adherence may be less important. Experts have not determined how strictly or for how long the diet should be followed or what complications may arise by following it.

A strict gluten-free diet can initially be an overwhelming undertaking in addition to being expensive. Gluten is a thickener; many processed foods use gluten-containing grains, additives, or preservatives. Gluten is not only in food products; beer, cosmetics, and postage stamps also contain gluten. All fresh fruits and vegetables, dairy products, and fresh meats—beef, chicken, fish, lamb, pork, are naturally gluten-free. The gluten-free diet can be well-balanced if foods are chosen wisely (e.g., more legumes and foods with lower energy density). Consumption of more fruits and vegetables, gluten-free whole grains, nuts, and seeds can help improve the nutritional value. A gluten-free diet may lead to reductions in beneficial gut bacteria. Probiotics can be especially helpful to increase gut bacteria and reduce symptoms of digestive irritation. Dietary fiber from whole foods, gluten-free sources (chia seeds, ground flaxseeds, rice bran, fruit, and vegetables) help strengthen and soothe the gastrointestinal tract.

Many gluten-free foods are not fortified or enriched. Nutrients added in enrichment are lacking in whole-grain cereals. The diet may be lacking iron, calcium, fiber, thiamin, riboflavin, niacin, folate, and vitamin D. Evidence strongly suggests that if patients are left on their own, a variety of macro- and micronutrient deficiencies can develop.[16] Gluten-free products may become healthier overall as manufacturers develop ways to fortify them. Extra sugar and fat are added to simulate the texture and fluffiness that gluten imparts, making many gluten-free products higher in fat and sugar than other products.

New high-quality gluten-free products are introduced on the market almost daily. Food manufacturers label foods "gluten-free" that are naturally free of gluten. In 2013, the FDA published a regulation for voluntary labeling of "gluten-free" foods. Foods bearing that label cannot contain more than 20 parts per million (ppm) of gluten. (Lower amounts could not be reliably detected.)

It is believed that even gluten-containing crumbs can damage the intestinal mucosa in celiac patients. Certain grains, such as oats, can be contaminated with wheat during growing and processing. Wheat flour can remain airborne for hours (especially in bakeries) and contaminate exposed preparation surfaces and utensils or uncovered gluten-free products, such as fruits. Cross-contamination can also occur at home if foods are prepared on common surfaces or with appliances or utensils that are not thoroughly cleaned after being used to prepare gluten-containing foods, for example, the toaster, microwave, or flour sifter.

Close to 2.7 million Americans are currently on a gluten-free craze, following a gluten-less diet, either believing it is healthier or may help with weight loss. There is nothing inherently healthy about a gluten-free diet. When patients with celiac disease follow a gluten-free diet, some gain, some lose, but for most, weights remain the same. Gluten-free foods may be less nutritious than their gluten-containing counterparts, as they tend to be more heavily processed, are high in refined carbohydrates, and contain fewer vitamins and minerals and less fiber. Evidence does not indicate that gluten is harmful to healthy people without a gluten-related disorder. A significant reduction in consumption of wheat-containing products has partially been attributed to individuals choosing gluten-free or multigrain products.

For most individuals, wheat gluten may impart some healthy benefits: (a) lower blood lipids and reduced risk of cardiovascular disease (CVD); (b) lower blood pressure; (c) improved immune system; (d) healthier composition of colonic bacteria; and (e) protection from some cancers. Because gluten-free flours, such as rice flour and cornstarch, typically cause a higher rise in blood sugars compared to wheat-based flours, a gluten-free diet may exacerbate insulin resistance, glucose intolerance, and weight gain. Americans on a gluten-free diet may be exposed to higher levels of arsenic and mercury.[17] A gluten-free diet may adversely affect gut health in those without celiac disease or gluten sensitivity. A gluten-free diet is necessary for those with celiac disease or gluten intolerance but may not be healthy for people without those conditions.

CASE APPLICATION FOR THE DENTAL HYGIENIST

Mr. A complains that he can hardly talk because his mouth is dry and sticky. Sores in his mouth make his dentures very uncomfortable. He states he does not leave his home often because he is unable to easily find liquids to prevent his tongue from sticking to the sides and roof of his mouth. He also complains that eating is difficult. Mr. A reports that his health care provider prescribed a diuretic for his hypertension.

Nutritional Assessment

- Recent change in weight
- Dietary intake
- Preferred fluids, frequency of intake
- Food preparation techniques
- Medications taken
- Oral examination to determine the condition of the underlying tissues
- Fit of dentures
- Willingness to learn and change habits

Nutritional Diagnosis

Knowledge deficit of the effects of diuretics on hydration of the body related to lack of information and understanding.

Nutritional Goals

The patient will continue taking the diuretic. His nutrient intake will improve to prevent further weight loss, and his fluid intake will increase to 8 to 10 glasses of fluid a day.

Continued

CASE APPLICATION FOR THE DENTAL HYGIENIST—cont'd

Nutritional Implementation

Intervention: Discuss the importance of adequate salivary flow for maintenance of soft tissues, taste functions, and teeth. If indicated and desired, suggest products designed to relieve xerostomia to provide temporary comfort as needed.

Rationale: Xerostomia has severe deleterious effects on a patient's ability to talk and on integrity of oral tissues.

Intervention: Review the importance of meticulous oral hygiene and periodically removing dentures.

Rationale: Xerostomia promotes plaque formation, which can lead to further gingival irritations for this patient. Removal of dentures allows underlying tissue to become healthy again.

Intervention: Discuss that although diuretics may cause this condition, they are important for his health.

Rationale: To prevent other health problems, Mr. A must continue the medication as prescribed by his health care provider.

Intervention: Discuss ways he can increase his fluid intake to 8 to 10 glasses daily: (a) drink more fluid with meals; (b) carry fluids with him in a large covered thermal container.

Rationale: To replace fluids excreted because of the diuretic, adequate fluid intake is essential.

Intervention: Encourage increased intake of nutrient-dense liquid or semiliquid foods, such as milkshakes, cream soups, gravies, and sauces.

Rationale: These foods contain larger proportions of nutrients, which will help Mr. A to consume adequate amounts of nutrients and will prevent weight loss.

Intervention: Recommend tips to relieve the dryness in his mouth, such as ice chips or sugar-free mints and gum containing xylitol.

Rationale: The patient's comfort will be enhanced if his mouth is moist; oral complications associated with xerostomia will be minimized. Use of chewing gum or mints containing xylitol will stimulate salivary flow, reduce caries-causing bacteria, and assist with remineralization of any early carious lesions.

Evaluation

If the patient continues to take the prescribed diuretic, consumes a well-balanced diet, increases fluid intake, uses correct oral hygiene practices, maintains body weight, and can state why he was having all these problems, dental hygiene care was effective.

Student Readiness

1. Chart or diagram the gastrointestinal secretions, where they are produced, and their digestive actions on nutrients present in milk. Homogenized milk contains the following: lactose (a disaccharide), proteins, emulsified fats, calcium, riboflavin, and vitamins A and D. Where are the end products absorbed?
2. Define *alimentary canal, hydrolysis, enzyme,* and *residue.*
3. A patient has problems secreting too much hydrochloric acid. What types of food would you recommend a patient to avoid?
4. Cut a small hole (1 mm in diameter) in a piece of paper. Place the tip of your tongue through the hole. Looking in the mirror, count the number of taste buds. Compare your findings with other classmates of varying ages. Observe the number of taste buds on adolescent and older patients.
5. If caloric intake were equal, which of the following breakfasts would probably delay feelings of hunger longest? Explain your reason.
   a. Dry cereal with skim milk, toast with jelly, and coffee with sugar
   b. Egg with ham, toast with butter, and coffee with cream
6. What are absorbable products resulting from digestion of carbohydrates, proteins, and fats?
7. Within what section of the alimentary canal does most digestion and absorption take place?
8. Considering secretions and the functions of the gastrointestinal tract, discuss the fallacy of diets that claim only one type of food (e.g., fruits) should be eaten at a given time.
9. Could constipation be called a nutrient deficiency? Defend your answer.
10. What types of problems might be encountered when a patient does not chew one's food well? Discuss dental issues that can lead to decreased ability to masticate food.
11. View http://www.foodinsight.org/Resources/Detail.aspx?topic=Foods_for_Health_Eating_for_Digestive_Health. Summarize the information from the video. What information can you personally use?

CASE STUDY

An 85-year-old man reports with several new caries. He complains that his mouth is always dry because he sleeps with his mouth open due to his sinus problems. He states he is having problems eating because the food becomes a dry lump in his mouth.

1. What information should you provide the patient to address the caries incidence?
2. Do you think his problem is due to his mouth breathing or lack of fluids?
3. What information can you provide regarding his diet?
4. Can you provide some suggestions to address the dryness at meals?
5. Discuss between appropriate meal snacks to prevent additional caries.

References

1. Davis C. The gut microbiome and its role in obesity. *Nutr Today.* 2016;51(4):167–174.
2. Kobyliak N, Conte C, Cammarota G, et al. Probiotics in prevention and treatment of obesity: a critical view. *Nutr Metab.* 2016; 13:14.
3. Eloe-Fadrosh CA, Brady A, Crabtree J, et al. Functional dynamics of the gut microbiome in elderly people during probiotic consumption. *MBio.* 2015;6(2):e00231–15.
4. Hill C, Gaurner F, Reid G, et al. Expert consensus document. The International Scientific Association for probiotics and prebiotics consensus statement on the scope and appropriate use of the term probiotic. *Nat Rev Gastroenterol Hepatol.* 2014;11(8):506–514.

5. Consumer. Lab. Product Review: Probiotics (for Adults, Children and Pets) and Kefirs. Initial Posting November 2015. Accessed September 27, 2016. https://www.consumerlab.com/reviews/Probiotic_Supplements_Lactobacillus_acidophilus_Bifidobacterium/probiotics/.
6. Gruner D, Paris S. Schwendicke F: Probiotics for managing caries and periodontitis: systematic review and meta-analysis. *J Dent.* 2016;48:16–25.
7. Scariya L, Nagarathna DV, Varghese M. Probiotics in periodontal therapy. *Int J Pharm Bio.* 2015;6(1):242–250.
8. Burton JP, Wescombe PA, Macklaim JM, et al. Persistence of the oral probiotic *Streptococcus salivarius* M18 is dose dependent and megaplasmid transfer can augment their bacteriocin production and adhesion characteristics. *PLoS ONE.* 2013;8(6):e65991. Jun 13.
9. Cenit MC, Codoner-Franch R, Sanz Y. Gut microbiota and risk of developing celiac disease. *J Clin Gastroenterol.* 2016;50(suppl 2):Proceedings from the 8th Probiotics, Prebiotics and New Foods for Microbiota and Human Health meeting held in Rome, Italy on September 13-15, 2015: S148-S152.
10. US Preventive Services Task Force. Screening for celiac disease: US Preventive Services Task Force recommendation statement. *JAMA.* 2017;317(12):1252–1257.
11. Kim HS, Patel KG, Orosz E, et al. Time trends in the prevalence of celiac disease and gluten-free diet in the US population. *JAMA Intern Med.* 2016;176(11):1716–1717.
12. US. Preventive Services Task Force. Screening for celiac disease: US Preventive Services Task Force recommendation statement. *JAMA.* 2017;317(12):1252–1257.
13. Paul SP, Kirkham EN, John R, et al. Coeliac disease in children—an update for general dental practitioners. *Br Dent J.* 2016;220(9): 481–485.
14. Karlin S, Karlin E, Meiller T, et al. Dental and oral considerations in pediatric celiac disease. *J Dent Child (Chic).* 2016;83(2):67–70.
15. Leonard MM, Weir DC, DeGroote M, et al. Value of IgA tTg in predicting mucosal recovery in children with celiac disease on a gluten free diet. *J Pediatr Gastroenterol Nutr.* 2016;64(2):286–291.
16. Vici G, Belli L, Biondi M, et al. Gluten free diet and nutrient deficiencies: a review. *Clin Nutr.* 2016;35(6):1236–1241.
17. Bulka CM, Davis MA, Karagas MR, et al. The unintended consequences of a gluten-free diet. *Epidemiology.* 2017;doi:10.1097/EDE.0000000000000640. Feb 1, [Epub ahead of print].

EVOLVE RESOURCES

Please visit http://evolve.elsevier.com/Stegeman/nutritional for additional practice and study support tools.

4

Carbohydrate: The Efficient Fuel

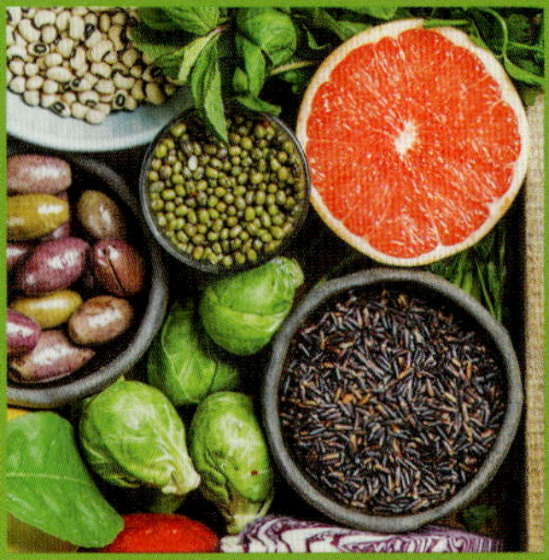

STUDENT LEARNING OUTCOMES

Upon completion of this chapter, the student will be able to achieve the following student learning outcomes:

1. Discuss various concepts related to the classification of carbohydrates, including:
   - Identify major carbohydrates in foods and in the body.
   - Differentiate among monosaccharides, disaccharides, and polysaccharides.
   - Describe ways glucose can be used by the body.
   - Summarize the functions of dietary carbohydrates.
   - Explain the importance of dietary carbohydrates.
   - Recognize dietary sources of lactose, other sugars, and starches.
   - Summarize the role and sources of dietary fiber.
2. Discuss the physiologic role of carbohydrates.
3. Discuss the acceptable macronutrient distribution range (AMDR) as related to carbohydrates, as well as sources of various types of carbohydrates.
4. Compare and contrast concepts related to hyperstates and hypostates, such as carbohydrate excess, obesity, cardiovascular disease (CVD), carbohydrate deficiency, and dental caries. In addition, formulate recommendations for patients concerning carbohydrate consumption to reduce risk for dental caries.
5. Discuss the use of nonnutritive sweeteners and sugar substitutes.

KEY TERMS

Anticariogenic
Cariogenic
Cariostatic
Complex carbohydrates
Dental erosion
Dextrin
Dietary fiber
Fermentable carbohydrate
Functional fiber
Hyperglycemia
Hypoglycemia
Ketosis
Lipogenesis
Nondigestible
Phenylketonuria
Plaque biofilm
Resistant starch
Soluble dietary fibers
***Streptococcus mutans* (*S. mutans*)**
Synergistic
Total fiber

TEST YOUR NQ

1. **T/F** Raw sugar is nutritionally superior to white sugar.
2. **T/F** Fructose is the principal carbohydrate in honey.
3. **T/F** All caloric sugars can be metabolized by plaque biofilm.
4. **T/F** The desire for sweetness in the diet is an acquired taste.
5. **T/F** Fiber tends to regulate the rate foods pass through the gastrointestinal tract.
6. **T/F** Carbohydrates are absorbed as monosaccharides.
7. **T/F** Excessive consumption of carbohydrates is the main cause of obesity.
8. **T/F** Glucose is the same as table sugar.
9. **T/F** Eliminating sucrose from the diet prevents development of dental caries.
10. **T/F** Natural sugars in foods can be just as cariogenic as added sugars.

Carbohydrates have been the major source of energy for people since the dawn of history. Worldwide, carbohydrates are the most important source of energy, furnishing 80% to 90% of calories for some African and Asian nations. Nutrition experts universally recommend that carbohydrates should represent 50% of total energy intake. Carbohydrate foods add variety and palatability to the diet and are the most economical form of energy.

As discussed in Chapter 2, carbohydrates contain carbon, hydrogen, and oxygen. During photosynthesis, carbon dioxide and water result in formation of carbohydrates and release of oxygen. Because glucose and other carbohydrates are essentially hydrogen (and oxygen) atoms bound to a carbon backbone, a carbohydrate could also be referred to as a "hydrated carbon." Carbohydrates have been falsely accused of numerous properties—for example, mysterious "fattening" power, causing abdominal obesity and weight gain—these claims are unfounded. Carbohydrates acquired a bad reputation in popular books in the 1950s and accusations continue in best-selling books, with one author recently claiming that modern grains are silently destroying your brain![1] Critics have labeled sugar as "toxic" and "addictive." Naturally, these unscientific statements affect food consumption patterns. Popular low-carbohydrate, high-protein weight-reduction diets have regularly caused the pendulum to swing away from choosing carbohydrate foods. Many of these diets are nutritionally unbalanced, providing inadequate amounts of nutrients known to help protect against several chronic diseases.

The first edition of the *Dietary Goals for the United States* in 1977 encouraged Americans to consume more complex carbohydrates (fruits, vegetables, legumes, and whole-grain products) to reduce their risk of various chronic diseases. Food supply data indicate that 48% of total calories come from carbohydrates for men, and 50.7% for women.[2] Americans consume less than eight servings of grain products daily and less than one serving of whole grains.[3] Even if people are consuming an adequate number of servings of grains, the types of foods chosen need to be adjusted to improve fiber intake.

Additionally, the amount of added sugars (those added to foods during processing or at the table) needs to be reduced to improve the quality of intake. Because most high-carbohydrate food choices are sugar-sweetened beverages (SSBs), cakes, cookies, pastries, and pies, intake of fat as well as sugar is detrimentally affected. Mean intakes of caloric sweeteners decreased for all age groups between 2003 and 2004 and 2011 to 2012 (from 21.0 tsp to 18.4 tsp). This reduction in added sugars occurred at the same rate as reduction in calorie intake, resulting in Americans consuming less added sugars today than 15 years ago.[4] Some misconceptions surrounding the intake of sugars include: (a) sugar is the cause of tooth decay, (b) food with a high sugar concentration is more dangerous to the teeth, and (c) avoidance of sticky sweets prevents tooth decay. With water fluoridation, the incidence of caries has decreased in industrialized countries despite increased sugar consumption. All dental practitioners must be knowledgeable about the effect of carbohydrates on soft and hard tissues in the oral cavity and about chronic health problems caused by low-carbohydrate, high-fat diets. Dental professionals need to educate patients about ways to modify carbohydrate consumption and intake patterns that are consistent with overall good health.

Classification

Chapter 2 and the Evolve website provide detailed information regarding the metabolism of carbohydrates. Generally, the chemical components of carbohydrates are in these proportions: $C_n(H_2O)_n$. An empirical formula such as $C_6H_{12}O_6$ or $C_{12}H_{22}O_{11}$ can readily be identified as a carbohydrate. The number of carbon atoms in the molecule is used to classify carbohydrates. Monosaccharides are simple sugars containing two to six carbon atoms. Disaccharides are composed of two simple sugars joined together and contain 12 carbon atoms. Polysaccharides are **complex carbohydrates** containing a minimum of 10 units of various simple sugars. - 26 carbons

Monosaccharides and disaccharides contribute to the palatability of a food because of their sweetness. Temperature, pH, and the presence of other substances influence the sweetness of a food. Relative sweetness of sugars is measured by subjective sensory tasting; sucrose is used as the standard of comparison (Table 4.1).

TABLE 4.1 Caloric Value and Relative Sweetness of Sugars and Sweeteners

Sugar or Sweetener	cal/g	Relative Sweetness[a]
Fructose	4	170
High-fructose corn syrup-90	4	160
Agave syrup	4	150
High-fructose corn syrup-55	4	120
Honey (fructose and glucose)	4	110
High-fructose corn syrup-42	4	110
Sucrose	4	100
Coconut palm sugar	4	100
Molasses (sucrose and invert sugar)	2.4	100
Brown sugar (sugar and molasses)	3.8	100
Coconut palm sugar	4	100
Dextrose/glucose (corn syrup)	4	75
Lactose	4	15
Reduced Calorie Sweeteners		
Xylitol	2.4	100
Tagatose	1.5–2.4	75–92
Erythritol	0.2	70
Sorbitol	2.6	55
Mannitol	1.6	50
Hydrogenated starch hydrolysates (mixture of several sugar alcohols)	3.0	40
Nonnutritive Sweeteners		
Acesulfame K	0	200
Aspartame	0	200
Lu han guo (monk fruit)	0	300
Neotame	0	8000
Rebaudioside A (Truvia, Stevia)	0	300
Saccharin	0	300
Sucralose	0	600

[a]Relative to sucrose (= 100).

Data from Sugar-and-Sweetener-Guide. Sweetener values, including calories and glycemic index. Accessed October 26, 2016. http://www.sugar-and-sweetener-guide.com/sweetener-values.html

Monosaccharides

The simplest carbohydrates, monosaccharides, are absorbed without further digestion. The monosaccharides of greatest significance in foods and body metabolism are glucose, fructose, and galactose. Fig. 2.3 in Chapter 2 identifies slight differences between these three six-carbon sugars and glucose.

Glucose

Also called dextrose or corn sugar, glucose is naturally abundant in many fruits, such as grapes, oranges, and dates, and in some vegetables, including fresh corn. It is prepared commercially as corn syrup or by special processing of starch. Glucose is the principal product formed by the digestion of disaccharides and polysaccharides. It provides energy for cells via the bloodstream. Glucose is the only sugar transported through the bloodstream that can nourish all cells in the body.

Fructose

Fructose, also known as levulose, is found naturally in honey and fruits. It is the sweetest of the monosaccharides and is a product of the digestion of sucrose. Fructose can be manufactured from glucose.

High-fructose corn syrup (HFCS) is made from corn starch; however, corn products contain only glucose molecules. HFCS is industrially produced by changing some glucose molecules into fructose, making the syrup sweeter than sucrose. It is available in several different concentrations for different products and has become a popular component of processed foods, especially soft drinks, because of its lower cost. HFCS-42 contains approximately the same amount of fructose as honey, and some natural fruit juices have twice as much fructose as glucose. The most frequently used concentration of HFCS in foods (principally beverages) is HFCS-55. Since its introduction in the food supply in 1968, consumption of HFCS gradually increased, along with rising consumption of all sugars, until 1999 when both HFCS and sugar intake began decreasing (Fig. 4.1).

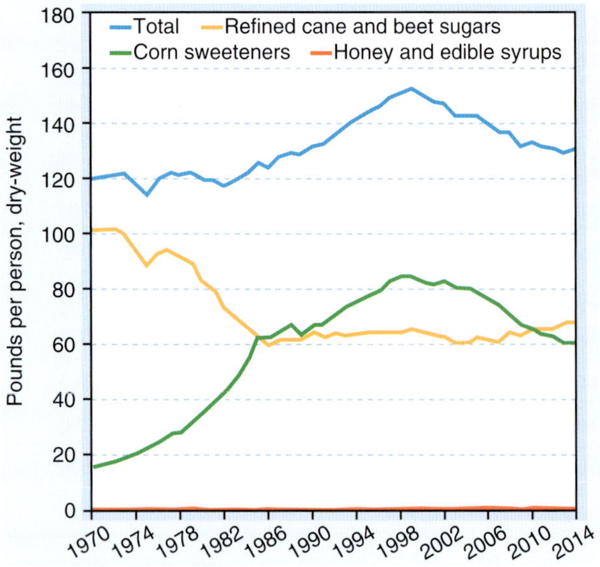

• **Figure 4.1** United States per capita sweetener availability, 1970 to 2014.

Galactose

Galactose, another six-carbon sugar, is a product of lactose digestion (milk sugar). Galactose is rarely found free in nature. Physiologically, it is a constituent of nerve tissue and is produced from glucose during lactation.

Sugar Alcohols

Sugar alcohols are formed from or converted to sugar. Sugar alcohols may appear naturally in foods or be added by a manufacturer. The most common polyols include sorbitol, xylitol, and mannitol.

For a given quantity, xylitol and tagatose (a naturally occurring monosaccharide) add about the same amount of sweetness as glucose but furnish fewer calories. Xylitol is found in fruits and vegetables (lettuce, carrots, and strawberries). As a food additive, it is more expensive than other sugar alcohols but has no aftertaste.

The benefit of sorbitol is that it is absorbed and metabolized more slowly than sucrose. Sorbitol, the most commonly used sugar alcohol, is the least expensive. Mannose is a six-carbon sugar found in some legumes. Mannitol, derived from mannose, is found in foods.

Incomplete absorption of sugar alcohols produces a laxative effect—soft stools or diarrhea—by causing an osmotic transfer of water into the gastrointestinal tract. Sugar alcohols are not considered sugars, and their use by food manufacturers is expected to increase in their attempts to comply with the *Dietary Guidelines* for reducing sugar intake. Sugar alcohols do not cause sudden increases in blood glucose levels and they do not contribute to tooth decay.

Disaccharides

Intact disaccharides cannot be metabolized by the body, but they contribute to body functions after digestion. As discussed in Chapter 2, monosaccharides are absorbed from the gastrointestinal tract with no further action, but disaccharides and polysaccharides or complex carbohydrates must be broken down into their constituent monosaccharides before they can be absorbed (Fig. 4.2).

Sucrose

Granulated table sugar is the most common form of sucrose, which is a combination of one molecule of glucose and one molecule of fructose, as shown in Fig. 2.4. Commercially, sucrose is produced from sugar cane or sugar beets (not to be confused with red beets). It is also found in molasses, maple syrup, and maple sugar. Some fruits (apricots, peaches, plums, raspberries, honeydew, cantaloupe) and vegetables (beets, carrots, parsnips, winter squash, peas, corn, sweet potatoes) naturally contain varying amounts of sucrose.

Lactose

The sugar found in milk is lactose. Lactose, which contains galactose and glucose (see Fig. 2.5) is unique to mammalian milk. In the fermentation of milk, some of the lactose is converted to lactic acid, giving buttermilk and yogurt their characteristic flavors.

Maltose

Maltose, shown in Fig. 2.4, contains two molecules of glucose. Also called *malt sugar*, maltose does not occur naturally. It is created in making bread and brewing beer and is present in some processed cereals and baby foods.

DENTAL CONSIDERATIONS

- Assess patients with an increased risk of dental caries for frequency of sugar intake, including sources of natural and added sugars.
- Newborns exhibit a preference for sweetness; thus, it is not considered an acquired taste. Although infants and young children typically select the most intensely sweet foods, the pleasure response to sweetness is observed across individuals of all ages, races, and cultures.
- A judgmental attitude or criticism by the dental hygienist is not beneficial in modifying a patient's use of carbohydrates or sugars.
- All caloric sugars and starches, whether they are naturally occurring in foods or added to foods, have some cariogenic effect.

NUTRITIONAL DIRECTIONS

- Sugar alcohols are not fermented alcohols and do not need to be restricted by individuals suffering with alcoholism.
- All disaccharides contain the same caloric and nutrient content. The body cannot distinguish between natural honey, refined table sugar, or HFCS; absorption and metabolism are similar to their component sugars.
- Encourage use of hard candies and chewing gum containing sugar alcohols (xylitol and sorbitol) to prevent caries. However, inform patients that using more than three to four pieces of sugar alcohol–containing items daily may cause gastrointestinal distress.

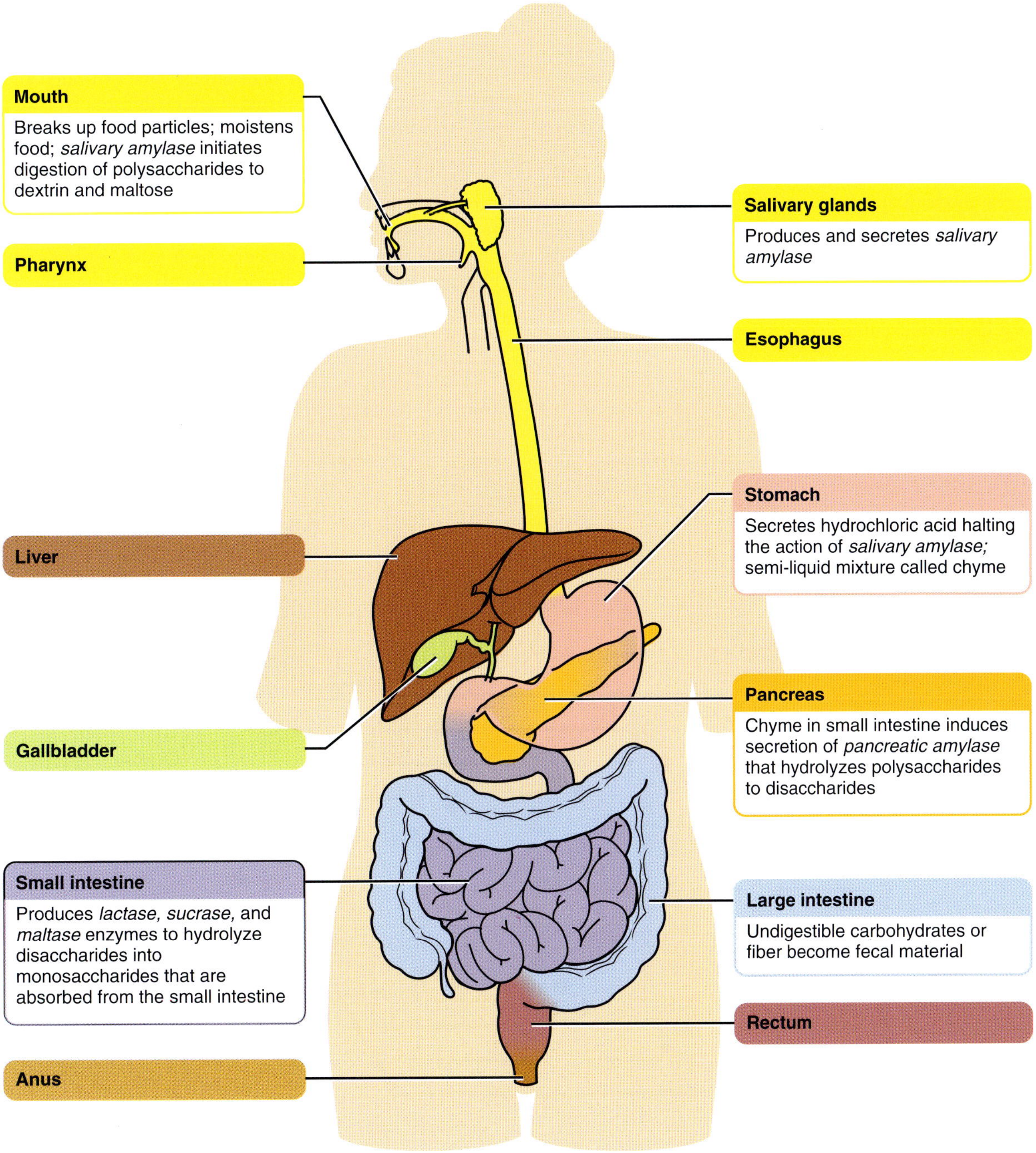
Mouth
Breaks up food particles; moistens food; *salivary amylase* initiates digestion of polysaccharides to dextrin and maltose
Pharynx
Liver
Gallbladder
Small intestine
Produces *lactase, sucrase,* and *maltase* enzymes to hydrolyze disaccharides into monosaccharides that are absorbed from the small intestine
Anus
Salivary glands
Produces and secretes *salivary amylase*
Esophagus
Stomach
Secretes hydrochloric acid halting the action of *salivary amylase;* semi-liquid mixture called chyme
Pancreas
Chyme in small intestine induces secretion of *pancreatic amylase* that hydrolyzes polysaccharides to disaccharides
Large intestine
Undigestible carbohydrates or fiber become fecal material
Rectum

• **Figure 4.2** Summary of carbohydrate digestion. Note: enzymes are in *italics*.

Polysaccharides or Complex Carbohydrates

Complex carbohydrates, also called polysaccharides, contain more than 10 monosaccharides (see Fig. 2.7). Some polysaccharides have a role in energy storage and are digestible. Dietary fiber is largely indigestible by intestinal enzymes in humans.

Starch

Starches are composed of many long-chain or branched glucose units. Most food sources of complex carbohydrates are in the form of starch from cereal grains, roots, vegetables, and legumes. The amount of starch present in a vegetable increases with its maturity. For example, corn tastes much sweeter immediately after it is picked than it does several days later because the simple sugars in corn have not developed into starch. In contrast, the amount of starch in fruit decreases as it ripens—that is, complex carbohydrates are broken down during the ripening process into simple sugars. In digestion, complex carbohydrates are broken down into **dextrin** (long glucose chains) molecules until the end product, glucose, is absorbed (Fig. 4.3).

A cell wall, or cellulose, surrounding the starch granule causes starch to be insoluble in cold water. Cellulose is composed of long, straight chains of glucose units attached in a very strong bonding to provide great mechanical strength with limited flexibility. Cooking facilitates digestion by causing granules to swell, rupturing the cell wall so that digestive enzymes have access to the starch inside the cell. In cooking, this swelling is referred to as thickening, as occurs in making gravy. Industrially, food starch is modified by chemicals to produce a better thickening agent.

Glucose Polymers

Industrially produced carbohydrate supplements are composed of glucose, maltose, and dextrins. Dextrins are intermediate products of digestive enzymes on starch molecules or long glucose chains split into shorter ones. In the process of toasting bread, dextrins are produced. Consistent with other carbohydrate products, glucose polymers provide energy equivalent to 4 cal/g.

Glycogen

Glycogen is the carbohydrate storage form of energy in humans (see Fig. 2.7). Stored in the muscle and liver, glycogen is readily available as a source of glucose and energy. Carbohydrates are frequently consumed in excess of immediate energy needs. Excess glucose is converted to glycogen until the limited glycogen storage capacity is filled; simultaneously, glucose is converted into fats and stored as adipose tissue. The total amount of glycogen stores is relatively small, only enough to meet energy demands for less than a day.

Dietary Fiber

Fiber refers to nondigestible components of food that nevertheless have desirable health effects. **Nondigestible** means that enzymes in the human gastrointestinal tract cannot digest and absorb the substance; plant cells remain largely intact through the digestive process. **Dietary fiber** consists of several different types of nondigestible carbohydrates and lignin that occur naturally in plants (thus, grains, fruits, and vegetables are good sources of fiber).

Dietary fiber includes polysaccharides, lignin, and associated substances in plants, such as whole grains, legumes, vegetables, fruits, seeds, and nuts (Table 4.2). Sources of dietary fiber usually contain other macronutrients, such as digestible carbohydrates and protein, normally found in foods. During food processing, many added compounds have the same physiologic effect as naturally occurring fiber but may not have other health benefits, such as vitamins and minerals.

Soluble dietary fibers become viscous (sticky, thick) in solution. Insoluble dietary fibers, or the structural part of the plant, do not dissolve in fluids. Insoluble and soluble fibers have different physiologic functions in the body.

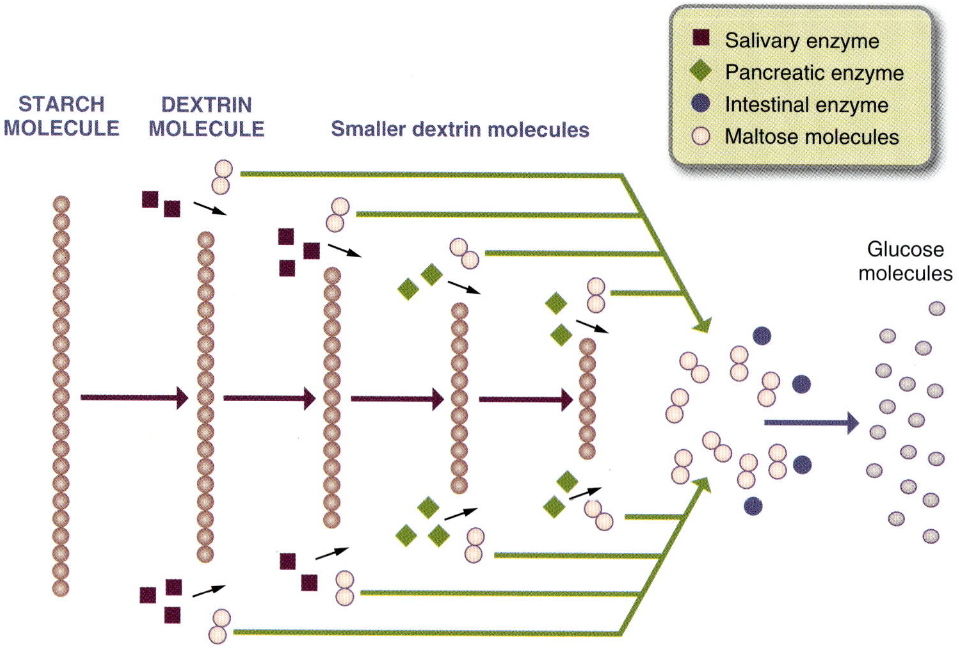

• **Figure 4.3** The gradual breakdown of large starch molecules into glucose by digestion enzymes. (Reproduced with permission from Mahan LK, Escott-Stump S, Raymond JL. *Krause's Food and the Nutrition Care Process*. 14th ed. St Louis: Saunders Elsevier; 2017.)

TABLE 4.2 Synopsis of Dietary Fibers

Type of Fiber	Dietary Fiber Sources	Physiologic Effects
Insoluble Fiber		
Cellulose and hemicellulose	Whole grains, bran, plant foods (stalks and leaves of vegetables); dried beans	Laxation (increases fecal volume and decreases gut transit time); beneficial effect on serum cholesterol levels
Lignin (noncarbohydrate)	Fruits with edible seeds (strawberries, flaxseeds) mature vegetables (broccoli stems)	Antioxidant; beneficial effect on serum cholesterol levels; fermentation produces short-chain fatty acids, thus functioning as a prebiotic; binds with minerals (calcium, iron, and zinc), which are then excreted
Soluble Fiber		
Gums	Oats, dried beans, legumes, barley, guar	Beneficial effect on blood glucose and serum lipids; aids satiety
Mucilages (psyllium)	Psyllium seeds, high-fiber cereals	Laxation (increases fecal volume and decreases gut transit time); binds water; beneficial effect on blood glucose and serum lipids; aids satiety
Pectin	Plant foods (apples, citrus fruits, berries, carrots)	Beneficial effect on serum cholesterol levels

Resistant starch is a form of dietary fiber that cannot be digested. It delivers some of the health benefits of soluble and insoluble fibers. Resistant starches are not absorbed; thus, they function as a prebiotic by providing fatty acids for bacteria in the colon. Resistant starches trap water and add bulk to the stool, helping with regularity.

Fiber added during the manufacturing process is called **functional fiber.** Functional fiber consists of isolated, nondigestible carbohydrates that have beneficial physiologic effects in humans. Various types of fiber from carbohydrate sources are added in the manufacturing process because of their functional properties, such as thickening or emulsifying. Many of these substances, including carrageenan and guar gum, are common food additives.

Total fiber is the sum of dietary fiber and functional (added) fiber. Many fibers can be classified either as dietary fiber or functional fiber depending on whether they are a natural component of the food or added to the food during processing. Plant-based foods are a good source of dietary fiber, but commercially developed functional fibers for use in processed foods also have a beneficial role in health. Various types of fibers have distinct properties resulting in different physiologic effects (see Table 4.2). The Nutrition Facts label reflects naturally occurring dietary fiber and added isolated or synthetic fibers the Food and Drug Administration has determined have a beneficial physiologic effect on health (beta-glucans soluble fiber, psyllium husk, cellulose, guar gum, pectin, locust bean gum, and hydroxypropylmethylcellulose).

Physiologic Roles

Energy

The principal role of absorbed sugars is to provide a source of energy for body functions and activity and for heat to maintain body temperature. Glucose is the preferred source of energy for the brain and central nervous system, red blood cells, and lens of the eye. When carbohydrate intake is restricted, fat and protein stores may be used as an energy source. Although many organs can use fats for energy, glucose is the preferred fuel. A carbohydrate, whether it was originally from a sugar or a starch, provides 4 cal/g. Because of incomplete absorption, sugar alcohols contribute varying amounts of calories (see Table 4.1). Glycogen stores are a readily available source of glucose for tissues.

Fat Storage

Sugars in the blood ensure replenishing of glycogen stores; however, excessive intake of energy from any source results in converting glucose to fats in a process known as **lipogenesis**. When carbohydrates are eaten in excess of needs, lipogenesis results in increased fat stores.

Conversion to Other Carbohydrates

Monosaccharides are important constituents of many compounds that regulate metabolism. Examples include heparin, which prevents blood clotting; galactolipins, which are constituents of nervous tissue; and dermatan sulfate, present in tissues rich in collagen (especially skin).

Conversion to Amino Acids

The liver can use part of the carbon framework from the sugar molecule and part of a protein molecule contributed by the breakdown of an amino acid to produce nonessential amino acids. These are physiologically essential but are not required in the diet.

Normal Fat Metabolism

Oxidation of fats requires the presence of some carbohydrates. When carbohydrate intake is low, the body relies on energy from fat intake or stores. As detailed in Chapter 2, when fats are metabolized faster than the body can oxidize them, intermediate products, called ketone bodies, may accumulate. Ketones are normal products of lipid metabolism in the liver; muscles can use ketones for energy only if adequate amounts of glucose are available. An accumulation of ketones in the blood, or incompletely oxidized fatty products, results in **ketosis**.

Protein Sparers

Carbohydrates, by furnishing energy in the diet, are said to be protein sparing. Energy is an essential physiologic requirement. With insufficient carbohydrate intake, the body burns protein for fuel. If carbohydrate intake is adequate, protein can be used to build and repair tissue.

Intestinal Bacteria

Dietary fiber remains in the gastrointestinal tract longer than other nutrients. Undigestible fibers—such as lignin, cellulose, and hemicellulose—may be fermented by microflora in the large intestine. Fermentation produces gas and volatile fatty acids; cells lining the colon use these fatty acids for energy. Undigestible fiber functions as a prebiotic by encouraging growth of bacteria that synthesize some of the B-complex vitamins and vitamin K.

Gastrointestinal Motility

Dietary and certain functional fibers, particularly those that are poorly fermented, improve fecal bulk and laxation, ameliorate constipation, and perform various other functions (see Table 4.2). Dietary fiber and functional fibers *accelerate* transit rate (the time it takes for waste products to move through the intestine) in individuals with a slow transit time (constipation). Soluble fiber *decreases* transit rate in individuals with a rapid transit time (diarrhea). The ability of fiber to bind water in the intestine and increase bulk from nondigestible substances decreases the length of time waste products are in the alimentary tract. An increased transit time lengthens the duration of tissue exposure to cancer-causing nitrogenous waste products.

An added benefit of fiber is its stool-softening ability, which helps prevent constipation. Fiber in the colon increases stool bulk, exercising digestive tract muscles by increasing the radius of the colon and preventing the muscle from being chronically contracted. As muscle tone is maintained and colonic pressure declines, the gut is able to resist bulging out into pouches known as diverticula (Fig. 4.4).

Soluble dietary fibers include pectins, gums, psyllium, mucilages, and algal polysaccharides; they influence the physiology of the upper gastrointestinal tract. Soluble fibers are physiologically important for their gel-forming ability, resulting in increased viscosity of chyme and delayed gastric emptying. They bind bile acids, decrease serum cholesterol levels, and may improve glucose tolerance. Physiologic benefits of dietary fiber are listed in Box 4.1.

Fiber-rich foods are not energy dense and are retained longer in the stomach. They may cause one to feel full on a fewer number of calories. Whether fiber plays a significant role in weight management has yet to be determined.

Other Nutrients

Carbohydrates are normally accompanied by other nutrients. Starchy foods are especially important for their contribution of protein, minerals, and B vitamins. Whole-grain products are superior because they contain fiber plus other nutrients (see Table 1.5); enriched products should always be used in preference to products that are processed but not enriched.

• BOX 4.1 Benefits of a High Dietary Fiber Diet

1. Digested slowly
2. Reduced mortality rate
3. Helps reduce risk of type 2 diabetes
4. Helps control weight
5. May protect against metabolic syndrome
6. Reduced risk of cardiovascular disease—lower cholesterol levels and blood pressure, and stroke
7. Reduced risk of cancer

Data from Zong G, Gao A, Hu FB, Sun Q. Whole grain intake and mortality from all causes, cardiovascular disease, and cancer. A meta-analysis of prospective cohort studies. Circulation. 2016;133:2370–2380; Aune D, Keum N, Giovannucci E, et al. Whole grain consumption and risk of cardiovascular disease, cancer, and all cause and cause specific mortality: systematic review and dose–response meta-analysis of prospective studies. BMJ. *2016;353:i2716; Chen GC, Tong X, Xu JY, et al. Whole-grain intake and total, cardiovascular, and cancer mortality: a systematic review and meta-analysis of prospective studies. Am J Clin Nutr 2016;104(1):164–172.*

DENTAL CONSIDERATIONS

- Carbohydrate metabolism requires an adequate supply of B vitamins, phosphorus, and magnesium. Usually, adequate amounts of these nutrients accompany carbohydrate intake. However, this may not be true if refined sugars and breads are predominantly chosen.
- Ketosis can occur in patients with uncontrolled diabetes or in individuals who have inadequate carbohydrate intake, such as those who are ill or are following a high-protein, very-low-carbohydrate regimen because they are burning fat rather than carbohydrate. Among other concerns, ketosis creates a disturbance in the patient's acid–base balance. Question patients with acetone or fruity-smelling breath about their recent dietary intake.
- Increasing dietary fiber may reduce risk of gingivitis and periodontal disease.[5,6]
- Table 4.3 provides guidelines for assisting patients in increasing dietary fiber.
- Some fibers added to foods by manufacturers have not been proven beneficial to human health and cannot be included in the total amount of dietary fiber on the Nutrition Facts label.
- Concerns are not about consumption of individual types of sugar but rather about overconsumption of added sugar. Recommendations should focus on choosing nutrient-dense foods.
- Increasing dietary fiber without increasing total energy intake may lead to improvements in gastrointestinal health and blood pressure, reduced body fat stores, and lower risk of cardiovascular disease (CVD) and type 2 diabetes.[7,8]

NUTRITIONAL DIRECTIONS

- Fiber tends to regulate the transit rate of foods in the gastrointestinal tract. The best source of dietary fiber to relieve constipation is bran, but it must be initiated slowly to avoid severe gas and bloating.
- An excessive amount of bran (50–60 g) yields negative benefits, such as diarrhea and decreased mineral and vitamin absorption.
- Some vegetables and fruits (e.g., bananas, white potatoes, and apples) are high in pectin, which binds water. They are frequently used to control diarrhea but also can help relieve constipation by softening the stool.
- Even when an individual strives to reduce caloric intake, carbohydrates are important, especially vegetables, fruits, and whole-grain breads and cereals, to provide vital nutrients.
- Carbohydrates supply 4 cal/g of energy and are a less-concentrated source of energy than fats (9 cal/g).

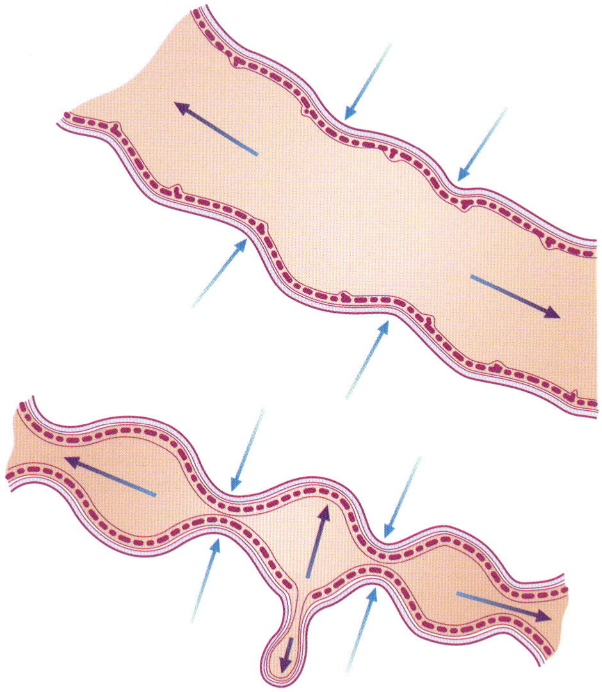

• **Figure 4.4** Mechanism by which low-fiber, low-bulk diets might generate diverticula. Where colon contents are bulk (*top*), muscular contractions exert pressure longitudinally. If lumen is smaller (*bottom*), contractions can produce occlusion and exert pressure against the colon wall, which may produce a diverticular "blowout." (Reproduced with permission from Peckenpaugh NJ. *Nutrition Essentials and Diet Therapy*, 11th ed. St Louis, MO: Saunders Elsevier; 2010.)

Requirements

The acceptable macronutrient distribution range (AMDR) for carbohydrates is based on providing energy for the body, particularly brain cells. The brain is the only organ that requires glucose. The AMDR for digestible carbohydrates is 130 g per day for adults and children (see p. iii). Generally, men typically consume 200 to 330 g per day and women consume 180 to 230 g per day to meet energy requirements without exceeding acceptable levels of fat and protein. Research studies do not indicate a requirement for a specific amount of starch or sugar.

The AMDR for carbohydrates is limited to no less than 45% (to prevent excess fat intake) and no more than 65% (to ensure required nutrients from protein and fats that also provide essential micronutrients). The American diet currently furnishes approximately 50% of the calories from carbohydrates. The dietary reference intakes compiled by the National Academy of Medicine (formerly the Institute of Medicine) suggest a maximum intake of 25% or less of energy from added sugars.

As discussed in Chapter 1, the *Dietary Guidelines* recommend less than 10% of total calories for the day from added sugars. This is not due to scientific evidence that sweeteners contribute to chronic diseases but rather to meet nutrient needs within caloric limits. For most individuals, after consuming the appropriate amounts of foods from all the food groups, less than 20% of their daily calories is available for added sugars and fats. For an individual consuming 2000 cal per day, the maximum amount of added sugars, or 10% of total caloric intake, would be 11 tsp of added sugars (200 cal). The American diet contains approximately 12% of total calories from added sugars.[9] As shown in Fig. 4.1, there

TABLE 4.3 Guidelines for Developing a High-Fiber Diet

Principles	Guidelines
Before recommending any changes, evaluate the patient's fiber and fluid intake. For patients ≤ 50 years old, the recommended level of dietary fiber is 38 g for men and 25 g for women; for patients ≥ 51 years old, the optimal level of dietary fiber is 30 g for men and 21 g for women.	Fiber normalizes bowel movements to once or twice a day by moderating the transit rate of food through the gastrointestinal tract. Cooking and freezing only slightly decrease fiber content; vegetables (e.g., mushrooms, peppers, onions, tomatoes) can be added to various dishes (meatloaf, spaghetti, chili, omelets, or scrambled eggs). Grinding or pureeing foods (as in smoothies) significantly decreases fiber content.
Foods containing soluble and insoluble fibers are the preferred way to increase fiber rather than fiber supplements.	Recommend choosing a rainbow of colorful foods: 2–4 servings daily of fruits, especially those with skins and edible seeds 3–5 servings of vegetables daily Combine raw vegetables with low-fat dip as appetizers or snacks, and include in brown-bag lunches. Add leafy greens, tomatoes, bell peppers, and cucumbers to sandwiches. Substitute fresh fruits and vegetables or plain popcorn for fried chips and cookies. Incorporate beans into soups, casseroles, nachos, or salads. Experiment with brown rice, rye flour, barley, buckwheat, millet, whole-wheat pasta, and bulgur. Ancient grains such as quinoa, teff, and farro may not be enriched.
Adequate fluids are important to keep the intestinal contents moving because fiber absorbs water in the intestines.	Ensure intake of 10–12 cups of decaffeinated fluids a day to avoid problems such as fecal impactions.
Increase high-fiber foods gradually. Begin with 5- to 10-g increments to avoid adverse side effects. At least 6–8 weeks should be allowed for adaptation to prevent flatulence, abdominal cramping, and diarrhea/constipation.	Dietary fiber comes principally from whole-grain products. Choose breads and cereals with at least 2 g of fiber (5 g is ideal), but no more than 2 g of fat per serving. Add bran, bran flakes, wheat germ, chopped nuts, seeds, or oatmeal to mixed meat dishes, casseroles, salads, cooked cereal, cookies, breads, muffins, and pancake batter or for a crispy coating on meats or fish.
Increase intake of oat bran, beans, barley, and psyllium to help reduce cholesterol levels.	Use dried beans and peas as the main dish (in place of meat) at least once a week along with an overall low-fat diet.

has been a sustained downward trend in added sugar intake, resulting in an average of 3300 cal per day. Higher intake of added sugars is associated with various sociodemographic and behavioral characteristics (younger age, less education, lower income, less physically active, and smokers).[10]

The comprehensive report by the World Health Organization (WHO) on nutrition recommends limiting added sugar intake to less than 10% of total energy intake (e.g., 12 tsp of added sugars for 2200 cal).[11] They further recommended that a reduction below 5% (or roughly 25 g [6 tsp] per day) would provide additional health benefits. The WHO decision was based on economic, social, and political issues—not on scientific evidence—to prevent and control chronic health problems, especially obesity.

Adequate total fiber intake is 14 g per 1000 cal per day, or 38 g for men and 25 g for women daily. That calculation is based on the amount needed to prevent CVD. Dietary fiber intake has remained relatively stable despite efforts to encourage consumers to increase intake and a significant increase of whole-grain products on the market. More than 90% of adults and children fall short of meeting daily fiber recommendations, yet approximately 60% meet daily intake goals for total grain intake, and only 8% consume the recommended amount of whole grains (Fig. 4.5).[12] Mean dietary fiber intake was 16 g per day for 2009 to 2010 and 15.9 g per day for 2007 to 2008.[13] Determining total dietary fiber intake is tedious, since the fruit and vegetable groups along with foods from the grains group contribute to total fiber intake.

Sources

Carbohydrates are furnished by the following food groups: milk, grain, fruits, and vegetables. The only animal foods supplying significant quantities of carbohydrate are milk and milk products, which contain the disaccharide lactose. In cheese making, lactose is removed as a by-product. Consequently, most cheeses contain only trace amounts of lactose.

Other sugars are furnished from table sugar, syrups, jellies, jams, and honey. Sugars are incorporated into many popular foods (e.g., candy, beverages, cakes and desserts, chewing gum, and ice cream). Only about 25% of the sugar that Americans consume is added to foods in homes, institutions, and restaurants. The remainder is added to foods during processing, for example, canning; freezing; breakfast cereals; condiments and salad dressings; SSBs; cookies, crackers, and candies; flavored extracts and syrups; flour and bread products; and milk and dairy products.

Approximately 18% of caloric intake is from naturally occurring sugars in fruits and vegetables. (This amount does not include sugar in milk.) Sugars, mainly glucose and fructose, are furnished by fruits and vegetables in varying amounts that depend on their maturity (ripe bananas contain more simple sugars than green bananas) and their water content (spinach contains less carbohydrate than potatoes).

Because there is no physiologic requirement for added sugars, *MyPlate* does not include a separate section for sugars; added sugars are included in the discretionary calories. Eating sugar in moderation implies a proper balance among foods and nutrients, which should be the primary consideration in food selection. Eating lower amounts does not necessarily guarantee that a diet meets nutritional requirements nor does high sugar consumption mean a poorer-quality diet.

Complex carbohydrates, or starches, are furnished by grain products (wheat, corn, rice, oats, rye, barley, buckwheat, and millet). Some vegetables, especially root and seed varieties (potatoes, sweet

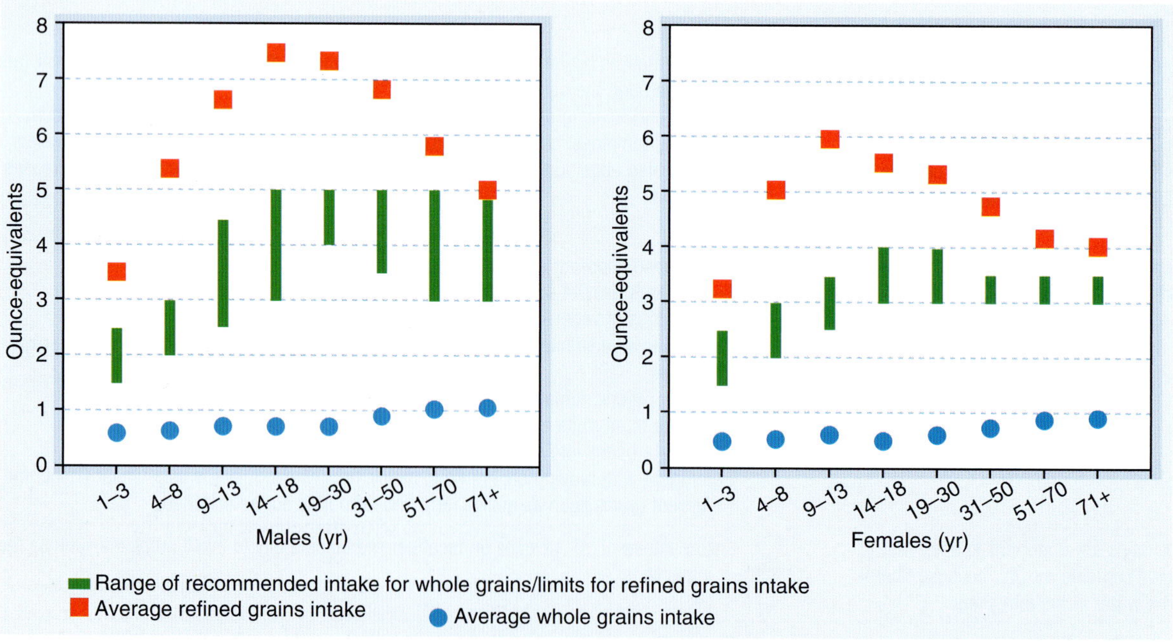

• **Figure 4.5** Average whole and refined grain intakes in ounce-equivalents per day by age-sex groups, compared to ranges of Recommended Daily Intake for whole grains and limits for refined grains* (Data Sources: What We Eat in America, National Health and Nutrition Examination Survey 2007–2010 for average intakes by age-sex group. Healthy U.S.-Style Food Patterns, which vary based on age, sex, and activity level, for recommended intake ranges. From US Department of Health and Human Services and U.S. Department of Agriculture. *2015–2020 Dietary Guidelines for Americans*. 8th ed. December 2015. http://health.gov/dietaryguidelines/2015/guidelines/.)

potatoes, beets, peas, and winter squashes), also contain considerable amounts of starch. Legumes, or dried beans and peas, are excellent sources of complex carbohydrates. Table 4.4 shows the complex carbohydrate and sugar content of the sample menu from Fig. 1.4 in Chapter 1.

Some dietary fiber, especially hemicellulose and cellulose and other indigestible compounds, is furnished by whole-grain breads and cereals and legumes. Cellulose is found principally in the stems, roots, leaves, and seed coverings of plants; unpeeled fruits and leafy vegetables are good sources. Legumes are also a good source of dietary fiber (see Table 4.2). The pectin contributed by fruits and vegetables is an important source of soluble fiber. A popular American snack food, popcorn (preferably without butter and salt), is also a whole-grain food. Table 4.4 lists the fiber content of foods in the sample menu from Fig. 1.4.

The fiber in whole grains provides important contributions to health (see Box 4.1). Consumers equate whole-grain label statements with claims about fiber content and choose products containing whole grains, expecting to increase fiber intake. The fiber content of foods claiming "whole grain" varies significantly and is very low (< 3 g) in many cases. "Made with whole grains" may contain principally refined flour with a small amount of whole grain. A product containing less than 3 g dietary fiber cannot be considered a "good" source of fiber. A product listing "whole grains" first in the ingredient list would be a healthful choice. This consumer confusion is likely caused by unclear and inconsistent labeling for whole-grain–containing products, the need for a universally accepted definition of whole-grain foods, and lack of consumer education encouraging label reading (Box 4.2).

DENTAL CONSIDERATIONS

- Assess total sugar intake and frequency, form, and time of day for carbohydrate intake (see Chapter 18).
- The number of teaspoons of sugar in a food product can be determined from the label (see Fig. 1.8). Four grams of sugar is equivalent to 1 level teaspoon of sugar. A product containing 16 g of sugar is 4 tsp of sugar. Measuring the number of teaspoons of sugar in a product is a valuable visual aid for patients.
- To determine the percentage of sugar in a serving of a food, (a) multiply the number of grams of added sugar in a product by 4 (cal/g), (b) divide this number by the total number of calories per serving, and (c) multiply by 100 to establish the percentage of calories as sugar. Using the example of the label shown in Fig. 1.8:

$$10 \text{ g sugar} \times 4 \frac{\text{cal}}{\text{g}} = 40 \text{ cal from sugar}$$

$$\frac{40 \text{ cal sugar}}{230 \text{ cal/serving}} = 0.17 \times 100\% = 17\%$$

- Fiber helps reduce constipation, diverticulosis, heart disease, and the risk of some cancers (see Table 4.3 for ideas to enhance fiber intake).
- A diet with adequate amounts of carbohydrate helps to maintain glycogen reserves, while a diet high in fat and very low in carbohydrate results in poor glycogen reserves. Glycogen stores in the heart are critical for continuous functioning of the heart muscle.
- Sugar increases palatability and may improve choices of certain foods otherwise disliked. Combining sugar with other nutritious foods, as in milk used for pudding, may increase the variety of foods consumed and enjoyed.

• BOX 4.2 Tips for Following the *Dietary Guidelines* for Carbohydrates

- Be aware of the amount of sugars in processed foods. Sugar may be identified as any of the following on food labels: sucrose, fructose, corn sweetener, cane sugar, evaporated cane juice, honey, molasses, high-fructose corn syrup, raw sugar, and maple syrup. Try to avoid foods if one of these is the first ingredient listed.
- Choose water and other beverages that contain little or no added sweeteners.
- Pay attention to nutrition labels, not only for the amount of added sugars but also for the amount of fiber in a serving. Because fiber is not absorbed, it does not contribute any calories. A product with 25 g of carbohydrate may have only 80 cal if at least 5 g of the carbohydrate is from fiber.
- Choose fruits in place of foods with added sugars.
- Look for breads and cereals that list "whole grain" or "whole wheat" first in the ingredients list. A more promising sign is "100% whole grain." Brown color is no guarantee of whole-grain content.
- Popular whole-grain foods include black, brown, and wild rice; whole wheat, corn, barley, buckwheat, millet, oats, quinoa, rye, sorghum, and spelt. Many of the ancient grains, becoming more popular, are also whole-grain foods.
- Balance caloric intake to achieve an appropriate weight.
- Choose nutrient-dense foods to provide adequate amounts of required nutrients.

NUTRITIONAL DIRECTIONS

- A tablespoon of honey has more calories than a tablespoon of sugar and only trace amounts of other nutrients. (Honey is not appropriate for children younger than 1 year old because of the risk of botulism.) Its retentive nature makes honey more cariogenic than refined sugar.
- Encourage patients to adhere to the *Dietary Guidelines* by discussing information from Box 4.2.

Hyperstates and Hypostates

The role of carbohydrates in nutritional health and behavior continues to be misrepresented by the press and some professionals. Many stories published in the media link sugar to practically every modern-day illness, including malnutrition, hypoglycemia, diabetes mellitus, blood lipid abnormalities, hyperactivity, criminal behavior, obesity, malabsorption syndrome, allergies, gallstones, and cancer. The public's perception of sugar consumption continues to be at odds with scientific facts.

Normal physiologic conditions and disease states affect carbohydrate metabolism, which is reflected in serum glucose levels. For individuals with diabetes, a blood glucose level that is greater than 130 mg/dL before meals or greater than 180 mg/dL 2 hours after meals indicates **hyperglycemia**; a blood glucose level less than 70 mg/dL indicates **hypoglycemia**.[14] Other factors concerning too much or too little carbohydrate are discussed later.

Carbohydrate Excess

As previously mentioned, there has been quite a bit of controversy regarding how much carbohydrate (mainly sucrose) is excessive. The preponderance of evidence based on scientific literature indicates

TABLE 4.4 Carbohydrate, Dietary Fiber, and Added Sugars Content of the Sample Menu

Sample Menu	Carbohydrate (g)	Dietary Fiber (g)	Added Sugars (g)
Breakfast			
1½ c Frosted Mini-Wheat cereal	67	9	14
12 oz skim milk	18	0	0
12 oz black coffee	0	0	0
Mid-Morning Snack			
12 oz water	0	0	0
1 oz dry roasted almonds, unsalted	6	3	0
1 medium orange	15	3	0
Lunch			
Sandwich with			
1 c tuna salad with egg, low-calorie mayonnaise	17	1	6
¼ c thin-sliced cucumber	1	0	0
3 thin slices tomato	1	0	0
2 medium lettuce leaves	0	0	0
2 thin slices 100% wheat bread	20	3	2
8 baby carrots	6	2	0
1 medium applesauce cookie	9	0	3
1 cup grapes	27	1	0
12 oz water	0	0	0
Mid-Afternoon Snack			
8 oz low-fat vanilla yogurt	31	0	15
12 oz herbal tea with nonnutritive sweetener	1	0	0
Dinner			
3 oz pot roast beef with	0	0	0
¼ c sauteed mushrooms	2	1	0
1 c white and wild rice blend with margarine	35	1	0
½ c vegetable juice	2	0	0
2 c tossed salad with lettuce, avocado, tomatoes, and carrots	3	1	0
¼ c shredded low-fat Muenster cheese	1	0	0
2 tbsp vinaigrette salad dressing	4	0	3
⅛ medium cantaloupe	6	1	0
12 oz iced tea with low-calorie sweetener	1	0	0
Evening Snack			
3 c low-fat microwave popcorn	16	3	0
12 oz water	0	0	0
TOTALS[a]	289	29	43

[a]Totals may vary due to rounding.
From nutrient data SuperTracker. https://www.supertracker.usda.gov/default.aspx. Accessed April 17, 2017.

that sugar consumption at the level recommended in the *Dietary Guidelines* does not directly contribute to any chronic health or behavioral problems. Avoiding excessive amounts of calories from sugars is prudent, but the scientific basis for optimal levels for preventing and controlling chronic diseases remains unsettled.[15] Excessive sugar consumption leading to energy imbalance may contribute to weight gain. Added sugars (> 25% of total energy) may result in an inadequate intake of foods containing necessary micronutrients. Intake of nutrients at most risk for inadequacy (vitamins A, D, E, and C, and magnesium, potassium, dietary fiber, choline, and calcium) decrease as added sugars increase above 5% to 10% of total calories. But the predominant issue is the low-quality and overall high-energy intake of United States diets, regardless of sweetener content. Weight gain occurs resulting from excess caloric intake, not physiologic or metabolic consequences of sucrose or any specific sugar. Americans need to reduce added sugar intake, but the average amount of 13% of total calories per day in the United States is not above the level presumed by the National Academy of Medicine to be inadequate or to contribute to chronic diseases if total energy intake is appropriate (Fig. 4.6).

A principle concern in the *Dietary Guidelines* is consumption of adequate amounts of vitamins and minerals without consuming excess energy. Sweeteners contain no other nutrients (vitamins or minerals) and, when consumed as SSBs and hard candies, provide nothing other than pleasure and energy. Consumers are drinking enormous amounts of calories in liquid form. As shown in Fig. 4.7, SSBs, fruit drinks with added sugar, and sports and energy drinks contribute 39% of all sugar intake. On a positive note, soft drink consumption has been declining recently from about 53 gallons per capita in 1998 to approximately 40.6 gallons in 2015.[16,17]

Obesity

A common misperception is that sugar is uniquely fattening. Because the taste of sugar is so pleasant, some rationalize that sugar becomes irresistible to the point of overconsumption or addiction. However, most individuals have a limit as to how sweet they prefer their foods and how much they can consume in a given period.

Four leading scientific and health organizations—the Food and Agriculture Organization, WHO, the National Academy of Medicine, and the Academy of Nutrition and Dietetics—have all concluded that dietary sugars are not associated with causing illness or chronic diseases, including obesity. The evidence available to date continues to show no direct connection between total sugar intake and obesity.[18] Current findings indicate that food energy density and pleasures derived from eating promote excessive energy intake.[15,18]

Some studies indicate an association between higher intake of whole grains (minimum of three servings daily) with healthier body weights and fat stores. However, data from National Health and Nutritional Examination Surveys found no correlation between whole-grain intake and body mass index, but whole grains were related to positive nutrient profiles and chronic disease risk factors. The *Dietary Guidelines* recommend a fiber-rich diet to help in the management of obesity as it provides bulk, which may help with satiety while reducing calories consumed.

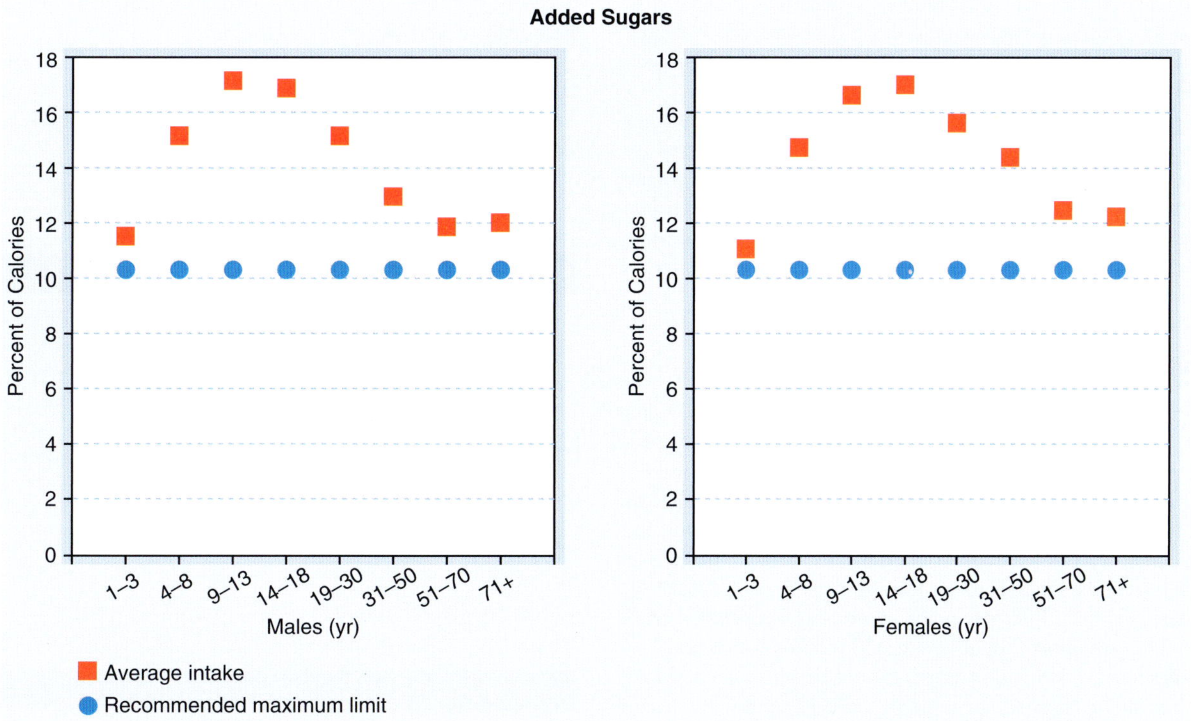

• **Figure 4.6** Average intakes of added sugars as a percent of calories per day by age-sex group, in comparison to the *Dietary Guidelines* maximum limit of less than 10% of calories. (Data Source: What We Eat in America, National Health and Nutrition Examination Survey 2007–2010 for average intakes by age-sex group. From U.S. Department of Health and Human Services and US Department of Agriculture. *2015–2020 Dietary Guidelines for Americans*. 8th ed. December 2015. http://health.gov/dietaryguidelines/2015/guidelines/)

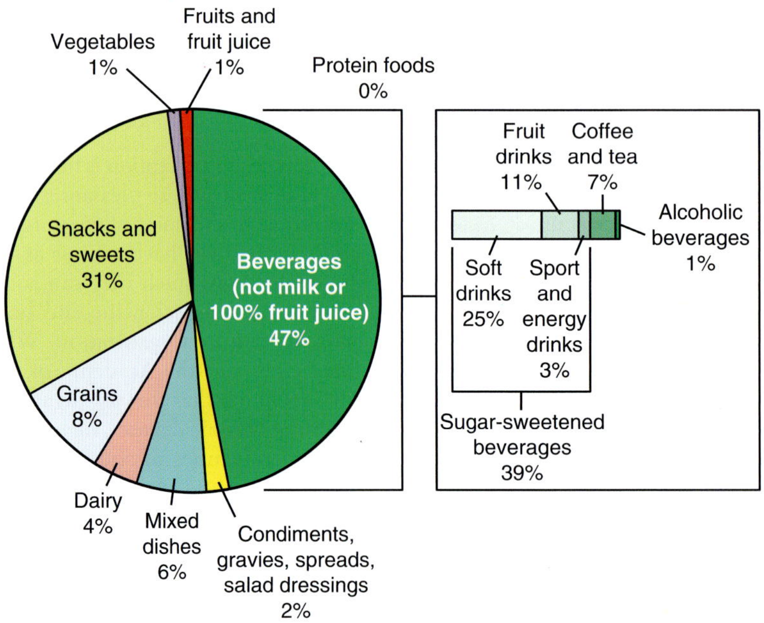

• **Figure 4.7** Food category sources of added sugars in the U.S. population ages 2 years and older. (Data Source: What We Eat in America (WWEIA) Food Category analyses for the 2015 Dietary Guidelines Advisory Committee. Estimates based on day 1 dietary recalls from WWEIA, National Health and Nutrition Examination Survey 2009–2010.)

Excessive caloric intake leads to obesity, whether from carbohydrates, proteins, fats, or alcohol. Although excessive energy intake from sugar may lead to obesity, epidemiologic studies and several studies have shown that obese patients actually consume less sugar than thin patients. Many sweet foods contain large amounts of fat. Excessive carbohydrates, including sugars, are likely to be consumed when fat is severely restricted and overall food intake is not restricted to some degree.

Altering the proportion of dietary carbohydrate is less important in weight management than the total caloric intake. Only when sugar consumption interferes with or replaces a well-balanced intake does the diet become inadequate. When that occurs, sugar warrants the designation of "empty calorie," indicating that it is inadequate in vitamins, minerals, and trace elements. Fortification of foods has a positive effect on nutrient density of the diet.

Cardiovascular Disease

The claim that sugar intake causes chronic diseases (especially diabetes and CVD) has been widely researched and continues to be controversial. Some research studies are refuted by other well-designed studies.[15] Whereas numerous studies have found an association between diets rich in added sugars (17%–21% or more of calories) or SSBs and the onset of heart disease risk factors (hypertension, stroke, and higher triglyceride levels), the biologic mechanism underlying this association is not understood.[19,20] Other systematic reviews and controlled trials using moderate amounts of sugar have not found this correlation.[21–23] Many studies focus only on consumption of SSBs; although SSBs are the most prevalent form of sugar intake, they may not be a true reflection of an individual's total sugar intake.

Carbohydrate Deficiency

Frequently, carbohydrates are eliminated in an effort to lose weight. When carbohydrates are severely restricted, protein and fat intake usually increase. Very-high-protein, low-carbohydrate diets do not necessarily lead to greater weight loss than traditional diets, and care must be taken to prevent elevated lipid levels that may accompany higher fat intake. Extremely-low-carbohydrate diets may lead to ketosis.

When complex carbohydrates are eliminated, an insufficient intake of B vitamins, iron, and fiber may occur. Vitamins and minerals are necessary for the body to use glucose, but these nutrients do not need to be present in the same foods.

DENTAL CONSIDERATIONS

- Scientific studies do not support the claim that sugars interfere with bioavailability of vitamins, minerals, or trace nutrients, or the notion that dietary imbalances are preferentially caused by increased sugar consumption. Do not assume that because a patient is obese, increased sugar intake is the culprit.
- Scientific consensus to date shows that (a) the link between sugar intake and obesity is inconsistent, (b) sugar intake alone does not cause diabetes, and (c) sugar intake is not an independent risk factor for CVD.[15,20,23]

NUTRITIONAL DIRECTIONS

- Encourage a well-balanced diet containing adequate nutrients with appropriate amounts of fruits, vegetables, and milk and dairy products.
- Several organs depend on glucose to function. A minimal-carbohydrate, high-protein, high-fat diet may result in an inadequate intake of numerous nutrients and cognitive impairment.

Dental Caries

For many years, sucrose, the most frequently consumed form of sugar, has been considered the "archvillain" in dental caries formation. Many health professionals and consumers mistakenly believe that removing sucrose from the diet would largely eliminate dental caries. The American Dental Association (ADA) recognizes that carbohydrates provide energy required for optimal nutrition. The ADA acknowledges that "sucrose-free chewing gum (containing either xylitol only or polyol combinations) or xylitol lozenges are useful adjunct therapies for caries prevention."[24]

Sucrose and other disaccharides and monosaccharides (glucose, fructose, maltose, and lactose) have unusual biochemical properties that promote bacterial growth. The presence of sucrose and other carbohydrates in the mouth increases the volume and formation rate of plaque biofilm. Even low amounts of sucrose promote production of polysaccharides (glucans) by ***Streptococcus mutans (S. mutans)***, the bacteria that facilitate adherence of plaque biofilm to teeth. These glucans help provide a matrix, supporting communities of microorganisms collectively referred to as **plaque biofilm**. A **fermentable carbohydrate** (i.e., carbohydrates that can be metabolized by bacteria in plaque biofilm, including all sugars and cooked or processed starches) that can reduce salivary pH to less than 5.5 is referred to as being **cariogenic**.

Glucose, available from sucrose or any other carbohydrate food, can be used for energy by oral bacteria in plaque biofilm. These sugars lower the pH of plaque biofilm, hastening the dissolution of hydroxyapatite crystals of the enamel. **Dental erosion** is the chemical removal of minerals from the tooth structure that occurs when an acidic environment causes enamel to gradually dissolve. In laboratory tests, the rate that fructose and glucose lowers plaque biofilm pH is similar to sucrose; they are considered as cariogenic as sucrose. Therefore, substituting glucose or fructose for sucrose is not significantly effective in reducing caries rates. Lactose is less cariogenic than other sugars. The kind of sugar is not significant; the concentration or quantity of sugar in a foodstuff is not critical to its cariogenic potential. The total amount of fermentable carbohydrate seems to be of less importance than the form in which it is eaten and the frequency of consumption. This may be related to variables influencing the length of time that the carbohydrate is in contact with teeth and its potential for promoting growth of caries-forming, acid-producing bacteria. (See Chapter 18 for further discussion.)

SSBs and energy drinks contain fermentable carbohydrates and are highly acidic (Table 4.5). Despite differences in the carbohydrate content of SSBs, fruit drinks, 100% fruit juice (approximately 10% carbohydrates), sport drinks (approximately 46%–48% carbohydrates), energy drinks (approximately 9%–10% carbohydrates), flavored coffees and teas, and powdered drinks, all of these beverages seem to have similar cariogenic potential.

In addition to their sugar content, SSBs, fruit juices, and sport drinks are very acidic, with pH ranges below 4.0. Dental erosion can occur with frequent exposure to any liquid with a pH below 4.2. Citrus juices contain citric acid, which is especially damaging to tooth enamel; the citrate binds with calcium in saliva, reducing its potential to remineralize the tooth. Deleterious effects of 100% fruit juices can be minimized with chemical modification or calcium fortification.[25] Sour sweets and acidic products, even if they are sugar free, may increase the probability of dental erosion.[26] SSBs, acid snack/sweets and natural acidic fruit and juices increase erosion occurrence while milk and yogurt have a protective effect.[27] Research suggests the extent of enamel erosion caused by various beverages occurs in the following order (from greatest to least): energy drinks, sports drinks, regular soda, and diet soda.[28]

No definite relationship has been shown between total carbohydrate consumption and caries. Cooked starches can cause acid production in plaque biofilm due to their high retentiveness in the mouth. Some foods—such as potato chips or crackers, containing a high-carbohydrate, low-sugar content—can contribute to the caries process when salivary amylase hydrolyzes complex carbohydrate to simple sugars. Starch molecules are large and cannot penetrate into plaque biofilm. Cooked and refined cereal grains are readily hydrolyzed by salivary amylases to produce maltose, which can lower pH and demineralize enamel. Some foods high in sugar are removed more quickly and do not lower the pH of plaque biofilm as much as starchy foods with less sugar. Starches, such as breads and pasta, are considered less cariogenic than sugars, but they tend to prolong the caries attack after it has

TABLE 4.5 Drinks That Eat Teeth

Beverages	pH[a]	Sugar (tsp in 12 oz)
Lemon juice	2.00–2.60	–
Pepsi	2.49	9.8
Coke Classic	2.53	8.9
Orange juice (Minute Maid)	2.80	11.2
Mellow Yellow	2.80	10.1
Diet Cherry Coke	2.80	0
Squirt	2.85	9.5
Dr. Pepper	2.92	9.5
Gatorade	2.95	5.5
Grapefruit juice	3.00	7.4
Pepsi One	3.05	0
Fresca	3.20	0
Mountain Dew	3.22	11.0
Diet Mountain Dew	3.34	0
Diet Coke	3.39	0
Apple juice	3.40	4.8
Diet Dr. Pepper	3.41	0
Sprite	3.42	9.0
Tomato juice	4.10–4.60	0
Brewed coffee, black	5.51	0
Milk, skim	6.80	3.5
Water	7.0	0
Tea (brewed)	7.2	0

[a]Neutral pH 7. Because the pH scale is logarithmic, one unit change in pH is associated with a 10-fold change in the acidity. For example, lemon juice has a pH of 2.0, whereas grapefruit juice has a pH of 3.0; lemon juice is therefore more than 100 times as acidic as grapefruit juice.

Data from 21st Century Dental: Drinks that eat teeth. https://www.21stcentury dental.com/ph_drinks.html. Accessed November 7, 2016.

been initiated (especially when sugar is added, as in sweet breads and cookies).

Some popular snack products contain sweeteners that are less cariogenic than sucrose. Sugar alcohols may decrease the risk of dental caries through any of the following mechanisms: (a) inhibiting the growth of *S. mutans,* (b) not promoting synthesis of plaque biofilm, or (c) not lowering plaque biofilm pH. Studies evaluating evidence for an anticariogenic effect of sugar-free chewing gum concluded that it has a caries-reducing effect, but more well-designed, randomized studies are recommends to confirm the findings.[29,30] The ADA has approved the use of its seal on sugarless gums by several gum manufacturers and recommended chewing gum after each meal for at least 20 minutes to reap the most benefits if oral hygiene cannot be performed.

Sorbitol causes only a slight pH decrease in plaque biofilm. Bacteria in plaque biofilm are able to ferment sorbitol and mannitol but only at a very slow rate over several weeks. After a period of adaptation, however, acid production increases.

The anticariogenic effect of xylitol has been accepted globally, as it exhibits both passive and active anticaries effects and directly inhibits the growth of *S. mutans.*[31] An **anticariogenic** substance reduces caries risk by preventing bacteria from recognizing a cariogenic food. Oral bacteria lack the enzymes to ferment xylitol; it does not lower plaque biofilm pH. The anticariogenic effect of xylitol-containing chewing gum may be enhanced by the chewing process. Xylitol stimulates secretion of saliva, which contains a large number of bicarbonate ions to neutralize acid. Additionally, xylitol promotes remineralization of early lesions on tooth enamel.

Erythritol is another sugar alcohol that may improve oral health by decreasing adherence of bacteria to tooth surfaces, inhibiting growth and activity of *S. mutans,* and reducing the overall number of dental caries. In studies testing the efficacy of erythritol and xylitol candy, compared with sorbitol candy, fewer dental caries developed in the erythritol group than in the xylitol or control groups.[32,33]

Lactitol cannot be metabolized by bacteria in plaque biofilm and may provide a protective effect for teeth. However, it is only about one-third as sweet as sucrose. Saccharin inhibits tooth decay in rats. Aspartame does not support the growth of *S. mutans*, acid production, or plaque biofilm formation.

DENTAL CONSIDERATIONS

- Approximately 90% of commonly consumed snack foods contain fermentable carbohydrates (sugars or cooked starch or both). Frequently consumed fermentable carbohydrates include chewing gum, chewable tablets, lozenges, mints, and snack foods such as gummy bears.
- Snacks contribute significantly to the nutritional intake of young children and teenagers who need larger amounts of energy for growth.
- Patients unable to tolerate adequate amounts at meals require snacks to promote healing and avoid loss of lean tissue.
- Although sucrose is a major factor in caries risk, provide factual information without overemphasizing sugar's role in caries formation.
- Some foods—such as milk, yogurt, and aged cheese—actually protect teeth by increasing oral pH and inhibiting acid production.
- Assess patient consumption of acidic beverages. Patients with frequent consumption of acidic beverages, decreased salivary flow, prolonged holding habits, or mouth breathing may be at increased risk for dental erosion.
- Excessive intake (more than 20 g per day) of sugar alcohol-containing gum and sweets may lead to unintended weight loss as a result of chronic diarrhea. One stick of sugar-free gum contains about 1.25 g sorbitol.
- Polyol-based, sugar-free products may cause dental erosion if they contain acidic flavoring.
- The association between eating and weight status is not the result of a single eating pattern but rather is from a combination of food choices that are interrelated and cumulative in their effect.
- The most important cause of dental caries is frequency of consuming fermentable carbohydrates that supply substrate to caries-producing oral bacteria.
- The potential for caries risk exists every time a carbohydrate is eaten because most foods promote acid formation if no procedures are taken to remove food debris or plaque biofilm, to buffer the acid produced, or to interfere with acid production.
- The amount of carbohydrate in a food is unrelated to its caries-forming potential; all carbohydrate foods are potentially cariogenic. Proteins and fats are **cariostatic**, or cannot be metabolized by microorganisms in plaque biofilm, and are caries inhibiting.
- Natural sugars, primarily fructose and glucose, in unprocessed foods, such as bananas and raisins, are potentially as cariogenic as sucrose.

NUTRITIONAL DIRECTIONS

- If snacks are needed when oral hygiene cannot be performed, suggest low-fat milk products, aged cheese, or yogurt; or chew xylitol-containing gum.
- Xylitol and erythritol may cause less gastrointestinal distress than other sugar alcohols.[34]
- Complete and permanent elimination of sweets is unrealistic. The best advice is to (a) use sugar in moderation, (b) limit the frequency of sugar exposure, (c) consume sweets with a meal, and (d) brush the teeth after consuming sugar-containing products. If oral hygiene cannot be performed, chew xylitol, sorbitol, or xylitol-sorbitol chewing gum.
- Encourage patients to brush their teeth before consuming acidic foods and chew sugar-free gum as brushing their teeth afterward may increase dental erosion.
- Vegetables such as lettuce, celery, and broccoli contain a minimal amount of carbohydrate (5 g per serving) and do not cause acid production or demineralization of enamel in humans.
- Sugar alcohols are less likely to promote caries; xylitol may prevent caries formation.
- Highly acidic foods may prevent bacterial fermentation but cause enamel erosion.
- Replace potentially cariogenic snacks with foods such as fresh fruits and vegetables; low-fat cottage cheese, cheese, and yogurt (flavored with nutmeg, cinnamon, or fresh fruit); peanuts; or low-fat popcorn to decrease caries risk and promote other health-conscious nutritional habits.
- Use a straw with beverages such as carbonated drinks or lemonade to reduce contact with teeth and lessen caries risk.
- Consumption of SSBs should be limited to 8 oz or less daily with a meal.
- Complex unrefined carbohydrates are high in fiber and other nutrients.

Nonnutritive Sweeteners/Sugar Substitutes

The practice of flavoring foods without additional calories is one of many approaches to the problems of excess energy intake and a sedentary lifestyle. Nonnutritive sweeteners, also called artificial sweeteners, add sweetness but contain no or minimal carbohydrates (or energy) and do not raise blood sugars. Most are synthesized compounds from fruits, herbs, or sugar itself. The use of sugar substitutes also has beneficial ramifications for dental hygiene. The desire to decrease sugar consumption is being met through widespread and increasing use of numerous nonnutritive sweeteners. Consumption of low-caloric and noncaloric sweeteners is increasing faster than that of caloric sweeteners.[35]

Nonnutritive sweeteners are used principally for their sweetening power, making some foods more palatable. The large variety of sweeteners is desirable because each has certain advantages and limitations. Because each sweetener has different properties, the availability of various products helps satisfy various flavor and texture requirements in foods and beverages. Sweeteners may be combined because of their **synergistic** effect—that is, when combined, sweeteners yield a sweeter taste than that provided by each sweetener alone.

These sweeteners have the potential to reduce sugar and energy intakes, but Americans' BMIs have risen parallel to the rise in use of nonnutritive sweeteners. Although taste buds may be fooled by their sweetness, nonnutritive sweeteners do not produce a prolonged feeling of satiety. Concerns have been expressed that nonnutritive sweeteners may promote energy intake and contribute to obesity. The preponderance of evidence from human randomized controlled studies indicates that nonnutritive sweeteners do not increase energy intake or body weight and may even reduce intake and weight.[36,37]

Currently, data is insufficient to conclusively determine whether the use of nonnutritive sweeteners replacing caloric sweeteners reduces added sugars or carbohydrate intakes, or has an effect on appetite, energy balance, body weight, or other risk factors. Nevertheless, the American Heart Association concluded that nonnutritive sweeteners could be used in a structured diet to replace added sugars, thereby resulting in decreased total energy and weight loss/weight control, and promoting beneficial effects on related metabolic parameters.[38] Individuals who use nonnutritive sweeteners may choose a healthier eating pattern and engage in better lifestyle habits.[39]

Whether use of these nonnutritive sweeteners decreases total caloric intake depends on other food choices. Making compensatory food choices, such as drinking a diet carbonated beverage to permit a piece of cheesecake, is ineffective in weight control, whereas replacing a high-calorie food with a low-calorie food, watching other food intake, and engaging in some form of exercise may be beneficial.

Many consumers question the safety of these products. All products on the market have been extensively researched and are safe for most people if consumed in moderation except for aspartame. Aspartame is safe in moderate amounts for everyone except individuals who have **phenylketonuria**, a genetic disorder characterized by an inability to metabolize the amino acid phenylalanine. Table 4.6 summarizes information regarding sugar substitutes.

DENTAL CONSIDERATIONS

- Sugar substitutes can reduce energy content and decrease cariogenicity of a product. Used in moderation, nonnutritive sweeteners are beneficial for many people, especially patients with diabetes.
- Because aspartame contains phenylalanine, aspartame-containing products are labeled to warn patients with phenylketonuria to avoid their use.
- Use of sugar substitutes is advocated for between-meal snacks to decrease tooth exposure to sugar. For individuals who do not need to decrease energy intake, sugar alcohols may be recommended.
- Nonnutritive sweeteners are not fermentable and do not promote caries formation; antimicrobial activity has not been observed. Saccharin and aspartame exhibit microbial inhibition and caries suppression.
- Dental professionals are often asked to provide advice regarding the importance of diet and the role of sugars and nonnutritive sweeteners in caries formation and weight control. A reduction of fermentable sugars and carbohydrates coupled with good oral hygiene practices will reduce incidence of dental decay.

NUTRITIONAL DIRECTIONS

- Nonnutritive sweeteners have been deemed safe and their use is supported by many reputable health agencies.
- Although nonnutritive sweeteners may not have cariogenic potential, bulking ingredients that allow them to pour and measure more like sugar (and other constituents of a product) may have cariogenic potential if they contain fermentable carbohydrates.
- Nonnutritive sweeteners do nothing to appease the appetite, but they do provide the pleasure of sweetness. They may enable patients to choose a wide variety of foods or improve taste appeal of healthy products, such as oatmeal, while managing caloric or cariogenic intake.
- When evaluating the amount of nonnutritive sweeteners a client (especially relevant for a child) is consuming, refer to Table 4.7. These acceptable daily intake limits are excessively high, but indicate amounts that may be harmful. Other nutritional requirements have not been factored into this (e.g., consuming adequate amounts of required nutrients). Remember that children need energy for growth and development.
- Combinations of sweeteners can produce a sweet taste more similar to that of sugar than can a single high-intensity sweetener.
- During pregnancy, saccharin is not recommended because it is known to cross the placenta. Refer a pregnant patient to her obstetrician for counseling about use of any nonnutritive sweeteners.

TABLE 4.6 Noncaloric Sugar Substitutes (Nonnutritive Sweeteners)*

	Acesulfame K (Sweet One, Sweet & Safe, Sunette)	Aspartame† (NutraSweet, Equal, Sugar Twin)	Stevia (Truvia, Rebinana, PureVia, SweetLeaf, Sun Crystals)	Saccharin (Sweet and Low, Sweet Twin, NectaSweet)	Sucralose (Splenda)
Description	200% sweeter than sucrose	200% sweeter than sucrose Made from 2 amino acids—phenylalanine and aspartic acid	250% sweeter than sucrose	300% sweeter than sucrose	600% sweeter than sucrose Made from sucrose
Facts	No aftertaste Non-cariogenic Heat stable Works synergistically with other sweeteners	No aftertaste Intensifies flavors Non-cariogenic	Natural, from stevia leaves Works synergisticaly with other sweeteners Readily soluble in water	Works synergistically with other sweeteners Slight aftertaste	No aftertaste Heat stable Replaces sugar in equal amounts Non-cariogenic

*Data from Firch C, Keim KS. Position of the Academy of Nutrition and Dietetics. Use of nutritive and nonnutritive sweeteners. *J Acad Nutr Diet.* 2012;112(5):739–758.
†Not recommended for patients with phenylketonuria.

HEALTH APPLICATION 4

Lactose Intolerance

Some patients are unable to digest specific carbohydrates because of insufficient amounts of disaccharide-degrading enzymes. When those carbohydrates are eaten, the disaccharide is fermented by intestinal bacteria rather than being broken down into simple sugars. Lactase, an intestinal enzyme responsible for lactose digestion, is the only disaccharidase whose activity is reduced in a significant proportion of older children and adults. Per the National Institute of Diabetes and Digestive and Kidney Diseases, lactase deficiency occurs when the small intestine produces low levels of lactase and cannot digest much lactose.[40] Lactase deficiency may cause lactose malabsorption, in which undigested lactose passes to the colon, leading to lactose intolerance. Symptoms (diarrhea, abdominal cramps, flatulence, and halitosis) usually begin 30 minutes to 2 hours after consuming milk or milk products.

Not all people with lactase deficiency and lactose malabsorption have digestive symptoms. Symptoms of lactose intolerance generally do not occur until lactase production is less than 50%.

With rare exceptions, all infants of every racial and ethnic group can successfully digest the lactose in human milk and infant formulas. In most patients, the production of lactase declines following weaning (age 2 years) unless milk and milk products are consumed routinely.[41] Lactose intolerance primarily affects African Americans, Hispanic Americans, Native Americans, Asian Americans, Alaskan Natives, and Pacific Islanders. For most people, lactase deficiency appears to be genetically determined. It may also be a temporary condition caused by gastrointestinal diseases or intestinal mucosa damage. Occasionally, an infant has a lactase deficiency at birth because of an inborn error of metabolism. Lactose intolerance can be diagnosed based on the results of a hydrogen breath test or stool acidity test ordered by a health care provider.

Nutritional Care

Lactase deficiency is easily treated by reducing lactose-containing foods in one's diet. Because milk provides significant amounts of calcium, vitamin D, phosphorus, riboflavin, and sometimes protein, elimination is not advisable. The ability to digest lactose is not an all-or-nothing phenomenon; most patients with lactose intolerance can tolerate some lactose. The amount of dairy products is reduced to a patient's tolerance level (Box 4.3). Most adults and adolescents with lactose malabsorption can tolerate at least 12 to 18 g of lactose.[38] Larger doses may be tolerated when dairy products are ingested with other nutrients. Milk is tolerated better when taken with a meal and limited to 8 oz at a time. Whole milk is better tolerated than skim milk.

Individuals who avoid dairy products may exacerbate their risk for osteoporosis. Calcium is necessary for adequate bone accretions and optimal peak bone mass. When children's and teenagers' diets are deficient in calcium and/or vitamin D, bone accretion may be affected and optimal peak bone mass may not occur. Patients should be taught the approximate calcium composition of milk products and other calcium-rich foods (see Chapter 9, Table 9.2) to achieve adequate intake.

Fermented dairy products—especially yogurt, buttermilk, aged cheese, and sour cream—are often better tolerated by lactase-deficient individuals than other dairy products. Because it contains active lactase and less lactose, yogurt made with the organisms *Lactobacillus bulgaricus* or *Streptococcus thermophilus* is better tolerated than nonfermented dairy products. Most commercially available unflavored yogurt can be beneficial to lactose-intolerant patients. Pasteurization of frozen yogurts decreases the lactase activity and kills lactose-producing bacteria; thus, most frozen yogurts are not well tolerated by lactose-intolerant patients.

Commercially available lactase in tablet or liquid form can be beneficial. Lactase tablets, taken with a lactose-containing food, are effective in the stomach's acidic environment for approximately 45 minutes. Liquid lactase is effective in a neutral pH and, when added to milk, the lactose is hydrolyzed before ingestion. Specialized lactose-reduced products are also commercially available.

TABLE 4.7 Acceptable Daily Intake (ADI) of Nonnutritive Sweeteners

	Acesulfame K	Aspartame	Sucralose	Stevia Glycosides
ADI mg/kg body weight	0–15	0–50	0–5	0–4 as steviol
Packets/day	23	75	23	9
Servings of 12 oz (350 ml) sodas/day	25	18	15	16

From http://www.fda.gov/Food/IngredientsPackagingLabeling/FoodAdditivesIngredients/ucm397725.htm. Accessed April 12, 2017.

• BOX 4.3 Suggestions for Lactose-Intolerant Patients

- Adequate amounts of calcium are needed even when dairy products must be avoided. Because of different tolerance levels, each patient needs to experiment to determine which method is most effective for providing necessary nutrients without discomfort. Consume small amounts of lactose-containing foods with meals several times a day.
- Consume fermented dairy products—yogurt,[a] kefir,[b] and buttermilk—that contain probiotics (live bacteria).
- Choose aged cheeses (e.g., Swiss, Colby, and Longhorn) that naturally contain less lactose.
- Try small amounts of whole-milk dairy products.
- Buy lactose-reduced or lactose-free products.
- Read ingredient labels for "hidden" lactose (whey, milk by-products, nonfat dry milk powder, malted milk, buttermilk, and dry milk solids). Also, check for lactose in prescription and over-the-counter drugs.
- Drink or eat calcium-fortified foods, such as fruit juices, soy or almond milk, and cereals.
- Use over-the-counter lactase enzymes available in tablet or liquid form to hydrolyze the lactose in milk products or consume lactose-hydrolyzed commercially available milk.
- Increase consumption of other calcium-containing foods, such as salmon and sardines canned with bones, vegetables (collards; spinach; kale; turnip, mustard, and dandelion greens; broccoli), beans, and nuts and seeds.
- Consider commercially available nutrition supplements, such as Resource (Novartis/Sandoz Nutrition) and Boost and Sustacal (Nestle Health Science).
- If these suggestions are not feasible to maintain an adequate intake of 1000–1200 mg of calcium, consult a health care provider or dietitian for calcium supplements that are well absorbed. These supplements may also need to include vitamin D.

[a]*Unflavored yogurt is usually best tolerated.*
[b]*Kefir is a fermented milk beverage that contains different bacteria than yogurt.*

CASE APPLICATION FOR THE DENTAL HYGIENIST

A healthy patient needs information on how to eat less refined sugar and more complex carbohydrates. He knows this regimen is encouraged but does not know all the health reasons. Fiber intake is also important to him, but he is not knowledgeable about the types of food needed or the benefits.

Nutritional Assessment

- Willingness/motivation to learn
- Usual dietary habits; focus especially on carbohydrate
- Basic knowledge of carbohydrate and carbohydrate principles
- Usual food/nutrient intake
- Financial status, employment status, and where most of the food is consumed
- Support system—family, friends, coworkers
- Use of community resources
- Food shopping practices

Nutritional Diagnosis

Health-seeking behavior related to lack of knowledge concerning carbohydrate and carbohydrate principles for optimal nutrition.

Nutritional Goals

The patient will consume a high-fiber food and complex carbohydrate foods daily, and state three principles concerning carbohydrate.

Nutritional Implementation

Intervention: Explain that (a) the main function of carbohydrates is to provide energy for the body; (b) that excessive amounts of carbohydrates by themselves do not cause obesity but excessive overall caloric intake increases body fat (and consequently weight); and (c) the role of carbohydrates in the dental caries process and enhancing plaque biofilm formation.

Rationale: Knowledge corrects misinformation.

Intervention: (a) Follow suggestions in Table 4.3. (b) Explain the importance of fiber. Recommend 30 to 38 g of fiber daily and help the patient plan a diet that will provide this amount, incorporating his food preferences. Stress the importance of adequate fluid intake.

Rationale: These suggestions increase fiber in the diet. Fiber increases stool bulk, exercising digestive tract muscles and preventing them from being chronically contracted. Muscle tone is maintained, colonic pressure is diminished, and the gut is able to resist bulging out into pouches. Additionally, fiber slows starch hydrolysis and delays glucose absorption.

Intervention: Explain sources of complex carbohydrates and fiber sources and provide the patient with a list of these foods. Emphasize the importance of increasing fiber intake gradually and increasing noncariogenic, noncaloric fluid intake when increasing fiber.

Rationale: The patient's increased knowledge will encourage him to increase consumption of complex carbohydrate and fiber.

Intervention: (a) Recommend substituting nonnutritive sweeteners for sugar, especially at snack time. (b) Read a label with the patient to show him how to recognize sugars (they usually end in *-ose*). (c) Recommend substituting fresh fruit for juices to increase fiber. (d) Instruct him to limit products that contain complex carbohydrates and sugar, such as cookies and pastries.

Continued

CASE APPLICATION FOR THE DENTAL HYGIENIST—cont'd

Rationale: He wanted to reduce refined sugar intake; these measures will help meet this personal goal.
Intervention: Refer him to an RDN and county extension agencies.
Rationale: These will provide expert knowledge and community resources for continued compliance.
Intervention: Review labeling: (a) "no sugar added" means sugar was not added, although the product may naturally contain sugar; (b) "sugar-free" means the product contains no added sucrose but may have other sugars added, such as sorbitol; (c) a high-fiber food has been defined as containing 5 g or more per serving; (d) incorporate foods with 3 g or more of fiber per serving.
Rationale: Knowing the meaning of these terms facilitates making healthy food choices.

Evaluation

The patient consumes a bran muffin, beans, or other high-fiber foods daily and verbalizes that carbohydrates provide energy and fiber, carbohydrate has several roles in maintaining gut functioning, and most sugars end in *-ose.* Other indicators of success include reading a label correctly, modifying intake of refined sugars, and using the community resources.

Student Readiness

1. Differentiate between the three classes of carbohydrates.
2. Identify sources of complex carbohydrates in the diet.
3. What are the main sources of fiber in the American diet? What are the main sources of starch?
4. List three of your favorite foods high in added sugar. What realistic modifications can you make to your diet with respect to these high-sugar foods?
5. Explain the functions of sugars and fiber in the diet in terms a patient can understand.
6. From cereal boxes at the local grocery store, identify some of the products that claim to be high in fiber: (a) evaluate the source of fiber on the ingredient label to determine if those are soluble or insoluble fibers, and (b) rank the cereals according to the amount of dietary fiber they contain. Which would you recommend?
7. Based on ready-to-eat cereals available at the grocery store, identify five that list a whole grain as the first ingredient.
8. Role play: To a patient consuming a very low-carbohydrate diet, discuss why this diet is neither healthy nor wise.
9. Role play: Advise a mother who has been told she should never give her infant anything that contains sugar because the infant will develop a sweet tooth.
10. What is the basis for the WHO's recommendation of 10% or less of calories from sugars? Why is the National Academy of Medicine recommendation of 25% or less of energy intake different?
11. Match the carbohydrates on the left with the appropriate answer in the right column.

Dextrose	Cannot be used by the body
Glycogen	Milk
Fructose	Sweetest sugar
Lactose	Glucose
Cellulose	Storage form of carbohydrate in the body

CASE STUDY

A 22-year-old African American man presents with four carious lesions acquired since his last dental hygiene recare appointment. While questioning the patient, you learn that he frequently skips meals and relies heavily on snacks to get him through the day.

1. What further information about his dietary intake do you need?
2. Could the patient's snacking habits be related to his increase in dental caries?
3. Which types of foods should be suggested as snack foods and why?
4. What other precautions could the patient practice that might be helpful in preventing further caries problems?

CASE STUDY

A 22-year-old Asian woman reports a history of lactose intolerance. She is concerned about her calcium intake because she has eliminated all dairy products from her diet.

1. What should be included in dietary recommendations made by the dental hygienist?
2. Can this patient consume dairy products?
3. Which dairy products are best tolerated by lactose-deficient individuals?
4. When should lactase tablets be taken?
5. What symptoms may the patient report that are associated with lactose intake?
6. Why should she include dairy products?

References

1. Perlmutter D. *Grain Brain: The Surprising Truth about Wheat, Carbs and Sugar—Your Brain's Silent Killers.* New York: Little, Brown & Co.; 2013.
2. Centers for Disease Control and Prevention, National Center for Health Statistics. Diet/Nutrition. Dietary intake for adults 20 years of age and over. Health, United States, 2016 (Table 56). Hyattsville, MD, 2016. https://www.cdc.gov/nchs/fastats/diet.htm.
3. US Department of Health and Human Services and US Department of Agriculture. 2015-2020 *Dietary Guidelines for Americans.* 8th ed. December 2015, accessed November 8, 2016. https://health.gov/dietaryguidelines/215/guidelines. Accessed August 14, 2017.
4. Powell ES, Smith-Taille LP, Popkin BM. Added sugars across the distribution of US children and adult consumers 1977-2012. *J Acad Nutr Diet.* 2016;116(10):1548–1550.
5. Woelber JP, Bremer K, Vach K. An oral health optimized diet can reduce gingival and periodontal inflammation in humans—a randomized controlled pilot study. *BMC Oral Health.* 2016;17(1):28.
6. Nielsen SJ, Trak-Fellermeier A, Joshipura K, et al. Dietary fiber intake is inversely associated with periodontal disease among US adults. *J Nutr.* 2016;146(12):2530–2536.
7. Chen C, Zeng Y, Xu J, et al. Therapeutic effects of soluble dietary fiber consumption on type 2 diabetes mellitus. *Exp Ther Med.* 2016;12(2):1232–1242.
8. Jenkins DJ, Jones PJ, Frohlich J, et al. The effect of a dietary portfolio compared to a DASH-type diet on blood pressure. *Nutr Metab Cardiovasc Dis.* 2015;25(12):1132–1139.

9. Bowman SA, Friday JE, Clemens JC, et al. A Comparison of Food Patterns Equivalents Intakes by Americans: *What We Eat in America.* NHANES 2003-2004 and 2011-2012. Food Survey Research Group. Dietary Data Brief No. 16, Sept. 2016. Accessed August 16, 2017. https://www.ars.usda.gov/ARSUserFiles/80400530/pdf/DBrief/16_Food_Patterns_Equivalents_0304_1112.pdf.
10. Park S, Thompson FE, McGuire LC, et al. Sociodemographic and behavioral factors associated with added sugars intake among US adults. *J Acad Nutr Diet.* 2016;116(10):1589–1598.
11. World Health Organization. Guideline. Sugars Intake for Adults and Children. Geneva Switzerland, 2016, www.who.int/nutritionpublications/guidelines/sugars_intake/en/. Accessed November 8, 2016.
12. Haile R. Whole grains slowly gaining. Tufts University Health & Nutrition Letter, Apr 2016. www.nutritionletter.tufts.edu/issues/12-4/todays-newsbites/Whole-Grains-Slowly-Gaining-1926-1.html. Accessed July 10, 2017.
13. Hoy MK, Goldman JP. Fiber Intake of the US Population: *What We Eat in America*, NHANES 2009-2010. Food Surveys Research Group, Agricultural Research Service. Dietary Data Brief No. 12. September 2014. https://www.ars.usda.gov/ARSUserFiles/80400530/pdf/DBrief/12_fiber_intake_0910.pdf. Accessed April 14, 2017.
14. American Diabetes Association. Standards of Medical Care in Diabetes–2017. *Diabetes Care.* 2017;40(suppl 1):S11–S24.
15. Rippe JM, Sievenpiper JL, Lê KA, et al. What is the appropriate upper limit for added sugars consumption? *Nutr Rev.* 2017;75(1):18–36.
16. Kell J. Soda consumption falls to 30-year low in the US. March 29, 2016. http://fortune.com/2016/03/29/soda-sales-drop-11th-year/. Accessed October 31, 2016.
17. Holodny E. The epic collapse of American soda consumption in one chart. March 10, 2016. http://www.businessinsider.com/americans-are-drinking-less-soda-2016-3. Accessed October 31, 2016.
18. Markus CR, Rogers PJ, Brouns F, et al. Eating dependence and weight gain; no human evidence for a 'sugar-addiction' model of overweight. *Appetite.* 2017;114:64–72.
19. Dhurandhar NV, Thomas D. The link between dietary sugar intake and cardiovascular disease mortality: an unresolved question. *JAMA.* 2015;313(9):959–960.
20. Yang Q, Zhang Z, Gregg EW, et al. Added sugar intake and cardiovascular diseases mortality among US adults. *JAMA Intern Med.* 2014;174(4):516–524.
21. Angelopoulos RJ, Lowndes J, Sinnett S, et al. Fructose containing sugars at normal levels of consumption do not effect adversely components of the metabolic syndrome and risk factors for cardiovascular disease. *Nutrients.* 2016;8(4):179.
22. Kelishadi R, Mansourian M, Heidari-Beni M. Association of fructose consumption and components of metabolic syndrome in human studies: a systematic review and meta-analysis. *Nutrition.* 2014;30(5):503–510.
23. Tasevska N, Park Y, Jiao L, et al. Sugars and risk of mortality in the NIH-AARP diet and health study. *Am J Clin Nutr.* 2014;99(5):1077–1088.
24. Hayes C. Nonfluoride caries preventive agents show varied effectiveness in preventing dental caries. *J Evid Based Dent Pract.* 2012;12(2):79–80.
25. Stefański T, Postek-Stefańsk L. Possible ways of reducing dental erosive potential of acidic beverages. *Aust Dent J.* 2014;59(3):280–288.
26. Søvik JB, Skudutyte-Rysstad R, Tveit AB, et al. Sour sweets and acidic beverage consumption are risk indicators for dental erosion. *Caries Res.* 2015;49(3):243–250.
27. Salas MM, Mascimento GG, Vargas-Ferreira F. Diet influenced tooth erosion prevalence in children and adolescents: Results of a meta-analysis and meta-regression. *J Dent.* 2015;43(8):865–875.
28. Owens BM, Kitchens M. The erosive potential of soft drinks on enamel surface substrate: an in vitro scanning electron microscopy investigation. *J Contemp Dent Pract.* 2007;8(7):11–20.
29. Riley P, Moore D, Ahmed F, et al. Xylitol-containing products for preventing dental caries in children and adults. *Cochrane Database Syst Rev.* 2015;(3):CD010743.
30. Dodds MW. The oral benefits of chewing gum. *J Ir Dent Assoc.* 2012;58(5):253–261.
31. Hashiba T, Takeuchi K, Shimazaki Y, et al. Chewing xylitol gum improves self-rated and objective indicators of oral health status under conditions interrupting regular oral hygiene. *Tohoku J Exp Med.* 2015;235(1):39–46.
32. de Cock P, Mäkinen K, Honkala E, et al. Erythritol is more effective than xylitol and sorbitol in managing oral health endpoints. *Int J Dent.* 2016;2016:9868421.
33. Falony G, Honkala S, Runnel R, et al. Long-term effect of erytritol on dental caries development during childhood: a posttreatment survival analysis. *Caries Res.* 2016;50(6):579–588.
34. Mäkinen KK. Gastrointestinal disturbances associated with the consumption of sugar alcohols with special consideration of xylitol: scientific review and instructions for dentists and other health-care professionals. *Int J Dent.* 2016;2016:5967907.
35. Sylvetsky AC, Rother KI. Trends in the consumption of low-calorie sweeteners. *Phys Behavior.* 2016;164(Pt B):446–450.
36. Azad MB, Abou-Setta AM, Chauhan BF, et al. Nonnutritive sweeteners and cardiometabolic health: a systematic review and meta-analysis of randomized controlled trials and prospective cohort studies. *CMAJ.* 2017;189(28):E929–E939.
37. Rogers PJ, Hogenkamp PS, de Graaf C, et al. Does low-energy sweetener consumption affect energy intake and body weight? A systematic review, including meta-analyses, of the evidence from human and animal studies. *Int J Obes (Lond).* 2016;40(3):381–394.
38. American Heart Association. Non-nutritive sweeteners (artificial sweeteners). Updated March 18, 2014. http://www.heart.org/HEARTORG/HealthyLiving/HealthyEating/Nutrition/Non-Nutritive-Sweeteners-Artificial-Sweeteners_UCM_305880_Article.jsp#.WCD4PslUO_g. Accessed August 14, 2017.
39. Drewnowski A, Rehm CD. Consumption of low-calorie sweeteners among U.S. adults is associated with higher Healthy Eating Index (HEI 2005) scores and more physical activity. *Nutrients.* 2014;6(10):4389–4403.
40. National Institute of Diabetes and Digestive and Kidney Disease. Lactose intolerance. https://www.niddk.nih.gov/health-information/health-topics/digestive-diseases/lactose-intolerance/pages/ez.aspx. Accessed November 9, 2016.
41. Deng Y, Misselwitz B, Dai N, et al. Lactose intolerance in adults: biological mechanism and dietary management. *Nutrients.* 2015;7(9):8020–8035.

EVOLVE RESOURCES

Please visit http://evolve.elsevier.com/Stegeman/nutritional for additional practice and study support tools.

5

Protein: The Cellular Foundation

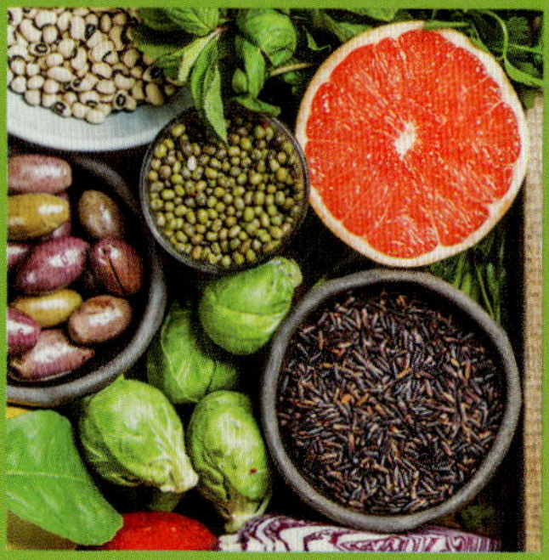

STUDENT LEARNING OUTCOMES

Upon completion of this chapter, the student will be able to complete the following student learning outcomes:

1. Explain the possible fates of amino acids.
2. Categorize amino acids as indispensable or dispensable; categorize foods as sources of high-quality or low-quality proteins.
3. List and describe the seven categories of the physiologic functions of proteins.
4. Discuss protein requirements for health, and plan individualized menus to meet the recommended protein level for a diet containing animal foods, a vegetarian diet, and a vegan diet containing only plant proteins.
5. Discuss the following related to underconsumption and overconsumption of protein:
   - List the problems associated with protein deficiency or excess.
   - Appraise a patient's protein consumption to determine protein deficiency or excess.
   - Explain how protein foods can be used to complement one another.
   - Discuss how protein energy malnutrition affects oral health in children.
   - Identify and explain nutrition principles regarding food intake to prevent a patient consuming too much or inadequate amounts of protein.

KEY TERMS

Ad libitum
Bioavailability
Collagen
Complementary foods
Conditionally indispensable amino acids
Dipeptide
Dispensible amino acids
Erythema
Flexitarians
High-quality protein
Immune response
Immunocompromised
Immunoglobulins
Indispensable amino acids
Interstitial
Kwashiorkor
Lactovegetarian
Low-quality proteins
Marasmus
Necrosis
Necrotizing ulcerative gingivitis (NUG)
Nitrogen balance
Noma
Ovolactovegetarian
Ovovegetarian
Periodontium
Protein-energy malnutrition (PEM)
Sarcopenia
Secretory immunoglobulin A (sIgA)
Thermogenesis
Vegan
Vegetarian

TEST YOUR NQ

1. **T/F** A protein deficiency during childhood may lead to increased caries susceptibility related to alterations in tooth development and diminished salivary flow.
2. **T/F** Despite poor nutrition, malnourished children have a decreased rate of caries because they do not consume much sugar.
3. **T/F** Gelatin is a good source of high-quality protein.
4. **T/F** Older patients require less protein than younger adults.
5. **T/F** High protein intake strengthens tooth enamel.
6. **T/F** Excessive protein intake will contribute to the risk of developing diabetes.
7. **T/F** Amino acids are the building blocks of proteins.
8. **T/F** Marasmus is a protein-deficiency disorder.
9. **T/F** Protein requirements are based on the assumption that indispensable amino acids and calories are provided in adequate amounts.
10. **T/F** Positive nitrogen balance occurs during periods of growth.

Until the middle of the 19th century, many scientists thought all life was composed of a single basic chemical: protein. Protein is present in every living cell, making up almost half of the dry weight of a cell. Second to water, protein is the most plentiful substance in the body. The United States is a nation of meat eaters, consuming more meat per capita than any other nation. Most Americans are unable or unwilling to plan a balanced meal without a meat entree. High-protein diets have been increasingly popular for weight reduction for many years, contributing to increased protein consumption. Meat consumption declined for nearly a decade, but United States per capita meat consumption rose at a higher rate in 2015 than any other year over the past four decades, with Americans averaging 193 pounds of meat per person. Over the past few decades, beef consumption has trended downward as chicken's popularity has increased dramatically (Fig. 5.1).[1] Most likely, the increase in poultry consumption was based on economic reasons rather than health concerns (cost of poultry has decreased). But the American culture continues to value animal protein above other protein sources.

Amino Acids

Individuals consume meats, eggs, milk and milk products, dried beans and peas, and nuts—all of which provide the essential nutrient, protein. As described in detail in Chapter 2 and on the Evolve website, proteins are very large molecular structures containing the elements carbon, hydrogen, oxygen, and nitrogen, and sometimes sulfur and phosphorus. Proteins consumed are hydrolyzed by enzymes in the small intestine into individual amino acids for absorption and utilization (Fig. 5.2).

All the billions of proteins associated with life are made from combinations of 20 different amino acids. Amino acids are similar to letters of the alphabet used in different sequences and combinations to make billions of words. An amino acid contains a basic, or amino, grouping (–NH_2) and an acidic, or carboxyl, grouping (–COOH). Fig. 5.3 shows the general design of an amino acid.

The distinguishing feature of amino acids is the amine group, which is the body's source of nitrogen. The fundamental constituent of the protein molecule, called the side chain (R group), is the part of the structure that varies to form the many different amino acids.

Amino acids combine with each other to make long chains. As shown in Fig. 5.3, two amino acids together form a **dipeptide**. Several amino acids bound together form a polypeptide. Food and body proteins contain polypeptides. The number of amino acids in a protein varies greatly (from 100 to 300), but each protein has a specific number. The protein chain adopts a compact, folded, three-dimensional structure (see Chapter 2, Fig. 2.9) which is essential to perform its basic function.

Classification

A prerequisite for life and health are the 20 amino acids, the building blocks of protein. These amino acids, listed in Table 5.1, can be classified as indispensable, dispensable, or conditionally indispensable. (These classifications were previously known as essential, nonessential, and conditionally essential, respectfully). Nine **indispensable amino acids** are required in the diet. **Dispensable amino acids** are essential for the body, but they can be produced from indispensable amino acids so are not required in normal conditions. In certain nutritional or disease states, or stages of development, several dispensable amino acids become indispensable; these are classified as **conditionally indispensable**.

If any one of the indispensable amino acids is not available when needed for protein synthesis, the protein cannot be produced.

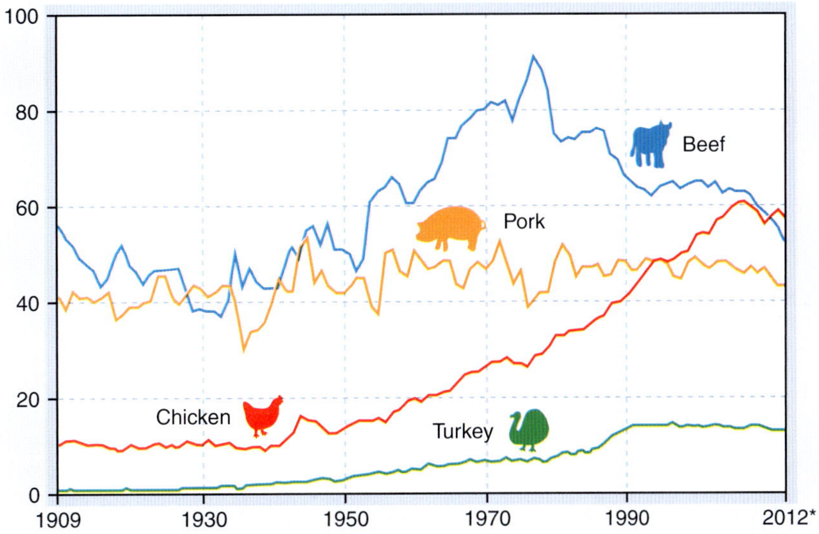

• **Figure 5.1** U.S. meat consumption per person, in pounds. Americans have been eating less beef and a lot more chicken. (From Earth Policy Institute. Wong, A/NPR: *A nation of meat of eaters: see how it all adds up*. June 27, 2012. Accessed November 22, 2016. http://www.npr.org/blogs/thesalt/2012/06/27/155527365/visualizing-a-nation-of-meat-eaters.)

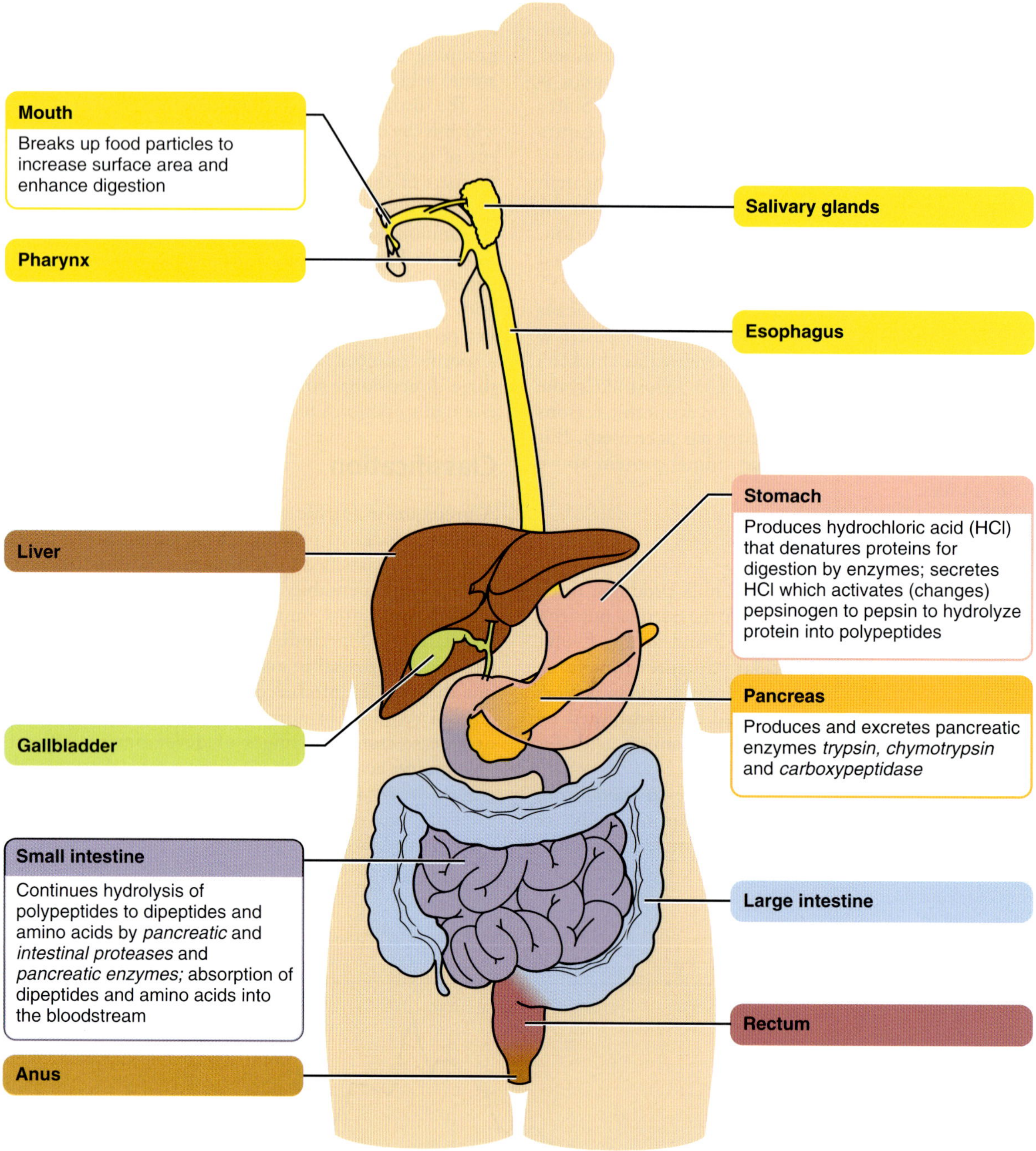
Mouth
Breaks up food particles to increase surface area and enhance digestion
Pharynx
Salivary glands
Esophagus
Stomach
Produces hydrochloric acid (HCl) that denatures proteins for digestion by enzymes; secretes HCl which activates (changes) pepsinogen to pepsin to hydrolyze protein into polypeptides
Liver
Pancreas
Produces and excretes pancreatic enzymes *trypsin, chymotrypsin* and *carboxypeptidase*
Gallbladder
Small intestine
Continues hydrolysis of polypeptides to dipeptides and amino acids by *pancreatic* and *intestinal proteases* and *pancreatic enzymes;* absorption of dipeptides and amino acids into the bloodstream
Large intestine
Rectum
Anus

• **Figure 5.2** Summary of protein digestion. Note: active enzymes are in *italics*.

The body is able to make adequate amounts of dispensable amino acids if a sufficient amount of protein is available to furnish the nitrogen needed and enough calories are present to allow the catabolism (breakdown) of amino acids.

The amount of indispensable amino acids furnished by a food determines its ability to support growth, maintenance, and repair. A food with all the indispensable amino acids present is identified as a "complete" protein. When the nine indispensable amino acids are provided from a food in amounts adequate to maintain nitrogen balance and permit growth, the food is said to provide **high-quality protein**. High-quality protein foods have all the indispensable amino acids present in balanced amounts for human physiologic requirements. Foods providing high-quality proteins include meats (e.g., chicken, pork, beef, lamb, veal, goat, rabbit), poultry (chicken, turkey, duck, wild game birds), and all types of seafood.

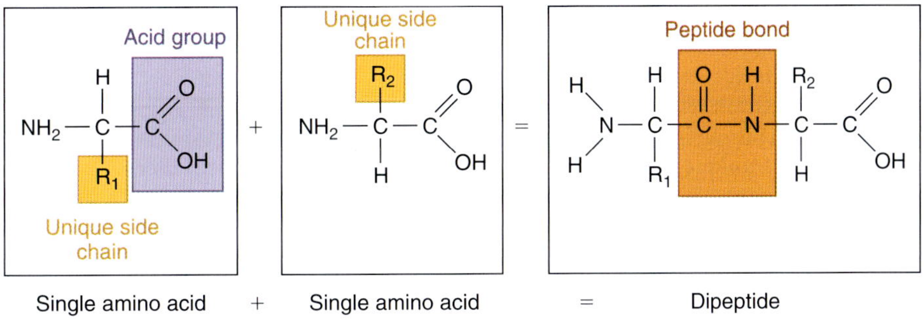

• **Figure 5.3** Structure of amino acids. (Modified from Mahan LK, Escott-Stump, S, Raymond JL. *Krause's Food and the Nutrition Care Process*. 13th ed. St. Louis, MO: Saunders Elsevier; 2012.)

TABLE 5.1 Amino Acids in the Human Diet

Indispensable	Dispensable[a]	Conditionally Indispensable[b]
Histidine[c]	Alanine	Arginine
Isoleucine	Aspartic acid	Cysteine
Leucine	Asparagine	Glutamine
Lysine	Glutamic acid	Glycine
Methionine	Serine	Proline
Phenylalanine		Tyrosine
Threonine		
Tryptophan		
Valine		

[a]Required in the diet when the body cannot produce enough to meet metabolic needs.
[b]Required in the diet when the body is unable to synthesize adequate amounts for metabolic functions for special pathophysiologic conditions.
[c]Although histidine is considered indispensable, unlike the other eight indispensable amino acids, it does not fulfill the criteria of reducing protein deposition and inducing negative nitrogen balance promptly upon removal from the diet.
Data from Food and Nutrition Board, Institute of Medicine. *Dietary Reference Intakes for Energy, Carbohydrate, Fiber, Fat, Fatty Acids, Cholesterol, Protein, and Amino Acids (Macronutrients)*. Washington, DC: National Academy Press; 2002.

• BOX 5.1 Nitrogen Balance[a]

N balance: body protein constant
N intake = N excretion
Positive N balance: increase in body protein
N intake > N excretion
Negative N balance: decrease in body protein
N intake < N excretion

Positive N Balance	Negative N Balance
Growth	Inadequate protein intake (e.g., fasting, gastrointestinal tract diseases)
Pregnancy or lactation	Inadequate energy intake
Recovery from illnesses, surgery, or trauma	Illnesses (e.g., fevers, infections, or wasting diseases)
Medications	Routine intake of glucocorticoids
Athletic training	Injury or immobilization
	Deficiency of indispensable amino acids
	Accelerated protein loss (e.g., albuminuria, protein-losing gastroenteropathy)
	Burns
	Increased secretion of thyroxine and glucocorticoids

[a]*Because nitrogen is a unique component of protein metabolism, measurements of nitrogen and nitrogenous constituents in the blood and urine assess protein equilibrium in the body. Although "nitrogen balance" means that the output is equal to input, the amount of excreted nitrogen atoms is usually not the same as that ingested. For nitrogen equilibrium, not only must the diet contain the required amounts of protein, but also energy intake must be adequate to prevent protein being used for energy.*

If the quantity of one or more of the indispensable amino acids in a food is insufficient for optimal protein synthesis, the food is a source of low-quality protein. **Low-quality proteins**, if the only protein source consumed, support life but not normal growth. These include proteins found in legumes, nuts, and grains. The amino acid in short supply relative to need is referred to as the "limiting amino acid."

Nitrogen balance refers to the balance of reactions in which protein substances are broken down or destroyed and rebuilt (Box 5.1). Healthy individuals excrete (in feces and urine, and from skin) the same amount of nitrogen as is consumed from their food. A patient with a burn or illness excretes more nitrogen than is ingested. In periods of growth, as in a child or pregnant woman, the body is in positive nitrogen balance (more protein is retained than is lost daily).

DENTAL CONSIDERATIONS

- Inquire about the patient's use of amino acid supplements because toxicity and amino acid imbalances may occur when an excess of one amino acid is ingested. Additionally, supplements may contain toxic contaminants. For example, when large doses of tryptophan are taken, toxic metabolites build up, causing an unusual autoimmune disorder. Refer patients who take protein supplements regularly to their health care provider or registered dietitian nutritionist (RDN).

NUTRITIONAL DIRECTIONS

- Protein from animals and fish (except for gelatin) are high-quality proteins but are not essential to an adequate diet.

Physiologic Roles

Individual indispensable amino acids act as metabolic signals influencing protein synthesis, inflammation responses and satiety, among other metabolic functions.[2] Leucine (an indispensable amino acid prevalent in animal proteins) has a unique role in stimulating skeletal muscle protein synthesis and may improve satiety and insulin use. In older adults and physical inactivity (bed rest, surgery, trauma), efficiency of indispensable amino acids for muscle synthesis is reduced, which may increase the amount of protein needed. Resistance exercise appears to increase the efficiency of indispensable amino acids for muscle anabolism, suppress muscle protein catabolism, and promote positive nitrogen balance.[3]

Proteins are the principal source of nitrogen for the body and are fundamental components of every human cell. Although proteins are an essential part of a diet, performing many important physiologic roles, other nutrients are also essential for the body to fully utilize available protein. Proteins are necessary for many physiologic functions, which can be classified into the following seven categories:

1. *Generation of new body tissues.* Because protein is a constituent of all cells, it is necessary for growth. During periods of increased growth (infancy, childhood, adolescence, and pregnancy) and in periods of wound healing or recovery (illness, surgery, burns, or fever), the need for protein to build new tissues is increased. Moderately high protein consumption may stimulate muscle protein growth, favoring retention of lean muscle mass while improving metabolism, especially in individuals who are physically active (Fig. 5.4).
2. *Repair of body tissues.* Body proteins are continuously being broken down, necessitating their replacement.
3. *Production of essential compounds.* Amino acids and proteins are constituents of regulatory enzymes, hormones, and other body secretions. The structural compound **collagen** is a protein substance in connective tissue that helps support body structures, such as skin, bones, teeth, and tendons. Low protein intake may affect all of these compounds.
4. *Regulation of fluid balance.* Protein dissolved in water forms a colloidal solution; in other words, it attracts water. Blood albumin (a protein) draws water from **interstitial** (space between tissue cells) fluid or cells to maintain blood volume. During protein deficiency, a decreased amount of protein in the blood causes a loss of osmotic balance, resulting in an accumulation of interstitial fluid (edema).
5. *Resistance to disease.* Antibodies, or **immunoglobulins**, the body's main protection from disease, are proteins. Low protein levels may negatively affect an individual's **immune response**, resulting in an inability to fight bacteria and other harmful organisms.
6. *Transport mechanisms.* Proteins enable insoluble fats to be transported through the blood.
7. *Energy.* After the nitrogen grouping is removed, the remaining carbon skeleton can be used for energy, furnishing 4 cal/g. Although this is not one of its main functions, protein is used in this manner when caloric intake from carbohydrate and fat is inadequate and indispensable amino acids are not available for synthesis of proteins.

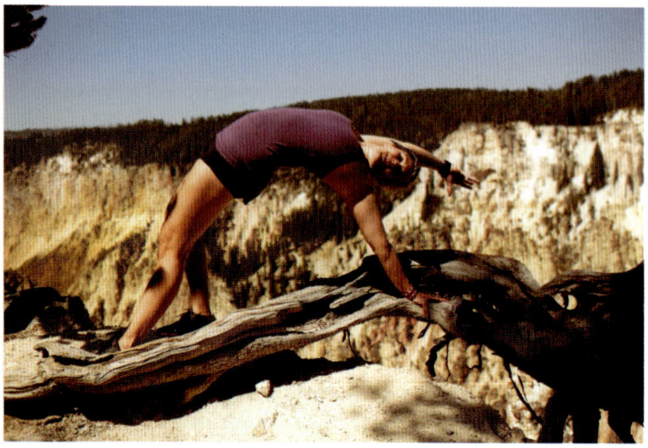

• **Figure 5.4** Protein is important to stimulate muscle growth and lean muscle mass and for physical strength and activity. (Reprinted with permission of D2 Studios, www.d2studios.net.)

Requirements

Protein requirements for health are based on body size and rate of growth. The body requires more protein during growth periods as well as for maintenance and repair of a larger body mass. To a certain extent, the better the quality of protein (amount of indispensable amino acids), the less quantity is required. Protein requirements are based on the assumption that indispensable amino acids and calories are provided in adequate amounts.

The recommended dietary allowances (RDAs) for protein vary proportionately for different ages and stages of life to adjust for growth rates (Table 5.2). The National Academy of Medicine (formerly the Institute of Medicine) determined that the daily minimum requirement of protein for adults is approximately 0.6 g/kg (see p. ii). Using 0.6 g/kg, a person weighing 150 lb (68.2 kg) would require 41 g of protein. Because RDAs provide a margin of safety, the National Academy of Medicine established 0.8 g/kg daily as the RDA. With this standard, a patient weighing 150 lb (68.2 kg) requires 56 g of protein. Ideally, protein needs are based on body weight, not energy intake. In comparison, the World Health Organization recommends 0.75 g of protein per kilogram of lean body weight, which translates to 45 g of protein daily for an average woman and 56 g for an average man.

When any condition of health or disease causes a significant protein loss, an increased protein intake (greater than the RDA) prevents excessive loss of tissue and plasma proteins. Although these conditions increase protein requirements, RDAs have not been established for them. Providing additional amounts through supplementation with high-quality proteins can help prevent protein malnutrition and shorten recovery periods.

Very few individuals consume protein amounts close to the highest acceptable macronutrient distribution range of 35% for their age-sex group. The acceptable macronutrient distribution range (AMDR) allows a lot of flexibility in protein intake, between 10% and 35% of total caloric intake. The flexibility within the AMDR is beneficial since a growing body of literature suggests that current dietary reference intakes (DRIs) may not be sufficient to promote optimal muscle health in all populations (see Underconsumption and Health-Related Problems section). Moderate evidence indicates that diets containing more than 35% of total calories from protein are generally no more effective at building muscle mass than 25% to 35%.

TABLE 5.2 Protein Recommendations

Life Stage/Gender	Age (years)	RECOMMENDED DIETARY ALLOWANCES Protein (g/kg)	Protein (g/d)	% Calories
Infants	0–6 mo	1.52	9.1[a]	5–10
	7–12 mo	1.2	11	5–10
Children	1–3	1.05	13	5–10
	4–8	0.95	19	10–30
Males	9–13	0.95	34	10–30
	14–18	0.85	52	10–30
	19–70	0.80	56	10–35
Females	9–13	0.95	34	10–30
	14–18	0.85	46	10–30
	19–70	0.80	46	10–35
Pregnant	All ages	1.1	71 (+25 g/day)	10–35
Lactating	All ages	1.3	71 (+25 g/day)	10–35

[a]Adequate Intake, based on 0.8 g protein/kg body weight for reference body weight. For healthy, breastfed infants, the adequate intake is the mean intake.
Data from Institute of Medicine of the National Academies: *Dietary Reference Intakes For Energy, Carbohydrates, Fiber, Fat, Protein, and Amino acids.* Washington, DC: National Academy Press; 2002.

The *Dietary Guidelines* indicate that more than half the United States population is meeting or exceeding the protein foods recommendation.[4] The *Dietary Guidelines* encourage a healthy eating pattern that includes a variety of protein-rich foods and maintaining a healthy body weight. Nutrient-dense foods should be a primary focus, limiting protein foods with high amounts of fats, especially saturated fats (Box 5.2). The *Dietary Guidelines* encourage meeting nutritional needs primarily from foods, not protein or amino acid supplements. The *Healthy Pattern* includes oz-eq weekly recommendations for three subgroups: seafood; meats, poultry, eggs; and nuts, seeds, and soy products.

Ordinarily, dietary protein is restricted only in some physiologic disease states affecting the liver and kidney because these organs are heavily involved in protein metabolism and excretion of protein waste products. If the liver and kidney are diseased, excessive amounts of protein cannot be properly handled without further organ damage.

An increasing number of Americans are becoming vegetarians (see *Health Application 5*). **Vegetarians** purposefully do not eat meat (beef, pork, poultry, seafood, other animal flesh, and sometimes by-products of animals). The *Dietary Guidelines* endorses a vegetarian diet as a healthy eating pattern. For some vegetarians, intake is at the lower level or around 10% of calories recommended by the AMDR.

Sources

Foods with a high protein content are readily available in the United States. Table 5.3 lists the average protein content of some foods. Meat and milk food groups furnish most of the protein. (Although milk products are excellent sources of protein, they are not included in the protein group because of their nutrient profile—providing less iron, niacin, vitamins E or B_6 than other protein-rich foods). A variety of high-protein foods should be included, as each food has distinct nutritional contributions in addition to protein (Table 1.6). While Americans are consuming

• BOX 5.2 Implementation of *2015–2020 Dietary Guidelines* Related to Protein

- Choose a healthy eating pattern that includes a variety of protein foods in nutrient-dense forms: seafood, lean meat, poultry, eggs, soy products, nuts and seeds, legumes (beans and peas).
- Use the recommended amounts of foods from the *Healthy Pattern* (see Table 1.1) for the appropriate caloric level to maintain a desirable weight.
- Choose the designated amount of nutrient-dense lean or low-fat meats, poultry, and fish:
  - Opt for lean meats, such as white meat of chicken, loin and round cuts of beef and pork that are trimmed, flank or strip steak, and ground beef that is 90% lean or leaner.
  - Remove visible fat from meats.
  - Remove skin from chicken.
- Limit the amounts of processed meats and poultry because of the added sodium and sugars.
- Prepare without additional fats (i.e., frying).
- Use sauces and gravies with additional fat, salt, or sugar sparingly.
- Choose unsalted nuts, seeds, and soy products at least 2 times a week, as indicated for the appropriate caloric level.
- Choose small portions of nuts and seeds because they are high in calories.
- Choose seafood (not fried) at least twice a week in the amount indicated for the appropriate caloric level.
- Eat more beans and peas, which are a natural source of fiber and protein. (If counted as a protein food, do not count as a vegetable.)
- Choose legumes (beans or peas) or tofu for the protein food at least once a week, or substitute beans for at least half of the beef, chicken, or pork in chili, burritos, pasta, or stir-fry dishes.
- Choose nonfat or low-fat dairy product in the amounts indicated for the appropriate caloric level.

TABLE 5.3 Protein Content of Select Foods

Food	Quantity	Protein (g)
Chicken, light meat, cooked	1 oz	9
Milk, whole, reduced fat, or low fat	1 cup	8–9
Pork chop, lean, cooked	1 oz	8
Beef, cooked, lean cuts	1 oz	8
Nonfat dried skim milk powder	⅓ cup	8
Chicken, dark meat, cooked	1 oz	7
Cheddar cheese	1 oz	7
Egg, hard boiled	1	7
American processed cheese	1 oz	7
Peanut butter	2 Tbsp	7
Thick milkshake	11 oz	7
Cottage cheese	¼ cup	6
Cod fish, cooked	1 oz	6
Macaroni, cooked	1 cup	6
Oatmeal, cooked	1 cup	6
Rice, brown, cooked	1 cup	5
Ice cream	1 cup	5
Pinto beans, cooked	¼ cup	4
Rice, white, cooked	1 cup	4
Corn muffin, small	1	2
Enriched white bread	1 slice	2
Vegetables	½ cup	1–2
Fruits	½ cup	0.1–1

Data from U.S. Department of Agriculture, Agricultural Research Service, Nutrient Data Laboratory. USDA National Nutrient Database for Standard Reference, Release 28. September 2015, slightly revised May 2016. https://www.ars.usda.gov/northeast-area/beltsville-md/beltsville-human-nutrition-research-center/nutrient-data-laboratory/docs/usda-national-nutrient-database-for-standard-reference/. Accessed July 12, 2017.

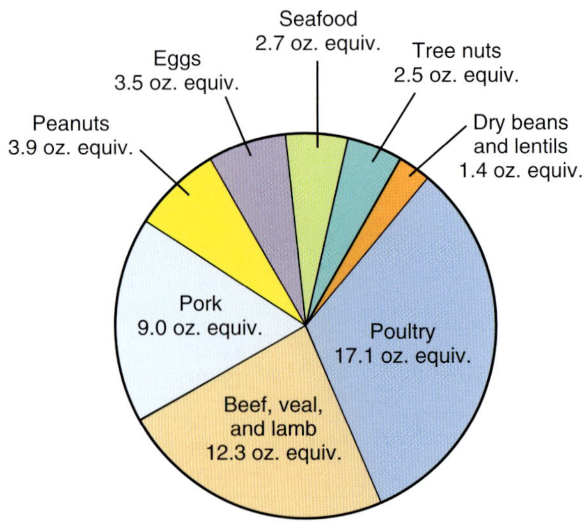

Note: oz. equiv. = ounce equivalent. One ounce of meat, poultry, or fish; ¼ cup of cooked beans; 1 egg; 1 tablespoon of peanut butter; ½ ounce of nuts or seeds is equal to 1 ounce equivalent from the Protein Foods group.
Source: USDA, Economic Research Service, Loss-Adjusted Food Availability data.

• **Figure 5.5** Seafood was one of the least consumed protein foods on a weekly per capita basis in 2014 Note: oz equiv. - ounce equivalent. One ounce of meat, poultry, or fish; ¼ cup of cooked beans; 1 egg; 1 tablespoon of peanut butter; ½ ounce of nuts or seeds is equal to 1 ounce equivalent from the Protein Foods group. (From Kantor L. Americans' seafood consumption below recommendations. *Amber Waves,* October 3, 2016. Accessed November 22, 2016. https://www.ers.usda.gov/amber-waves/2016/october/americans-seafood-consumption-below-recommendations/.)

adequate amounts of protein, they are not meeting recommendations for the subgroups within the protein foods group. As shown in Fig. 5.5, seafood is one of the least consumed protein foods. Compared to some other protein sources, seafood is nutrient dense and relatively low in calories and saturated fat.[5] The American Heart Association and *Dietary Guidelines* recommend that adults eat two fish meals a week, but the average intake is one 4-oz serving weekly. A seafood-rich diet is beneficial in lowering the risk of cardiovascular disease (CVD) and may help with weight control. Legumes (beans and peas) are also considered part of the protein foods group (but one serving can be counted only once—either in the protein or vegetable group). Soy is a good source of protein and has other health benefits. Consumption of cereal products also boosts protein intake. The protein content of items from the sample menu presented in Fig. 1.4 is shown in Fig. 5.6.

Depending on sex, size, and activity level, *MyPlate* and the *Healthy Eating Pattern* recommend 5½ to 6½ oz of cooked lean meat, poultry, or fish daily for adults. Protein foods, the purple portion of the plate, covers only ¼ of the plate (see Fig. 1.6a). The *Healthy Pattern* has designated the amount considered one serving (Table 5.4). About 3 tbsp of chopped/ground meat, or the size of a small matchbox, equals 1 oz of meat; a small chicken drumstick or thigh is equivalent to 2 oz of meat; and a deck of cards or the size of your palm is approximately a 3-oz; ½ cup of beans, or the amount that can fit in a cupped hand, or 1 tbsp of peanut butter (size of a ping-pong ball) can be substituted for 1 oz of meat. Not to be overlooked, dairy is not optional, even though it is located above the plate where a glass is normally placed. The *Dietary Guidelines* recommend 3 cups of fat-free or low-fat milk and dairy products daily for Americans 9 years of age and older, 2 to 2½ cups for children 4 to 8 years, and 2 cups for children ages 2 to 3 years. Three cups of milk provide 24 g of protein as well as other essential nutrients.

In most cases, digestibility and nutritional value are favorably affected by cooking procedures. Proper cooking sometimes facilitates digestion and use. Cooking makes egg albumin more readily digestible, and cooking soybeans increases amino acid bioavailability. **Bioavailability** indicates the amount of nutrient available to the body after absorption. Processing affects proteins in cereal by binding lysine (an amino acid), making it unusable by the body.

Sample Menu	Protein (g)	Ovolactovegetarian Menu	Protein (g)
Breakfast			
1 ½ c Frosted Mini-Wheat cereal	7	1 c Complete wheat bran flakes cereal	4
12 oz skim milk	12	12 oz skim milk	12
12 oz black coffee	0	1 hard boiled egg	6
Mid-Morning Snack			
12 oz water	0	12 oz water	0
1 oz dry roasted almonds, unsalted	6	1 oz dry roasted almonds, unsalted	6
1 medium orange	1	1 medium orange	1
Lunch			
Sandwich with			
1 c tuna salad with egg, low-calorie mayonnaise	28 0	Sandwich wrap with vegetables and rice	13
¼ c thin-sliced cucumber		¼ c thin-sliced cucumber	0
3 thin slices tomato	0	3 thin slices tomato	0
2 medium lettuce leaves	0	2 medium lettuce leaves	0
2 thin slices 100% wheat bread	6		
8 baby carrots	1	8 baby carrots	1
1 medium applesauce cookie	1	1 medium applesauce cookie	1
1 c grapes	1	1 c grapes	1
12 oz water	0	12 oz water	0
Mid-Afternoon Snack			
8 oz low-fat vanilla yogurt	11	8 oz low-fat vanilla yogurt	11
12 oz herbal tea with nonnutritive sweetener	0	12 oz herbal tea with nonnutritive sweetener	0
Dinner			
3 oz pot roast beef with	26	1 c vegetarian baked beans	12
¼ c sauteed mushrooms	1	½ c sauteed mushrooms	1
1 c white and wild rice blend cooked with cooked margarine and	4	1 c white and wild rice blend with margarine	4
½ c vegetable juice	1	½ c vegetable juice	1
2 c tossed salad with lettuce, avocado, tomatoes, and carrots	2	2 c tossed salad with lettuce, avocado, tomatoes, and carrots	2
¼ c shredded low-fat Muenster cheese	7	¼ c shredded low-fat Muenster cheese	7
2 tbsp vinaigrette salad dressing	0	2 tbsp vinaigrette salad dressing	0
⅛ medium cantaloupe	1	⅛ medium cantaloupe	1
12 oz iced tea with low-calorie sweetener	0	12 oz iced tea with low-calorie sweetener	0
Evening Snack			
3 c low-fat microwave popcorn	3	3 c low-fat microwave popcorn	3
12 oz water	0	12 oz water	0
TOTALS[a]	119		87

[a]Totals may vary due to rounding.

From nutrient data Super Tracker Accessed April 17, 2017:

https://www.supertracker.usda.gov/default.aspx

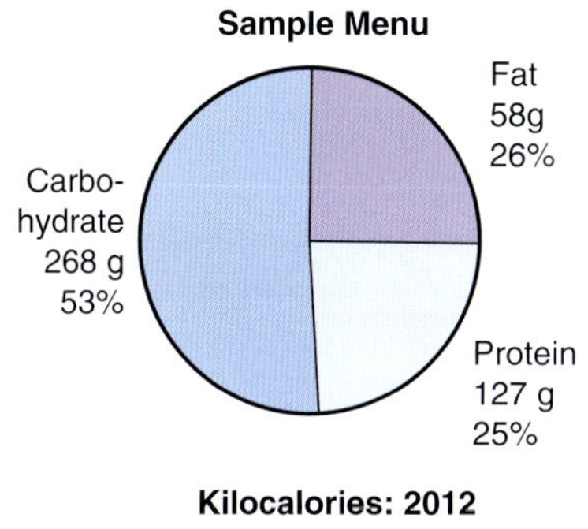

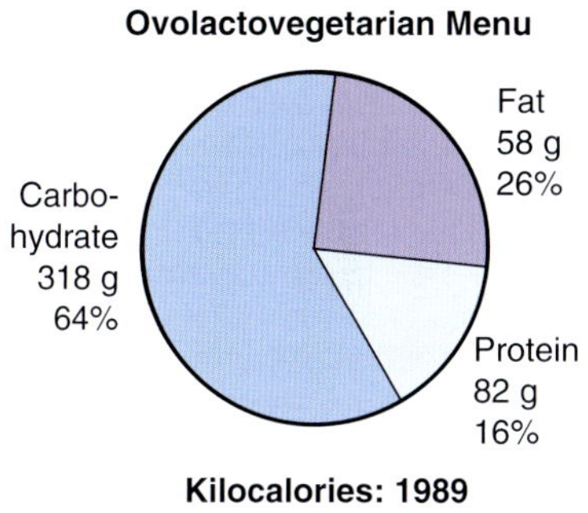

• **Figure 5.6** Protein content of sample menu and modifications for ovolactovegetarian diet. (U.S. Department of Agriculture's Food and Nutrient Database for Dietary Studies, 5.0 [2012] was used to calculate nutrient values, using the SuperTracker.)

TABLE 5.4 Portions for 1 Serving of Protein Foods

Protein Food	Serving Size
Seafood	1 oz
Meats	1 oz
Poultry	1 oz
Eggs	1
Nuts	½ oz
Seeds	½ oz
Soy products (tofu)	¼ c
Legumes (beans and peas)	¼ c
Peanut butter	1 tbsp

DENTAL CONSIDERATIONS

- Most Americans consume almost twice as much protein as recommended in the RDAs.
- Consuming approximately 1.0 to 1.6 g/kg per day is above the RDA, but within the AMDR for protein. Routine consumption of 1.5 g/kg or more for protein is considered a high-protein diet.
- When nutrient-dense protein sources (such as fried or high-fat meats) are not chosen, meeting the RDAs for other nutrients is difficult.
- An inadequate protein intake could affect any or all of the physiologic functions of protein. If dietary intake seems inadequate, evaluate the patient's status in the areas described in the Physiologic Roles section and refer the patient to an RDN or health care provider.
- Assessing protein intake of patients with periodontal issues is especially important. Protein deficiencies may compromise the physiologic systemic response to inflammation and infection, and periodontal problems may increase the protein requirement to promote healing in patients with inadequate or marginal protein intake.
- Collagen is a protein substance in connective tissue that helps support body structures, such as skin, bones, teeth, and tendons.
- The DRIs indicate that protein should provide 10% to 35% of caloric intake. If protein intake seems inappropriate, determine caloric or protein intake or both. The adequacy of intake can be established by using one of two methods. As an example, assuming consumption of 2200 cal per day, the amount of protein based on total energy intake is calculated as follows:

  2200 cal × 0.35 (maximum recommended % of total cal from protein) = 770 cal from proteins or less

  770 cal ÷ 4 (cal/g protein) = 193 g or less of protein.

  An intake of 193 g protein is the highest level recommended. Because 35% is the upper limit, protein consumption above this level may jeopardize adequate intakes of nutrients available from other food sources.
- A second method of calculating percentage of protein intake based on actual protein intake: Protein intake of 55 g with cal intake of 2200 cal:

  55 (g protein) × 4 (cal/g protein) = 220 cal from protein

  220 (cal from proteins) ÷ 2200 (total cal intake) × 100(%) = 10% of total cal from protein

  Because 10% is the lower limit, this patient's protein may be inadequate, and professional counseling may be warranted. Refer the patient to an RDN.
- Do not overemphasize animal sources of protein to patients on restricted incomes (e.g., elderly, homeless, and impoverished individuals). Too much emphasis on high-protein foods may result in inadequate amounts of other nutrients in the diet, especially when the food budget is low. Complementary sources of protein (described in *Health Application 5*), which are less expensive, can provide adequate protein.
- Evaluate food intake by comparing data from the patient with the recommended servings from *MyPlate* for the stage of growth, and DRIs for calorie and protein requirements (see p. ii).

NUTRITIONAL DIRECTIONS

- Protein supplements are unnecessary for healthy adults participating in endurance or resistance exercise.[6] However, high levels of protein by athletes has not proven to be harmful.[7] The amount of protein needed by an athlete should be determined by a Board Certified Specialist in Sports Dietetics or an RDN specializing in sports nutrition.
- Protein requirements should be met by foods from several sources (including different animal protein foods) because of other nutrients that accompany the protein. For example, pork is an excellent source of thiamin, while red meats furnish a significant amount of iron. In contrast, too many egg yolks in the diet contribute excessive cholesterol.
- Animal sources of protein are generally the most expensive. When patients have limited resources, counsel them to (a) eat protein in adequate but not excessive amounts, (b) use a variety of proteins of lower quality (which are less expensive), and (c) purchase less expensive kinds of protein foods.
- Emphasize that for people with adequate protein intake, amino acid supplements are not beneficial and could be harmful.

Underconsumption and Health-Related Problems

Although protein foods in the United States are plentiful and drastic protein deficiency is uncommon, several groups of individuals are susceptible to insufficient intakes: (a) elderly individuals, (b) individuals with low income, (c) strict vegetarians or vegans, (d) individuals with a lack of education or who are unwilling to shop wisely, and (e) patients who are chronically ill or hospitalized (e.g., patients with acquired immune deficiency syndrome, anorexia nervosa, or cancer). Intentionally restricting dietary protein to improve bone health is unwarranted. Dietary protein works synergistically with calcium to improve calcium retention and bone metabolism.[8] A systematic review and meta-analysis indicated positive trends on bone mineral density with higher protein intake.[9]

Fewer than 10% of Americans over 70 years of age get less than the recommended 0.8 g/kg body weight per day. Lower consumption of protein by older Americans may be related to cost, inability to prepare nutritious meals, depression, difficulty chewing, or concerns about the fat and cholesterol content of meats. Inadequate amounts of dietary protein contribute to sarcopenia. **Sarcopenia** is the progressive loss of muscle mass and strength with aging, a condition many believe is normal for elderly individuals. For the older population, a moderate increase in dietary protein intake (above the RDA of 0.8 g/kg) may be beneficial to maintain muscle mass and bone density, while still falling within the safe and acceptable range for protein consumption.[10]

Based on numerous studies, many researchers are questioning the adequacy of the RDAs. Scientific studies substantiate benefits of higher protein intakes at amounts approximately double the RDA, but less than the AMDR maximum of 35% of calories.[11] Specifically, higher-quality protein intake appears to be beneficial in promoting and maintaining muscle mass,[12–15] maintaining mobility,[16] managing body weight, preventing sarcopenia and osteoporosis,[17–19] and reducing and treating chronic diseases (e.g., type 2 diabetes and cardiovascular disease [CVD]).[20–22] Therefore, some researchers believe that overweight, obese, and older Americans may benefit by consuming up to 35% of their calories from protein and engaging in physical activity. In healthy, resistance-trained men, a high-protein diet (> 3 g/kg/d) did not adversely affect blood lipids, liver and kidney function, nor cause weight gain.[7] It would seem prudent, however, to include a significant proportion of the protein from vegetable sources.

Increasing evidence points to the importance of a fairly equal distribution of protein intake throughout the day (20 to 30 g/meal).[15,23] When protein intake is provided at all feedings throughout the day, body weight and appetite are better managed and progressions of sarcopenia in older adults may be reduced.[11,21]

Certain physiologic conditions and impaired digestion or absorption cause excessive protein losses, especially with individuals undergoing kidney dialysis, and may precipitate **protein-energy malnutrition (PEM)**. Although PEM is uncommon in the United States, malnutrition in these conditions is frequently unrecognized and is usually accompanied by other nutritional deficiencies. Separating effects of different nutrient deficiencies by observing clinical symptoms is often difficult. PEM affects the whole body, including every component of the orofacial complex.

The occurrence of PEM during critical developmental stages, including prenatal and postnatal periods, may affect developing tissues or lead to irreversible changes in oral tissues. During tooth development, mild-to-moderate protein deficiency results in smaller molars, significantly delayed eruption, and retardation during development of the mandible. Smaller salivary glands result in diminished salivary flow; this saliva is different in its protein composition and amylase and aminopeptidase activity, compromising the immune function of saliva.

Poor nutrition results in delayed eruption and exfoliation of deciduous teeth. Although malnourished children have an increased rate of caries, the peak caries experience is delayed by approximately 2 years. The increase in caries rate may simply be related to length of time a tooth is in the oral cavity; if the delay in exfoliation is greater than delay in eruption, the tooth is in the mouth longer and thus is exposed to caries-producing bacteria longer. Children with malnutrition (e.g., in developing countries and in many urban and rural areas in developed countries) have different dietary habits overall and oral environments that are not conducive to dental caries. However, teeth in these populations are highly susceptible to dental caries. Increased caries susceptibility may be related to alterations in structure of tooth crowns and diminished salivary flow, or changes in saliva composition may be related to malnutrition issues.

Epithelium, connective tissue, and bone also may be poorly developed. An increase in acid solubility associated with chemical alterations of the exposed enamel surface may contribute to increased caries susceptibility.

The **periodontium** includes hard and soft tissues surrounding and supporting the teeth: gingiva, alveolar mucosa, cementum, periodontal ligaments, and alveolar bone. An insufficient intake of protein creates negative nitrogen balance, decreasing nitrogen reserves and blood protein levels, and resistance of the periodontium to infections. In addition, ability of the periodontium to withstand the stress of injury or surgery is reduced and recovery periods are longer. In malnourished children, **secretory immunoglobulin A (sIgA)** levels are depressed. sIgA is the predominant immunoglobulin, or antibody, in oral, nasal, intestinal, and other mucosal secretions, providing the first line of defense in the oral cavity. Low sIgA levels in malnourished children probably play a role in their increased susceptibility to mucosal infections.

PEM may be a major reason for increased incidence of **noma** and **necrotizing ulcerative gingivitis (NUG)**, conditions strongly associated with depressed immune responses caused by nutritional deficiencies, stress, and infection (see Chapter 19, Fig. 19.8). Noma is a progressive **necrosis** (degeneration and cellular death) that usually manifests as a small ulcer on the gingiva that spreads to produce extensive destruction of lips, cheeks, and tissues covering the jaw with an accompanying foul odor. NUG is characterized by **erythema** (marginated redness of mucous membranes caused by inflammation) and necrosis of the interdental papillae. This painful gingivitis is generally accompanied by a metallic taste and foul oral odor. Cratered papillae often remain after treatment of the disease.

NUG occasionally occurs among college students who are under a great deal of psychological stress and have poor eating habits. It also can be observed in individuals who live in developed countries and are severely debilitated or **immunocompromised** (having an immune response weakened by a disease or pharmacologic agent) or in children 2 to 6 years old who live in developing countries, are malnourished, and have recently experienced a stressful event, such as viral disease.

NUG can be precipitated by emotionally stressful situations that affect eating patterns, leading to acute deficiencies and

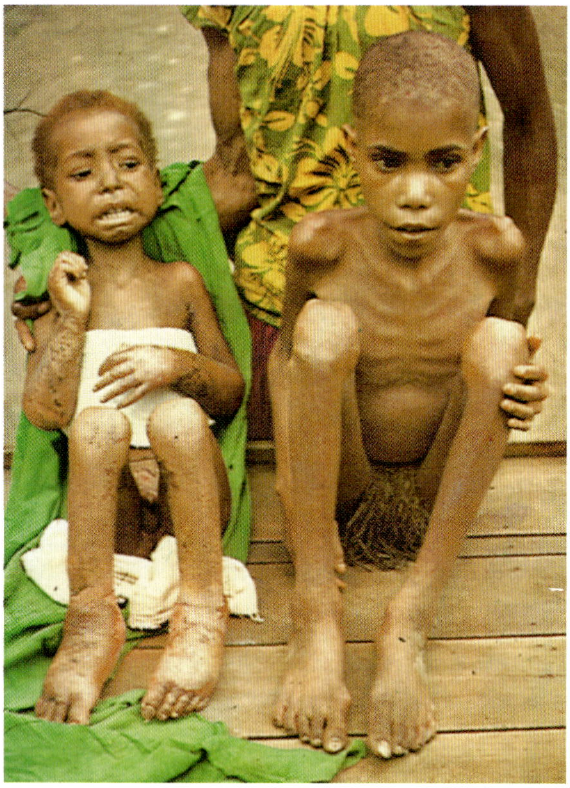

• **Figure 5.7** Kwashiorkor and marasmus in brothers. The younger brother, on the left, has kwashiorkor with generalized edema, skin changes, pale reddish yellow hair, and an unhappy expression. The older child, on the right, has marasmus, with generalized wasting, spindly arms and legs, and an apathetic expression. (Reproduced with permission from Peters W, Pasvol G, eds. *Tropical Medicine and Parasitology*. 5th ed. London: Mosby; 2006.)

depressed immune response to bacteria normally found in the oral cavity. Decreased host resistance to infection may permit gingival lesions to spread rapidly into adjacent tissues, producing extensive necrosis and destruction of orofacial tissues, whereas in a healthy individual, the lesion is limited to the gingiva alone. Wound healing is also delayed (see Chapter 19 for further discussion).

In other areas of the world, where quantities of high-quality protein and calories are insufficient, PEM is commonly seen. **Kwashiorkor** develops when young children consume adequate calories and inadequate high-quality protein (Fig. 5.7). It is almost exclusively seen in association with famine in the tropics. It usually appears after the child has been weaned from breast milk. **Marasmus** occurs in infants when both protein and calories are deficient in the diet.

Kwashiorkor and marasmus are very serious health problems that have received much attention by the United Nations and the World Health Organization. Incaparina (a high protein food made from maize, cottonseed and sorghum flours fortified with minerals and vitamins), skim milk powder, and the addition of lysine to cereal products have been used to improve nutritional status in developing countries. However, most of these efforts to improve the nutritional status worldwide have not been well accepted for various reasons, and protein-energy problems in the world still exist.

DENTAL CONSIDERATIONS

- The protein requirement of older adults is the same as that of young adults; however, older adults are frequently less motivated to choose a healthy eating pattern due to physical, social, and financial reasons. Decreased protein intake is common as a result of ill-fitting dentures or edentulousness. Closely assess protein intake of older patients.
- Overweight, obese, and older Americans may benefit by consuming up to 35% of their calories from protein and engaging in some physical activity.
- Consuming 20 to 30 g of protein per meal optimizes skeletal muscle synthesis; this amount three times daily is below current estimates for safe upper levels for protein or indispensable amino acids for healthy persons.
- Older adults and individuals trying to lose weight may benefit by distributing their protein intake throughout the day and to especially not omit protein at breakfast. (Bacon is not a protein-rich food.)
- When assessing for marasmus or kwashiorkor, remember that the main difference between the two conditions is the presence of some subcutaneous fat tissue in individuals with kwashiorkor and edema, especially in the abdomen, feet, and legs. Fat stores and edema are absent in marasmus. Assess the patient's financial status because poverty is a major cause of PEM and has been identified in rural and urban inner-city areas in the United States. To assess for inadequate protein intake, look for frequent or extended periods of fasting, medications that cause anorexia, abnormal food intake, nausea and vomiting, and problems with hair (dull, dry, brittle, breaks easily), skin (flaky and dry), or fingernails (dry and cracked, spoon-shaped).
- Treatment of malnutrition requires referral to a health care provider or an RDN.
- Malnourished patients take longer to heal and regain strength and are at risk for frequent infections. Adequate infection control procedures are particularly important for these patients.
- In the United States, noma-like lesions may occur in patients with cancer whose immune systems have been severely impaired by chemotherapy or advanced acquired immune deficiency syndrome.

NUTRITIONAL DIRECTIONS

- Suggest Meals on Wheels or community senior centers for older patients with an inadequate diet and refer them to a social worker.
- Supplement dietary protein by adding skim milk powder to milk, soups, or mashed potatoes (if the patient is not lactose intolerant) and by adding cheese to foods.
- A high-protein breakfast may help improve attempts toward weight management (prevention of body fat gain and increased satiety).[21]

Overconsumption and Health-Related Problems

An upper limit for safe levels of protein intake has not been determined. Most patients believe that no upper limits for protein exist. Americans frequently eat 150% to 200% of the RDA for protein. Numerous studies have shown that a higher protein intake does not have an adverse effect on bone health except in a context of inadequate calcium supply.

When protein intake is excessive, fluid imbalances may occur in all age groups but especially in infants. Metabolism of 100 cal of protein requires 350 g of water compared with 50 g of water for a similar amount of carbohydrates or fats. Water requirements are increased as well as end products of protein metabolism in the bloodstream.

Whether popular high-protein diets are excessive in protein content is controversial. Usually, a high-protein diet refers to 25% to 35% of calories coming from protein foods. Regardless, this trend stimulated scientific research that expanded scientific knowledge in this realm. Higher-protein diets support weight control by enhancing loss of body fat with less muscle loss and improved control of blood glucose levels. Dietary protein may aid in weight loss by increasing satiation; increasing muscle mass, which burns more calories; increasing **thermogenesis** (production of body heat); and decreasing energy efficiency. Protein intake generally increases satiety to a greater extent than carbohydrate or fat and may facilitate a reduction in **ad libitum** (as desired) energy consumption.

Obtaining adequate protein, or within the upper range of recommended amounts, is an important dietary concern, especially for weight loss or management, or for physical strength and activity. To maximize weight loss using a high-protein diet, the goal should be 120 g of high-quality protein daily, distributed evenly throughout the day.[8] Other macronutrients also need to be considered. If the principal source of protein is red meat and regular dairy products, intake of saturated fat and cholesterol content is high, which raises the risk of CVD, including stroke. If carbohydrates are severely restricted by choosing primarily protein foods, high-fiber foods are limited. High-fiber plant foods help lower blood lipids. Restriction of plant-based carbohydrate foods limits nutrients that offer protection against cancer and other diseases and causes problems such as constipation and diverticulosis.

Although high-protein intake is not associated with diminished kidney function in individuals with healthy kidneys, high-protein diets may be harmful to the kidneys in individuals with preexisting metabolic renal dysfunction.[24,25] When renal function is impaired, the American Diabetes Association recommends limiting protein intake to less than 20% of total calories (100 g protein for a 2000-cal diet).[26]

DENTAL CONSIDERATIONS

- Protein intake should be fairly equally distributed throughout the day.
- Good choices of high-protein, low-fat foods include fish, skinless chicken, low-fat dairy products, and lean beef and pork.

NUTRITIONAL DIRECTIONS

- Extremely high protein intake is especially undesirable in infants.
- Because proteins must be metabolized by the liver and filtered by the kidneys, excessive amounts (more than 200% of the RDA) result in additional work by or stress on these organs.

HEALTH APPLICATION 5

Vegetarianism

Despite the fact that protein is not limited in the United States food supply, some people choose plant sources of protein for health reasons or because of philosophical, ecological, or religious convictions. Large numbers of vegetarian cookbooks and meatless "veggie" burgers and sausage-style products would lead one to believe vegetarianism is a growing consumer movement. The Vegetarian Resource Group indicates that approximately 3.3% of the population are true vegetarians, or approximately 9 million Americans.[27]

Technically, variations of vegetarian diets differ in the types of foods included, as shown in Box 5.3. "Self-described" vegetarians are not true vegetarians because they occasionally eat fish and poultry. When milk and cheese products are included, they complement plant foods and enhance the amino acid content of the diet. If adequate quantities of eggs, milk, and milk products are consumed, all nutrients are more likely to be provided in sufficient quantities. Strict supervision is unnecessary for all types of vegetarians with the exception of vegans. The strict vegetarian diet does not include any food of animal origin (e.g., meat, milk, cheese, eggs, and butter). Approximately 2% of the United States population follows this strict plant-based diet.[28]

A *Healthy Vegetarian Eating Pattern* (*Vegetarian Pattern)* was developed to provide recommendations that meet the *Dietary Guidelines* for individuals who choose to omit meat. The pattern can be adapted by vegans by substituting soy beverages for dairy products. The *Vegetarian Pattern* is the same as the *Healthy Pattern* except for protein foods (Table 5.5). Nutritionally, this pattern is similar to the *Healthy Pattern,* providing a little more calcium and fiber, and lower in vitamin D.[4]

Textured vegetable products, or meat substitutes, are produced from vegetable proteins, usually soybeans. Protein in textured vegetable protein products is of good quality, but these products may have high sodium content. The protein in the *Vegetarian Pattern* is provided by eggs, legumes, soy products, and nuts and seeds. The number of servings per week are designed to provide optimum nutrition using nutrient-dense choices.

Indispensable amino acids can be provided by plants, but larger amounts of these plant products must be consumed to match protein obtained from animal sources. Indispensable amino acids present in low levels in grains are abundant in other plants, such as legumes. Beans are low in methionine and tryptophan, and corn is low in lysine and threonine. When eaten together, as in pinto beans and cornbread, they are said to be **complementary foods**, and less volume is required.

Protein from a single source is seldom consumed alone. Foods are usually combined without awareness that they are complementary to each other (e.g., beans are usually combined with rice, bread, or crackers [wheat], or tortillas or cornbread [corn]). When a combination of plant proteins is eaten throughout the day, the amino acids provided by each complement each other; that is, the deficiencies of one are offset by the adequacies of another. Additionally, small amounts of high-quality proteins can be combined with plant foods, as in macaroni and cheese or cereal and milk, to provide adequate amounts of indispensable amino acids. If caloric intake is adequate, protein requirements are met when a variety of protein-containing foods are eaten throughout the day. Foods providing complementary amino acids do not have to be consumed simultaneously.

With some basic nutrition knowledge, patients following a vegetarian pattern are frequently healthier than those who choose to eat meat. Foods can be nutritionally balanced without meats, by providing protein from different sources. *My Vegan Plate* (Fig. 5.8) is designed specifically to address nutrient inadequacies and reduced mineral bioavailability of vegetarian and vegan diets. Table 5.5 indicates the number of servings from the food groups to meet nutrient recommendations for various caloric levels. By using a variety of principally unrefined foods and enough calories to promote good health, protein quantity and other nutrients can be adequate for most individuals.

Vegetarian diets generally result in lower dietary intake of saturated fat and cholesterol, and high levels of dietary fiber, magnesium, potassium, vitamins C and E, and folate. Key nutrients that may fall short of the DRIs in the vegan diet and less often in the vegetarian diet include zinc, calcium, iron, iodine, vitamins D and B_{12}, and long-chain n-3 fatty acids.[29]

Persons following a vegan diet must pay closer attention to food choices and will need supplementation or fortification of vitamins B_{12} and D, and

Continued

Vegetarianism—cont'd

possibly zinc and iodine. Vitamin B_{12} deficiency rates are especially high for pregnant women, adolescents, older adults, and those who have adhered to a vegetarian diet since birth. Vegans who do not utilize vitamin B_{12} supplements are especially at high risk of deficiency.[30] Commonly available fortified foods (e.g., fortified breakfast cereals and nondairy soymilks) are emphasized to ensure good sources of vitamins B_{12} and D and calcium. Because of difficulties consuming adequate volumes of food to meet nutritional needs, the vegan diet is not recommended for infants, children, or pregnant/lactating women. More information can be found at http://www.theveganrd.com/food-guide-for-vegans. During periods of rapid growth, vegans should be referred to an RDN.

Much can be said of the healthy aspects of vegetarian diets. Vegetarian diets can meet the DRIs as long as variety and amounts of foods are adequate. That vegetarian diets and lifestyles seem to be conducive to good health is exemplified by vegetarians exhibiting reduced risk of numerous health problems, including heart disease, type 2 diabetes, hypertension, certain types of cancer, and obesity.[29] A vegetarian diet rich in healthier plant foods is associated with substantially lower CVD risk as opposed to a vegetarian diet that includes principally less healthy plant foods.[31] Health advantages are not attributed solely to avoidance of meat products but rather benefits from phytochemical-rich plant foods. For instance, beans, legumes, and whole-grain products help with blood glucose control; plant foods are associated with a lower risk of CVD.

When working with vegetarian or vegan patients, keep lines of communication open by respecting their decision, unless eating habits are potentially harmful. Patients who have an interest in pursuing a vegetarian diet should be encouraged to do so. All patients should be encouraged to have more meatless meals (see http://www.meatlessmonday.com/) and to consume more plant proteins.

TABLE 5.5 Healthy Vegetarian Eating Patterns: Recommended Amounts of Food From Each Food Group for 4 Calorie Levels

Calorie Level of Pattern[a]	1200	1800	2200	2800
Food Group	**Daily Amount**[b] of Food From Each Group (vegetable and protein foods subgroup amounts are per week)			
Vegetables	**1½ oz-eq**	**2½ c-eq**	**3 oz-eq**	**3½ c-eq**
Dark-Green Vegetables (c-eq/wk)	1	1½	2	2½
Red and orange vegetables (c-eq/wk)	3	5½	6	7
Legumes (beans and peas (c-eq/wk)	½	1½	2	2½
Starchy vegetables (c-eq/wk)	3½	5	6	7
Other vegetables (c-eq/wk)	2½	4	5	5½
Fruits	**1 c-dq**	**1½ c-eq**	**2 c-eq**	**2½ c-eq**
Grains	**4 oz-eq**	**6½ oz-eq**	**7½ oz-eq**	**10½ oz-eq**
Whole grains[c] (oz-eq/day)	2	3½	4	5½
Refined grains (oz-eq/day)	2	3	3½	5
Dairy	**2½ c-eq**	**3 c-eq**	**3 c-eq**	**3 c-eq**
Protein Foods	**1½ oz-eq**	**3 oz-eq**	**3½ oz-eq**	**5 oz-eq**
Eggs (oz-eq/wk)	3	3	3	4
Legumes (beans & peas, oz-eq/wk)[d]	2	6	6	10
Soy products (oz-eq/wk)	3	6	8	11
Nuts and seeds (oz-eq/wk)	2	6	7	10
Oils	**17 g**	**24 g**	**29 g**	**36 g**
Limit on Calories for Other Uses, Calories (% of Calories)[e]	**170 (14%)**	**190 (11%)**	**330 (15%)**	**400 (14%)**
Total Legumes (Beans & Peas) (c-eq/wk)	**1**	**3**	**3½**	**5**

[a]Food intake patterns below 1400 calories (see Evolve website for more caloric levels) are designed to meet the nuritional needs of 2- to 8-year-old children. Patterns from 1600 to 3200 calories are designed to meet the nutritional needs of children 9 years and older and adults. If a child 4 to 8 years of age needs more calories and, therefore, is following a pattern at 1600 calories or more, that child's recommended amount from the dairy group should be 2.5 cups per dy. Children 9 years and older and adults should not use caloric patterns below 1400 calories.

[b]Food group amounts shown in cup-equivalents (c-eq) or ounce-equivalents (oz-eq), as appropriate for each group, based on caloric and nutrient content. Oils are shown in grams (g).

[c]Amounts of whole grains in the Patterns for children are less than the minimum of 3 oz-eq in all Patterns recommended for adults.

[d]About half of total legumes are shown as vegetables, in cup-eq, and half as protein foods, in oz-eq. Total legumes in the Patterns, in cup-eq, is the amount in the vegetable group plus the amount in protein foods group (in oz-eq) divided by 4.

[e]All foods are assumed to be in nutrient-dense forms; lean or low-fat; and prepared without added fats, sugars, refined starches, or salt. If all food choies to meet food group recommendations are in nutrient-dense forms, a small number of calories remain within the overall calorie limit of the Pattern (i.e., limit on calories for other uses). The number of these calories depends on the overall calroie limit in the Pattern and the amounts of food from each food group required to meet nutritional goals. Calories from protein, carbohydrates, and total fats should be within the acceptable macronutrient distribution ranges (AMDRs).

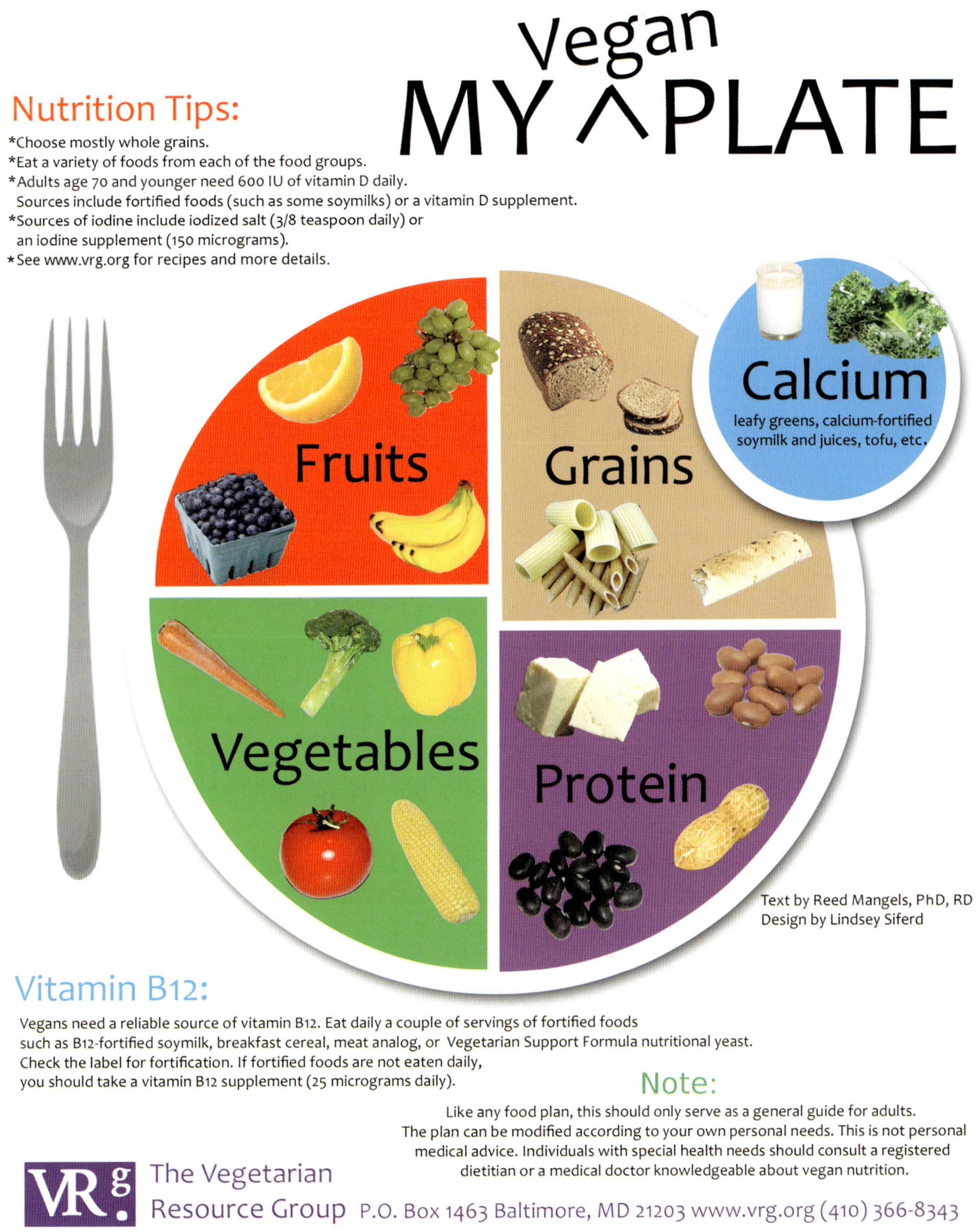
MY Vegan PLATE
Nutrition Tips:
*Choose mostly whole grains.
*Eat a variety of foods from each of the food groups.
*Adults age 70 and younger need 600 IU of vitamin D daily.
Sources include fortified foods (such as some soymilks) or a vitamin D supplement.
*Sources of iodine include iodized salt (3/8 teaspoon daily) or
an iodine supplement (150 micrograms).
*See www.vrg.org for recipes and more details.
Fruits
Grains
Calcium
leafy greens, calcium-fortified soymilk and juices, tofu, etc.
Vegetables
Protein
Text by Reed Mangels, PhD, RD
Design by Lindsey Siferd
Vitamin B12:
Vegans need a reliable source of vitamin B12. Eat daily a couple of servings of fortified foods
such as B12-fortified soymilk, breakfast cereal, meat analog, or Vegetarian Support Formula nutritional yeast.
Check the label for fortification. If fortified foods are not eaten daily,
you should take a vitamin B12 supplement (25 micrograms daily).
Note:
Like any food plan, this should only serve as a general guide for adults.
The plan can be modified according to your own personal needs. This is not personal
medical advice. Individuals with special health needs should consult a registered
dietitian or a medical doctor knowledgeable about vegan nutrition.
VRg The Vegetarian Resource Group P.O. Box 1463 Baltimore, MD 21203 www.vrg.org (410) 366-8343

• **Figure 5.8** My Vegan Plate. (From The Vegetarian Resource Group, Baltimore, MD. Accessed August 17, 2013. http://www.vrg.org/nutshell/MyVeganPlate.pdf.)

• BOX 5.3 Terminology for Different Types of Vegetarian Diets

Flexitarian	Do not regularly eat meat, but occasionally eat fish and poultry
Vegetarian	Plant proteins, but may or may not include egg or dairy products
Lactovegetarian	Plant proteins plus dairy products
Ovolactovegetarian	Plant proteins plus milk, cheese, and eggs
Ovovegetarian	Plant proteins plus eggs
Vegan	Plant proteins only

◆ CASE APPLICATION FOR THE DENTAL HYGIENIST

A single mother of two children comes to the clinic complaining about sensitivity to hot and cold foods and bleeding gums. She has recently lost her job and child support payments are irregular. She is very concerned about the limited amount of protein foods she is able to purchase with her food stamps. Based on her diet diary, her caloric intake is 1800 cal per day, and protein is approximately 50 g. Food intake is principally pastas, tortillas, chips, sweet pastries, and sodas.

Nutritional Assessment

- Willingness to learn
- Knowledge base of protein, carbohydrate, and fat principles for optimal nutrition
- Cultural beliefs
- Recent percentage of calories from protein (11%)
- Types of protein intake and total nutrient intake
- Overall nutrient intake
- Carbonated beverage intake

Nutritional Diagnosis

Altered health maintenance and limited nutrition knowledge related to insufficient funds to purchase foods to provide adequate nutrients.

Nutritional Goals

The patient will verbalize three principles concerning protein as well as the benefits from other nutrients. The patient will consume foods providing complementary protein and incorporate some fruits and dairy products into her menus.

Nutritional Implementation

Intervention: Discussion points: (a) the seven functions or roles of protein, (b) the difference between indispensable amino acids and dispensible amino acids, (c) the difference between high-quality and lower-quality protein, and (d) how to incorporate complementary protein into menus.

Rationale: Knowledge corrects inaccurate information.

Intervention: Discuss cheaper sources of protein.

Rationale: Good sources of protein do not have to be high-priced meats.

Intervention: Encourage the use of milk and milk products.

Rationale: Dairy products are an excellent source of protein and provide other nutrients important to maintain health.

Intervention: Encourage incorporating fruits and vegetables into the menus.

Rationale: Protein is not the only nutrient needed to maintain good oral health. In addition, consumption of more fruits and vegetables models healthy eating to her children.

Intervention: Refer her to a social worker.

Rationale: The social worker will be knowledgeable about local and federal programs she is eligible for and can direct her to local food banks and other resources.

Evaluation

The patient should understand that protein is important, but also realize it is possible to purchase cheaper sources of protein that provide all the indispensable amino acids. To determine this, have the patient repeat three of the principles she remembers from your teaching. The patient should also express her intention to use complementary proteins to provide adequate amounts of amino acids, which will provide other nutrients necessary for health, and purchase some dairy products, fruits, and vegetables each week.

◆ Student Readiness

1. Define bioavailability, kwashiorkor, sarcopenia, nitrogen balance, high-quality protein, and complementary proteins for a patient.
2. List and explain the functions of proteins.
3. Using your desirable body weight, how many grams of protein should you consume?
4. Given a patient weighing 180 lb who has a caloric intake of 2500 cal, if the diet averages 15% protein, how many calories are provided by protein? How many grams of protein is this? How does this compare with the RDA for this patient?
5. What would you tell a strict vegetarian (vegan) parent about feeding her infant?
6. What are the oral effects of too much protein in the diet? What are the oral effects of too little protein in the diet?
7. Explain the relationship between calories and protein.
8. What are two methods of obtaining the indispensable amino acids from vegetarian foods? List two food combinations for each type of vegetarian diet that would provide adequate amounts of indispensable amino acids.
9. How do high-protein diets help with weight loss or maintenance?
10. Using the Internet or a reputable sports magazine, identify a professional athlete who is vegan. Note what is said about his/her health, strength, and types and amounts of foods consumed.
11. Determine the cost of the protein in the following items to determine which one is the wisest choice economically:
    a. One jumbo-size egg contains 8 g protein; 1 cup milk contains 8 g protein.
    b. ¾ cup dried pinto beans provides 20 g protein (cooked); 3½ oz canned tuna provides 20 g protein.
    c. 3¼ oz raw chicken breast with bone and skin provides 20 g protein; 3½ oz raw beef liver provides 20 g protein.
    d. 4 oz sliced American cheese provides 20 g protein; 3½ chicken wings provides 20 g protein
    e. 4 oz boneless ham provides 20 g protein; 3¾ oz raw ground turkey provides 20 g protein

References

1. Tufts University. Reversing trend, US meat eating jumps. Tufts Health & Nutrition Letter. November 2016. http://www.nutritionletter.tufts.edu/issues/12_11/todays-newsbites/Reversing-Trend-US-Meat-Eating-Jumps_2039-1.html. Accessed July 11, 2017.
2. Layman DK, Anthony TG, Rasmussen BB, et al. Defining meal for protein to optimize metabolic roles of amino acids. *Am J Clin Nutr.* 2015;101(6):1330S–1338S.
3. Phillips SM. The impact of protein quality on the promotion of resistance exercise-induced changes in muscle mass. *Nutr Metab (Lond).* 2016;13:64.
4. US Department of Health and Human Services and US Department of Agriculture. 2015–2020 Dietary Guidelines for Americans. 8th edition. December 2015. Available at http://health.gov/dietaryguidelines/2015/guidelines/.
5. Kantor L. Americans' seafood consumption below recommendations. Amber Waves. Oct 3 2016. https://www.ers.usda.gov/amber-waves/2016/october/americans-seafood-consumption-below-recommendations/. Accessed December 21, 2016.
6. Thomas DT, Erdman KA, Burke LM. Position of the Academy of Nutrition and Dietetics, Dietitian of Canada, and the American College of Sports Medicine: Nutrition and athletic performance. *J Acad Nutr Diet.* 2016;16(3):501–528.
7. Antonio J, Ellerbroak A, Silver T, et al. A high protein diet has no harmful effects: A one-year crossover sudy in resistance-trained males. *J Nutr Metab.* 2016;2016:9104792. [Epub Oct 11, 2016].
8. Phillips SM, Chevalier S, Leidy HJ. Protein 'requirements' beyond the RDA: implications for optimizing health. *Appl Physiol Nutr Metab.* 2016;41(5):565–572.
9. Shams-White MM, Chung M, Du M, et al. Dietary protein and bone health: a systematic review and meta-analysis from the National Osteoporosis Foundation. *Am J Clin Nutr.* 2017;105(6):1528–1543.
10. Kim JE, O-Connor LE, Sands LP, et al. Effects of dietary protein intake on body composition changes after weight loss in older adults: a systematic review and meta-analysis. *Nutr Rev.* 2016;74(3):210–224.
11. Rodriguez NR, Miller SL. Effective translation of current dietary guidance: understanding and communicating the concepts of minimal and optimal levels of dietary protein. *Am J Clin Nutr.* 2015;101(6):1353S–1358S.
12. Lancha AH Jr, Zanella R Jr, Tanabe SG, et al. Dietary protein supplementation in the elderly for limiting muscle mass loss. *Amino Acids.* 2017;59(1):33–47.
13. Phillips SM. The impact of protein quality on the promotion of resistance exercise-induced changes in muscle mass. *Nutr Metab (Lond).* 2016;13:64.
14. Longland TM, Oikawa SY, Mitchell CJ, et al. High compared with lower dietary protein during an energy deficit combined with intense exercise promotes greater lean mass gain and fat mass loss: a randomized trial. *Am J Clin Nutr.* 2016;103(3):738–746.
15. Paddon-Jones D, Campbell WW, Jacques PF, et al. Protein and healthy aging. *Am J Clin Nutr.* 2015;101(6):1339S–1345S.
16. Isanejad M, Mursu J, Sirola J, et al. Dietary protein intake is associated with better physical function and muscle strength among elderly women. *Br J Nutr.* 2016;115(7):1281–1291.
17. Oh C, Jeon BH, Storm R, et al. The most effective factors to offset sarcopenia and obesity in the older Korean: physical activity, vitamin D, and protein intake. *Nutrition.* 2017;33:169–173.
18. Bonjour JP. The dietary protein, IGF-1, skeletal health axis. *Horm Mol Biol Clin Investig.* 2016;28(1):39–53.
19. Langsetmo L, Shikany JM, Cawthon PM, et al. The association between protein intake by source and osteoporotic fracture in older men: a prospective cohort study. *J Bone Miner Res.* 2017;32(3):592–600.
20. Astrup A, Raben A, Geiker N. The role of higher protein diets in weight control and obesity-related comorbidities. *Int J Obes (Lond).* 2015;39(5):721–726.
21. Leidy HJ, Clifton PM, Astrup A, et al. The role of protein in weight loss and maintenance. *Am J Clin Nutr.* 2015;101(6):1320S–1329S.
22. Arentson-Lantz E, Clairmont S, Paddon-Jones D, et al. Protein: A nutrient in focus. *Appl Physiol Nutr Metab.* 2015;40(8):755–761.
23. Arciero PF, Edmonds R, He F, et al. Protein-pacing caloric restrictions enhances body composition similarly in obese men and women during weight loss and sustains efficacy during long-term weight maintenance. *Nutrients.* 2016;8(8):pii:E476.
24. Ko GJ, Obi Y, Tortorici AR, et al. Dietary protein intake and chronic kidney disease. *Curr Opin Clin Nutr Metab Care.* 2017;20(1):77–85.
25. Wang M, Chou J, Chang Y, et al. The role of low protein diet in ameliorating proteinuria and deferring dialysis initiation: what is old and what is new. *Panminerva Med.* 2017;59(2):157–165.
26. Standards of Medical Care in Diabetes—2017. Microvascular complications and foot care. *Diabetes Care.* 2017;40(suppl 1):S88–S98.
27. Vegetarian Resource Group. The vegetarian resource group asks in a 2016 national poll conducted by Harris Poll. www.vrg.org/nutshell/polls/2016_adults_veg.htm. Accessed November 21, 2016.
28. Fields H, Ruddy B, Wallace MR, et al. How to monitor and advise vegans to ensure adequate nutrient intake. *J Am Osteopath Assoc.* 2016;116(2):96–99.
29. Posthauer MEE, Malone A, Sabate J. Position of the Academy of Nutrition and Dietetics: vegetarian diets. *J Acad Nutr Diet.* 2016;116(12):1970–1980.
30. Pawlak R, Lester SE, Babatunde T. The prevalence of cobalamin deficiency among vegetarians assessed by serum vitamin B_{12}: a review of literature. *Eur J Clin Nutr.* 2014;68(5):541–548.
31. Satija A, Shilpa NB, Spiehelman D, et al. Healthful and unhealthful plant-based diets and the risk of coronary heart diease in U.S. adults. *J Am Coll Cardiol.* 2017;70(4):411–422.

e EVOLVE RESOURCES

Please visit http://evolve.elsevier.com/Stegeman/nutritional for additional practice and study support tools.

6 Lipids: The Condensed Energy

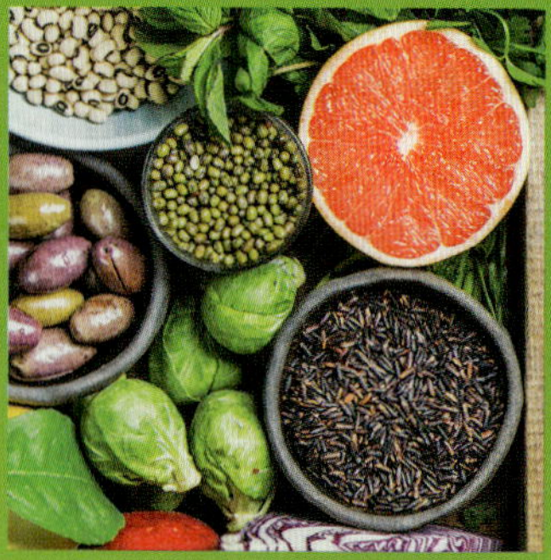

STUDENT LEARNING OUTCOMES

Upon completion of this chapter, the student will be able to achieve the following student learning outcomes:

1. Related to the classification, chemical structure, and characteristics of lipids:
   - Describe how fatty acids affect the properties of fat.
   - Explain the function of fat in the body.
   - Discuss the chemical structure of lipids.
   - Describe the characteristics of lipids.
2. Describe the function of various compound lipids, and identify foods that contain each. Also, discuss the function and sources of cholesterol.
3. List and describe the physiologic roles of lipids in the body.
4. Discuss the effects of dietary fats on oral health.
5. Related to dietary requirements of lipids:
   - Calculate the recommendation for a person's consumption of dietary fat.
   - Evaluate a patient's food intake for appropriate amounts of saturated fats.
   - Suggest appropriate foods when dietary modification of fat intake has been recommended to a patient.
   - Compare the types of fatty acids in various fats and oils.
6. Discuss nutritional directions for various patient issues related to the overconsumption and underconsumption of fat.

KEY TERMS

Adipose tissue
α-Linolenic acid
Atherosclerosis
Calorie-dense foods
Cardiovascular disease (CVD)
Compound lipids
Docosahexaenoic acid (DHA)
Eicosapentaenoic acid (EPA)
Essential fatty acid (EFA)
Hyperlipidemia
Interesterified fats
Lipoproteins
Long-chain fatty acids
Medium-chain fatty acids
Omega-3 fatty acids
Omega-6 fatty acids
Phospholipids
Plant sterols
Protein sparing
Short-chain fatty acids
Structural lipids
***Trans* fatty acid**

TEST YOUR NQ

1. **T/F** All foods containing more than 35% of their calories from fat are not considered healthy.
2. **T/F** Fats containing vitamin E deteriorate and become rancid rapidly.
3. **T/F** A product containing more unsaturated fatty acids than saturated fatty acids is a healthier food choice than one containing a higher proportion of saturated fatty acids.
4. **T/F** Dietary fat intake should be less than 20% of total calories.
5. **T/F** Bananas and avocados contain cholesterol.
6. **T/F** Oils are less fattening than solid fats.
7. **T/F** Fat intake has been linked more frequently to cancer than any other dietary factor.
8. **T/F** Nuts and cheeses are nutritious foods that should be recommended as snacks to all patients because they reduce the rate of caries.
9. **T/F** Fats contain 9 kcal/g.
10. **T/F** Omega-3 fatty acids are polyunsaturated fatty acids.

Unsweetened coconut, mayonnaise, sour cream, blue cheese, salad dressing, almonds, pecans, olives, avocados, and sausages—what do all these foods have in common? More than 50% of the calories in each of these foods come from fat, a vital nutrient in our diet.

Added fats and oils provide more calories in the average American diet than any other food group. Examination of the United States food supply trends between 2000 and 2010 indicates that total fat intake remains at a high level with a slight increase in fats provided by vegetable oils and a decrease in consumption of saturated fats, principally due to fewer *trans* fats.[1] Approximately 70% of Americans consume more saturated fat than is recommended in the *Dietary Guidelines* and 70% to 75% consume less oil (polyunsaturated fats) than recommended.[2] Consumers have become more aware of healthy food choices, but making changes in eating patterns is difficult. Food manufacturers, producers, and grocers have responded

TABLE 6.1 Common Food Sources and Physiological Actions of Fatty Acids

Fatty Acids/Classification	Common Food Sources	Physiologic Action
Saturated Fatty Acid (SFA)		
Lauric, myristic, palmitic, stearic; palmitic; carprylic, and capric acids	Animal sources (meats, eggs, butter, lard, beef tallow); processed food products containing saturated vegetable oils; coconut oil, palm and palm kernel oil; cocoa butter, fully hydrogenated vegetable oils	Raises total and LDL (except stearic acid)
Monounsaturated Fatty Acid (MUFA)		
Cis configuration (oleic and palmitoleicacid)	Olive and canola oil; avocados, almonds; macadamia nuts; lesser amounts in beef tallow, lard	Decreases total and LDL cholesterol and triglycerides; increases HDL cholesterol when substituted for SFAs and carbohydrate, but not when replacing PUFAs
Trans configuration (elaidic acid)	Partially hydrogenated vegetable oils	Raises total and LDL cholesterol similar to SFAs, decreases HDL more than saturated fatty acids. Increases CVD and diabetes risk factors
Trans configuration (vaccenic acid)	Dairy fat, meat from ruminating animals (beef, lamb)	No significant differences in blood lipids or lipoproteins observed. May have beneficial health effects, especially vaccenic acid; more research needed
Polyunsaturated Fatty Acid (PUFA)		
n-6 Fatty Acids		
Linoleic acid	Soybean oil, corn oil, shortening	Decreases total and LDL cholesterol
Arachidonic acid	Meat, poultry, eggs	Precursor for important biologically active substances; substrate for synthesis of a variety of proinflammatory compounds
Conjugated linoleic acid	Ruminant meat and dairy	May help reduce body fat deposits and improve immune function
n-3 Fatty Acids		
α-Linolenic acid	Flaxseed, chia, canola oil, walnuts	Decreases cardiovascular risk
Eicosapentaenoic acid (EPA); docosapentaenoic acid (DPA); docosahexaenoic acid (DHA)	Fish and seafood	Decreases risk of sudden death from cardiovascular conditions; beneficial effects on nervous system development and health; potentially potent anti-inflammatory agents

HDL, High-density lipoprotein; LDL, low-density lipoprotein.
Adapted from Vannice G, Rasmussen H. Position of the Academy of Nutrition and Dietetics: dietary fatty acids for healthy adults. *J Acad Nutr Diet.* 2014;114(1):136-153.

to concerns by (a) trimming fat from meats, (b) providing leaner cuts of beef and pork, (c) replacing tropical oils and *trans* fats in processed foods, and (d) manufacturing foods containing less fat. Additionally, some consumers have increased their consumption of fish and poultry and substituted lower-fat milk for whole milk. Fat content of very lean beef and pork cuts currently compares favorably with a skinless chicken breast. The functions of fatty acids are shown in Table 6.1.

Classification

Dietary fats should actually be called lipids. Lipids contain the same three elements as carbohydrates: carbon, hydrogen, and oxygen. Lipids contain less oxygen in proportion to hydrogen and carbon than carbohydrates. The structure of lipids is covered in detail in Chapter 2 and on the Evolve website. Because of their structure, they provide more energy per gram than either carbohydrates or proteins.

The two classes of water-insoluble substances are (a) simple lipids, or triglycerides, which occur in foods and in the body; and (b) **structural lipids**, which are produced by the body for specific functions. The structural component of lipids is fatty acids. Triglycerides with one or more of the fatty acids replaced with carbohydrate, phosphate, or nitrogenous compounds are called **compound lipids**. Dietary lipids used physiologically include triglycerides, fatty acids, phospholipids, and cholesterol. Lipoproteins are found solely in the body.

Chemical Structure

Triglycerides are composed of fatty acids and glycerol, as shown:

Monoglycerides = glycerol + one fatty acid

Diglycerides = glycerol + two fatty acids

Triglycerides = glycerol + three fatty acids

A fatty acid is a chain of carbon atoms attached to hydrogen atoms with an acid grouping on one end. Glycerol is the alcohol portion of a triglyceride to which fatty acids attach. Triglycerides

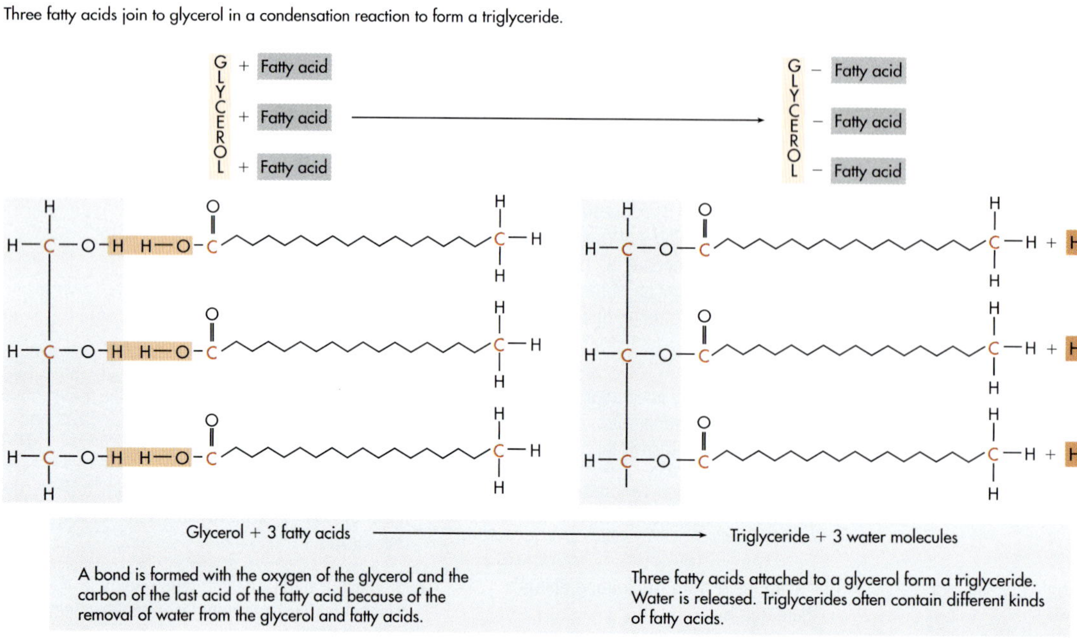
Three fatty acids join to glycerol in a condensation reaction to form a triglyceride.
GLYCEROL
Fatty acid
Fatty acid
Fatty acid
GLYCEROL
Fatty acid
Fatty acid
Fatty acid
H2O
H2O
H2O
Glycerol + 3 fatty acids
Triglyceride + 3 water molecules
A bond is formed with the oxygen of the glycerol and the carbon of the last acid of the fatty acid because of the removal of water from the glycerol and fatty acids.
Three fatty acids attached to a glycerol form a triglyceride. Water is released. Triglycerides often contain different kinds of fatty acids.

• **Figure 6.1** Formation and structure of a triglyceride. (Reproduced with permission from Grodner M, Escott-Stump S, Dorner S. *Nutritional Foundations and Clinical Applications*, 6th ed. St Louis: Mosby Elsevier; 2016.)

are the most common fat present in animal or protein foods (Fig. 6.1). Monoglycerides and diglycerides are found in the small intestine and result from the breakdown of triglycerides during digestion (Fig. 6.2). Free fatty acids, monoglycerides, and glycerol can cross cell membranes.

Each of the three fatty acids attached to the triglyceride can be different: they can be long, medium, or short, and saturated or unsaturated. Medium-chain and short-chain fatty acids are readily digested and absorbed, but most fats in foods (especially vegetable fats) contain predominantly long-chain fatty acids. **Short-chain fatty acids** contain less than six carbon atoms, **medium-chain fatty acids** contain 6 to 10 carbon atoms, and **long-chain fatty acids** contain 12 or more carbon atoms.

Saturated Fatty Acids

As discussed in Chapter 2, fatty acids are classified according to their degree of saturation. Saturation of a fatty acid depends on the number of hydrogen atoms attached to the carbon chain. Saturated fatty acids (SFAs) contain only single bonds, with each carbon atom having two hydrogen atoms attached to it (see Fig. 2.15). Palmitic and stearic acids (see Table 2.4), the two most prevalent SFAs, are structural components of tooth enamel and dentin.

Monounsaturated Fatty Acids

When adjacent carbon atoms are joined by a double bond because two hydrogen atoms are lacking, there is a gap between the hydrogen atoms in the chain; it is called an unsaturated fatty acid. Monounsaturated fatty acids (MUFAs) contain only one double bond (see Fig. 2.14). The most abundant MUFA is oleic acid. Oleic acid is also a structural component of the tooth.

Trans Fatty Acids

Hydrogenation is a commercial process in which vegetable oil is converted to a solid margarine or shortening by adding hydrogen. This process results in naturally unsaturated vegetable oils being changed to an SFA by changing unsaturated bonds to saturated bonds. The hydrogenation process not only increases the proportion of SFAs but also changes the shape of the fatty acid. When the hydrogen atoms are rotated so that they are on opposite sides of the bond, in the "*trans*" position (see Fig. 2.16), the fatty acid is called a ***trans* fatty acid**. Partial hydrogenation results in large numbers of fatty acids having this altered shape. A common *trans* fatty acid is elaidic acid, found in partially hydrogenated vegetable oils, such as tub margarine and cooking oils. A naturally occurring *trans* fatty acid, vaccenic acid, with double bonds on adjacent carbons, is present in small amounts in milk and meat of ruminants (cows, sheep, and deer).

Polyunsaturated Fatty Acids

When carbons in a fatty acid are connected by two or more double bonds, the fatty acid is polyunsaturated (see Fig. 2.14). Linoleic acid and arachidonic acid are polyunsaturated fatty acids (PUFAs), also known as **omega-6 fatty acids** (or n-6 PUFAs). Their first double bond is on the sixth carbon from the omega (terminal) end.

Omega-3 fatty acids, or α-linolenic acids, make up another class of PUFAs. As shown in Fig. 2.15, these fatty acids are unique because the first double bond is located three carbon atoms from the omega end of the molecule; thus, they are called omega-3s or *n-3*s. Omega-3 fatty acids include **α-linolenic acid**, which has 18 carbon atoms and two double bonds, and **eicosapentaenoic acid (EPA)**, which has 20 carbon atoms and five double bonds.

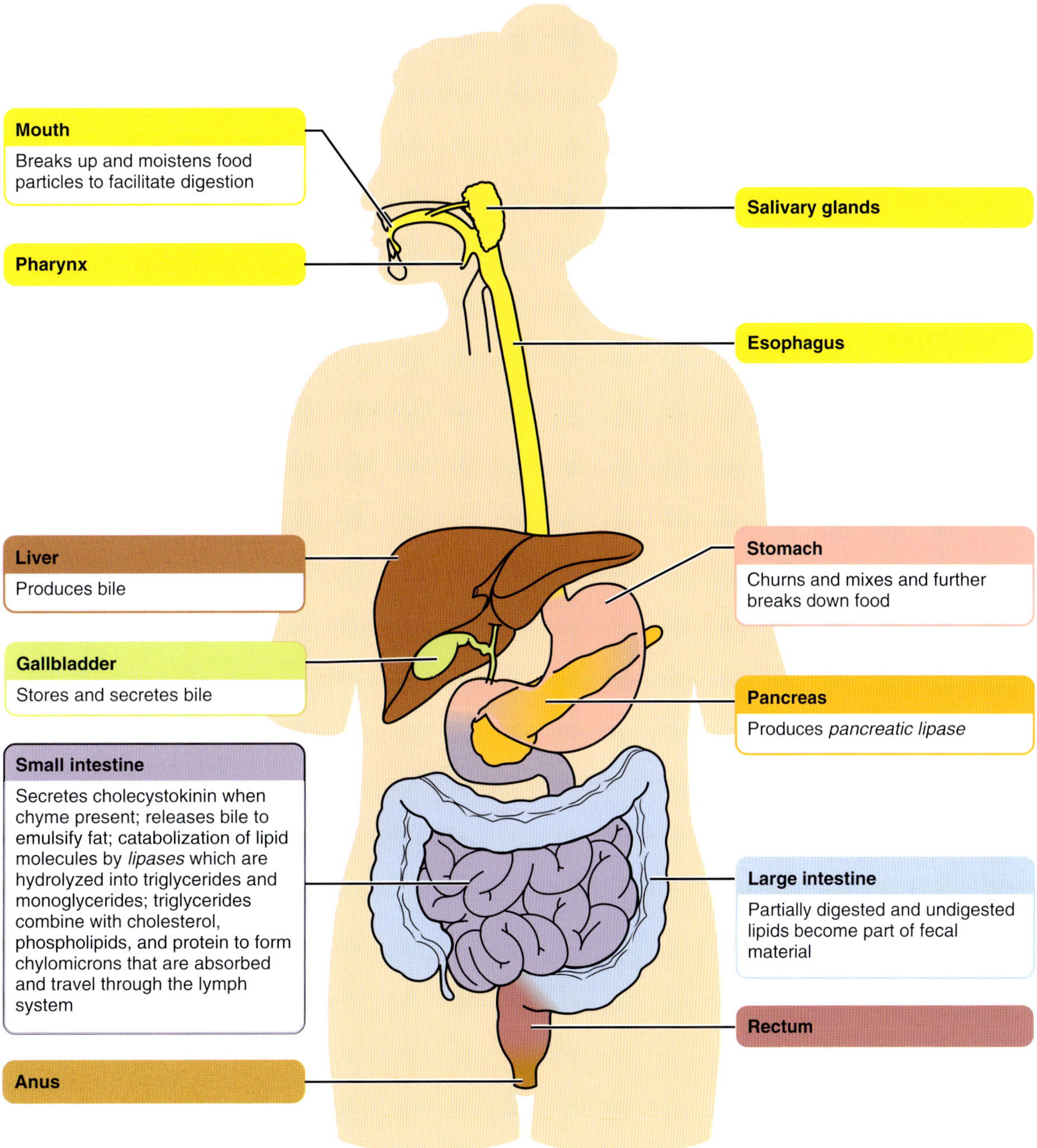
Mouth
Breaks up and moistens food particles to facilitate digestion
Pharynx
Salivary glands
Esophagus
Liver
Produces bile
Stomach
Churns and mixes and further breaks down food
Gallbladder
Stores and secretes bile
Pancreas
Produces *pancreatic lipase*
Small intestine
Secretes cholecystokinin when chyme present; releases bile to emulsify fat; catabolization of lipid molecules by *lipases* which are hydrolyzed into triglycerides and monoglycerides; triglycerides combine with cholesterol, phospholipids, and protein to form chylomicrons that are absorbed and travel through the lymph system
Large intestine
Partially digested and undigested lipids become part of fecal material
Rectum
Anus

• **Figure 6.2** Summary of lipid digestion. NOTE: Enzymes are in *italics*.

Characteristics of Fatty Acids

The carbon chain length and degree of saturation determine various properties of fats, including their flavor and hardness, or melting point (the temperature at which a product becomes a liquid). Most SFAs are solid at room temperature; for example, animal fats, being solid at room temperature, are predominantly saturated fats. Short-chain fatty acids (6 carbon atoms or less), MUFAs, and PUFAs that are liquid at room temperature are oils. Milk fat contains a large amount of short-chain SFAs.

Fats with a high proportion of unsaturated fatty acids may deteriorate or become rancid, resulting in unpleasant flavors and odors. Fats become rancid when subject to high temperatures and light, causing oxidation and decomposition of fats. The decomposition results in peroxides that may be toxic in large amounts. Vitamin E, a fat-soluble vitamin, is an antioxidant and, to some degree, protects the oil to which it is added. However, in doing so, vitamin E is inactivated and cannot be used by the body.

DENTAL CONSIDERATIONS

- Lipids are an integral part of many foods and are important physiologically.
- The primary form of fat in the body is triglyceride, not cholesterol.

NUTRITIONAL DIRECTIONS

- Frying foods at low temperatures causes the food to absorb excessive amounts of fats, whereas frying at very high temperatures results in decomposition of some fats, which can be irritating to the intestine, causing gastrointestinal discomfort after meals containing fried foods.
- The relatively small amounts of *trans* fatty acids occurring naturally in meat and dairy products do not appear to be harmful.
- Butylated hydroxyanisole (BHA) and butylated hydroxytoluene (BHT) are antioxidants added to processed foods to retard or prevent spoilage.

Compound Lipids

Phospholipids

Phospholipids contain phosphorus and a nitrogenous base in addition to fatty acids and glycerol. Detail on the biochemistry of phospholipids can be found on the Evolve website. Fats from plant and animal foods contain phospholipids but are not required in the diet because the body produces adequate amounts of phospholipids. These substances cannot be absorbed intact; they are broken down into their chemical components before absorption. As a structural component of cell membranes, tooth enamel, and dentin, they are the second most prevalent form of fat in the body. As such, these substances are not used for energy, even in a state of severe starvation. Although the mechanism is not fully understood, phospholipids are involved in the initiation of calcification and mineralization in teeth and bones. They are present in higher amounts in the enamel matrix of teeth than in dentin.

Phospholipids are important in fat absorption and transport of fats in the blood. Phospholipids mix with either fat-soluble or water-soluble ingredients to transport these products across membrane barriers. Phospholipids include lecithin, cephalin, and sphingomyelins. Phospholipids, especially lecithin, are used as additives in commercial products to prevent fat and water components from separating.

Lecithin, the most widely distributed phospholipid, is present in all cells. Lecithin supplements have been marketed for reducing the risk of **atherosclerosis** (a complex disease of the arteries in which the interior lining of arteries becomes roughened and clogged with fatty deposits that hinder blood flow; Fig. 6.3), weight loss, and other chronic health conditions. However, the value of lecithin in this role is questionable because lecithin is digested before its absorption.

Cephalin is present in thromboplastin, which is necessary for blood clotting. Sphingomyelins are important constituents of brain tissue and the myelin sheath around nerve fibers.

Lipoproteins

Lipoproteins are produced by the body to transport insoluble fats in the blood. Lipoproteins are compound lipids composed of triglycerides, phospholipids, and cholesterol combined with protein (see Fig. 2.20). The liver and intestinal mucosa produce lipoproteins. Four different types of lipoproteins are present in the blood: high-density lipoproteins (HDLs), low-density lipoproteins (LDLs), very-low-density lipoproteins (VLDLs), and chylomicrons.

The ratio of lipid to protein in lipoproteins varies widely; these variations affect their density. Density increases as lipids decrease and protein increases. Lipoproteins can be classified according to their density and composition, as shown in Fig. 6.4. Phospholipids in lipoproteins are present in approximately the same proportions in all individuals.

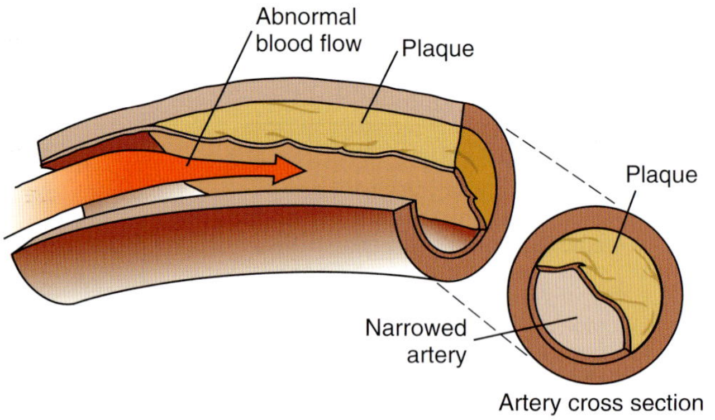

• **Figure 6.3** Atherosclerosis. An artery narrowed by the buildup of plaque. (Reproduced with permission from Workman ML, LaCharity L, Kruchko SL. *Understanding Pharmacology*. 2nd ed. St. Louis, Saunders; 2016.)

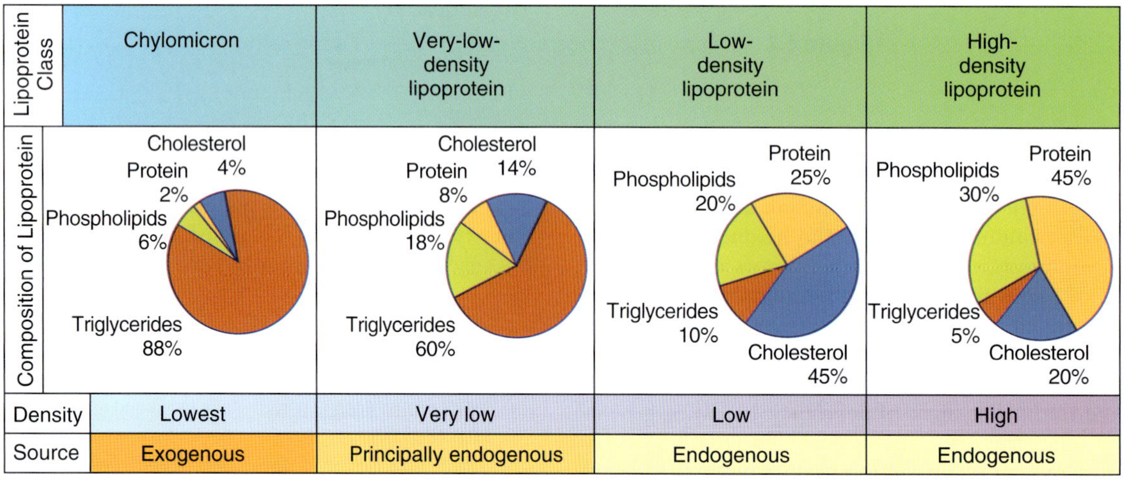

Lipoprotein Class
Chylomicron
Very-low-density lipoprotein
Low-density lipoprotein
High-density lipoprotein
Composition of Lipoprotein
Cholesterol 4%
Protein 2%
Phospholipids 6%
Triglycerides 88%
Cholesterol 14%
Protein 8%
Phospholipids 18%
Triglycerides 60%
Protein 25%
Phospholipids 20%
Triglycerides 10%
Cholesterol 45%
Protein 45%
Phospholipids 30%
Triglycerides 5%
Cholesterol 20%
Density
Lowest
Very low
Low
High
Source
Exogenous
Principally endogenous
Endogenous
Endogenous

• **Figure 6.4** Characteristics of lipoproteins.

HDLs contain greater amounts of protein and less lipid. LDL cholesterol typically constitutes 60% to 70% of the total blood cholesterol and is considered the main agent in elevated serum cholesterol levels, or the "bad" cholesterol. Serum LDL is causally related to CVD morbidity and mortality,[3] as discussed in *Health Application 6*.

Cholesterol

Cholesterol is a fat-like, waxy substance classified as a sterol derivative with a complex ring structure (see Fig. 2.19 and on the Evolve website). Because the body frequently produces more cholesterol than it absorbs, cholesterol intake is not essential. Cholesterol has important functions as a constituent of the brain, nervous tissue, and bile salts; a precursor of vitamin D and steroid hormones; and a structural component of cell membranes and teeth. Lipoproteins transport cholesterol in the blood.

Physiologic Roles

Energy

Dietary fats are a concentrated source of energy, furnishing 9 cal/g. Foods high in fats are generally referred to as calorie dense, a beneficial quality in some cases. **Calorie-dense foods** are high in fats (or fat and sugar) and low in vitamins, minerals, and other nutrients. A characteristic of calorie-dense foods is that less volume of food is needed to furnish energy requirements. As an energy source, fats are also referred to as **protein sparing** because they allow protein to be used for the important functions of building and repairing tissues.

Satiety Value

Dietary fats are important for their satiety value. Fats have a higher satiety value than carbohydrates or protein because digestion of high-fat meals is slower than other energy-containing nutrients. The higher the fat content of a meal, the longer the food remains in the stomach. Nevertheless, approximately 95% of ingested fats are absorbed. Soft fats that are liquids at body temperature (e.g., margarine) are digested more quickly than hard fats (e.g., meat fats).

Palatability

Fats contribute to the palatability and flavor of foods. In cooking, they improve texture. A receptor on the tongue and a potential pathway for detection of a "fatty taste" has been identified, which may affect food preferences.[4] Preference for high-fat foods develops at an early age and persists through adulthood.

Complementary Relationships

Fat-soluble vitamins and essential fatty acids are generally found in foods containing fat. The absorption of fat-soluble vitamins is facilitated by the presence of fats in the gastrointestinal tract.

Linoleic acid, an omega-6 fatty acid with 18 carbon atoms and two double bonds, cannot be synthesized by the body and must be supplied from dietary sources (see Table 6.1). If linoleic acid is not furnished in the diet, signs of deficiency, including growth retardation, skin lesions, and reproductive failure, result. For this reason, linoleic acid is an **essential fatty acid (EFA)**. Linoleic acid may be a protective factor against heart disease.

Arachidonic acid (18-carbon chain with four double bonds) and linolenic acid (18-carbon chain with three double bonds) are also considered EFAs, but healthy individuals can produce them from sufficient quantities of linoleic acid (see Fig. 2.15). Linolenic acid can be converted into omega-3 fatty acids in the body, but the process is affected by numerous factors, including genetics and dietary and lifestyle factors. Studies suggest that less than 10% of linolenic acid is converted to EPA or **docosahexaenoic acid (DHA)** is another omega-3 fatty acid present in fish, especially in fatty fish. Omega-3 fatty acids are very important, participating in many interactions in the body to improve health, as shown in Box 6.1. Because of their importance in building and maintaining a healthy body, it is no wonder omega-3 fatty acid supplements have become so popular. However, in numerous studies, supplementation has not been associated with either lower risk of all-cause mortality or major cardiovascular disease (CVD) outcomes.[5] Studies indicate that dietary intake of fatty fish is more effective than supplements. Supplements may be beneficial after a heart attack.[6]

Fat Storage

Adipose tissue, or body fat, has several roles: (a) it provides a concentrated energy source, (b) protects internal organs, and (c) maintains body temperature.

Energy

Excess dietary carbohydrates and protein are converted to fat and stored in adipose tissue. Fatty acids can be used as an energy source by all cells except red blood cells and central nervous system cells. People can survive total starvation for 30 to 40 days with only water to drink.

Protection of Organs

Fatty tissue surrounds vital organs and provides a cushion, protecting them from traumatic injury and shock.

Insulation

The subcutaneous layer of fat functions as an insulator that preserves body heat and maintains body temperature. Excessive layers of fat can also deter heat loss during hot weather.

• BOX 6.1 Health Effects of Omega-3 Fatty Acids

Omega-3 fatty acids (eicosapentanoic acid [EPA] and docosahexanoic acid [DHA] serve many purposes.

Produce compounds that:

- Regulate blood pressure
- Improve immune response
- Regulate gastrointestinal secretions
- Prevent heart arrhythmias
- Promote development of brains and nerve tissues in fetal and neonatal development and ongoing cognitive development in children
- Protect neurons in neurodegenerative conditions

Reduces or ameliorates:

- Blood pressure
- Elevated triglyceride levels (leads to coronary heart disease)
- Blood coagulation (relates to clogged arteries leading to atherosclerosis)
- Inflammation in conditions such as rheumatoid arthritis
- Symptoms of depression and other mental health disorders in some individuals
- Serious eye problems, such as macular degeneration
- Risks/symptoms associated with Parkinson and Alzheimer disease

Dietary Fats and Dental Health

Dietary fats are essential for oral health because they are incorporated into the tooth structure. Epidemiologic and laboratory studies indicate that fats may have a cariostatic effect. Individuals whose diet may contain 80% fat from animal and seafood sources (e.g., Alaskan natives) have a very low incidence of dental caries, but this could possibly be a result of their low carbohydrate intake. Dietary fats probably have local rather than systemic influence because fats added to foods protect the teeth more than foods naturally high in fat. Precisely how fats reduce the caries rate is unknown; however, several hypotheses have been explored, as follows:

1. Some fatty acids, specifically oleic acid, are growth factors for lactic acid bacteria, whereas streptococcal organisms are inhibited by lauric acid (Lauricidin). About 50% of the fatty acids in coconut oil is lauric acid, a saturated fat.
2. Long-chain fatty acids may reduce dissolution of hydroxyapatite by acids.
3. Oral food retention is reduced by fat intake.
4. Fats may lubricate the tooth surface and prevent penetration of acid to the enamel (i.e., the "greased" tooth is impervious to acid, protecting caries-susceptible areas).
5. Fats may produce a film on food particles and prevent partial digestion of food particles in the mouth.
6. Dietary fat delays gastric emptying, enhancing fluoride absorption, and increasing tissue fluoride concentration.

Bacterial inflammation and systemic immune response are believed to play a central role in the initiation and propagation of atherosclerosis. Periodontal diseases (including gingivitis and periodontitis) are oral conditions caused by bacteria (and poor oral hygiene) that are risk factors contributing to cardiovascular disease. **Cardiovascular disease (CVD)**, also referred to as coronary heart disease or coronary artery disease, is a condition involving the heart and blood vessels and producing various pathologic effects. When bacteria are allowed to grow rampantly in the mouth, inflammation may occur throughout the body. Bacteria from dental plaque biofilm can cause blood clots when they escape into the bloodstream and become involved in inflammation of the lining of blood vessels and atherosclerosis. This inflammation may serve as a base for development of arterial atherosclerotic plaques, but—contrary to some concerns—omega-6 fatty acids do not promote inflammation in humans.[7] Research studies show that the inflammatory process can be attenuated by n-3 fatty acids.[8–10] However, omega-3 fatty acid from fatty fish is more effective than supplements.[6] A study including more than 15,000 heart disease patients from 39 countries concluded that every increased level of tooth loss was associated with roughly 15% higher risk of cardiovascular mortality.[11] This established a link, not a cause-and-effect relationship, between dental health and heart health. Periodontal health may be promoted by reducing saturated fat intake and increasing MUFA and PUFA.[12]

DENTAL CONSIDERATIONS

- Although fat intake may have a positive effect on dental health, the patient's medical history needs to be considered when providing nutrition education.
- Lipids as a source of energy provide 9 cal/g, whereas carbohydrates and proteins provide 4 cal/g.
- Fish consumption may have a favorable effect on blood platelets and other blood-clotting mechanisms, reducing the risk of clot formation.
- The only proven benefit and suggested use of lecithin supplements is for individuals taking niacin to treat high cholesterol levels.
- Tooth loss could be an easy and inexpensive way to identify patients at higher risk of CVD needing more intense prevention efforts (diet and lifestyle changes).
- Because omega-3 fatty acids may be beneficial to health, determine the patient's frequency of fish consumption and supplement use. An increase in fish consumption is recommended for most patients, but some fish, especially mackerel and tuna, should be consumed in moderation because of their mercury content.
- Fish oils are beneficial for many conditions, but they may have a negative effect on patients taking anticoagulants or aspirin. Do not advocate indiscriminate use of omega-3 fatty acid supplements. Scientific evidence does not indicate that fish oil supplements prevent heart disease. Patients should consult their health care provider or a registered dietitian nutritionist (RDN) before taking an omega-3 fatty acid supplement.
- Krill oil (a type of fish oil) contains omega-3 fatty acids but is more expensive than other omega-3 supplements. Studies have not shown convincing evidence that health benefits of krill oil are superior to those of regular fish oil.
- Educate patients on how to read labels of omega-3 fatty acid supplements; those made from liver should be avoided because high levels of pesticides or heavy metals may be present.
- Both saturated and *trans* fats have an undesirable effect on CVD. Especially encourage patients with periodontal disease to include *more* fish and foods containing MUFA and PUFA (and less saturated fat) to improve oral status.

NUTRITIONAL DIRECTIONS

- Fats act as a lubricant in the intestines, decreasing constipation.
- Although digestion of fried foods takes longer, the process is as complete as that of other foods in most individuals if food is fried at the proper temperature.
- Fatty fish and some oils contain omega-3 fatty acids and should be included in the diet at least 2 times a week as part of the U.S.-Pattern.
- Omega-3 fatty acids are better absorbed with a high-fat meal rather than on an empty stomach.
- Intake of more than 3 g of omega-3 fatty acid supplements should be supervised by a health care provider.
- The potential relationship between periodontal disease and heart disease emphasizes important health reasons for good dental hygiene and following the U.S.-Pattern.

Dietary Requirements

A certain amount of fat is needed to provide adequate amounts of fat-soluble vitamins and EFAs. The acceptable macronutrient distribution range for fat is between 20% to 35% of energy intake for adults (see p. iii). The lower limit for fat intake was established to minimize the increase in blood triglyceride levels and decrease in HDL cholesterol levels that occur with higher intakes of refined carbohydrates. The upper limit of 35% calories from fat was based on information indicating that higher fat intake is associated with a greater intake of energy and SFA, which may be detrimental to health. Box 6.2 shows a method for calculating the National Academy of Medicine (formerly the Institute of Medicine) recommendation for dietary fat. The World Health Organization also recommends a range of 20% to 35% of total calories from fats.

The *Dietary Guidelines* do not indicate a specific amount of fat but rather indicate that fat intake should be limited based on an individual's caloric requirement to achieve/maintain a healthy weight. The *Dietary Guidelines* and dietary reference intakes (DRIs) also recommend that SFA and *trans* fatty acid intakes be as low as possible while consuming a diet providing an adequate intake of all essential nutrients. The *Dietary Guidelines* recommend less than 10% of calories from saturated fats, replacing them with MUFAs and PUFAs. Currently, approximately 16% of the calories from fats consumed by Americans are saturated.[2] Studies do not support substituting saturated fats with refined carbohydrate foods, but modifying the type of fat seems to provide better protection against CVD.[13–15]

The recommendation for oils in the U.S.-Pattern for a 2000-calorie intake is 27 g (about 5 tsp) daily. Average intakes of oils are not far from recommendations, but almost all individuals are slightly below the recommendations.[2]

Adequate intake established for linoleic acid is 0.6% of energy intake or 17 g per day for men and 12 g per day for women 19 to 50 years, and 14 g per day for men and 11 g per day for women older than 51 years (see p. iii). A dietary reference intake has not been established for omega-3 fatty acids (EPA and DHA); more information is needed to establish an amount necessary to maximize cardiac health.[16] Many scientists think that the target should be between 250 and 500 mg per day; current daily intake is around 130 mg.[17]

• BOX 6.2 Calculating Total Daily Fat Recommendations for Specific Caloric Levels[a]

To calculate dietary fat:

1. Determine caloric level of the diet (see Dietary Reference Intake for Energy for Active Individuals, p. ii) (e.g., patient needs 2000 cal).
2. Multiply the calories by 0.35 to determine the number of calories of fat the diet can contain (e.g., 2000 cal × 0.35 [% of total calories] = 700 cal from fat).
3. Divide the answer by 9 to determine the grams of fat allowed daily (e.g., 700 cal from fat ÷ 9 cal/g of fat = 77.7 g of fat).

Calorie Level	Grams of Fat per Day
1200	< 46
1500	< 58
1800	< 70
2000	< 78
2200	< 86
2400	< 93

[a]*Total fat intake limited to less than 35% of the total daily calories.*

An adult can produce all the cholesterol needed; thus, no dietary requirement is necessary. On the other hand, the National Academy of Medicine recommends individuals eat as little dietary cholesterol as possible by utilizing the U.S.-Pattern.

Sources

As already discussed, foods contain a combination of fatty acids; each of the fatty acids attached to the glycerol may be different, resulting in different proportions of SFA, MFA, or PUFA. The *Dietary Guidelines* emphasize that rather than attempting to reduce fat intake, the focus should be on fewer calories and less saturated fat intake. Fig. 6.5 compares the types of fatty acids in various fats and oils; those with higher amounts of PUFA and MUFA should be encouraged. For example, corn oil, with approximately 57% PUFA, 29% MUFA, and 14% SFA, is considered a good source of PUFA. On the other hand, coconut and palm kernel oil (technically solids at room temperature, thus they are not an oil) contain more than 85% to 90% SFA and negligible amounts of PUFA.

Table 6.2 itemizes selected animal products containing SFAs, MUFAs, and PUFAs. Of the food groups (excluding fats and oils), animal products (meat and milk) contribute the largest proportion of saturated fat, although their share has been declining. SFAs are found in animal fats, butter fat, coconut oil, cocoa butter, coffee creamers, and fully hydrogenated vegetable oils. As shown in Fig. 6.6, the biggest food contributors of saturated fat consumed by Americans are mixed dishes (particularly those containing cheese, meat, or both—including burgers, sandwiches, tacos, pizza, and other meat, poultry, and seafood dishes) and snacks and sweets. Animal products and canola and olive oils supply approximately 50% of MUFAs. Oleic acid, the most prevalent MUFA, is present in most fats, oils, nuts, seeds, and avocados.

PUFAs from the n-6 series are derived from land plants, especially foods from the grain group, and additional fats and oils (see Fig. 6.5). Linoleic acid is the most prevalent PUFA in the food supply. Cottonseed, soybean, and corn oils provide the most PUFA; food sources are nuts and seeds. Most oils are consumed in packaged foods, such as salad dressings, mayonnaise, prepared vegetables, snack chips, and nuts and seeds. Almost 80% of all vegetable oil consumed in the United States is soybean oil. It is also the principal source of omega-3 fatty acids in the American diet. Conjugated linoleic acids are natural components of beef, lamb, and dairy products. Linolenic acid is present in plant products—flaxseed, canola, and soybean oils; soybeans; walnuts; flaxseed; and wheat germ. Table 6.3 indicates the amount of saturated fat, monounsaturated fat, and polyunsaturated fat in the sample menu introduced in Fig. 1.4.

Long-chain omega-3 fatty acids (EPA and DHA), provided from seafood, include fatty fish such as mackerel, salmon, herring, and albacore tuna, and fish oils. Most shellfish contain very little omega-3s except the rich source found in oysters. These foods are also low in saturated fat. The *Dietary Guidelines* and American Heart Association (AHA) recommend consumption of fish at least two times a week or at least 8 oz-eq/week. Well-controlled studies substantiate that fish intake containing EPA and DHA is associated with reducing CVD.[18]

In 2003 to 2004, approximately 52% of the soybean oil used in the United States was partially hydrogenated; currently, liquid soybean oil does not contain any *trans* fat.[19] *Trans* fats may still be present in some margarines, snack foods, and prepared desserts and processed foods, such as in microwave popcorn,

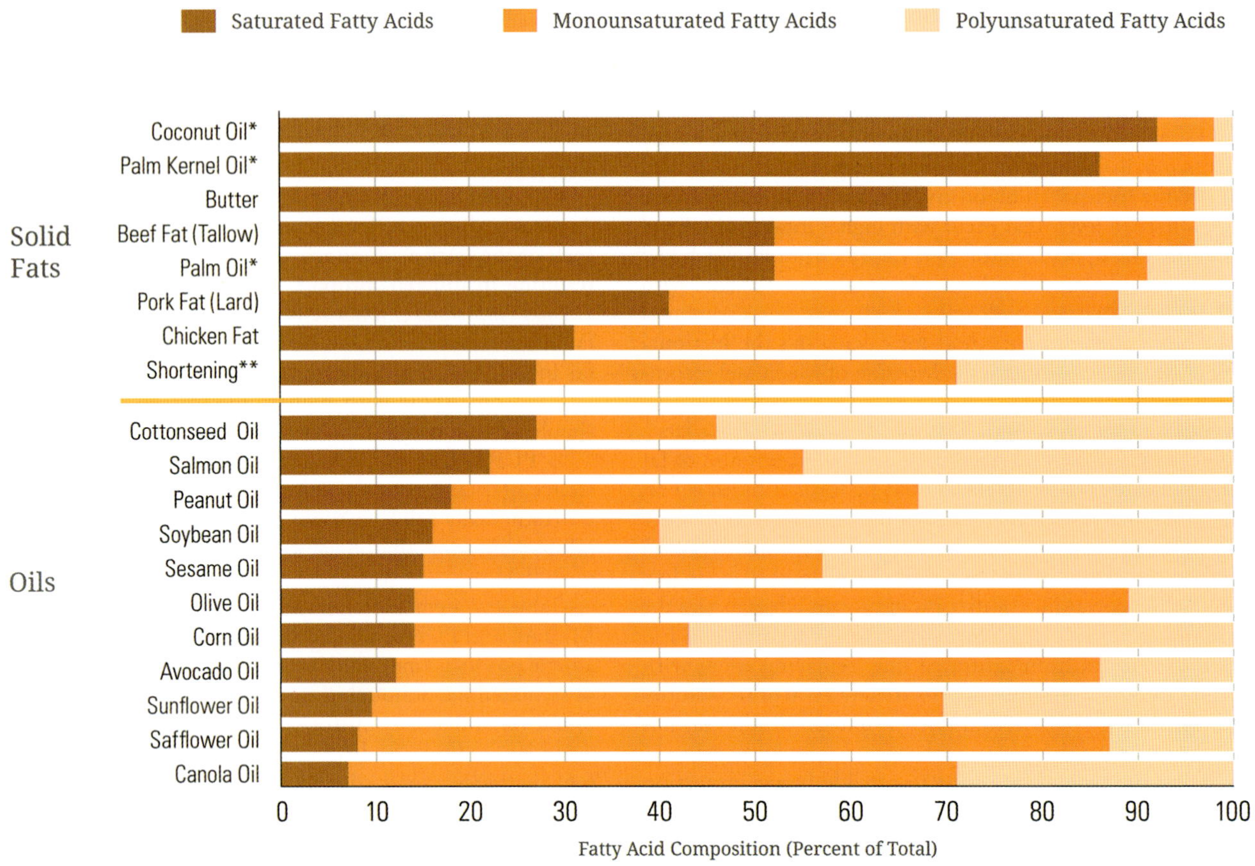

* Coconut, palm kernel, and palm oil are called oils because they come from plants. However, they are solid or semi-solid at room temperature due to their high content of short-chain saturated fatty acids. They are considered solid fats for nutritional purposes.

** Shortening may be made from partially hydrogenated vegetable oil, which contains *trans* fatty acids.

DATA SOURCES: U.S. Department of Agriculture, Agricultural Research Service, Nutrient Data Laboratory. USDA National Nutrient Database for Standard Reference. Release 27, 2015. Available at: http://ndb.nal.usda.gov/. Accessed August 31, 2015.

• **Figure 6.5** Fatty acid profiles of common fats and oils.

TABLE 6.2 Fatty Acids and Cholesterol Content of Selected Foods (per 100 g)

Food	Total Fat (g)	SFA (Saturated Fatty Acids) (g)	MUFA (Monounsaturated Fatty Acids) (g)	PUFA (Polyunsaturated Fatty Acids [Total]) (g)	Cholesterol (mg)
Cheese, cheddar	33.3	18.9	9.3	1.4	99
Cheese, Monterey	30.3	19.1	8.8	0.90	89
Cottage cheese, 2%	2.3	1.2	0.5	0.08	12
Cream cheese	34.4	20.2	8.9	1.48	101
Ice cream, vanilla	11.0	6.8	3.0	0.45	44
Yogurt, low fat	1.3	0.8	0.3	0.04	5
Milk, 1%	1.0	0.63	0.3	0.04	5
Milk, 2%	1.98	1.23	0.6	0.07	8
Milk, whole, 3.7%	3.25	1.86	0.8	0.20	10

TABLE 6.2 **Fatty Acids and Cholesterol Content of Selected Foods (per 100 g)—cont'd**

Food	Total Fat (g)	SFA (Saturated Fatty Acids) (g)	MUFA (Monounsaturated Fatty Acids) (g)	PUFA (Polyunsaturated Fatty Acids [Total]) (g)	Cholesterol (mg)
Beef, lean ground (85%/15%)	15.3	5.81	6.6	0.48	89
Beef liver	4.7	2.5	1.1	1.02	381
Chicken breast, skinless	3.2	1.0	1.2	0.79	116
Chicken breast, with skin	7.8	2.2	3.0	1.7	84
Chicken thigh, skinless	15.8	4.4	6.2	3.5	91
Egg, large whole	9.51	3.1	3.71	1.91	372
Egg white	0.2	0	0	0	0
Pork chop, center loin, lean only	11.1	3.5	4.2	1.4	84
Salmon, canned	5.0	0.9	1.2	1.42	55
Salmon, chinook	13.4	3.2	5.7	2.7	84
Shrimp, mixed species	1.7	0.52	0.4	0.6	211
Veal loin, lean only	4.4	1.7	2.1	0.26	78

Data from U.S. Department of Agriculture (USDA), Agricultural Research Service, Nutrient Data Laboratory. USDA National Nutrient Database for Standard Reference, Release 28 (Slightly revised May 2016). https://www.ars.usda.gov/ba/bhnrc/ndl Accessed December 12, 2016.

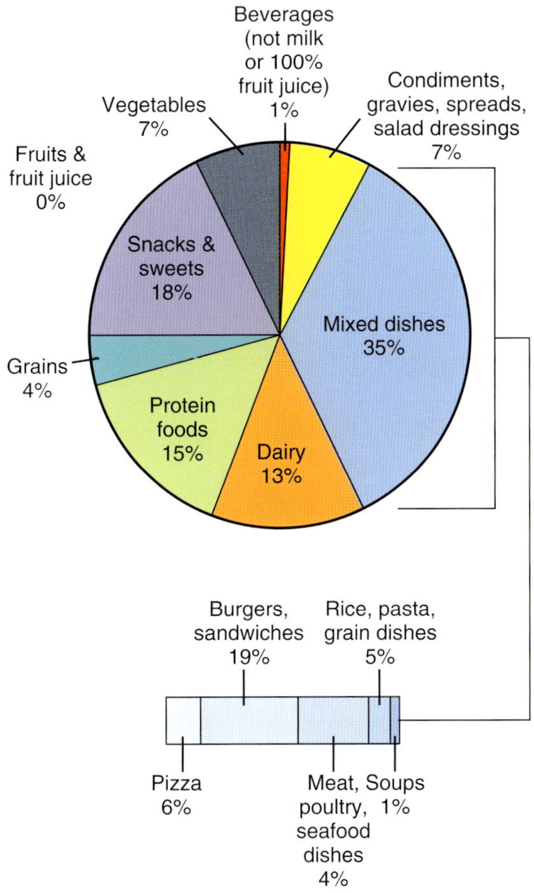

• **Figure 6.6** Food category sources of saturated fats in the U.S. population ages 2 years and older. (Data Source: What We Eat in American (WWEIA) Food Category analyses for the 2015 Dietary Guidelines Advisory Committee. Estimated based on day 1 dietary recalls from WWEIA, National Health and Nutrition Examination Survey (NHANES) 2009–2010. From U.S. Department of Health and Human Services and U.S. Department of Agriculture. *2015–2020 Dietary Guidelines for Americans*. 8th ed. December 2015. https://health.gov/dietaryguidelines/2015/guidelines/.)

frozen pizza, and coffee creamers. Box 6.3 details how to limit the total amount of fat in the diet, focusing on reducing foods high in saturated and *trans* fats and choosing more foods containing unsaturated fats.

Only animal products contain cholesterol; it is not found in egg whites or plant foods (e.g., vegetable oils). Cholesterol is highest in egg yolks, liver, and other organ meats. Since foods higher in saturated fats also contain cholesterol, when saturated fats are within the recommended lower amounts, cholesterol will necessarily be limited. The average amount of cholesterol intake in the United States is slightly above 300 mg; this amount is felt to be in a healthy range.

Food Choices

The percentage of fat by weight is widely used on food labels and in advertising. Although this information is correct, it is misleading and confusing. The recommendation limiting fat to 35% refers to the percentage of fat based on total calories in the total diet.

TABLE 6.3 **Saturated Fat, Monosaturated Fat, and Polyunsaturated Content of the Sample Menu**

Sample Menu	Saturated fat (g)	Monounsaturated fat (g)	Polyunsaturated fat (g)
Breakfast			
1½ c Frosted Mini-Wheat cereal	0	0	1
12 oz skim milk	0	0	0
12 oz black coffee	0	0	0
Mid-Morning Snack			
12 oz water	0	0	0
1 oz dry roasted almonds, unsalted	1	9	4
1 medium orange	0	0	0
Lunch			
Sandwich with			
1 c tuna salad with egg, low-calorie mayonnaise	2	3	4
¼ c thin-sliced cucumber	0	0	0
3 thin slices tomato	0	0	0
2 lettuce leaves	0	0	0
2 thin slices 100% wheat bread	0	0	1
8 baby carrots	0	0	0
1 medium applesauce cookie	1	1	0
1 c grapes	0	0	0
12 oz water	0	0	0
Mid-Afternoon Snack			
8 oz low-fat vanilla yogurt	2	1	0
12 oz herbal tea with nonnutritive sweetener	0	0	0
Dinner			
3 oz pot roast beef with	4	5	0
¼ c sauteed mushrooms	0	0	0
1 c white and wild rice blend with margarine and cooked in	1	2	1
½ c vegetable juice	0	0	0
2 c tossed salad with lettuce, avocado, tomatoes, and carrots	0	0	0
¼ c shredded low-fat Muenster cheese	3	1	0
2 tbsp vinaigrette salad dressing	1	2	3
⅛ medium cantaloupe	0	0	0
12 oz iced tea with low-calorie sweetener	0	0	0
Evening Snack			
3 c low-fat microwave popcorn	0	1	1
12 oz water	0	0	0
TOTALS[a]	15	25	15

[a]Totals may vary due to rounding.
From nutrient data SuperTracker. https://www.supertracker.usda.gov/default.aspx. Accessed April 17, 2017.

• BOX 6.3 Wise Choices of Dietary Fats

Purchasing and Planning

- Read nutrition labels on foods to determine the amount of fat and saturated fat in a serving. Low fat is less than 3 g fat per serving.
- Choose fats and oils with 2 g or less saturated fat per tablespoon, such as tub margarines and vegetable oils (e.g., canola, corn, safflower, sunflower, and olive oil). Liquid vegetable oil should be listed as the first ingredient. Avoid saturated fats such as butter, lard, and palm and coconut oils.
- Avoid foods containing partially hydrogenated fats because they contain *trans* fatty acids. Foods containing partially hydrogenated fats may have some redeeming factors if they consist of canola or soybean oil that contain trace amounts of partially hydrogenated oil.
- Watch for reformulated products with zero *trans* fats.
- Substitute plain low-fat Greek-style yogurt for mayonnaise or sour cream or purchase light sour cream (compare fat content on labels).
- Purchase fresh fruits, vegetables, and nuts for snacks rather than sugar-sweetened beverages, chips, pastries, and high-calorie baked goods (e.g., muffins, doughnuts).
- Choose two or three servings of lean meat, skinless poultry, or fish, with a daily total of about 6 oz.
- Choose a vegetarian entree (e.g., dry beans and peas) at least once a week.
- Include fish (not fried) at least twice a week.
- Include a variety of fresh meats (not processed); producers breed animals to produce leaner beef and pork.
- Choose "select" grade beef rather than "choice" because it contains fewer calories as a result of less fat marbling. Fat content of meats also depends on the type of cut; leaner cuts include flank steak, sirloin or tenderloin, loin pork chops, and 85% or greater lean ground beef.
- Choose lean turkey or chicken sausage, or turkey bacon.
- Use low-fat ground turkey or extra-lean ground beef in casseroles, spaghetti, and chili.
- Moderate the use of egg yolks (maximum of four egg yolks weekly) and organ meats (liver, brain, and kidney).
- Choose tuna packed in water, not in oil (compare fat content on labels).
- Select fat-free or low-fat milk and dairy products. Choose cheeses with 6 g or less of fat per ounce (90% of the calories in cream cheese are from fat).

Food Preparation

- Use fats and oils (e.g., olive, canola, corn, sunflower, or cottonseed) sparingly in cooking (roast, bake, grill, or broil when possible). Baste meats with broth or stock.
- Use nonstick cookware and an aerosol cooking spray.
- Prepare and eat smaller portions.
- Use the paste method for making gravy or sauces: add flour or cornstarch to cold liquids slowly and blend well.
- Season with herbs, lemon juice, or stock rather than lard, bacon, ham, margarine, or fatty sauces.
- Remove skin from poultry and visible fat from beef and pork products.
- Skim fat from homemade soups or stews by chilling and removing the fat layer that rises to the top.
- A small amount of olive or canola oil in salads increases absorption of antioxidants and fat-soluble vitamins.
- Include olives and healthful fats, such as flaxseed oils, nuts, and avocados.
- Rely on mustard, salad greens, shredded carrots, tomato slices, sweet peppers, and red onions to add moisture to sandwiches rather than fat-laden spreads.
- Top a baked potato with salsa and a dollop of fat-free Greek yogurt instead of butter or sour cream.
- Substitute two egg whites for one whole egg.
- Prepare broth-based chicken, vegetable, or bean-based soups rather than cream soups made with high-fat dairy products.
- Marinate leaner cuts of meat in lemon juice, flavored vinegars, or fruit juices.
- Sauté with olive oil instead of butter.
- Sprinkle slivered nuts, flaxseed, or sunflower seeds on salads instead of bacon bits.
- Choose a handful of nuts rather than chips or crackers.
- Place meat or poultry on a rack to allow the fat to drain.
- Steam, simmer, boil, broil, bake, grill, or microwave foods rather than frying them.
- Use smaller servings of oil-based or low-fat salad dressings.
- Use whole-grain flours to enhance the flavor of baked goods made with less fat.
- Choose nonhydrogenated peanut butter or other nut-butter spreads on celery, banana, or rice or popcorn cakes.
- Add avocado slices rather than cheese to a salad or sandwich.

TABLE 6.4 Analysis of Fat Content of Milk

Type of Milk	Calories per 245 g (1 cup)	Total Fat (g)	Percentage of Fat by Weight	Percentage of Fat by Calories
Whole milk (3.25%)	149	7.9	3.3	48
Low-fat milk (2%)	125	4.7	1.9	34
Low-fat milk (1%)	105	2.4	1	21
Skim milk	83	0.20	0.1	2

Data from U.S. Department of Agriculture (USDA), Agricultural Research Service, Nutrient Data Laboratory. USDA National Nutrient Database for Standard Reference, Release 28 (Slightly revised). May 2016. https://www.ars.usda.gov/ba/bhnrc/ndl Accessed December 12, 2016.

As shown in Table 6.4, the percentage of fat in whole milk is 48% of the total calories, not 3.25% as the label indicates.

The Nutrition Facts label on foods (see Fig. 1.8) indicates the grams and % Daily Value for fat, saturated fat, and *trans* fats in a serving. All *trans* fats, including those from ruminant animals, are included on the Nutrition Facts label. Since 2006, when the U.S. Food and Drug Administration (FDA) began requiring the amount of *trans* fats on the Nutrition Facts label, the amount of *trans* fats in foods has declined significantly. In 2013, the FDA determined that partially hydrogenated oils (the major source of commercially produced *trans* fats) were no longer "generally recognized as safe" based on its being a contributing factor to CVD. The FDA allowed food manufacturers a 3-year compliance period to eliminated *trans* fatty acids from their products. The key to knowing whether the product contains any *trans* fats is to read the ingredient label; "partially hydrogenated" oil is an indicator that the product contains at least small amounts of this unhealthy ingredient.

For most people, a decrease in red meat consumption is probably desirable, but complete elimination is unnecessary. In recent years, through improvements in breeding and feeding livestock, these products are lower in fat, saturated fat, calories, and cholesterol. Important nutrients are present in beef, pork, and lamb; moderate consumption of these products is encouraged for everyone. Loin (sirloin, tenderloin, or center loin) and round cuts (top, bottom, eye, or tip) and lean or extra lean ground beef contain the least amount of fat. More important than the fat content of any product is its saturated and *trans* fatty acid content that are related to CVD.

DENTAL CONSIDERATIONS

- Use Box 6.2 when determining fat recommendations.
- Interview the patient to evaluate total fat intake. Everyone needs adequate amounts of fat to allow protein to perform its functions of building and repairing. If total energy intake is inadequate, healing is slower. Also, inadequate fat intake could lead to secondary deficiencies of fat-soluble vitamins.
- Assess patients' intake of dairy and meat products; they frequently consume more fat than they realize because of the inherent "invisible" fats. Foods having a higher fat content are more calorie dense. For example, 1 oz of peanuts and 45 medium-size baby carrots have the same number of calories (160 cal). Carrots have only a trace of fat; peanuts contain 14 g of fat per 1 oz (28 g). Knowledge of fat content of foods is necessary to assess fat intake.
- Have patients read a Nutrition Facts label to determine whether the product is a good buy as well as a healthy choice with regard to fat.
- Foods such as nuts and certain cheeses (cheddar, Monterey Jack, Swiss) may protect teeth against acid attack, especially when consumed after fermentable carbohydrates. Even though they are generally considered nutritious foods, they have a relatively high fat content and may not be appropriate for all people.
- Teach patients to read labels and understand that the percentage of fat should be determined based on the total calories, not the weight, of the food. To determine fat content, use either of the following formulas:
  - Grams of fat $\times$ 9 = calories provided by fat, or
  - Calories of fat $\div$ total calories of the product $\times$ 100 = % fat content of the product.
  - Encourage intake of fruits and vegetables, whole-grain foods, and low-fat dairy products, and discourage intake of fatty meats, fried foods, and processed foods that are low in fiber and high in saturated and *trans* fats.

NUTRITIONAL DIRECTIONS

- Butter contains more saturated fats than most margarines; it also contains cholesterol, whereas soft margarines do not. However, butter does not contain *trans* fatty acids.
- An easy way to determine whether a food is low in fat is to hold up one finger for every 50 cals in the food (based on the food label); if the total number of fingers you are holding is more than the total fat grams on the label, the item is low fat; if the total number of fingers you are holding is less than the total fat grams, the item is high fat.
- Purchase processed foods that contain more PUFAs and MUFAs than SFAs. If the food label only lists the total fat, saturated fat, and *trans* fat content, subtract the total number of grams of saturated fat and *trans* fat from the total fat. For example, if the product contains 8 g of fat with 2 g of saturated fat and 1 g of *trans* fat, the 5 g of MUFAs and PUFAs is more than the 3 g from saturated and *trans* fats. This product is acceptable, but if there is another similar product that contains less than 3 g of saturated and *trans* fats, that product would be a wiser choice.
- Fully hydrogenated fats contain almost no *trans* fats.
- Tropical oils—including palm, palm kernel, and coconut oils—are saturated fats and their consumption should be limited. In transitioning away from *trans* fats, it is important to avoid reverting to alternatives, such as palm or coconut oils, which are saturated fats and are associated with increased risk of CVD.[20]
- Fruits, vegetables, and whole-grain foods should be used to replace high-fat foods.
- A few fruits and vegetables (plants) contain a small amount of fat (actually considered an oil). Bananas contain a trace of fat (0.55 g or 0.5% fat by weight and 6% of the calories); avocados contain 31 g of fat (15% by weight and 86% of the calories). Over 75% of the fat in avocados is MUFA with a small amount being PUFA. Both bananas and avocados are good sources of several vitamins and minerals.
- Increasing intake of dietary sources of omega-3 fatty acids is recommended over taking supplements.
- Fats and oils (100% fat) are necessary to provide adequate PUFAs and fat-soluble vitamins; food items are averaged together to determine if an item exceeding 35% fat would cause the overall intake to exceed the maximum 35% desired fat level.
- Children younger than age 2 years grow rapidly; fat restriction is potentially unsafe for this age group because of uncertainties about the amounts of energy, cholesterol, and EFAs required for growth. After age 2 years, the *Dietary Guidelines* are applicable.

Overconsumption and Health-Related Problems

Some conditions related to fat intake are observed in dental hygiene practice. The following conditions may suggest alteration of the type or possibly the amount of dietary fat: obesity, diabetes mellitus, **hyperlipidemia** (elevated concentrations of any or all of the blood lipids, especially triglycerides and LDL cholesterol), fatty infiltration of the liver, and certain types of cancer.

Obesity

Excessive fat stores are a common disorder in the United States (as discussed in Chapter 1, *Health Application 1*). Although the cause is usually overconsumption of all energy nutrients, calories from fat are so concentrated that relatively small quantities may rapidly increase caloric intake.

Blood Lipid Levels

Elevated blood lipids are related to diet and other risk factors. Hyperlipidemia is associated with CVD. Many factors can affect blood lipid levels; the strongest dietary determinant of blood cholesterol is saturated and *trans* fats. Total dietary fat content also affects serum lipid levels but to a lesser extent than saturated fatty acids. Reduction of total dietary fat content helps to reduce saturated fat content. Based on results of metabolic and epidemiologic studies, as little as a 2% increase in *trans* fatty acids can raise the risk of CVD as much as 29%. PUFAs are encouraged not only to reduce the risk of CVD, but they also are associated with lower risk of death from all causes.[21]

Stearic acid, a saturated fat in beef and cocoa butter, has no detrimental effect on serum cholesterol, but two saturated fatty acids (lauric acid and myristic acid) in coconut and palm kernel oils and butterfat are associated with higher risk of CVD.[22]

Because of new FDA regulations, commercially produced *trans* fatty acids should virtually disappear from the food supply.[23] Preserving the structural characteristics and palatability of some food products without *trans* fats is difficult. A relatively new industrial process is used to produce customized fats, which are called **interesterified fats**, with properties suitable for commercial preparation. Highly saturated hard fats are blended with oils to produce fats with intermediate characteristics. Many of the *trans* fatty acid alternatives, especially those made from tropical fats containing SFA, have not been thoroughly researched and may not have a desirable effect on blood lipids.[24,25] Interesterified fats may negatively affect blood lipids but not as severely as *trans* fats. Needless to say, more research is needed to determine the potential consequences of the replacement products. Factors and dietary modifications influencing serum lipid levels are discussed in more detail in *Health Application 6*.

Coconut oil recently has been touted as being "near miraculous," protecting against cancer and melting away excess body fat. Despite all the hype, these claims—especially for improving conditions such as autism, cancer, diabetes, or thyroid dysfunction—have not been supported by large, well-controlled human studies published in peer-reviewed journals demonstrating their health benefits.[26] Limited animal research studies suggest that some of the natural components of coconut oil may support health through antioxidant and an antiinflammatory action. Coconut oil, containing 60% medium-chain triglycerides, is a solid at room temperature and does not deteriorate rapidly. Natural coconut products and virgin coconut oil affect blood lipid levels differently even though they contain the same saturated fats. More importantly, saturated fatty acids in processed coconut oil (refined, bleached, and deodorized) are proven to increase total and LDL cholesterol (unhealthy) as well as HDL levels (beneficial).[26,27] Processed coconut oil consistently raises cholesterol levels. Some epidemiologic studies on indigenous populations that consume coconut flesh or coconut cream have not shown a negative effect.[28] Possibly, the harsh processing may destroy some of its natural components. Coconut products, including oil, can be consumed as part of a daily eating plan and/or in food preparation within the context of the U.S.-Pattern. However, 1 T virgin coconut oil contains 13.6 g of saturated fat, contributing a significant portion of the recommended total daily saturated fat limit of less than 7% of energy. Thus, it must be used sparingly, especially by patients who would benefit from reductions in total and LDL-cholesterol levels.

Cancer

A large portion of deaths caused by cancer in the United States each year can be attributed to diet and physical activity. Research continues to examine whether the association between high-fat diets and various cancers is attributable to the total amount of fat, the particular type of fat, the calories contributed by fat or some other factor associated with high-fat foods. Increased body weight and weight gain are associated with higher risk of breast and ovarian cancer. MUFAs, omega-3 fatty acids, and other PUFAs have not been associated with increased risk of cancer. Different mechanisms may be involved in tumor development at different sites and stages of cancer. Despite many uncertainties about a relationship between dietary fat and cancer risk, experts agree it is best to limit total fat intake by increasing the consumption of fish and lean meat, fruits, vegetables, and whole grain products while decreasing high-fat meats and foods, especially those high in saturated fats. These are important concepts of the Mediterranean Diet that have been shown to reduce the risk of postmenopausal breast cancer.[29,30]

DENTAL CONSIDERATIONS

- To distinguish obesity from edema, when the skin of an obese subject is palpated, it has a flabby consistency, in contrast to the mushy or spongy consistency found in edematous skin.
- Ask adult patients if they know their blood lipid levels. A high serum HDL level is considered desirable to prevent heart disease, whereas elevated levels of cholesterol, triglycerides, LDL, and VLDL increase the risk of heart disease.
- Inquire about a family history of CVD and other risks associated with heart disease.
- Stay current on research differentiating health effects of commercially produced and naturally occurring *trans* fatty acids.
- Teach patients to read the Nutrition Facts label for saturated and *trans* fats to avoid substituting one unhealthy fat for another and prevent significantly increasing carbohydrate intake.
- Guide patients toward a whole-foods-based diet that focuses on the quality food shown to have health benefits.
- Coconut oil cannot be assumed to have the same health effects as other oils and should not replace a significant amount of other plant oils.
- Coconut oil is not low in calories nor can it be considered a healthy food (does not contain less than 15% of calories from fat).

NUTRITIONAL DIRECTIONS

- Ten percent of total caloric intake should be from linoleic acid. Serum cholesterol can be reduced by increasing intake of MUFAs and PUFAs (see Table 6.1 and Fig. 6.5).
- Limit dietary cholesterol intake to around 300 mg daily by limiting high-fat meats and whole milk and cheese.
- "Low cholesterol" on a food label can be misleading. A cholesterol-free product, such as stick margarine, can still be high in saturated and *trans* fatty acids that elevate blood cholesterol.
- Choosing foods containing soluble fibers may decrease serum cholesterol.
- Wise food choices to prevent heart disease include unsaturated fats found in liquid vegetable oils, nuts, and seeds; and omega-3 unsaturated fats from fatty fish, such as salmon, sardines, and shellfish.
- Interesterified fat may be listed on food labels as fully hydrogenated oil.

Underconsumption and Health-Related Problems

Overconsumption of fat is a primary concern in health care, whereas underconsumption of fats is virtually nonexistent in the United States without medical or dietary intervention. However, clinical symptoms of fat deficiency may occur, especially in patients with malabsorption syndromes such as cystic fibrosis or patients in later stages of acquired immunodeficiency syndrome. EFA deficiency results in poor growth, dermatitis, reduced resistance to infection, and poor reproductive capacity.

When overall food intake, including fats, is poor, patients lose weight, depleting subcutaneous fat stores needed to maintain body temperature. Patients with anorexia nervosa are especially of concern (see Chapter 17).

DENTAL CONSIDERATIONS

- If a patient has poor reserves of subcutaneous fat, monitor temperature closely. These patients are unable to regulate body temperature as effectively as patients who have subcutaneous fat reserves.
- A patient with inadequate fat intake is thin, has dry skin and dull hair, and is sensitive to cold temperatures. If these signs and symptoms are noted, suggest an examination by a health care provider.

NUTRITIONAL DIRECTION

- Although much attention is given to the problems with fat consumption, fats have important physiologic functions, and a certain amount must be provided in the diet.

Fat Replacers

As a result of health concerns regarding dietary fats, numerous foods are being manufactured containing less fat. Fat replacers may be helpful in reducing fat and energy consumption. Most of the formulations to replace fat are carbohydrate and protein based, but lipid-based materials are available. Each of these fat replacers possesses diverse sensory, functional, and physiologic properties that affect their incorporation into various types of products (Table 6.5). Low-calorie salad dressing, low-fat yogurt, and imitation margarine are made by using modified starches and gums to reduce the oil or fat in the product.

By substituting fat replacers for fats, total fat intake can be reduced, and some weight loss may be achieved. However, an overall weight-loss program is still needed to effect weight loss. By consuming large portions of lower-fat products, an individual can potentially negate the caloric and fat savings of the replacement foods. Fat substitutes seem to pose little risk to health, but data are sparse regarding possible benefits under conditions of normal consumer use.

DENTAL CONSIDERATIONS

- Assess the use of fat replacers.
- Evaluate overall dietary habits because a patient may think that using fat replacers will make a desirable change in health without considering other aspects of the diet.
- If a patient exhibits symptoms such as gastrointestinal distress after consuming a product containing a fat substitute, recommend avoidance of that fat substitute.

NUTRITIONAL DIRECTIONS

- Patients allergic to eggs or cow's milk could be at risk for an allergic reaction to Simplesse because it is made from egg white and milk protein.
- Intake of fat replacers needs to be balanced with variety and moderation in food choices to achieve an overall healthy, nutritious diet.

TABLE 6.5 Fat Replacers

Generic Name (Trade Name)	kcal/g	Appropriate Uses
Carbohydrate Based		
Cellulose	0	Dairy-type products, sauces, frozen desserts, salad dressings
Dextrins	4	Salad dressings, puddings, spreads, dairy-type products, frozen desserts
Fiber	0	Baked goods, meats, spreads, extruded products
Gums	0	Salad dressings, desserts, processed meats
Inulin	1–1.2	Yogurt, cheese, frozen desserts, baked goods, icings, fillings, whipped cream, dairy products, fiber supplements, processed meats
Maltodextrin	4	Baked goods, dairy products, salad dressings, spreads, sauces, frostings, fillings, processed meats, frozen desserts
Nu-Trim	4	Baked goods, milk, cheese, ice cream
Oatrim	1–4	Baked goods, fillings and frostings, frozen desserts, dairy beverages, cheese, salad dressings, processed meats, confections
Polydextrose	1	Baked goods, chewing gums, confections, salad dressings, frozen dairy desserts, gelatins, puddings
Polyols	1.6–3	Bulking agent
Starch and modified food starch	1–4	Processed meats, salad dressings, baked goods, fillings and frostings, sauces, condiments, frozen desserts, dairy products
Z-Trim	0	Baked goods, burgers, hot dogs, cheese, ice cream, yogurt

TABLE 6.5 Fat Replacers—cont'd

Generic Name (Trade Name)	kcal/g	Appropriate Uses
Protein-based		
Microparticulated protein (Simplesse)	1–2	Dairy products (e.g., ice cream, butter, sour cream, cheese, yogurt), salad dressings, margarine- and mayonnaise-type products, baked goods, coffee creamers, soups, sauces
Modified whey protein concentrate		Milk and dairy products (e.g., cheese, yogurt, sour cream, ice cream), baked goods, frostings, salad dressings, mayonnaise-type products
Fat Based		
Emulsifiers	9	Cake mixes, cookies, icings, vegetable dairy products
Esterified propoxylated glycerol (EPG)[a]		Formulated products, baking and frying
Olestra (Olean)	0	Salty snacks, crackers, fried products
Salatrim	5	Confections, baked goods, dairy products
Sorbestrin[a]	1.5	Fried foods, salad dressings, mayonnaise, baked goods

[a]May require U.S. Food and Drug Administration approval.
Data from Calorie Control Council. *Glossary of fat replacers.* Copyright © 2016 Calorie Control Council. http://www.caloriecontrol.org/glossary-of-fat-replacers/. Accessed December 17, 2016.

HEALTH APPLICATION 6

Hyperlipidemia

Despite years of research and copious studies, CVD is still a major concern in the United States. Costs for CVD are expected to double from $555 billion in 2016 to $1.1 trillion in 2035.[31] *Healthy People 2020* established 50 objectives for heart disease and stroke. CVDs include hypertension, heart disease, stroke, congenital cardiovascular defects, myocardial ischemia, congestive heart failure, and many other anomalies. Dietary issues were addressed, that is, obesity and types of fats consumed. CVD prevalence in the United States has declined overall; mortality has decreased because of improvements in treatment and a reduction in risk factors. One of the *Healthy People 2020* objectives to lower the rate of deaths from heart disease from 129.2 per 100,000 in 2007 exceeded the 2020 target; in 2013, deaths from heart disease was 102.6.[32] CVD accounted for approximately 23.4% of deaths (< 1 of every 4) in the United States in 2014. The most common kind of CVD is coronary atherosclerosis, the leading cause of death in the United States. Heart disease remains the number one leading cause, and stroke is the fifth leading cause of death.[33]

Hyperlipidemia, or increased plasma cholesterol and LDL levels, appears to be a major risk factor for CVD. The Committee that compiled the *Third Report of the Expert Panel (NCEP) on Detection, Evaluation, and Treatment of High Blood Cholesterol in Adults* (ATP III)[34] and the AHA routinely re-evaluate guidelines and update recommendations for health care professionals to help prevent CVD. Continual scientific research provides more information allowing refinement of recommendations on detection and management of established risk factors, including evidence of the safety and efficacy of interventions previously considered promising. The leading risk factor for death and disability in the United States is suboptimal diet quality, which contributed to 318,656 deaths in 2012.[35] Most CVD is preventable through the adoption of healthy diet and lifestyles, basically adhering to the *Dietary Guidelines* and choosing more fruits and vegetables, nuts/seeds, whole grains, and seafood, and reducing sodium intake.

The AHA and National Cholesterol Education Program (NCEP) encourage a fasting lipoprotein profile screening (total cholesterol, LDL and HDL cholesterol, and triglycerides) for all adults older than age 20 years every 5 years along with an assessment of risk factors. More than 100 million (about 13%) Americans over age 20 years have total cholesterol levels greater than 200 mg/dL and almost 31 million greater than or equal to 240 mg/dL.[36] Average blood cholesterol values have declined since about 1960. LDL levels less than 100 mg/dL throughout life are associated with a very low risk for CVD; LDL greater than 100 mg/dL is the primary target of therapy. Reducing LDL cholesterol at early stages produces favorable outcomes for coronary lesions and reduces the likelihood of acute coronary syndromes.[3] Table 6.6 shows levels that are considered desirable or optimal. Fortunately, in 2011 to 2012, LDL levels decreased from 126 mg/dL to 111 mg/dL in 2013 in 2014.[37] This improvement may be attributed to changes in *trans* fatty acids in the food supply, use of statin medications, or overall dietary changes. Further reduction mandates would be expected with total elimination of *trans* fats; this should help lower the risk of CVD in adults. Higher levels of HDL have been thought to be a protective factor for CVD, but recent large studies have shown that increased HDL have not improved CVD outcomes.[38,39]

Beginning in 1988, the National Heart, Lung, and Blood Institute introduced two diets designed to lower blood cholesterol based on the individual's lipoprotein profile. This has been updated two times. The latest NCEP (ATP III) report focuses on a healthy body weight, diet, physical activity, and other controllable risk factors.[34] The Therapeutic Lifestyle Changes were written and amended by the American College of Cardiology and the AHA (Box 6.4).[40] Maintaining a healthy diet and lifestyle offers the greatest potential of all known approaches for reducing the risk of CVD in the general public. For all individuals without CVD risk equivalents whose LDL cholesterol is less than 100 mg/dL, adoption of healthy life habits (including cigarette smoking cessation or abstinence, following the *Dietary Guidelines* for a healthy food pattern, weight control, and increased physical activity), is recommended, as well as routine medical checkups for blood pressure and cholesterol. If the lipoprotein profile does not normalize after implementing these guidelines, drug treatment may be added.

Specific dietary recommendations are similar to those mentioned in Box 6.3. Natural food sources generally are recommended for nutrients rather than supplements. Other diets and lifestyle changes recommended in the *Dietary Guidelines* have been successful in reducing CVD, namely, the

Continued

HEALTH APPLICATION 6

Hyperlipidemia—cont'd

Mediterranean diet,[29,30] which promotes vegetables, monounsaturated fats, and nuts (Fig. 6.7), and Dietary Approaches to Stop Hypertension (DASH) regime (see Chapter 12).

Many other dietary factors have been proposed to help reduce the risk of CVD. Some of these are generally unproven or have uncertain effects on CVD. Although naturally occurring antioxidants in foods seem to prevent CVD, antioxidant supplements or other supplements such as selenium are inconclusive and have not shown major benefits in CVD prevention.[41-43] Phytochemicals found in fruits and vegetables may be important in reducing the risk of atherosclerosis. Foods containing antioxidants from a variety of fruits and vegetables, whole grains, and vegetable oils, and spices such as turmeric, garlic, and cinnamon, are recommended. Until more is known about the mode of action of these compounds, the most prudent practice to ensure optimum consumption of bioactive compounds is by increasing intake of fruits and vegetables and replacing salt with spices.

Plant sterols are bioactive compounds found in all vegetable foods, which inhibit cholesterol absorption. Small quantities of sterols are present in a variety of foods, including fruits, vegetables, nuts, seeds, cereals, and legumes. Consumption of soy protein–rich foods, a source of plant sterols, may indirectly reduce CVD risk if they replace products containing saturated fat and cholesterol. Plant sterols may lower LDL-C up to 10%.[44,45] In the United States, sterols are added to margarine spread, orange juice, and other products. A low-fat diet increases the effectiveness of these products.

The AHA recommends patients without CVD eat a variety of fish, preferably fatty fish, at least twice a week. Individuals who already have CVD are advised to consume at least 1 g of EPA and DHA daily, preferably from fatty fish. Of all the dietary changes recommended, cholesterol intake probably has the least effect on plasma cholesterol concentrations in most individuals because of less endogenous cholesterol production in response to cholesterol absorption. Consuming an egg daily does not increase risk for CVD.[46] One large egg contains less than 200 mg cholesterol. The *Dietary Guidelines* recommend limiting cholesterol to less than about 300 mg per day. AHA recommendations do not limit the number of eggs as long as total dietary cholesterol is about 300 mg per day. Most studies have found that reducing total dietary fat reduces serum cholesterol. Because fat consumption generally coincides with decreased saturated fat intake, changes in blood lipids appear to be related more to the type of fat consumed rather than total fat. However, a low-cholesterol, low-fat diet rarely reduces cholesterol more than 15%, and medications may be needed to reduce blood lipids further. A diet that limits fat to 35% of calories with 5% to 10% from PUFAs and 10% from SFAs and *trans* fatty acids reduces total and LDL cholesterol concentrations in most patients with hyperlipidemia. Replacing saturated and *trans* fats with PUFA may benefit lipid profiles, but replacing them with refined carbohydrate foods increases risk factors. By replacing some SFAs with MUFAs and some PUFAs and decreasing total fat, LDL is lowered without decreasing HDL concentrations. These changes result in a more palatable diet that is better received by Americans.

Because of Americans' high intake of sugar, which exceeds discretionary calorie allowances, especially in the form of sugar-containing beverages, concurrent with the *Dietary Guidelines,* the AHA recommends reducing added sugar intake. A high intake of refined carbohydrates negatively affects lipid profile (decreases HDL, increases triglyceride and LDL). A prudent upper limit of the discretionary calorie allowance from added sweeteners is 170 cal for an 1800-cal diet and 280 cal for a 2200-cal diet, consistent with the U.S.-Pattern.

One of the most important facts for decreasing the risk of CVD is the types of foods chosen to replace saturated fat intake. When a decrease in saturated fats is recommended, suggestions should be made regarding what types of foods/fats should be chosen to replace those calories. Overall dietary quality includes (a) carbohydrate quality (whole vs. refined grains, and dietary fiber); (b) intake of specific individual fatty acids; (c) inclusion of a variety of healthful foods such as fruits, vegetables, nuts, fish, dairy products, and vegetable oils; (d) limited amounts of sugar-sweetened beverages and processed meats and foods; and (e) energy balance. Recommendations will continue to change as research leads to knowledge about the effect of specific fatty acids on lipid profiles and CVD.

TABLE 6.6 Desirable/Optimal Blood Lipid Levels

Lipid	Desirable/Optimal Level (mg/dL)
Total cholesterol	< 200
LDL	< 100
HDL	> 60
Triglyceride	< 150

Data from National Cholesterol Education Program (NCEP): *Third report of the National Cholesterol Education Program (NCEP) on detection, evaluation, and treatment of high blood cholesterol in adults (Adult Treatment Panel III), final report.* Publication No. 02-5125. Bethesda, MD, 2002, National Institutes of Health, National Heart, Lung, and Blood Institute, and American Heart Association: *What your cholesterol means.* https://www.nhlbi.nih.gov/files/docs/guidelines/atp3xsum.pdf. Accessed December 17, 2016.

BOX 6.4 Lifestyle Management Guidelines

The optimal goal for all Americans, regardless of risk for CVD, is to follow these recommendations:

- Consume a dietary pattern that emphasizes intake of vegetables, fruits, and whole grains; this includes low-fat dairy products, poultry, fish, legumes, nontropical vegetable oils and nuts; and limits intake of sweets, sugar-sweetened beverages, and red meats.
  - Adapt this dietary pattern to appropriate calorie requirements, personal and cultural food preferences, and nutrition therapy for other medical conditions (including diabetes mellitus).
  - Achieve this pattern by following plans such as the Mediterranean pattern, DASH dietary pattern, the USDA Food Pattern, or the AHA diet.
- Aim for a dietary pattern that achieves 5% to 6% of calories from saturated fat
- Reduce percent of calories from saturated fat.
- Reduce percent of calories from *trans* fat.
- Engage in aerobic physical activity 3 to 4 sessions a week, lasting 40 minutes per session, on average, and involving physical activity of moderate to vigorous intensity.

AHA, American Heart Association; DASH, Dietary Approaches to Stop Hypertension; USDA, U.S. Department of Agriculture.

Adapted from Eckel RH, Jakicic JM, Ard JD, and other Expert Work Group Members. 2013 AHA/ACC Guideline on lifestyle management to reduce cardiovascular risk. J Am Coll Cardiol. *2014;63(25 Pt B):2960–2984.*

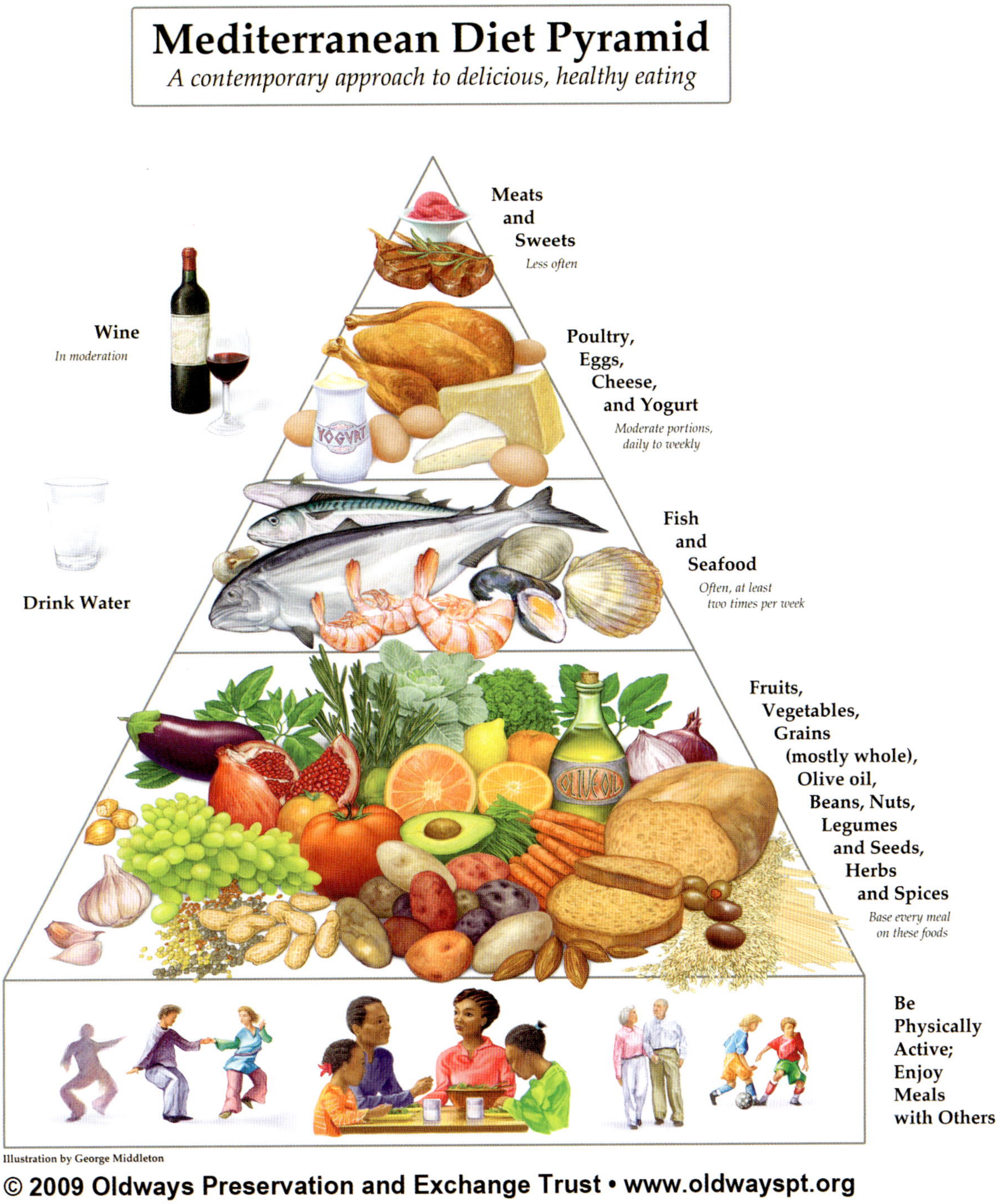

Mediterranean Diet Pyramid
A contemporary approach to delicious, healthy eating
Meats and Sweets
Less often
Wine
In moderation
Poultry, Eggs, Cheese, and Yogurt
Moderate portions, daily to weekly
YOGURT
Fish and Seafood
Often, at least two times per week
Drink Water
Fruits, Vegetables, Grains (mostly whole), Olive oil, Beans, Nuts, Legumes and Seeds, Herbs and Spices
Base every meal on these foods
OLIVE OIL
Be Physically Active; Enjoy Meals with Others
Illustration by George Middleton
© 2009 Oldways Preservation and Exchange Trust • www.oldwayspt.org

• **Figure 6.7** Mediterranean Diet Pyramid. The Traditional Healthy Mediterranean Diet Pyramid. (Courtesy Oldways Preservation and Exchange Trust. Accessed December 14, 2016. www.oldwayspt.org.)

CASE APPLICATION FOR THE DENTAL HYGIENIST

A 50-year-old patient complains to his dental hygienist that he has recently been having chest pain. He says a recent testing at his grocery store indicated his blood cholesterol level was elevated. A health care provider told him several years ago his cholesterol was slightly elevated and that he probably should lower his fat intake. No formal medical nutrition treatment was ordered and no follow-up work has been done. His blood pressure is 145/90 mm Hg.

He continues to eat anything he wants. He realizes some foods are high in fat and should be avoided, but he is unable to identify these foods. When questioned about fat requirements and different types of fat, he says that he does not understand all of those big medical terms. He also indicates his parents ate what they wanted without all these problems and concerns.

Nutritional Assessment

- Readiness/willingness to learn
- Knowledge level concerning fat principles and how these relate to his diagnosis

Continued

CASE APPLICATION FOR THE DENTAL HYGIENIST—cont'd

- Total amount of fat intake
- Typical foods eaten
- Type of dietary habits: who purchases and prepares the food, where he lives, where most meals are eaten
- Blood pressure
- Serum lipids, if known
- Family medical history (parents still living, cause of death)

Nutritional Diagnosis

Altered health maintenance related to lack of knowledge of fat principles; diet and how it relates to the condition.

Nutritional Goals

The patient will adhere to a low-fat, low-cholesterol diet; list foods high and low in fat; and state how the disease may improve or deteriorate with diet.

Nutritional Implementation

Intervention: Emphasize the importance of having a thorough examination annually by a health care provider and a confirmation of laboratory work with a complete fasting lipid profile.

Rationale: Dietary changes and lifestyle changes are probably indicated; however, the best individuals to diagnose and prescribe treatment are a health care provider and RDN.

Intervention: Explain how diet and lifestyle affect his condition: (a) saturated and *trans* fats increase the rate of fatty deposits in the arteries; (b) high cholesterol intake also adversely affects this process; (c) physiologic roles of fat (see p. 105); (d) smoking increases the risk of heart disease; and (e) maintaining a body mass index within normal range decreases risk.

Rationale: Knowledge increases compliance.

Intervention: Explain the difference between PUFAs and SFAs: (a) use actual Nutrition Facts labels; (b) provide a list of foods high and low in these two types of fat; (c) keep fat intake to less than 35% of total calories; less than 10% of caloric intake from SFAs and *trans* fatty acids, up to 20% from MUFAs, and up to 10% from PUFAs.

Rationale: If the patient knows the difference between the two types of fat, he can make informed choices to help reduce the likelihood of heart disease.

Intervention: Explain the difference between the types of lipids and cholesterol: (a) provide a list of foods high and low in cholesterol; (b) limit daily cholesterol intake to 300 mg or less; (c) explain that "cholesterol free" does not mean "fat free."

Rationale: Reducing serum cholesterol levels may help slow the effects of heart disease.

Intervention: Inquire at each recare appointment if the patient has had a blood lipid profile check recently (HDL > 35 mg/dL for men; LDL < 100 mg/dL for men). Use these as motivators to stay on a healthy diet.

Rationale: These values can provide concrete evidence for motivation and compliance.

Intervention: Monitor blood pressure values at each recare appointment. Inform the patient that hypertension is another risk factor for heart disease. Refer to the health care provider for elevated values.

Rationale: If the patient is aware of his blood pressure and the harmful effects of blood pressure elevation, he will make attempts to lower it.

Intervention: Teach the patient how to read nutrition labels (use an actual food label for teaching); use a margarine brand that lists the first ingredient as liquid oil. Explain the different claims on labels, such as "fat free," "low fat," and "reduced fat." (See Box 1.4.)

Rationale: Labels can be confusing. Accurate information can promote healthy food choices and reduce the incidence of heart disease.

Intervention: Suggest that the patient decrease the amount of dietary fat and saturated fats: advise him to (a) eat smaller servings of meat; (b) trim visible fat from meats; (c) consume more skinless poultry and fatty fish; (d) avoid fried foods; and (e) use less salad dressing, change the type of fat (use olive oil), or reduce the amount of fat in the salad dressing (fat free or low fat).

Rationale: These are all ways to decrease fat intake, thereby decreasing the progression of atherosclerosis. The use of more fish increases intake of omega-3 fatty acids.

Evaluation

If the patient lists foods higher and lower in fat and makes better choices to consume a low-fat, low-cholesterol diet, dental hygiene care was effective. In addition, dental hygiene care was successful if the patient can identify the healthiest low-fat, low-cholesterol choices from three food labels; state how fat and cholesterol can lead to further deterioration of his disease; and verbalize that fat speeds up the accumulation of fatty deposits. Other factors to evaluate include whether (a) blood lipid levels improve, (b) blood pressure is within normal values, and (c) the patient has begun a smoking cessation program.

Student Readiness

1. Describe the following terms: *lipoproteins, hyperlipidemia, structural lipids,* and *EFA.*
2. A patient wants to know which foods to consume to (a) increase PUFAs, (b) increase MUFAs, and (c) decrease SFAs. Name three sources of each.
3. In observing physical properties of fats, how could you estimate the polyunsaturated and saturated fat content of a food?
4. What unsaturated fatty acid is essential in the diet? What are the functions of unsaturated fatty acids in the body?
5. Compare the Nutrition Facts labels of three brands of stick margarine, three brands of tub margarine, two brands of diet margarine, and two brands of spray margarine. How do they differ in their polyunsaturated-to-saturated fat ratio? List the first ingredient of each.
6. Describe the functions of fat in the diet.
7. Evaluate one day of your intake for types of foods consumed and amounts of cholesterol, *trans* fatty acid, and saturated fat. If that day represented your average cholesterol and saturated fat intake over an extended period, determine whether the cholesterol or saturated fat content of intake should be reduced. List some simple, realistic suggestions for decreasing their intake.
8. Describe the role of cholesterol in the body.
9. Calculate the caloric value of the following items:
   2 slices bacon (8 g of fat, 4 g of protein)
   1 tbsp margarine (12 g of fat)
   1 tbsp whipped margarine (8 g of fat)
   1 tbsp mayonnaise (6 g of fat)
   1 tbsp lard (13 g of fat)
10. A patient asks if it is possible to lose or gain 1 lb of body fat every day. What would you say?
11. Calculate the grams of fat a patient could consume on (1) a 1500-cal diet and (2) a 2000-cal diet to meet the *Dietary Guidelines.*
12. List five points you think a patient should know about fats in general.

References

1. Wang DD, Leung CW, Li Y, et al. Trends in dietary quality among adults in the United States, 1999 Through 2010. *JAMA Intern Med.* 2014;174(10):1587–1595.
2. U.S. Department of Health and Human Services and U.S. Department of Agriculture. *2015-2020 Dietary Guidelines for Americans.* 8th ed. 2015. https://health.gov/dietaryguidelines/2015/guidelines/. Accessed July 12, 2017.
3. Griffin BA. Serum low-density lipoprotein as a dietary responsive biomarker of cardiovascular disease risk: consensus and confusion. *Nutr Bull.* 2017;42(3):266–273.
4. Zhou X, Shen Y, Parker JK, et al. Effects of sensory modalities and importance of fatty acid sensitivity on fat perception in a real food model. *Chemosens Percept.* 2016;9:105–119.
5. Writing Group for the AREDS2 Research Group, Bonds DE, Harrington M, et al. Effect of long-chain ω-3 fatty acids and lutein + zeaxanthin supplements on cardiovascular outcomes: results of the Age-Related Eye Disease Study 2 (AREDS2) randomized clinical trial. *JAMA Intern Med.* 2014;174(5):763–771.
6. Heydari B, Abdullah S, Pottala JV, et al. Effect of omega-3 acid ethyl esters on left ventricular remodeling after acute myocardial infarction. The OMEGA-REMODEL Randomized Clinical Trial. *Circulation.* 2016;134:378–391.
7. Fritsche KL. The science of fatty acids and inflammation. *Adv Nutr.* 2015;6(3):293S–301S.
8. Azzi DV, Viafara JA, Zangeronimo MG, et al. n-3 ingestion may modulate the severity of periodontal disease? Systematic review. *Crit Rev Food Sci Nutr.* 2017;1–6. [Epub ahead of print].
9. Woelber JP, Bremer K, Vach K, et al. An oral health optimized diet can reduce gingival and periodontal inflammation in humans—a randomized controlled pilot study. *BMC Oral Health.* 2016;17(1):28.
10. Sun M, Zhou Z, Dong J, et al. Antibacterial and antibiofilm activities of docosahexaenoic acid (DHA) and eicosapentaenoic acid (EPA) against periodontopathic bacteria. *Microb Pathog.* 2016;99:196–203.
11. Vedin O, Hagström E, Budaj A, et al. Tooth loss is independently associated with poor outcomes in stable coronary heart disease. *Eur J Prev Cardiol.* 2016;23(8):839–846.
12. Varela-López A, Giampieri F, Bullón P, et al. Role of lipids in the onset, progression and treatment of periodontal disease. A systematic review of studies in humans. *Int J Mol Sci.* 2016;17(8).
13. Wang DD, Li Y, Chiuve SE, et al. Association of specific dietary fats with total and cause-specific mortality. *JAMA Intern Med.* 2016;176(8):1134–1145.
14. Li Y, Hruby A, Bernstein AM, et al. Saturated fats compared with unsaturated fats and sources of carbohydrates in relation to risk of coronary heart disease: A prospective cohort study. *J Am Coll Cardiol.* 2015;66(14):1538–1548.
15. Farvid MS, Ding M, Pan A, et al. Dietary linoleic acid and risk of coronary heart disease: a systematic review and meta-analysis of prospective cohort studies. *Circulation.* 2014;130(18):1568–1578.
16. Flock MR, Harris WS, Kris-Etherton PM. Long-chain omega-3 fatty acids: time to establish a Dietary Reference Intake. *Nutr Rev.* 2013;71(10):692–707.
17. International Food Information Council (IFIC) EPA and DHA: Time to establish a Dietary Reference Intake level? Food Insight. Last updated September 19, 2014. http://www.foodinsight.org/articles/epa-and-dha-time-establish-dietary-reference-intake-level. Accessed December 7, 2016.
18. Alexander DD, Miller PE, Van Elswyk ME, et al. A meta-analysis of randomized controlled trials and prospective cohort studies of eicosapentaenoic and docosahexaenoic long-chain omega-3 fatty acids and coronary heart disease risk. *Mayo Clin Proc.* 2017;92(1):15–29.
19. United Soybean Board. Soybean Oil Facts: Conventional Soybean Oil. http://www.soyconnection.com/sites/default/files/2016_Conventional%20Soybean%20Oil_Final.pdf. Accessed December 12, 2016.
20. Doheny K. Palm oil: the new fat under fire. WebMD. February 9, 2017. http://www.webmd.com/food-recipes/news/20170209/palm-oil-the-new-fat-under-fire#1.
21. Marklund M, Leander K, Vikström M, et al. Polyunsaturated fat intake estimated by circulating biomarkers and risk of cardiovascular disease and all-cause mortality in a population-based cohort of 60-year-old men and women. *Circulation.* 2015;132(7):586–594.
22. Zong G, Li Y, Wanders AJ, et al. Intake of individual saturated fatty acids and risk of coronary heart disease in U.S. men and women: two prospective longitudinal cohort studies. *BMJ.* 2016;355:i5796.
23. FDA Consumer Health Information. FDA Cuts Trans Fat in Processed Foods. U.S. Food and Drug Administration. June 2015. http://www.fda.gov/ForConsumers/ConsumerUpdates/ucm372915.htm. Accessed December 12, 2016.
24. Mills CE, Hall WL, Berry SEE. What are interesterfied fats and should we be worried about them in our diet? *Nutr Bull.* 2017;42(2):153–158.
25. Afonso MS, Lavrador MSF, Koike MK, et al. Dietary interesterified fat enriched with palmitic acid induces atherosclerosis by impairing macrophage cholesterol efflux and eliciting inflammation. *J Nutr Biochem.* 2016;32:91–100.
26. Lockyer S, Stanner S. Coconut oil—a nutty idea? *Nutr Bull.* 2016;41(1):42–54.
27. Eyres L, Eyres MF, Chisholm A, et al. Coconut oil consumption and cardiovascular risk factors in humans. *Nutr Rev.* 2016;74(4):267–280.
28. Feranil AB, Duazo PL, Kuzawa CW, et al. Coconut oil is associated with a beneficial lipid profile in premenopausal women in the Philippines. *Asia Pac J Clin Nutr.* 2011;20(2):190–195.
29. van den Brandt PA, Schulpen M. Mediterranean diet adherence and risk of postmenopausal breast cancer: results of a cohort study and meta-analysis. *Int J Cancer.* 2017;140(10):2220–2231.
30. Romagnolo DF, Selmin OI. Mediterranean diet and prevention of chronic diseases. *Nutr Today.* 2017;52(5):208–222.
31. Khavjou O, Phelps D, Leib A. *Projections of Cardiovascular Disease Prevalence and Costs, 2015–2035.* Research Triangle Park: RTI International; 2016.
32. National Center for Health Statistics. Chapter 21: Heart Disease and Stroke. Healthy People 2020 Midcourse Review. Hyattsville, MD. 2016. https://www.cdc.gov/nchs/data/hpdata2020/HP2020MCR-C21-HDS.pdf. Accessed July 12, 2017.
33. Center for Disease Control and Prevention. Injury prevention & control: data & statistics (WISQARS™). https://www.cdc.gov/injury/wisqars/pdf/leading_causes_of_death_by_age_group_2014-a.pdf. Accessed December 14, 2016.
34. National Cholesterol Education Program (NCEP). *Third report of the National Cholesterol Education Program (NCEP) expert panel on detection, evaluation, and treatment of high blood cholesterol in adults. NIH Publication No. 02-5215.* Bethesda, MD: National Institutes of Health; 2002. Web site: https://www.nhlbi.nih.gov/files/docs/guidelines/atp3xsum.pdf. Accessed December 13, 2016.
35. Micha R, Peñalvo JL, Cudhea F, et al. Association between dietary factors and mortality from heart disease, stroke, and Type 2 diabetes in the United States. *JAMA.* 2017;317(9):912–924.
36. Mozaffarian D, Benjamin EJ, Go AS, et al. Heart disease and stroke statistics—2016 update. A report from the American Heart Association. *Circulation.* 2015;132(4):447–454.
37. Rosinger A, Carroll MD, Lacher D, et al. Trends in total cholesterol, triglycerides, and low density lipoprotein in U.S. adults, 1999–2014. *JAMA Cardiol.* 2017;2(3):339–341.
38. Siddiqi HK, Kiss D, Rader D. HDL-cholesterol and cardiovascular disease: rethinking our approach. *Curr Opin Cardiol.* 2015;30(5):536–542.
39. Hovingh GK, Rader DJ, Hegele RA. HDL re-examined. *Curr Opin Lipidol.* 2015;26(2):127–132.
40. Eckel RH, Jakicic JM, Ard JD, other Expert Work Group Members. 2013 AHA/ACC Guideline on lifestyle management to reduce cardiovascular risk. *J Am Coll Cardiol.* 2014;63(25 Pt B):2960–2984.

41. Siscovick DS, Barringer TA, Fretts AM, et al. Omega-3 polyunsaturated fatty acid (fish oil) supplementation and the prevention of clinical cardiovascular disease: A science advisory from the American Heart Association. *Circulation*. 2017;[Epub ahead of print].
42. Freeman AM, Morris PB, Barnard N, et al. Trending cardiovascular nutrition controversies. *J Am Coll Cardiol*. 2017;69(9):1172–1187.
43. Benstoem C, Goetzenich A, Kraemer S, et al. Selenium and its supplementation in cardiovascular disease—what do we know? *Nutrients*. 2015;7(5):3094–3118.
44. Gylling H, Plat J, Turley S, et al. Plant sterols and plant stanols in the management of dyslipidaemia and prevention of cardiovascular disease. *Atherosclerosis*. 2014;232(2):346–360.
45. Ras RT, Geleijnse JM, Trautwein EA. LDL-cholesterol-lowering effect of plant sterols and stanols across different dose ranges: a meta-analysis of randomised controlled studies. *Br J Nutr*. 2014;112(2): 214–219.
46. Richard C, Cristall L, Fleming E, et al. Impact of egg consumption on cardiovascular risk factors in individuals with type 2 diabetes and at risk for developing diabetes: a systematic review of randomized nutritional intervention studies. *Can J Diabetes*. 2017;41(4): 453–463.

EVOLVE RESOURCES

Please visit http://evolve.elsevier.com/Stegeman/nutritional for additional practice and study support tools.

7

Use of the Energy Nutrients: Metabolism and Balance

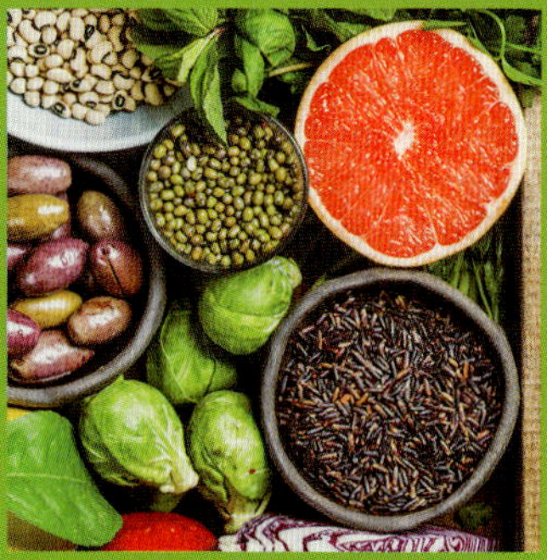

STUDENT LEARNING OUTCOMES

Upon completion of this chapter, the student will be able to achieve the following student learning outcomes:

1. Discuss the roles of the liver and the kidneys in metabolism. In addition, describe carbohydrate metabolism.
2. Discuss protein metabolism.
3. Discuss lipid metabolism, alcohol metabolism, metabolic relationships, and metabolic energy.
4. Identify factors affecting the basal metabolic rate.
5. Calculate energy needs according to a patient's weight and activities.
6. Assess factors affecting energy balance; explain physiologic and psychologic sources of energy.
7. Discuss the following related to inadequate energy intake:
   - Summarize the effects of inadequate energy intake.
   - Explain the principles for and importance of regulating energy balance to a patient.
   - Individualize dental hygiene considerations to patients regarding energy metabolism.
   - Relate nutritional directions to meet patients' needs regarding energy metabolism.

KEY TERMS

Appetite
Basal energy expenditure
Basal metabolic rate (BMR)
Calorimeter
Catecholamines
Cofactor
Glycemic index
Glycogenesis
High-energy phosphate compounds
Hunger
Indirect calorimetry
Ketoacidosis
Ketonuria
Kilocalorie (kcal)
Lipolysis
Normoglycemic
Pedometer
Postabsorptive state
Renal failure
Thermic effect

TEST YOUR NQ

1. **T/F** Insulin is a hormone that decreases blood glucose levels.
2. **T/F** Even during sleep, the body requires energy.
3. **T/F** BMR stands for blood malnutrition reaction.
4. **T/F** A malnourished patient would have a low BMR.
5. **T/F** The hypothalamus controls hunger and satiety.
6. **T/F** Hunger is the same as appetite.
7. **T/F** Fats are a good source of quick energy.
8. **T/F** The kidneys play an important role in maintaining nutrient balance within the body.
9. **T/F** Ketoacidosis can occur as a result of strict carbohydrate restriction.
10. **T/F** Vitamins are a source of energy.

After foods are chewed and digested, the macronutrients (carbohydrate, protein, fat, and alcohol) supplying physiologic energy for the body are converted to glucose, fatty acids, and amino acids. These basic nutrient units are delivered to cells where, at the direction of specific enzymes, they can be used.

Recall from earlier chapters that no single nutrient can be isolated from the others because nutrients are concurrently distributed in foods and share many points of interaction in digestion, absorption, and metabolism. Metabolism encompasses the continuous processes whereby living organisms and cells convert nutrients into energy, body structure, and waste.

Metabolism

In metabolic activity, the two major chemical reactions are catabolism and anabolism. Catabolism is splitting complex substances into simpler substances; anabolism is using absorbed nutrients to build or synthesize more complex compounds (see Chapter 2 or online at Evolve for more detail). Anabolism and catabolism are continuous reactions in the body. Cells in the epithelial lining of the oral and gastrointestinal mucosa are replaced approximately every 3 to 7 days. Despite this rapid turnover, the rate of catabolism is usually equal to that of anabolism in a healthy adult. During certain stages of life, such as growth periods or pregnancy, more anabolism is occurring than catabolism. Conversely, when illness or stress occurs, excessive catabolism is evident.

Other phases of metabolism include delivery of nutrients to the cells where they are needed and delivery of waste products to sites where they can be excreted. After absorption of the macronutrients, glucose, fatty acids, and amino acids can be used to yield energy via a common pathway within the mitochondria of cells (Fig. 7.1). The catabolic end products of carbohydrates, proteins, and fats are carbon dioxide, water, and energy. Nitrogen is an additional end product of protein.

The Krebs cycle (also called citric acid cycle or tricarboxylic acid [TCA] cycle) converts glucose, fatty acids, and amino acids to a usable form of energy, requiring many enzymes. Additional information on the TCA cycle can be found in Chapter 2 and online at Evolve. For activation of some enzymes, vitamins or minerals or both must be available. An enzyme needing vitamins for activation is called a coenzyme. Thiamin, riboflavin, and niacin are B vitamins essential as coenzymes in the TCA cycle. An enzyme may also require a cofactor. A **cofactor** functions in the same way as coenzymes, but the molecule required is a mineral or electrolyte.

Anabolic processes require energy. Examples of anabolism are the building of new muscle tissue or bone and the secretion of cellular products such as hormones. Hormones are "messengers" produced by a group of cells that stimulate or retard the functions of other cells. Hormones principally control different metabolic functions that affect secretions and growth. Anabolism involves the use of glucose, amino acids, fatty acids, and glycerol to build various substances that comprise the body itself and other substances necessary for proper functioning. All nutrients are intertwined in

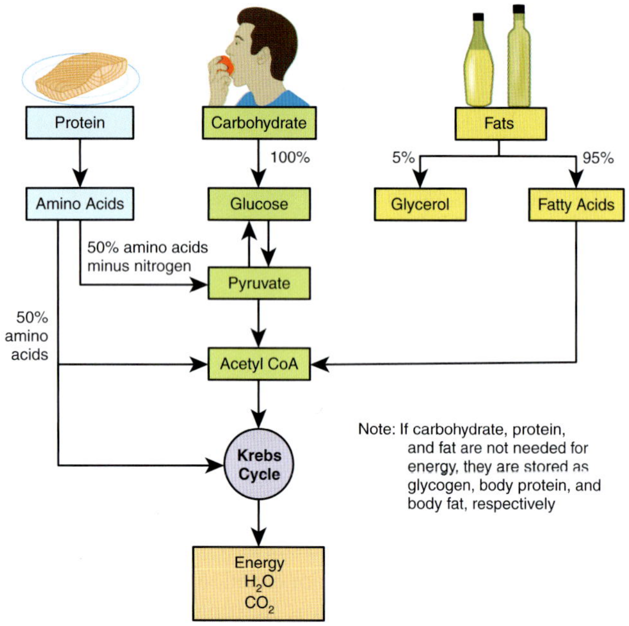

• **Figure 7.1** Metabolic pathways. (Modified from Peckenpaugh NJ: *Nutrition Essentials and Diet Therapy*, 11th ed. St. Louis, MO: Saunders; 2010.)

this process. For instance, dispensable amino acids are ordinarily used to build proteins, but glucose can be the basis for anabolism of amino acids and fatty acids.

Role of the Liver

The liver plays a major regulatory role by controlling the kinds and quantities of nutrients in the bloodstream. All monosaccharides are converted to glucose in the liver to provide an energy supply for the cells. Glycogen, a polysaccharide, also can be broken down to glucose and released into the circulating blood as needed. Other end products of digestion may be oxidized to provide energy; converted to glucose, protein, fat, or other substances; or released to circulate at prescribed levels in the blood for use by all the cells.

Role of the Kidneys

Kidneys perform the important metabolic task of removing waste products from the blood and, along with the liver, control the levels of many nutrients in the blood. Metabolic end products from cells, unnecessary substances absorbed from the gastrointestinal tract, potentially harmful compounds that have been detoxified by the liver, and drugs are removed from the blood by the kidneys.

Kidneys accomplish this task by a process of filtration and reabsorption. Glucose, amino acids, vitamins, water, and various minerals are reabsorbed or excreted by the kidneys depending on the body's need. Excess nitrogen from protein catabolism also is excreted by the kidneys. Kidneys help maintain nutrient balance within the body. Other routes of excretion of waste products are through the bowel; the skin, which excretes water and electrolytes; and the lungs, which remove carbon dioxide and water.

DENTAL CONSIDERATIONS

- The goal of nutrition in a dental setting is to promote anabolism for growth or healing.
- Uncontrolled blood glucose levels may cause numerous complications, such as poor wound healing and increased risk of infection for patients with diabetes.
- The kidneys' ability to reabsorb nutrients may be altered by certain medications, especially diuretics, or a kidney disorder. Function also depends on fluid balance.

NUTRITIONAL DIRECTIONS

- The liver is a vital organ for metabolism of food and drugs.
- The kidneys help the body dispose of waste products and drugs. Adequate fluid intake (9–11 cups per day) facilitates this process.
- If the kidneys are not working properly, drugs and nutrients may be retained or lost. Both are undesirable.

Carbohydrate Metabolism

Monosaccharides are transported through the portal vein to the liver for **glycogenesis**, a process of glycogen formation. During this process, sugars—including fructose, galactose, sorbitol, and xylitol—may be stored as glycogen. Glucose, the circulating sugar in the blood, is the major energy supply for cells. The level of circulating glucose is closely monitored by the liver and is constantly maintained at a **normoglycemic** level (normal blood glucose range), between 70 and 100 mg/dL. Insulin is a hormone that lowers blood glucose levels. Blood glucose levels peak at 140 mg/dL 30 to 60 minutes after a meal and return to normal within 3 hours in individuals with normal secretion and use of insulin. This consistent blood glucose level is significant, indicating the necessity of a certain amount of glucose in the blood for normal functioning of body tissues (Fig. 7.2). Hyperglycemia (elevated blood glucose) and hypoglycemia (decreased blood glucose) are very serious conditions that can be fatal; the precipitating cause for either should be identified. Many patients with diabetes who take insulin or an antidiabetic medication that can cause hypoglycemia, or both, may exhibit symptoms related to hypoglycemia, particularly if they have not eaten within a 4- to 5-hour time span. These patients need to be treated with a carbohydrate source before continuing treatment (see *Health Application 7*).

Carbohydrate foods and beverages are digested and absorbed at different rates. Individuals with diabetes often respond differently to different carbohydrate sources. **Glycemic index (GI)** measures the effect of different carbohydrate foods on blood glucose levels. The thought is that a food with a high GI will raise blood glucose to a greater extent than a food with a low GI. In general, dairy products, legumes, pasta, fruits, and sugars have a low GI. Breads, cereals, and rice can have either a low or high GI. There is no standardized definition for low-, high- or moderate-GI foods.[1,2] The American Diabetes Association reports little difference in consumption of low GI and high GI foods for glycemic control.[1] For weight loss measures, the Academy of Nutrition and Dietetics does not recommend a low-GI diet since it is ineffective.[3] The recommendation for all individuals, including those with diabetes, includes increasing intake of whole grains, legumes, fruits, and vegetables while limiting intake of refined carbohydrates and added sugars.

A complex hormonal system maintains a constant blood glucose level. Insulin is the primary hormone that lowers blood glucose levels. When hyperglycemia occurs, insulin is secreted to decrease blood glucose levels. Conversely, hypoglycemia elicits the secretion of several hormones (thyroid, epinephrine, glucagon, and growth hormone) to increase blood glucose levels. The liver can elevate blood glucose levels by converting amino acids from protein and glycerol from fats to glucose. The process of synthesizing glucose from noncarbohydrate sources is known as gluconeogenesis (see Chapter 2 or online at Evolve for additional details).

Dietary carbohydrates ensure optimal glycogen stores and are digested faster than other energy nutrients. The liver can degrade

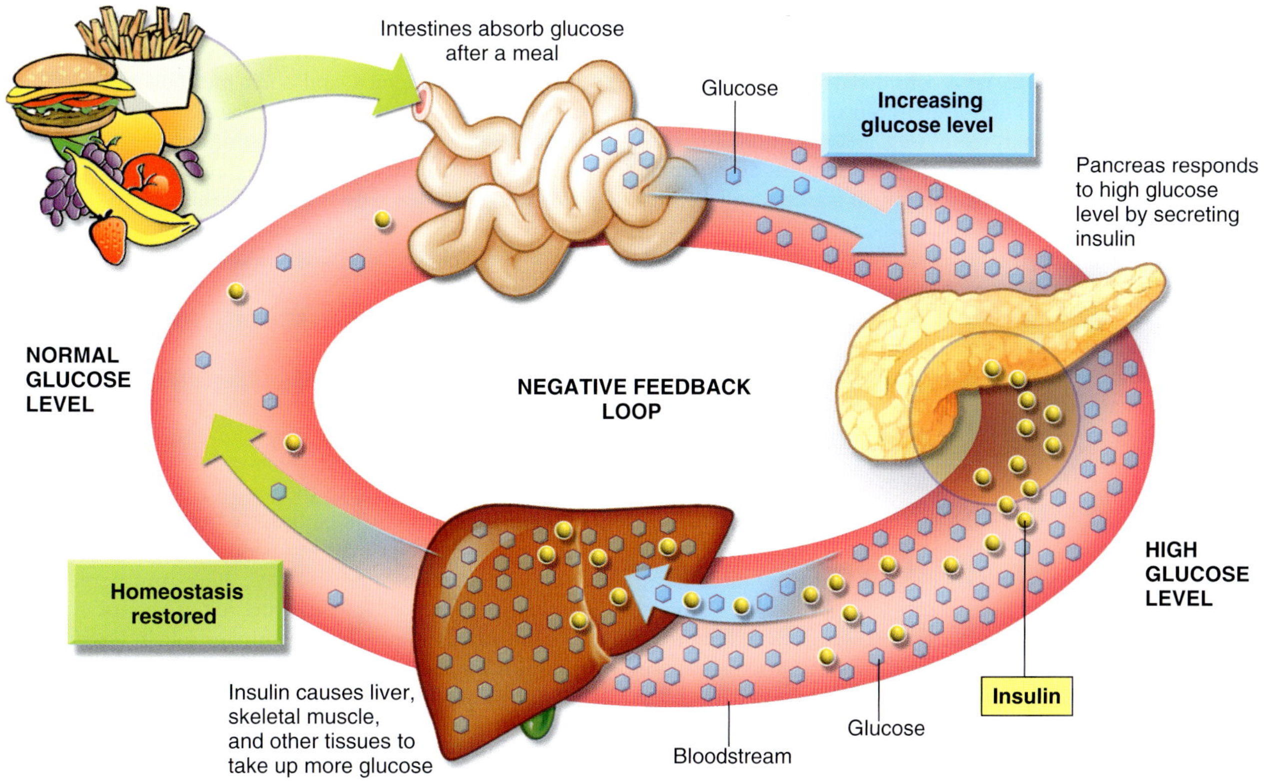

• **Figure 7.2** Role of insulin. Insulin operates in a negative feedback loop that prevents blood glucose concentration from increasing too far above the normal (or setpoint) level. Insulin promotes uptake of glucose by all cells of the body, enabling them to catabolize or store it, or both. The liver and skeletal muscles are especially well adapted for storage of glucose as glycogen. Excess glucose is removed from the bloodstream. If the glucose level falls below the setpoint level, hormones such as glucagon promote the release of glucose from storage into the bloodstream. (Reproduced with permission from Thibodeau GA, Patton KT. *Anatomy and Physiology*. 9th ed. St. Louis, MO: Mosby Elsevier; 2016.)

glycogen to glucose. The amount of energy available from glycogen stores is generally less than a day's energy expenditure or approximately 1200 to 1800 cal. Red blood cells and cells in the heart, brain, and renal medulla prefer glucose as their energy source.

Protein Metabolism

Amino acids are transported through the portal vein into the liver. The liver is an "aminostat," monitoring the intake and breakdown of most of the amino acids. Individual amino acids are released by the liver to enter the general circulation at specific levels so that each amino acid is available as needed to synthesize each individual protein. Amino acids transported in the blood are rapidly removed for use by cells. If individual amino acids increase above a specific level in the blood, they are removed and oxidized for energy.

Protein metabolism is in a constant dynamic state, with catabolism and anabolism occurring continuously to replace worn-out proteins in cells. Even during anabolic periods, such as growth, muscle catabolism is elevated as each cell remodels itself. Anabolic and catabolic processes are controlled by the liver and hormones. Insulin, thyroxine, and growth hormone stimulate protein synthesis.

Anabolism

A small reservoir of amino acids, which is called the *amino acid metabolic pool,* is available for anabolism and to maintain the dynamic state of equilibrium. This metabolic pool, containing approximately 70 g of amino acids, is less than what most Americans consume in a day and could hardly be classified as a large storage of protein. Increasing muscle size is considered an increase in body mass, not protein storage. High-protein diets are neither safe nor effective as a means to increase muscle mass without physical activity or exercise to promote muscle development. To maintain a satisfactory protein status, a daily supply of essential amino acids obtained from the diet is necessary.

Anabolism depends on the presence of all essential amino acids simultaneously. It is not a stepwise process in which the synthesis of a protein can be started at one point and completed when the needed amino acid appears later.

Protein synthesis is also affected by caloric intake. If caloric intake is inadequate, tissue proteins are used for energy, resulting in increased nitrogen excretion. This process requires the B vitamin pyridoxine.

Catabolism

Amino acids are catabolized principally in the liver, but metabolism also occurs to some extent in the kidneys and muscles. Removal of the nitrogen grouping from amino acids, a process requiring the B vitamins pyridoxine and riboflavin, yields carbon skeletons and ammonia. The carbon skeletons can be (a) used to make nonessential amino acids, (b) used to produce energy via the Krebs cycle, or (c) converted to fats and stored as fatty tissue. Not all ingested protein is used to build muscle.

When amino acids are not needed for protein anabolism and energy is not needed, they are converted to fat and stored in the body. If caloric intake is inadequate, proteins are used for energy rather than to build or repair lean body mass or produce essential protein-based compounds.

Urea is the major waste product of protein catabolism. Ammonia is a toxic substance the liver converts to urea to be excreted by the kidneys. The levels of urea and ammonia vary directly with dietary protein levels.

Lipid Metabolism

Hormones involved in carbohydrate metabolism also control fat metabolism. Insulin increases fat synthesis, whereas thyroxine, epinephrine, growth hormone, and glucocorticoids increase fat mobilization. The liver is the principal regulator of fat metabolism and lipoprotein synthesis. Fatty acids can be hydrolyzed or modified by shortening, lengthening, or adding double bonds before their release from the liver into the circulation. The liver produces cholesterol, removes it from the blood, and uses it to make bile acid.

Metabolism of chylomicrons in the liver results in triglycerides being transported to the tissues for energy or other uses or carried to adipose tissue to be stored. Serum triglycerides are the result of not only absorption from foods but also the conversion of carbohydrates and proteins into fats. Triglycerides can be synthesized in the intestinal mucosa, adipose tissue, and liver. Fats are synthesized in the process of lipogenesis and broken down during **lipolysis** (the splitting or decomposition of fat). These continual processes are in equilibrium when energy needs are balanced.

The process of hydrolyzing triglycerides into two-carbon entities to enter the Krebs cycle for energy production is known as oxidation. A discussion of oxidation can be found in Chapter 2 and online at Evolve. During oxidation, 1 lb of fat results in the release of 3500 cal for energy—more than most individuals use in a 24-hour period. When excessive amounts of fats are oxidized for energy, the liver is overwhelmed, and acidic metabolic products, or ketones, are formed. Ketones are not oxidized in the liver but rather are carried to the skeletal and cardiac muscles, where, under normal circumstances, they are rapidly metabolized.

If the glucose supply is reduced, the capacity of the tissues to use ketone bodies may be exceeded. Accumulation of ketone bodies is known as **ketosis**. Ketosis may lead to ketoacidosis (acidic condition due to accumulation of large quantities of ketone bodies in the blood). The signs and symptoms of ketoacidosis include nausea, vomiting, and stomach pain. Ketoacidosis can be a dangerous condition for several reasons. Bases must neutralize these strong acids (ketones) to maintain acid–base balance in the blood. Ketones are excreted in the urine, a condition known as **ketonuria**, along with sodium. If adequate amounts of base are not available, acidosis may result. In addition to the loss of sodium ions, large amounts of water are lost, which can lead to dehydration (or rapid weight loss for an individual reducing caloric intake). When blood glucose levels remain low for several days, brain and nerve cells adapt to use ketones for some of their fuel requirements.

Carbohydrates play a predominant role in heavy exercise when the muscle's oxygen supply is limited, but triglycerides provide about half the energy with continued exercise. Although fats can be stored as adipose tissue in virtually inexhaustible amounts, their slower rate of metabolism makes them a less efficient source of quick energy. The amount of energy available is highly variable in individuals, but usually at least 160,000 cal are available from body fat stores.

Alcohol Metabolism

Although alcohol is considered a drug, the calories it provides can be used by the body for energy, providing approximately

7 cal/g. When consumed in excessive amounts, alcohol is a toxin. Caloric content of alcoholic beverages can be calculated by using the equations in Box 7.1. Alcoholic beverages contain negligible nutrients.

Alcohol is metabolized primarily by the liver. Alcohol provides an alternative fuel that is oxidized instead of fat; this may result in accumulation of lipids in the liver. Not much is known about safe amounts of alcohol consumption without risk of liver damage.

A well-balanced diet accompanied by habitual consumption of alcoholic beverages in excess of energy needs can be a risk factor for weight gain. However, excessive amounts of alcohol in a person who is an alcoholic tend to result in poor appetite for food and may lead to weight loss and malnutrition. In addition to causing liver damage, alcohol can interfere with the transport, activation, catabolism, and storage of almost every nutrient. There may be protective effects of moderate alcohol consumption on cardiovascular events; however, heavy use has a marked effect.[4]

The *Dietary Guidelines* advise moderation in alcohol consumption: one drink a day for women and no more than two drinks a day for men. (An alcoholic beverage is defined as 12 oz of regular beer, 5 oz of wine, or 1.5 oz of 80-proof distilled spirits.) Alcoholic beverages should be avoided by women who may become pregnant, are pregnant, or breastfeeding.

Metabolic Interrelationships

The body is an overwhelmingly complex system. Whether excessive food intake is in the form of protein, carbohydrate, fat, or alcohol, most excess energy intake is stored as adipose tissue (Fig. 7.3). Glycogen is another storage form of energy; however, the amount of glycogen stored in the body is limited.

Protein from the metabolic pool of amino acids and in lean muscle mass is generally not considered a good source of energy, but it can be used for energy if caloric intake is below caloric expenditure. Fat is a good source of energy, but carbohydrate is the preferred fuel. However, the body cannot metabolize excessive quantities of fat without some side effects—ketoacidosis, hyperlipidemia, and accumulation of fat in the liver.

Carbohydrates can be used in forming nonessential amino acids. Proteins contribute to synthesis of some lipids (e.g., lipoproteins). Although lipids do not contribute significantly to the synthesis of amino acids, glycerol from triglycerides can be used for synthesis of carbohydrates. Fatty acids and some amino acids can be converted to glucose.

Catabolism of all classes of foodstuffs involves oxidation through the TCA cycle to produce energy. The quantity of calories in the diet from carbohydrate or lipids influences protein metabolism. In some situations, one nutrient can be substituted for another because of their interrelationship. For example, a decrease in carbohydrate intake increases lipolysis; protein excess can be used for energy. Because the body can easily adapt to shifts in either carbohydrate or fat as the main source of energy and in view of substantial body fat stores, large variations in macronutrient intake (energy sources) and energy expenditure are well tolerated.

In addition to energy-providing nutrients, vitamins and minerals are essential for digestion, absorption, and metabolism of carbohydrate, protein, and fat. Although vitamins and minerals are not required in the large quantities that macronutrients are, their presence is just as important. When a deficiency occurs, reactions do not proceed normally. For example, although protein may be consumed alone (as in liquid protein supplements), many other nutrients, including vitamins and minerals, must be present for the protein to be used by cells. Each nutrient has its specific function; all nutrients must be present simultaneously for optimal benefits.

A detailed discussion of metabolic interrelationships is beyond the scope of this text. These interrelationships are important, and for optimal use of nutrients, food sources of all the nutrients should be consumed. The easiest way to obtain optimal nutrition is to include a variety of foods from all the food groups.

• BOX 7.1 Calculation of Energy Value of Alcoholic Beverages

The equation for determining energy (caloric) value of liquors is as follows:

Ounces of beverage × proof × 0.8 cal/proof/1 oz

Example: 1.5 oz × 86 proof × 0.8 cal/proof/1 oz = 103.2 cal

The equation for determining energy (caloric) value of beer and wines is as follows:

Ounces of beverage × % of alcohol × 1.6

Example: 12 oz × 5% × 1.6 = 96 cal

Reproduced with permission from Gastineau CF. Nutrition note: alcohol and calories. Mayo Clin Proc. *1976;51(2):88.*

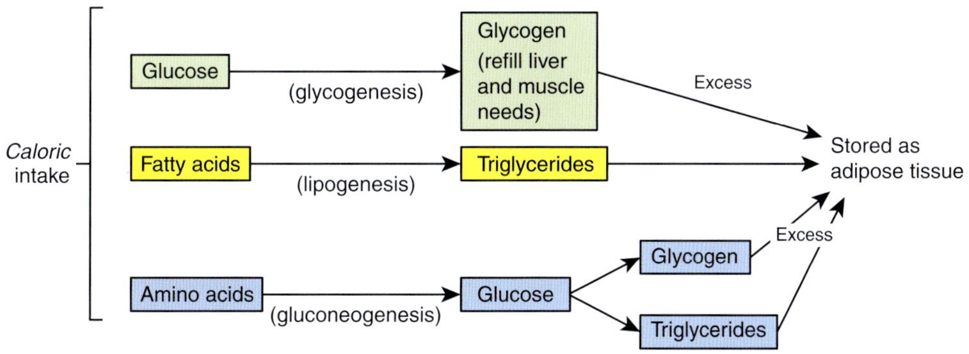

• Figure 7.3 Metabolic pathways of excess energy. (Modified from Nix S. *Williams' Basic Nutrition and Diet Therapy*. 15th ed. St Louis, MO: Mosby Elsevier; 2017.)

DENTAL CONSIDERATIONS

- Glycogen stores are depleted with a carbohydrate-poor diet even when high levels of fat and protein are eaten. A patient who ingests a carbohydrate-poor diet has decreased energy reserves and is prone to prolonged healing periods and fatigue.
- Insulin deficiency can cause slow glycogenesis, low glycogen storage, decreased glucose catabolism and increased blood glucose.
- Blood glucose concentrations are increased only slightly when fructose, sorbitol, or xylitol is given because these sugars are absorbed more slowly; less insulin is required for their metabolism. Caution with portion size is still a consideration for individuals with diabetes.
- Patients with compromised liver or renal function may postpone progression of their condition by avoiding excessive amounts of protein.
- Ketoacidosis does not result from rapid breakdown of adipose tissue alone; severe curtailment of carbohydrate intake must occur simultaneously. Ensure that patients consume an adequate amount of carbohydrate.
- Ketoacidosis frequently occurs in patients with uncontrolled diabetes mellitus (see *Health Application 7*) or who are fasting (as a result of illness or weight reduction) because the body is burning fat rather than carbohydrate. Question patients with fruity-smelling breath about recent food and fluid intake, weight loss, and conditions such as diabetes mellitus.
- High ketone levels may be associated with starvation or high-protein, low-carbohydrate, low-calorie diets. These result in decreased appetite and occasionally nausea, which can worsen the condition.
- Symptoms of hypoglycemia include weakness or light-headedness; confusion; irritability; pale color; sweating; and rapid, shallow breathing. Or the patient may experience hypoglycemic unawareness, yet have low blood glucose levels.

NUTRITIONAL DIRECTIONS

- A diet high in protein without limiting total energy intake may convert excess protein to fat stores.
- Increasing protein intake does not necessarily (or may not) increase muscle tissue and may lead to dehydration.
- High-protein, low-carbohydrate diets have been promoted as an effective way of reducing calories by creating a state of ketoacidosis to lose weight. The amount of calories lost may be insignificant when considering the risk involved.
- The National Institute on Alcohol Abuse and Alcoholism defines binge drinking as 4 drinks for women and 5 drinks for men within 2 hours. The Substance Abuse and Mental Health Services Administration (SAMHSA) defines binge drinking as 5 or more alcoholic beverages on the same occasion on at least 1 day in the past 30 days. SAMHSA defines heavy drinking as 5 or more alcoholic beverages on the same occasion on each of 5 or more days in the past 30 days.[5]

Metabolic Energy

Without energy from chemical reactions, people could not bat an eye, wiggle a toe, or think a thought. Energy is required for all physiologic functions. Energy from food is converted into forms the body can use: electrical for the brain and nerves, mechanical for muscles, thermal for body heat, and chemical for synthesis of new compounds.

The potential energy value of foods and energy exchanges within the body are expressed in terms of the kilocalorie. A **kilocalorie (kcal)** is the amount of heat required to increase the temperature of 1 kg of water 1°C. A kilocalorie is 1000 times larger than the small calorie. Although kilocalorie is the proper term, it is commonly used interchangeably with calorie (cal) or Calorie (Cal).

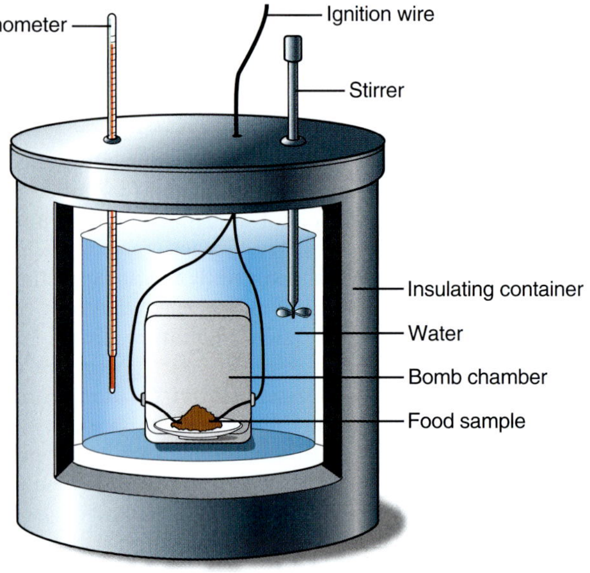

• **Figure 7.4** Cross section of a bomb calorimeter. To determine energy, a dried portion of food is burned inside a chamber charged with oxygen that is surrounded by water. As the food is burned, it gives off heat. The heat raises the temperature of the water surrounding the chamber. The increase in water temperature indicates the number of cal contained in the food. One cal equals the amount of heat needed to raise the temperature of 1 kg of water by 1°C. (Reproduced with permission from Grodner M, Escott-Stump S, Dorner S. *Nutritional Foundations and Clinical Applications. A Nursing Approach*. 6th ed. St. Louis, MO: Mosby Elsevier; 2016.)

Carbohydrate, fat, protein, and even alcohol provide energy for humans. Vitamins and minerals are not energy sources but are necessary for energy-producing reactions. Physiologic energy values commonly used are 4 cal/g carbohydrate, 9 cal/g fat, 4 cal/g protein, and 7 cal/g alcohol.

Measurement of Potential Energy

The amount of energy, or calories, available in a food may be precisely calculated by placing a weighed amount of food inside a device used to measure calories, called a **calorimeter** (Fig. 7.4). As a food is burned, an increase in water temperature indicates the heat given off or potential (free) energy of that food.

Energy Production

The metabolism of basic nutrients results in production of cellular energy, which is stored as adenosine triphosphate (ATP). ATP is an instant source of cellular energy for mechanical work, transport of nutrients and waste products, and synthesis of chemical compounds generated from the Krebs cycle. ATP units, also called **high-energy phosphate compounds**, are the currency, or "money," that the body uses for energy. Because ATP can be metabolized without oxygen, the reaction is classified as anaerobic. The body must always have a supply of ATP, and several systems ensure a constant supply in the body. A more detailed discussion of ATP can be found in Chapter 2 and online at Evolve.

Increasing caloric intake from carbohydrates and fats would not produce optimal energy without adequate protein intake. Energy use is remarkably sensitive to the quantity and the quality of dietary protein.

Basal Metabolic Rate

Even during sleep, the body requires energy for the basic minimum tasks of respiration and circulation and for many intricate activities within each cell. **Basal metabolic rate (BMR)** indicates energy required for involuntary physiologic functions to maintain life, including respiration, circulation, and maintenance of muscle tone and body temperature. The BMR is lowest while lying down, awake, rested, and relaxed in a comfortable environment, not having eaten for 12 to 15 hours. The BMR can be measured in a clinical setting using **indirect calorimetry**, which indirectly measures the rate of oxygen used while the person is resting. Because digestion and absorption require energy, the BMR is the amount of energy required when the body is in a **postabsorptive state** (digestion and absorption are minimal).

Factors Affecting the Basal Metabolic Rate

Various factors can increase or decrease the BMR, which determines energy needs.

Sleep

Metabolic rate is lowest after a few hours of sleep because muscles are more relaxed. Approximately 10% less energy is needed for the BMR during this relaxed state.

Age

From birth through age 2 years, growth results in the highest BMR, which then decreases until the puberty growth spurt and is followed by a gradual decline for the rest of the life cycle (Fig. 7.5).

Pregnancy and Lactation

During the last trimester of pregnancy, the BMR increases approximately 15% to 30%. The amount of energy necessary to produce milk for lactation can increase the BMR as much as 40%.

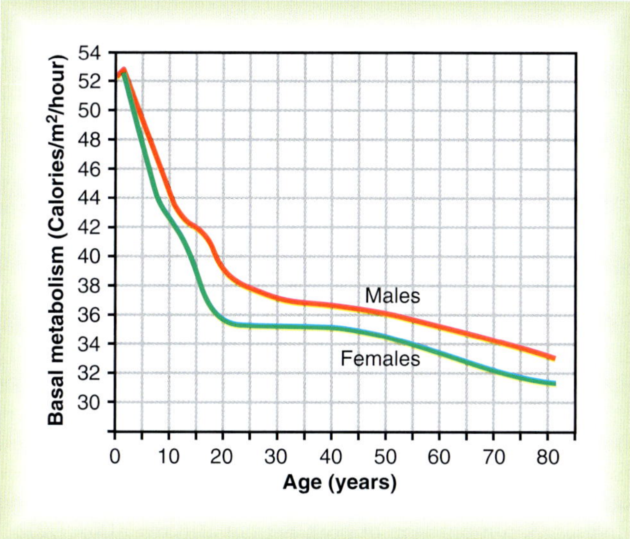

• **Figure 7.5** Normal basal metabolic rates at different ages for each sex. (Reproduced with permission from Guyton AC, Hall JE. *Textbook of Medical Physiology*. 13th ed. Philadelphia, PA: Elsevier; 2016.)

Surface Area and Size

The more body surface area, the greater the BMR. Because of greater surface area, a tall, thin person requires more energy than a short one of similar weight.

State of Health

Illnesses and diseases may increase or decrease the BMR. Patients recovering from a wasting illness require extra energy to build new tissue. Additionally, the activity level may be influenced by such conditions as lack of sleep, exhaustion, tenseness, fatigue, or depression.

Body Composition and Gender

In adults, lean body mass is the best single predictor of the BMR. Because cells in muscles and glands are more active than cells in bone and fat, body composition influences the BMR. The amount of muscle versus fat tissue in adults is a distinguishing factor; normally, women have more fat tissue and use fewer calories. Differences in the BMR may be primarily related to typical variations in body composition rather than directly related to gender.

Muscle tone is an important factor in metabolism; the state of tension or relaxation also has an effect. An athlete who has better muscle tone than a sedentary individual of similar size and shape requires more calories.

Endocrine Glands: Chemical Messengers

Thyroxine, the iodine-containing hormone secreted by the thyroid gland, has a greater influence on the rate of metabolic processes than secretions from any other gland.

Adrenal glands affect metabolism to a lesser degree. Stimulations by fright, excitement, or even joy can cause a temporary increase in the BMR by releasing **catecholamines**, particularly epinephrine. Catecholamines are obtained from tyrosine or phenylalanines. The pituitary gland accounts for about a 15% to 20% increase in the BMR during growth of children and adolescents.

Temperature

The BMR can be affected by body temperature or climate. The BMR is slightly higher in cooler climates to maintain normal body temperature. A fever will increase the BMR.

Fasting and Starvation

Individuals who are undernourished or fasting for long periods have a lower than normal BMR. This is a result of decreased muscle mass and an adaptive body process to conserve energy. Numerous studies indicate that the body responds to dieting the way it does to famine, by decreasing the BMR.

Total Energy Requirements

Basal energy expenditure includes calories necessary to maintain BMR plus additional calories needed for thermic effect, voluntary activities, and any increased needs from catabolic processes (e.g., disease states or fever) or anabolic processes (e.g., growth or pregnancy) for a 24-hour period. The **thermic effect** of food refers to increased energy expenditure resulting from the consumption of food or the number of calories needed for digestion.

BMR can be estimated using several methods based on a patient's age, gender, and body size. For most individuals, the BMR accounts for 65% to 70% of the body's total energy requirement. Calculations determining a patient's BMR are inexact, but many general guidelines have been formulated. One quick guideline for adults is as follows:

$$10 \times \text{ideal weight (lb)} = \text{calories needed for BMR daily}$$

Food digestion requires energy. The thermic effect of a mixed diet is estimated to be approximately 10% of the energy required for BMR. Many times, this factor is omitted in calculations determining total energy expenditure.

Voluntary Work and Play

The most variable factor affecting total energy needs is muscle activity, which is influenced by the physical activity level (Table 7.1). Mental activity uses almost no extra energy (approximately 3 to 4 cal per hour). Activity level normally accounts for 20% to 30% of the daily energy requirement.

The *Dietary Guidelines* and *MyPlate* guidelines address the need for regular physical activity. Along with these sources, the Physical Activities Guidelines from the U.S. Department of Health and Human Services recommends 2.5 hours per week of moderate intensity activities for substantial health benefits.[6] Not only does physical activity help with heart disease, weight control and physical strength, but reductions in mortality risks and blood pressure are observed with even small increaes in activity.[7,8] Leisure-time physical activity has been associated with lower risks of many types of cancer.[9] The exercise or activity should be one the individual enjoys to enhance the likelihood of consistent participation. Inactive individuals may need to gradually increase the duration and intensity of exercise.

Estimated Energy Requirements

The estimated energy requirements established by the National Academy of Medicine (formerly the Institute of Medicine) indicate the daily calorie intake needed to maintain energy balance in healthy individuals of a specific age, gender, weight, height, and level of physical activity (see p. ii). These levels are recommended to sustain body weights in the desired range for good health (body mass index [BMI] 18.5–25 kg/m^2), while maintaining a lifestyle with adequate levels of physical activity. A Recommended Dietary Allowance was not established because energy intakes greater than the estimated energy requirement could result in weight gain. Weight gain resulting in a BMI greater than 25 kg/m^2 is associated with an increased risk of early mortality. Numerous studies substantiate a morbidity risk of type 2 diabetes, hypertension, CVD, stroke, gallbladder disease, osteoarthritis, and some types of cancer for BMIs greater than 25 kg/m^2. The National Academy of Medicine suggests that at the end of adolescence, BMI should be around 22 kg/m^2 to allow for a moderate weight gain in midlife without exceeding the 25 kg/m^2 threshold.[10]

DENTAL CONSIDERATIONS

- Encourage intake of adequate amounts of the macronutrients and energy to spare protein for growth or healing, as needed. If energy is insufficient, healing is prolonged.
- Low-carbohydrate diets are not as effective in supporting high activity levels as a high intake of complex carbohydrates. For athletic patients, advise increased intake of complex carbohydrates.
- For healthy men, the BMR usually ranges from about 1580 to 1870 cal daily, whereas approximately 1150 to 1440 cal is needed for women. If energy intake is inadequate, physical status may deteriorate. A referral to a health care provider or registered dietitian nutritionist (RDN) is needed to improve nutrient intake.
- Increased thyroxine activity (hyperthyroidism) may double the BMR and can cause vitamin deficiencies because the quantity of many enzymes is increased. Unless physical activity is above average, the BMR represents the largest proportion of a patient's energy requirement. Determination of the BMR can be used to evaluate adequacy of caloric intake.
- Encourage inactive adults to engage in some leisure time physical activity and do not discourage adults who already participate in high activity levels.

NUTRITIONAL DIRECTIONS

- The BMR may be elevated or depressed. A high BMR requires more calories; fewer calories are needed for a low BMR.
- Because the BMR decreases about 2% every 10 years after age 25 years, many patients gain weight because previous eating habits are maintained without increasing activity.
- A naturally higher BMR is a reason why children and pregnant women do not feel as cold as adults under the same weather conditions. Do not overdress children based on an adult's perception.

Energy Balance

The proper energy balance for stable weight is maintained when caloric intake equals the amount of energy needed for body processes and physical activities (Fig. 7.6). Energy balance is maintained when the calorie intake equals the amount of energy needed for body processes and physical activities. This statement sounds simple, but very few Americans are able to maintain energy balance at an appropriate body weight. Many factors help create this unbalanced equation; because it is a complex system, there are no easy answers. The government recommendation is 1600 cal/day for women and 2200 cal/day for men. Dental professionals, in collaboration with dietetic professionals, can play a role in health promotion efforts to educate patients in the prevention and management of obesity.

Many healthy patients are able to control energy intake to balance energy output with little effort; their **appetite**, or desire to eat, controls food intake to balance energy expenditure. **Hunger**, or the physiologic drive to eat, is regulated by a complex network of factors (see Fig. 7.6). Appetite is frequently used in the same sense as hunger, but it usually implies desire for specific types of food and is related to the pleasurable sensation of eating.

Hunger and appetite greatly affect weight balance. When more calories are consumed than the body needs, the excess is stored as fat, resulting in weight gain. One pound of body fat is equivalent to 3500 cal. Overweight patients have a very difficult time losing extra pounds and maintaining their energy balance to keep off unwanted pounds. Weight control can be approached by either decreasing the number of calories consumed or increasing physical activities. A combination of both is most effective (Box 7.2).

Intake is generally regarded as the key to weight regulation. A patient's weight tends to remain stable for long periods with only a 1- to 5-lb gain or loss of adipose tissue over a year. Even small

TABLE 7.1 Energy Expenditure During Various Activities

Activity (1 Hour)	130 lb	155 lb	180 lb
Aerobics, general	384	457	531
Aerobics, low impact	295	352	409
Carpentry, general	207	246	286
Cleaning, dusting	148	176	204
Construction, exterior, remodeling	325	387	449
Cycling, 14 to 15.9 mph, vigorous bicycling	590	704	817
Cycling, <10 mph, leisure bicycling	236	281	327
Diving, springboard or platform	177	211	245
Downhill snow skiing, moderate	354	422	490
Downhill snow skiing, racing	472	563	654
Electrical work, plumbing	207	246	286
Fishing, general	177	211	245
Football or baseball, playing catch	148	176	204
Football, competitive	531	633	735
Football, touch, flag, general	472	563	654
Frisbee playing, general	177	211	245
Golf, walking and carrying clubs	266	317	368
Handball	708	844	981
Health club exercise	325	387	449
Hiking, cross country	354	422	490
Horseback riding	236	281	327
Housework, light	148	176	204
Judo, karate, jujitsu, martial arts	590	704	817
Marching, rapidly, military	384	457	531
Mowing lawn, walk, power mower	325	387	449
Painting	266	317	368
Polo	472	563	654
Pushing stroller, walking with children	148	176	204
Racquetball, playing	413	493	572
Raking lawn	254	303	351
Rowing machine, light	207	246	286
Rowing machine, vigorous	502	598	695
Running, 5 mph (12-minute mile)	472	563	654
Running 6 mph (9-minute mile)	590	704	817
Running, 7 mph (8.5-minute mile)	679	809	940
Walking 2.0 mph	177	211	245
Walking 3.0 mph, moderate	195	232	270
Walking 4.0 mph, very brisk	295	352	409

Adapted from NutriStrategy Software. Calories are calculated based on research data from *Medicine and Science in Sports and Exercise,* The Official Journal of the American College of Sports Medicine. Copyright © 2015 by NutriStrategy. http://www.nutristrategy.com/activitylist4.htm. Accessed December 14, 2016.

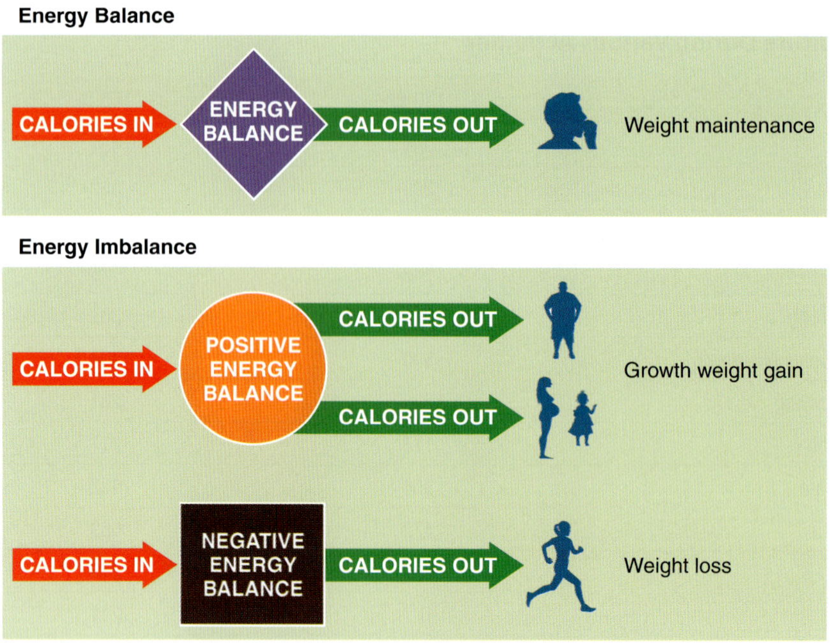

• **Figure 7.6** Factors affecting energy balance.

• BOX 7.2 Equation for Weight Loss

The total energy expenditure for a sedentary individual 67 inches tall who weighs 191 lb (BMI = 30) is 2235 cal.

For 1 lb weight loss per week, decrease caloric intake by 500 cal/day:

2235 − 500 = 1735 cal/day

The result of a 500-cal deficit in 1 week:

500 × 7 = 3500 cal

A calorie reduction combined with exercise to lose 2 lb/week can be accomplished by increasing caloric expenditure by 500 cal/day.

Cycling at a rate of 15 mph or running at a rate of 10 minutes/mile for 45 minutes = 525 cal:

525 × 7 = 3675 cal

This would result in a weight loss of 2 lb/week or 8 lb/month.

daily deviations can result in gradual yet significant fluctuations in fat stores. For instance, an additional 100 cal daily would result in a 10-lb weight gain over 1 year and a 100-lb gain over 10 years.

Physiologic Factors

The hypothalamus, located in the middle of the brain, is especially important in controlling hunger. A satiety center and a hunger (or feeding) center are present within the hypothalamus.

Stimulation of the hunger center causes insatiable hunger; damage to this area results in no desire for food. Stimulation of the satiety center results in complete satiety. If the satiety center of the hypothalamus is destroyed, the appetite becomes voracious, resulting in obesity. The feeding center stimulates the drive to eat, whereas the satiety center inhibits the feeding center.

Usually, the body discerns food characteristics such as sweetness and viscosity to gauge intake. The body may use this information to determine how much food is needed to meet its caloric requirements. High intensity sweeteners may reduce calorie intake short-term, but whether they are effective as a long-term weight management strategy is unknown.[11] Several mechanisms affect the amount eaten at a particular meal. Distention of the stomach results in inhibitory signals that suppress the feeding center, reducing the desire to eat. Cholecystokinin in response to fat in the duodenum has a strong direct effect on the feeding center, causing the person to cease eating. Food in the stomach and duodenum causes the secretion of glucagon and insulin, both of which suppress the feeding center.

The hypothalamus is also responsive to body temperature. Cold temperatures lead to increased food intake, resulting in a higher metabolic rate and more fat stores for insulation.

The relationship between exercise and food intake is unclear. Exercise has been reported to increase, decrease, or have no effect on appetite. These findings cannot be explained but may be related to the timing or duration of the exercise, individual metabolic differences, or some unknown reason. Generally, acute exercise decreases food intake after the activity, but regular exercise promotes increased energy intake.

Nutrient and hormonal signals affect the brain and liver to stimulate satiety and feeding centers (Table 7.2). Numerous studies have shown that physiologic control of energy intake is unreliable. Energy balance must be adjusted through some other mechanism.

Psychological Factors

Appetite is affected by the fact that eating is rewarding or pleasurable and makes us feel good. The eating behavior of obese individuals is thought to be influenced more by external cues—including time, taste, smell, and sight of food—than it is in individuals of normal weight. Greater weight usually means that the individual is responding to feelings and emotions rather than actual hunger. Boredom and stress are factors that frequently affect eating habits of obese individuals.

Energy Expenditure

Contrary to popular opinion, obese women have a similar or higher metabolic rate than thinner women. The effect of this is less weight

TABLE 7.2 Stimuli Affecting Food Intake

	FOOD INTAKE	
Signal	**Increased**	**Decreased**
Food odors	Pleasant	Repulsive
Taste	Desirable	Offensive
Climate (temperature)	Cold	Hot
Gastrointestinal	Hunger pains	Distention Cholecystokinin Glucagon
Glucose level	Low	High
Lipoprotein	High	Low
Nutrient stores	Decreased	Increased

Reproduced with permission from Davis JR, Sherer K. *Applied Nutrition and Diet Therapy for Nurses*, 2nd ed. Philadelphia, PA: Saunders; 1994.

gain for a given increase in caloric intake. Genetics may also play a role in the BMR. Some families have low metabolic rates, but not all individuals with a low BMR are obese.

Exercise tolerance of obese individuals is less than normal, but any activity uses more calories because of the amount of additional mass to be moved. Not all inactive patients are obese; thus, activity level does not seem to be a principal determinant in development of obesity. Because of differences in body composition (percentage of muscle and fat), the BMR affects energy expenditure for various activities. Weight loss resulting from a specific energy deficit is invariably smaller than expected. Conversely, overconsumption fails to produce weight gains anticipated. Adjustments in energy expenditure seem to be adaptive.

Because food is abundant in the United States and most Americans enjoy eating, increased physical activity is needed to balance energy intake. Walking is a physical activity that has been emphasized because it is inexpensive and convenient, and most individuals are physically able to walk, even if they initially need to walk at a slow rate. Numerous studies have shown that using a **pedometer** (a small meter worn at the waist that monitors the number of steps a person takes) results in a significant increase in the number of steps per week.[12-14] Usually, the goal is 10,000 steps a day, but individuals are encouraged to start at a comfortable pace and distance, gradually increasing intensity and distance.

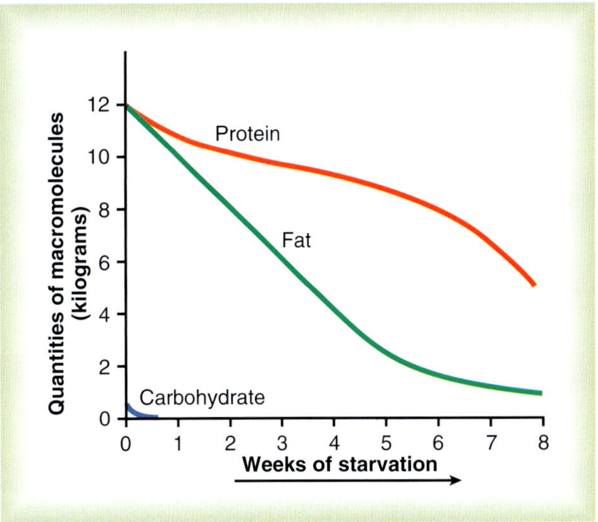

• **Figure 7.7** Effects of starvation on the body. Three major macromolecules serve as primary energy sources: carbohydrates, fats, and proteins. During starvation, the carbohydrate stores (glycogen) are rapidly depleted. However, stored lipids can mobilize and provide much of a person's energy needs for several weeks. Eventually, lipid stores run low and the body starts using proteins as a major source of energy, causing the breakdown of muscle and other protein-rich tissues. Muscle damage during starvation usually leads to death. (Reproduced with permission from Guyton AC, Hall JE. *Textbook of Medical Physiology*. 13th ed. Philadelphia, PA: Elsevier; 2016.)

Inadequate Energy Intake

A deficiency in energy intake may result in a depressed rate of growth in children and weight loss in adults. Intentional weight loss may be helpful or harmful, depending on the methods used for losing weight. Decreased fat stores are normally the goal, but loss of muscle may be an undesirable side effect (Fig. 7.7).

Inadequate energy intake may result in malnutrition and become a serious problem in the face of a physiologically stressful situation. Inadequate intake may be intentional, as in the case of anorexia nervosa (discussed in Chapter 17), a psychological disorder in which undernourishment is not perceived by the individual. Inadequate intake causes a vicious downward spiral in which metabolic imbalances decrease hunger and may become life-threatening without proper treatment.

DENTAL CONSIDERATIONS

- Observe emotional factors. Depression and stress as well as other emotional factors result in overeating and decreased activity in some patients. Referral to a health care provider may be indicated.
- A positive energy balance is desirable during periods of growth; a proportionately larger amount of energy is needed by pregnant and lactating women, and by children.
- Be aware of the complexities of maintaining energy balance and be understanding of patients who have problems managing their weight.
- When nutrient stores decrease, the feeding center of the hypothalamus becomes active, and the patient becomes hungry. When nutrient stores are abundant, the patient feels satiated and loses the desire to eat. If the hypothalamus is injured in any way (as in a head injury or stroke), hunger and satiety may be altered.
- If calories are underestimated, the body must use stored energy (fat and protein), putting the patient at risk for malnutrition. If excessive calories are consumed, the body converts excess calories to fat.
- A patient with a BMI between 18.5 kg/m^2 and 25 kg/m^2 has approximately 13 to 44 lb of body fat, which could provide 50,000 to 200,000 cal.
- It is acceptable for the dental professional to promote healthy weight loss behaviors and strategies. It is out of the scope of practice for the dental hygienist to assess and counsel patients on weight loss. Refer patients to an RDN.

NUTRITIONAL DIRECTIONS

- Exercise may enhance the BMR by increasing the amount of lean body mass, which uses more energy than fat.
- To gain 1 lb of fat, a patient must consume 3500 cal more than are used.
- To lose 1 lb of weight, energy intake must be 3500 cal less than the number of calories used.
- A decrease from prior activity level or additional caloric intake may result in weight gain.
- Large variations from energy balance are well tolerated but may be reflected in gains or losses of fat.
- Although quitting smoking is linked to an increased risk of weight gain, encourage patients who smoke to enroll in a smoking cessation program along with a weight-loss program. Remind the patient that the benefits of not smoking outweigh the potential risk factors of weight gain associated with quitting smoking (see *Health Application 19* in Chapter 19).

HEALTH APPLICATION 7

Diabetes Mellitus

Diabetes mellitus is a heterogeneous group of metabolic abnormalities in which carbohydrates, proteins, fats, and insulin are ineffectively metabolized, leading to disturbances in fluid and electrolyte balances (Fig. 7.8). It is a chronic, lifelong disease. Diabetes mellitus is specifically related to hormonal pancreatic secretions but involves the entire endocrine system.

Diabetes mellitus is presently one of the most common disorders, with rates increasing at an alarming pace, especially in children and adolescents. African Americans, Hispanic Americans, and Native Americans have the highest incidence of diabetes mellitus of all cultural population groups. In addition to metabolic complications secondary to diabetes mellitus, life expectancy is approximately 70% to 80% that of the general population. The Centers for Disease Control and Prevention estimates that more than 21 million individuals in the United States have diabetes mellitus, 86 million have prediabetes, and an additional 8.1 million have diabetes but are not aware of it.[15] Type 2 diabetes mellitus (T2DM) can be prevented or delayed by changes in lifestyles by high-risk individuals. Exercise improves the body's sensitivity to insulin and helps the body metabolize glucose better, preventing development of diabetes in individuals who are at high risk.

The two most prevalent types of diabetes mellitus are characterized by different metabolic defects and can appear to be very different conditions (Table 7.3). Type 1 diabetes mellitus (T1DM), which affects 5% to 10% of individuals with the disease, is distinguished by little or no endogenous insulin production and autoimmune β-cell destruction. Diagnostic values can be found in Table 7.4. This condition most commonly manifests in young people but can occur at any age. T1DM was formerly known as juvenile or insulin-dependent diabetes; the name was changed because adults also develop type 1 diabetes and those with T2DM can be on insulin. Onset is sudden, with all the clinical symptoms associated with this condition. Patients are prone to ketosis and must receive exogenous insulin for life.

Approximately 90% to 95% of Americans with diabetes have T2DM, which results from insulin resistance, usually with a relative insulin deficiency. Family history, age, history of gestational diabetes, obesity (BMI > 27 kg/m^2), and sedentary lifestyle are risk factors associated with diabetes. For obese patients, increased fat stores cause some degree of insulin resistance. In many cases, insulin is secreted in adequate or higher-than-normal amounts, but glucose uptake by body cells (except for the brain) is decreased.

Abnormalities in insulin levels precipitate clinical manifestations. Insulin deficiency or defects in insulin action or both result in hyperglycemia, the main manifestation of T2DM. Diagnostic values can be found in Table 7.4. Symptoms of hyperglycemia include thirst, frequent urination, hunger, blurry vision, fatigue, frequent infections, and dry, itchy skin; or the patient can be asymptomatic.

Prediabetes occurs when blood glucose levels are higher than normal, but not yet high enough to be diagnosed as diabetes. Comparison of diagnostic values can be found in Table 7.4. It is also known as impaired glucose tolerance or impaired fasting glucose, depending on the test used when it was detected. Those individuals with prediabetes are at risk of the long-term complications associated with T2DM. Changes to lifestyle behaviors, such as weight reduction, watching portion sizes, and exercise, can return blood glucose levels to normal ranges.

Treatment should be implemented as soon as possible after diagnosis to prevent complications of metabolic alterations secondary to diabetes mellitus. Elevated blood glucose levels can damage almost every major organ of the body. Early, tight control of diabetes can postpone and minimize many of these severe complications. Chronic complications develop slowly over long periods as body tissues are adversely exposed to hyperglycemia and hypoglycemia. Hyperglycemia in T2DM causes macrovascular and microvascular disease (involving large and small vessels) and can damage almost every major organ of the body. Patients with uncontrolled diabetes experience slow wound healing, frequent abscesses, periodontal disease, a predisposition to bacterial infections, a compromised immune system, skin irritations, pruritus (itching), numbness and tingling of the extremities, and visual disturbances. The American Diabetes Association defines uncontrolled blood glucose levels as three consecutive readings of 200 mg/dL or greater and/or an A_{1C} of 9% or greater.[16] Because of the increased risks of hyperglycemia in the oral cavity, the patient may need to be rescheduled for dental visits when the patient's blood glucose levels are in a safe range (70 to 200 mg/dL).

Obtaining a blood glucose level using a glucose monitoring system (a personal meter used to monitor capillary blood glucose levels) provides a day-to-day, minute-to-minute reading. It is a "snapshot" of the blood glucose level at the time it is taken. This is valuable information to obtain prior to a dental procedure because blood glucose levels can vary throughout the day. It is measured in milligrams per deciliter (mg/dL) or millimoles per liter (mmol/L). For patients not diagnosed with diabetes but with multiple risk factors, the American Diabetes Association suggests that screening be carried out in a health care setting. However, further research is needed to investigate the feasibility and effectiveness of screening in a dental environment.[16]

Another valuable reading is the glycosylated hemoglobin (A_{1C}) assay, a widely accepted and reliable measure of a blood glucose level over the past 3 months. It provides a guide for long-term planning and possible adjustments to diabetes treatment. However, hemoglobin A_{1C} does not show the ups and downs in a given day, just a 3-month average level. This reading helps evaluate metabolic control and determines whether the target range is maintained.[16]

Changes in capillary membranes can occur with uncontrolled blood glucose levels and result in renal complications (leading to **renal failure**, the inability of kidneys to excrete toxic waste materials), obstruction of circulation in the extremities (leading to gangrene), and progressive blood vessel damage in the retina of the eye (leading to blindness). Neuropathy, or deterioration of nervous tissue, also is frequently seen in patients with diabetes mellitus. Abnormalities of the gastrointestinal tract causing nausea, early satiety, and frequent vomiting interfere with food intake and absorption.

Hypoglycemia, or low blood glucose levels (< 70 mg/dL) can occur when a patient is taking insulin or an antidiabetic medication whose side effect is hypoglycemia. Symptoms include rapid heartbeat, hunger, shakiness, blurry

HEALTH APPLICATION 7

Diabetes Mellitus—cont'd

vision, sweating, fatigue, dizziness, and irritability. However, the patient may be unaware of these symptoms (hypoglycemia unawareness); as a precautionary measure, obtain blood glucose readings before treatment to prevent a medical emergency. A patient whose blood glucose level is less than 70 mg/dL should be treated with 10 to 15 g of a carbohydrate source, such as 3 glucose tablets, 1 tube of glucose gel, 8 hard candies (disk), 4 oz of regular soda, or 4 oz of fruit juice. Wait 15 minutes and retest. If the blood glucose level is still less than 70 mg/dL or symptoms remain, repeat. When the blood glucose level is greater than 70 mg/dL, continue with treatment, and offer a meal or snack within 30 minutes. If the patient is experiencing severe hypoglycemia (e.g., being uncooperative, unable to take fluids, or unconscious), administer glucagon to bring the blood glucose value into an appropriate range. Call the community emergency medical services for assistance.

Medical nutrition therapy is the cornerstone for preventing hyperglycemia and hypoglycemia and decreasing chronic complications. No single dietary plan can be appropriate for all individuals with different personalities and lifestyles. The objective of a meal plan is to empower patients to maintain good control of their diabetes or to promote near-normal blood glucose, lipid, and blood pressure levels. Additionally, food choices should promote overall health by providing optimal nutrition and allowing physical activity; achieving or maintaining an ideal body weight; and preventing or delaying development or progression of periodontal disease, cardiovascular, renal, retinal, neurologic, and other complications associated with diabetes, insofar as these are related to metabolic control. The meal plan should be flexible to allow personal and cultural preferences and lifestyles, while respecting the individual's wishes and willingness to make changes. Table 7.5 list some of the specific nutrition recommendations by the American Diabetes Association.

Not only are food choices important to the diabetes meal pattern, but spacing of meals and portion sizes are important concepts to also consider. Carbohydrate consumption during the day should be spaced to every 4 to 5 hours, allowing for addition of nutrient-dense snacks throughout the day. The use of food scales plus measuring cups and spoons will help with portion size. Dental professionals need to understand and respect the role nutrition plays in diabetes in order to support the patient's efforts and emphasize healthful eating patterns.

Carbohydrate counting, consistent with the *Dietary Guidelines* and *MyPlate,* focuses on total carbohydrate consumption. Because carbohydrate is the major factor in blood glucose fluctuations, the given amount of carbohydrate affects insulin requirements more than the protein and fat content.

For individuals with a healthy weight and normal lipid profile, the American Diabetes Association recommends the same guidelines as advocated by the National Cholesterol Education Program, discussed in Chapter 6. Because many patients with diabetes have undesirable lipid levels, a moderate increase in monounsaturated fat with a moderate intake of carbohydrate is recommended.

Certified Diabetes Educator

All individuals with diabetes or at risk of diabetes should be referred to a certified diabetes educator (CDE) for education. A CDE is the diabetes expert. As defined by the credentialing organization, the National Certification Board for Diabetes Educators, a CDE is "a health professional who possesses comprehensive knowledge of and experience in prediabetes, diabetes prevention, and management. The CDE educates and supports people affected by diabetes to understand and manage the condition. A CDE promotes self-management to achieve individualized behavioral and treatment goals that optimize health outcomes."[17] Physicians, nurses, pharmacists, and dietitians are examples of health professionals who are invited to complete the rigorous requirements needed to become a diabetes expert. In 2014, the National Certification Board for Diabetes Educators expanded the opportunity to dental professionals with a minimum of a master's degree in a health-related area of study. Dental professionals can now equally and thoughtfully join other health care colleagues in the pursuit of an improved quality of life for dental patients with diabetes.

TABLE 7.3 Comparison of Type 1 and Type 2 Diabetes Mellitus

	Type 1	Type 2
Prevalence	Approximately 5% to 10% of cases	90% to 95% of cases (1 in 5 adults > 65 years old)
Age at onset	Most frequently during childhood or puberty, but may occur at later ages	Frequently > 40 years, but occurring more frequently in overweight children and adolescents
Precipitating cause	Genetic, autoimmune destruction of the pancreatic cells that produce insulin	Obesity and inactivity
Type of onset	Sudden, but may develop slowly in adults	Usually gradual; may go undetected for years
Family history of diabetes	Frequently positive	Usually positive
Nutritional status at time of onset	Normal weight with recent weight loss, but occasionally obese	Usually overweight (BMI > 25) with increased percentage of body fat predominantly in the abdominal region
Symptoms	Polydipsia, polyphagia, ketoacidosis, weight loss	Glycosuria without ketonuria; absent or mild polyuria and polydipsia
Blood glucose stability	Fluctuates widely in response to changes in insulin, diet, exercise, infection, and stress	Fluctuations less marked
Control of diabetes	Difficult	Easy, especially if diet is followed

Continued

TABLE 7.3 Comparison of Type 1 and Type 2 Diabetes Mellitus—cont'd

	Type 1	Type 2
Ketosis	Frequent	Seldom
Plasma insulin	Negligible or absent	May be low (not absent) or high, with insulin resistance
Vascular complications and degenerative changes	Occurs after diabetes is present for approximately 5 years	Increased risk of macrovascular and microvascular complications
Medical nutrition therapy	Required	May eliminate need for hypoglycemic agents or insulin or both
Medication	Insulin required for all	Usually can be controlled with hypoglycemic agents; insulin may be necessary for some

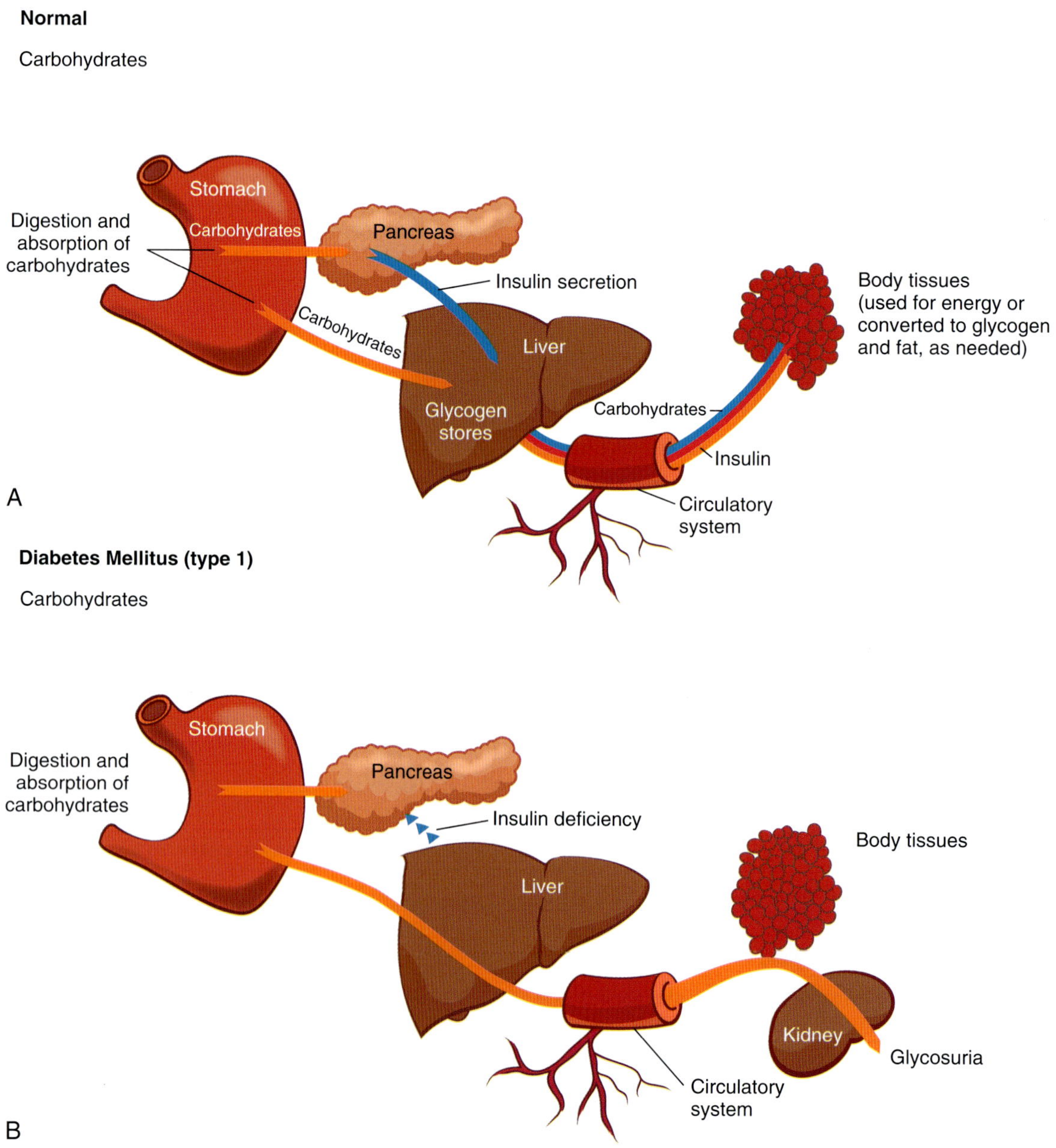

• **Figure 7.8** Comparison of carbohydrate use in patients without diabetes (A) and patients with diabetes (B). (Adapted from *What Is diabetes?* Indianapolis, IN: Eli Lilly & Co.; 1973.)

TABLE 7.4 American Diabetes Association Comparison of Diagnostic Values

Result	Fasting Plasma Glucose	2-hour Plasma Glucose	A_{1c}
Normal	< 100 mg/dl	< 140 mg/dl	< 5.7%
Prediabetes	100–125 mg/dl	140–199 mg/dl	5.7%–6.4%
Diabetes	126 mg/dl or higher	200 mg/dl or higher	6.5% or higher

Data From Diabetes is diagnosed based on the plasma glucose levels. American Diabetes Association. Classification and diagnosis of diabetes. Sec. 2 In Standards of Medical Care in Diabetes—2017. Diabetes Care 40(suppl. 1):S11–S24, 2017.

TABLE 7.5 American Diabetes Association Medical Nutrition Therapy Recommendations

A to C, E Rating[a]	Recommendation
Effectiveness of Nutrition Therapy	
A	An individualized nutrition program, preferably provided by a registered dietitian, is recommended for all people with T1DM or T2DM.
Energy Balance	
A	Modest weight loss achievable by the combination of lifestyle modification and the reduction of energy intake benefits overweight or obese adults with T2DM as well as those at risk for diabetes. Intervention programs to facilitate this process are recommended.
Protein	
A	
B	In individuals with T2DM, ingested protein appears to increase insulin response without increasing plasma glucose concentrations. Therefore, carbohydrate sources high in protein should not be used to treat or prevent hypoglycemia.
Dietary Fat	
B	Whereas data on the ideal total dietary fat content for people with diabetes are inconclusive, an eating plan emphasizing elements of a Mediterranean-style diet rich in monounsaturated fats may improve glucose metabolism and lower cardiovascular disease risk and can be an effective alternative to a diet low in total fat but relatively high in carbohydrates.
Eating Patterns and Macronutrient Distribution	
E	As there is no single ideal dietary distribution of calories among carbohydrates, fats, and proteins for people with diabetes, macronutrient distribution should be individualized while keeping total calorie and metabolic goals in mind.
B	Carbohydrate intake from whole grains, vegetables, fruits, legumes, and dairy products, with an emphasis on foods higher in fiber and lower in glycemic load, should be advised over other sources, especially those containing sugars.
B, A	People with diabetes and those at risk should avoid sugar-sweetened beverages in order to control weight and reduce their risk for cardiovascular disease and fatty liver **(B)** and should minimize the consumption of sucrose-containing foods that have the capacity to displace healthier, more nutrient-dense food choices **(A).**
Micronutrients and Herbal Supplements	
C	There is no clear evidence that dietary supplementation with vitamins, minerals, herbs, or spices can improve diabetes, and there may be safety concerns regarding the long-term use of antioxidant supplements.
Alcohol	
C	Adults with diabetes who drink alcohol should do so in moderation (no more than one drink/day for adult women and no more than two drinks/day for adult men).
B	Alcohol consumption may place people with diabetes at increased risk for delayed hypoglycemia, especially if taking insulin or diabetes medications in which hypoglycemia is a side effect. Education and awareness regarding the recognition and management of delayed hypoglycemia are warranted.
Sodium	
B	As for the general population, people with diabetes should limit sodium consumption to <2300 mg/day, although further restriction may be indicated for those with both diabetes and hypertension.
Nonnutritive Sweeteners	
B	The use of nonnutritive sweeteners has the potential to reduce overall calorie and carbohydrate intake if substituted for caloric sweeteners and without compensation by intake of additional calories from other food sources. Nonnutritive sweeteners are generally safe to use within the defined acceptable daily intake levels.

[a]ABC rating—evidence based on research criteria: **A**, strong supporting evidence; **B**, some supporting evidence; **C**, limited supporting evidence; **E**, based on expert consensus.
Data from American Diabetes Association. Standards of Medical Care in Diabetes—2017. *Diabetes Care* 2017;40(Suppl 1):S33–S43.

◆ CASE APPLICATION FOR THE DENTAL HYGIENIST

On a routine recare appointment, Ronnie, who is 10 years old, reports that he was diagnosed with type 2 diabetes about a year ago. He appears to be about 100 lb overweight. After talking with him, you learn that he does not want to be labeled as "different" from his friends, so he eats when and what they eat. Typically, they eat cheeseburgers, pizza, french fries, shakes, and regular sodas throughout the day. He says he does not have time to eat breakfast. He does not floss his teeth, has numerous caries, and has bleeding on probing.

Nutritional Assessment

- Observe height, weight, BMI, and age
- Knowledge of diabetes guidelines
- Motivation level
- Food/nutrient intake
- Eating habits
- Support from family and friends
- Activity level

Nutritional Diagnosis

Altered nutrition: Body requirements less than calorie intake in relation to energy expenditure.

Nutritional Goals

The patient will have gradual weight loss until a BMI for age is below the 85th percentile.

Nutritional Implementation

Intervention: Give Ronnie and his parents the name of preferably a CDE or an RDN who can provide necessary nutritional counseling.

Rationale: Well-balanced food choices that naturally contain a large amount of vitamins and minerals, rather than high-calorie foods, are needed to maintain his health and promote growth. The knowledge of nutrition and expertise of an RDN or CDE in counseling is recommended to provide adequate nutrients safely and effectively without affecting his linear growth.

Intervention: Explain that some of his food choices are not good for his overall physical or oral health.

Rationale: Consuming too many carbohydrates at meals and snacks affects his blood glucose level and increases the risk of caries.

Intervention: Explain that carbohydrates, proteins, and fats all provide calories, but fats are the most concentrated source of energy.

Rationale: To maintain his weight while still growing, wise food choices are advisable. Foods high in fat and sugar will not help him in his attempts to look handsome and may worsen his diabetes status.

Intervention: Stress the importance of consuming complex carbohydrate and fiber, and reducing intake of fat and calories.

Rationale: Complex carbohydrate and fiber intake is effective in helping maintain a lower caloric intake without excessive hunger. Fat reduction enhances weight maintenance because a lower fat intake may help reduce energy intake and decrease risk of developing heart disease.

Intervention: Discuss the benefits of eating at routine times.

Rationale: This is important for control of his diabetes and may allow him time to brush his teeth after eating, reducing his risk of caries.

Intervention: Discuss the importance of a plan incorporating diet, exercise, and behavior modification.

Rationale: This combination of therapies has proven more effective for long-term weight control.

Intervention: Explain that good oral hygiene is very important for patients with diabetes because of an exaggerated response to plaque bacteria.

Rationale: Knowledge may help increase compliance.

Intervention: Suggest becoming involved in some sports, increasing his activity level by walking to friends' homes, or participating in some recreational activity, such as skating.

Rationale: Weight and diabetes control is improved when energy expenditure is increased along with decreased caloric intake. Additionally, physical activity helps increase muscle mass and improves strength.

Evaluation

The patient consulted with the RDN and did not gain any weight before the next recall visit. Also, no new caries developed.

◆ Student Readiness

1. Define the terms *energy*, *thermogenic effect*, *basal metabolism*, and *basal energy expenditure*.
2. Calculate your total caloric needs for 1 day (BMR plus estimated voluntary energy expenditures plus thermogenic effect).
3. Assuming that height and weight are the same, is the BMR higher or lower in:
   A man or a woman?
   An athlete or a sedentary person?
   A 40-year-old or a 20-year-old?
   A woman who is not pregnant or a woman who is pregnant?
4. How many calories of protein, fat, and carbohydrate are in 1 cup of homogenized milk that contains 8.5 g of protein, 8.5 g of fat, and 12 g of carbohydrate?
5. A boxer achieved a dramatic weight loss of about 18 kg (39.6 lb) in approximately 60 days. A strict diet, heavy exercise, thyroid supplements, and a diuretic drug produced significant weight loss. His defeat in a boxing match shocked some of his fans. What happened to his physical condition? Explain.

◆ CASE STUDY

Jay G. is a 16-year-old high school athlete on the football and baseball teams. He recently developed three dental caries. His classmates have encouraged him to eat a high-protein, low-carbohydrate diet. His mother is concerned about this and talks to her best friend, who is a dental hygienist.

1. What points do you think the dental hygienist should mention to this mother?
2. For increased energy expenditure, what should be the primary source of nutrients?
3. Would decreasing dietary carbohydrate content have a positive effect on the rate of dental caries?
4. What is the effect of high-protein intake?
5. On a high-protein, low-carbohydrate diet (approximately 120 g of protein, 80 g of carbohydrate, 2800 cal), where would most of his energy requirements come from? Is this good or bad?
6. Which vitamins are important in the production of energy?
7. Is the diet varied? Does the diet provide recommended amounts of fruits, vegetables, grains, and other nutrients?

References

1. American Diabetes Association. Standards of Medical Care in Diabetes—2017. *Diabetes Care*. 2017;40(suppl 1):S11–S24.
2. Academy of Nutrition and Dietetics. Nutrition Care Manual. Glycemic index. https://www.nutritioncaremanual.org/topic.cfm?ncm_toc_id=272751. Accessed December 20, 2016.
3. Raynor HA, Champagne CM. Position of the Academy of Nutrition and Dietetics. Interventions for the treatment of overweight and obesity in adults. *J Acad Nutr Diet*. 2016;116(1):129–147.
4. Mostofsky E, Chahal HS, Mukamal KJ, et al. Alcohol and immediate risk of cardiovascular events. A systematic review and dose–response meta-analysis. *Circulation*. 2016;133(10):979–987.
5. National Institute on Alcohol Abuse and Alcoholism. Drinking levels defined. https://www.niaaa.nih.gov/alcohol-health/overview-alcohol-consumption/moderate-binge-drinking. Accessed December 13, 2016.
6. U.S. Department of Health and Human Services. 2008 Physical Activity Guidelines for Americans. https://www.health.gov/paguidelines/guidelines/default.aspx. Accessed December 14, 2016.
7. Pescatello LS, MacDonald HV, Ash GI, et al. Assessing the existing professional exercise recommendations for hypertension: a review and recommendations for future research priorities. *Mayo Clin Proc*. 2015;90(6):801–812.
8. Ekelund U, Ward HA, Norat T, et al. Physical activity and all-cause mortality across levels of overall and abdominal adiposity in European men and women: The European Prospective Investigations into Cancer and Nutrition Study. *Am J Clin Nutr*. 2015;101(3):613–621.
9. Moore SC, Lee IM, Weiderpass E, et al. Association of leisure-time physical activity with risk of 26 types of cancer in 1.44 million adults. *JAMA Intern Med*. 2016;17(6):816–825.
10. Institute of Medicine (IOM), National Academy of Sciences. *Dietary Reference Intakes for Energy, Carbohydrates, Fiber, Fat, Protein and Amino acids (Macronutrients)*. Washington, DC: National Academy Press; 2002.
11. U.S. Department of Health and Human Services and U.S. Department of Agriculture. 2015-2020 Dietary Guidelines for Americans. 8th ed. December 2015. https://health.gov/dietaryguidelines/2015/guidelines/ Accessed August 17, 2017.
12. Belanger-Gravel A, Godin G, Bilodeau A, et al. The effect of implementation intentions on physical activity among obese older adults: a randomized control study. *Psychol Health*. 2013;28(2):217–233.
13. Huberty J, Beets M, Beighle A. Effects of a policy-level intervention on children's pedometer-determined physical activity: preliminary findings from Movin' Afterschool. *J Public Health Manag Pract*. 2013;19(16):525–528.
14. Eather N, Morgan PJ, Lubans DR. Social support from teachers mediates physical activity behavior change in children participating in the Fit-4-Fun intervention. *Int J Behav Nutr Phys Act*. 2013;10:68.
15. Centers for Disease Control and Prevention. *National Diabetes Fact Sheet: General Information and National Estimates on Diabetes in the United States, 2014*. Atlanta, GA: U.S. Department of Health and Human Services.; 2014. https://www.cdc.gov/diabetes/data/statistics/2014statisticsreport.html. Accessed December 15, 2017.
16. American Diabetes Association. Standards of Medical Care in Diabetes—2017. *Diabetes Care*. 2017;40(suppl 1):S11–S24.
17. National Certification Board for Diabetes Educators. http://www.ncbde.org/. Accessed December 15, 2017.

EVOLVE RESOURCES

Please visit http://evolve.elsevier.com/Stegeman/nutritional for additional practice and study support tools.

8

Vitamins Required for Calcified Structures

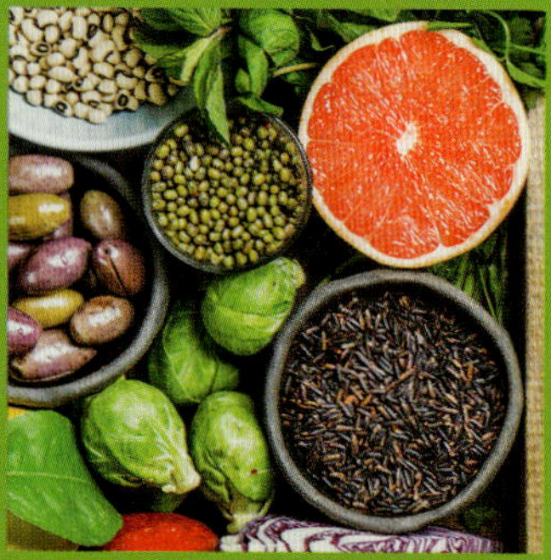

STUDENT LEARNING OUTCOMES

Upon completion of this chapter, the student will be able to achieve the following student learning outcomes:

1. Discuss the following related to vitamins:
   - Discuss requirements and deficiencies of vitamins.
   - List the fat-soluble vitamins, as well as the water-soluble vitamins.
   - Compare the characteristics of water-soluble vitamins with those of fat-soluble vitamins.
2. Discuss the following related to vitamin A:
   - Identify functions, deficiencies, surpluses, toxicities, and oral symptoms for vitamin A.
   - Select food sources for vitamin A.
   - Individualize dental hygiene considerations for patients regarding vitamin A.
   - Relate nutritional directions to meet patients' needs regarding vitamin A.
3. Discuss the following related to vitamin D:
   - Identify functions, deficiencies, surpluses, toxicities, and oral symptoms for vitamin D.
   - Select food sources for vitamin D.
   - Individualize dental hygiene considerations for patients regarding vitamin D.
   - Relate nutritional directions to meet patients' needs regarding vitamin D.
4. Discuss the following related to vitamin E:
   - Identify functions, deficiencies, surpluses, toxicities, and oral symptoms for vitamin E.
   - Select food sources for vitamin E.
   - Individualize dental hygiene considerations for patients regarding vitamin E.
   - Relate nutritional directions to meet patients' needs regarding vitamin E.
5. Discuss the following related to vitamin K:
   - Identify functions, deficiencies, surpluses, toxicities, and oral symptoms for vitamin K.
   - Select food sources for vitamin K.
   - Individualize dental hygiene considerations for patients regarding vitamin K.
   - Relate nutritional directions to meet patients' needs regarding vitamin K.
6. Discuss the following related to vitamin C:
   - Identify functions, deficiencies, surpluses, toxicities, and oral symptoms for vitamin C.
   - Select food sources for vitamin C.
   - Individualize dental hygiene considerations for patients regarding vitamin C.
   - Relate nutritional directions to meet patients' needs regarding vitamin C.

KEY TERMS

Alopecia
Ameloblasts
Anticoagulant
Calcitonin
Collagen
Diplopia
Enamel hypoplasia
Epiphyses
Fibroblasts
Follicular hyperkeratosis
Hematopoiesis
Hypercarotenemia
Hypervitaminosis A
Leukoplakia
Lysosomes
Meta-analysis
Night blindness
Odontoblasts
Osteoblasts
Osteocalcin
Osteoclasts
Osteodentin
Osteomalacia
Petechiae
Prostaglandins
Prothrombin
Retinoic acid
Rhodopsin
Scorbutic
Secondary deficiency
Tocopherols
Tocotrienols
Xeroderma
Xerophthalmia

TEST YOUR NQ

1. **T/F** Fat-soluble vitamins are stored in the body.
2. **T/F** Vitamins do not provide energy.
3. **T/F** Vitamin E is found in vegetable oils and green leafy vegetables.
4. **T/F** Fat-soluble vitamins include A, D, E, and K.
5. **T/F** Animal foods are the principal dietary source of beta-carotene.
6. **T/F** Xerophthalmia occurs with a deficiency of vitamin A.
7. **T/F** The liver and kidney help convert vitamin D to its active form.
8. **T/F** An excess of vitamin D causes rickets.
9. **T/F** Vitamin K is essential for regulation of blood calcium and phosphorus levels.
10. **T/F** Vitamin C is needed for wound healing.

Overview of Vitamins

Nutrients never work single-handedly but rather in partnership with each other. Vitamins are catalysts for all metabolic reactions using proteins, fats, and carbohydrates for energy, growth, and cell maintenance. Because only small amounts of these chemical substances obtained from food facilitate millions of processes, they may be regarded as "miracle workers."

Eating fats, carbohydrates, and proteins without enough vitamins means the energy from these nutrients cannot be used. The opposite is also true. Vitamins do not provide energy, and they cannot be used without an adequate supply of fats, carbohydrates, proteins, and minerals. Most vitamins come in several forms; each form may perform a different task. Vitamins are easily destroyed by the heat, oxidation, and chemical processes used in their extraction. In this text, water-soluble vitamins, fat-soluble vitamins, and minerals are presented based on their function in calcified structures (teeth and periodontium) or their role in oral soft tissues (oral mucous membranes and salivary glands) to familiarize the dental hygienist with nutrients that might be involved when oral changes are observed. Most dental hygiene students are well aware of the role of several minerals in calcified structures in the oral cavity, but vitamins presented in this chapter are also important for healthy teeth and the periodontium (Box 8.1).

Most nutrients have various functions; some are involved in both calcified and soft oral tissues. Oral physiologic roles for these nutrients are presented in appropriate chapters, but information such as requirements and food sources is found only when the vitamin is first discussed. Fat-soluble and water-soluble vitamins differ in many ways, but a basic understanding of their fundamental similarities can facilitate learning.

Requirements

Although vitamins are vital to life, they are required in minute amounts. Vitamins are similar to hormones because of their potent effects, but they must come from an outside source because they either cannot be produced by the body or cannot be produced in adequate amounts to meet physiologic needs. Each vitamin is essential, although the amount needed may vary from 2.4 μg per day for vitamin B_{12} to 550 mg per day for choline.

Although the dietary reference intakes (DRIs) list the amounts of vitamins for different ages and sexes, many factors (e.g., smoking; use of alcohol, caffeine, or drugs; and stress) modify an individual's requirements. Periods of rapid growth; pregnancy or lactation; fever; and recovery from accidents, disease, surgery, and burns are all considered stressful. Requirements for most vitamins, especially water-soluble vitamins, are increased during periods of stress because of elevated metabolic activity.

• BOX 8.1 Vitamins Required for Calcified Structures

Fat-Soluble Vitamins	Water-Soluble Vitamins
Vitamin A	Vitamin C
Vitamin D	
Vitamin E	
Vitamin K	

• BOX 8.2 Groups at Potential Risk of Nutritional Deficiencies

- Older adults
- Impoverished, low income
- Vegans
- Chronic disease states
- Alcoholics
- Inadequate intake
- Smokers
- Excessive caffeine use
- Polypharmacy
- Physiologic stress
- Periods of rapid growth
- Pregnancy
- Lactation
- Infants, children, adolescents
- Medical conditions causing
  - Inadequate absorption
  - Inadequate use
  - Excessive excretion
  - Destruction
- Physical stress
- Surgery
- Accidents
- Disease
- Burns
- Fever

Deficiencies

If adequate amounts of the nutrient are unavailable to sustain biochemical functions, a nutritional deficiency occurs. A nutritional deficiency as a result of decreased intake is called a primary deficiency. A vitamin deficiency caused by inadequate absorption or use, increased requirements, excretion, or destruction is called a **secondary deficiency**. Nutrients are codependent; a deficiency of one may cause deficiency symptoms of another.

Although specific vitamin deficiency syndromes are rare in the United States, several groups are at risk (Box 8.2). Vitamin levels in the blood are often unmeasurable; thus, a nutritional deficiency may be identified on the basis of clinical signs and symptoms and their response to vitamin supplementation. However, one of the peculiarities of vitamins is that the symptoms of a deficiency frequently resemble the symptoms caused by an overdose, making definitive diagnosis difficult.

Characteristics of Fat-Soluble Vitamins

Although the four fat-soluble vitamins (A, D, E, and K) differ in function, use, and sources, they have several similar characteristics: (a) they are soluble in fat or fat solvents; (b) they are fairly stable to heat, as in cooking; (c) they are organic substances (contain carbon); (d) they do not contain nitrogen; (e) they are absorbed in the intestine along with fats and lipids in foods; and (f) they require bile for absorption.

Fat-soluble vitamins are different from water-soluble vitamins mainly because larger amounts can be stored in the body. Vitamins A and D are stored for long periods; thus, minor shortages may not be identified until drastic depletion has occurred. For example, vitamin A can be stored in the liver to meet basic needs for at least 1 year. Observable signs and symptoms of a dietary deficiency are often not identified until they are in an advanced state. Dietary deficiencies occur when foods consumed do not provide necessary amounts of a nutrient.

Because several forms of each of the fat-soluble vitamins can be used by the body, vitamins A, D, and E were previously measured by their biologic activity based on the growth of animals. International units (IU) reflect this biologic activity in animal studies and do not always represent absorption rates in humans. Because of this, the retinol activity equivalents (RAEs) standard was created for vitamin A. The recommended dietary allowances (RDAs) for vitamins A and E were determined based on the biologic effectiveness of each form because the different forms of these vitamins have varying activity levels. After measurement of all active forms of the vitamins, the quantity is converted to micrograms or milligrams and totaled to indicate the amount of vitamin in that food. RAEs reflect vitamin A activity of foods. Although previous food tables listed IUs, more accurate weight measurements in micrograms or milligrams are now used.

Characteristics of Water-Soluble Vitamins

B-complex vitamins and vitamin C are water soluble and are organic substances. In contrast to vitamin C and fat-soluble vitamins, B-complex vitamins contain nitrogen. Water-soluble vitamins have vital roles as coenzymes, which are necessary for almost every cellular reaction in the body. Vitamin C is discussed in this chapter with the fat-soluble vitamins because of its vital role as a structural component of teeth; it is also important in oral soft tissues. B-complex vitamins are discussed in Chapter 11.

Most water-soluble vitamins are readily absorbed in the jejunum. High concentrations of these vitamins result in decreased absorption efficiency. The body stores very small amounts of each of these vitamins; few water-soluble vitamins produce toxic symptoms. Because of their limited storage, daily intake is important.

DENTAL CONSIDERATIONS

- Assessment is crucial to determine requirements for vitamins. Assess for the following: smoking, alcohol use, excessive caffeine use, medications, physiologic stress, or surgery. If any of these is present, vitamin requirements in the diet may need to be altered.
- Dietary and physical assessments are more diagnostic for vitamin deficiencies than laboratory values. A combination of the three assessments provides the greatest amount of information on an individual's nutrition status.
- Patients with mobile teeth, ill-fitting dentures and/or partials, and those with edentulous areas are at greater risk of vitamin deficiencies.
- Evaluate nutrient intake of groups at high risk for developing nutritional deficiencies, such as older adults, impoverished/low-income patients, patients with chronic diseases, and those with physiologic disorders that interfere with food consumption. If indicated, refer the patient to a registered dietitian nutritionist (RDN).

NUTRITIONAL DIRECTIONS

- No vitamin contains calories, but some vitamins, especially the B-complex vitamins, are essential to the production of energy.
- The use of mineral oil as a laxative can interfere with absorption of fat-soluble vitamins.

Vitamin A (Retinol, Carotene)

Retinol is the dietary source of vitamin A from animal sources, and beta-carotene is the principal carotenoid present in plant pigments. Retinoic acid is the most biologically active form of vitamin A.

Physiologic Roles

Vitamin A has many hormone-like roles in the body. It is also required for normal bone growth and development and facilitating the transcription of DNA into RNA.

Vision

Retinol is converted to retinal in the eye. Retinal combines with opsin, a protein in the eye, to form the visual pigment, **rhodopsin**. **Night blindness** may result from inadequate vitamin A to permit rhodopsin production. This condition takes years to develop in adults, but occurs much sooner in children because they have fewer body stores.

Growth

Vitamin A is necessary for growth of soft tissues and bones. In skeletal tissue, vitamin A is necessary for resorption of old bone and synthesis of new bone. **Retinoic acid**, produced by the body from retinal, is the form of vitamin A involved in development of teeth, especially in formation of **ameloblasts** (enamel-forming cells) and **odontoblasts** (dentin-forming cells) along with growth of bone. Vitamin A deficiency during preeruptive stages of tooth development leads to enamel hypoplasia and defective dentin formation. Vitamin A also is involved with normal teeth spacing and promotes osteoblast function of alveolar bone.

Cancer

Vitamin A and carotene have consistently been associated with cancer prevention because of their importance in development and integrity of cells. The antioxidant role of vitamin A is discussed in *Health Application 8*. Antioxidants prevent cell membrane damage by free radicals that are produced by cells and tissues using free oxygen. Unchecked by an antioxidant, free radicals can damage the structure and impair the function of cell membranes. Research is inconclusive in regard to use of beta-carotene to prevent cancer. Studies suggest that vitamin A and beta-carotene may resolve oral leukoplakia, but relapse is common.[1] **Leukoplakia** (see Figs. 17.11 and 17.16) is a white plaque that forms on oral mucous membranes that cannot be wiped away. It has the potential to become cancerous. Whether beta-carotene or some other components in fruits and vegetables can help to resolve leukoplakia has not been determined. Supplementation is not advised other than increasing consumption of fruits and vegetables because some studies show an increased risk of lung cancer among smokers using beta-carotene supplements.[2] The American Cancer Society does not support vitamin A

TABLE 8.1 National Academy of Medicine Recommendations for Vitamin A

	EAR (µg/day)		RDA (µg/day)			
Life Stage	Male	Female	Male	Female	AI (µ/day)	UL (µg/day)[a]
0–6 months					400	600
7–12 months					500	600
1–3 years	210	210	300	300		600
4–8 years	275	275	400	400		900
9–13 years	445	420	600	600		1700
14–18 years	630	485	900	700		2800
> 18 years	625	500	900	700		3000
Pregnancy						
14–18 years		530		750		2800
19–50 years		550		770		3000
Lactation						
14–18 years		885		1200		2800
19–50 years		900		1300		3000

Data from Institute of Medicine (IOM), Food and Nutrition Board. *Dietary Reference Intakes For Vitamin C, Vitamin K, Arsenic, Boron, Chromium, Copper, Iodine, Iron, Manganese, Molybdenum, Nickel, Silicon, Vanadium, and Zinc.* Washington, DC: National Academy Press; 2000.
[a]Preformed vitamin A.

supplementation for cancer prevention, but recommends getting the vitamin through food sources.[2]

Requirements

As shown in Table 8.1, the RDA for vitamin A is 900 µg RAE for men and 700 µg RAE for women (1 RAE = 1 µg = 12 µg beta-carotene = 3.3 IU). The tolerable upper intake level (UL) is 3000 µg RAE per day. The need for vitamin A is increased during periods of rapid growth, when gastrointestinal problems affect its absorption or conversion (e.g., cystic fibrosis, celiac disease, Crohn disease, or chronic diarrhea), and in hepatic diseases that limit vitamin A storage or conversion of beta-carotene to its active form. Although no UL has been established for beta-carotene, the National Academy of Medicine (formerly the Institute of Medicine) does not advise supplements for healthy people.[3]

Average intake in the United States meets the RDA, and because vitamin A can be stored in the liver, most adults have sufficient quantities to maintain health. Inadequate intake occurs in lower socioeconomic groups as a consequence of inadequate vegetable and fruit intake.

Sources

Vitamin A, as preformed retinol, is found in organ meats, such as liver. It is also found in milk, cheese, butter, eggs, cod liver oil, and fortified foods (e.g., breakfast cereals). Sometimes retinol is added to skim milk and margarine. Beta-carotene or provitamin A is also present in yellow, orange, and green leafy vegetables (e.g., spinach, turnip greens, broccoli; Table 8.2). Although not as well absorbed as from animal sources and fortified foods, beta-carotene is still a valuable source of this vitamin. Beta-carotene is deep red in pure form and derives its name from carrots, from which it was first isolated. Chlorophyll disguises carotenoids in green vegetables. Most yellow, orange, and dark-green fruits and vegetables are high in carotene or vitamin A content. The deeper the color, the more vitamin A activity is present in a fruit or vegetable.

Absorption and Excretion

Absorption is optimal when body stores are depleted and when adequate amounts of other interrelated nutrients are present. The presence of vitamin E and the hormone thyroxine also enhances the use of vitamin A.

The liver stores approximately 90% of vitamin A, while smaller quantities are stored in the kidneys, lungs, and adipose tissue. Adequate serum proteins are necessary to mobilize vitamin A from the liver. Vitamin A is not readily excreted by the body, but a small amount is lost in urine.

Hyper States and Hypo States

Extreme levels of vitamin A (high or low) can cause serious problems, even resulting in death (Fig. 8.1).

Toxicity

When present in high concentrations, unbound vitamin A causes damage to cell membranes, especially in red blood cells and **lysosomes** (small bodies occurring in many types of cells). Large amounts of vitamin A supplements can exceed the storage capacity of the liver. If this occurs, free vitamin A

TABLE 8.2 **Food Sources of Vitamin A**

Food	Portion	Vitamin A (µg RAE)
Beef liver, cooked	1 slice	6421
Cod liver oil	1 tbsp	4080
Pumpkin, canned	1 cup	1906
Chicken liver, cooked	1 liver	1890
Sweet potato, baked	1 large	1799
Carrots, raw	½ cup sticks	1019
Butternut squash, baked	½ cup	572
Spinach, cooked	½ cup	472
Mustard greens, cooked	½ cup	433
Collard greens, cooked	½ cup	386
Turnip greens, cooked	½ cup	274
Cantaloupe	1 cup	270
Roamine lettuce, shredded	1 cup	205
Special K	1 cup	155
Skim milk, fortified	1 cup	150
Spinach, raw	1 cup	141
Apricots, dried	½ cup	117
Margarine	1 tbsp	116
Egg, hard boiled	1	75
Cheddar cheese	1 oz	75
Butter	1 tbsp	65
Broccoli, cooked	½ cup	60
Apricot, raw	1	34

Data from U.S. Department of Agriculture (USDA), Agricultural Research Service. *USDA National Nutrient Database for Standard Reference, Release 28.* 2016. https://ndb.nal.usda.gov/ndb/. Accessed December 19, 2016.

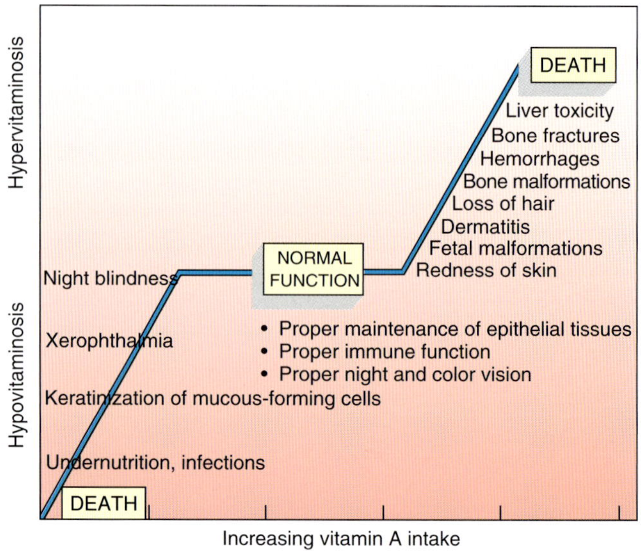

• **Figure 8.1** Vitamin A intake. This chart shows how changing the amount of vitamin A in the diet can lead to hypovitaminosis A or hypervitaminosis A. In the extreme, either condition can lead to death. (Reproduced with permission from Patton KT, Thibodeau GA. *Anatomy and Physiology*, 9th ed, St. Louis, MO: Mosby Elsevier; 2016.)

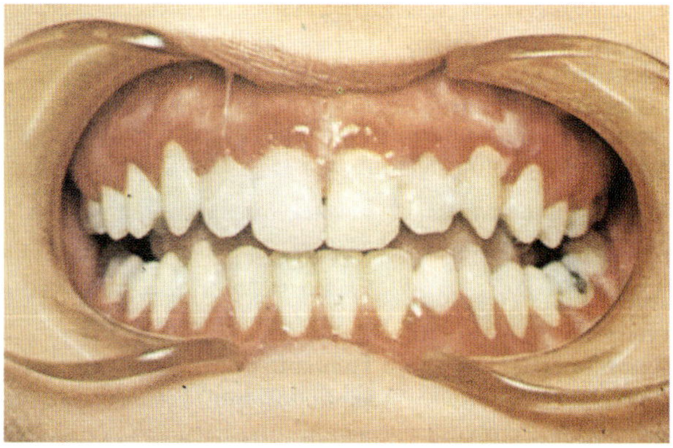

• **Figure 8.2** Hypervitaminosis A. Bright-red marginal discoloration of the gingiva shown here is characteristic. (Courtesy of Dr. M. D. Muenter. From McLaren DS. *A Colour Atlas and Text of Diet-Related Disorders*. 2nd ed. London: Mosby–Year Book; 1992.)

enters the bloodstream and exerts toxic effects on cell membranes. High levels of vitamin A in the body are referred to as **hypervitaminosis A**.

Maternal consumption of vitamin A supplements before conception and during the first trimester of pregnancy has been associated with fetal birth defects (see Table 13.3 for effects of vitamin A toxicity during pregnancy). Toxicity is evident in infants by bulging of the fontanelle as a result of increased cerebrospinal fluid pressure. Other clinical symptoms include headache; nausea and vomiting; **diplopia** (double vision); lethargy and irritability; **alopecia** (hair loss); dryness of the mucous membranes; reddened gingiva (Fig. 8.2); thinning of the epithelium; cracking and bleeding lips; and increased activity of **osteoclasts** (cells associated with bone resorption), which leads to decalcification, desquamation of oral mucosa, bone growth retardation, softening of the skull, and liver abnormalities.

Excess vitamin A (primarily in the form of retinol) may have a negative impact on bone health.[4] How this change in bone mineral density may affect alveolar bone is unknown.

Toxicity from excessive intake of vitamin A food source occurs occasionally, but most cases are a result of too much supplementation. Beta-carotene is much less toxic than vitamin A. The body converts only the amount of carotenoids it needs into vitamin A. Although beta-carotenes are not toxic, overconsumption may result in **hypercarotenemia**, yellow pigmentation of the skin occurring first on the palms of the hands and soles of the feet, which is

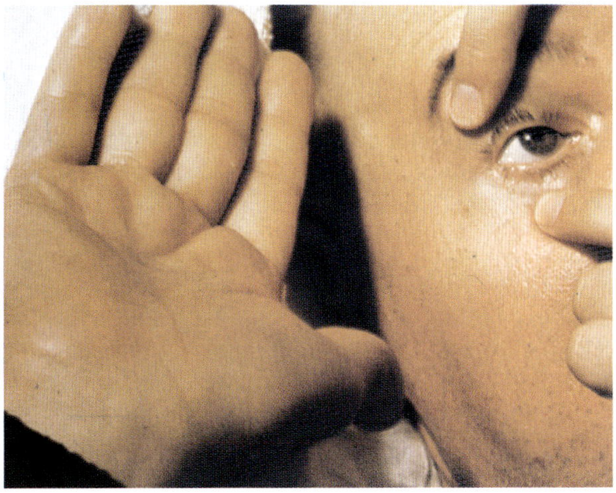

• **Figure 8.3** Hypercarotenosis. The face, eye, and palm of the hand. The sclerae remain clear, distinguishing the condition from jaundice. (Courtesy of Dr. I.A. Abrahamson, Sr. From McLaren DS. *A Colour Atlas and Text of Diet-Related Disorders*. 2nd ed. London: Mosby–Year Book; 1992.)

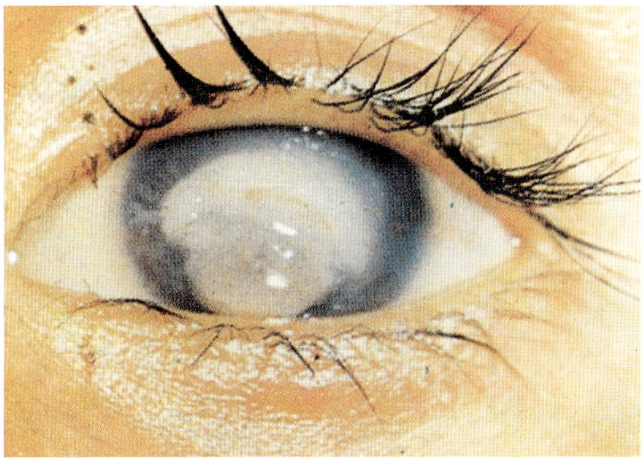

• **Figure 8.4** Xerophthalmia. (Reproduced with permission from McLaren DS. *A Colour Atlas and Text of Diet-Related Disorders*. 2nd ed. London: Mosby–Year Book; 1992.)

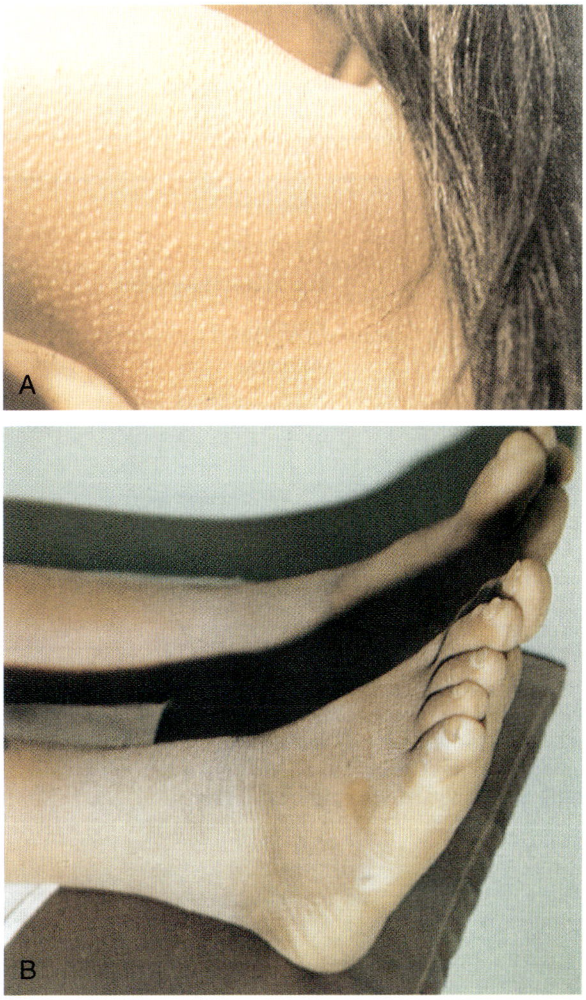

• **Figure 8.5** (A) Follicular hyperkeratosis caused by vitamin A deficiency. (B) Hyperkeratosis. The skin over parts of the body is thickened, dry, and wrinkled, associated with vitamin A deficiency. (Reproduced with permission from McLaren DS. *A Colour Atlas and Text of Diet-Related Disorders*. 2nd ed. London: Mosby–Year Book; 1992.)

caused by carotene storage in fatty tissue (Fig. 8.3). This condition subsides when ingestion of beta-carotene is reduced.

Deficiency

Inadequate dietary intake is the primary reason for vitamin A deficiency, found most commonly in children younger than 5 years of age. It also may result from chronic fat malabsorption or a high intake of alcohol. Vitamin A deficiency is rarely seen in the United States, but it is a major nutritional problem in developing countries. Mild vitamin A deficiency may contribute to a depressed immune response.

Inadequate vitamin A intake results in degeneration of epithelial cells in the eye and cessation of tear secretion. Lids are swollen and sticky with pus, and eyes are sensitive to light in **xerophthalmia**, sometimes resulting in permanent blindness. The first symptom of xerophthalmia is night blindness, followed by the occurrence of xerotic spots on the conjunctiva, called Bitot spots. These eye ulcerations may spread and result in blindness if left untreated (Fig. 8.4).

Degeneration of epithelial cells results in an inability to produce mucus. This occurs not only in epithelial cells, but also in the intestines and lungs. **Xeroderma** can progress until the whole body is covered with dry, flaky, scaly skin that is similar to dandruff. It is followed by **follicular hyperkeratosis**, in which the skin is thickened, dry, and wrinkled (Fig. 8.5). Keratinization may also affect the oral mucosa and the respiratory and gastrointestinal tracts. In these areas, degeneration of epithelial cells results in increased risk of infection and delayed or impaired wound healing.

Severe vitamin A deficiency may result in enamel hypoplasia and defective dentin formation in developing teeth. **Enamel hypoplasia** involves defects in the enamel matrix and incomplete calcification of the enamel, thereby inhibiting enamel formation. Odontoblasts lose their ability to arrange themselves in normal parallel linear formation, resulting in degeneration and atrophy of ameloblasts. The result is small pits or grooves in the crown (Fig. 8.6).

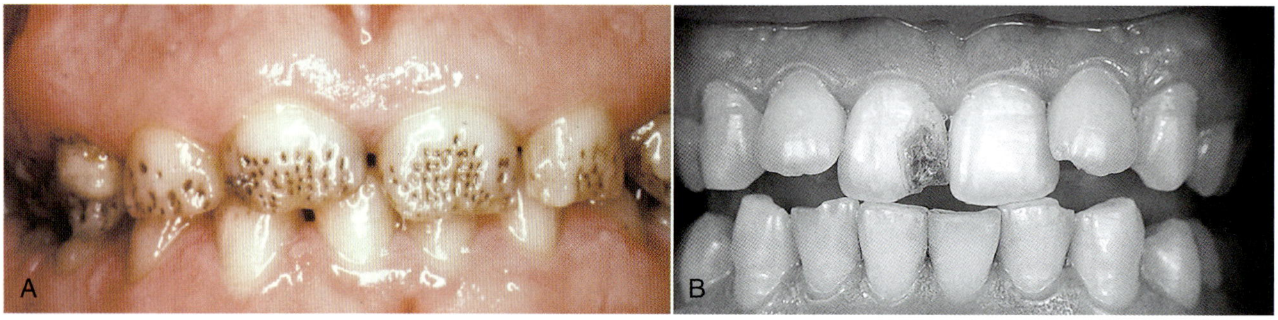

• **Figure 8.6** Enamel hypoplasia. Pitting occurred on the surfaces of the maxillary central and lateral incisors where the enamel is thin. (From Nelson SJ. *Wheeler's Dental Anatomy: Physiology and Occlusion.* 10th ed, St. Louis, MO: Saunders; 2014.)

DENTAL CONSIDERATIONS

- A deficiency of vitamin A is associated with increased risk of infection and poor wound healing.
- Vitamin A or beta-carotene supplements are not recommended for most healthy adults.
- Assess for signs of vitamin A deficiencies (loss of night vision, keratomalacia, corneal ulceration, or Bitot spots), especially in young and older patients. When in doubt, refer to a health care provider or RDN.
- In contrast to vitamin A, beta-carotene is not toxic, but large amounts can cause a temporary change in skin color. Hypercarotenemia may be distinguished from jaundice because the sclera retains its normal white color.
- Jaundice or any disorder affecting fat absorption also affects fat-soluble vitamin absorption, making these patients prone to vitamin A deficiency.
- Drugs such as orlistat (Xenical, Alli) used for weight loss and food components such as olestra negatively affect fat and fat-soluble vitamin absorption, especially the absorption of vitamin A and beta-carotene. Patients taking orlistat should follow a low-fat diet and take a multivitamin 2 hours before or after taking the drug.
- An alcoholic or alcoholic-cirrhotic patient may be deficient in vitamin A because of the effects of ethanol and impaired liver function.
- Vitamin A toxicity can be masked, especially when protein-energy malnutrition is present.
- Discourage patients from taking more than the RDA in over-the-counter vitamin preparations unless specifically advised to do so by a health care provider or RDN.
- Absorption of vitamin A may be decreased by excessive intake of either vitamin E or C. Do not encourage use of vitamin E and vitamin C supplements or vitamin E–rich or vitamin C–rich foods if the patient is at risk of vitamin A deficiency.

NUTRITIONAL DIRECTIONS

- Vitamin A from animal or fortified foods is used better by the body than beta-carotene.
- Vegans need to consume a minimum of five servings of dark-green, yellow, and orange fruits and vegetables daily to receive the recommended amount of vitamin A.
- Fortified foods and vitamin supplements should be used judiciously; severe, life-threatening liver damage or increased risk of hip fractures can result from chronic use in excess of the RDA.
- Recommend storing vitamins in a cool, dark place to prevent deterioration.
- Women of childbearing age need to limit intake of preformed vitamin A (retinol, retinyl, and retinoyl acetate)—found in liver, fortified foods (breakfast cereals), and dietary supplements—to about 100% of the Daily Value because of the increased risk of neural defects during the first trimester of pregnancy.

Vitamin D (Calciferol)

Although vitamin D has been called a vitamin, it is more appropriately classified as a hormone (a compound secreted by one type of cell that acts to control the function of another type of cell). Skin cells are able to make vitamin D when the precursor 7-dehydrocholesterol, present in the skin, is exposed to ultraviolet (UV) light or sunshine. Vitamin D from food, ergocalciferol (vitamin D_2), or cholecalciferol (vitamin D_3) is biologically inert. Further metabolism occurs in the liver with conversion of vitamin D_2 or vitamin D_3 into 25-hydroxycholecalciferol (calcidiol), and a final change to the active form of 1,25-dihydroxycholecalciferol (calciferol) primarily by the kidney. A special enzyme in the kidney, α-1-hydroxylase, activates calcidiol to produce calcitriol, the active form of vitamin D (Fig. 8.7). Individuals with kidney disease are often unable to convert vitamin D to its active form.

Until recently, vitamin D was viewed primarily as a protective agent against bone disease, such as rickets. Research has shown, however, that vitamin D receptors are present in approximately 36 different types of cells, and the hormone is involved in the maintenance of more than 200 human genes.[4,5] A flurry of reports from many nations have highlighted a variety of vitamin D insufficiency and deficiency diseases. More research is needed to learn about the impact of vitamin D on different stages of the life cycle and in racial and ethnic groups.[6]

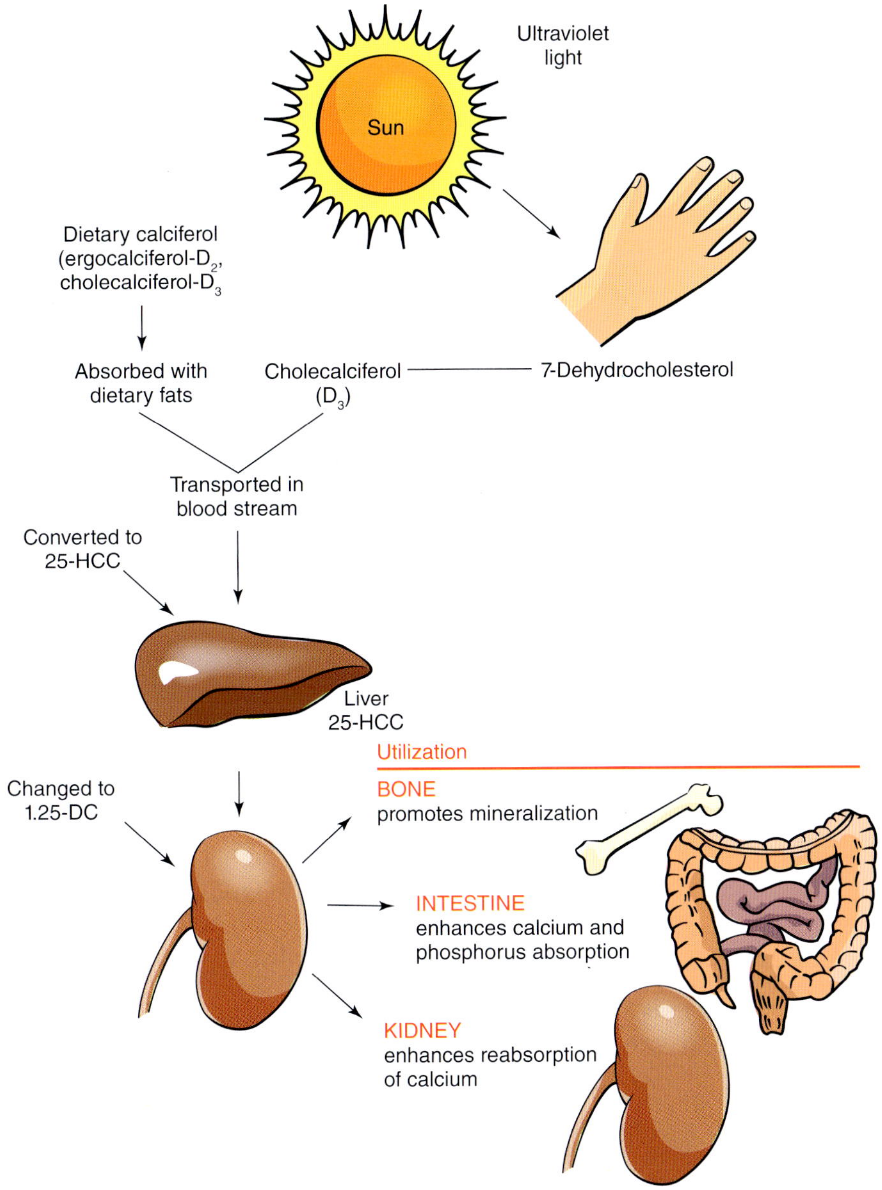

• **Figure 8.7** Vitamin D metabolism. 25-HCC, 25-hydrocalciferol [hydroxycholecalciferol (calcidiol)]; 1.25-DC, [dihydroxycholecalciferol (calciferol)] (Adapted from Kumar V, Abbas A, Aster J. *Robbins Basic Pathology.* 10th ed. Philadelphia: Saunders; 2017.)

Physiologic Roles

Vitamin D is intricately related to calcium and phosphorus, each being required for optimal use of the other. Vitamin D helps the body absorb and regulate calcium. The primary role of vitamin D is mineralization of bones and teeth and regulation of blood calcium and phosphorus levels. It functions with the parathyroid and thyroid (**calcitonin**) hormones to regulate intestinal absorption of calcium and phosphorus, enhance renal calcium and phosphorus reabsorption, and regulate skeletal calcium and phosphorus reserves (see Fig. 8.7).

Vitamin D may also be involved in the functioning of cells involved in **hematopoiesis** (formation of red blood cells), the skin, cardiovascular function, and immune responses. Its regulatory role helps keep serum calcium in the appropriate range to maintain cardiac and neuromuscular function. Calciferol (1,25-dihydroxycholecalciferol) interacts with **osteoblasts** (cells that help produce collagen and build and reform new bone) to increase the withdrawal of **osteocalcin** (calcium-binding noncollagen protein in bone) and other bone-building compounds, or interacts with parathyroid hormone to mobilize calcium stores from the skeleton when calcium is needed.

Requirements

The vitamin D requirement is difficult to determine, and there are widely varying recommendations. When sufficient sunlight is available, people may not require an exogenous dietary source of vitamin D. Because many North Americans have limited exposure to sunlight, however, and because many factors can interfere with

TABLE 8.3 National Academy of Medicine Recommendations for Vitamin D

Life Stage[a]	EAR μg/day (IU)	RDA μg/day (IU)	UL μg/day (IU)
0–6 months	10 μg/day (400 IU)	10 (400)	25 (1000)
7–12 months	10 (400)	10 (400)	37.5 (1500)
1–3 years	10 (400)	15 (600)	62.5 (2500)
4–8 years	10 (400)	15 (600)	75 (3000)
9–13 years	10 (400)	15 (600)	100 (4000)
14–18 years	10 (400)	15 (600)	100 (4000)
19–30 years	10 (400)	15 (600)	100 (4000)
31–50 years	10 (400)	15 (600)	100 (4000)
51–70 years	10 (400)	15 (600)	100 (4000)
> 70 years	10 (400)	20 (800)	100 (4000)
Pregnant and Lactating			
19–50 years	10 (400)	15 (600)	100 (4000)

EAR, Estimated average requirement; RDA, recommended dietary allowance; UL, upper intake level.

Data from Institute of Medicine (IOM), Food and Nutrition Board. *Dietary Reference Intakes for Calcium and Vitamin D.* Washington, DC: National Academy Press; 2011.

[a]All groups except pregnancy and lactation are males and females.

UV light–dependent synthesis of vitamin D in the skin, vitamin D is considered an essential dietary nutrient. Vitamin D is measured in micrograms (mcg or μg) or IU. One microgram is equivalent to 40 IU.

The National Academy of Medicine determined that an adequate intake of vitamin D for ages 1 to 70 years is 15 μg (600 IU); the recommended amount increases to 20 μg (800 IU) after age 70 (Table 8.3). The International Osteoporosis Foundation recommends 20 to 25 μg (800 to 1000 IU) for older adults to prevent fractures.[7] The National Osteoporosis Foundation urges adults older than age 50 years to get at least 800 to 1000 IU of vitamin D to prevent fractures; they recommend supplementation to get adequate amounts because of difficulty obtaining it from food sources, especially for individuals diagnosed with osteoporosis.[8] The U.S. Preventive Services Task Force found inconclusive evidence to support supplementation of vitamin D and does not recommend daily vitamin D supplements unless a deficiency exists (determined by laboratory data) or the patient is diagnosed with osteopenia or osteoporosis.[9] The nutrition label slated for release in 2018 will reflect an increase in the daily value (DV) for vitamin D to 20 μg (800 IU). Actual amounts of vitamin D are now required to be included on Nutrition Facts panels.

ULs for various life stages also were established for vitamin D. The estimated average requirement intake to prevent rickets is 10 μg or 400 IU. The American Academy of Pediatrics has recommended 10 μg (400 IU) of vitamin D for infants. Therefore, supplementation is needed for infants who are breastfed or consuming less than 1 L/day of formula. This practice should begin within the first few days following birth.[10]

Some medical researchers have expressed strong doubts in scientific journals about the adequacy of the current Dietary Reference Intake for vitamin D. One reason the National Academy of Medicine is hesitant to recommend further increases in intake is because of potential toxicity from vitamin D. More research is needed to validate the health benefits and appropriate level of vitamin D. Because United States residents comprise different ethnicities and locations and sensitivities, a "one-size-fits-all" recommendation may not be appropriate.

American and Canadian diets do not provide sufficient vitamin D.[6] A study involving healthy children and adolescents indicates that a low prevalence of vitamin D blood concentrations are related to low intake, race, and season.[6]

Sources

Sunlight

The body's ability to produce adequate amounts of vitamin D from sunlight is why the sun has been considered a source of health. UV radiation is the principal cause of sunburn and cellular damage that leads to skin cancer. UV radiation penetrates uncovered skin and converts a precursor of vitamin D to previtamin D_3, which becomes the active form of vitamin D_3, or calcitriol (see Fig. 8.7). Most people experience an increase in vitamin D levels during the summer months because changes in the angulation of the sun occur throughout the year. During summer months, 10 minutes a day without sunblock on hands and face can replete the body's supply.

Many people in the northern hemisphere (above a line approximately between the northern border of California and Boston), especially older adults and darker-skinned individuals, may lack sufficient exposure to UV radiation, especially mid-October through mid-March. Cloud cover, fog, haze, shade, and pollution can reduce the UV energy needed for vitamin D. UVB radiation does not penetrate glass. A broad spectrum sunscreen is protective from both UVA and UVB rays. Sunscreens also interfere with the formation of vitamin D_3. Dermatologists continue to advise sunscreen and clothing protection for anyone in the sun more than 20 minutes. Although sunscreen inhibits vitamin D production, its use and moderation in sun exposure are important to protect against skin cancer. By age 70 years, the skin generally produces only half the amount of vitamin D as a 20-year-old person.

Food

Although adequate quantities of vitamin D may be derived from exposure to sunlight, additional food sources are necessary in most cases. Naturally occurring vitamin D content in foods is variable; food tables do not normally list vitamin D content. This information has been added to the National Nutrient Database for Standard Reference (available at https://ndb.nal.usda.gov/ndb/).

Natural sources include oily fish such as salmon, sardines, and tuna, as well as cod liver oil and fish oils (Table 8.4). A diet composed of the best (unfortified) food sources of vitamin D may supply 2.5 μg (1000 IU) daily.

Because vitamin D deficiencies are prevalent in the United States, the U.S. Food and Drug Administration allows vitamin D fortification of orange juice and other foods, providing a good alternative source for people who do not drink milk. Other foods, such as margarine, infant formulas and cereals, prepared breakfast cereals, chocolate beverage mixes, and yogurt,

TABLE 8.4 Food Sources of Vitamin D

Food	Portion	Vitamin D (IU)
Cod liver oil	1 tbsp	1360
Salmon, cooked	3 oz	444
Total Raisin Bran	1 cup	189
Sardines, canned in oil, drained	3 oz	164
Orange juice, fortified with vitamin D	1 cup	100
Milk (skim, 1% or 2%), fortified with vitamin D	1 cup	98
Chocolate milk, low-fat, fortified with vitamin D	1 cup	98
Yogurt, nonfat, fortified with vitamin D	6 oz	88
American cheese, fortified with vitamin D	1 oz	85
Margarine, fortified	1 tbsp	60
Egg	1 large	44
Tuna fish, canned in water, drained	3 oz	40
Beef liver, cooked	1 slice	33

Data from U.S. Department of Agriculture (USDA), Agricultural Research Service. *USDA National Nutrient Database for Standard Reference, Release 28.* 2016. https://ndb.nal.usda.gov/ndb/. Accessed January 6, 2017.

also may be fortified with vitamin D (see Table 8.4). The food additive regulations were amended to allow companies to effectively double the amount of vitamin D to a maximum level of 200 IU/cup milk, 200 IU/cup plant-based milk alternatives (e.g. soy, almond beverage), and 151 IU/6 oz for plant-based yogurt alternatives.

Foods are not legally required to be fortified, but approximately 98% of the milk in the United States is fortified to provide 10 μg (400 IU) of cholecalciferol per quart. Vitamin D fortification of milk enhances absorption and utilization of the calcium and phosphorus inherent in milk and vice versa. Children especially benefit from vitamin D fortification of milk for bone growth. Vitamin D from fortified regular and low-fat cheeses is absorbed and metabolized well by the body. Because fortification is optional, it cannot be taken for granted.

Nutrition labels can be used to assess daily intake of vitamin D; this information plus the amount of exposure to sunlight must be considered to ensure adequate amounts of vitamin D. Vitamin D is in multivitamins, prenatal vitamins, calcium–vitamin D combinations, and individual vitamin D supplements. Most multivitamins provide 400 IU per dose. Vitamin D_3 is more effective at increasing calcidiol levels in the blood than vitamin D_2 (ergocalciferol).

Absorption

As with other nutrients, optimal absorption occurs when all closely interrelated nutrients (particularly calcium and phosphorus) are present in sufficient quantities. Conversely, diets high in fiber can result in less vitamin D absorption.

Hyper States and Hypo States

Toxicity

Vitamin D has the potential to become toxic at high levels. The risk for harm increases as the intake level exceeds the UL. When synthetic vitamin D supplements are taken orally in large amounts for 6 weeks, toxicity signs may occur. Nausea, vomiting, poor appetite, weight loss, constipation, dizziness, weakness, and tingling sensations in the mouth are signs of vitamin D toxicity. Vitamin D toxicity can also increase blood levels of calcium, causing mental changes, confusion, and heart rhythm abnormalities.[12] Calciferol excess can result in enhanced bone resorption, leading to deposition of calcium and phosphate in soft tissues and irreversible kidney and cardiovascular damage.[12] Unless symptoms are detected and the source of vitamin D is removed immediately, permanent damage results.

The most common reason for vitamin D toxicity is prolonged intake of excessive supplements or cod liver oil; otherwise, toxicity through diet is unlikely. Toxicity from excessive vitamin D intake may occur when a concentrated calciferol preparation is mistakenly given. For example, an infant given a commercial formula and a vitamin supplement can easily ingest vitamin D well above the adequate intake (AI) level.

Deficiency

Vitamin D research indicates that it may potentially protect against a wide variety of diseases.[13] In adults, vitamin D deficiency has been linked in research studies to conditions as diverse as asthma, cancer, cardiovasculardisease (CVD), hypertension, diabetes mellitus, depression, some infectious diseases, autoimmune disorders, and schizophrenia.[13,14] Many vitamin D researchers believe that by diligently shielding ourselves from sunlight, many benefits of this vitamin may be missed.[15,16] Also, the melanin pigment provides a natural protection against UV rays; thus, dark-skinned individuals are much more likely than fair-skinned individuals to have low levels of vitamin D. Nevertheless, dermatologists recommend sunscreen for all skin tones.

Vitamin D deficiency affects skeletal structure in children and adults. Signs of deficiency are commonly found in children because of increased requirements, decreased stores, decreased exposure to the sun, or use of sunscreens. In elderly patients, deficiencies are created by consuming inadequate diets with little exposure to the sun, reduced skin thickness, inability of the kidney to convert vitamin D to its active form, or inadequate absorption of vitamin D from the gastrointestinal tract. Plasma vitamin D is significantly lower in older patients than among the younger population; it is consistently higher for older men than women. A health care provider may recommend vitamin D and calcium supplements to older patients to prevent osteoporosis. When supplementation is recommended, care must be used to prevent toxic overdoses. Vitamin D deficiency is associated with muscle weakness, causing older individuals to tire easily and experience difficulty climbing stairs and rising from a chair. This muscle weakness frequently results in falls.

Rickets. Laboratory values indicating serum calcium or phosphorus above or below normal values, the failure of bones to grow properly in length, and radiographs showing abnormal **epiphyses** (the terminal end or growth points of bones) indicate deficiencies

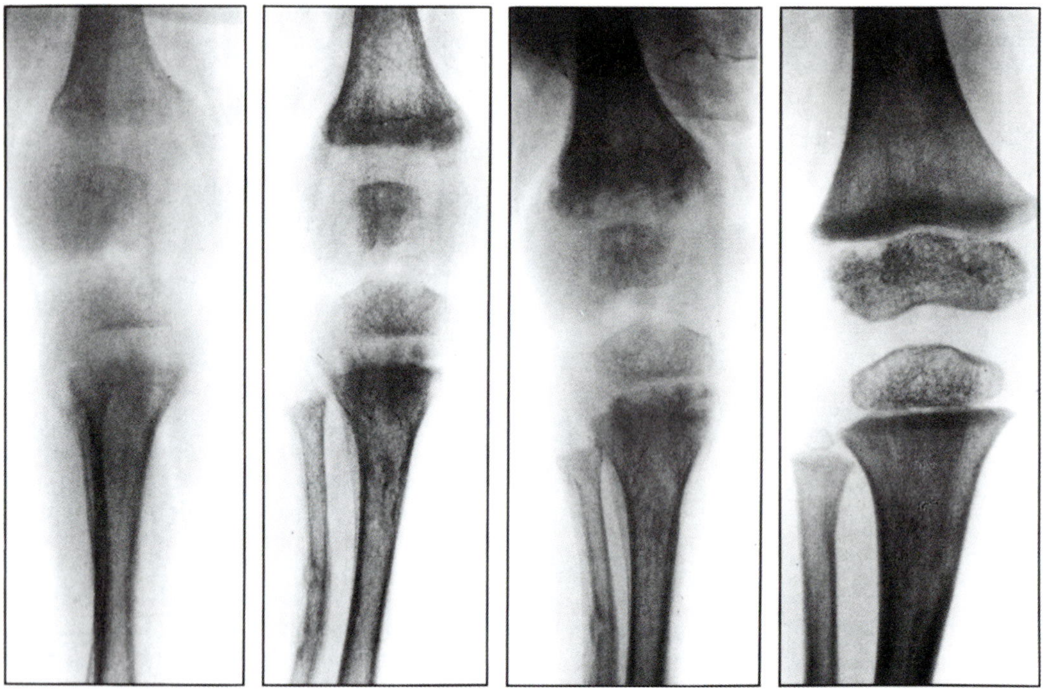

• **Figure 8.8** Active rickets of the knees. The metaphyses of the bones are concave and irregular, and the zone of uncalcified osteoid is enlarged. These radiographs show the progressive changes over 10 months, during which healing took place in this case. (Courtesy of Prof. A. Prader. From McLaren DS. *A Colour Atlas and Text of Diet-Related Disorders*. 2nd ed. London: Mosby–Year Book; 1992.)

(Fig. 8.8). Because vitamin D is intricately related to calcium and phosphorus functions, a change in any of these three nutrients affects the others.

The name *rickets* came from the word *wrikken,* meaning "to bend or twist." Rickets, caused by vitamin D deficiency, usually occurs in children 1 to 3 years old and is characterized by weak bones and skeletal deformities. Rachitic deformities such as bowlegs or knock-knees develop (Fig. 8.9A). The epiphyses of bones do not develop normally in children with this condition; thus, bones are twisted and warped. Other bone changes include a row of beadlike protuberances (rachitic rosary) on each side of the narrow, distorted chest (pigeon breast) at the juncture of the ribs and costal cartilage (Fig. 8.9B). A narrow pelvis, making future childbearing difficult in women, is also observed.

Rickets develops during a time of extremely rapid growth when children have had only a brief period to acquire vitamin D stores. Adequate intake of vitamin D during pregnancy and lactation is important because vitamin D is passed from the mother to the infant before birth and in breast milk. However, adequate vitamin D cannot be met solely by breastfeeding. Rickets is being diagnosed in the United States more frequently because of rising numbers of breastfed infants, lack of sun exposure, or use of sunscreens.[15,16]

The alveolar bone is affected similar to other bones in the body when rickets occurs. The trabeculae of the alveolar bone also weaken. Delayed dentition and small molars are observed in infants and children who are vitamin D deficient.

Enamel Hypoplasia and Dental Decay. A landmark study conducted in 1973 reported the possibility of increased risk of enamel hypoplasia in children of mothers experiencing vitamin D deficiency during pregnancy.[17] In addition, a few patients with evidence of rickets develop enamel hypoplasia as a result of a lack of vitamin D. Whether these teeth are more susceptible to dental caries is uncertain. The enamel does not seem to be weakened, but the rougher surface may facilitate adherence of dental biofilm and food residue. Finally, the research findings regarding an association between vitamin D status and dental decay indicate a possible association.[18-19]

Periodontitis. A deficiency in vitamin D could influence periodontal status. Studies suggest an association of adequate vitamin D intake with an overall healthier periodontium with less inflammation and a decreased risk of tooth loss.[20] Vitamin D inadequacy may also impact wound healing, causing negative treatment outcomes following periodontal surgery.[20]

Osteomalacia. Vitamin D deficiency in adults can lead to osteomalacia; it is also intricately related to calcium intake. Osteomalacia is characterized by decreased bone mineralization or softening of the bones, which may lead to deformities of the limbs, spine, thorax, and pelvis. The main symptoms are skeletal pain and muscle weakness, resulting in kyphosis, or an uneven gait. Oral manifestations include loss of the lamina dura around the roots of the teeth. The condition is more prevalent in women of childbearing age with calcium depletion because of multiple pregnancies or inadequate intake or in women who have little exposure to sun.

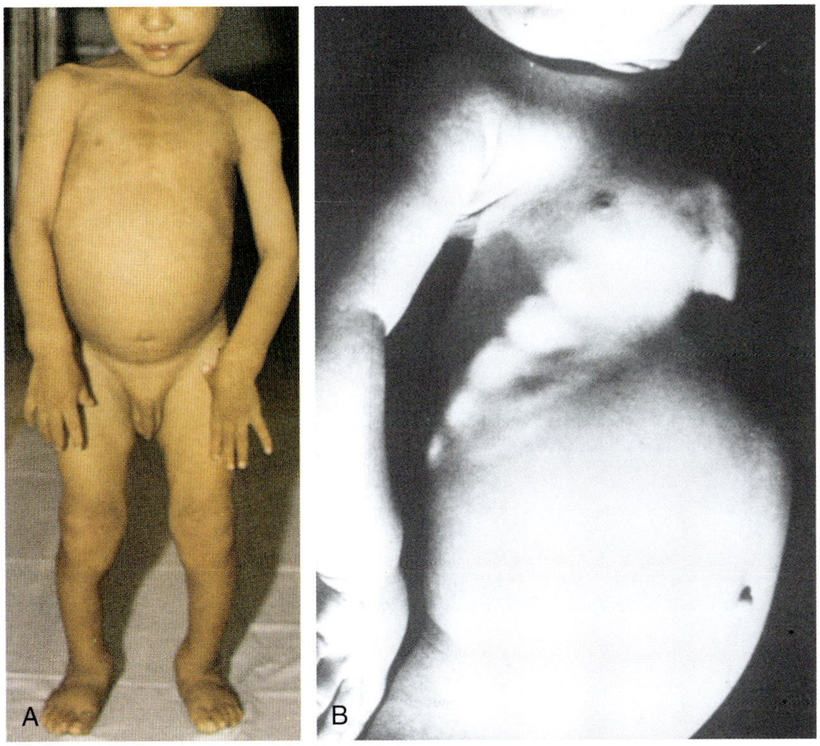

• **Figure 8.9** (A) Bowlegs in rickets. The typical lateral curvature indicates that the weakened bones have bent after the second year as a result of standing. (B) Rachitic rosary in a young infant. (A from McLaren DS. *A Colour Atlas and Text of Diet-Related Disorders*. 2nd ed. London: Mosby–Year Book; 1992. B from Kliegman RM, Stanton BMD, St. Geme J, Schor NF. *Nelson Textbook Of Pediatrics*. 20th ed, Philadelphia: Elsevier; 2016.)

A health care provider or RDN may recommend a vitamin D supplement and/or a calcium supplement with vitamin D to maximize absorption of calcium, especially for women who are at high risk for osteoporosis because of small frame size. Medication may also be prescribed to prevent further deterioration of bone mineral density.

Osteoporosis. Osteoporosis was previously thought to be a calcium deficiency, but research indicates that vitamin D levels are as important as calcium intake. As discussed previously, vitamin D deficiency interferes with mineralization of the skeleton, reducing bone density and increasing risk of bone fractures. Osteoporosis is a disease characterized by fragile bones and is associated with an increased incidence of bone fractures, especially the hip. Supplementation of vitamin D and calcium may lead to a reduction in the risk of future fractures and provides an even better protection to those at greatest risk of a deficiency of these nutrients.[21,22] Osteoporosis is discussed further in *Health Application 9*.

Cancer and Cardiovascular Risks. Laboratory, animal, and epidemiologic evidence suggests that vitamin D may be protective against some cancers. Numerous studies indicate that higher vitamin levels in blood are associated with reduced prostate, colon and colorectal cancers, and breast cancer.[23,24] The relationship of vitamin D and cancer is uncertain; evidence is based on limited data, and more studies are needed to determine optimal levels and intakes of vitamin D to reduce cancer risk.

Vitamin D may also be important for heart health. Evidence suggests that vitamin D may be related to a reduced risk of CVD. Individuals with lower blood levels of vitamin D had an increased risk of CVD. More research is needed to determine just how vitamin D affects these conditions and how much vitamin D is needed to prevent CVD.[25]

DENTAL CONSIDERATIONS

- Assess for vitamin D toxicity and deficiency, especially in young children, pregnant and lactating women, and older adults.
- Vitamin D supplements should be given only in prescribed amounts based on laboratory values because patients vary widely in their susceptibility to vitamin D toxicity. Do not recommend that patients buy vitamin D supplements. Refer them to a health care provider or RDN.
- If supplemental doses of vitamin D are used, cloudiness or a red color of the urine may indicate toxicity and should be brought to the health care provider's attention.
- Conditions leading to vitamin D deficiency include any abnormalities that (a) interfere with intestinal absorption (e.g., diarrhea, steatorrhea, celiac disease, Crohn disease, and cystic fibrosis), and (b) abnormalities in calcium balance and bone metabolism caused by disease states such as renal failure. Evaluate the patient's health status for risk of vitamin D deficiency.

DENTAL CONSIDERATIONS—cont'd

- Patients with minimal or no exposure to sunlight should be monitored for adequate vitamin D intake or supplementation or both to maintain adequate vitamin D stores. Question the patient regarding living environment or hobbies to determine exposure to sunlight.
- Determine the use of sunscreens. Consistent use of sunscreens may contribute to vitamin D deficiency in some patients. Sunscreens with a sun protection factor of 8 or greater block the UV rays from the sun necessary to produce vitamin D.
- Medications that have the potential to interact with vitamin D supplements include corticosteroids (e.g., prednisone), used to minimize inflammation; orlistat, used for weight loss; cholestyramine (e.g., Questran), used to lower cholesterol; and phenobarbital and phenytoin (e.g., Dilantin), used to prevent and control epileptic seizures.
- Calcitriol regulates the rate of calcium and phosphorus resorption from bone.
- Low skeletal bone mass may also be associated with periodontal bone loss and tooth loss.

NUTRITIONAL DIRECTIONS

- The bright sunlight between 11 AM and 2 PM offers maximum conversion. For light-skinned individuals, 10 to 20 minutes of daily sun exposure results in adequate conversion.
- Toxicity may result from excess intake of cod liver oil or from taking excessive vitamin D supplements.
- Older individuals, especially individuals living in a long-term care facility, are at high risk for vitamin D deficiency.
- Provide meal or snack ideas to include fortified cereal with fortified low-fat milk; raw vegetables with a fortified yogurt dip; or topping a salad with salmon.
- Encourage patients to consume adequate amounts of fruits and vegetables, exercise, discontinue tobacco use, and drink alcohol only in moderation for overall health.

TABLE 8.5 National Academy of Medicine Recommendations for α-Tocopherol[a]

Life Stage	EAR (mg/day)	RDA (mg/day)	AI (mg/day)	UL (mg/day)
0–6 months			4	ND[b]
7–12 months			6	ND[b]
1–3 years	5	6		200
4–8 years	6	7		300
9–13 years	9	11		600
14–18 years	12	15		800
19–70 years	12	15		1000
> 70 years	12	15		1000
Pregnancy				
≤ 18 years	12	15		800
19–50	12	15		1000
Lactation				
≤ 18 years	16	19		800
19–50 years	16	19		1000

AI, Adequate intake; EAR, estimated average requirement; RDA, recommended dietary allowance; UL, upper intake level.

Data from Institute of Medicine (IOM), Food and Nutrition Board. *Dietary Reference Intakes for Vitamin A, Vitamin K, Arsenic, Boron, Chromium, Copper, Iodine, Iron, Manganese, Molybdenum, Nickel, Silicon, Vanadium, and Zinc.* Washington, DC: National Academy Press; 2001.

[a]α-Tocopherol includes the only form of α-tocopherol that occurs naturally in foods and some of the forms that occur in fortified foods and supplements but not all forms because some that are used in fortified foods and supplements have not been shown to meet human requirements.

[b]ND: Not determinable because of lack of data of adverse effects in this age group and concern about lack of ability to handle excess amounts. Source of intake should be from food and formula to prevent high levels of intake.

Vitamin E (Tocopherol)

Eight different compounds are collectively called vitamin E: four **tocopherols** and four **tocotrienols**. Biologic activity of each form varies; α-tocopherol is the most active form and is used more efficiently by the body.

Physiologic Roles

Vitamin E is the most important fat-soluble antioxidant. Vitamin E protects the integrity of normal cell membranes and effectively prevents hemolysis of red blood cells. It also protects vitamins A and C, beta-carotene, and unsaturated fatty acids from oxidation. Vitamin E supplementation improves the immune response in healthy older adults; this effect may be mediated by increases in **prostaglandins**, which enhance growth of white blood cells. These functions promote resistance of the periodontium to inflammation. In larger amounts, vitamin E is an **anticoagulant**, or blood thinner. The role of vitamin E as an antioxidant is discussed further in *Health Application 8*.

Requirements

The DRIs for vitamin E (AI, RDA, and UL) are based solely on the α-tocopherol form because humans are unable to convert and use other forms. The RDA for vitamin E is 15 mg of α-tocopherol for healthy individuals 14 years old and older except for lactating women (Table 8.5). One milligram of α-tocopherol is the same as 1.5 IU. High intakes of polyunsaturated fatty acids increase the vitamin E requirement. Most polyunsaturated oils contain vitamin E, but chemical reactions may have rendered the antioxidant ineffective. If an individual's systemic stores are low, the vitamin E requirement is increased.

The daily UL is 1000 mg of α-tocopherol (1500 IU of natural vitamin E is equivalent to 1000 IU of synthetic vitamin E). The UL was established because of the adverse health effect of bleeding problems. Supplemental amounts in excess of the RDA should not be recommended.

Sources

Vitamin E is available from vegetable oils and margarine made from them; whole-grain or fortified cereals; wheat germ; nuts; green leafy vegetables; and some fruits. Meats, fish, and animal fats contain very little vitamin E. Milk may be fortified with vitamin E. Table 8.6 lists the amounts of vitamin E in some foods. Because vitamin E is widely distributed in foods, dietary deficiencies seldom occur if a well-balanced, varied diet is consumed.

TABLE 8.6 Food Sources of Vitamin E

Food	Portion	Vitamin E (mg)
Wheat germ oil	1 tbsp	20.3
Total whole-grain cereal	1 cup	18.0
Sunflower seeds	¼ cup	8.4
Almonds	1 oz	6.7
Special K cereal	1 cup	4.7
Safflower oil	1 tbsp	4.6
Hazelnuts	1 oz	4.3
Avocado	1 medium	4.2
Tomato sauce, canned	1 cup	3.5
Canola oil	1 tbsp	2.4
Peanut oil	1 tbsp	2.1
Peanut butter	2 tbsp	2.0
Peanuts	1 oz	2.0
Spinach, cooked	½ cup	1.9
Apricot, sliced	1 cup	1.5
Mango, cut	1 cup	1.5
Tomato juice, canned	1 cup	1.4
Margarine	1 tbsp	1.3
Mustard greens, cooked	½ cup	1.3
Sweet potato, baked	1 large	1.3
Soybean oil	1 tbsp	1.1
Ground beef, cooked	3 oz	0.0

Data from U.S. Department of Agriculture (USDA), Agricultural Research Service. *USDA National Nutrient Database for Standard Reference, Release 28*. 2016. https://ndb.nal.usda.gov/ndb/. Accessed January 13, 2017.

Absorption and Excretion

Absorption of vitamin E is inefficient, ranging from 20% to 80% in healthy individuals. Efficiency of absorption depends on the body's ability to absorb fat and seems to decline as the amount of dietary vitamin E increases.

Hyper States and Hypo States

Scientific studies suggest that this antioxidant may reduce the risk of CVD, some types of cancer, cataracts, age-related macular degeneration, and Parkinson and Alzheimer diseases. However, evidence is inconclusive that vitamin E reduces the risk of CVD and other chronic diseases. Vitamin E supplements do not seem to reverse any disease, including cancer.[26]

Higher doses of vitamin E may disturb the balance of beneficial, naturally occurring antioxidants. Individuals who may benefit from vitamin E supplementation are premature infants; infants, children, or adults who cannot absorb fats and oils because of diseases in the gastrointestinal tract; individuals with sickle cell anemia; smokers; and individuals consuming an extremely low-fat diet. Low vitamin E levels in the blood are associated with subsequent decline in physical function, but normal levels of vitamin E can be maintained by consuming vitamin E–rich foods.[27]

DENTAL CONSIDERATIONS

- Vitamin E may help the immune system function better; thus, assess intake of vitamin E in immunocompromised patients.
- Vitamin E supplementation may be of special concern for patients with vitamin K deficiency or with known coagulation defects, or for patients receiving anticoagulation therapy, which interferes with vitamin K activity, because it can increase risk for hemorrhaging.
- Naturally occurring α-tocopherol from foods is twice as potent as the synthetic form, making it a more desirable choice than synthetic supplements.
- In dietary supplements, synthetic vitamin E is labeled as "dl" α-tocopherol and "D" α-tocopherol to indicate a natural source of vitamin E.

NUTRITIONAL DIRECTIONS

- When oils are reused in frying, heavy losses of vitamin E occur.
- An increase in fruits and vegetables provides more low-fat sources of vitamin E.
- Because of widespread publicity of scientific studies linking vitamin E to decreased risk of heart disease, diabetes, cancer, Alzheimer disease, and cognitive decline, many patients may choose to use supplements. Advise patients to limit vitamin E supplements to the RDA unless they are instructed otherwise by their health care provider.
- Adverse effects of excessive amounts of vitamin E are associated with vitamin E supplements only; food sources of vitamin E are not associated with adverse reactions.
- If vitamin E supplements are recommended by a health care provider or RDN, they should be consumed with a meal containing fat to assist with absorption.[27]
- Vitamin E supplements cannot replace other proven and effective ways to reduce disease risks: not smoking, getting regular exercise, maintaining a healthy weight, and eating a well-balanced, healthy diet.

Vitamin K (Quinone)

Three forms of vitamin K, a fat-soluble vitamin, have been identified, all belonging to a group of chemical compounds known as quinones. The naturally occurring vitamins are K_1 (phylloquinone), which occurs in green plants, and K_2 (menaquinone), which is formed by *Escherichia coli* bacteria in the large intestine and is found in animal tissues. The fat-soluble synthetic compound menadione (vitamin K_3) is two to three times as potent as the natural vitamin.

Physiologic Roles

Vitamin K–dependent proteins have been identified in bone, kidney, and other tissues. Vitamin K_2 activates vitamin K-dependent proteins, activating osteocalciun (protein rquired to bind calcium to the mineral matrix), thus strengthening bone and may also slow

TABLE 8.7 National Academy of Medicine Recommendations for Vitamin K

	AI	
Life Stage	**Male (μg/day)**	**Female (μg/day)**
0–6 months	2	2
7–12 months	2.5	2.5
1–3 years	30	30
4–8 years	55	55
9–13 years	60	60
14–18 years	75	75
> 18 years	120	90
Pregnancy		
≤ 18 years		75
19–50 years		90
Lactation		
≤ 18 years		75
19–50 years		90

Data from Institute of Medicine (IOM), Food and Nutrition Board. *Dietary Reference Intakes for Vitamin A, Vitamin K, Arsenic, Boron, Chromium, Copper, Iodine, Iron, Manganese, Molybdenum, Nickel, Silicon, Vanadium, and Zinc.* Washington, DC: National Academy Press; 2001.

loss of bone. Vitamin K functions as a catalyst in synthesis of blood-clotting factors, primarily in maintaining **prothrombin** levels, which is the first stage in forming a clot. A low prothrombin level results in impaired blood coagulation.

Requirements

The RDA is 120 μg for men and 90 μg for women. No UL for vitamin K has been established (Table 8.7).

Sources

Although limited amounts of vitamin K are stored in the body, a shortage of vitamin K is unlikely because it is derived from food and microflora in the gut. Green leafy vegetables are high in vitamin K, but meats are also a source (Table 8.8).

Bacterial flora in the jejunum and ileum synthesize vitamin K and provide about half of the body's requirement. However, synthesis of vitamin K by intestinal bacteria does not provide adequate amounts of the vitamin; therefore, a restriction of dietary vitamin K can alter clotting factors.

Absorption and Excretion

Vitamin K absorption decreases with high levels of vitamin E supplementation. Some vitamin K is stored in the liver, and some becomes a component of lipoproteins. Ordinarily, 30% to 40% of the amount absorbed is excreted via bile into the feces as water-soluble metabolites, with approximately 15% excreted in the urine.

TABLE 8.8 Food Sources of Vitamin K

Food	Portion	Vitamin K (μg)
Kale, cooked	½ cup	531
Spinach, cooked	½ cup	444
Mustard greens, cooked	½ cup	415
Collard greens, cooked	½ cup	386
Broccoli, cooked	½ cup	110
Brussels sprouts, cooked	½ cup	109
Cabbage, raw	1 cup	53
Asparagus, cooked	½ cup	46
Ground beef, cooked	3 oz	2
Pot roast, cooked	3 oz	1.4

Data from U.S. Department of Agriculture (USDA), Agricultural Research Service. *USDA National Nutrient Database for Standard Reference, Release 28.* 2016. https://ndb.nal.usda.gov/ndb/. Accessed January 23, 2017.

Hyper States and Hypo States

No toxicity symptoms have been documented from oral intake of vitamin K. However, synthetic menadione (vitamin K_3) has caused toxic effects.

Primary vitamin K deficiency is uncommon, but disease or drug therapy may cause deficiencies. Effects of vitamin K deficiency are most pronounced in bone, cartilage, and arteries. Any condition of the biliary tract affecting the flow of bile prevents vitamin K absorption. Vitamin K deficiency is common in celiac disease and sprue, which affect absorption in the small intestine, and other diarrheal diseases (e.g., ulcerative colitis) as a result of malabsorption. In vitamin K deficiency or in patients taking anticoagulants, blood-clotting time is delayed, increasing the risk of bleeding problems. Newborns may develop hemorrhagic disease secondary to vitamin K deficiency because the gut is sterile during the first few days after birth. Newborns are usually given a single dose of vitamin K intramuscularly immediately after birth to prevent hemorrhage.

DENTAL CONSIDERATIONS

- Excessive amounts of vitamin A or E or both have a detrimental effect on vitamin K absorption.
- Mineral oil interferes with absorption of vitamin K and should not be consumed close to a meal.
- Vitamin K should never be confused with the symbol "K," which is used to designate potassium or kosher foods. If information is confusing or unclear, double-check with a health care provider or RDN.
- Vitamin K may be used prophylactically before any oral surgery to prevent prolonged bleeding in patients who have a condition that inhibits clotting.
- Frequently, blood-thinning agents may be discontinued for several days before any oral surgery to prevent excessive bleeding, or the patient may be hospitalized for a few days.

DENTAL CONSIDERATIONS—cont'd

- Cholestyramine prescribed for hyperlipidemia binds with bile salts. The presence of bile is required for vitamin K absorption. Patients taking cholestyramine are at risk of vitamin K deficiency; thus, assess for bleeding problems, such as **petechiae** (pinpoint, flat red spots) or ecchymosis (bruising).
- Antibiotic therapy inhibits vitamin K–producing intestinal microflora and seems to be a factor in the origin of vitamin K deficiency, especially with impaired hepatic or renal function.
- Patients receiving oral anticoagulants (usually warfarin) to prevent blood clots from forming may develop serious hemorrhaging problems. They should keep vitamin K intake consistent and should not consume vitamin K supplements.

NUTRITIONAL DIRECTIONS

- A lack of vitamin K may lead to bleeding problems.
- Vitamin K is stable to heat; cooking does not affect the vitamin K content of foods.

Vitamin C (Ascorbic Acid)

Physiologic Roles

As a coenzyme, vitamin C has numerous metabolic roles. It is important in the production of **collagen** (the primary structural protein in connective tissue, cartilage, and bone), which plays a vital role in wound healing. During the development of connective tissue, bones, and teeth, vitamin C is important in the formation of **fibroblasts** (collagen-forming cells), osteoblasts, and odontoblasts. Vitamin C strengthens tissues and promotes capillary integrity. Vitamin C facilitates development of red blood cells by enhancing iron absorption and use. It also aids the body in utilizing folate and vitamin B_{12}. It has a coenzymatic function in the metabolism of amino acids and biosynthesis of bile acids, thyroxine, epinephrine, and steroid hormones. Vitamin C can also affect immune responses because of its high concentration in white blood cells.

Vitamin C functions as an antioxidant in numerous physiologic reactions. In its role as an antioxidant, it protects cells and tissues against damage caused by free radicals, toxic chemicals, and pollutants. More details on the role of vitamin C as an antioxidant are found in *Health Application 8*.

Requirements

The RDA is established at 90 mg daily for men and 75 mg daily for women, increasing during pregnancy and lactation (Table 8.9). The requirement for vitamin C is increased under many situations in which it is directly involved (e.g., stress, healing, and infections). It is detrimentally affected by many drugs (e.g., tobacco, alcohol, oral contraceptives, and aspirin), which increase requirements, and is usually the first nutrient to be depleted. Smokers may benefit from an additional intake of 35 mg per day because they are more likely to experience biologic processes that damage cells and deplete vitamin C. The UL is 2000 mg per day.

TABLE 8.9 National Academy of Medicine Recommendations for Vitamin C

	EAR (mg/day)		RDA (mg/day)		AI (mg/day)		
Life Stage	Male	Female	Male	Female	Male	Female	UL (mg/day)
0–6 months					40	50	ND[a]
7–12 months					50	50	ND[a]
1–3 years	13	13	15	15			400
4–8 years	22	22	25	25			650
9–13 years	39	39	45	45			1200
14–18 years	63	56	75	65			1800
19–70 years	75	60	90	75			2000
> 70 years	75	60	90	75			2000
Pregnancy							
≤ 18 years		66		80			1800
19–50 years		70		85			2000
Lactation							
≤ 18 years		96		115			1800
19–50 years		100		120			2000

AI, Adequate intake; EAR, estimated average requirement; RDA, recommended dietary allowance; UL, upper intake level.
Data from Institute of Medicine (IOM), Food and Nutrition Board. *Dietary Reference Intakes for Vitamin C, Vitamin E, Selenium, and Carotenoids.* Washington, DC: National Academy Press; 2000.
[a]Not determinable because of lack of data on adverse effects in this age group and concern about lack of ability to handle excess amounts. Source of intake should be from food and formula to prevent high levels of intake.

TABLE 8.10 Food Sources of Vitamin C

Food	Portion	Vitamin C (mg)
Papaya	1 large	476
Red sweet pepper, raw	1 large	206
Tomato juice, canned	1 cup	170
Guava	1	126
Orange juice	1 cup	124
Mango	1	122
Strawberries, sliced	1 cup	98
Grapefruit	1	77
Orange	1	83
Pineapple, chunks	1 cup	59
Kiwi	1	64
Cantaloupe	1 cup	59
Broccoli, cooked	½ cup	51
Brussels sprouts, cooked	½ cup	48
Potato, baked	1 large	38
Sweet potato, baked	1 large	35
Cauliflower, cooked	½ cup	28
Cabbage, raw	1 cup	26
Tomato	1 large	25
Turnip greens, cooked	½ cup	20
Tomato sauce, canned	1 cup	17

Data from U.S. Department of Agriculture (USDA), Agricultural Research Service. *USDA National Nutrient Database for Standard Reference, Release 28.* 2016. https://ndb.nal.usda.gov/ndb/. Accessed January 23, 2017.

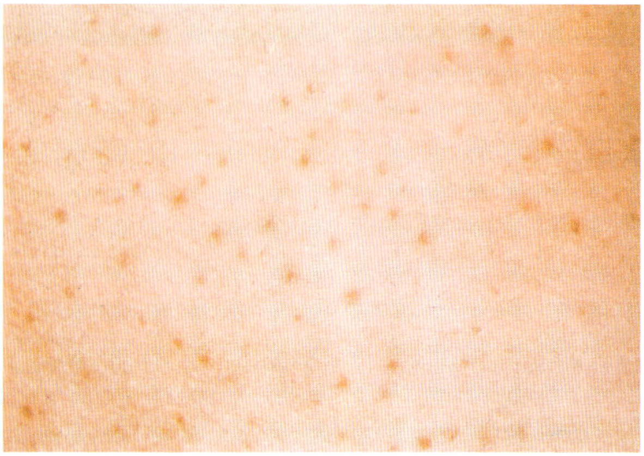

• **Figure 8.10** Perifollicular petechiae. Minimal bleeding into the hair follicles is often one of the earliest clinical manifestations of vitamin C deficiency. (Courtesy of Dr. H. H. Sandstead. From McLaren DS. *A Colour Atlas and Text of Diet-Related Disorders*. 2nd ed. London: Mosby–Year Book; 1992.)

Sources

The RDA can usually be met by choosing one serving daily of foods known as an excellent source of vitamin C (e.g., citrus fruits and juices, cantaloupe, green and red peppers, broccoli, kiwi, strawberries, and papaya). Good sources include peaches, cabbage, potatoes, sweet potatoes, and tomatoes; at least two servings of these sources a day may be required to meet the RDA (Table 8.10).

Hyper States and Hypo States

Intakes exceeding the UL of 2000 mg may result in stomach upset and diarrhea, and interfere with vitamin B_{12} absorption.

Health care professionals in the United States generally consider vitamin C deficiency, or scurvy, to be a disease of historical significance only. Many Americans exceed the RDAs for vitamin C. However, smokers have an elevated risk of vitamin C deficiency.

Scurvy, caused by vitamin C deficiency, can occur in 20 days. It is characterized by spontaneous gingival hemorrhaging perifollicular petechiae (see Fig. 8.10), follicular hyperkeratosis, diarrhea, fatigue, depression, and cessation of bone growth.

Inadequate amounts of vitamin C during tooth development may cause changes in ameloblasts and odontoblasts, resulting in **scorbutic** changes in the teeth or changes similar to those caused by scurvy. Atrophy of ameloblasts and odontoblasts leads to a decrease in their orderly polar arrangement in a vitamin C–deficient environment. Any new dentin deposits forming at this time are similar to **osteodentin** (dentin that resembles bone); the pulp also atrophies and is hyperemetic. Dentin deposits completely cease in severe vitamin C deficiency, with hypercalcification of predentin. Dentinal tubules also lack their normal parallel arrangement. In scorbutic adults, the dentin reabsorbs and is porotic.

Gingivitis, caused by ascorbic acid deficiency, also affects the periodontium, resulting in tooth mobility. This effect is probably related to weakened collagen secondary to vitamin C deficiency, which results in resorption of the alveolar bone (Fig. 8.11).

DENTAL CONSIDERATIONS

- Older patients (especially those who live alone or who avoid acidic foods to control gastroesophageal reflux), patients undergoing peritoneal dialysis or hemodialysis, smokers, and drug abusers are at greatest risk to become scorbutic. Assess for deficiency: periodontal disease, deep-red to purple gingiva, hyperplasia, bleeding on probing, reported nosebleeds, melena (stools containing blood), vomiting, and petechiae (especially lower legs and back).
- Adequate vitamin C intake can slow the progression of a common cold. There is no clear evidence that amounts above the RDA of vitamin C will reduce the frequency or severity of a cold.
- Vitamin C chewable tablets, syrup, or cough drops are associated with enamel erosion and dentin hypersensitivity.
- Steroids, antibiotics, and salicylates can increase excretion of vitamin C.
- Deficient vitamin C intake (5 mg or less per day) increases the propensity of the gingiva to become inflamed or bleed on probing, but serum levels and gingiva return to normal with an intake of 65 mg per day.[28]
- Evaluate vitamin C intake because low levels may affect the severity of periodontal disease.[29]

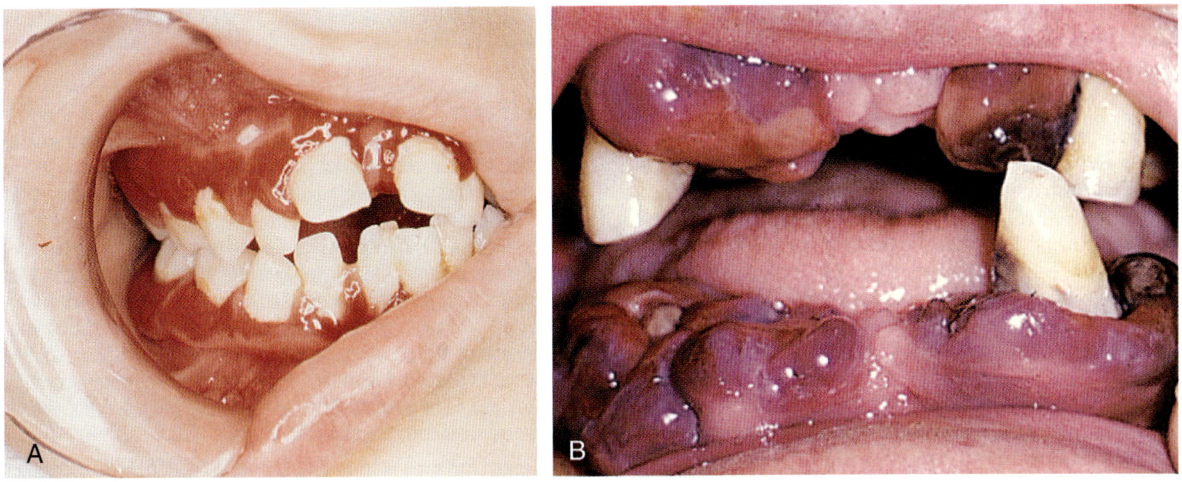

• **Figure 8.11** (A) Ascorbic acid deficiency. The gingiva is bright red and edematous. The earliest changes involve the interdental papillae, which swell and tend to bleed easily. (B) Effects on the periodontium result in tooth mobility (Note the bluish red gingiva). (Reproduced with permission from Swartz MH. *Textbook of Physical Diagnosis: History and Examination*. 7th ed. St Louis, MO: Saunders Elsevier; 2014.)

NUTRITIONAL DIRECTIONS

- Vitamin C requirements are readily available from small amounts of food. One cup of orange juice contains 124 mg of vitamin C, which is enough vitamin C for healthy nonsmoking adults.
- Patients who smoke need an additional 35 mg of vitamin C daily; a man who smokes should consume 125 mg instead of 90 mg of vitamin C each day. (Refer patients who smoke to a smoking cessation program, as discussed in Chapter 19, *Health Application 19*.)
- Deficiency symptoms may develop within 20 to 30 days after dietary elimination of vitamin C.
- Vitamin C is sensitive to heat, light, and oxidation. Proper storage is important to retain vitamin C.
- Fruit juices should be kept in an airtight container that is appropriate for the amount stored. For example, 2 cups of juice in a pint container with an airtight lid protects the vitamin C content better than 1 pint of juice in a gallon container.
- Cut fruits and vegetables in as large pieces as possible to decrease the surface area allowing nutrient loss. The pieces should be stored in a tightly covered container in the refrigerator. Minimize the time that they are exposed to air.
- Cook fruits and vegetables for a limited amount of time in a limited amount of water in a tightly covered device or steamed in a basket with the water below. The more water added for cooking, the more ascorbic acid leaches out of the fruit or vegetable.
- Use quick cooking methods, such as stir frying or a microwave.
- Ascorbic acid is another name for vitamin C.
- Acidic fruits and vegetables retain their ascorbic acid content better than nonacidic foods.
- Megadoses of vitamin C (2000 mg or greater per day) can interfere with vitamin B_{12} and copper use.

Apparently, the image of antioxidants as valiant warriors protecting the body from rampaging free radicals is too simplistic. The American Heart Association does not recommend antioxidant supplements, waiting for more convincing data.[30] Because of the lay press publicity surrounding the potential health benefits, many Americans are taking some form of antioxidant supplement to prevent chronic diseases.

High-intake levels of some antioxidants are well tolerated by most individuals, but several known factors must be considered before recommending supplements. Toxic effects occur with vitamin A; organ damage and deaths have been reported. Vitamin E supplements can antagonize vitamin K activity and enhance the effect of anticoagulant drugs. Adverse effects of vitamin C include diarrhea, increased risk of kidney stones, and decreased absorption of vitamin B_{12}. Although vitamin C increases iron absorption, large amounts decrease availability of vitamin B_{12} and copper. Erosion and hypersensitivity of tooth enamel are unique adverse effects of chewable vitamin C tablets. Simultaneous intake of carotenoids with α-tocopherol may inhibit the absorption of vitamin E. Possibly unexplored interactions may occur between large amounts of antioxidants and other nutrients. If a patient chooses to take vitamin C supplements, there is no benefit in taking more expensive ones, such as products containing bioflavonoids, over simple ascorbic acid.

Antioxidants may counteract the effects of cell damage produced by metabolic reactions and environmental factors such as pollution, smoking, and toxic chemicals in the diet. However, the health toll of a smoking habit is not corrected by simply eating right or taking vitamins (see Chapter 19, *Health Application 19*). Recommendations for supplemental amounts of these nutrients should be reserved for claims that have been well substantiated by clinical trials that prove cause and effect and explore related side effects. Patients should also be cautioned about taking megadoses of vitamins and minerals because side effects, nutrient–nutrient interactions, and drug–nutrient interactions can occur. Individuals who are seriously ill with cancer, CVD, or other conditions should talk with their health care provider about everything they put into their bodies, including vitamins, supplements, or herbs.

The *Dietary Guidelines* emphasize consumption of a varied diet to help prevent several chronic diseases. Dietary patterns high in fruits and vegetables are associated with a lower risk of disease. Advice to patients should be to eat a healthy diet that includes many fruits and vegetables, especially those that are high in vitamins C and E, and beta-carotene. A pill cannot provide what is available from a healthful diet—thus, the bottom line is to "eat your fruits and veggies." Antioxidant supplements cannot be expected to undo a

HEALTH APPLICATION 8

Antioxidants

Free radicals are highly unstable and reactive molecular fragments. They contain one or more unpaired electrons, which try to gain electrons to become more stable. During this process, the free radicals oxidize (damage) body cells. UV radiation from the sun, air pollution, ozone, and smoking are just a few conditions that can generate free radicals in the body. Antioxidants donate electrons to the free radicals to make them stable. This protects body cells from damage. The antioxidant is oxidized and destroyed. In some situations, an antioxidant can regain or regenerate an electron to allow it to function.

Although antioxidants have some properties in common, each one has unique properties. The best sources of antioxidants are beans (specifically small red, kidney, pinto, and black beans), fruits (particularly blueberries, cranberries, blackberries, plumes and prunes, raspberries, strawberries, apples, cherries, grapes, pears, bananas, kiwi, mangos, pomegranates, and pineapple), vegetables (especially potatoes, artichokes, okra, kale, and bell peppers), nuts (walnuts, pecans, pistachio, and almonds), dark chocolate, coffee and tea, and red wine.

Much has been learned about the functions of vitamins C and E, beta-carotene, and other phytochemicals (biologically active substances found in plants), and the minerals selenium, zinc, copper, and manganese in their roles as antioxidants. Numerous studies have suggested that antioxidants may be important in preventing CVD, cancer, age-related eye disease, and other chronic conditions associated with aging. Ascorbic acid is one of the strongest antioxidants and radical scavengers, serving as a primary defense against free radicals in the blood. However, the connections between vitamin C and these processes have yet to be established. Research has proven that vitamin C and other antioxidants in amounts greater than the RDA are desirable. This is especially true if increased levels are achieved by improving food choices.

Increased serum antioxidant concentrations are associated with a reduced risk of periodontitis. Research studies with antioxidants have indicated conflicting conclusions in regard to reduction of CVD and prevention of cancers. A systematic review and **meta-analysis** found no evidence to support antioxidant supplementation prevents mortality in healthy people or patients with CVD.[31] Neither vitamin E nor vitamin C supplementation reduced the risk of major CVD.[30]

Polyphenols are antioxidants that are naturally occurring compounds found in fruits (grapes, apples, pears, cherries and berries), vegetables, cereals, legumes, chocolate, and beverages (red wine, coffee, black and green tea). There has been much interest in the potential health benefits of plant polyphenols. Diets rich in polyphenols over a period of time may contribute to a reduction in risk of certain cancers, CVD, improving blood lipid levels, diabetes, osteoporosis, and neurodegenerative diseases. More research is needed to determine an optimal level of intake of polyphenols and the association with health benefits.[32]

CASE APPLICATION FOR THE DENTAL HYGIENIST

A healthy patient asks your advice about taking vitamin C supplements to prevent periodontal disease. She is unsure what foods to eat or what to look for if an excess or deficiency develops.

Nutritional Assessment

- Income
- Living arrangements, cooking and storage facilities
- Dietary assessment
- Tobacco and other drug use
- Knowledge level about vitamin C
- Beliefs about water-soluble vitamins
- Knowledge level about periodontal disease
- Physical status, especially any bleeding problems
- Use of over-the-counter or health care provider–prescribed supplements or medications
- Emotional state

Nutritional Diagnosis

Health-seeking behavior related to inadequate/insufficient knowledge about vitamin C and periodontal disease.

Nutritional Goals

The patient will consume foods high in vitamin C and state beliefs/information about vitamin C and periodontal disease.

Nutritional Implementation

Intervention: Teach the following about vitamin C: (a) functions, (b) requirements, and (c) sources. Teach the following about periodontal disease: (a) causes and (b) preventive factors.

Rationale: This provides the patient with a sound knowledge base about vitamin C and periodontal disease.

Intervention: Explain hyper- and hypo-vitamin C states.

Rationale: Large amounts of vitamin C decrease absorption of vitamin B_{12} and cause diarrhea, gastrointestinal distress, and kidney stones. Because vitamin C helps maintain capillary integrity, a vitamin C deficiency results in bleeding problems. Encourage food sources rather than supplements for increasing vitamin C.

Intervention: Provide oral hygiene instruction.

Rationale: The primary cause of periodontal disease is plaque biofilm. Providing education to effectively remove the plaque biofilm is essential. A vitamin deficiency does not cause periodontal disease, but it could exacerbate existing periodontal issues.

Evaluation

The patient should consume citrus fruits, strawberries, cantaloupes, and mangos. Additionally, the patient states that supplements are unnecessary for vitamin C, and large doses may interfere with absorption of other nutrients. She further states that if she does develop any bleeding problems, she will seek help. Last, the patient should verbalize information concerning excesses and deficiencies of vitamin C.

lifetime of unhealthy living. Adequate intake ideally should be in the form of improving dietary selections rather than supplements because as yet unidentified components present in food may be beneficial and protective. Beyond diet, decreased exposure to free radicals and increased physical activity are essential.

Student Readiness

1. How do water-soluble vitamins differ from fat-soluble vitamins? What do these differences mean as you choose foods for your own menu? What do these differences mean as you teach patients about nutrition?
2. Which fat-soluble vitamins are toxic? What are the symptoms of toxicity?
3. A patient asks why so many foods are now fortified with vitamin D. How would you respond?
4. Plan a one-day menu that meets the RDA for vitamin E.
5. Keep a record of your food intake for one day. Use a table of nutrient values of foods (http://www.ars.usda.gov/main/main.htm) or a nutrient analysis program (https://

www.supertracker.usda.gov/default.aspx) or Nutritrac (a link on the Evolve website) to determine your vitamin A intake. Was intake adequate? What are some wiser food choices to improve nutrients that were below the RDA?
6. Prepare a menu for one day that provides adequate amounts of vitamins A and D. Eliminate all sources of milk products and canned fish. What does this do to vitamin D intake? Now, remove various types of egg products, green leafy vegetables, and dark-yellow vegetables, and see the effect on the vitamin A content of the meal plan.
7. Justify the rationale of vitamin D supplementation of milk products in the United States. What age groups benefit most from vitamin D supplementation in milk?
8. What is the role of antioxidants in cancer prevention? What foods are advocated to prevent this condition?
9. Name the deficiency and toxicity conditions associated with vitamins A, D, K, and C.
10. Name five foods other than oranges that are good sources of vitamin C.
11. In a small group, discuss the pros and cons of the controversial issue of mandatory food labeling on nutrition supplements.

References

1. Franchini LG, Warnakulasuriya S, Varoni EM, et al. Interventions for treating oral leukoplakia to prevent oral cancer (review). *Cochrane Database Syst Rev*. 2016;(7):CD001829.
2. American Cancer Society Guidelines on Nutrition and Physical Activity for Cancer Prevention. February 5, 2016. http://www.cancer.org/healthy/eathealthygetactive/acsguidelinesonnutritionphysicalactivityforcancerprevention/. Accessed December 20, 2016.
3. Institute of Medicine (IOM), Food and Nutrition Board. *Dietary Reference Intakes for Vitamin A, Vitamin K, Arsenic, Boron, Chromium, Copper, Iodine, Iron, Molybdenum, Nickel, Silicon, Vanadium, and Zinc*. Washington, DC: National Academy Press; 2001.
4. Wacker M, Holick MF. Vitamin D-effects on skeletal and extraskeletal health and the need for supplementation. *Nutrients*. 2013;5:111–148.
5. Prentice RL, Pettinger MB, Jackson RD, et al. Health risks and benefits from calcium and vitamin D supplementation: Women's Health Initiative clinical trial and cohort study. *Osteoporos Int*. 2013;24(2):567–580.
6. Au LE, Rogers GT, Harris SS, et al. Associations of vitamin D intake with 25-hydroxyvitamin D in overweight and racially/ethnically diverse US children. *J Acad Nutr Diet*. 2013;113:1511–1516.
7. Dawson-Hughes B, Mithal A, Bonjour JP, et al. IOF position statement: vitamin D recommendations for older adults. *Osteoporos Int*. 2010;21:1151–1154.
8. National Osteoporosis Foundation. NOF responds to the U.S. Preventive Services Task Force Recommendations on Calcium and Vitamin D. https://www.nof.org/patients/treatment/calciumvitamin-d/get-the-facts-on-calcium-and-vitamin-d/. Accessed January 23, 2017.
9. U.S. Preventive Services Task Force. U.S. Preventive Services Task Force Issues Final Recommendation on Vitamin D and Calcium Supplements to Prevent Fractures. https://www.uspreventiveservicestaskforce.org/Page/Document/UpdateSummaryFinal/vitamin-d-and-calcium-to-prevent-fractures-preventive-medication. Accessed January 23 2017.
10. Perrine CG, Sharma AJ, Jefferds ED, et al. Adherence to vitamin D recommendations among US infants. *Pediatrics*. 2010;125(4):627–632.
11. Institute of Medicine (IOM), Food and Nutrition Board. *Dietary Reference Intakes: Calcium and Vitamin D*. Washington, DC: National Academy Press; 2011.
12. Cianferotti L, Cricelli C, Kanis JA, et al. The clinical use of vitamin D metabolites and their potential developments: a position statement from the European Society for Clinical and Economic Aspects of Osteoporosis and Osteoarthritis (ESCEO) and the International Osteoporosis Foundation (IOF). *Endocrine*. 2015;50:12–26.
13. Office of Dietary Supplements, National Institutes of Health. Dietary supplement fact sheet: Vitamin D. https://ods.od.nih.gov/factsheets/VitaminD-HealthProfessional/. Accessed January 23, 2017.
14. Paxton GA, Teale GR, Nowson CA, et al. Vitamin D and health in pregnancy, infants, children and adolescents in Australia and New Zealand: a position statement. *Med J Aust*. 2013;198(3):1–8.
15. Wall CR, Grant CC, Jones I. Vitamin D status of exclusively breastfed infants aged 2–3 months. *Arch Dis Child*. 2013;98:176–179.
16. Purvis RJ, Barrie WJ, MacKay GS, et al. Enamel hypoplasia of the teeth associated with neonatal tetany: A manifestation of maternal vitamin D deficiency. *Lancet*. 1973;2(7833):811–814.
17. Hujoel PP. Vitamin D and dental caries in controlled clinical trials. systematic review and meta-analysis. *Nut Rev*. 2013;71(2):88–97.
18. Schroth RJ, Rabbani R, Loewen G, et al. Vitamin D and dental caries in children. *J Dent Res*. 2016;95(2):173–179.
19. Jimenez M, Giovannucci E, Kaye EK, et al. Predicted vitamin D status and incidence of tooth loss and periodontitis. *Public Health Nutr*. 2014;17(4):844–852.
20. Harvey NC, Biver E, Kaufman JM, et al. The role of calcium supplememtation in healthy musculoskeletal ageing. *Osteoporos Int*. 2017;28(2):447–462.
21. Avenell A, Mak JC, O'Connell D. Vitamin D and vitamin D analogues for preventing fractures in post-menopausal women and older men. *Cochrane Database Syst Rev*. 2014;(4):CD000227.
22. Iniesta RR, Rush R, Paciarotti I, et al. Systematic review and meta-analysis: Prevalence and possible causes of vitamin D deficiency and insufficiency in pediatric cancer patients. *Clin Nutr*. 2016;35:95–108.
23. American Cancer Society. American Cancer Society guidelines on nutrition and physical activity for cancer prevention. http://www.cancer.org/healthy/eat-healthy-get-active/acs-guidelines-nutrition-physical-activity-cancer-prevention.html. Accessed January 25, 2017.
24. Lutsey PI, Michos ED. Vitamin D, calcium, and atherosclerotic risk: evidence from serum levels and supplementation studies. *Curr Atheroscler Rep*. 2013;15:293.
25. Russnes KM, Wilson KM, Epstein MM, et al. Total antioxidant intake in relation to prostate cancer incidence in the Health Professionals Follow-Up Study. *Int J Cancer*. 2014;134(5):1156–1165.
26. Borel P, Preveraud D, Desmarchelier C. Bioavailability of vitamin E in humans: an update. *Nutr Rev*. 2013;71(6):319–331.
27. Jacob RA, Omaye ST, Skala JH, et al. Experimental vitamin C depletion and supplementation in young men: nutrient interactions and dental health effects. *Ann N Y Acad Sci*. 1987;498:333–346.
28. Brock GR, Chapple ILC. The potential impact of essential nutrients vitamins C and D upon periodontal disease pathogenesis and therapeutic outcomes. *Current Oral Health Reports*. 2016;3(4):337–346.
29. American Heart Association. Scientific Position: Vitamin and Mineral Supplements. Updated August 17, 2015. http://www.heart.org/HEARTORG/HealthyLiving/HealthyEating/Nutrition/Vitamin-and-Mineral-Supplements_UCM_306033_Article.jsp#.WJddtXpuOZA. Accessed February 5, 2017.
30. Myung SK, Woong J, Cho B, et al. Efficacy of vitamin and antioxidant supplements in prevention of cardiovascular disease: systematic review and meta-analysis of randomized controlled trials. *Br Med J*. 2013;346:f10.
31. Somerville V, Bringnans C, Braakhuis A. Polyphenols and performance; a systematic review and meta-analysis. *Sports Med*. 2017;47(8):1589–1599.

EVOLVE RESOURCES

Please visit http://evolve.elsevier.com/Stegeman/nutritional for additional practice and study support tools.

9

Minerals Essential for Calcified Structures

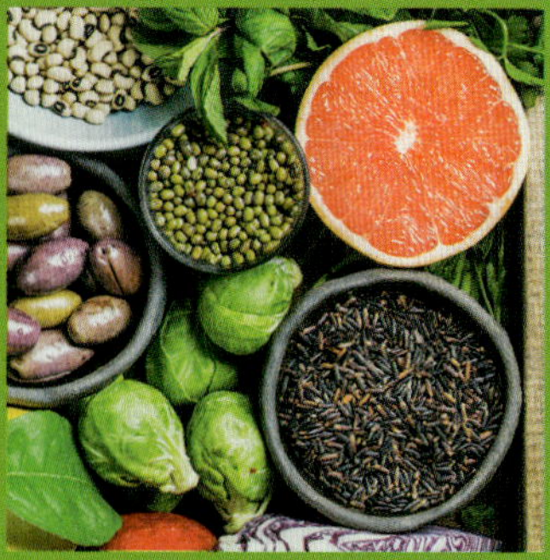

STUDENT LEARNING OUTCOMES

Upon completion of this chapter, the student will be able to achieve the following objectives:

1. Discuss the following related to bone mineralization and growth, formation of teeth, and the mineral elements of the body:
   - List the minerals found in collagen, bones, and teeth, and describe their main physiologic roles and sources.
   - List the three calcified tissues of which teeth are composed.
   - List and discuss major minerals and trace elements of the body.
2. Discuss the following related to calcium:
   - Describe the physiologic roles of calcium.
   - Discuss the RDA and estimated average requirement for calcium.
   - Discuss the importance of calcium balance in the body, and name common sources of calcium.
   - Individualize dental hygiene considerations to patients regarding calcium.
   - Discuss clinical conditions associated with excesses and deficiencies of calcium, and utilize nutritional directions to provide patient education regarding calcium.
3. Discuss the following related to phosphorus:
   - Describe the physiologic roles of phosphorus.
   - Discuss the RDA and Tolerable Upper Intake level for phosphorus.
   - Explain how dietary phosphorus is absorbed, and name common sources of phosphorus.
   - Individualize dental hygiene considerations to patients regarding phosphorus.
   - Discuss clinical conditions associated with excesses and deficiencies of phosphorus, and utilize nutritional directions to provide patient education regarding phosphorus.
4. Discuss the following related to magnesium:
   - Describe the physiologic roles of magnesium.
   - Discuss the RDA for magnesium.
   - Name common sources of magnesium.
   - Individualize dental hygiene considerations to patients regarding magnesium.
   - Discuss clinical conditions associated with excesses and deficiencies of magnesium, and utilize nutritional directions to provide patient education regarding magnesium.
5. Discuss the following related to fluoride:
   - Describe the physiologic roles of fluoride.
   - Discuss the average intake of fluoride for both men and women.
   - Name common sources of fluoride.
   - Individualize dental hygiene considerations to patients regarding fluoride.
   - Discuss clinical conditions associated with excesses and deficiencies of fluoride, and utilize nutritional directions to provide patient education regarding fluoride.
   - Discuss the role of water fluoridation in the prevention of dental caries.

KEY TERMS

Alveolar bone
Amorphous
Apatite
Bioavailability
Compressional forces
Fluorapatite
Fluorosis
Hydroxyapatite
Hypercalcemia
Hypercalciuria
Hypocalcemia
Mineralization
Osteoclasts
Osteoids
Osteoporosis
Periodontal disease
Phytochemicals
Remodeling
Rickets
Tensional forces
Tetany

TEST YOUR NQ

1. **T/F** Meats are good sources of phosphorus.
2. **T/F** The only nutrients essential for strong healthy bones are calcium and phosphorus.
3. **T/F** Tooth exfoliation may be an oral sign of osteoporosis.
4. **T/F** Systemic fluoride causes changes in tooth morphology that increase caries resistance.
5. **T/F** To obtain adequate calcium, a teenager needs to drink 2 cups of milk a day.
6. **T/F** Water fluoridation is economically inefficient because very little of the water is actually consumed.
7. **T/F** All women should take calcium supplements to prevent osteoporosis.
8. **T/F** Calcium absorption is increased when a sugar is present.
9. **T/F** Caffeine intake may decrease calcium loss.
10. **T/F** All bottled waters contain fluoride.

Bone Mineralization and Growth

Calcified structures in the body, which include bones and teeth, are composed of a matrix of organic and inorganic substances. Dentin, cementum, and bone originate with a protein matrix, or collagen deposition. Collagen is present throughout the periodontium as the primary connective tissue fiber in the gingiva and major organic constituent of alveolar bone. Collagen is continuously being remodeled (resorption and reformation of bone) throughout growth and development. Defective collagen synthesis affects formation of bones and teeth.

The organic matrix of bone is 90% to 95% collagen fibers, which are secreted by osteoblasts. Collagen formation requires the presence of a variety of substances, including protein; vitamin C; and the minerals iron, copper, and zinc. When collagen is formed, **apatite**, a calcium phosphate complex, automatically crystallizes adjacent to the collagen fibers.

In bones that have not undergone calcification, **osteoids** are formed rapidly. Most develop into the finished product, **hydroxyapatite** crystals (inorganic component of bones and teeth). The chemical formula for hydroxyapatite crystals is $Ca_{10}(PO_4)_6(OH)_2$.

Immediately after collagen formation, mineralization begins. **Mineralization** is the deposition of inorganic elements (minerals) on an organic matrix (mainly composed of protein in combination with some polysaccharides and lipids). In addition to calcium and phosphorus, numerous other minerals, especially magnesium, sodium, potassium, and carbonate ions, are incorporated into the mineral matrix.

Adequate nutritional components are necessary during collagen formation and mineral deposition phases to prevent structural imperfections. The crystalline mineral matrix provides great compressional strength, similar to marble. The combination of collagen and crystalline mineral matrix forms a material resembling reinforced concrete.

The skeleton is constantly growing, changing, and **remodeling** itself. Approximately 0.4% to 10% of total bone calcium remains in a shapeless or **amorphous** form. This calcium is a reserve source that can be rapidly used when serum calcium levels decrease. Osteoblasts deposit fresh calcium salts where new stresses have developed, and where **osteoclasts** (connected with absorption of bone) are removing calcium deposits. Bone absorption by osteoclasts is controlled by parathyroid hormone (PTH). The rate of osteoblast and osteoclast activity is normally in equilibrium, except during periods of growth. In older adults, bone resorption may exceed mineralization, causing osteoporosis.

This dynamic state accommodates changing demands of the body. Bone strength is adjusted in proportion to the degree of stress on the bone. Continual physical stress stimulates calcification and osteoblastic deposition of bone.

Formation of Teeth

Teeth are composed of three calcified tissues: enamel, dentin, and cementum. Enamel and dentin are principally composed of millions of hydroxyapatite crystals similar to those in bone. Approximately 30% of dentin, 50% of cementum, and 35% of alveolar bone is organic material, principally collagen; only 4% of the enamel is organic material. Dentin lacks the osteoblasts and osteoclasts found in bone; enamel and dentin do not contain blood vessels or nerves. As with bone, the mineral crystallization structure makes teeth extremely resistant to compressional forces; collagen fibers make teeth tough and resistant to tensional forces. Actions in which pressure attempts to diminish a structure's volume are referred to as **compressional forces**; **tensional forces** are actions in which pressure stretches or strains the structure.

After a tooth erupts, no more enamel is formed, but mineral exchanges occur slowly in response to the oral environment. Changes in mineral composition of enamel occur by exchange of minerals in saliva, rather than from the pulp cavity. Minerals—such as fluoride, sodium, zinc, and strontium—can replace calcium ions. Carbonate can be substituted for phosphate; carbonate and fluoride can be substituted for hydroxyl ions. These changes may alter the solubility of apatite. Despite changes that occur in enamel composition, enamel maintains most of its original mineral components throughout life.

The crystalline structure of enamel is one of the most insoluble and resistant proteins known. This special protein matrix, in combination with a crystalline structure of inorganic salts, makes enamel harder than dentin. In fact, it is the hardest structure in the body. It is comparable in hardness to quartz. Enamel is more resistant to acids, enzymes, and other corrosive agents than dentin.

Dentin, the main tissue of teeth, contains the same constituents as bone, but its structure is more dense. It is a hard, yellowish substance. Its principal component is hydroxyapatite crystals embedded in a strong meshwork of collagen fibers. Odontoblasts line the inner surface of dentin and provide nourishment for the dentin.

Cementum, which covers the dentin in the root area, is another bonelike substance, but because it contains fewer minerals, it is softer than bone. Just like dentin, it is also a hard, yellowish substance that contains many collagen fibers. The outer layer of cementum is lined with cementoblasts, capable of producing cementum throughout the life of the tooth. Compressional forces cause the cementum to become thicker and stronger. Cementum exhibits characteristics more typical of bone than enamel and dentin. Minerals are absorbed and deposited at rates similar to that of alveolar bone. The **alveolar bone** of the maxillae and mandible, comprised of the sockets for the teeth, is deposited next to the periodontal ligament.

Development of normal, healthy teeth is affected by metabolic factors, such as PTH secretion, and the availability of calcium, phosphate, vitamin D, protein, and many other nutrients. If these factors are deficient, calcification of teeth may be defective and abnormal throughout life.

Introduction to Minerals

Minerals are inorganic elements with many physiologic functions. Numerous inorganic elements in the body account for only about 4% of total body weight, or 6 lb for a 150-lb person. Minerals are subdivided into those required in larger amounts (major minerals) and those required in smaller amounts (micronutrients, also called trace elements) (Box 9.1). Despite the smaller amounts required, trace elements are just as important as major minerals.

• BOX 9.1 Mineral Elements in the Body

Major Minerals (> 100 mg/day)

Calcium (Ca)[a]
Phosphorus (P)[a]
Sodium (Na)[a]
Potassium (K)
Magnesium (Mg)[a]
Chlorine (Cl)[a]
Sulfur (S)

Trace Elements (< 100 mg/day)

Iron (Fe)[a]
Copper (Cu)[a]
Zinc (Zn)[a]
Manganese (Mn)[a]
Iodine (I)[a]
Molybdenum (Mo)[a]
Fluorine (F)[a]
Selenium (Se)[a]
Chromium (Cr)
Cobalt (Co)

Ultratrace Elements (No Recommended Dietary Allowances)

Boron (B)[a]
Arsenic (As)
Nickel (Ni)[a]
Silicon (Si)
Tin (Sn)
Vanadium (V)[a]
Cadmium (Cd)
Lead (Pb)
Bromide (Br)
Lithium (Li)
Aluminum (Al)

[a] *Tolerable Upper Intake Levels have been established.*

Calcium

Physiologic Roles

At least 99% of the body's calcium is found in the skeleton and teeth. Calcium is indispensable for skeletal function, which requires adequate dietary calcium to achieve full accretion of bone mass prescribed by genetic potential. Calcium (and phosphorus) in the bone, but not in the enamel of teeth, functions as a "savings account" for maintaining serum calcium levels. Only 1% of the body's calcium is found in blood, but as such, it controls body functions such as blood clotting, transmission of nerve impulses, muscle contraction and relaxation, membrane permeability, and activation of certain enzymes. Research indicates that calcium intake is important not only for bone health but also for reducing the risk of many other disorders, from hypertension to obesity to colon cancer.

Saliva is supersaturated with calcium; saliva is a source of calcium to mineralize an immature or demineralized enamel surface and reduce susceptibility to caries. Calcium and phosphate in saliva provide a buffering action to inhibit caries formation. This buffer prevents dissolution of minerals in the enamel by plaque biofilm.

Requirements

The National Academy of Medicine (NAM, formerly the Institute of Medicine) has established a recommended dietary allowance (RDA) and an estimated average requirement for calcium. The RDA is 1000 mg per day for ages 19 to 50 years. During growth periods, primarily from 9 to 18 years of age, the requirement is higher because peak bone mass appears to be related to calcium intake during periods of increased bone mineralization (Table 9.1). Peak bone mass occurs between 18 and 25 years of age.[1] Typically, calcium intake of teens between ages 13 and

TABLE 9.1 Adequate Intake for Calcium

Life Stage Group	EAR (mg/day)	RDA (mg/day)	AI (mg/day)	UL (g/day)
Infants (birth–6 months)			200	1.0
Infants (7–12 months)			260	1.5
Children (1–3 years)	500	700		2.5
Children (4–8 years)	800	1000		2.5
Adolescents (9–13 years)	1100	1300		3.0
Adolescents (14–18 years)	1100	1300		3.0
Adults (19–30 years)	800	1000		2.5
Adults (31–50 years)	800	1000		2.5
Adults (51–70 years)				
Males	800	1000		2.0
Females	1000	1200		2.0
> 70 years	1000	1200		2.0
Pregnancy and lactation		Same as for their age group		

AI, Adequate intake; EAR, estimated average requirement; RDA, recommended dietary allowance; UL, tolerable upper intake level.
Data from Institute of Medicine, Food and Nutrition Board. *Dietary Reference Intakes for Calcium and Vitamin D.* Washington, DC: National Academy Press; 2011.

19 years falls below the RDA for calcium. On the other hand, adequate intake of calcium is observed in ages 20 to 59 years for men but is inadequate for women.[2] Women may continue to increase bone growth and density through their 20s, but never achieve the bone mass levels observed in most men. From age 30 years until menopause, women tend to maintain bone mass; however, bone mass loss accelerates after menopause. The NAM recommends dietary intake of 1200 mg/day for females over 50 years of age.

Women are less likely than men to exceed their RDA. The estimated mean calcium intake for women over age 60 years during the 2009 to 2010 National Health and Nutrition Examination Survey was 842 mg per day compared with 966 mg/day for men in the same age category. Fortunately, when women in this age group include a calcium supplement, intake is boosted to 1629 mg/day, within their target range and surpassing men's intake of 1495 mg/day.[2]

Americans usually consume about 1029 mg of calcium per day.[2] Inadequate calcium intake can be attributed to (a) uninformed choices or not selecting adequate sources of calcium on a daily basis; (b) the mistaken beliefs that adults do not need milk or that milk contributes too many calories to the diet; (c) economic hardships, plus a lack of knowledge regarding inexpensive sources of calcium-rich foods; (d) lactose intolerance or allergies to dairy products; (e) access to and consumption of soda; and (f) dislike of calcium-rich foods.

Generally, inadequate calcium intake affects bone mass more than tooth structure. Inadequate calcium and vitamin D intake during tooth formation and maturation may result in hypomineralization of developing teeth. After tooth formation, dietary calcium does not affect caries rate.

Calcium Balance

Despite wide variations in calcium intake, serum calcium is relatively constant because each cell has a vital need for calcium. If the serum calcium level declines, bones are used as calcium reserves. Skeletal calcium turns over (transfers from in and out of bone) daily to promote bone homeostasis and maintain a constant serum calcium concentration. When calcium withdrawal from bones exceeds deposits, calcium imbalance occurs. Decreased bone density caused by insufficient calcium is a slow process.

Calcium–Phosphorus Balance

Serum levels of calcium and phosphorus are inversely related. If the calcium level increases, phosphorus levels decrease and vice versa. This relationship acts as a protective mechanism to prevent high combined concentrations, which can lead to calcification of soft tissue and stone formation or contraction of the heart muscle.

Absorption and Excretion

Calcium balance, achieved when intake equals excretion, does not solely depend on adequate calcium intake. Several hormones—including PTH, estrogen, glucocorticoids, and thyroid hormone—help to regulate calcium absorption. Under normal conditions, less than one-third of the calcium consumed is absorbed. Maximum calcium absorption occurs when it is consumed in small amounts and ingested several times throughout the day. In other words, individuals should consume 30% of the daily value or 300 mg per serving three or four times a day.

Absorption occurs in the small intestine and is affected by many factors, as shown in Fig. 9.1. Calcium absorption from various

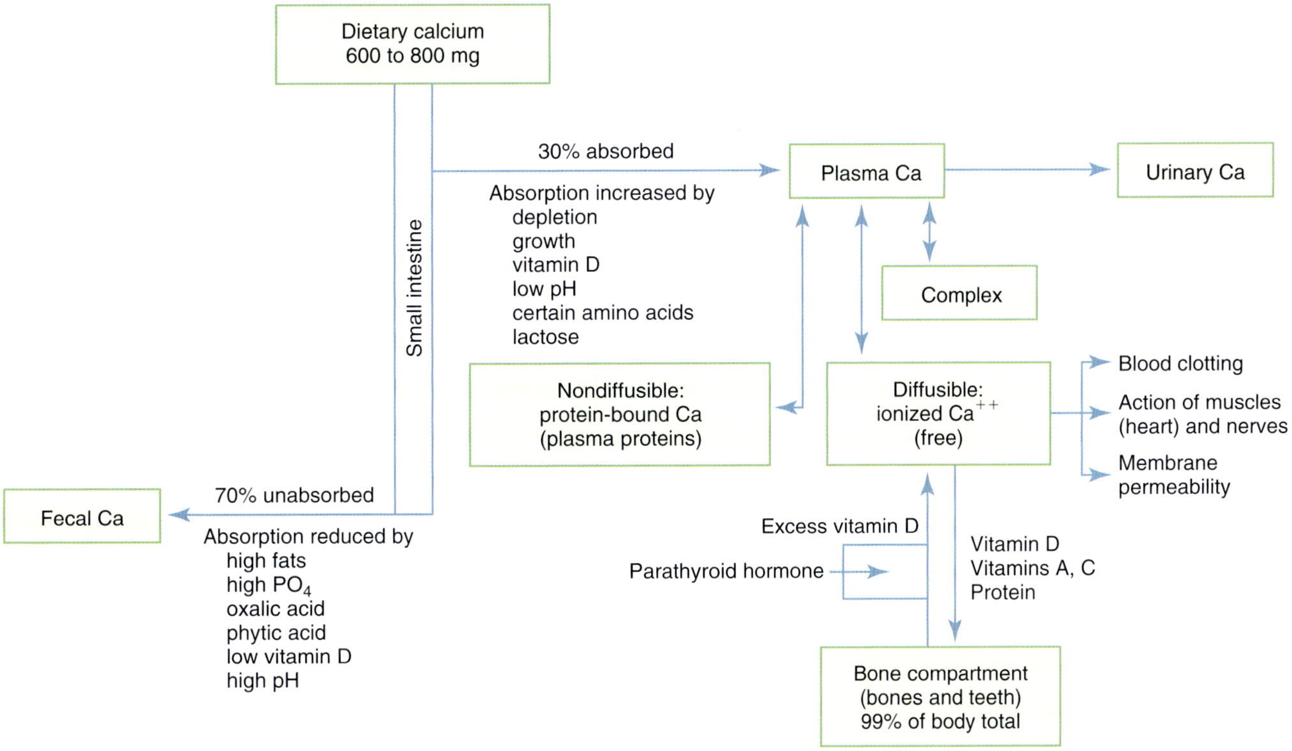

• **Figure 9.1** Calcium absorption and use. (Adapted from Schlenker ED, Gilbert J. *Williams' Essentials of Nutrition and Diet Therapy*. 11th ed. St. Louis, MO: Elsevier; 2015.)

dairy products is similar, whereas calcium present in many dark-green leafy vegetables is not readily absorbed. During periods of increased need—especially during growth, pregnancy, and lactation—calcium absorption increases. Calcium absorption decreases with age, probably because of decreased gastric acidity. The rate of absorption is lowest in postmenopausal women because of diminished estrogen levels.

Although several plant foods contain large amounts of calcium, absorption is poor. Oxalates (oxalic acid) in vegetables and phytates (phytic acid) from wheat bran bind with calcium in these foods to reduce absorption, but they do not interfere with calcium absorption from other foods. Dark-green leafy vegetables (e.g., kale, turnip greens) contain minimal amounts of oxalic acid, and calcium from these vegetables is readily absorbed. Excessive dietary fiber (more than 35 g/day) also interferes with calcium absorption.

High-protein intakes, typical in the United States, have a high phosphorus content. Phosphorus increases uptake of calcium by bone. The usual intake of protein and phosphorus does not cause calcium loss when intake is adequate, whereas a diet low in protein and phosphorus may have adverse effects on calcium balance with inadequate calcium intake. Generally, weight loss causes bone mineral loss. Stimulation of PTH results in the possible loss of bone mass to restore the levels to normal. PTH works concurrently with vitamin D to prevent calcium from being excreted and stimulates calcium release from bone when serum levels of calcium are low. Increasing synthesis of vitamin D by PTH also results in increased calcium absorption.

Sources

Milk and other dairy products supply the greatest amount of available calcium (Table 9.2). Not only are they preferred sources of calcium because of their high calcium content, but lactose and other nutrients in dairy products enhance calcium absorption. Milk also provides other essential nutrients. Box 9.2 lists portion sizes for various foods that provide approximately 300 mg of calcium.

• BOX 9.2 Calcium Equivalents[a]

The following foods contain approximately 300 mg of calcium:
1 cup milk
1 cup soymilk or coconut milk, fortified
1 cup almond milk
1 cup orange juice, fortified
1½ oz cheddar cheese
1½ oz mozzarella cheese
1½ oz American cheese
½ cup tofu
1 cup yogurt
2 cups ice cream
1½ cup spinach, cooked[b]
1¼ cup soybeans, cooked
1 serving cheese pizza

Data from U.S. Department of Agriculture (USDA), Agricultural Research Service. USDA National Nutrient Database for Standard Reference, Release 28. 2016. https://ndb.nal.usda.gov/ndb/. Accessed February 12, 2017.

[a]The RDA for calcium is 1000 mg for individuals 19 to 50 years old.

[b]Calcium from vegetable sources is not easily absorbed by the intestine and is not as effective in fulfilling calcium requirements.

TABLE 9.2 Calcium and Phosphorus Content of Selected Foods

Food	Portion	Calcium (mg)	Phosphorus (mg)
Total brand cereal	1 cup	1333	107
Romano cheese	1½ oz	452	323
Almond milk, vanilla	1 cup	451	19
Coconut milk, fortified	1 cup	451	0
Ice cream	2 cups	451	399
American cheese	1½ oz	444	273
Yogurt, nonfat plain	1 cup	388	306
Swiss cheese	1½ oz	378	244
Pizza, cheese	1 serving	356	356
Orange juice, calcium fortified	1 cup	349	117
Milk (1%, skim)	1 cup	314	245
Cheddar cheese	1½ oz	302	193
Soy milk, calcium fortified	1 cup	301	301
Buttermilk, low-fat	1 cup	284	218
Tofu, raw, firm, fortified	½ cup	253	152
Oats, instant, fortified	1 cup	187	180
Cottage cheese, low-fat	1 cup	187	358
Salmon, canned	3 oz	183	286
Cottage cheese, low-fat (1%)	1 cup	138	303
Soybeans, cooked	½ cup	130	142
Spinach, cooked	½ cup	122	50
Rice milk	1 cup	118	56
Fruit-flavored drink, fortified	1 cup	101	0
Hamburger bun	1	100	66
Turnip greens, cooked	½ cup	99	21
White beans, cooked	½ cup	65	151
Okra, cooked	½ cup	62	26
Spinach, raw	2 cups	59	29
Kale, cooked	½ cup	47	18
Broccoli, cooked	½ cup	31	52
Ground beef, cooked	3 oz	9	148
Cola	12 oz	4	33

Data from U.S. Department of Agriculture, Agricultural Research Service. 2016. *USDA National Nutrient Database For Standard Reference, Release 28.* https://ndb.nal.usda.gov/ndb/. Accessed February 12, 2017.

Since 1999, food manufacturers have been fortifying products such as fruit juices, fruit-flavored drinks, breakfast cereals, and breads with calcium. Numerous calcium-fortified foods introduced to the market have been well received. Food products containing natural or fortified calcium must use certain terminology on packaging, shown in Table 9.3.

An increasing percentage of the United States, population purchases supplements containing calcium. The U.S. Preventive Services Task Force found inconclusive evidence to support the use of a calcium supplement in men and premenopausal women.[3] Further, excessive calcium intake may increase the risk of cardiovascular disease (CVD).[4,5] Calcium supplements combined with vitamin D may result in small but significant reductions in bone loss and are effective in reducing falls and fractures.[6] This strong trend toward the use of calcium supplements is especially evident among older adults. Benefits may be less than expected, partly because of limited bioavailability of supplemental calcium. **Bioavailability** refers to the amount of a nutrient available physiologically and is based on its absorption rate.

A calcium supplement contains elemental calcium along with other substances, such as carbonate or citrate. The amount of elemental calcium varies among supplements. For example, calcium carbonate is 40% calcium by weight, whereas calcium citrate is 21% calcium. Some calcium supplements are better absorbed when taken with food, absorption being dependent on the availability of gastric acids. Others may be better absorbed when taken on an empty stomach. Calcium-citrate-malate, calcium lactate, calcium gluconate, and calcium sulfate are other forms of calcium in supplements or fortified foods. Choosing a supplement that has the United States Pharmacopeia (USP) designation means that the quantity in the supplement is more likely to be consistent with the label.

Hyper States and Hypo States

Clinical conditions are associated with excesses and deficiencies of calcium. Hypercalcemia (too much calcium) and hypocalcemia (too little calcium) are critical metabolic conditions that can lead to loss of consciousness, fatal respiratory failure, or cardiac arrest. These problems are seldom caused directly by calcium intake; however, loss of bone density can be related to intake.

TABLE 9.3 Food Labeling for Calcium

Daily Value (DV) of Calcium in a Food	FDA-Authorized Labeling Terms
10% DV of calcium	Calcium enriched Calcium fortified More calcium
10%–19% DV of calcium	Contains calcium Provides calcium Good source of calcium
≥ 20% DV of calcium	High in calcium Rich in calcium Excellent source of calcium

FDA, U.S. Food and Drug Administration.

Hypercalcemia

Hypercalcemia, or excessive levels of calcium in the blood, is rarely the result of dietary intake. Hypercalcemia can result in renal insufficiency, kidney stones or **hypercalciuria** (high levels of calcium in the urine). Idiopathic hypercalcemia is observed occasionally in infants 5 to 8 months old, sometimes with genetic causes. Overdoses of cholecalciferol or excessive amounts of vitamin D preparations can also cause hypercalcemia. Treatment involves providing a low-calcium diet with no vitamin D. Hyperparathyroidism, certain types of bone disease, vitamin D poisoning, sarcoidosis, cancer, and prolonged excessive intake of milk may cause adult hypercalcemia.

Hypocalcemia

Hypocalcemia, or deficient levels of serum calcium, results in **tetany**, a neuromuscular disorder of uncontrollable cramps and tremors involving the muscles of the face, hands, feet, and eventually the heart. Depressed serum calcium levels may be caused by hypoparathyroidism, some bone diseases, certain kidney diseases, and low serum protein levels.

Excessive Calcium Intake

Excessively high calcium intake may cause dizziness, flushing, nausea or vomiting, constipation, kidney stone formation, irregular heartbeat, tingling sensations, xerostomia, fatigue, and high blood pressure. It also may inhibit iron and zinc absorption.

Inadequate Calcium Intake

Rickets, discussed in Chapter 8 in connection with vitamin D deficiency, results in porous, soft bones. Rickets develops during childhood as a result of inadequate amounts of calcium being deposited in the bone. Calcium intake may be adequate, but absorption is poor because of inadequate vitamin D.

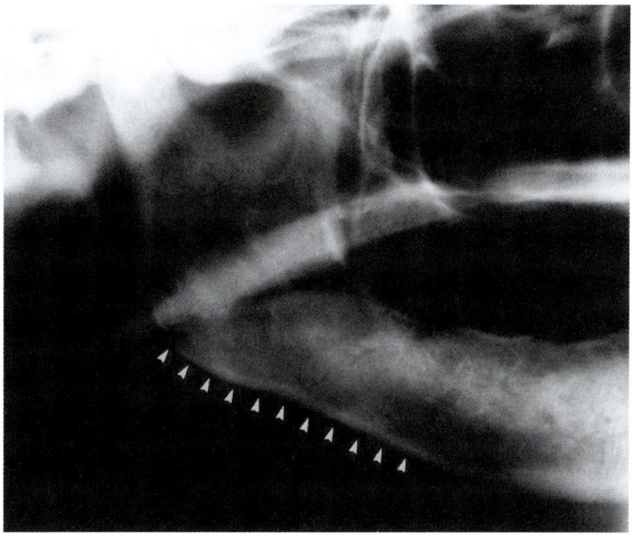

• **Figure 9.2** Radiographic appearance of osteoporosis affecting bone of the maxillofacial complex. This portion of a panoramic radiograph depicts thinning of the gonial and interior cortices of an edentulous mandible (*arrows*). A slight increase in the general size of marrow spaces is also apparent. (Courtesy of B. W. Benson, DDS, MS, Associate Professor, Department of Diagnostic Sciences, Texas A&M University College of Dentistry, Dallas, TX.)

Osteoporosis is an age-related disorder characterized by decreased bone mass, causing bones to be more susceptible to fracture. Numerous factors, including decreased estrogen, inadequate calcium or vitamin D intake, and lack of weight-bearing activity are implicated. The relationship of calcium intake to bone density indicates a protective effect in women reporting high lifetime calcium intake, but not in women who increased intake after menopause. Building bone during the formative years is the best insurance against osteoporosis.

An oral sign of osteoporosis is loss of calcium in the alveolar bone, contributing to tooth exfoliation (Fig. 9.2). The condition usually goes undetected, however, until pain or spontaneous fracture occurs. Osteoporosis is discussed further in *Health Application 9*. **Periodontal disease**, an inflammatory disease that leads to the destruction of the periodontium, can be exacerbated by calcium deficiency (see Chapter 19).[7]

DENTAL CONSIDERATIONS

- Physical inactivity results in bone depletion. In young individuals, recovery of calcium deposits is usually rapid, but older adults may never regain bone density.
- Inadequate calcium can lead to incomplete calcification of the tooth, abnormalities of the teeth and bones, periodontal disease, and early tooth loss.
- Patients with achlorhydria (the absence of hydrochloric acid in the stomach) may not absorb calcium supplements on an empty stomach and should take them with meals.
- Hyperparathyroidism induces bone loss. Alveolar bone is especially at risk, exhibiting extensive bone resorption.
- Patients who have had bariatric surgery for obesity are at risk of decreased bone mineral density.[8,9]
- Interventions for limiting or preventing further bone loss include encouraging exercise and foods rich in vitamin D and calcium.
- Patients who use excessive alcohol or caffeine, or smoke cigarettes, are at risk of calcium loss.
- Suggest alternatives for increasing calcium intake for patients with lactose intolerance (see Chapter 4, *Health Application 4*).
- Calcium supplements may interact with certain medications, including glucocorticoids, cellulose sodium phosphate (Calcibind), etidronate (Didronel), phenytoin (Dilantin), bisphosphonates, and tetracycline. Supplements should be taken 1 to 3 hours before or after the medication.
- Aluminum- and magnesium-containing antacids and corticosteroids increase urinary excretion of calcium.
- Mineral oil and some laxatives can decrease calcium absorption.
- Poor patient compliance may be expected if several tablets are necessary, the supplement is too expensive, or gastrointestinal problems (e.g., gas, bloating, diarrhea) occur. More than 500 mg of calcium per tablet may cause constipation.

NUTRITIONAL DIRECTIONS

- Adequate daily calcium, phosphorus, and vitamin D intake is important to support bone formation and maintenance. Try to consume adequate amount of the nutrients daily. Calcium supplement absorption can be enhanced by taking it with some form of sugar; lactose, dextrose, and sucrose enhance its absorption.
- Evaluate calcium supplements for their solubility, which affects absorption. For calcium to be absorbed from a supplement, the tablet must first dissolve. To measure how well a calcium tablet dissolves in the body, drop a tablet in a solution of 4½ oz water and 1½ oz vinegar to produce an environment similar to that of the stomach. Stir occasionally. At least two-thirds of a high-quality tablet dissolves within 30 minutes.
- Calcium supplements are available in tablets, gel capsules, liquids, and chewables.
- Compare the amount of elemental calcium provided (actual amount of calcium in the supplement) and cost per tablet. Refer patients who are appropriate candidates for calcium supplementation to a health care provider or RDN.
- Decreased calcium intake in women results in lower levels of estrogen production, which can be harmful to the bones. Estrogen enhances calcium absorption and enables more efficient use of calcium.
- Moderate alcohol intake enhances bone density mass as a result of less bone remodeling, but excessive amounts increase the risk of bone loss later in life.
- Weight-bearing exercise has a positive effect on calcium deposition in bone during childhood and adolescence. Weight-bearing exercise and resistance training prevent, and in some cases reverse, bone loss in adults.
- When daily calcium intake appears to be low, encourage increased consumption of dairy products. If the patient has an aversion to milk, powdered milk can be added to many items, or other high-calcium foods can be used.
- Green leafy sources of calcium that are low in oxalic acid include kale, turnip greens, rutabaga, and okra. Oxalates inhibit the absorption of calcium. This is particularly helpful information for vegans or those not consuming dairy products.
- Do not take calcium supplements within 1 to 2 hours of eating large amounts of fiber, especially foods containing large amounts of phytates and oxalates.
- After menopause, calcium and vitamin D supplements slow bone loss and reduce fractures when coupled with an approved osteoporosis-related therapy, such as estrogen replacement therapy or a bisphosphonate or both. If an adverse reaction to the osteoporosis medication is reported, encourage the patient to consult the health care provider before discontinuing it.

Phosphorus

Physiologic Roles

Phosphorus is the second most abundant mineral in the body, with approximately 85% in the skeleton and teeth. Its presence in all body cells is necessary for almost every aspect of metabolism, including (a) transfer and release of energy stored as adenosine triphosphate; (b) composition of phospholipids, DNA, and RNA; and (c) metabolism of fats, carbohydrates, and proteins. Phosphorus also helps regulate the acid–base balance in the body.

Requirements

The RDA of phosphorus for adults older than 18 years of age is 700 mg. Because phosphorus is more readily available than calcium in the United States food supply, intake is generally 1.5 times higher than calcium. Although harmful effects from excessive amounts of phosphorus have not been reported, the NAM established a tolerable upper intake level (UL) to reflect normal serum levels (Table 9.4). Note that pregnant and lactating women consume the same amount of phosphorus as nonpregnant women of the same age.

TABLE 9.4 National Academy of Medicine Recommendations for Phosphorus

Life Stage[a]	EAR (mg/day)	RDA (mg/day)	AI (mg/day)	UL (g/day)
Birth–6 months	—	—	100	ND
7–12 months	—	—	275	ND
1–3 years	380	460	—	3
4–8 years	405	500	—	3
9–18 years	1055	1250	—	4
19–70 years	580	700	—	4
> 70 years	580	700	—	3
Pregnancy				
≤ 18 years	1055	1250	—	3.5
19–50 years	580	700	—	3.5
Lactation				
≤ 18 years	1055	1250	—	4
19–50 years	580	700	—	4

AI, Adequate intake; EAR, estimated average requirement; RDA, recommended dietary allowance; UL, tolerable upper intake level.
[a]All groups except pregnancy and lactation include males and females.
Data from Institute of Medicine (IOM), Food and Nutrition Board. *Dietary Reference Intakes For Calcium, Phosphorus, Magnesium, Vitamin D, and Fluoride.* Washington, DC: National Academy Press; 1997.

Absorption and Excretion

Approximately 60% to 70% of dietary phosphorus is absorbed in the jejunum. Its absorption can be inhibited by the same dietary factors affecting calcium absorption: phytate, excessive fat, iron, aluminum, and calcium intake. The kidneys excrete excessive amounts of phosphorus to maintain optimal body levels.

Sources

Phosphorus is abundant in foods, which is the reason deficiencies have not been observed. A diet adequate in calcium and protein contains enough phosphorus because all three minerals are present in the same foods (see Table 9.2). In addition to milk products, meats are a good source of phosphorus. Dietary restriction of phosphorus is extremely difficult because of its wide use as a food additive in baked goods, cheese, processed meats, and soft drinks.

Hyper States and Hypo States

Both excesses and inadequacies of phosphorus can lead to medical complications, including impaired bone health. Hyperphosphatemia (serum level > 2.6 mg/dL) may occur in cases of hypoparathyroidism or renal insufficiency. Excessive amounts of phosphorus bind with calcium, resulting in tetany and convulsions.

Hypophosphatemia may occur with long-term ingestion of aluminum hydroxide antacids, which bind phosphorus, interfering with absorption, or it may occur in certain stress conditions in which the calcium-to-phosphorus balance is disturbed. Intestinal conditions, such as sprue and celiac disease, can result in phosphorus malabsorption and thus deficiencies. The principal clinical symptom of hypophosphatemia is muscle weakness. Even small phosphorus depletions may cause increased calcium excretion, resulting in a negative calcium balance and bone loss.

During tooth development, a phosphorus deficiency can result in incomplete calcification of teeth, failure of dentin formation, and increased susceptibility to caries.

DENTAL CONSIDERATIONS

- A phosphorus deficiency is more likely to develop or occur in alcoholics; older adults with inadequate dietary intake; patients with disordered eating, inappropriate weight loss, and long-term diarrhea; and patients taking aluminum-containing antacids or diuretics. Assess the phosphorus status and document any signs or symptoms of a deficiency for these patients. A referral to the health care provider or RDN may be needed.
- Low phosphate intake may lead to an increased rate of caries formation, but additional or supplemental phosphate may not be helpful in preventing dental caries.

NUTRITIONAL DIRECTIONS

- A high intake of phosphates, such as sodas and colas, may lead to an increase in caries rate and a decrease in bone density by reducing bone formation and increasing bone resorption.[10]
- Adequate intake of phosphorus from dairy products may be a factor in lower blood pressure.[11]
- Hyperphosphatemia can be a risk factor for CVD.[11]

Magnesium

Physiologic Roles

Bones contain almost two-thirds of the body's magnesium. It is the third most prevalent mineral in teeth, with dentin containing about two times more than enamel. Magnesium has an important function in maintaining calcium homeostasis and preventing skeletal abnormalities. Magnesium is involved in more than 300 enzymatic reactions, including energy metabolism, insulin activity, and glucose use. Magnesium is vital to the structural integrity of muscles, especially the heart muscle, and nerves. Magnesium balance is largely controlled by the kidney through urinary excretion. Its role in enzymes is fundamental to energy (adenosine triphosphate) production. It is also crucial in controlling blood pressure and preventing stroke.[1]

Requirements

The RDA for magnesium ranges from 240 mg per day for 9-year-old children to 420 mg per day for men (Table 9.5). Although it is impossible to get too much magnesium from food alone, excessive amounts can be obtained from supplements. The UL is provided for patients using supplements and other nonfood sources of magnesium.

Sources

Magnesium is widely distributed in plant and animal foods; however, whole-grain products, nuts, beans, and fortified foods are some of the best sources (Table 9.6). Magnesium (Mg) is part of the chlorophyll molecule (Fig. 9.3); therefore, green leafy vegetables are also good sources. In addition, bananas and chocolate are sources of magnesium. Although whole grains are good sources of magnesium, enrichment of refined grain products does not replace magnesium lost during processing. Varying amounts of magnesium can be found in tap, mineral, and bottled waters. Nonfood sources of magnesium include laxatives and antacids.

Hyper States and Hypo States

Because kidneys regulate plasma magnesium levels, toxicity has been associated with kidney failure or impaired renal function. This often results in diarrhea, nausea, and abdominal cramping while very high serum levels can lead to cardiac arrest. There is no evidence of harmful effects related to overconsumption of magnesium from food sources. A high dose of magnesium acts like a laxative (e.g., milk of magnesia).

In certain diseases or under stressful conditions, deficiencies may occur. Magnesium in bone is not available to replace serum magnesium deficits. A deficiency may result from numerous disease states, including gastrointestinal abnormalities with diarrhea, renal disease, general malnutrition, alcoholism, and medications interfering with magnesium conservation. Magnesium deficiency symptoms include fatigue, anorexia, nausea, neuromuscular dysfunction, personality changes, disorientation, muscle spasms, seizures, tremors, and cardiac arrhythmias.

TABLE 9.5 National Academy of Medicine Recommendations for Magnesium

	EAR (mg/day)		RDA (mg/day)		AI (mg/day)		
Life Stage[a]	**Male**	**Female**	**Male**	**Female**	**Male**	**Female**	**UL (mg/day)**
Birth–6 months	—	—	—	—	30	30	ND
7–12 months	—	—	—	—	75	75	ND
1–3 years	65	65	80	80			65
4–8 years	110	110	130	130			110
9–13 years	200	200	240	240			350
14–18 years	340	300	410	360			350
19–30 years	330	255	400	310			350
> 30 years	350	265	420	320			350
Pregnancy							
≤ 18 years		335		400			350
19–30 years		290		350			350
31–50 years		300		360			350
Lactation							
≤ 18 years		300		360			350
19–30 years		255		310			350
31–50 years		265		320			350

AI, Adequate intake; EAR, estimated average requirement; RDA, recommended dietary allowance; UL, tolerable upper intake level.
[a]All groups except pregnancy and lactation include males and females.
Data from Institute of Medicine (IOM), Food and Nutrition Board. *Dietary Reference Intakes For Calcium, Phosphorus, Magnesium, Vitamin D, and Fluoride*, Washington, DC: National Academy Press; 1997.

TABLE 9.6 Magnesium Content of Selected Foods

Food	Portion	Magnesium (mg)
Sesame seeds	1 oz	101
Hummus	½ cup	87
Spinach, cooked	½ cup	78
Cashew nuts	1 oz	77
Lima beans, cooked	½ cup	63
Shredded Wheat cereal	2 biscuits	61
Peanut butter	2 tbsp	54
Edamame, cooked	½ cup	50
Navy beans, cooked	½ cup	48
Brown rice, cooked	½ cup	40
Potato, baked	1 medium	47
Sunflower seeds	1 oz	36
Soymilk, vanilla	1 cup	36
Split peas, cooked	½ cup	35
Banana	1 medium	32
Dark chocolate	2⅗ oz bar	23
Bread, multigrain	1 slice	20
Broccoli, cooked	½ cup	16

Data from U.S. Department of Agriculture (USDA), Agricultural Research Service. *USDA National Nutrient Database for Standard Reference, Release 28.* 2016. https://ndb.nal.usda.gov/ndb/. Accessed March 1, 2017.

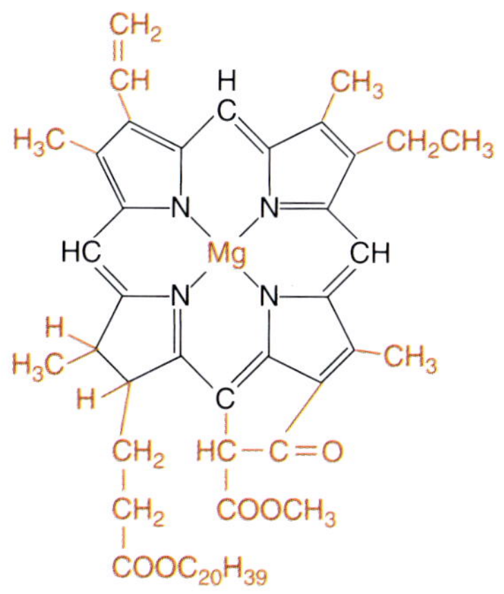

• **Figure 9.3** Structure of chlorophyll. All chlorophyll molecules are essentially alike; they differ only in details of the side chains. Magnesium is basic to all chlorophyll molecules.

Dietary deficiencies of magnesium may affect teeth and their supporting structures. Changes in ameloblasts and odontoblasts result in hypoplasia of the enamel and dentin during development. Alveolar bone formation may be reduced along with a widening of the periodontal ligament space and gingival hyperplasia.

DENTAL HYGIENE CONSIDERATIONS

- Decreased food intake, impaired magnesium absorption, or the use of certain diuretics may contribute to hypomagnesemia, or a below-normal blood serum concentration of magnesium. Encourage the patient to follow a healthy eating pattern as defined by the *Dietary Guidelines.*
- Supplements containing magnesium can decrease the absorption of oral bisphosphonates and interfere with the effectiveness of certain antibiotics. Encourage the patient to seek assistance from a pharmacist.

NUTRITIONAL DIRECTIONS

- Diets high in unrefined grains and vegetables provide more magnesium than diets that include a lot of refined foods, meats, and milk products.
- Magnesium plays a major role in blood pressure regulation; magnesium from foods is more effective than from supplements.[12]

Fluoride

Physiologic Roles

In a strict nutritional sense, fluoride is not a nutrient essential for health. Fluoride present in low concentrations in soft tissues does not have any known metabolic function. However, because of its benefits to dental and bone health, fluoride is considered a desirable element for humans. Varying amounts of fluoride in food and/or beverages remaining in the oral cavity after ingestion will be absorbed through the mucosa or become part of plaque biofilm and saliva.

Fluoride is also advantageous to dental health because of its systemic effects before tooth eruption and topical effects after tooth eruption (Fig. 9.4). The caries-preventing properties of systemic and topical fluoride are cumulative.

Fluoride ions can replace hydroxyl ions in the hydroxyapatite crystal lattice. This fluoridated hydroxyapatite, or **fluorapatite**, is less soluble and makes the tooth more resistant to acid demineralization. Additionally, it enhances remineralization when the tooth is subject to the caries process (Fig. 9.5). Calcium and phosphate are present in saliva and plaque at higher concentrations than fluoride. When small pits develop in the enamel, fluoride is believed to promote deposition of calcium phosphate to remineralize the enamel surface.

Primary teeth benefit from the presence of fluoride during tooth development beginning at 6 months of age. Fluoride is present in the inner part of the enamel and dentin at lower concentrations; this occurs mainly during the amelogenesis/odontogenesis stage. Enhanced concentration in the surface enamel occurs during the maturation stage of tooth development. Fluoride can be readily incorporated into the apatite crystal from topically available fluoride during the maturation stage, but this reversible process is superficial rather than fluoride being distributed throughout the enamel thickness.

The presence of fluoride in saliva interferes with the demineralization process, resulting in a less cariogenic environment. Topically available fluoride reduces dental caries by inhibiting demineralization, promoting remineralization, and interfering with formation and function of acidogenic bacteria. Higher concentrations of fluoride inhibit *Streptococcus mutans*, *Streptococcus sobrinus*, and

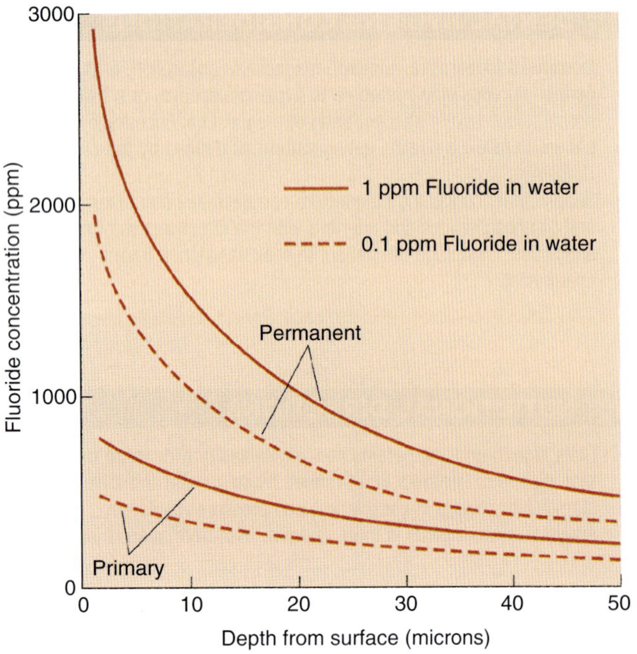

• **Figure 9.4** Concentration gradients of fluoride in outer enamel from permanent and deciduous teeth, from areas with 1 part per million (ppm) and 0.1 ppm of fluoride in the drinking water. (From Gron P: Inorganic chemical and structural aspects of oral mineralized tissues. In Shaw JH, editors: *Textbook of Oral Biology*, Philadelphia, 1978, Saunders, pp 484-507.)

Lactobacillus in plaque biofilm, and accelerate remineralization during early stages of enamel caries development.

Maximum protection by fluoride against caries occurs during the first 6 to 10 years of life, but adults and children continue to benefit from the presence of fluoride. Systemic fluoride uptake by calcified tissues is high from infancy until age 16 years, when mineralization of unerupted permanent teeth occurs. Compared with healthy enamel, demineralized enamel retains more fluoride.

Fluoride stimulates osteoblast growth and increases new mineral deposition in cancellous bone, improves bone integrity, and decreases bone resorption and bone solubility. Concurrent adequate intake of calcium, vitamin D, and fluoride is essential.

Requirements

Because of the risk of toxicity, adequate intake of fluoride has been established at 3 mg per day for all women and 4 mg per day for men (Table 9.7). Average intake in the United States is 0.9 mg per day in areas with nonfluoridated water and 1.7 mg per day in areas with fluoridation. The UL for healthy individuals age 9 years and older is 10 mg per day, including food, beverages, supplements, rinses, and toothpaste.

Absorption and Excretion

Most fluoride is absorbed in the stomach, with small amounts also absorbed in the intestine. The rate and degree of absorption depend

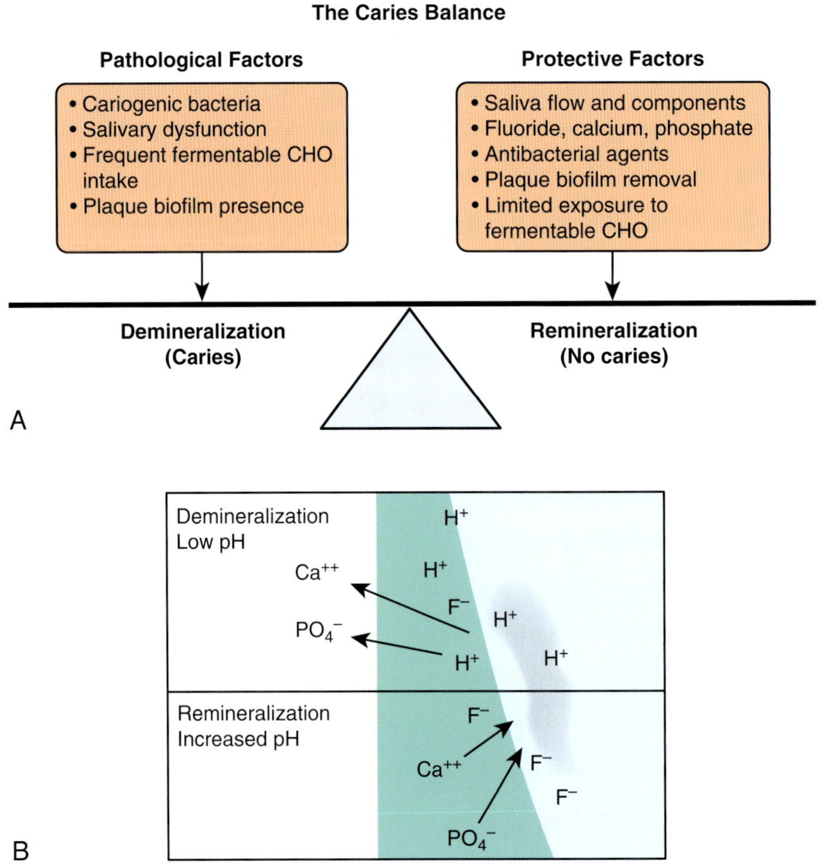

• **Figure 9.5** (A) The action of fluoride in the demineratization–remineralization process. (B) Fluoride ions replace hydroxyl ions. Fluoride promotes the deposition of calcium and phosphate to remineralize the enamel.

TABLE 9.7 National Academy of Medicine Recommendations for Fluoride

	AI (mg/day)		
Life Stage Group	Male	Female	UL
Birth–6 months	0.01	0.01	0.7
7–12 months	0.5	0.5	0.9
1–3 years	0.7	0.7	1.3
4–8 years	1	1	2.2
9–13 years	2	2	10
14–18 years	3	3	10
> 18 years	4	3	10
Pregnancy and Lactation			
≤ 50 years	—	3	10

AI, Adequate intake; UL, tolerable upper intake level.

Data from Institute of Medicine (IOM), Food and Nutrition Board. *Dietary Reference Intakes for Calcium, Phosphorus, Magnesium, Vitamin D, and Fluoride.* Washington, DC: National Academy Press; 1997.

on the solubility of the fluoride and amount ingested at a particular time. Absorption of fluoride from sodium fluoride in water is estimated to be 50% to 80%, depending on physiologic need. Incorporation of fluoride into bones and enamel is proportional to total intake and need. Children retain a larger percentage of fluoride in developing bones and teeth, whereas adults retain less in calcified structures. Protein-bound fluoride in foods is not as well absorbed.

A varying amount of fluoride intake is excreted by the kidneys, also depending on physiologic need. Aluminum (aluminum-containing antacids) and soy (soy-based foods) bind with fluoride and increase fluoride excretion in the feces. Calcium and fluoride supplements given at the same time inhibit absorption of both.

Sources

Water

The Centers for Disease Control and Prevention (CDC) recognizes water fluoridation as one of the most important public health measures.[13] Fluoride is available through community water supplies, food, beverages, dentifrices, and other fluoridated dental products. Fluoridation of community water contributes to fluoride intake and is a practical, cost-effective means of achieving significant decreases in the prevalence of dental caries. Approximately 80% of fluoride consumed is provided from tap and bottled water and water-based beverages, especially teas. To ensure everyone receives adequate amounts of fluoride, the U.S. Department of Health and Human Services and the U.S. Environmental Protection Agency (EPA) suggest drinking water contain approximately 0.7 parts per million (ppm) of fluoride (equivalent to 1 mg/L).[14] Scientists do not all agree on the maximum acceptable fluoride level. Several government agencies recommend no more than 2 ppm. Additional studies are currently being conducted to determine appropriate guidelines.[15,16] Home water purification and filtration systems can reduce the fluoride content of tap water.

Approximately 74% of the United States population has access to optimally fluoridated drinking water; the goal, as stated by *Healthy People 2020*, targets 79.6% of the population. The *Healthy People 2010* objective of 75% was met by only 27 states.[17] Water fluoridation is particularly beneficial for children and teens in economically depressed communities who have less access to oral health care and alternative fluoride resources. Children who do not regularly receive dental care or have no dental insurance are at high risk for dental caries.

Many households and businesses are using bottled water, water treatment systems, or water filters for various reasons, including taste preference and convenience. Bottled water may be chosen as a healthy alternative to soft drinks and alcoholic beverages. The U.S. Food and Drug Administration requires that fluoride be listed on the label of bottled water only if the manufacturer adds fluoride during processing. Fluoride amounts in bottled water may or may not be listed on the label. Bottled water containing 0.6 to 1.0 mg per liter of fluoride may state on the packaging, "Drinking fluoridated water may reduce the risk of tooth decay."

In some areas of the United States, the water supply naturally contains much higher levels of fluoride than the recommended amounts. Naturally occurring fluoride is found in soils and bedrock, which will dissolve into ground water. The EPA allows a maximum level of 4 mg per liter.[15] This level could possibly cause adverse health effects.

Food

Food is not a major source of fluoride for adults. All foods contain some fluoride, but the amounts provided in vegetables, meats, cereals, and fruits are insignificant (0.2–1.5 ppm of fluoride; Table 9.8). Seafood may contain 5 to 15 ppm of fluoride. Brewed tea provides approximately 1 to 6 ppm of fluoride per cup, depending on the amount of tea, brewing time, and amount of fluoride in the water, but herbal tea has negligible fluoride levels. The process of mechanically deboning poultry results in poultry containing a high concentration of fluoride. Carbonated beverages can be a significant source of fluoride if the water used in the bottling process is fluoridated. Foods prepared in fluoridated water will be also be a source.

Because of varied levels of fluoride in the water supply, the amount of fluoride in infant formulas was reduced in 1979. Components in soy bind fluoride; soy-based formulas usually contain some fluoride.

Topical

Topical applications of fluoride include gels, foams, varnishes, dentifrices, prophylactic paste (polishing paste), and mouth rinses. These high-concentration fluoride sources prevent demineralization when oral pH decreases. When used in combination with other fluoride sources, a decline in prevalence or severity of dental caries occurs.

Hyper States and Hypo States

Fluorosis and Bone Health

Mottling of tooth enamel results from overexposure (approximately three to four times the amount necessary to prevent caries) during tooth formation. Ameloblasts are extremely sensitive to excessive fluoride ingestion. Dental **fluorosis** (hypomineralization of enamel) is directly related to fluoride exposure during tooth development and cannot occur after tooth development is complete. Fluorosed enamel contains a total protein content similar to normal enamel,

TABLE 9.8 **Fluoride Content of Selected Foods**

Food	Fluoride (μg/100 g)
Black tea, brewed	373
Instant tea	335
Raisins	234
Crab, canned	210
Wine	202
Shrimp, canned	201
Grape juice	138
Coffee, brewed	91
Oysters, cooked	63
Cola	57
Potatoes, boiled	50
Carrots, cooked	48
Rice, white, cooked	33
Cheese, American, processed	35
Tomato sauce	35
Cottage cheese	32

Data from U.S. Department of Agriculture (USDA), Agricultural Research Service. *USDA National Nutrient Database for Standard Reference, Release 28.* 2016. https://ndb.nal.usda.gov/ndb/. Accessed March 1, 2017.

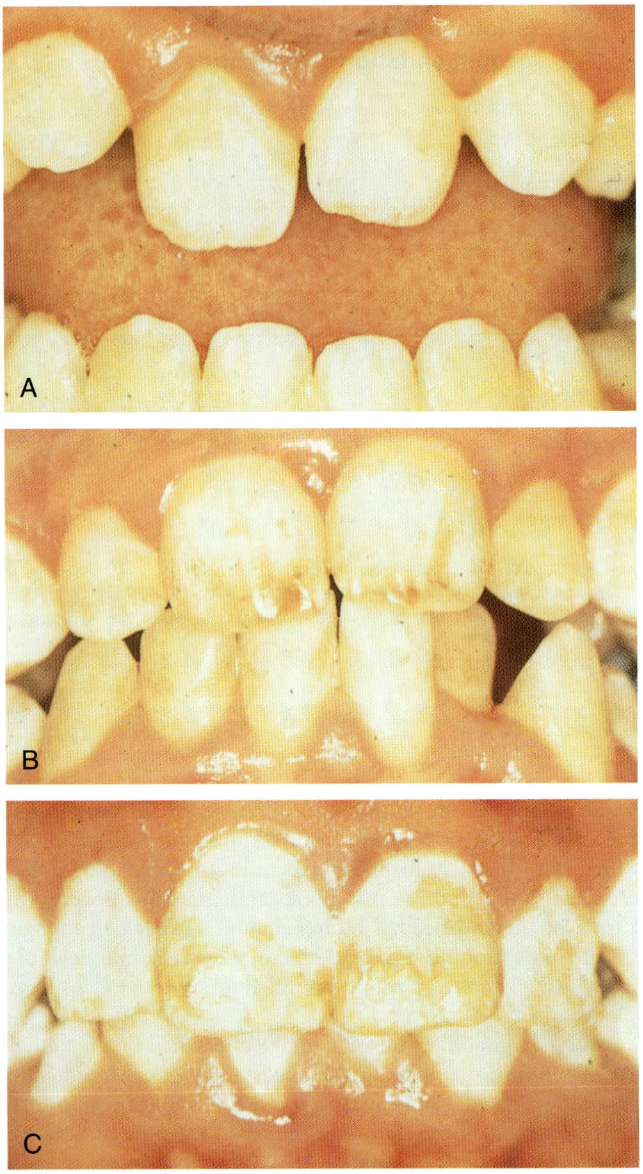

• **Figure 9.6** (A) Mild fluorosis: white opaque areas in the enamel over less than 50% of the tooth. (B) Moderate fluorosis all enamel surfaces of the teeth are affected; a brown stain is frequently present. (C) Severe fluorosis: hypoplasia affecting the general shape of the tooth; widespread brown stains, corroded-like appearance of teeth. (Courtesy of Alton McWhorter, DDS, MS, Associate Professor, Department of Pediatric Dentistry, Texas A&M University College of Dentistry, Dallas, TX.)

but it contains a relatively high proportion of immature matrix proteins. Mild to moderate enamel fluorosis on early forming enamel surfaces was strongly associated with use of infant formula before 1979. Frequent brushing with fluoridated toothpaste was encouraged, and fluoride supplements were used.

Dental fluorosis varies from very mild cases characterized by whitish opaque flecks to white or brown staining (Fig. 9.6A), to severe dental fluorosis with secondary, extrinsic, brownish discoloration and varying degrees of enamel pitting (Fig. 9.6C). When drinking water contains 2 ppm or more of fluoride, teeth appear extremely white; brown stains appear when the fluoride level is greater than 4 ppm. Mild to moderate fluorosis is primarily cosmetic, but teeth are caries-resistant; severe dental fluorosis can result in increased caries rate.

Excessive fluoride intake for adults can result in adverse effects on skeletal tissue and kidney function. These changes may gradually increase in severity, eventually resulting in a general increase in bone fractures and calcification of ligaments in the neck and vertebral column.

Dental Caries. A lack of fluoride may result in increased dental caries.[18] The protective effect against caries is greatest during tooth formation. The American Dental Association and the American Academy of Pediatrics recommend exposure of the teeth to fluoride until calcification of all teeth is completed (about age 16 years). Dosages for fluoride supplements for children are presented in Table 14.2. Various conditions warrant topical fluoride treatment in adults, such as hypersensitivity, exposed root surfaces, white spot lesions, xerostomia, use of smokeless tobacco, and radiation therapy.

Continued use of fluoridated water by adults is beneficial in maintaining the integrity of teeth. Posteruption, systemic fluoride is present in saliva and plaque, creating an environment that inhibits demineralization and enhances remineralization of tooth surfaces.

Safety

The addition of fluoride in the United States water supply continues to be opposed by a small but vocal and aggressive minority of people. Antifluoridation groups have attempted to link water fluoridation to cancer, acquired immunodeficiency syndrome, Alzheimer disease, mental illness, lowered IQ in children, CVD, fertility, and Down syndrome, but scientific evidence to support these allegations has not been provided. Regardless, a handful of communities in the United States have banned the addition of fluoride to their water.

Fluoridation is one of the most thoroughly researched health issues in recent history. No negative trends have been identified that could be attributed to the introduction or duration of fluoride in drinking water. In contrast, almost all professional health organizations have concluded that results of numerous long-term community trials of adding fluoride to public water supplies at optimal levels verify the effectiveness, safety, and cost-benefit of this public health measure in reducing the prevalence of dental caries. Water fluoridation is the most cost-effective method of preventing dental caries, providing the greatest benefit to individuals who can least afford preventive and restorative dentistry.

DENTAL HYGIENE CONSIDERATIONS

- Educate patients about the purpose and value of fluoridation to oral and bone health.
- Go to the CDC website, My Water's Fluoride (https://nccd.cdc.gov/DOH_MWF/), or contact the state or local health department to determine the fluoride content of the water system in the area. Encourage patients to send samples of well water or home water treatment systems to their state health department to determine fluoride content.
- The ESPE FluoriCheck Water Analysis System (3M) can also be used to determine the fluoride content of drinking water.
- Request the content of fluoride in bottled water from the manufacturer.
- Long-term use of infant formulas, particularly powdered formulas reconstituted with fluoridated water, can be a factor for mild fluorosis.
- Carefully estimate the total amount of fluoride the patient consumes daily in foods and water. Because fluoride is available from multiple sources, the possibility of toxic levels should be considered when recommending fluoride supplements or providing treatment, especially for children. Consider the number of carbonated beverages consumed and consumption of all beverages using fluoridated water. The fluoride content is not listed on the label, making it difficult to approximate the amount of fluoride being consumed.
- Educate patients about the caries process. Encourage patients to practice optimal oral hygiene. Plaque biofilm is the primary factor in caries formation. Appropriate oral hygiene when using topical fluorides at home also increases their effectiveness.
- Recommend fluoride supplements only when the fluoride level of the home water supply is known to be deficient.
- Fluoride supplements can be in liquid or tablet form. Tablet forms that dissolve slowly in the mouth also provide a topical effect.[19]
- An adequate fluoride intake is beneficial during development of skeletal tissue and teeth. Encourage fluoride-fortified foods, water, or supplements for breastfed infants and fluoridated water for children and adolescents, if applicable.
- Growth of cariogenic bacteria is reduced by the presence of fluoride. Suggest use of dentifrices or mouthwashes with fluoride for oral self-care for individuals older than 3 years.
- Caution parents of children between 2 to 6 years of age to (a) use only small (pea size) amounts of fluoridated dentifrices, (b) minimize swallowing toothpaste, (c) avoid using fluoride mouth rinse, (d) keep fluoride products out of the reach of children, and (e) use a nonfluoridated toothpaste for children age 2 years and younger. Fluoride levels in children's toothpastes often equal the levels in adult fluoridated toothpastes.
- If fluoride and calcium supplements are given concurrently, absorption of both is decreased.
- For individuals living in an area where the fluoride content of water is naturally 2 to 4 ppm, recommend drinking bottled water without fluoride or using commercially available filters that can reduce the fluoride to safer levels.
- There is no risk of fluorosis after enamel has developed.
- Dental professionals need to be alert and active in their communities and prepared to present factual information to governing bodies.

NUTRITIONAL DIRECTIONS

- A 2.2-mg amount of sodium fluoride contains 1 mg of fluoride ion.
- To provide maximum benefits, systemic fluoride is important before tooth eruption, when development of unerupted permanent teeth is occurring.
- Fluoride supplementation is recommended for patients 6 months to 16 years old with less than 0.6 ppm of fluoride in their water source (home, childcare settings, school, or bottled) if there is no other significant source of fluoride.
- Fluoride supplements are not recommended during pregnancy.
- If a child receives suboptimal levels of fluoride, an increase in dental caries may occur. Exposure to multiple sources of fluoride increases the risk of excess fluoride, causing fluorosis.
- Fluoride supplements are inappropriate for individuals living in areas where the fluoride content of drinking water is optimal.
- Topical availability of fluoride at low concentrations on a daily basis after tooth eruption is important to deter development of dental caries.
- If caries susceptibility is high, professionally applied and self-applied home fluoride therapies may be an integral component of dental hygiene care.
- When bottled water is being used, obtain the fluoride content from the distributor or the label.
- Studies have found no association between fluoride supplementation and cancer in humans.
- Aluminum antacids decrease fluoride absorption.
- High levels of calcium can interfere with the absorption of fluoride.

HEALTH APPLICATION 9

Osteoporosis

Osteoporosis is a serious, common, and costly disease, increasing in prevalence in men and women. This condition is partly genetically determined. Ten million Americans are affected by osteoporosis and another 34 million have low bone mass (osteopenia). Approximately 80% of individuals with osteoporosis are women (one in two women older than age 50 years); however, osteoporosis will also affect one in four men older than age 50 years.[1]

Osteoporotic bone is characterized as porous with reduced mineralization and density. Fig. 9.7 shows the enlargement of cancellous bone combined with a reduced and weakened trabecular bone. Osteoporotic bones are fragile and fracture easily.

Osteoporosis is more likely to develop in individuals with at least some of the risk factors listed in Box 9.3. The incidence of osteoporosis is greatest in white, Asian, Hispanic, and African American women, especially those who are small and thin. A woman's risk of osteoporosis starts around menopause (age 50 years or older). Women can lose 20% of their bone mass within 5 to 7 years after menopause. Bone loss in men increases after age 65 years. Men who fall and break a hip are twice as likely to die within a year after the incident.[1] For individuals at risk for osteoporosis, an objective of treatment is to slow or stop disease progression before irreversible structural changes have occurred. The National Osteoporosis Foundation recommends steps for preventing osteoporosis:[20,21]

1. Get the daily recommended amounts of calcium and vitamin D. Dietary modifications for patients at risk of developing osteoporosis should include at least two portions of dairy products daily (to provide 75% of RDAs). For patients who have inadequate intake of milk or milk products (including patients who are lactose intolerant), inclusion of calcium and vitamin D supplements may be indicated.
2. Engage in regular weight-bearing and muscle-strengthening exercise.
3. Avoid tobacco use and excessive alcohol.
4. Talk to a health care provider about bone health and supplement use.
5. Take steps to prevent falling, such as regular vision and hearing exams, investigate neurologic problems, and improve safety concerns at home.
6. Have a bone mineral density (BMD) test and take medication when appropriate. Specialized tests to assess BMD should be conducted on women older than 65 years, men older than 70 years, those older than 50 years with risk factors for osteoporosis, and all individuals who have broken a bone after age 50 years.

The oral cavity (teeth, maxilla, and mandible) can be affected by osteoporosis. When identifying periodontal issues, such as tooth mobility or loss, resorption of alveolar bone, temporomandibular disorders, and clinical attachment loss, a relationship to osteoporosis should be considered.[22] Advise patients with osteoporosis about the importance of regular oral hygiene care to reduce the risk of these dental issues also explaining development of periodontitis may be faster and more severe.

Postmenopausal women treated with estrogen for osteoporosis have been found to be at a lower risk of periodontitis.[23]

To date, osteoporosis cannot be cured, but medications can help prevent or deter bone loss. Medications used to slow bone loss include estrogen hormone, bisphosphonates (alendronate, alendronate plus D, ibandronate, risedronate, risedronate with 500 mg of calcium carbonate and zoledronic acid), calcitonin, estrogen agonists/selective estrogen receptor modulators, and PTH. A significant dental consideration for the use of bisphosphonates, particularly following intravenous bisphosphonate treatment for patients with cancer, is the risk for the development of osteonecrosis of the jaw.[24] Commonly used medications for other conditions have a documented effect on bone mineralization. Thiazide diuretics, principally used for blood pressure control, positively affect bone mineralization. Glucocorticoids, used to reduce inflammation, adversely affect bone mineralization. Antiandrogenic drugs for prostate cancer may lead to bone loss.

An adequate calcium intake is important at all stages of life, with a daily intake of a minimum of 1000 mg for all healthy adults and 1200 mg for women older than 51 years. Adequate exposure to sunlight and vitamin D intake are also important. The action of these two nutrients is complementary; calcium supports bone formation and repair, and vitamin D helps with calcium absorption. Other nutritional considerations include B vitamins and vitamin K, which may reduce fracture risk by improving BMD. Several studies have reported a positive association between the use of phytochemicals (plant chemicals) and preventing bone loss. Diets high in fruits, vegetables, and whole grains contribute nutrients that may reduce calcium excretion. However, high fiber intake (including oxalates and phytates) should be paired with increased calcium intake. High levels of phosphorus, sodium, or caffeine intake may increase calcium loss in urine.[25] **Phytochemicals**, natural components of foods, found in soy products and flaxseed, stimulate estrogen secretion, which may boost BMD.[26] A health care provider or RDN can tailor the osteoporosis regimen to meet the patient's needs.

• BOX 9.3 Risk Factors for Osteoporosis

Certain people are more likely to develop osteoporosis than others. Factors that increase the likelihood of developing osteoporosis and broken bones are called "risk factors." These risk factors include:

- Being female
- Older age
- Family history of osteoporosis or broken bones
- Being small and thin (low body mass index)
- Certain races/ethnicities such as white, Asian, or Hispanic/Latino, although African Americans are also at risk
- History of broken bones
- Low sex hormones
  - Low estrogen levels in women, including menopause
  - Missing periods (amenorrhea)
  - Low levels of testosterone and estrogen in men
- Diet
  - Low calcium intake
  - Low vitamin D intake
  - Excessive intake of protein, sodium, and caffeine
- Inactive lifestyle
- Smoking
- Excessive alcohol (3 or more drinks/day)
- Certain medications such as steroid medications, anticonvulsants, anticoagulants (heparin), chemotherapeutic drugs and others. Potential risks should be explained.
- Certain diseases and conditions such as anorexia nervosa, bulimia, athletic amenorrhea, premature menopause (< 40 years), rheumatoid arthritis, gastrointestinal diseases, cystic fibrosis and others

Data from National Osteoporosis Foundation. Prevention and healthy living. http://www.nof.org/learn/prevention. Accessed March 13, 2017.

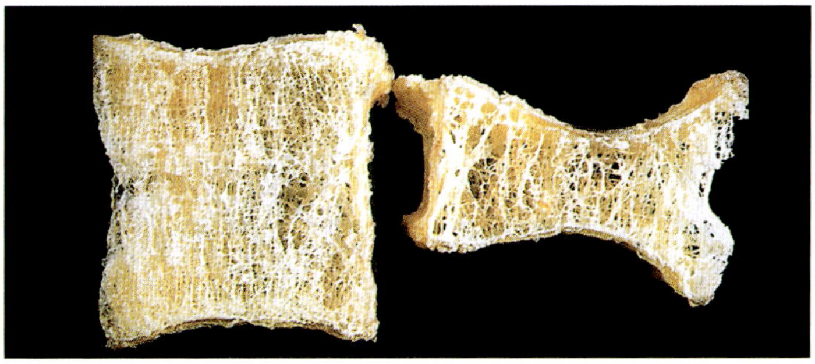

A

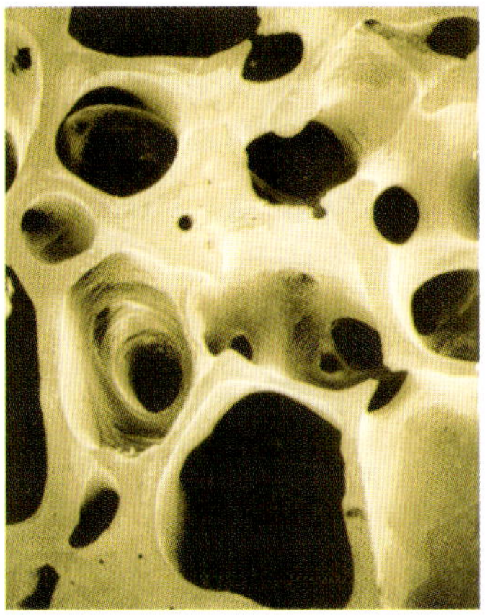

B

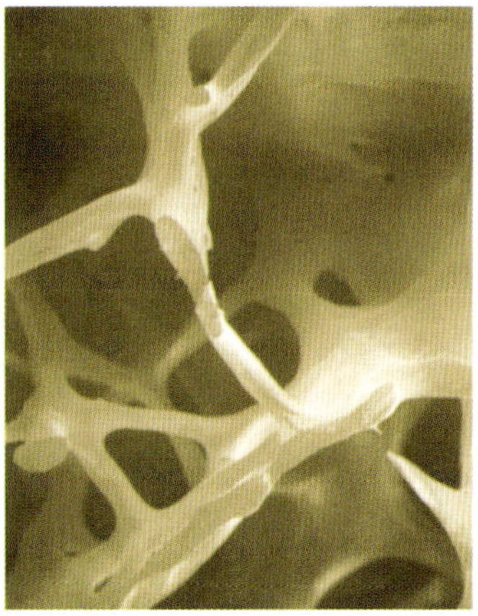

C

• **Figure 9.7** Osteoporosis. (A) Compare the normal vertebral body (*left*) with the osteoporotic specimen (*right*). Note that the osteoporotic vertebral body has been shortened by compression fractures. (B) Microscopic normal bone. (C) Microscopic osteoporotic bone. Note the loss of trabecular bone and appearance of enlarged pores caused by osteoporosis. (Modified from Patton KT, Thibodeau GA. *Anatomy and Physiology*. 9th ed, St. Louis, MO: Elsevier; 2016.)

CASE APPLICATION FOR THE DENTAL HYGIENIST

During Annie's routine dental examination, her mother asked the dental hygienist whether she should start Annie (age 5 years) on a fluoride supplement. Annie's examination revealed a caries-free mouth. She had been brushing her teeth twice a day.

Nutritional Assessment

- Food consumption pattern
- Frequency of carbohydrate intake
- Fluoride content of water consumed; average amount of water/water-based beverages consumed
- Type and amount of toothpaste used

Nutritional Diagnosis

Health-seeking behaviors related to inadequate knowledge about fluoride supplementation.

Nutritional Goals

The patient will practice good oral self-care and receive adequate fluoride to prevent dental caries.

Nutritional Implementation

Intervention: Explain the benefits of fluoride.

Rationale: Fluoride is advantageous to dental health because of its systemic effect before tooth eruption and its topical effects after tooth eruption. The caries-preventive properties of systemic and topical fluoride are additive.

Intervention: Discuss the toxic effects of fluoride.

Rationale: Dental fluorosis is directly related to the level of fluoride exposure during tooth development. It can also have adverse effects on bone structure.

Intervention: Assess current fluoride consumption from (a) food, (b) water supply, (c) carbonated beverages, and (d) fluoridated dentifrices and mouth rinses.

Rationale: (a) All foods contain some fluoride, but the amounts provided in vegetables, meats, cereals, and fruits are insignificant unless large amounts of seafood, tea, or deboned poultry are consumed; (b) water is usually the main source of fluoride, but some municipal water supplies and bottled waters may contain negligible amounts of fluoride; and (c) fluoride is added to 90% of all dentifrices in the United States. Because younger children swallow most of the toothpaste used, they should be provided with a dentifrice without fluoride.

Intervention: Show Annie and her mother how much toothpaste to use, and discuss the importance of not swallowing it.

Rationale: Because fluoride in toothpaste can be readily absorbed, toothpaste should not be swallowed to prevent the harmful effects of systemically available fluoride.

Intervention: Encourage the patient and her mother to consume a well-balanced diet with limited amounts of fermentable carbohydrates at snack time.

Rationale: Not only is fluoride important, but also other nutrients are essential for dental health. Snacks, especially carbohydrate-containing foods, increase risk for dental caries.

Continued

◆ CASE APPLICATION FOR THE DENTAL HYGIENIST—cont'd

Intervention: Suggest fluoride supplements only if fluoride intake seems to be low.
Rationale: In many cases, total fluoride exposure seems to be higher than necessary to prevent tooth decay. No more than the amount of fluoride necessary to provide the desired effect should be used.
Intervention: Recommend parental supervision and assistance for Annie's tooth brushing and flossing.
Rationale: Monitoring the child's brushing technique and assisting with flossing will ensure that effective biofilm removal occurs once a day.

Evaluation

If the patient and her mother can demonstrate the toothbrushing procedure, the patient says she will brush her teeth after every meal and will try to eat the foods her mother provides, and dental caries continues to be minimal, dental hygiene care was effective.

◆ Student Readiness

1. A patient claims that she dislikes milk. How would you advise her to obtain the calcium she needs?
2. What are the main physiologic roles of calcium, phosphorus, magnesium, and fluoride?
3. How do minerals differ from vitamins?
4. How would you respond to a remark that milk is only for babies?
5. Discuss three dietary factors that affect calcium absorption.
6. Determine the level of fluoride in your community's drinking water.
7. If an adult patient (weight about 75 kg) is drinking only bottled water that does not contain fluoride, and the patient dislikes fish and tea, how much topical fluoride would be necessary to furnish the recommendation for fluoride?
8. List five types of over-the-counter calcium supplements available. Evaluate these items for primary sources of calcium and elemental calcium per unit consumed. Find how many tablets or units would have to be consumed daily to receive 1000 mg of elemental calcium.
9. Discuss how to deal with a patient who is opposed to community water fluoridation.
10. Why would you advise patients to obtain their mineral requirement from food sources rather than mineral supplements (unless ordered by the health care provider)?

◆ CASE STUDY

Mrs. J. M., a 69-year-old woman, fell and fractured her hip 6 months ago. She admits she is taking calcium supplements occasionally, when she can afford them. She does not like milk and has been unable to walk much since her fall.

1. What additional questions would you ask to clarify the situation?
2. What nutritional advice could you give her about her osteoporosis?
3. What is her RDA for calcium?
4. What foods could you suggest she consume to increase her calcium intake?
5. When should she take her calcium supplement to maximize its absorption?
6. What oral changes might you expect to find in your assessment?
7. What effect would increased vitamin D intake have on her condition?

References

1. National Osteoporosis Foundation. Bone health basics: get the facts. https://www.nof.org/preventing-fractures/general-facts/. Accessed March 13, 2017.
2. U.S. Department of Agriculture, Agricultural Research Service. What we eat in America, NHANES 2009–2010; 2014. http://www.ars.usda.gov/ba/bhnrc/fsrg. Accessed February 6, 2017.
3. U.S. Preventive Services Task Force. U.S. Preventive Services Task Force issues final recommendation on vitamin D and calcium supplements to prevent fractures. https://www.uspreventiveservicestaskforce.org/Page/Document/UpdateSummaryFinal/vitamin-d-and-calcium-to-prevent-fractures-preventive-medication. Accessed February 13, 2017.
4. Xiao Q, Murphy RA, Houston DK, et al. Dietary and supplemental calcium intake and cardiovascular disease mortality. *JAMA Intern Med.* 2013;173(8):639–646.
5. Reid IR. Cardiovascular effects of calcium supplements. *Nutrients.* 2013;5:2522–2529.
6. Committee to Review Dietary Reference Intakes for Vitamin D and Calcium, Food and Nutrition Board, Institute of Medicine. *Dietary Reference Intakes for Calcium and Vitamin D.* Washington, DC: National Academy Press; 2010.
7. Farela-Lopez A, Giampiere F, Bullon P, et al. A systematic review on the implication of minerals in the onset, severity and treatment of periodontal disease. *Molecules.* 2016;21:doi:10.3390/molecules21091183. www.mdpi.com/journal/molecules. Accessed February 13, 2017.
8. Liu C, Wu D, Zhang J-F, et al. Changes in bone metabolism in morbidly obese patients after bariatric surgery: a meta-analysis. *Obes Surg.* 2016;26:91–97.
9. Brzozowska MM, Sainsbury A, Eisman JA, et al. Bariatric surgery, bone loss, obesity and possible mechanisms. *Obes Rev.* 2013;14(1):52–67.
10. Goodson JM, Ping S, Mumena CH, et al. Dietary phosphorus burden increases cariogenesis independent of vitamin D uptake. *J Steroid Biochem Mol Biol.* 2017;167:33–38.
11. Takeda E, Yamamoto H, Yamanaka-Okumura H, et al. Dietary phosphorus in bone health and quality of life. *Nutr Rev.* 2012;70(6):311–321.
12. Larsson SC, Orsini N, Wolk A. Dietary magnesium intake and risk of stroke: a meta-analysis of prospective studies. *Am J Clin Nutr.* 2012;95(2):362–366.
13. Centers for Disease Control and Prevention. Division of Oral Health. 2014 water fluoridation statistics. https://www.cdc.gov/fluoridation/statistics/2014stats.htm. Accessed March 2, 2017.
14. U.S. Department of Health and Human Services Agency, U.S. Environmental Protection Agency. Public Health Service recommendation for fluoride concentration in drinking water for prevention of dental caries. https://www.federalregister.gov/documents/2015/05/01/2015-10201/public-health-service-recommendation-for-fluoride-concentration-in-drinking-water-for-prevention-of. Accessed March 2, 2017.

15. Environmental Protection Agency. Review of the fluoride drinking water regulation; 2011. https://www.epa.gov/dwsixyearreview/review-fluoride-drinking-water-regulation. Accessed March 13, 2017.
16. National Research Council, Committee on Fluoride in Drinking Water. Fluoride in drinking water: a scientific review of EPA's standards; 2006. Washington, DC: National Academies Press.
17. Healthy People 2020. Oral Health 2020 Topics and Objectives. http://www.healthypeople.gov/2020/topicsobjectives2020/objectiveslist.aspx?topicId=32. Accessed March 13, 2017.
18. Iheozor-Ejiofor Z, Worthington HV, Walsh T, et al. Water fluoridation for the prevention of dental caries. *Cochrane Database Syst Rev.* 2015;(6):CD010856. doi:10.1002/14651858.CD010856.pub2. Accessed March 13, 2017.
19. Palmer CA, Gilbert JA, Academy of Nutrition and Dietetics. Position of the Academy of Nutrition and Dietetics: the impact of fluoride on health. *J Acad Nutr Diet.* 2012;112(9):1443–1453.
20. Prentice RL, Pettinger MB, Jackson RD, et al. Health risks and benefits from calcium and vitamin D supplementation: Women's Health Initiative clinical trial and cohort study. *Osteoporos Int.* 2013;24(2): 567–580.
21. Cosman F, de Beur SJ, LeBoff MS, et al. Clinician's guide to prevention and treatment of osteoporosis. *Osteoporos Int.* 2014;http://link.springer.com. Accessed March 13, 2017.
22. Chambrone L. Current status of the influence of osteoporosis on periodontology and implant dentistry. *Curr Opin Endocrinol Diabetes Obes.* 2016;23(6):435–439.
23. Passos-Soares J, Vianna MIP, Gomes-Filho IS, et al. Association between osteoporosis treatment and severe periodontitis in post-menopausal women. *Menopause.* 2017;24(7):1.
24. Grgic O, Kovacey-Zavisic B, Veljovic T, et al. The influence of bone mineral density and bisphosphonate therapy on the determinants of oral health and changes on dental panoramic radiographs in post-menopausal women. *Clin Oral Investig.* 2016;21:151–157.
25. De Franca NAG, Camargo MBR, Lazaretti-Castro M, et al. Dietary patterns and bone mineral density in Brazilian postmenopausal women with osteoporosis: a cross-sectional study. *Eur J Clin Nutr.* 2016;70:85–90.
26. Leitzmann C. Characteristics and health benefits of phytochemicals. *Forsch Komplementmed.* 2016;23(2):69–74.

EVOLVE RESOURCES

Please visit http://evolve.elsevier.com/Stegeman/nutritional for additional practice and study support tools.

10

Nutrients Present in Calcified Structures

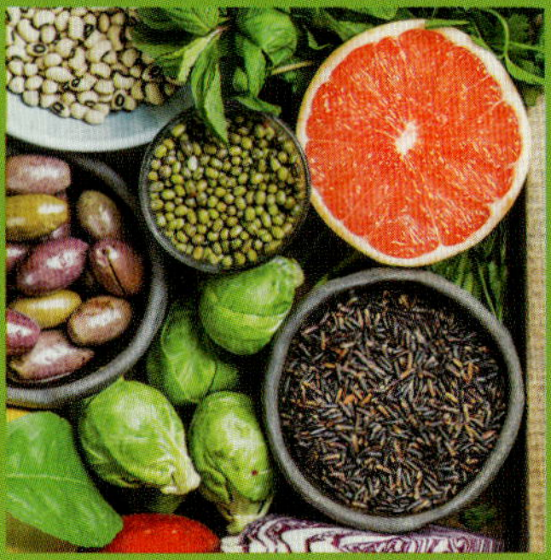

STUDENT LEARNING OUTCOMES

Upon completion of this chapter, the student will be able to achieve the following student learning outcomes:

1. Discuss the following related to copper:
   - Describe the physiologic roles of copper and how they apply to oral health, state the recommended dietary allowance (RDA) for copper, and list sources of copper.
   - Discuss hyper states and hypo states related to copper, and apply dental considerations for when either occurs.
2. Discuss the following related to selenium:
   - Describe the physiologic roles of selenium and how they apply to oral health, state the RDA for selenium, and list sources of selenium.
   - Discuss hyper states and hypo states related to selenium, and apply dental considerations for when either occurs.
3. Discuss the following related to chromium:
   - Describe the physiologic roles of chromium and how they apply to oral health, state the RDA for chromium, and list sources of chromium.
   - Discuss hyper states and hypo states related to chromium, and apply dental considerations for when either occurs.
4. Discuss the following related to manganese and molybdenum:
   - Describe the physiologic roles of manganese and molybdenum and how they apply to oral health, state the RDA for manganese and molybdenum, and list sources of manganese and molybdenum.
   - Discuss hyper states and hypo states related to manganese and molybdenum, and apply dental considerations for when either occurs.
5. List ultratrace elements present in the body.

KEY TERMS

Enteral feedings
Kayser-Fleischer ring
Keshan disease
Manganese madness
Neurotransmitters
Osteodystrophy
Stannous
Total parenteral nutrition (TPN)

TEST YOUR NQ

1. **T/F** The National Academy of Medicine (formerly the Institute of Medicine) has established tolerable upper intake levels (ULs) for copper, manganese, chromium, and molybdenum.
2. **T/F** Lead in dental enamel can be used to determine environmental exposure to lead.
3. **T/F** Copper is important in the formation of collagen.
4. **T/F** Aluminum toxicity causes Alzheimer disease.
5. **T/F** Selenium functions as an antioxidant.
6. **T/F** Refined foods are good sources of trace minerals.
7. **T/F** Aluminum is cariogenic.
8. **T/F** The function of many trace elements present in enamel and dentin is unknown.
9. **T/F** Sugar is a good source of chromium.
10. **T/F** Selenium supplements are a good way to increase longevity.

Very small amounts of several minerals are essential for optimal growth and development. Many of these ultratrace elements (Table 10.1) are found in enamel and dentin. The role of minerals may not be obvious as you clinically assess patients; nevertheless, patients with inadequate amounts may exhibit deficiency symptoms.

Tolerable upper intake levels (ULs) have not been established for several of these nutrients because of the lack of data. The requirement for these nutrients should be obtained from food sources because even small amounts may be toxic. Available evidence suggests that ultratrace minerals—especially arsenic, boron, nickel, and silicon—may be physiologically essential. Because no human

TABLE 10.1 Trace Element Concentrations in Human Enamel and Dentin

	Enamel[a] (ppm)	Dentin[a] (ppm)
Aluminum	1.5–700	10–100
Boron	0.5–39	1–10
Cadmium	0.3–10	
Chromium	< 0.1–100	1–100
Copper	0.1–130	0.2–100
Iron	0.8–200	90–1000
Lead	1.3–100	10–100
Lithium	0.23–3.40	
Manganese	0.8–20	0.6–1000
Molybdenum	0.7–39	1–10
Nickel	10–100	10–100
Selenium	0.1–10	10–100
Strontium	26–1000	90-1000
Sulfur	130–530	
Tin	0.03–0.9	
Vanadium	0.01–0.03	1–10
Zinc	60–1800	

ppm, parts per million
[a]μg/g dry weight.
Adapted from Gron P. Inorganic chemical and structural aspects of oral mineralized tissues. In Shaw JH, eds. *Textbook of Oral Biology.* Philadelphia, Saunders; 1978; 484–507.

TABLE 10.2 National Academy of Medicine Recommendations for Copper

	EAR (μg/day)		RDA (μg/day)		
Life Stage	Male	Female	Male	Female	AI (μg/day)
Birth–6 months	—	—	—	—	200
7–12 months	—	—	—	—	220
1–3 years	260	260	340	340	
4–8 years	340	340	440	440	
9–13 years	540	540	700	700	
14–18 years	685	685	890	890	
> 18 years	700	700	900	900	
Pregnancy					
14–18 years		785		1000	
19–50 years		800		1000	
Lactation					
14–18 years		985		1300	
19–50 years		1000		1300	

AI, Adequate intake; EAR, estimated average requirement; RDA, recommended dietary allowance.
Data from Institute of Medicine (IOM), Food and Nutrition Board. *Dietary Reference Intakes for Vitamin A, Vitamin K, Arsenic, Boron, Chromium, Copper, Iodine, Iron, Manganese, Molybdenum, Nickel, Silicon, Vanadium, and Zinc.* Washington, DC: National Academy Press; 2001.

deficiencies have been determined, their importance in humans can only be inferred from results of animal studies. Human requirements have not been quantified. If they are required, the amounts needed are easily met by naturally occurring sources in food, water, and air. Other elements present in calcified structures, such as cadmium, lead, and tin, have no known function and may be contaminants.

Copper

Physiologic Roles

Copper is the third largest trace element found in the human body, following iron and zinc. Copper is essential for formation of red blood cells and connective tissue. Its function as a catalyst is important in the formation of collagen from a precollagenous stage. Copper is a component of many enzymes that function in oxidative reactions, and copper-containing enzymes encourage production of **neurotransmitters** (including norepinephrine and dopamine), which transmit messages through the central nervous system. Two other roles are nutrient metabolism and immune function.

Copper is readily incorporated into tooth enamel. Radiographic fluorescence imaging of teeth shows an increased concentration of copper in carious portions of the tooth. Therefore, a copper deficiency may induce caries. However, copper may be cariostatic by reducing the acidogenicity of plaque.

Requirements

The National Academy of Medicine (formerly the Institute of Medicine) established the recommended dietary allowance (RDA) for copper as 900 μg per day for adults. The UL has been set at 10 g per day for adults (Table 10.2).

Absorption and Excretion

Approximately one-third of dietary copper is absorbed, occurring primarily in the stomach and duodenum. Absorption is enhanced by a low pH and is diminished by large amounts of calcium and zinc. Copper is stored mostly in the liver and muscle and is excreted through bile in feces.

Sources

Copper is widely distributed in foods. The richest sources include shellfish, oysters, crabs, liver, nuts, sesame and sunflower seeds, soy products, legumes, and cocoa.

Hyper States and Hypo States

Copper toxicity is seldom encountered. Copper taken orally is an emetic; 10 mg of oral copper can produce nausea. Serum copper levels are elevated in patients with rheumatoid arthritis, myocardial

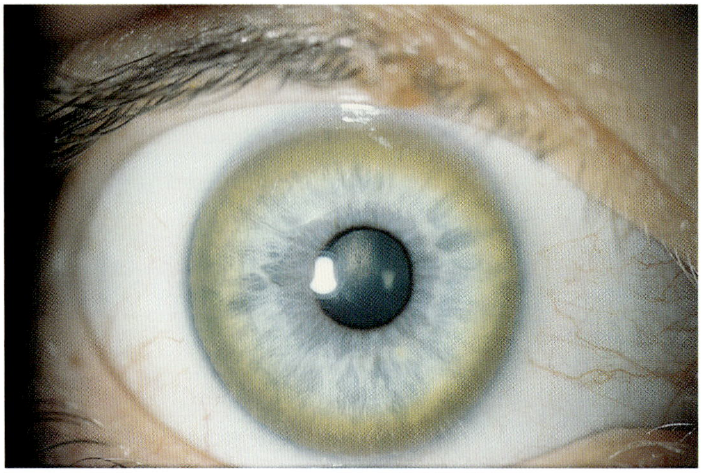

• **Figure 10.1** Cornea in Wilson disease. Copper deposits in the corneal periphery produce the characteristic Kayser-Fleischer ring. This is a complete or incomplete brown-to-green ring near the cornea, best seen in early stages of the disease. (Reproduced with permission from Swartz MH. *Textbook of Physical Diagnosis: History and Examination*. 7th ed. St. Louis, MO: Elsevier; 2014.)

infarction, conditions requiring administration of estrogen, and pregnancy.

Wilson disease is a special metabolic disorder in which large amounts of copper accumulate in the liver, kidney, brain, and cornea. The body cannot release copper from the liver at a normal rate due to a genetic abnormality. Copper concentrates in the cornea, causing a characteristic brown or green ring called the **Kayser-Fleischer ring** (Fig. 10.1).

Most copper deficiencies have been detected under unusual conditions, such as with zinc supplementation, malnutrition, malabsorption disorders, or in patients receiving **total parenteral nutrition** (**TPN**, delivery of all nutritional needs intravenously). Copper deprivation results in profound effects on the bones, brain, arteries, and other connective tissues; decreased hair and skin pigmentation; and hematologic abnormalities, such as a low white blood cell count. Seemingly, all these effects are ultimately caused by an inadequate supply of copper, which is required for enzyme synthesis and activity.

Copper deficiency causes a variety of lesions within connective tissues and bone, resulting in failure to grow (in children), spontaneous fractures, osteoporosis, arthritis, arterial disease, and ultimately marked bone deformities. These lesions have been attributed to abnormal formation of cross-linkages in collagen and elastin.[1]

DENTAL CONSIDERATIONS

- Anemia that cannot be corrected with iron supplements may be caused by copper deficiency.
- High doses of zinc supplements decrease copper absorption, possibly leading to anemia-related fatigue.

NUTRITIONAL DIRECTIONS

- High-fiber intake increases the dietary requirement for copper.
- Large amounts of vitamin C supplements decrease serum bioavailability of copper.
- Excess molybdenum produces a copper deficiency.

Selenium

Physiologic Roles

Selenium functions mainly as a cofactor for an antioxidant enzyme that protects membrane lipids, proteins, and nucleic acids from oxidative damage. It also has an impact on skeletal integrity and contributes to the maintenance of normal immune function. Selenium works hand in hand with vitamin E as an antioxidant; a deficiency of either nutrient increases the requirement for the other.

Selenium is present in tooth enamel and dentin. It is probably incorporated into the enamel during amelogenesis. Large amounts during tooth formation may be detrimental to the mineralization process.

Requirements

The RDA establishes the adult requirement at 55 μg. The UL is 400 μg per day for adults (Table 10.3). Typical intake in the United States is 60 to 220 μg daily.

Sources

Animal products—especially seafood, kidney, liver, and other meats—are rich in selenium. Selenium intake correlates closely with caloric and protein consumption. Selenium in dairy products and eggs is more readily absorbed than selenium from other foods. Whole-grain products, nuts, and mushrooms are also good sources.

Hyper States and Hypo States

Toxicity and deficiency symptoms have occurred in animals from irregular distribution of selenium in soil, but these are rarely seen in humans. Routine ingestion of 2 to 3 mg of selenium can cause toxic symptoms, including nausea and vomiting, weakness, dermatitis, hair loss, white blotchy nails, mottled teeth, metallic taste, and garlic-smelling breath. Cirrhosis of

TABLE 10.3 National Academy of Medicine Recommendations for Selenium

Life Stage	EAR (μg/day)	RDA (μg/day)	AI (μg/day)
0–6 months			15
7–12 months			20
1–3 years	17	20	
4–8 years	23	30	
9–13 years	35	40	
> 13 years	45	55	
Pregnancy			
≤ 14–50 years	49	60	
Lactation			
≤ 14–50 years	59	70	

AI, Adequate intake; EAR, estimated average requirement; RDA, recommended dietary allowance.
Data from Institute of Medicine (IOM), Food and Nutrition Board. *Dietary Reference Intakes For Vitamin C, Vitamin E, Selenium, and Carotenoids.* Washington, DC: National Academy Press; 2000.

the liver also may develop. A moderate intake of selenium has been linked to reduced risk of cancers of the prostate, lung, and colon and reduced risk of heart disease because of its role as an antioxidant.

Excessive selenium may promote dental caries when given before eruption, whereas moderately high levels seem to have some cariostatic effects. Increased dental caries rates have been observed in areas where food and water contain higher levels of selenium. Whether this increase in caries is caused by a topical effect on plaque biofilm or by an effect on the structural composition of teeth is unknown.

In parts of China, an endemic cardiomyopathy called **Keshan disease** is associated with severe selenium deficiency. Oral selenium prophylaxis is extremely effective in reducing Keshan disease but not in eradicating it. A deficiency of selenium may also occur in patients undergoing dialysis or those living with human immunodeficiency virus.

DENTAL CONSIDERATIONS

- Decreased selenium levels may cause heart damage, resulting in a heart attack.
- Selenium is essential for health, but it can also be toxic.

NUTRITIONAL DIRECTIONS

- Because of increased risk of toxicity, selenium supplements should not be taken by patients with cancer, cardiovascular disease (CVD), arthritis, and human immunodeficiency virus, unless recommended by a health care provider.
- Gastrointestinal disorders, such as Crohn disease, can impair selenium absorption.

TABLE 10.4 National Academy of Medicine Recommendations for Chromium

	AI (μg/day)	
Life Stage Group	Male	Female
Birth–6 months	0.2	0.2
7–12 months	2.2	2.2
1–3 years	11	11
4–8 years	15	15
9–13 years	25	21
14–18 years	35	24
19–50 years	35	25
> 50 years	30	20
Pregnancy		
14–18 years		29
19–50 years		30
Lactation		
14–18 years		44
19–50 years		45

AI, Adequate intake.
Data from Institute of Medicine (IOM), Food and Nutrition Board. *Dietary Reference Intakes for Vitamin A, Vitamin K, Arsenic, Boron, Chromium, Copper, Iodine, Iron, Manganese, Molybdenum, Nickel, Silicon, Vanadium, and Zinc.* Washington, DC: National Academy Press; 2001.

Chromium

Physiologic Roles

Chromium is an odorless and tasteless metallic element. Chromium is involved in carbohydrate and lipid metabolism. In the use of glucose, chromium may potentiate the action of insulin; however, there is limited evidence to support the use of chromium supplements for glycemic control in individuals with type 2 diabetes.[2] There is no known association with the oral cavity.

Requirements

The adequate intake (AI) of a healthy adult has been estimated as 20 to 35 μg per day. No UL has been set (Table 10.4). The National Academy of Medicine reports the average chromium content in well-balanced diets as 13.4 μg/1000 cal. Chromium is poorly absorbed; whether intestinal absorption compensates for increased demand is unclear. Chromium status decreases with age, suggesting that older adults may have an increased risk of deficiency.

Sources

Chromium is found in meats, whole-grain cereals, wheat germ, nuts, mushrooms, green beans, broccoli, brewer's yeast, beer, wine, and tap water. The refining process depletes chromium from grains and cereal. The Safe Drinking Water Act (2010) required the U.S. Environmental Protection Agency (EPA) to determine the level of contaminants in drinking water at which no adverse effects are likely to occur. This reevaluation indicated current limitations of chromium in water were appropriate. A number of systems are used to monitor for harmful levels of chromium in drinking water. The current EPA standard for chromium in public water systems is not to exceed 100 parts per billion (ppb).[3] Chromium supplements are available as picolinate, nicotinate, or chloride (the form provided in most multivitamin–mineral supplements).

Hyper States and Hypo States

Chromium deficiencies result in decreased insulin sensitivity, impaired glucose intolerance, neuropathy, and elevated plasma free fatty acid concentration. Patients on TPN are at risk of a chromium deficiency. Chromium toxicity has been caused by use of chromium supplements and by industrial exposure, resulting in liver damage and lung cancer.

DENTAL CONSIDERATIONS

- Assess patients employed in industrial settings or artists using supplies with high chromium content for chromium toxicity.
- Serum chromium levels decline with age.
- Chromium supplements may cause serious renal impairment when taken in excess.

NUTRITIONAL DIRECTION

- Do not take chromium supplements unless instructed by a health care provider. Currently, the evidence is unclear as to whether any type of supplemental chromium can help with fat loss or enhance lean body mass.

Manganese

Physiologic Roles

Manganese is essential in several enzyme systems and is important for optimal bone matrix development; prevention of osteoporosis; insulin production; and amino acid, cholesterol, and carbohydrate metabolism. It is absorbed in the small intestine, transported to the liver, and excreted in bile.

Requirements

As shown in Table 10.5, an adequate intake is 1.8 to 2.3 mg per day for adults. The absorption of iron and manganese is inversely proportional, so a large amount of one reduces absorption of the other. The UL has been established as 11 mg per day for adults. Median intake in the United States is 2.1 to 2.3 mg per day for men and 1.6 to 1.8 mg per day for women.

Sources

Foods high in manganese include whole-grain cereals, legumes, nuts, tea, leafy greens, and infant formula. The bioavailability of manganese from meats, milk, and eggs makes these important sources despite their smaller quantities.

TABLE 10.5 National Academy of Medicine Recommendations for Manganese

	AI (mg/day)	
Life Stage Group	**Male**	**Female**
Birth–6 months	0.003	0.003
7–12 months	0.6	0.6
1–3 years	1.2	1.2
4–8 years	1.5	1.5
9–13 years	1.9	1.6
14–18 years	2.2	1.6
> 18 years	2.3	1.8
Pregnancy		
14–50 years		2
Lactation		
14–50 years		2.6

AI, Adequate intake.
Data from Institute of Medicine (IOM), Food and Nutrition Board. *Dietary Reference Intakes for Vitamin A, Vitamin K, Arsenic, Boron, Chromium, Copper, Iodine, Iron, Manganese, Molybdenum, Nickel, Silicon, Vanadium, and Zinc.* Washington, DC: National Academy Press; 2001.

Hyper States and Hypo States

Manganese dust can be an environmental hazard. Manganese miners and welders have developed a syndrome similar to Parkinson disease called "**manganese madness**." Manganese miners are exposed to large amounts of manganese fumes, but other groups are at risk for manganese poisoning as well, including workers in factories manufacturing dry alkaline batteries and workers in facilities making manganese alloys. Symptoms of toxic exposure include ataxia, headache, fatigue, anxiety, hallucinations, psychosis, and a syndrome similar to Parkinson disease (marked by memory loss, tremors, and rigid body posture). In addition, elevated concentrations of manganese in salivary plaque and enamel are associated with increased caries.

Manganese deficiencies have never been reported in individuals consuming a normal diet. Signs of deficiency include abnormal formation of bone and cartilage, growth retardation, congenital malformations, hypercholesterolemia, impaired glucose tolerance, and poor reproductive performance.

DENTAL CONSIDERATIONS

- Inhaling manganese dust can be toxic. Patients whose occupations expose them to increased inhalation of manganese (i.e., factory workers, welders, or manganese miners) may exhibit psychotic symptoms or Parkinson-like symptoms.

NUTRITIONAL DIRECTIONS

- Phytate and fiber in bran, tannins in tea, and oxalic acid in spinach inhibit absorption of manganese.
- Consistent low iron intake results in more manganese absorption.
- Excess manganese can produce iron-deficiency anemia.[4]
- Manganese should not be confused with magnesium.

Molybdenum

Physiologic Roles

Molybdenum functions as an enzyme cofactor. Molybdenum, a trace element present in teeth, may inhibit caries formation.

Requirements

The RDA for molybdenum is 45 μg per day for adults. The UL is set at 2000 μg per day for adults (Table 10.6).

Sources

Legumes, whole-grain cereals, and nuts are the best sources; milk, liver, and many vegetables are poor sources.

Hyper States and Hypo States

Except for deficiency reported during administration of TPN, molybdenum deficiency has not been documented in the United States.

DENTAL CONSIDERATIONS

- Consumption of large quantities of molybdenum may result in copper deficiency, making the patient prone to anemia and risk of gout.[4]

NUTRITIONAL DIRECTIONS

- Legumes (e.g., lentils, beans, peas), nuts, and whole grains are good sources of molybdenum.

TABLE 10.6 National Academy of Medicine Recommendations for Molybdenum

	EAR (μg/day)		RDA (μg/day)		
Life Stage	Male	Female	Male	Female	AI (μg/day)
Birth–6 months	—	—	—	—	2
7–12 months	—	—	—	—	3
1–3 years	13	13	17	17	
4–8 years	17	17	22	22	
9–13 years	26	26	34	34	
14–18 years	33	33	43	43	
> 18 years	34	34	45	45	
Pregnancy					
14–50 years		40		50	
Lactation					
14–18 years		35		50	
19–50 years		36		50	

AI, Adequate intake; EAR, estimated average requirement; RDA, recommended dietary allowance.
Data from Institute of Medicine (IOM), Food and Nutrition Board. *Dietary Reference Intakes for Vitamin A, Vitamin K, Arsenic, Boron, Chromium, Copper, Iodine, Iron, Manganese, Molybdenum, Nickel, Silicon, Vanadium, and Zinc.* Washington, DC: National Academy Press; 2001.

Ultratrace Elements

Many ultratrace elements have been studied for their potential influence on dental caries. Results of research investigations are complicated by many factors. Nevertheless, some studies suggest relationships between some ultratrace elements and the development of caries in humans or animals. Further research is warranted to determine the mechanism of their effects.

More attention has been given to ultratrace elements as contaminants in the environment and foods. Some are considered to have no harmful effects and are used therapeutically, such as aluminum in antacids.

Boron

Boron may have an effect on metabolism of calcium, phosphorus, magnesium, or vitamin D, and may be needed to maintain membrane structure. Inadequate amounts of vitamin D increase the boron requirement. Boron, along with fluoride, is necessary for development and maintenance of strong, healthy bones. Dietary intake may also have an association with inflammation.[5] Boron is principally present in foods of plant origin, especially fruits, vegetables, nuts, legumes, and wine.

Boron deficiency affects mineral metabolism. Patients with disturbed mineral metabolic disorders of unknown etiology, such as osteoporosis, may be deficient in boron.

Nickel

The physiologic role of nickel is still unclear. It may be involved in the metabolism of vitamin B_{12} and folic acid. Nickel deficiency results in suboptimal growth in animals. Inadequate nickel alters trace-element composition of bone and impairs iron use. Good sources of nickel include dried beans and peas, grains, nuts, and chocolate.

Silicon

Silicon contributes to the structure and resilience of collagen, elastin, and polysaccharides. Silicon is present in tooth enamel in larger amounts than most other trace elements, but its function, if any, is unknown. Deficiencies in animal studies result in depressed collagen in bone and long bone abnormalities, resulting in malformed joints and defective bone growth. Whole grains and root vegetables are good food sources.

Tin

Tin has no known function in development or maintenance of bone, but it may affect bone metabolism because tin accumulates in bone. The absorption of tin can alter use of calcium and zinc, affecting bone growth and maintenance.

Most Americans consume minimal amounts of tin daily because most foods contain trace amounts of tin. Foods packed in tin cans that are totally coated with lacquer contain very little tin, but acidic foods, such as pineapple and orange juice and tomato sauce, packed in cans that are not coated with lacquer contain significant amounts of tin. Other sources of tin include **stannous** (chemical term for tin) chloride, approved for use as a food additive, and fluoride, the active ingredient in some self-applied dentifrices and mouth rinses.

Aluminum

Aluminum probably is not an essential nutrient; its presence in the body seems to be harmful. Under normal conditions, very little aluminum is absorbed; the kidneys excrete about the same amount as is absorbed.

Aluminum accumulates in bone and has been observed to cause **osteodystrophy** (defective bone formation) in patients who have received aluminum from routes other than through the gastrointestinal tract. Water used in intravenous solutions and dialysis fluid is sometimes contaminated with aluminum. The kidneys are frequently unable to remove the daily load of aluminum present in these fluids, causing undesirable effects. Aluminum content of these fluids has been reduced, but may still be high because of naturally occurring aluminum in the water used to make the solutions. Aluminum accumulation can occur through oral ingestion of aluminum hydroxide antacids and from the diet.

Aluminum is also present in all dental tissues. Dental caries may be reduced because aluminum enhances the uptake and retention of fluoride and enhances the cariostatic activity of fluoride. Solubility of enamel is decreased, and plaque biofilm formation and acidogenicity are inhibited by aluminum.

Lead

Much information is available about the harmful effects of lead in the body, but little is known about its beneficial role or its essentiality. As a result of implementation of aggressive public health measures, blood lead levels have decreased markedly since the late 1970s.

Lead is more readily absorbed from the gastrointestinal tract during infancy and early childhood than in adulthood, meaning children are more susceptible to lead exposure. Lead is ingested from toddlers' normal hand-to-mouth activities; in older children, playing with dirt or lead-contaminated objects may result in lead ingestion. Milk intake results in reduced lead absorption. Nutritional status can influence susceptibility to lead toxicity. Lead is also a contaminant in water, most commonly resulting from corroding lead pipes. Therefore, it cannot be directly detected. The EPA requires water systems to control the level of lead to less than 15 ppb.[6]

Inorganic lead can have detrimental effects on children. Even low levels of lead exposure may impair intellectual performance. With elevated serum lead levels, general cognitive, verbal, and perceptual abilities are increasingly affected by slower learning aptitudes, which appear to be irreversible. Lead toxicity is most pronounced in children and fetuses because it can damage the central nervous system and kidneys. Lead also decreases normal production of red blood cells.

A large proportion of absorbed lead is incorporated into the skeleton and teeth. Lead deposited in the enamel matrix has been associated with pitting hypoplasia. The amount of lead in shed deciduous teeth can be used as an index of lead exposure. The effects of lead stored in the bones and teeth are unknown. Elevated levels of lead in the blood may be associated with periodontitis.

Lithium

Lithium is another ultratrace element found in calcified structures. As lithium accumulates in animal bones, calcium content decreases. When this substitution is made in apatite of bone and teeth, the structure and solubility properties are changed.

Vanadium

Studies on the essentiality of vanadium have been inconsistent in their findings. Most research has not found that vanadium deficiency consistently impairs any biologic function in animals. Vanadium is readily incorporated into areas of rapid mineralization of bones and tooth dentin, but its role in bones and teeth is unknown.

The cariostatic effect of vanadium has been studied with inconclusive results. It has been hypothesized that vanadium may exchange for phosphorus in the apatite tooth substance. Shellfish, mushrooms, and parsley contain small amounts of vanadium.

Mercury

Mercury is not a nutrient, but this toxic substance is often found in the food and water supply either naturally in the environment or emitted by industrial pollution. Even a trace amount of mercury can cause neurologic and developmental problems in infants and young children. It is also harmful to the kidney and cardiovascular system. The U.S. Food and Drug Administration (FDA) monitors the presence of contaminants in food and water, issuing warnings as needed. In 2001, the FDA advised women of childbearing age, pregnant and nursing women, and young children to avoid shark, swordfish, mackerel, and tilefish because of the high levels of methylmercury (MeHg) in them. The FDA and EPA recommends potentially vulnerable consumers (i.e., young children and pregnant and nursing women) limit their intake of albacore tuna to less than 6 oz per week because of its mercury content.[7]

DENTAL CONSIDERATIONS

- Boron deficiency signs may be related to abnormalities in vitamin D, calcium, phosphorus, or magnesium levels.
- Aluminum is a cariostatic agent, especially in combination with fluoride.
- Seafood is a good source of important nutrients, including omega-3 fats that promote neurodevelopment. The American Heart Association and the *Dietary Guidelines* recommend at least two servings of fish each week. Encourage fish and shellfish with lower mercury levels, such as salmon, clams, sardines, crab, tilapia, scallops, shrimp, catfish, perch, whitefish, and cod. Large, older fish higher on the food chain—such as shark, swordfish, king mackerel, orange roughy, tuna, and tilefish, contain higher levels of mercury (see Fig. 13.4). For example, a scallop may have a mercury concentration of 0.003 ppm while tilefish may have 1.123 ppm.

NUTRITIONAL DIRECTIONS

- A diet low in boron increases calcium excretion; thus, patients with osteoporosis should be encouraged to consume recommended amounts of fresh fruits and vegetables.
- Acidic foods and foods with high nitrate content, such as tomatoes, can accumulate very high levels of tin if left in unlaquered, opened cans in the refrigerator for more than 3 days. Once opened, these foods should be stored in glass or plastic containers.
- Consumption of a variety of foods and fluids helps people obtain trace minerals and avoid excessive amounts.
- Unrefined foods generally provide more trace minerals than highly refined foods.
- Supplements of these trace elements are not encouraged.
- Some bone meal and oyster shell used for calcium supplementation may contain dangerous amounts of lead.
- Patients who use well water can contact the local health department or water system for information on contaminants or they may have the water tested for contaminants.

HEALTH APPLICATION 10

Alzheimer Disease

Identified more than 100 years ago, Alzheimer disease is the most common type of dementia in individuals, comprising 60% to 80% of dementia cases. An estimated 5.3 million Americans have Alzheimer disease; 5.1 million of those individuals are older than 65 years. About half of those with Alzheimer disease may be undiagnosed. Alzheimer disease is the sixth leading cause of death. Direct and indirect health care costs together exceed $226 billion. The incidence increases with age, with the greatest risk at age 65 or older. It is estimated that someone in the United States develops the disease every 67 seconds. However, Alzheimer disease is not a normal part of aging and those younger than 65 years can develop the disease.[8] It is a slowly progressive disease, characterized by deterioration of judgment, orientation, memory, personality, and intellectual capability, typically with a period of 8 to 10 years between onset and death. Individuals progress through the disease at varying rates.

Known risk factors for developing Alzheimer disease include age, family history of Alzheimer disease, head trauma, and genetic disposition. Currently, there is no treatment available to delay or stop progressive deterioration of brain cells in Alzheimer disease. Research suggests that the health of the brain is a key to preventing Alzheimer disease. The Alzheimer's Association has compiled a list of ways to "Maintain Your Brain" (Box 10.1).

Although much has been learned about the disease, a specific cause has not been determined. Different types of nerve cells in the brain degenerate and die. Similarities observed between aluminum toxicity and Alzheimer disease led to the hypothesis that dietary or environmental aluminum might be involved. As a result, the public was inaccurately advised that aluminum cookware could be toxic. Chelation therapy was advocated to remove aluminum from the body as an unorthodox treatment for Alzheimer disease. However, brain lesions and neurotransmitter changes seen in aluminum toxicity and Alzheimer disease are different. In contrast to the subtle cognitive changes associated with Alzheimer disease, aluminum toxicity manifests with motor dysfunction.

A key element of disease management is early diagnosis to initiate therapy. Some causes of dementia can be treated, and some of the symptoms can possibly be reversed. A series of evaluations are used to make a clinical diagnosis of Alzheimer disease, including medical and behavioral assessments. Often, reports from family members and friends provide valuable information regarding mental status of the individual. The Alzheimer's Association has developed "warning signs" for detection of Alzheimer disease (Box 10.2).

The FDA has approved five medications to improve cognitive symptoms of Alzheimer disease.[9] Behavioral and psychiatric symptoms—such as physical or verbal outbursts, restlessness, hallucinations, and delusions—are treated either with medications prescribed to control symptoms or with nondrug treatments. Vitamin E supplementation is sometimes prescribed by the health care provider because it is an antioxidant and may protect nerve cells. Although vitamin E may slightly delay the loss of ability to perform daily activities, it should only be used under the supervision of a health care provider. A health care provider may suggest a multivitamin and monitor blood glucose and lipid levels in order to achieve normal values.

Many herbal remedies, vitamins, and other nutrition supplements are promoted as memory enhancers or treatments. Studies involving these alternative therapies have not substantiated these claims. Currently, promoters of ginkgo biloba (a plant extract), huperzine A (a moss extract), coenzyme Q10 (an naturally occurring antioxidant in the body), coral calcium, omega-3 fatty acids, tramiprosate (an amino acid), coconut oil, and phosphatidylserine (a phospholipid) claim that these products can cure or prevent Alzheimer disease.[10] Further scientific studies are required not only to determine the effectiveness of alternative nutritional therapies but also to observe their interaction with other drugs and nutrients.

Alzheimer disease has significant effects on nutrition and hydration status. Initially, individuals with Alzheimer disease may have problems with food purchasing and meal preparation. Appetite and food intake fluctuate with mood swings and increasing confusion. Forgetting when they last ate, they may skip some meals, eat twice, or forget about food cooking on the stove. Changes in food preferences may be tied to a decline in olfactory function. Sweet and salty foods are preferred.

During the middle phase of the illness, individuals with Alzheimer disease often become agitated and may pace all night, increasing caloric expenditure. Weight loss is common. Energy requirements may increase up to 1600 cal per day and frequent snacking is necessary to maintain body weight. Because of abnormal sleep patterns, caffeine may need to be discontinued to avoid further stimulation of the central nervous system.

Appetite is usually good, but caloric intake may be inadequate to maintain body weight unless snacks or liquid nutritional supplements or both are provided. Food hoarding (to accumulate or stash food) or failure to chew food sufficiently increases the risk of choking. Ability to use utensils deteriorates. Finger foods may be more appropriate to allow continuation of self-feeding. Foods should be cut up and offered in bite-size pieces. Serving foods one at a time helps decrease confusion. A larger meal at midday, when cognitive abilities are at their peak, is recommended.

During the final stage, which is characterized by severe intellectual impairment, food may not be recognized and may be refused. The individual also may forget how to swallow. **Enteral feedings** (the provision of nutrients through a tube placed in the nose, stomach, or small intestine) may be indicated to maintain nutritional status as a result of impaired cognition.

• BOX 10.1 Maintain Your Brain

- Stay physically active. Physical exercise is essential for maintaining good blood flow to the brain as well as to encourage new brain cells. It also can significantly reduce the risk of heart disease, stroke, and diabetes, thereby protecting against those risk factors for Alzheimer disease.
- Adopt a brain-healthy diet. Research suggests that high cholesterol may contribute to stroke and brain cell damage. A low-fat, low-cholesterol diet is advisable. There is growing evidence that antioxidants may help protect brain cells.
- Remain socially active. Social activity not only makes physical and mental activity more enjoyable, it can reduce stress levels, which helps maintain healthy connections among brain cells.
- Stay mentally active. Mentally stimulating activities strengthen brain cells and the connections between them, and may even create new nerve cells.

Data from Alzheimer's Association: Brain health. *www.alz.org/we_can_help_brain_health_maintain_your_brain.asp. Accessed March 14, 2017.*

• BOX 10.2 Warning Signs of Alzheimer Disease

- Memory loss that disrupts daily life
- Challenges in planning or solving problems
- Difficulty performing familiar tasks
- Confusion with time or place
- Trouble understanding visual images and spatial relationships
- New problems with words in speaking or writing
- Misplacing things or losing the ability to retrace steps
- Decreased or poor judgment
- Withdrawal from work or social activities
- Changes in mood or personality

Data from Alzheimer's Association: Symptoms of Alzheimer's. *http://www.alz.org/alzheimers_disease_symptoms_of_alzheimers.asp. Accessed March 14, 2017.*

◆ CASE APPLICATION FOR THE DENTAL HYGIENIST

A young female executive confides in you that she always feels tired and sometimes finds it difficult to get through the day. When you bring up the subject of nutrition, she tells you that she read a book about the importance of minerals and began taking supplements approximately 1 year ago. These self-prescribed supplements include selenium and zinc. She also takes a vitamin C supplement daily. She is concerned about a lack of energy, which she relates to her poor eating habits. Meals are frequently missed or eaten at her desk.

Nutritional Assessment

- Willingness to learn
- Knowledge level regarding food consumption guidelines, such as the *MyPlate* and the *Dietary Guidelines*
- Desire for improving nutritional and general health
- Cultural or religious influences
- Knowledge of the physiological roles of vitamins and minerals
- Recognition of the interactive effects of vitamins and minerals, especially when taken in excess of RDAs

Nutritional Diagnosis

Health-seeking behaviors related to inadequate knowledge of optimal nutrition, healthy eating habits, and the deleterious effects associated with consumption of excess vitamins and minerals.

Nutritional Goals

The patient will use the *Dietary Guidelines* and *MyPlate* to improve her eating pattern and dietary intake of nutrient-dense foods. The patient will recognize the health risks associated with improper supplementation and will decrease reliance on nutritional supplements.

Nutritional Implementation

Intervention: Review the *Dietary Guidelines* and discuss how these guidelines support healthy eating habits and disease prevention.

Rationale: Healthy dietary practices can improve energy reserves and overall nutritional status.

Intervention: Encourage consumption of a variety of foods from each of the five main food groups.

Rationale: A nutritious diet is composed of a variety of foods that together supply all the essential nutrients needed for good health.

Intervention: Review serving sizes and emphasize more servings of nutrient-dense foods. Encourage a meal timetable that is planned according to her daily schedule.

Rationale: Eating an inadequate number of calories from foods that are limited in nutrients can contribute to fatigue and poor nutrition. Scheduled mealtimes throughout the day help to supply an adequate number of calories when appropriate serving sizes of nutritious food are selected.

Intervention: Describe the body's metabolic need for vitamins and minerals. Inform the patient that a well-balanced diet can supply all the nutrients needed without supplementation.

Rationale: Vitamins and minerals are required for normal metabolic and physiologic functions. When supplements are taken in excess of the RDAs, some nutrients can be harmful.

Intervention: Describe how zinc supplements interact with copper absorption and relate to fatigue. Inform the patient that large amounts of vitamin C in excess of the RDAs may decrease the availability of copper in the blood. List the toxic effects of selenium.

Rationale: Because most minerals are supplied by a varied diet, supplementation can result in toxic levels and harmful nutrient interactions.

Intervention: Advise the patient to see her health care provider if fatigue persists or worsens.

Rationale: Poor dietary intake may act as a contributing factor to fatigue when the actual cause may be related to a systemic disease or condition.

Evaluation

The patient will improve dietary habits by planning meals and snacks each day. Meal planning will accommodate the patient's work schedule. The patient will use *MyPlate* and the *Dietary Guidelines* to improve the nutritional quality and quantity of her diet. The patient can state the symptoms associated with large quantities of zinc, selenium, and vitamin C, and will stop taking supplements. Persistent or worsening symptoms of fatigue will prompt the patient to seek the advice of a health care provider.

Student Readiness

1. List all nutrient interactions indicated in this chapter that decrease the absorption or alter the metabolism of another nutrient. Why would a dental hygienist advise a patient to obtain mineral requirements from food sources rather than mineral supplements (unless ordered by a health care provider)?
2. Which trace minerals incorporated into enamel are beneficial? Which weaken the tooth or make it more susceptible to tooth decay?
3. Which element is involved in insulin metabolism?
4. If a patient is concerned about obtaining adequate amounts of trace elements, what are some suggestions that a dental hygienist can make?
5. Name some minerals that may be useful as well as toxic to patients.

References

1. Medeiros DM. Copper, iron, and selenium dietary deficiencies negatively impact skeletal integrity: a review. *Exp Biol Med.* 2016; 241:1316–1322.
2. Costello RB, Dwyer JT, Bailey RL. Chromium supplements for glycemic control in type 2 diabetes: limited evidence of effectiveness. *Nutr Rev.* 2016;74(7):455–468.
3. U.S. Environmental Protection Agency. Chromium Drinking Water Standard. https://www.epa.gov/dwstandardsregulations/chromium-drinking-water. Accessed March 15, 2017.
4. Keenan KP, Wallig MA, Haschek WM. Nature via nurture: effect of diet on health, obesity, and safety assessment. *Toxicol Pathol.* 2013;41(2):190–209.
5. Hunt CD. Dietary boron: progress in establishing essential roles in human physiology. *J Trace Elem Med Biol.* 2012;26:157–160.
6. U.S. Environmental Protection Agency. Drinking water requirements for states and public water systems. Lead and copper rule. https://www.epa.gov/dwreginfo/lead-and-copper-rule. Accessed March 15, 2017.
7. Cusack LK, Smit E, Kile ML, et al. Regional and temporal trends in blood mercury concentrations and fish consumption in women of child bearing age in the United States using NHANES data from 1999–2010. *Environ Health.* 2017;16(10):http://ehjournal.biomedcentral.com/articles/10.1186/s12940-017-0218-4. Accessed March 14, 2017.
8. Alzheimer's Association Report. 2015 Alzheimer's disease facts and figures. *Alzheimers Dement.* 2015;11:332–384.
9. Kumar A, Singh A. A review on Alzheimer's disease pathophysiology and its management: an update. *Pharmacol Rep.* 2015;67: 195–203.
10. Alzheimer's Association. Alternative treatments. http://www.alz.org/alzheimers_disease_alternative_treatments.asp. Accessed March 15, 2017.

EVOLVE RESOURCES

Please visit http://evolve.elsevier.com/Stegeman/nutritional for additional practice and study support tools.

11 Vitamins Required for Oral Soft Tissues and Salivary Glands

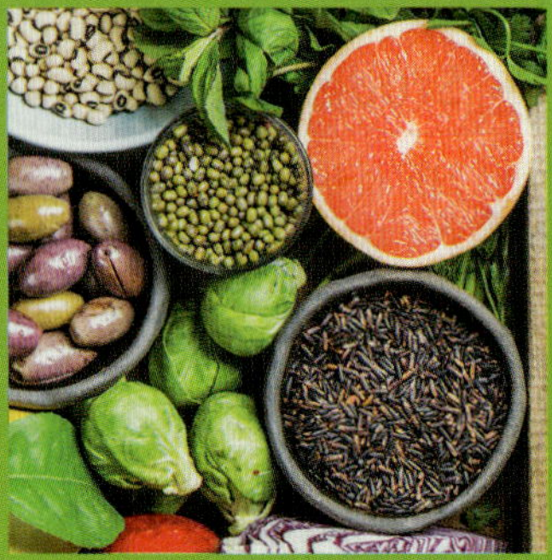

STUDENT LEARNING OUTCOMES

Upon completion of this chapter, the student will be able to achieve the following student learning outcomes:

1. Describe the physiology of soft tissues.
2. Discuss the following related to thiamin (Vitamin B_1):
   - Describe the physiologic roles of thiamin, as well as list the Recommended Dietary Allowance (RDA) and sources of thiamin.
   - Identify dental considerations and nutritional directions for hypo states related to thiamin.
3. Discuss the following related to riboflavin (Vitamin B_2):
   - Describe the physiologic roles of riboflavin, as well as list the Recommended Dietary Allowance (RDA) and sources of riboflavin.
   - Identify dental considerations and nutritional directions for hypo states related to riboflavin.
4. Discuss the following related to niacin (Vitamin B_3), pantothenic acid (Vitamin B_5), and Vitamin B_6 (Pyridoxine):
   - Describe the physiologic roles of each vitamin, as well as list the Recommended Dietary Allowance (RDA) and sources of each.
   - Identify dental considerations and nutritional directions for hyper and hypo states related to each vitamin.
5. Discuss the following related to folate/folic acid, vitamin B_{12} (Cobalamin), and biotin (vitamin B_7):
   - Describe the physiologic roles of each vitamin, as well as list the Recommended Dietary Allowance (RDA) and sources of each.
   - Explain to a patient who is vegan why vitamin B_{12} is important.
   - Identify dental considerations and nutritional directions for hyper and hypo states related to each vitamin.
6. Discuss the importance of vitamins C, A, and E in oral soft tissues and salivary glands.

KEY TERMS

Achlorhydria
Antigenic
Ariboflavinosis
Ataxia
Avidin
Beriberi
Bradycardia
Candida
Cheilosis
Cholinergic
Circumvallate lingual papillae
Epithelialization
Filiform papillae
Foliate papillae
Fungating
Fungiform papillae
Glossitis
Glossopyrosis
Hypotonic
Intrinsic factor
Keratinized epithelium
Megaloblastic anemia
Myelin
Neoplasia
Neural tube defects
Nystagmus
Parasympathetic autonomic nerves
Pellagra
Periodontal disease
Pernicious anemia
Pyogenic
R-binder
Sensory neuropathy
Signs
Squamous metaplasia
Stomatitis
Sympathetic autonomic nerves
Symptoms
Tachycardia
Thiaminase

TEST YOUR NQ

1. **T/F** Milk is a good source of riboflavin.
2. **T/F** Vitamin B_6 is the sunshine vitamin.
3. **T/F** Beriberi is caused by niacin deficiency.
4. **T/F** Vegans may be prone to vitamin B_{12} deficiency.
5. **T/F** Complaints of flushing and intestinal disturbances are symptoms of thiamin toxicity.
6. **T/F** A smooth purplish red or magenta tongue may be observed in patients with vitamin B_6 deficiency.
7. **T/F** Enriched breads and cereals are good sources of thiamin.
8. **T/F** Carrots are a good source of folate.
9. **T/F** Thiamin requirement is determined by one's energy requirement.
10. **T/F** The first signs of a nutritional deficiency often occur in the oral cavity.

Physiology of Soft Tissues

The oral cavity can reflect systemic disease before other **signs** (noticeable to the clinician) and **symptoms** (perceived by the patient) become evident; the condition in the oral cavity may also cause systemic problems by affecting the patient's nutrient intake. The oral cavity is the site of a wide variety of systemic disease manifestations for several reasons: (a) it has a rapid cellular turnover rate, (b) it is under constant assault by microorganisms, and (c) it is a trauma-intense environment.

The systemic circulation provides nutrients and removes metabolic waste products from underlying structures and the salivary glands via the blood supply. Fig. 11.1 shows healthy gingiva; changes in color, size, shape, texture, and functional integrity of the oral tissues often reflect systemic nutritional disorders. Signs and symptoms in soft oral tissues can be caused by deficiencies of many of the B-complex vitamins, vitamins C and E, iron, and protein (Box 11.1). Nutritional deficiencies result in similar oral signs and symptoms, such as pain, erythema, atrophy of tissues, and infection. **Pyogenic** (producing pus) and **fungating** (skin lesions with ulcerations, necrosis, and foul smell) microorganisms cause local infections in cracked epithelial surfaces. Approximately 90% of saliva is produced and secreted by three paired sets of major salivary glands: the parotid, submandibular, and sublingual glands (Fig. 11.2). Additionally, the lips and inner lining of the cheeks are equipped with hundreds of minor salivary glands.

Saliva keeps surfaces of the oral cavity healthy and lubricated and is necessary to maintain functional integrity of taste buds. Solid substances first must be dissolved in saliva to be tasted. Healthy adults produce approximately 1 to 1.5 L/day of saliva. **Sympathetic autonomic nerves** stimulate the body in times of stress and crisis; sympathetic impulses influence salivary composition. **Parasympathetic autonomic nerves** balance or slow down impulses from sympathetic nerves; parasympathetic stimulation increases the amount of saliva secreted.

Compared with plasma, saliva is hypotonic, with its main constituent being water. **Hypotonic** solutions have a lower solute concentration than plasma. Saliva contains more than 20 proteins and glycoproteins along with many electrolytes, including sodium, potassium, calcium, chloride, bicarbonate, inorganic phosphate, magnesium, sulfate, iodide, and fluoride. Saliva functions as a buffer to maintain the oral pH. Buffering substances increase their acid or alkali content to change the pH of the solution. The pH of unstimulated saliva is approximately

• BOX 11.1 Vitamins and Minerals Required for Healthy Oral Soft Tissues

Water-Soluble Vitamins
- B Vitamins
  - Thiamin
  - Riboflavin
  - Niacin
  - Vitamin B_6
  - Folate
  - Vitamin B_{12}
  - Pantothenic acid
  - Biotin
- Vitamin C

Fat-Soluble Vitamins
- Vitamin A
- Vitamin E

Minerals
- Iron
- Zinc
- Iodine

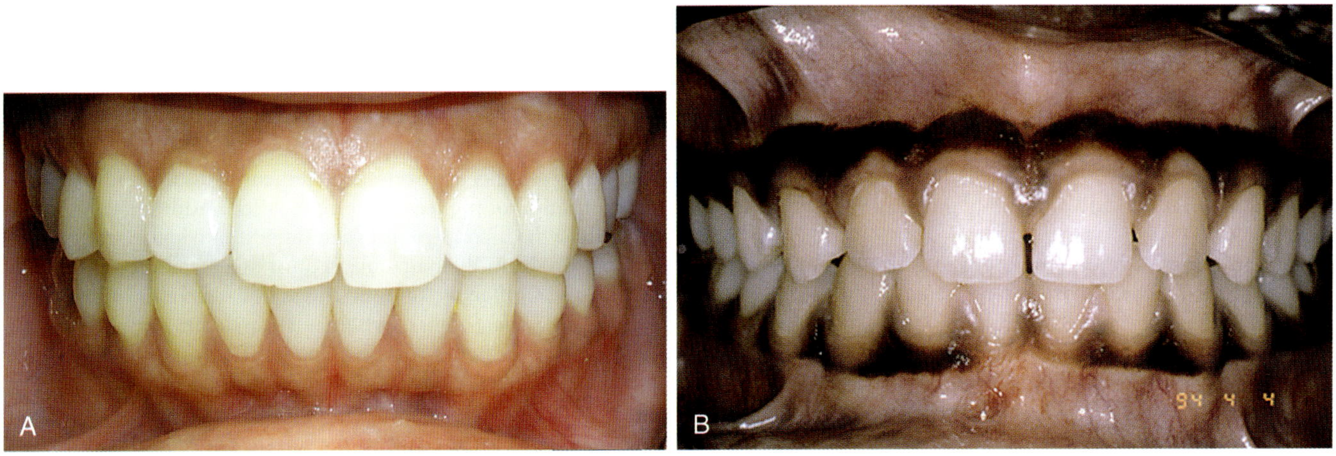

• Figure 11.1 Healthy gingiva. (A) Light-skinned individual. (B) Physiologic pigmentation in gingiva of dark-skinned individual. (From Perry DA, Essex G: *Periodontology for the dental hygienist*, ed 4, Philadelphia, 2014, Elsevier Saunders.)

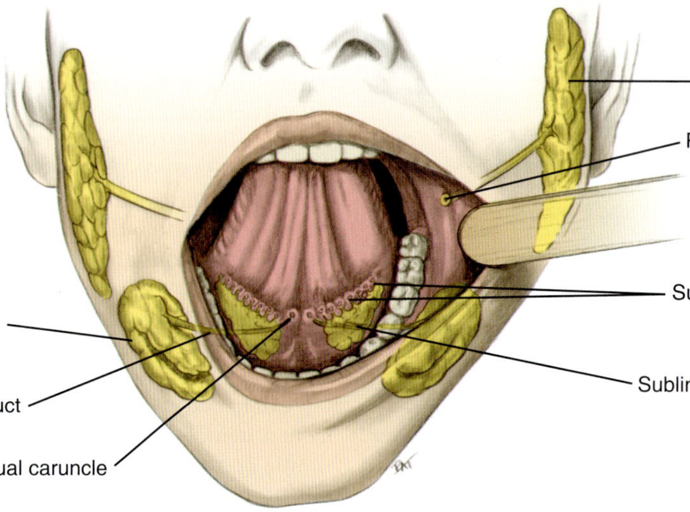

• **Figure 11.2** The major salivary glands and associated structures. (Reproduced with permission from Fehrenbach MJ, Herring SW. *Illustrated Anatomy of the Head and Neck*. 4th ed. Philadelphia, PA: Elsevier Saunders; 2012.)

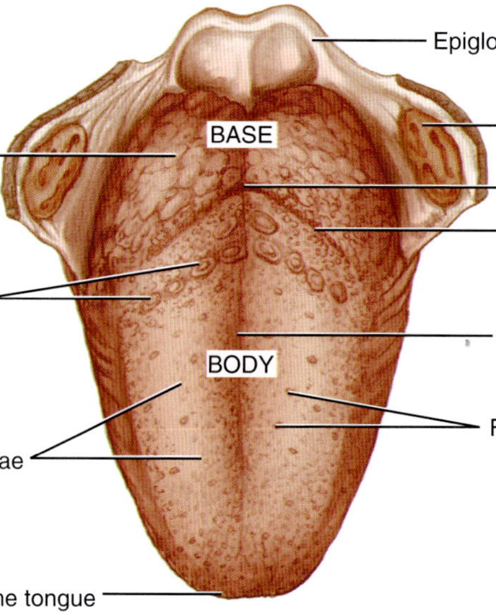

• **Figure 11.3** Papillae on the tongue with its landmarks noted. (Reproduced with permission from Fehrenbach MJ, Herring SW. *Illustrated Anatomy of the Head and Neck*. 4th ed. Philadelphia, PA: Elsevier Saunders; 2012.)

6.1, but this can rise to 7.8 at high flow rates. Antimicrobial properties of saliva provide protection and remove toxins, such as tobacco smoke.

The oral cavity is lined with nonkeratinized mucosa except for the hard palate, dorsum of the tongue, and gingiva surrounding the teeth, which are covered with a **keratinized epithelium** (a protein, the main component of the epidermis and horny tissues). The oral cavity may contain **antigenic** (capable of inducing an immune response with specific antibodies) substances; the oral mucosa separates a potentially adverse environment from underlying connective tissue.

Mucosal cells have a very rapid turnover rate, resulting in complete turnover in 3 to 5 days. Rapid generation of new cells in the oral epithelia provides replacement tissue for trauma resulting from friction of the teeth and mastication. Additionally, hundreds of cells in the filiform papillae and fungiform papillae are in constant transition, from their anabolism until their catabolism (Fig. 11.3). **Filiform papillae** are smooth, threadlike structures on the dorsum surface of the tongue, whereas **fungiform papillae** are red, mushroom-shaped structures scattered throughout the filiform papillae. There are greater numbers of fungiform papillae at the apex (tip) of the tongue.

Taste buds are located on the **foliate papillae** (vertical grooves located on the lateral borders of the tongue), **circumvallate lingual papillae** (large, mushroom-shaped distinct structures forming a V) on the dorsal surface, and the fungiform papillae of the tongue.

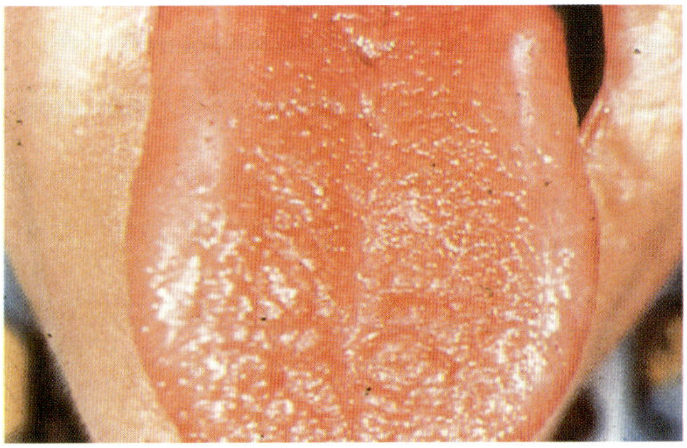

• **Figure 11.4** Glossitis associated with thiamin deficiency. (Reproduced with permission from the American Dental Association Council on Dental Therapeutics: *Oral Manifestations of Metabolic and Deficiency Changes*. Chicago, IL.)

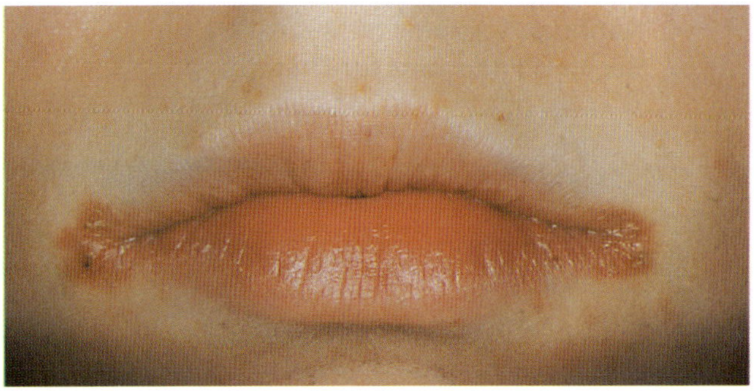

• **Figure 11.5** Angular cheilitis. (Reproduced with permission from Ibsen OAC, Phelan JA. *Oral Pathology for the Dental Hygienist*. 6th ed, St. Louis, MO: Elsevier Saunders; 2014.)

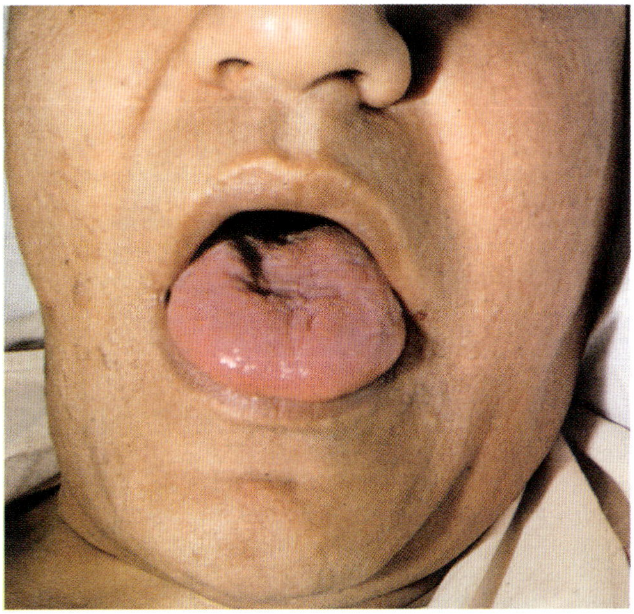

• **Figure 11.6** Glossitis associated with severe riboflavin deficiency. (Reproduced with permission from McLaren DS: *A Colour Atlas and Text of Diet-Related Disorders*. 2nd ed. London: Mosby-Year Book; 1992.)

Atrophy of fungiform and foliate papillae leads to loss of taste buds and changes in taste acuity.

Many filiform papillae cover the anterior two-thirds of the tongue. If the filiform papillae become denuded or atrophied, the tongue appears red and pebbled, giving it a strawberry-like appearance. Fungiform papillae are bright red because of a rich vascular supply. Keratinized cells normally cover the fungiform papillae on the tongue surface. Chronic severe nutrient deficiencies result in loss of fungiform papillae and a smooth red tongue.

DENTAL CONSIDERATIONS

- Because of rapid turnover rate of oral tissues, the first signs of nutritional deficiency are frequently evident in the oral cavity. The glossal epithelium is usually the first to be affected, followed by areas around the lips. Assess patients for oral signs of nutritional deficiencies.
- The tongue may become edematous as a result of disease or nutritional deficiency.
- Angular cheilitis or **cheilosis** (cracks around the corners of the mouth; Fig. 11.5) and **glossitis** (inflammation of the tongue; Figs. 11.4 and 11.6) are commonly associated with deficiencies of several B-complex vitamins.
- Saliva aids in the ability to speak properly, and taste and swallow foods.
- The composition of saliva affects taste and can be a determining factor in food choices.
- Xerostomia may result in increased incidence of caries, **stomatitis** (inflammation of oral mucosa), gingival inflammation, and greater susceptibility to oral infections (see Chapter 19).
- Saliva may be used to diagnose some local and systemic diseases and heavy-metal toxicity, such as mercury toxicity.
- Salivary secretion is controlled primarily by **cholinergic** (nerves stimulated by acetylcholine) parasympathetic (autonomic) nerves; patients taking anticholinergic medications (which usually contain atropine) exhibit decreased salivary flow. These medications may be prescribed for **bradycardia** (low heart rate), diarrhea, peptic ulcers, and occasionally asthma.

NUTRITIONAL DIRECTIONS

- Saliva helps maintain integrity of the teeth, tongue, and mucous membranes of the oral and oropharyngeal areas.
- Nutritional abnormalities affect oral soft tissues in a variety of ways (e.g., angular cheilitis and glossitis).
- The RDA is higher than the average need for an individual. If the amount consumed is slightly under the listed RDA, most individuals will still be healthy. However, the lower the requirement of a vitamin or mineral, the greater the risk of a deficiency.

Thiamin (Vitamin B_1)

Physiologic Roles

Thiamin functions as a coenzyme in metabolism of energy nutrients via the tricarboxylic acid cycle (or Krebs or citric acid cycle) to produce energy. This role makes it crucial for normal functioning of the brain, nerves, muscles, and heart. However, the main effects

TABLE 11.1 National Academy of Medicine Recommendations for Thiamin

	EAR (mg/day)		RDA (mg/day)		
Life Stage	Male	Female	Male	Female	AI (mg/day)
0–6 months					0.2
7–12 months					0.3
1–3 years	0.4	0.4	0.5	0.5	
4–8 years	0.5	0.5	0.6	0.6	
9–13 years	0.7	0.7	0.9	0.9	
14–18 years	1	1	1.2	1	
≥ 19 years	1	0.9	1.2	1.1	
Pregnancy					
14–50 years		1.2		1.4	
Lactation					
14–50 years		1.2		1.4	

AI, Adequate Intake, EAR, Estimated Average Requirement; RDA, Recommended Dietary Allowance.

Data from Institute of Medicine (IOM), Food and Nutrition Board: *Dietary Reference Intakes for Thiamin, Riboflavin, Niacin, Vitamin B_6, Folate, Vitamin B_{12}, Pantothenic Acid, Biotin, and Choline.* Washington, DC: National Academy Press; 1998.

TABLE 11.2 Thiamin Content of Selected Foods

Food	Portion	Thiamin (mg)
Total, whole grain	1 cup	2.0
Wheaties cereal	1 cup	1.0
Lean pork chop, broiled	3 oz	0.79
Trail mix, tropical	1 cup	0.63
Bagel, enriched	3½–4 inches	0.60
Spaghetti, enriched, cooked	1 cup	0.42
Green peas, cooked	½ cup	0.26
White rice, enriched, cooked	1 cup	0.26
Sweet potato, baked	1 cup	0.21
Bread, pita, enriched	1 medium	0.17
Pinto beans, cooked	½ cup	0.17
Bread, whole-wheat	1 slice	0.13
Peanuts, dry roasted	1 oz	0.04

Data from U.S. Department of Agriculture (USDA), Agricultural Research Service. 2016. *USDA National Nutrient Database for Standard Reference, Release 28.* Nutrient Data Laboratory Home Page. https://ndb.nal.usda.gov/ndb/. Accessed March 16, 2017.

of thiamin deficiency are disturbances of carbohydrate metabolism, which is impossible without thiamin. Thiamin is a component necessary for the synthesis of niacin, and it also helps regulate appetite. It is a constituent of enzymes that degrade sucrose to organic acids that can ultimately dissolve tooth enamel.

Requirements

Thiamin is involved in using carbohydrates for energy; the requirement is based on total caloric need. The Recommended Dietary Allowance (RDA) for men (≥ 14 years old) is 1.2 mg per day and for women (≥ 19 years old) is 1.1 mg per day (Table 11.1). Participation in rigorous physical activity uses more energy, which requires more thiamin. Also, requirements are increased by pregnancy and lactation, hemodialysis or peritoneal dialysis, fever, hyperthyroidism, cardiac conditions, alcoholism, and the use of loop diuretics. No known adverse effects are evident from excessive thiamin intake, including supplements. Although a Tolerable Upper Intake Level (UL) is not established for thiamin, care should be taken when consumption routinely exceeds the RDA.

Sources

Thiamin is widely distributed in foods, and intake of a variety of foods, including enriched grains or whole grains, can ensure adequate amounts (Table 11.2). Approximately 40% of thiamin intake is provided by enriched breads, cereals, and pasta. (Because of enrichment, enriched breads may contain almost twice as much thiamin as whole grains.) In the meat group, pork is an exceptionally good source. Other good sources include nuts and legumes. Following the recommendations of *MyPlate* and the *Dietary Guidelines*, which both emphasize eating a variety of foods, ensures adequate intake.

Hypo States

Thiamin is required for metabolism of carbohydrates, proteins, and fats; insufficient intake adversely affects most organ systems. Primary dietary deficiency usually occurs in developing countries where polished rice is the staple diet. In developed countries, thiamin deficiency is secondary to alcoholism, ingestion of raw fish containing microbial **thiaminase** (an enzyme that inactivates thiamin), chronic febrile states, and total parenteral nutrition (TPN). Cooking deactivates thiaminase.

Thiamin is called the "morale vitamin" because short-term deficiency causes patients to become depressed, irritable, anorexic, fatigued, and unable to concentrate. The brain and central nervous system, almost entirely dependent on glucose for energy, are seriously impaired when thiamin is unavailable.

Severe thiamin deficiency results in **beriberi**, which causes extensive damage to the nervous and cardiovascular systems. Beriberi means "I cannot"; patients with this severe thiamin deficiency cannot move easily. The classic chronic form of beriberi manifests with impairment of sensory and motor function without involvement of the central nervous system. Other symptoms include muscular wasting (dry beriberi), edema (wet beriberi), deep muscle pain in the calves, peripheral paralysis, **tachycardia** (rapid heartbeat), and an enlarged heart.

A thiamin deficiency in infancy may result in less calcified and smaller percentage of inorganic material in enamel.[1] Whether or not a thiamin deficiency is evident in oral tissues is controversial. Some clinicians have associated a flabby, red, and edematous tongue with thiamin deficiency (see Fig. 11.4). The fungiform papillae become enlarged and hyperemic (engorged with blood).

Wernicke-Korsakoff syndrome is another thiamin deficiency disease, typically associated with alcoholism, which is characterized by mental confusion, **nystagmus** (involuntary rapid movement of the eyeball), and **ataxia** (a gait disorder characterized by uncoordinated muscle movements). These symptoms occur most frequently in malnourished alcoholics. Alcohol intake increases thiamin requirement, yet total nutrient intake is usually poor in alcoholics. Early diagnosis is essential to initiate thiamin therapy early in the course of the disease to prevent permanent damage and death.

DENTAL CONSIDERATIONS

- A careful medical, social, and dietary history—including a clinical assessment of the oral cavity, alcohol consumption, and activity level—helps identify early stages of thiamin deficiency.
- Risk of alcohol abuse or dependence is based on how much and how often an individual drinks. Moderation is considered 4 to 14 drinks per week for men and 3 to 11 drinks per week for women; 5 or more drinks per occasion is considered excessive for any adult.
- Vitamin deficiencies seldom occur in isolation. If a deficiency is suspected, symptoms of other vitamin B deficiencies also may be present.
- Because thiamin is essential for carbohydrate metabolism, a thiamin deficiency is closely linked to aberrations of brain function. For patients who are confused or have altered thought processes, assess nutrient intake.
- Carbohydrate loading or a very-high-carbohydrate diet and high physical activity slightly increase the thiamin requirement. (Generally, increased food intake results in increased thiamin consumption.)
- Thiamin deficiency has been reported in patients after gastrectomy and bariatric surgery (gastric bypass) related to decreased absorption.
- Although immediate clinical response to thiamin therapy is often dramatic, ultimate recovery may be incomplete and relapses may occur, especially if precipitating factors persist.
- Massive amounts (1000 times greater than the RDA) of thiamin suppress the respiratory system and cause death.

NUTRITIONAL DIRECTIONS

- Raw fish contains an active enzyme, thiaminase, which destroys thiamin.
- Baking soda added to cooking water to enhance the color of vegetables destroys thiamin.
- Overcooking and high temperatures destroy thiamin.
- Antacids reduce use of thiamin.
- Some diuretics can increase thiamin excretion.

Riboflavin (Vitamin B_2)

Physiologic Roles

Riboflavin functions as a coenzyme in metabolism of carbohydrate, protein, and fat to release cellular energy. Closely related to the metabolism of protein, all conditions requiring increases in protein (e.g., growth spurts or burns) lead to additional riboflavin requirements. Riboflavin is also essential for healthy eyes and skin and maintenance of mucous membranes. Along with thiamin, riboflavin is necessary for synthesis of niacin.

Requirements

As shown in Table 11.3, the National Academy of Medicine (formerly the Institute of Medicine) recommends an intake of 1.3 mg per day for men (14 years old and older) and 1.1 mg per day for women (19 years old and older). This level is influenced by individual energy requirements. Additionally, when nitrogen balance is positive, more riboflavin is retained. No UL has been established.

TABLE 11.3 National Academy of Medicine Recommendations for Riboflavin

	EAR (mg/day)		RDA (mg/day)		
Life Stage	Male	Female	Male	Female	AI (mg/day)
0–6 months					0.3
7–12 months					0.4
1–3 years	0.4	0.4	0.5	0.5	
4–8 years	0.5	0.5	0.6	0.6	
9–13 years	0.8	0.8	0.9	0.9	
14–18 years	1.1	0.9	1.3	1	
≥ 19 years	1.1	0.9	1.3	1.1	
Pregnancy					
14–50 years		1.2		1.4	
Lactation					
14–50 years		1.3		1.6	

AI, Adequate Intake, EAR, Estimated Average Requirement; RDA, Recommended Dietary Allowance.

Data from Institute of Medicine (IOM), Food and Nutrition Board: *Dietary Reference Intakes for Thiamin, Riboflavin, Niacin, Vitamin B_6, Folate, Vitamin B_{12}, Pantothenic Acid, Biotin, and Choline*. Washington, DC: National Academy Press; 1998.

Sources

Although milk and milk products are excellent sources of riboflavin, approximately 30% of the dietary intake is furnished by foods in the grain group (Table 11.4). Meat, poultry, and fish also provide about one-fourth of the dietary requirement.

Hypo States

The body carefully guards its limited riboflavin stores. Even in severe deficiency, one-third of the normal amount is present in the liver, kidney, and heart. Primary riboflavin deficiency is uncommon but is encountered in patients with multiple nutrient deficiencies as a result of poor nutrient absorption or use. Because riboflavin is essential in vitamin B_6 and niacin functions, riboflavin deficiency leads to symptoms related to secondary deficiency of these nutrients.

Symptoms associated with riboflavin deficiency, or **ariboflavinosis**, include angular cheilitis (see Fig. 11.5), glossitis (see Fig. 11.6), dermatitis, and anemia with pale oral mucosa. With consistently inadequate intake, these symptoms may be observed within 8 weeks. Along with angular cheilosis, the lips may become extremely red and smooth. Fungiform papillae become swollen and slightly flattened and mushroom shaped during early stages of riboflavin deficiency; the tongue has a pebbly or granular appearance. Severe chronic deficiencies lead to progressive papillary atrophy and patchy, irregular denudation of the tongue. The tongue may become purplish red or magenta in color because of vascular proliferation and decreased circulation. In more advanced cases, the entire tongue may become atrophic and smooth (see Fig. 11.6). These symptoms, especially glossitis and dermatitis, may be secondary to vitamin B_6 deficiency.

TABLE 11.4 **Riboflavin Content of Selected Foods**

Food	Portion	Riboflavin (mg)
Beef liver, braised	1 slice	2.30
Total, whole grain	1 cup	2.28
Wheaties cereal	1 cup	1.12
Custard, egg	1 cup	0.68
Egg, hard boiled	1	0.51
Chicken breast, meat only, roasted	3 oz	0.50
Yogurt, low-fat, plain	8 oz	0.49
Milk, skim	1 cup	0.45
Cottage cheese, low-fat	1 cup	0.37
Bagel, enriched	3½–4 inches	0.36
Spinach, cooked	½ cup	0.21
Pork loin, lean only, broiled	3 oz	0.29
Spaghetti, enriched, cooked	1 cup	0.23
Cornbread	1 piece	0.19
Trail mix, tropical	1 cup	0.16
Salmon, cooked	3 oz	0.14

Data from U.S. Department of Agriculture (USDA), Agricultural Research Service. 2016. *USDA National Nutrient Database for Standard Reference, Release 28.* Nutrient Data Laboratory Home Page. https://ndb.nal.usda.gov/ndb/. Accessed March 16, 2017.

DENTAL CONSIDERATIONS

- Hyperthyroidism, fevers, the added stress of injuries or surgery, excessive alcohol consumption, and malabsorption syndromes increase riboflavin requirements. Assess patients with these conditions for signs of deficiency: cheilitis, papillary atrophy, glossitis, and dermatitis.
- Congenital facial abnormalities may occur if the mother is deficient in riboflavin at the time of conception.
- Bilateral cheilosis may not be due to riboflavin deficiency; consider improperly constructed dentures, fungal (candidiasis) or yeast infection, and aging that may contribute to cheilosis.
- Some antibiotics may increase excretion of riboflavin; thus, monitor for a deficiency in patients on long-term therapy.

NUTRITIONAL DIRECTIONS

- Enriched products provide more riboflavin than their whole-grain counterparts.
- Lighted display cases have the potential to cause decomposition of riboflavin when milk is marketed in translucent plastic containers.
- A mixed diet that contains a pint of low-fat milk and 4 to 6 oz of meat daily ensures adequate riboflavin intake.
- Vegans and those who consume minimal or no dairy products (e.g., patients who are lactose intolerant) are at risk of developing riboflavin deficiency.
- Riboflavin is not known to be toxic, but there is no benefit from high doses.
- A riboflavin deficiency typically does not occur in isolation but rather is a result of a variety of vitamin B-complex deficiencies.

Niacin (Vitamin B_3)

Physiologic Roles

The term *niacin* is loosely used to refer to two compounds, nicotinic acid and nicotinamide. Both compounds are used by the body. Niacin is crucial as a coenzyme in energy (adenosine triphosphate) production. It functions with riboflavin in glucose production and metabolism and is involved in lipid and protein metabolism. Niacin also functions in enzymes involved in microbial degradation of sucrose to produce organic acids.

Requirements

The body obtains niacin not only directly from food but also indirectly from conversion of an amino acid, tryptophan, and from synthesis by intestinal microorganisms. RDAs are given in terms of niacin equivalents, which include dietary sources of niacin plus its precursor, tryptophan. Approximately 1 mg of niacin may be formed from 60 mg of dietary tryptophan. Niacin requirements are related to caloric intake. The RDA niacin equivalents for adults are 14 to 16 mg daily (Table 11.5). The UL for adults is 35 mg daily. Naturally occurring niacin in foods has not been shown to cause adverse effects.

Sources

Niacin is widely distributed in plant and animal foods. Good sources include meats, cereals, legumes, seeds, and nuts (Table 11.6). Approximately 65% of the niacin in the United States diet is obtained from meat and milk. Tryptophan is found mainly in milk and meats. The RDA for niacin equivalents is easily met by consuming foods high in niacin and foods containing tryptophan.

Hyper States and Hypo States

Effects of excessive nicotinamide from supplements has been observed, but not from food or beverage sources. The use of 50 mg of niacin taken daily can function as a vasodilator, producing flushing of the skin, itching, tachycardia, nausea and vomiting, and severe liver damage. Extended-release niacin is associated with few gastrointestinal symptoms without increasing liver damage. Because the body is able to store some niacin, larger doses associated with supplements may lead to serious problems, including abnormal liver function and gout. Supplemental doses of nicotinic acid (1 to 3 g/day) are a treatment option for reducing low-density lipoprotein cholesterol and triglycerides, while increasing high-density lipoprotein cholesterol. (Nicotinamide does not function in this role.) Larger supplemental doses of niacin should be closely monitored by a health care provider.

Niacin deficiency is usually associated with a maize (corn) diet because corn products contain all the essential amino acids except tryptophan. This diet increases the body's requirements for tryptophan and niacin. A deficiency is also seen in chronic alcoholism, malnutrition, and poverty, but is unlikely in individuals who consume adequate protein. Niacin deficiency results in degeneration of the skin, gastrointestinal tract, and nervous system, a condition known as **pellagra**. Symptoms of pellagra have been referred to as "the 4 Ds"—dermatitis, diarrhea, depression or dementia, and death. The term *pellagra* is derived from the Latin word for animal hide; the skin may become rough and resemble goose flesh. The

TABLE 11.5 Institute of Medicine Recommendations for Niacin

	EAR (mg/day)[a]		RDA (mg/day)			
Life Stage	**Male**	**Female**	**Male**	**Female**	**AI (mg/day)[b]**	**UL (mg/day)**
0–6 months					2	ND[c]
7–12 months					4	ND[c]
1–3 years	5	5	6	6		10
4–8 years	6	6	8	8		15
9–13 years	9	9	12	12		20
14–18 years	12	11	16	14		30
≥ 19 years	12	11	16	14		35
Pregnancy						
14–18 years		14		18		30
≥ 19 years		14		18		35
Lactation						
14–18 years		13		17		30
≥ 19 years		13		17		35

AI, Adequate Intake; EAR, Estimated Average Requirement; RDA, Recommended Dietary Allowance; UL, Tolerable Upper Intake Level.
[a]Niacin equivalents.
[b]Preformed niacin.
[c]ND—not determinable because of lack of data of adverse effects in this age group and concern with regard to lack of ability to handle excess amounts. Source of intake should be from food and formula to prevent high levels of intake.
Data from Institute of Medicine (IOM), Food and Nutrition Board: *Dietary Reference Intakes for Thiamin, Riboflavin, Niacin, Vitamin B_6, Folate, Vitamin B_{12}, Pantothenic Acid, Biotin, and Choline.* Washington, DC: National Academy Press; 1998.

TABLE 11.6 Niacin Content of Selected Foods

Food	Portion	Niacin (mg)	Food	Portion	Niacin (mg)
Total, whole-grain cereal	1 cup	26.68	Bagel, enriched	3½–4 inches	4.74
Wheaties cereal	1 cup	13.32	Peanuts, dry roasted	1 oz	4.07
Beef liver, braised	1 slice	11.92	Potato, white, baked	1 med	2.64
Chicken breast, skinless, cooked	3 oz	8.19	Rice, enriched white, cooked	1 cup	2.33
Turkey, whole, cooked	3 oz	8.08	Mushrooms, raw	½ cup	1.73
Halibut, broiled	3 oz	6.72	Lentils, boiled	½ cup	1.05
Salmon, cooked	3 oz	6.61	Pinto beans, boiled	½ cup	0.27
Sunflower seeds	½ cup	5.84	Milk, skim	1 cup	0.23
Tuna, white, canned in water	3 oz	4.93			

Data from U.S. Department of Agriculture (USDA), Agricultural Research Service. 2016. *USDA National Nutrient Database for Standard Reference, Release 28.* Nutrient Data Laboratory Home Page. https://ndb.nal.usda.gov/ndb/. Accessed March 16, 2017.

most striking and characteristic sign of pellagra is a reddish skin rash—especially on the face, hands, or feet—which is always bilaterally symmetrical (i.e., appears on both sides of the body at the same time; Fig. 11.7A). It flares up when skin is exposed to strong sunlight. Neurologic symptoms include depression, apathy, headache, fatigue, and loss of memory. If untreated, it may lead to death.

Deficiency also affects mucous membranes: (a) painful stomatitis causes diminished food intake, and (b) lesions in the gastrointestinal tract result in diarrhea and less vitamin absorption. Pellagrous glossitis begins with swelling of the papillae at the tip and lateral borders of the tongue. The tongue becomes painful, scarlet, and edematous (Fig. 11.7B). Atrophic changes involve loss of filiform and fungiform papillae, and the tongue becomes smooth and shiny.

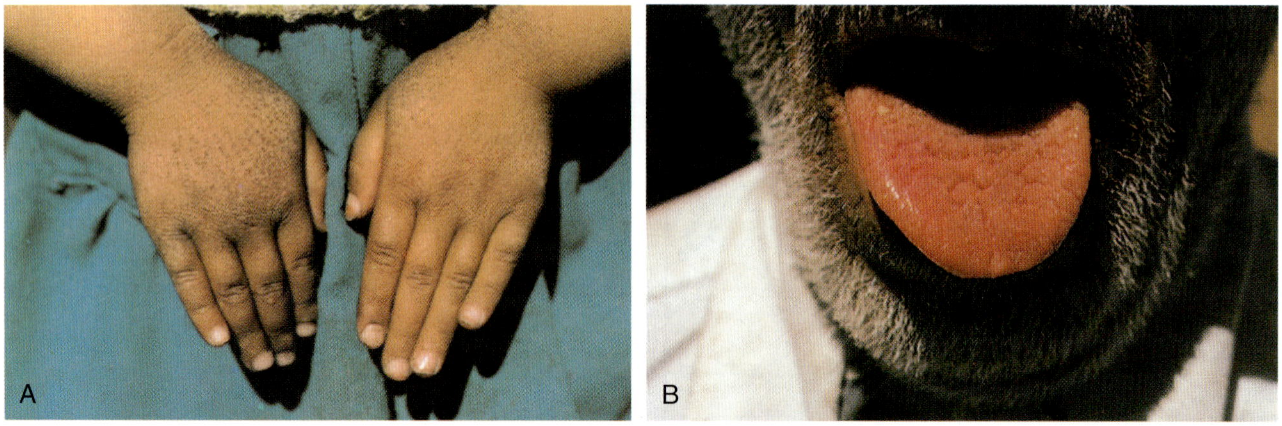

• **Figure 11.7** (A) Symmetrical chapping of the dorsum of the hands. This is a common site for the skin changes of pellagra to occur. A careful history and full examination permit the diagnosis to be made. (B) Scarlet tongue. The tongue in pellagra is frequently scarlet in appearance and extremely painful. However, this may occur in many nonnutritional conditions; other signs, especially those in the skin, have to be present to make the clinical diagnosis. Fissuring of the tongue alone is not significant. (Reproduced with permission from McLaren DS: *A Colour Atlas and Text of Diet-Related Disorders*. 2nd ed. London: Mosby-Year Book; 1992.)

The mucosa is also reddened. Fissures occur in the epithelium and along the sides of the tongue; these become infected rapidly. The gingiva may become inflamed, resembling ulcerative gingivitis. Corners of the lips are initially pale; fanlike fissuring occurs that radiates into the perioral epithelium and may leave permanent scars.

DENTAL CONSIDERATIONS

- Assess patients—especially those consuming excessive amounts of alcohol, who are malnourished, or those with a heavy dependence on corn or maize—for oral signs of niacin deficiency. Symptoms to watch for include complaints of a nonspecific burning sensation throughout the oral cavity; a smooth, shiny, bright-red tongue swollen at the tip and lateral margins; stomatitis; and red and inflamed marginal and attached gingiva.
- Prolonged treatment with isoniazid for tuberculosis may lead to niacin deficiency. Niacin supplements may be prescribed by the health care provider to prevent deficiency.

NUTRITIONAL DIRECTIONS

- Patients should understand that a frequent side effect of a therapeutic dose of nicotinic acid is flushing (i.e., feeling warm; redness; itching or tingling of the face, neck, arms or upper chest). This should be discussed with the health care provider.
- Nicotinic acid, nicotinamide, and niacinamide are correct terms for niacin and should not be confused with nicotine.

Pantothenic Acid (Vitamin B_5)

Physiologic Roles

Pantothenic acid is similar to other B vitamins in its metabolic roles. Pantothenic acid plays a key role in carbohydrate, fat, and protein metabolism. Additionally, it is important in synthesis and degradation of triglycerides, phospholipids, and sterols and in formation of certain hormones and nerve-regulating substances.

TABLE 11.7 National Academy of Medicine Recommendations for Pantothenic Acid

Life Stage	AI (mg/day)
0–6 months	1.7
7–12 months	1.8
1–3 years	2
4–8 years	3
9–13 years	4
14–18 years	5
≥ 19 years	5
Pregnancy	
14–50 years	6
Lactation	
14–50 years	7

AI, Adequate intake.
Data from Institute of Medicine (IOM), Food and Nutrition Board: *Dietary Reference Intakes for Thiamin, Riboflavin, Niacin, Vitamin B_6, Folate, Vitamin B_{12}, Pantothenic Acid, Biotin, and Choline*. Washington, DC: National Academy Press; 1998.

Requirements

The Estimated Average Requirement (EAR), RDA, or UL has not been determined for pantothenic acid for any age group. The Adequate Intake (AI) for adults is 5 mg per day (Table 11.7).

Sources

Pantothenic acid is synthesized by most microorganisms and plants. It is particularly abundant in animal foods and whole-grain cereals (Table 11.8). Bacteria in the digestive tract also produce pantothenic acid.

TABLE 11.8 Pantothenic Acid Content of Selected Foods

Food	Portion	Pantothenic Acid (mg)
Total, whole-grain cereal	1 cup	10
Beef liver, cooked	3 oz	8.3
Sunflower seeds	½ cup	4.7
Trout, cooked	1 filet	1.4
Pork loin chop, broiled	3 oz	1.0
Chicken, skinless, cooked	3 oz	1.0
Yogurt, low-fat, plain	6 oz	1.0
Egg, poached	1	0.8
Corn, canned	1 cup	0.7
Salmon, cooked	3 oz	0.7
Cottage cheese	½ cup	0.63
Orange juice	1 cup	0.5
Rice, enriched, cooked	1 cup	0.5
Mushrooms, raw	½ cup	0.3
Mixed nuts	1 oz	0.3

Data from U.S. Department of Agriculture (USDA), Agricultural Research Service. 2016. *USDA National Nutrient Database For Standard Reference, Release 28.* Pantothenic acid (mg) content of selected foods per common measure. https://ndb.nal.usda.gov/ndb/. Accessed March 16, 2017.

Hypo States

Naturally occurring dietary deficiency of pantothenic acid is very rare. A deficiency results in dysfunctional lipid synthesis and energy production. Symptoms include burning sensations in the feet, depression, fatigue, insomnia, and weakness.

DENTAL CONSIDERATIONS

- Pantothenic acid deficiency rarely occurs alone but may occur along with other B-vitamin deficiencies.
- Pantothenic acid may help in wound healing; thus, encourage patients undergoing oral or periodontal surgery to eat a well-balanced diet.

NUTRITIONAL DIRECTIONS

- Distribution of pantothenic acid is widespread.
- Diets including whole-grain unprocessed foods contain more pantothenic acid.

Vitamin B_6 (Pyridoxine)

Vitamin B_6 is the term commonly used for a group of three compounds: pyridoxine, pyridoxal, and pyridoxamine. All three forms can be used by the body in their role as coenzymes.

Physiologic Roles

Several essential roles for vitamin B_6 have been identified. In addition to (a) its role as a coenzyme in protein metabolism, vitamin B_6 plays a part in (b) conversion of tryptophan to niacin, (c) hemoglobin synthesis, (d) synthesis of unsaturated fatty acids from essential fatty acids, (e) energy production from glycogen, (f) production of antibodies and immune cells, and (g) proper functioning of the nervous system, including synthesis of neurotransmitters.

Requirements

The current RDA for vitamin B_6 ranges from 1.1 to 1.7 mg daily for adults (Table 11.9). The requirement for vitamin B_6 increases with protein intake because of its major role in amino acid metabolism. Limited amounts of vitamin B_6 are produced by microorganisms in the digestive tract. The UL has been determined to be 100 mg per day for adults. Teenagers, women of childbearing age, smokers, non-Hispanic African American men, and individuals who are underweight are frequently deficient in vitamin B_6.

Sources

Meat, poultry, and fish are good sources of vitamin B_6. Other good sources include some fruits, nuts, fortified cereals, whole-grain products, and vegetables (Table 11.10). Vitamin B_6 from animal sources has greater bioavailability than that provided by plants. Pyridoxine in some plants (potatoes, spinach, beans, and other legumes) is frequently bound to proteins, resulting in low bioavailability. Canning, roasting, boiling, or stewing meat and various food-processing techniques can reduce pyridoxine content of food, as the vitamin is leached into the liquid.

Absorption and Excretion

Absorption of vitamin B_6 differs from other B-complex vitamins. All three forms of the vitamin are converted to an absorbable form by an intestinal enzyme. Body stores are small and repletion is gradual.

Hyper States and Hypo States

Numerous studies suggest possible benefits of supplemental amounts of vitamin B_6 in cardiovascular disease (CVD), sickness during pregnancy, premenstrual syndrome, asthma, carpal tunnel syndrome, and neuropathies. Because of inconsistent findings, supplemental amounts beyond the UL are not currently recommended. Acute pyridoxine toxicity is uncommon; however, routine supplementation with megadoses has documented side effects, including ataxia and severe **sensory neuropathy** (impairment of the ability to feel) and, in some instances, bone pain and muscle weakness. In most cases, complete recovery occurs with discontinuation of megadose supplementation.

Deficiency rarely occurs alone; vitamin B_6 deficiency is most commonly observed along with deficiency of several other B vitamins. Individuals with poor-quality diets in addition to overall low nutrient intake (e.g., alcoholism and older adults) may experience a deficiency. Clinical signs include central nervous system abnormalities or convulsions, dermatitis with cheilosis and glossitis, impaired immune responses, and anemia. Pyridoxine deficiency–induced glossitis is denoted by pain, edema, and papillary changes. Initially, the tongue has a scalded sensation, followed by reddening

TABLE 11.9 **National Academy of Medicine Recommendations for Pyridoxine/Vitamin B_6**

	EAR (mg/day)		RDA (mg/day)			
Life Stage	**Male**	**Female**	**Male**	**Female**	**AI (mg/day)**	**UL (mg/day)[a]**
0–6 months					0.1	ND[b]
7–12 months					0.3	ND[b]
1–3 years	0.4	0.4	0.5	0.5		30
4–8 years	0.5	0.5	0.6	0.6		40
9–13 years	0.8	0.8	1	1		60
14–18 years	1.1	1	1.3	1.2		80
19–50 years	1.1	0.9	1.3	1.3		100
≥ 51 years	1.4	1.3	1.7	1.5		100
Pregnancy						
14–18 years		1.6		1.9		80
≥ 19 years		1.6		1.9		100
Lactation						
14–18 years		1.7		2		80
≥ 19 years		1.7		2		100

AI, Adequate Intake, EAR, Estimated Average Requirement; RDA, Recommended Dietary Allowance; UL, Tolerable Upper Intake Level.
[a]Vitamin B_6 as pyridoxine.
[b]ND—not determinable because of lack of data of adverse effects in this age group and concern with regard to lack of ability to handle excess amounts. Source of intake should be from food and formula to prevent high levels of intake.
Data from Institute of Medicine (IOM), Food and Nutrition Board: *Dietary Reference Intakes for Thiamin, Riboflavin, Niacin, Vitamin B_6, Folate, Vitamin B_{12}, Pantothenic Acid, Biotin, and Choline.* Washington, DC: National Academy Press; 1998.

and hypertrophy of filiform papillae at the tip, margins, and dorsum (Fig. 11.8).

Stores of vitamin B_6 in a mother's body are critical to the well-being of her newborn infant. Oral contraceptive agents (OCAs) taken before conception may reduce maternal vitamin B_6 levels during pregnancy and in breast milk. An increase in dietary intake of vitamin B_6 may be recommended for women taking OCAs, especially if a pregnancy is planned in the near future.

DENTAL CONSIDERATIONS

- Patients may present with pain of the tongue, which precedes redness and swelling of the tip of the tongue. Eventually, atrophy of papillae results in a smooth, purplish tongue. Angular cheilitis, oral ulcers, and stomatitis also may be noted.
- Encourage foods high in vitamin B_6, and monitor for deficiency signs and symptoms, especially in women of childbearing age, excessive alcohol intake, and older adults.
- Use of drugs affecting vitamin B_6 metabolism warrants supplementation to avoid secondary vitamin B_6 deficiency. These drugs include isoniazid and cycloserine (for tuberculosis), penicillamine (for Wilson disease, lead poisoning, kidney stones, and arthritis), and theophylline (for asthma).
- Excessive pyridoxine can reduce clinical benefits of levodopa therapy in patients with Parkinson disease or other neurologic problems. Encourage these patients to limit intake of foods fortified with vitamin B_6 and to avoid vitamin B_6 supplements. If desired effects of the drug are not seen, or if over-the-counter supplements are being taken, refer the patient to the health care provider.

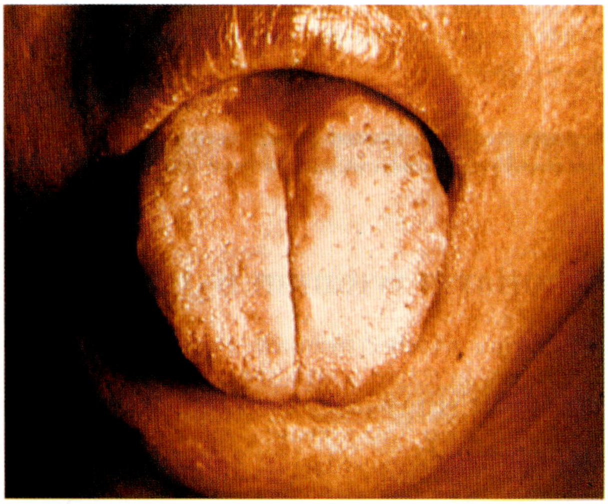

• **Figure 11.8** Fungiform papillary hypertrophy. The condition can be seen and felt as a tongue blade is drawn lightly over the anterior two-thirds of the tongue. The tongue may have a berrylike appearance. (Courtesy of Dr. H. H. Sandstead. McLaren DS: *A Colour Atlas and Text of Diet-Related Disorders*. 2nd ed. London: Mosby-Year Book; 1992.)

TABLE 11.10 Pyridoxine (Vitamin B_6) Content of Selected Foods

Food	Portion	Pyridoxine (mg)
Total, whole-grain cereal	1 cup	2.67
Wheaties cereal	1 cup	1.33
Beef liver, braised	1 slice	0.69
Turkey, cooked	3 oz	0.55
Halibut, broiled	3 oz	0.54
Sunflower seeds	¼ cup	0.47
Salmon, cooked	3 oz	0.47
Banana	1 med	0.43
Potato, white, baked	1 med	0.37
Chicken, meat only, roasted	3 oz	0.27
Pinto beans, cooked	1 cup	0.23
Spinach, cooked	½ cup	0.22
Tuna, white, canned in water	3 oz	0.18
Lentils, boiled	½ cup	0.18
Peanuts, dry roasted	1 oz	0.13
Brown rice, cooked	½ cup	0.12
Tomato, raw	1 med	0.10

Data from U.S. Department of Agriculture (USDA), Agricultural Research Service. 2016. *USDA National Nutrient Database For Standard Reference, Release 28.* Nutrient Data Laboratory Home Page. https://ndb.nal.usda.gov/ndb/. Accessed March 16, 2017.

NUTRITIONAL DIRECTIONS

- Vitamin B_6 supplements should not be taken unless ordered by a health care provider.
- If supplements are needed, signs and symptoms improve within 1 week.
- Adequate daily intake of pyridoxine is important.
- Vitamin B_6 is removed during grain processing and not replaced during enrichment; whole-grain breads and cereals are better sources.

Folate/Folic Acid (Vitamin B_9)

The generic term *folate* encompasses several compounds that have nutritional properties similar to those of folic acid. Several different metabolically active forms have been identified. The terms *folate*, *folic acid*, and *folacin* are used interchangeably. Folate is the natural form found in foods, whereas folic acid is a synthetic form used in vitamin supplements and food fortification. The body converts folic acid to folate.

Physiologic Roles

Folate functions as a coenzyme for approximately 20 enzymes. As such, the methylenetetrahydrofolate reductase (MTHFR) enzyme is involved in synthesis of RNA and DNA. MTHFR is important for numerous chemical reactions involving folate and is required for the process of converting the amino acid hymocysteine to methionine. (This amino acid is used to make proteins and other important compounds). It functions in conjunction with vitamins B_{12} and C in maintaining normal levels of mature red blood cells (RBCs). Folate has an important role in proper formation of the neural tube during the first month of fetal development.

Requirements

As shown in Table 11.11, the RDA is 400 μg for adults. Folate can be expressed as dietary folate equivalents, which are equivalent to 1 μg of folate. Requirements for folate are increased during periods of growth and development, such as adolescence, pregnancy, and lactation, because of its role in DNA formulation. The National Academy of Medicine (formerly the Institute of Medicine) established a UL for the synthetic forms of folic acid available in dietary supplements and fortified foods, but the UL does not pertain to folate from food because a high intake from food sources has not been reported to cause adverse effects.

Sources

Rich sources of folate include liver, green leafy vegetables, fortified cereals and grain products, legumes, and some fruits (e.g., grapefruit and oranges; Table 11.12).

In 1996, the U.S. Food and Drug Administration (FDA) mandated the addition of specific amounts of folic acid to all enriched cereals and grain products. Since then, folate intake and serum folate levels have been monitored because of potential risks of some individuals consuming excessive amounts.

Absorption and Excretion

Dietary folate must undergo changes to be absorbed. The intestinal enzyme that accomplishes this requires a slightly acidic pH and is activated by the presence of zinc. Folic acid from supplements and fortified foods is actually absorbed almost twice as well as that from naturally occurring folate in foods. Individuals needing larger amounts, especially menstruating women who may become pregnant, may need a supplement in addition to fortified folate-rich foods.

Hyper States and Hypo States

A high folic acid intake may be harmful for some people. Prolonged intake of excessive folic acid can cause kidney damage and mask symptoms of vitamin B_{12} deficiency, resulting in neurologic and cognitive symptoms. Although an increased risk of cognitive decline has been suggested in older adults taking folic acid supplements, evidence-based research indicates only a causal relationship between high folic acid intake and risk of developing dementia.[2] Therefore, additional studies need to be conducted.

Abundant intake of folate-rich foods may protect against some common cancers, particularly colorectal cancer. A meta-analysis of scientific studies found no significant effect of folic acid supplementation on incidence of cancer of the large intestine, prostate, lung, breast, or any other specific site.[3,4] The UL of 1000 μg per day for adults is applicable to supplements and fortified foods, not to naturally occurring folate in food.

TABLE 11.11 National Academy of Medicine Recommendations for Folate[a]

Life Stage	EAR (µg/day) Male	EAR (µg/day) Female	RDA (µg/day) Male	RDA (µg/day) Female	AI (µg/day)	UL (µg/day)[b]
0–6 months					65	ND[c]
7–12 months					80	ND[c]
1–3 years	120	120	150	150		300
4–8 years	160	160	200	200		400
9–13 years	250	250	300	300		600
14–18 years	330	330	400	400		800
≥ 19 years	320	320	400	400		1000
Pregnancy						
14–18 years		520		600		800
≥ 19 years		520		600		1000
Lactation						
14–18 years		450		500		800
≥ 19 years		450		500		1000

[a]Dietary folate equivalents.
[b]Folate from fortified foods or supplements.
[c]ND—not determinable because of lack of data of adverse effects in this age group and concern with regard to lack of ability to handle excess amounts. Source of intake should be from food and formula to prevent high levels of intake.
EAR, Estimated Average Requirement; RDA, Recommended Dietary Allowance; AI, Adequate Intake; UL, Tolerable Upper Intake Level.
Data from Institute of Medicine (IOM), Food and Nutrition Board: *Dietary Reference Intakes for Thiamin, Riboflavin, Niacin, Vitamin B_6, Folate, Vitamin B_{12}, Pantothenic Acid, Biotin, and Choline.* Washington, DC: National Academy Press; 1998.

• BOX 11.2 Drugs That May Negatively Affect Folate Status

Anticonvulsants
Oral contraceptives
Analgesics
Metformin (antihyperglycemic)
Sulfasalazine (antiinflammatory, antiarthritic)
H_2-receptor blockers (decreased gastric acid secretion)
Antacids
Triamterene (diuretic)
Methotrexate (antiarthritic, antineoplastic)
Alcohol

Folate deficiency, the most common vitamin deficiency among the B-complex vitamins, usually occurs with other nutrient deficiencies. Folate inadequacy may occur secondary to excessive alcohol consumption, malabsorptive disorders, pregnancy and lactation, kidney disease, inadequate dietary intake, or taking medications that interfere with folate absorption or metabolism (Box 11.2). Folate deficiencies are also associated with a mutation in the MTHFE gnen. Variations in the MTHFR gene are common in many populations woldwide. While individuals with neural tube defects have this genetic variation, many people with a gene variation in MTHFR do not have neural tube defects, nor do their children. MTHFR gene variations have been implicated as possible risk factors for a variety of common conditions, including CVD, preeclampsia, glaucoma, psychiatric disorders, and certain types of cancers.

Folate deficiency can produce soreness and shallow ulcerations on the tongue and oral mucosa as well as swelling of the tongue. Glossitis is usually present in individuals with folic acid deficiency. The tongue becomes fiery red and papillae are absent (Fig. 11.9). Folic acid deficiency impairs immune responses and resistance of the oral mucosa to penetration by pathogenic organisms such as ***Candida***.

Deficiency symptoms first appear in rapidly dividing cells, such as in the gastrointestinal tract, RBCs, and white blood cells. RBCs do not develop normally; they become pale and extremely large (megaloblastic) but cannot transport oxygen to cells, a condition known as **megaloblastic anemia**.

Folic acid deficiency during pregnancy, which may be caused by MTHFR variation, is associated with an increased risk of spina bifida and other **neural tube defects** (birth defects of the skull, brain, and spinal cord), cleft palate and lip, low birth weight, and premature birth. More than 300,000 infants are born each year with neural tube defects worldwide. Before fortification, approximately 4130 babies had neural tube defects each year in the United States, and nearly 1200 died. After folic acid fortification, the yearly number of pregnancies affected by neural tube defects dropped to approximately 3000 and the related deaths declined to 840.[5]

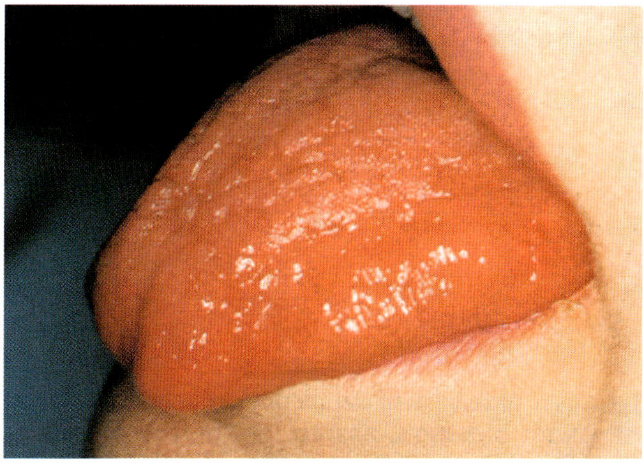

• **Figure 11.9** Folic acid deficiency. Fiery red tongue completely devoid of papillae. (Courtesy of Dr. W. R. Tyldesley. McLaren DS: *A Colour Atlas and Text of Diet-Related Disorders*. 2nd ed. London: Mosby-Year Book; 1992.)

DENTAL CONSIDERATIONS

- Evaluate oral status for folate deficiency. Observe for swelling and pallor or reddening of the tip of the tongue (depending on the degree of anemia) with atrophy of filiform papillae, reddening of the fungiform papillae at the tip and lateral border, and formation of small ulcers. Posterior progression eventually leads to complete atrophy of the filiform papillae and formation of bright red spots (fungiform papillae). Angular cheilitis (see Fig. 11.5) and painful ulcerations of the buccal mucosa and palatal and gingival epithelia may also occur.
- Factors increasing metabolic rate, such as infection and hyperthyroidism, or cellular turnover rate, such as a malignancy, increase folate requirement. Assess folate intake by questioning about dietary intake.
- Folic acid supplementation may improve resistance to periodontal inflammation in patients deficient in folate.
- A low serum folate level is associated with **periodontal disease** (infections and lesions affecting tissues that form the attachment apparatus of the teeth). Encourage patients to consume adequate intakes of folate-rich foods, along with meticulous oral hygiene.
- Folate is one of the most common nutrient deficiencies after bariatric surgery.[6] Encourage patients who have had this procedure to adhere to strict eating behavior guidelines and supplements as recommended by their health care providers.
- Folate absorption is lower when folate is given to individuals taking anticonvulsants and OCAs.
- Methotrexate (drug used for chemotherapy and arthritis) interferes with the conversion of folate to the active form used by cells. Heavy supplementation of folic acid could reduce the therapeutic efficacy of the drug and should be taken under the supervision of the health care provider.
- Increased gingival inflammation has been associated with OCAs; encourage women taking OCAs to increase their consumption of folate-rich foods.
- Phenytoin (Dilantin) is associated with gingival overgrowth (see Fig. 17.13. Studies have shown that folate supplementation reduces severity and incidence of this overgrowth. However, patients taking anticonvulsants should be closely monitored if folate supplements are prescribed because high intakes can decrease effectiveness of the medication.

TABLE 11.12 Folate Content of Selected Foods

Food	Portion	Folate (DFE; µg)
Total, whole-grain cereal	1 cup	901
Wheaties cereal	1 cup	449
Spaghetti, enriched, cooked	1 cup	185
Lentils, boiled	½ cup	179
Pinto beans, cooked	½ cup	172
Liver, beef, braised	1 slice	172
Bagel, enriched	3½–4 inches	171
Asparagus, cooked	½ cup	134
Spinach, cooked	½ cup	131
Navy beans	½ cup	127
Turnip greens, cooked	½ cup	85
Broccoli, cooked	½ cup	84
Corn bread	1 piece	77
Potato, white, baked	1 med	66
Romaine lettuce	1 cup	64
Trail mix, tropical	1 cup	59
Bread, pita, enriched	1 small	48
Orange	1 med	48
Orange juice	1 cup	47
Egg, hard-boiled	1	44
Peanuts, dry roasted	1 oz	41
Grapefruit	1 med	26
Banana	1 med	24
Tomato	1 med	18
Brown rice, cooked	1 cup	18
Bread, whole-wheat	1 slice	13

DFE, dietary folate equivalent.

Data from U.S. Department of Agriculture (USDA), Agricultural Research Service. 2016. *USDA National Nutrient Database For Standard Reference, Release 28.* Nutrient Data Laboratory Home Page. https://ndb.nal.usda.gov/ndb/. Accessed March 16, 2017.

NUTRITIONAL DIRECTIONS

- Folate may be called folic acid or folacin.
- Prolonged cooking destroys folate.
- Folate is easily destroyed by food processing; raw vegetables provide more folate than cooked ones.
- Adequate folic acid is important in the periconceptual period (400 µg/day before conception and 600 µg/day for pregnant women).The critical time for neural tube formation is the first month of pregnancy and cleft palates and/or lips develop in weeks 7 to 11.
- There is also an association between adequate intake of foods fortified with folic acid and a reduction of congenital heart defects at birth.[7]
- Orange juice is a good source of folate because vitamin C protects it from deterioration. Choosing fortified cereals and crackers also enhances folate intake.

TABLE 11.13 National Academy of Medicine Recommendations for Vitamin B_{12}

	EAR (µg/day)		RDA (µg/day)		
Life Stage	Male	Female	Male	Female	AI (µg/day)
0–6 months					0.4
7–12 months					0.5
1–3 years	0.7	0.7	0.9	0.9	
4–8 years	1	1	1.2	1.2	
9–13 years	1.5	1.5	1.8	1.8	
≥ 14 years	2	2	2.4	2.4	
Pregnancy					
14–50 years		2.2		2.6	
Lactation					
14–50 years		2.4		2.8	

AI, Adequate intake, EAR, estimated average requirement; RDA, recommended dietary allowance.
Data from Institute of Medicine (IOM), Food and Nutrition Board: *Dietary Reference Intakes For Thiamin, Riboflavin, Niacin, Vitamin B_6, Folate, Vitamin B_{12}, Pantothenic Acid, Biotin, and Choline.* Washington, DC: National Academy Press; 1998.

TABLE 11.14 Vitamin B_{12} Content of Selected Foods

Food	Portion	Vitamin B_{12} (µg)
Beef liver, braised	1 slice	48.0
Total, whole-grain cereal	1 cup	8.0
Wheaties cereal	1 cup	4.0
Salmon, cooked	3 oz	3.8
Beef, ground (90/10), broiled	3 oz	2.2
Shrimp	3 oz	1.4
Yogurt, low-fat, plain	8 oz	1.3
Skim milk	1 cup	1.2
Lean pork chop, broiled	3 oz	0.7
Cottage cheese	½ cup	0.5
Chicken breast, roasted	3 oz	0.3
Egg, hard-boiled	1	0.3

Data from U.S. Department of Agriculture (USDA), Agricultural Research Service. 2016. *USDA National Nutrient Database for Standard Reference, Release 28.* Nutrient Data Laboratory Home Page. https://ndb.nal.usda.gov/ndb/. Accessed March 16, 2017.

Vitamin B_{12} (Cobalamin)

Vitamin B_{12}, or cobalamin, is a complex group of compounds that contains cobalt. (The only known physiologic function of cobalt is as an integral component of vitamin B_{12}.) It is the only vitamin that contains a mineral.

Physiologic Roles

Vitamin B_{12} functions as a coenzyme in conjunction with folate metabolism in DNA synthesis. It also functions in metabolism of certain amino acids, fatty acids, carbohydrates, and folate. Vitamin B_{12} is essential in formation and regeneration of RBCs, myelin synthesis, and cognitive function. **Myelin** is the lipid substance that insulates nerve fibers and affects transmission of nerve impulses. It is essential for a normal functioning nervous system.

Requirements

The RDA for adults is 2.4 µg daily (Table 11.13). A high vitamin B_{12} intake results in accumulation in the liver with increasing age, but this may be desirable because serum vitamin B_{12} levels decline in elderly individuals due to lower absorption rates. No UL has been established, but caution against excessive intake is warranted.

Sources

Microorganisms (bacteria, fungi, and algae) can synthesize vitamin B_{12}. Vitamin B_{12} is not found in plants unless they are fortified or contaminated by microorganisms (legumes and root vegetables). Fortified soymilk and sea vegetables (e.g., dulse, kelp, alaria, laver, sea lettuce) are vegan sources. More than 80% of dietary vitamin B_{12} is provided by meat and animal products (Table 11.14). Gastrointestinal flora produce small amounts of absorbable vitamin B_{12}.

Absorption and Excretion

Vitamin B_{12} from food is released from its protein bond by hydrochloric acid and enzymes in the stomach and intestine. Free vitamin B_{12} combines with salivary **R-binder** (protein produced by the salivary glands) in the stomach. In the small intestine, trypsin (pancreatic enzyme) removes the R-binder, and vitamin B_{12} combines with **intrinsic factor**, a glycoprotein secreted by the parietal cells in the stomach. Absorption of vitamin B_{12} occurs at specific receptor sites in the ileum and is possible only if it is bound to intrinsic factor. The vitamin is recycled from bile and other intestinal secretions. Excessive amounts are bound to a protein and stored for 3 to 4 years in the liver or are excreted.

Hyper States and Hypo States

Excessive intake of folic acid from supplements delays the diagnosis of, or exacerbates the effects of, vitamin B_{12} deficiency by correcting the anemia but not the cognitive impairment. Injections of vitamin B_{12} are popular treatments for a deficiency related to malabsorption because this delivery bypasses potential barriers to absorption. Oral administration of vitamin B_{12} is not as effective as intramuscular administration in correcting the deficiency since the vitamin may not be absorbed. Vitamin B_{12} deficiency is rarely caused by insufficient dietary sources, unless strict vegan diets are followed over a long period. Lack of intrinsic factor, R-binder, or an enzyme needed for absorption of vitamin B_{12}, is the primary

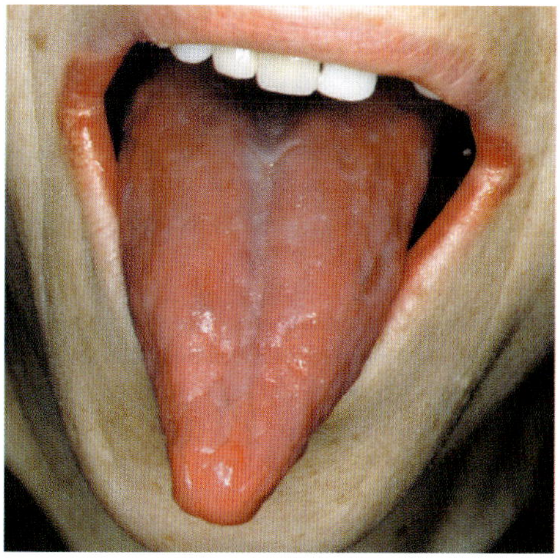

• **Figure 11.10** Pernicious anemia. (Reproduced with permission from Ibsen OAC, Phelan JA. *Oral Pathology for the Dental Hygienist*. 6th ed, St. Louis, MO: Elsevier Saunders; 2014.)

cause of deficiency. **Pernicious anemia**, which is characterized by abnormally large RBCs, glossitis, gastrointestinal disturbances, weakness, and neurologic manifestations, occurs frequently in older patients relative to **achlorhydria** (decreased hydrochloric acid production in the stomach) and decreased synthesis of intrinsic factor by the parietal cells. Rapid neuropsychiatric decline occurs with severe vitamin B_{12} deficiency; however, supplementation with vitamin B_{12} may not improve cognitive ability. More research is needed.[8]

Cobalamin malabsorption is caused by inability to release vitamin B_{12} from food so that it cannot be taken up by intrinsic factor for absorption. Patients develop a lemon-yellow tint of the skin and eyes as a result of concurrent anemia and jaundice from inability to produce RBCs; a smooth, beefy red tongue; and neurologic disorders. Deficiency symptoms develop very slowly.

Initial oral symptoms of vitamin B_{12} deficiency include **glossopyrosis** (unexplained pain of the tongue), followed by swelling and pallor with eventual disappearance of the filiform and fungiform papillae. The tongue may be completely smooth, shiny, and deeply reddened with a loss or distortion of taste (Fig. 11.10). Bright red, diffuse, excruciatingly painful lesions may occur in the buccal and pharyngeal mucosa and undersurface of the tongue. An oral examination may reveal stomatitis or a pale or yellowish mucosa, xerostomia, cheilosis, hemorrhagic gingiva, and bone loss.

Neurologic symptoms, such as numbness or tingling, occur as a consequence of demyelination of the nerves. Deficiency symptoms are rapidly corrected with vitamin B_{12} supplements or intramuscular injections. The crystalline form of vitamin B_{12} found in supplements does not require gastric acid or enzymes for initial digestion, and large oral doses (containing more than 200 times the RDA) can reverse biochemical signs of vitamin B_{12} deficiency in older adults.

Children with vitamin B_{12} deficiency (e.g., vegans) may have growth challenges. Other symptoms include anorexia (loss of appetite), altered taste sensation, abdominal pain, and general weakness. A vitamin B_{12} deficiency is also associated with poor cognitive performance.[9]

DENTAL CONSIDERATIONS

- Assess for oral signs of deficiency; signs and symptoms of vitamin B_{12} deficiency are similar to those of folic acid deficiency except that burning tongue pain precedes physical signs of vitamin B_{12} deficiency.
- Without R-binder, absorption of vitamin B_{12} is drastically reduced.
- Patients with xerostomia may have poor absorption of vitamin B_{12}.
- Patients older than age 50 years are encouraged to choose fortified sources of vitamin B_{12} to meet their needs because the synthetic form is better absorbed than naturally occurring vitamin B_{12} in foods.
- Concomitant ingestion of megadoses of ascorbic acid via foods or supplements can destroy substantial amounts of vitamin B_{12} and produce vitamin B_{12} deficiency. Patients prone to or who have vitamin B_{12} deficiency and take large amounts of vitamin C supplements should be advised to decrease vitamin C intake gradually to approximately the RDA level. Refer them to their health care provider and/or RDN for guidance.
- Patients who have had permanent gastric surgery or ileal damage require other forms of vitamin B_{12} for life. Vitamin B_{12} injections and nasal gel do not require intrinsic factor.
- Because of profound changes in digestive physiology after gastric bypass surgery, vitamin B_{12} is one of the nutrients of concern.
- Vitamin B_{12} deficiency is associated with metformin (an antihyperglycemic medication) therapy in patients with diabetes. Patients with diabetes taking metformin may need a supplement. Levels of vitamin B_{12} should be monitored by the health care professional and/or RDN in those patients at increased risk of a deficiency.[10,11]
- Some antiulcer medications decrease the production of acid by the parietal cells, inhibiting vitamin B_{12} absorption. Histamine receptor antagonists (H_2 blockers; ranitidine [Zantac EFFERdose], famotidine [Pepcid], and cimetidine [Tagamet]) do not affect vitamin B_{12} status, but prolonged use of proton-pump inhibitors (esomeprazole [Nexium], lansoprazole [Prevacid], omeprazole [Prilosec OTC], pantoprazole [Protonix], and rabeprazole [AcipHex]) by older adults negatively affects vitamin B_{12} status. Oral supplementation with recommended amounts of vitamin B_{12} does not prevent this decline. Encourage patients taking these medications to consult their health care provider and/or RDN.

NUTRITIONAL DIRECTIONS

- Because vitamin B_{12} is found only in animal products, vegans (strict vegetarians) require vitamin B_{12}–fortified foods or a daily supplement.
- One cup of fortified cereal will provide the daily requirement for vitamin B_{12}. The synthetic form of the vitamin is easily absorbed by individuals who have limited stomach acid.
- Vitamin B_{12} shots are not a panacea for "tired blood."

Biotin (Vitamin B_7)

Physiologic Roles

Biotin functions as a coenzyme in metabolism of carbohydrates, proteins, and fats. It has an important biochemical role in every living cell in maintaining metabolic homeostasis. Biotin also plays

TABLE 11.15 National Academy of Medicine Recommendations for Biotin

Life Stage	AI (μg/day)
0–6 months	5
7–12 months	6
1–3 years	8
4–8 years	12
9–13 years	20
14–18 years	25
> 18 years	30
Pregnancy	
14–50 years	30
Lactation	
14–50 years	35

AI, adequate intake.
Data from Institute of Medicine (IOM), Food and Nutrition Board: *Dietary Reference Intakes for Thiamin, Riboflavin, Niacin, Vitamin B_6, Folate, Vitamin B_{12}, Pantothenic Acid, Biotin, and Choline.* Washington, DC: National Academy Press; 1998.

an important role in regulating gene transcription (synthesis of DNA and RNA) and metabolically functions closely with folic acid, pantothenic acid, and vitamin B_{12}.

Requirements

Because of insufficient data, only an adequate intake for biotin has been established for all age groups (Table 11.15). Intakes of 10 to 200 μg/day are considered safe and adequate. No UL has been established for biotin.

Sources

Although biotin is widely distributed in foods, its availability is low compared with that of other water-soluble vitamins. Rich sources of biotin include egg yolk, liver, and cereals. The microflora in the gastrointestinal tract probably provides part of the body's needs. Biotin is included in many dietary supplements, infant formulas, and baby foods. Food composition tables usually do not report biotin content of food.

Hypo States

Biotin deficiency can be produced by the ingestion of **avidin**, the protein found in raw egg whites. Avidin is denatured by heat; cooked egg white does not present a problem. Twelve to 24 raw egg whites per day can produce anorexia, nausea, vomiting, glossitis, pallor, depression, and dry scaly dermatitis.

Oral signs of biotin deficiency are pallor of the tongue and patchy atrophy of the lingual papillae. Although the pattern resembles geographic tongue, it is confined to the lateral margins or is generalized to the entire dorsum.

DENTAL CONSIDERATIONS

- Assess patients for signs of deficiency: glossitis, pallor of the mucosal tissue, and papillary atrophy.
- Antibiotics reduce the production of biotin by intestinal bacteria along with some antiseizure, antipsychotic, and antidepressant drugs.

NUTRITIONAL DIRECTIONS

- Drinking or eating large amounts of raw egg whites over a long period may lead to biotin deficiency.
- Eggs should be cooked to decrease avidin's binding capacity and to minimize the danger of *Salmonella* poisoning.
- A balanced diet that includes a variety of foods contains adequate amounts of biotin.

Other Vitamins

As you have already learned, most nutrients perform more than one physiologic function. Although one nutrient may appear to be more important in calcified structures and of lesser importance in oral soft tissues, its roles actually are equally important. The following nutrients have been discussed in previous chapters, but they have important functions in soft oral tissues that the dental hygienist should not overlook.

Vitamin C

Vitamin C is involved in improving the host defense mechanism by ensuring optimal activity of white blood cells. It has an important role in protecting soft oral tissues from infections caused by bacterial toxins and antigens and protecting tooth enamel from plaque microorganisms.

The role of vitamin C in collagen formation is well known. Vitamin C deficiency causes weakened collagen, leading to gingivitis and poor wound healing (see Fig. 8.11,A).

Vitamin A

Vitamin A, necessary for maintaining the integrity of epithelial tissues, is a significant factor in the development and maintenance of salivary glands. Large amounts of vitamin A have an antikeratinizing effect on epithelial cells. Vitamin A increases synthesis of cellular proteins that stimulate growth and influence metabolism.

Vitamin A deficiency produces **squamous metaplasia** (change in cell structure in the oral cavity) with keratin production in the duct cells of salivary glands. This results in decreased salivary secretion and xerostomia. Oral and oropharyngeal cancers have been associated with vitamin A deficiency in humans.

Vitamin E

As discussed in Chapter 8, cell membranes contain polyunsaturated fatty acids that are susceptible to peroxidation. Vitamin E plays a major role as an antioxidant to neutralize free radicals, especially in membranes that contain a large proportion of unsaturated fatty acids. It not only prevents inflammation of the periodontium but also promotes integrity of cell membranes of the mucosa.

DENTAL CONSIDERATIONS

- One of the first signs of vitamin C deficiency is increased susceptibility to infections. During later stages, the gingiva becomes reddened and swollen, and bleeds easily with an increased risk of candidiasis and petechiae. Also, the collagenous structure is weakened and wound healing is slow.
- When a deficiency exists, vitamin C supplementation decreases permeability of the sulcular epithelium and increases collagen synthesis.
- Parotid gland enlargement is associated with deficiencies of vitamins A and C and protein malnutrition.
- Vitamin A deficiency may result in retarded **epithelialization** (natural healing), impaired wound healing and tissue regeneration, and increased risk of candidiasis.

NUTRITIONAL DIRECTIONS

- Foods rich in antioxidants (vitamins E and carotene) may suppress chemically induced **neoplasia** (abnormal growth of tissue) in the mouth, esophagus, and stomach. However, a meta-analysis indicated an increased risk of mortality related to supplementation of these nutrients. Encourage individuals with these neoplasias to choose nutrient-dense foods that are rich in vitamin E and beta-carotenes.
- Vitamin C functions in maintaining periodontal health. A varied and adequate diet including at least one vitamin C–rich food (see Table 8.10) daily provides adequate amounts.

HEALTH APPLICATION 11

Vitamin and Mineral Supplements

Approximately one-half of the U.S. population consumes vitamin and mineral dietary supplements. One-third use a multivitamin-multimineral (MVM) supplement on a daily basis. Approximately 65% of adults aged 62 to 85 years used dietary supplements in 2003 to 2006.[12] An estimated $37 billion was spent on dietary supplements in 2014, including $14 billion for all vitamin and mineral supplements plus $6 billion for multivitamin supplements.[13] Less than 25% of supplements were recommended by a health care provider. These supplements are subject to misrepresentation and misuse because they are misunderstood by most consumers.[12] The five most popular products are fish oil, multivitamins, vitamin D, calcium, and CoQ10. Most adults are taking dietary supplements to optimize their health and well-being (e.g., enhance cognition and physical performance, increase energy); prevent chronic diseases, cancer in particular; and as nutritional "insurance" to cover lifestyle choices.[14] Interesting is the fact that people who take dietary supplements generally are consuming more nutrient-dense foods, resulting in higher nutrient intakes than those who do not take a supplement.[15]

Rates of vitamin–mineral deficiencies involve less than 10% of the general population. The nutrients and their rates of deficiency are vitamin B_6 (10%); iron (9.5%); vitamin D (8.1%); vitamin C (6%); vitamin B_{12} (2%); and vitamins A and E, and folate (< 1%).[16] MVM supplements usually contain 100% of the recommended intake for 10 vitamins and 10 minerals except for calcium (100% Reference Daily Intake for calcium makes the pill too large). There is no standard or regulation governing which vitamins and minerals or how much are included in an MVM supplement.

Vitamin and mineral supplements are drugs, but they are not subject to the same regulations as standard drugs. The *Dietary Supplement Health and Education Act* (DSHEA) of 1994 defines dietary supplements (or dietary ingredients) as vitamins, minerals, amino acids, sports nutrition and weight loss supplements, homeopathic medicines, herbs and botanicals (see Health Application 15), and other products such as enzymes, organ tissues, and metabolites to supplement dietary intake. In other words, a dietary supplement is any product not meant for use as a conventional food or as a sole item of a meal or diet. The DSHEA restricted the FDA's ability to regulate products marketed as "dietary supplements." This act allows supplement manufacturers to market products without proving purity, strength, or effectiveness of supplements to the FDA. Manufacturers are responsible for ensuring that products are safe before they put them on the market. Once a product is marketed, the FDA is responsible for showing that a dietary supplement is "unsafe" before taking action to restrict the product's use or removal from the marketplace. Manufacturers of dietary supplements must record, investigate, then forward to the FDA any reports they are aware of; however, a great majority of the adverse events (Box 11.3) that occur annually remain unreported. In summary, the FDA does not review dietary supplement products for safety and effectiveness before they are marketed. Therefore, it is essential for consumers and health care providers to report adverse effects to the FDA.

In 2007, the FDA implemented good manufacturing practices to ensure that supplements are produced in a quality manner, do not contain contaminants or impurities, and are labeled truthfully. The new mandate was intended to ensure that products are free of contamination and impurities. The FDA has determined that many dietary supplements contain undeclared active pharmaceutical ingredients. Of particular concern are supplements contaminated with prescription medications, controlled substances, experimental compounds, or drugs rejected by the FDA because of safety concerns. Some products on the market contain ingredients used for patients with diabetes, high cholesterol, dementia, or insomnia. Most of the products containing potentially hazardous ingredients are those promising sexual enhancement, optimal athletic performance, and weight loss.

Because there are no uniform manufacturing rules for these products, MVM supplements may not contain what the bottle claims, could be contaminated with something from the manufacturing plant, or may have tainted ingredients. ConsumerLab.com, often called the "watchdog" of the supplement industry, is a private organization that provides independent evaluations of dietary products. In a recent evaluation, more than 30% of multivitamins tested contained significantly more or less of an ingredient than claimed, were contaminated with lead, or did not dissolve fast enough for maximum absorption.[17]

Manufacturers can legally make three types of claims for a dietary supplement: health claims, structure/function claims, and nutrient content claims. Claims can describe the link between a food substance and disease or a health-related condition; intended benefits of using the product; or the amount of a nutrient or dietary substance present. The label on a product sold as a dietary supplement and promoted as a treatment, prevention, or cure for a specific disease or condition would not be allowed. Manufacturers must notify the FDA if they want to make a claim on the product and must include evidence of the product's effectiveness and safety.

If the FDA finds that supplements do not contain ingredients claimed, the agency can consider the products adulterated or misbranded. In minor cases, the FDA may ask the manufacturer to remove an ingredient or revise

Continued

HEALTH APPLICATION 11

Vitamin and Mineral Supplements—cont'd

its label. In more serious cases, it could seize the product, file a lawsuit, or seek criminal charges.

The United States Pharmacopeia (USP), the National Sanitation Foundation International (NSF), and ConsumerLab.com (CL) are nonprofit groups that verify whether companies offer contamination-free products and use good manufacturing practices. The presence of a USP, NSF, or CL symbol on the label helps to ensure quality of a product because the symbols mean that the product has been tested to disintegrate and dissolve in the gastrointestinal tract, contains uniform quality (potency and purity), and contains ingredients as listed on the packaging. These organizations require an expiration date on the packaging. The symbols do not indicate that the supplement is safe for everyone or has any benefits. Not every brand has the seals; some manufacturers may not submit their products for testing.

In most instances, evidence does not indicate a need for most MVM supplements, but use of supplementation is endorsed when there is a demonstrated vitamin or mineral deficiency based on laboratory tests. Some nutrients are more likely to be inadequate during particular phases of life, as follows:

- Iron and folic acid—for adolescent girls and women during childbearing years, especially during pregnancy (see Chapter 13)
- Vitamin B_{12}—for people who are older than age 50 years (see Chapter 15)
- Vitamin D—for older adults, people with heavily pigmented skin, and people exposed to inadequate ultraviolet-B radiation (see Chapter 8)

Additionally, during specific circumstances, typical nutritional needs or eating patterns change; thus, health care professionals should assess and determine whether a nutrient supplement is appropriate. Low-calorie food intake patterns (< 1200 kcal daily) are typically inadequate in vitamins and minerals. Supplements may be used to prevent, treat, or manage disease or other conditions. This would include supplementation with calcium and vitamin D for osteoporosis and electrolyte replacement to treat acute diarrhea. Individuals who limit the variety of foods in their diet may need an MVM supplement, especially if whole food groups are omitted. Examples include vegans (inadequate amounts of calcium, iron, zinc, and vitamins D and B_{12}); people who eliminate all dairy foods (lack of calcium and vitamin D); and patients who severely restrict food choices because of allergies and food intolerances, such as celiac disease (malabsorption and elimination of grain-based foods). In general, unless a health care provider specifically indicates a need for more than 100% of the RDA of a particular nutrient, supplementation is probably not wise.

Patients may be taking amino acid and folic acid supplements, unconventional items, or herbal products described as "natural." These supplements may be deemed safe and desirable, but may adversely affect an existing medical condition or interact with other supplements or prescribed medications. Heroin, cocaine, and tobacco also can be considered "natural" plant-based substances but lead to obvious health issues and are unsafe.

Megadoses of vitamins with intakes of 20 to 600 times the RDAs are sometimes advocated. Vitamin megadosage is defined as a dosage that is more than 10 times the RDA. A megadose of a vitamin is actually a misnomer because, at these levels, the vitamin is functioning as a drug rather than a nutrient. This practice is dangerous and should be supervised by a health care provider to ensure that toxicities do not occur. A well-established principle of pharmacologic therapy is that all substances are potentially toxic at large enough doses. Taking more than the National Academy of Medicine's UL means that risks likely outweigh benefits.

The body processes essential nutrients from food differently than pill form, probably because substances in foods interact with each other in a way that may affect nutrient absorption and utilization. High-dose dietary supplements may not only fail to prevent chronic disease but may actually do harm. For example, kidney stones may occur with high doses (500 mg/day) of vitamin C.

Patients become their own diagnosticians by self-prescribing MVMs or single supplements without consulting their health care provider. The potencies of these self-prescribed supplements vary widely, containing from insignificant amounts to more than 5000% of the Dietary Reference Intake. Consumers use dietary supplements to achieve their self-care goals. Dietary supplements are, in their opinion, an easy means to ensure good health; treat and prevent serious illnesses, colds, and flu; increase mental acuity; and alleviate depression. These individuals may delay seeking medical attention for various health problems. Dietary supplements are not intended to treat disease. Many patients consider vitamins safe to take in any amount. However, each year, thousands of supplement toxicities occur, especially in children.

Public health nutrition would be served best by insisting on a scientifically sound basis for dietary supplementation. Many research and observational studies have shown little or no evidence of protection regarding associations of MVM use for incidence of cardiovascular disease or cancer.[18]

Despite consensus of public opinion, healthy patients do not need dietary supplements if they eat a well-balanced diet 80% to 90% of the time using a variety of foods. Vitamin and mineral supplements are not recommended as a preventive measure in a well-nourished population. Foods are the best source of nutrients. Only a few supplements are likely to help, some may do more harm than good, and many are expensive disappointments. U.S. Poison Control Centers has received a significant increase in the rate of calls regarding dietary supplement exposures since 2000. Approximately 70% of dietary supplement exposures were unintentional, occurring in the home, among children younger than age 6.[19]

The long-term impact of supplementation is unknown. Supplements do not replace or improve the benefits of eating fruits and vegetables, and they may cause unwanted health consequences. In most situations, money is better spent on fresh fruits and vegetables. Obtaining nutrients from dietary sources rather than supplements reduces risk for nutrient deficiencies, excesses, and potential interactions with other drugs or medical conditions. A vast body of observational and epidemiologic studies has associated an increased dietary intake of antioxidants from fruits and vegetables with reduced risks of a range of diseases, including cancer.[20]

Conservative, evidence-based information is often hard to balance against dramatic claims for health in a pill. Whereas the scientific community has reached a consensus about the overall lack of scientific evidence for healthy Americans needing a supplement, several cautions, shown in Box 11.4, are offered for decision making.

One of the biggest dangers is the effect that supplements may have on people's attitudes: "I'm taking vitamins; I don't have to exercise, I can continue to smoke, and I can eat however I like." For patients who choose to self-prescribe supplements, low levels of nutrients that do not exceed the RDA are recommended. Amounts greater than 100% of the RDA should be limited to treatment of specific circumstances under medical supervision.

Store brands of vitamins are often identical to name brands; expensive supplements are no better than less costly supplements. Except for vitamin E, "natural" vitamins are no more beneficial than synthetic vitamins. (An all-natural vitamin E should contain only d-α-tocopherol.) Also, food folate is not as well absorbed as synthetic folic acid, and some individuals have difficulty absorbing naturally occurring vitamin B_{12}. Other components in foods, however, may help with the absorption and use of some nutrients.

Daily MVM supplements are most effective when taken with a meal. It takes longer for a full stomach to empty, allowing more time for the supplement to dissolve and be absorbed. Some nutrients may compete with

HEALTH APPLICATION 11

Vitamin and Mineral Supplements—cont'd

or block the action or absorption of another nutrient; taking single supplements at different meals may be necessary to avoid potential interactions. Chelated supplements are marketed to have superior absorption ability, but they are broken down by gastric acids and absorbed in a manner similar to other supplements. Most supplements marked "timed release" also have no value. The body does not need to maintain a constant level of vitamins as it does for some medications, such as antibiotics.

A medical history should include specific queries about dietary and herbal supplements because many patients typically do not inform health care professionals of their usage. Document the type of supplement, amount, potential interactions, and dental implications (Box 11.5). By asking additional questions to determine why the patient is taking the supplement, the dental hygienist can discuss the benefits of a balanced diet, fluids, exercise, and smoking cessation (see Chapter 19, *Health Application 19*). More important, a careful investigation of peer-reviewed literature and use of scientifically based, current, quality research with valid clinical trials, a systematic review, or meta-analysis would provide dental hygienists with accurate information to help assess a patient's intake and provide advice.

All health professionals are responsible for reporting any damaging effects or illness resulting from nutritional supplements to the FDA (https://www.safetyreporting.hhs.gov/) and submitting complaints to the Federal Trade Commission regarding misleading advertising (http://www.ftc.gov/ftc/complaint.htm). Dental hygienists must consider whether their academic training and scope of practice qualifies them to provide advice regarding dietary supplement usage. Promoting healthy eating patterns and lifestyles according to national guidelines is appropriate advice to provide to patients. A complete nutritional assessment of the patient needs to be conducted to validate the use of a supplement.

• BOX 11.3 Adverse Events Related to Dietary Supplements to Report to the FDA

- Itching, rash, hives, throat/lip/tongue swelling, wheezing
- Low blood pressure, fainting, chest pain, shortness of breath, palpitations, irregular heart beat
- Severe, pesistent nausea, vomiting, diarrhea, or abdominal pain
- Difficulty urinating, decreased urination, dark urine
- Fatigue, appetite loss, yellowing skin/eyes
- Severe joint/muscle pain
- Slurred speech, one-sided weakness of face, arm, leg, vision
- Abnormal bleeding from nose or gingiva
- Blood in urine, stool, vomit, or sputum
- Marked mood, cognitive, or behavioral changes, thoughts of suicide
- Visit to emergency department or hospitalization

FDA, U.S. Food and Drug Administration.

From U.S. Food and Drug Administration. Dietary supplements—how to report a problem. Updated January 10, 2017. https://www.fda.gov/Food/DietarySupplements/ReportAdverseEvent/default.htm. Accessed March 27, 2017.

• BOX 11.4 Buyer Beware!!

- Beware of extravagant claims; if it sounds too good to be true, it is usually not true.
- Beware of testimonials and endorsements, especially from celebrities. Even the most sincere, all-meaning success stories offered by friends and relatives without financial incentives cannot establish a product's safety or efficacy.
- Beware of the idea that if a little is good, more is better. Although vitamin A is essential for health, for example, doses that exceed the UL (3000 IU a day) increase risk of fractures. Also, a high intake of folic acid may increase risk for certain tumors.
- Beware of meaningless terms such as all-natural, antioxidant-rich, clinically proven, antiaging, and other vague but seductive claims that a product will promote heart health, prostate health, sexual prowess, energy, weight loss, fat loss, muscle power, and the like.
- Beware of interactions between supplements and medication. Always inform all health care providers, including pharmacists, about supplements taken, and ask specifically about potential interactions with prescription and over-the-counter medications.
- Beware of adulterated products. Do not assume that all supplements are safe. More than 140 products laced with undisclosed pharmaceutical ingredients have been recalled because of U.S. Food and Drug Administration (FDA) intervention. Products touted for sexual performance, weight loss, and athletic performance are most likely to be contaminated with medications.
- Beware of products that do not contain the amounts indicated on the label (more than or less than). In general, products that have been approved by the United States Pharmacopeia or National Sanitation Foundation International are safest.
- Beware of overconsumption of nutrients. In spite of all the publicity regarding the need for calcium to prevent osteoporosis, several recent studies have linked high-dose calcium supplements with cardiovascular health. Estimate how much calcium and vitamin D is provided from usual food intake, then determine if supplementation is needed. Calcium from food is the ideal way of obtaining calcium.
- Beware of products marketed via the Internet. Whereas FDA oversight is seen by many as overly obtrusive, other countries have no regulations for manufacturing dietary supplements. Most of the recalled supplements are produced in other countries.

Adapted from Harvard Men's Health Watch: Supplements: a scorecard. *Harvard Health Publications Harvard Medical School. April 2012. http://www.health.harvard.edu/newsletters/Harvard_Mens_Health_Watch/2012/April/supplements-a-scorecard. Accessed March 27, 2017.*

Continued

HEALTH APPLICATION 11

Vitamin and Mineral Supplements—cont'd

• BOX 11.5 "ABCD" Approach to Asking Patients about Use of Dietary Supplements

Ask

- What do you take: what form, what brand, what dose, and what else?
- How long have you been taking it, how much do you take, and how often?
- Why do you take it, why was it recommended, and by whom?
- Does it do what you thought it would?

Be

- Wary of any single nutrient used (e.g., vitamin C, E, or B_{12}) not recommended by a health care provider or RDN, and of doses exceeding the National Academy of Sciences, National Academy of Medicine, Food and Nutrition Board Dietary Reference Intakes.
- Sure to look up supplements used in a reliable resource.

Communicate

- Any concerns or risks about safety, drug–nutrient interactions, toxicity to the patient.

Document

- Supplements used, risks of concern, communication with patient, interaction.

Do

- Not get into the supplement business; when in doubt or wanting to refer a patient, contact the credentialed nutrition professional, an RDN.

RDN, registered dietitian nutritionist.

Reproduced with permission from Touger-Decker R. Vitamin and mineral supplements: what is the dentist to do? J Am Dent Assoc. *2007;138(9):1222–1226.*

CASE APPLICATION FOR THE DENTAL HYGIENIST

A young mother of a 3-year-old says she has heard that she should be taking folate supplements because she is considering discontinuing her birth control pills. She is concerned about the effects of the birth control pills on her nutritional status and their effect on a fetus should she become pregnant.

Nutritional Assessment

- Types of foods consumed
- Knowledge base of foods rich in folate
- Current use of any dietary supplements
- Motivation to change eating habits
- Knowledge of physiologic values and absorption of folate

Nutritional Diagnosis

Health-seeking behavior related to nutritional status and effects on fetus.

Nutritional Goals

The patient will consume foods rich in folate and ask her health care provider about the need to take a multivitamin supplement or a folate supplement.

Nutritional Implementation

Intervention: Evaluate the oral area for symptoms of folate or other nutrient deficiencies.

Rationale: This will help determine whether she is currently deficient and help determine whether she should consult her health care provider immediately.

Intervention: Teach the following about folate: (a) different names used, (b) functions, (c) requirements, and (d) sources.

Rationale: This provides the patient with a sound base of knowledge about folic acid.

Intervention: Discuss symptoms of folate deficiency and harmful effects of too much folic acid.

Rationale: Although the patient needs to consume adequate amounts of folic acid to prevent neural tube defects, too much can also be harmful.

Intervention: Discuss the stability of folate during cooking and processing.

Rationale: Knowing that folate can easily be destroyed during food preparation allows the patient to make decisions based on her eating habits and to determine whether her diet provides adequate amounts of folate.

Intervention: Explain that her requirement for folic acid is increased because of the birth control pills and because of the needs of the fetus and other physiologic changes occurring early during pregnancy.

Rationale: This knowledge will help her realize the importance of changing dietary patterns and maintaining the new healthful diet.

Evaluation

The patient should increase her intake of folate-rich foods (cereal and grain products that are fortified with folate, oranges, legumes, liver, green leafy vegetables). Additionally, she should consult her health care provider before she discontinues the OCA and begins taking a multivitamin. She can state why she has an increased requirement for folic acid and why it is important not to take excessive amounts.

Student Readiness

1. Name the two water-soluble vitamins most involved in the metabolism of fats, proteins, and carbohydrates to form energy (adenosine triphosphate) through the Krebs cycle.
2. Match the conditions associated with the appropriate vitamin deficiency:

Thiamin	Ariboflavosis
Riboflavin	Scurvy
Niacin	Pellagra
Vitamin B_{12}	Megaloblastic anemia
Ascorbic acid	Beriberi
	Pernicious anemia
	Wernicke-Korsakoff syndrome
	Neutral tube defects

3. Why is it important that water-soluble vitamins be consumed daily?

4. Define "vitamin megadose." What are the disadvantages of taking vitamin megadoses?
5. Name three foods that are good sources of each of the following nutrients: thiamin, riboflavin, vitamin B_{12}, and folate.
6. What would you teach a vegan about vitamin B_{12}?
7. Discuss why signs and symptoms of deficiencies of water-soluble vitamins appear periorally. List signs and symptoms of deficiencies you should be alert for and list vitamins that might be implicated.
8. What recommendations could you offer to a patient to ensure the availability of folate? Why is folate so important before and during pregnancy?
9. Evaluate five of the stress or megavitamin supplement preparations in a drugstore or health food store. List the amounts of vitamin C, niacin, and vitamin B_6 (pyridoxine) in them, and compare those amounts with the RDAs for children younger than 10 years old, men 19 to 24 years old, and women 25 to 50 years old.

CASE STUDY

A 32-year-old man presents with the following symptoms: swollen tongue with reddening at the tip, small oral ulcerations, and gingival hyperplasia. The patient is being treated with long-term anticonvulsant medication.

1. Is a dietary assessment indicated? Explain your answer.
2. What are possible effects of the patient's medication on his nutritional and oral status?
3. If a deficiency exists, which vitamins/minerals are most likely lacking? Why?
4. Which types of foods and food preparation methods should be suggested? Why?
5. What advice should you give regarding oral care?

References

1. Moskovitz M, Dotan M, Zilberman U. The influence of infantile thiamine deficiency on primary dentition. *Clin Oral Investig.* 2017;21(4):1309–1313.
2. Horvat P, Gardiner J, Kubinova R, et al. Serum folate, vitamin B-12 and cognitive function in middle and older age: the HAPIEE study. *Exp Gerontol.* 2016;76:33–38.
3. Vollset SE, Clarke R, Lewington S, et al. Effects of folic acid supplementation on overall and site-specific cancer incidence during the randomised trials: meta-analyses of data on 50,000 individuals. *Lancet.* 2013;381(9871):1029–1036.
4. Colapinto CK, O'Connor DL, Sampson M, et al. Systematic review of adverse health outcomes associated with high serum or red blood cell folate concentrations. *JPublic Health.* 2015;38(2): 84–97.
5. Centers for Disease Control and Prevention (CDC). Global initiative to eliminate folic acid-preventable neural tube defects. Division of Birth Defects, National Center on Birth Defects and Developmental Disabilities, Centers for Disease Control and Prevention, Atlanta GA. Last updated November 14, 2011. http://www.cdc.gov/ncbddd/folicacid/global.html. Accessed March 24, 2017.
6. Saltzman E, Karl JP. Nutrient deficiencies after gastric bypass surgery. *Ann Rev Nutr.* 2013;33:183–203.
7. Liu S, Joseph KS, Luo W, et al. Effect of folic acid food fortification in Canada on congenital heart disease subtypes. *Circulation.* 2016;134:647–655.
8. Zhang D-M, Ye J-X, Mu J-S, et al. Efficacy of vitamin B supplementation on cognition in elderly patients with cognitive-related diseases: a systematic review and meta-analysis. *J Geriat Psychiatry Neurol.* 2017;30(1):50–59.
9. Moore E, Mander A, Ames D, et al. Cognitive impairment and vitamin B_{12}: a review. *Int Psychogeriatr.* 2012;24(4):541–556.
10. Aroda VR, Edelstein SL, Goldberg RB, et al. Long-term metformin use and vitamin B_{12} deficiency in the Diabetes Prevention Program Outcomes Study. *J Clin Endocrinol Metab.* 2016;101(4):1754–1761.
11. Chapman LE, Darling AL, Brown JE. Association between metformin and vitamin B_{12} deficiency in patients with type 2 diabetes: a systematic review and meta-analysis. *Diabetes Metab.* 2016;42:316–327.
12. Kantor ED, Rehm CD, Mengmeng D, et al. Trends in dietary supplement use among US adults from 1999–2012. *JAMA.* 2016;316(14):1464–1474.
13. Bradley J. The US supplement industry is $37 billion, not $12 billion. *Nutr Bus J.* 2015; http://www.nutraingredients-usa.com/content/view/print/1125262. Accessed March 27, 2017.
14. Bailey RL, Gahche JJ, Miller PE, et al. Why US adults use dietary supplements. *JAMA Intern Med.* 2013;173(5):355–361.
15. Moshfegh AJ. Monitoring the U.S. population's diet: the third step—the national "What We Eat in America" survey. *Agric Res.* 2012;60(3):16–21. http://www.ars.usda.gov/is/AR/archive/mar12/diet0312.htm. Accessed March 27, 2017.
16. Centers for Disease Control and Prevention (CDC). CDC's second nutrition report: a comprehensive biochemical assessment of the nutrition status of the U.S. Population (Paris). 2012;http://www.cdc.gov/nutritionreport/. Accessed March 27, 2017.
17. ConsumerLab. Multivitamin and multimineral supplements review. Updated February 22, 2017. https://www.consumerlab.com/reviews/review_multivitamin_compare/multivitamins/. Accessed March 27, 2017.
18. Schwingshackl L, Boeing H, Stelmach-Mardas M, et al. Dietary supplements and risk of cause-specific death, cardiovascular disease, and cancer: a systematic review and meta-analysis of primary prevention trials. *Adv Nutr.* 2017;8:27–39.
19. Rao N, Spiller HA, Hodges NL, et al. An increase in dietary supplement exposures reported to US Poison Control Centers. *J Med Toxicol.* 2017;doi:10.1007/s13181-017-0623-7. [Epub ahead of print].
20. Fulton SL, McKinley MC, Youg IS, et al. The effect of increasing fruit and vegetable consumption on overall diet: a systematic review and meta-analysis. *Crit Rev Food Sci Nutr.* 2016;56:802–816.

EVOLVE RESOURCES

Please visit http://evolve.elsevier.com/Stegeman/nutritional for additional practice and study support tools.

12

Fluids and Minerals Required for Oral Soft Tissues and Salivary Glands

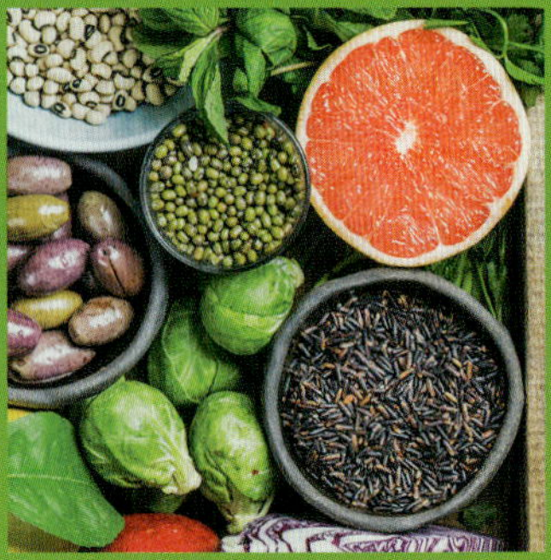

STUDENT LEARNING OUTCOMES

Upon completion of this chapter, the student will be able to achieve the following student learning outcomes:

1. In relation to fluids:
   - Describe the physiologic roles of fluid, and list the fluid requirements for both men and women. Also, identify factors that may affect those requirements.
   - List and discuss the various sources of fluid.
   - Discuss hyper and hypo states related to fluid imbalances in the body, identify oral signs and symptoms of fluid imbalances, and discuss areas of nutritional concern with patients who have fluid imbalances.
2. Explain how electrolytes affect hydration status.
3. Pertaining to sodium and chloride:
   - Describe the physiologic roles of sodium and chloride, and list the sodium and chloride requirements for both men and women.
   - List and discuss the various sources of sodium and chloride, and discuss with patients how to decrease dietary sources of sodium.
   - Discuss hyper and hypo states related to sodium and chloride imbalances in the body, identify oral signs and symptoms of sodium imbalances, and discuss areas of nutritional concern with patients who have sodium imbalances.
   - Identify diseases and medications associated with restriction of sodium intake.
4. In relation to potassium:
   - Describe the physiologic roles of potassium, and list and potassium requirements for both men and women.
   - List and discuss the various sources and potassium, and discuss with patients how to increase dietary sources of potassium.
   - Discuss hyper and hypo states related to potassium imbalances in the body, identify oral signs and symptoms of potassium imblanaces, and discuss areas of nutritional concern with patients who have potassium imbalances.
5. Related to iron:
   - Describe the physiologic roles of iron, and list the iron requirements for both men and women.
   - List and discuss the various sources of iron.
   - Discuss hyper and hypo states related to iron imbalances in the body, identify oral signs and symptoms of iron imblanaces, and discuss areas of nutritional concern with patients who have iron imbalances.
6. Related to zinc and iodine:
   - Describe the physiologic roles of zinc and iodine, and list the zinc and iodine requirements for both men and women.
   - List and discuss the various sources of zinc and iodine, and discuss with patients how to increase dietary sources of zinc and iodine.
   - Discuss hyper and hypo states related to zinc and iodine imbalances in the body, identify oral signs and symptoms of zinc and iodine imblanaces, and discuss areas of nutritional concern with patients who have zinc and iodine imbalances.

KEY TERMS

Aldosterone
Anions
Antidiuretic hormone (ADH)
Cations
Cretinism
Ergogenic
Essential hypertension
Extracellular fluid (ECF)
Fluid volume deficit (FVD)
Fluid volume excess (FVE)
Goiter
Goitrogens
Guarana
Heme iron
Hemochromatosis
Hyperkalemia
Hypernatremia
Hypodipsia
Hypokalemia
Hyponatremia
Interstitial fluid
Intracellular fluid (ICF)
Longitudinal fissures
Myxedema
Nonheme iron
Osmoreceptors
Peripheral edema
Quercetin
Renin
Solutes
Solvent
Taurine
Transferrin

TEST YOUR NQ

1. **T/F** Thirst is the primary regulator of fluid intake.
2. **T/F** Meats are more than half water.
3. **T/F** Water is the most abundant component in the body.
4. **T/F** Heme iron is provided by meat sources and is more readily absorbed than iron from vegetable or grain products.
5. **T/F** Normal fluid requirements are eight 8-oz cups of total water daily.
6. **T/F** The Recommended Dietary Allowance (RDA) for sodium is 5000 mg/day.
7. **T/F** Taste alteration is a symptom of zinc deficiency.
8. **T/F** Potassium is principally found in extracellular fluid.
9. **T/F** Milk is a good source of potassium.
10. **T/F** Oral pallor is associated with iodine deficiency.

Water and several mineral elements are essential for maintenance of healthy oral tissues, including tooth enamel. Visual signs of these nutrient deficiencies in the gingiva, mucous membranes, and salivary glands are less obvious than signs observed with the B vitamin complex and vitamin C deficiencies discussed in Chapters 9 and 11. Nevertheless, water and several minerals have a significant effect on integrity of the oral cavity and, ultimately, nutritional status. Oral problems associated with hyper states or hypo states of the minerals discussed in this chapter are slow to develop and may not be evident immediately. Chronically decreased salivary flow attributable to inadequate body fluids may lead to rampant tooth decay and eventually loss of teeth.

Fluids

Water is the most abundant component in the body. At birth, water constitutes approximately 75% to 80% of body weight. Because such a large percentage of the infant's body weight consists of water, fluid loss is more significant in infants than in adults. Total body water decreases with age, representing 50% to 60% of an adult's body weight. Adipose tissue contains less water than muscle; a person with a large amount of fat has a lower percentage of total body water. Women's bodies, with inherently larger fat stores, contain less water than men's bodies, which have a higher percentage of lean muscle tissue.

Body fluids are distributed in compartments, separated by semipermeable membranes. **Intracellular fluid (ICF)**, which constitutes 60% of the body's fluid weight, includes all the fluid within cells (chiefly in muscle tissue; Fig. 12.1). **Extracellular fluid (ECF)** consists of fluid outside the cells, including fluid in plasma and lymph and the **interstitial fluid** that fills the space between cells. These fluids help control movement of water and electrolytes through the body. Membranes serve as barriers by preventing movement of certain substances from one compartment to another; however, they do not completely isolate the compartments. Water is essentially unrestricted in its movement from compartment to compartment. Certain dissolved substances, or **solutes**, such as glucose, amino acids, and oxygen, also cross membranes freely. Cellular membranes allow maintenance of solute concentration by their selectivity.

When two compartments are separated by semipermeable membranes and movement of some solutes is restricted, osmosis occurs. Osmotic pressure within the body equalizes the solute concentration of ICFs and ECFs by shifting small amounts of water in the direction of higher concentration of solute, as shown in Chapter 3, Fig. 3.5.

Physiologic Roles

Water has several important physiologic roles: (a) it acts as a **solvent** (fluid in which substances are dissolved), enabling chemical reactions to occur by entering into reactions, such as hydrolysis; (b) it maintains stability of all body fluids, as principal component and medium for fluids (blood and lymph), secretions (saliva and gastrointestinal fluids), and excretions (urine and perspiration); (c) it enables transport of nutrients to cells and provides a medium for excretion of waste products; (d) it acts as a lubricant between cells to permit movement without friction; and (e) it regulates body temperature by evaporating as perspiration from skin and vapor from the mouth and nose. Negative fluid balance has serious

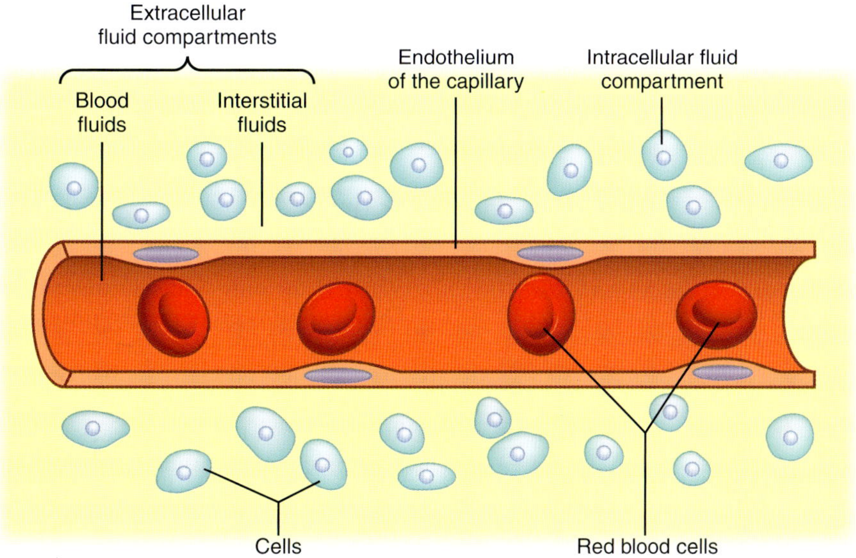

• **Figure 12.1** Water is a key component of the fluid compartment inside (intracellular) and outside (extracellular) cells.

detrimental effects on many physiologic functions. A few days without water can be fatal.

Requirements and Regulation

Fluid requirements are based on experimentally derived intake levels that are expected to meet nutritional needs of a healthy population. To maintain normal hydration, the National Academy of Medicine (formerly the Institute of Medicine) established an Adequate Intake (AI) for total fluid (beverages, water, and food). As shown in Table 12.1, men require 3.7 L/day (125 oz), and women require 2.7 L/day (91 oz). Daily fluid intake averaged 117 oz/day for men and 93 oz for women in 2009 to 2012.[1] No Tolerable Upper Intake Level (UL) is established for water, although water intoxication does occur occasionally.

Overconsumption and underconsumption of fluids can occur over short periods. However, if adequate amounts of fluids are available, consumption matches physiologic needs over an extended period. Individuals who consume a high-protein or high-fiber diet, have diarrhea or vomiting, or are physically active or exposed to warm or hot weather, require more fluids.

Water is lost by a variety of routes: (a) urination, (b) perspiration, (c) expiration, and (d) defecation. Urine production depends on the amount of fluid intake and type of diet eaten. However, waste products must be kept in solution; minimum urine output to eliminate waste products is 400 to 600 mL/day.

Water losses in the form of sweat can vary greatly. An increase in body temperature (fever) is accompanied by increased sweating and respiration. Strenuous exercise can greatly affect the amount of water lost through the skin. Vapor in expired air varies with the rate of respiration. The presence of inflammation also elevates respiration rate. Approximately 100 to 200 mL of water is lost each day in feces; this dramatically increases with diarrhea.

Water losses result in stimulation of water (thirst) and decreased kidney output to maintain fluid balance. Saliva also may help maintain water balance because saliva flow is reduced in dehydration, leading to drying of the mucosa and sensation of thirst.

Normal fluid requirements (Fig. 12.2) can be drastically changed in different climatic environments, with various exercise levels, diet, and social activities, and with illnesses accompanied by diarrhea or vomiting. The body cannot store water, so the amount lost must be replaced.

In healthy adults, thirst is the earliest sign of the body's need for fluids but is often mistaken for hunger (Fig. 12.3). The ability to regulate water balance is not as precise in infants and older adults. Older patients often have a reduced sensation of thirst. When 2% of body water is lost, osmoreceptors are stimulated, creating a physiologic desire to ingest liquids. **Osmoreceptors** are neurons in the hypothalamus sensitive to changes in serum osmolality levels. Stimulation of osmoreceptors not only causes thirst but also increases release of **antidiuretic hormone (ADH)** from the pituitary gland. ADH causes the body to retain fluid by decreasing urinary output (see Fig. 12.2). Conversely, ADH secretion is inhibited when fluid accumulates and excess water is eliminated.

Decreased blood pressure also stimulates release of the enzyme **renin**, which ultimately leads to increased release of the hormone **aldosterone** by the adrenal cortex. This release of aldosterone results in retention of sodium and water by the kidneys and excretion of potassium and hydrogen ions, causing blood pressure to increase.

TABLE 12.1 National Academy of Medicine Recommendations for Water

	AI[a]	
Life Stage	Male (L/day)[b]	Female (L/day)[b]
0–6 months	0.7[c]	0.7[c]
7–12 months	0.8[d]	0.8[d]
1–3 years	1.3[e]	1.3[e]
4–8 years	1.7[f]	1.7[f]
9–13 years	2.4[g]	2.1[h]
14–18 years	3.3[i]	2.3[g]
> 18 years	3.7[j]	2.7[k]
Pregnancy		
14–50 years		3[l]
Lactation		
14–50 years		3.8[m]

[a]AI (Adequate Intake) *The AI is not equivalent to a Recommended Dietary Allowance.*
[b]L = liter; 1 L = 4.2 cups.
[c]Assumed to be from human milk.
[d]Assumed to be from human milk, complementary foods, and beverages. This includes ~0.6 L (~3 cups) as total fluid, including formula or human milk, juices, and drinking water.
[e]Total water. This includes ~0.9 L (~4 cups) as total beverages, including drinking water.
[f]Total water. This includes ~1.7 L (~5 cups) as total beverages, including drinking water.
[g]Total water. This includes ~1.8 L (~8 cups) as total beverages, including drinking water.
[h]Total water. This includes ~1.6 L (~7 cups) as total beverages, including drinking water.
[i]Total water. This includes ~2.6 L (~11 cups) as total beverages, including drinking water.
[j]Total water. This includes ~3 L (~13 cups) as total beverages, including drinking water.
[k]Total water. This includes ~2.7 L (~9 cups) as total beverages, including drinking water.
[l]Total water. This includes ~3 L (~10 cups) as total beverages, including drinking water.
[m]Total water. This includes ~3.1 L (~13 cups) as total beverages, including drinking water.
Data from Institute of Medicine (IOM), Food and Nutrition Board: *Dietary Reference Intakes for Water, Potassium, Sodium, Chloride, Chloride, and Sulfate.* Washington, DC: National Academies Press; 2005.

Absorption

No digestion is necessary for water absorption; it is transported easily in both directions across the intestinal mucosa by osmosis (see Chapter 3, Fig. 3.5). Within an hour, 1 L can be absorbed from the small intestine. Normally, almost all fluid is absorbed, with a small amount excreted in feces.

Sources

Water

Water is the only liquid nutrient essential for body hydration. During the process of metabolism, liquids and solid foods provide water. Some fruits and vegetables have a higher percentage of water than does milk, and meats are more than half water (Table 12.2). Regardless of its source, fluids act the same physiologically. Water liberated in the process of metabolism is also available. Metabolism of fat produces approximately twice as much water as the metabolism of protein or carbohydrate; metabolism of these macronutrients supplies about 300 to 350 mL daily.

Plain tap water is the most natural source of fluids, best for quenching thirst, most economical, and healthiest. About 30% to 34% of fluid intake comes from water.[1] Many Americans have

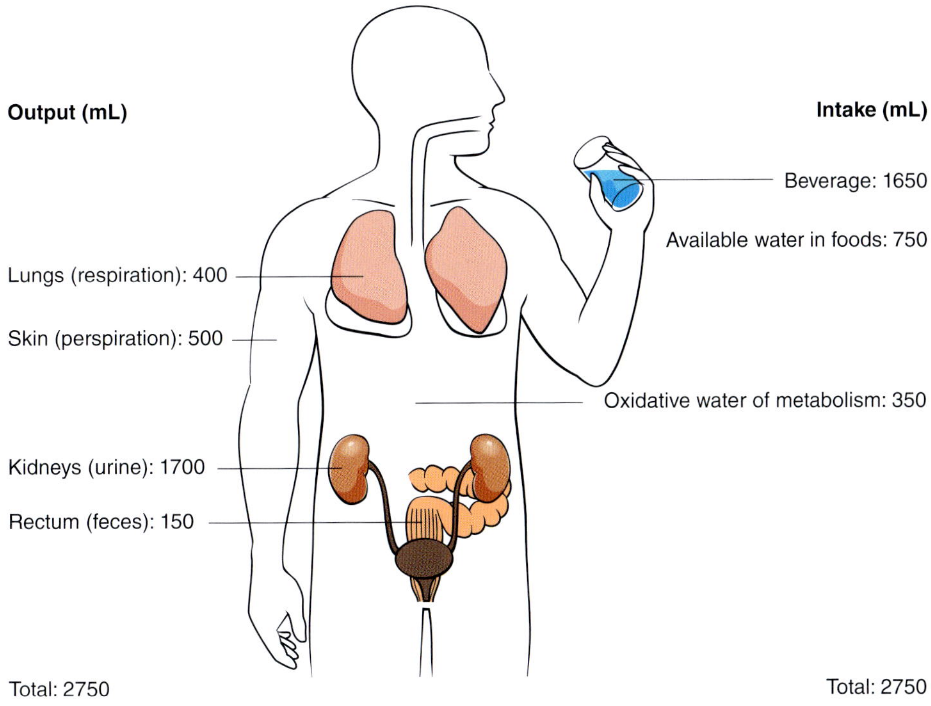

• **Figure 12.2** The role of osmoreceptors and antidiuretic hormone in fluid balance.

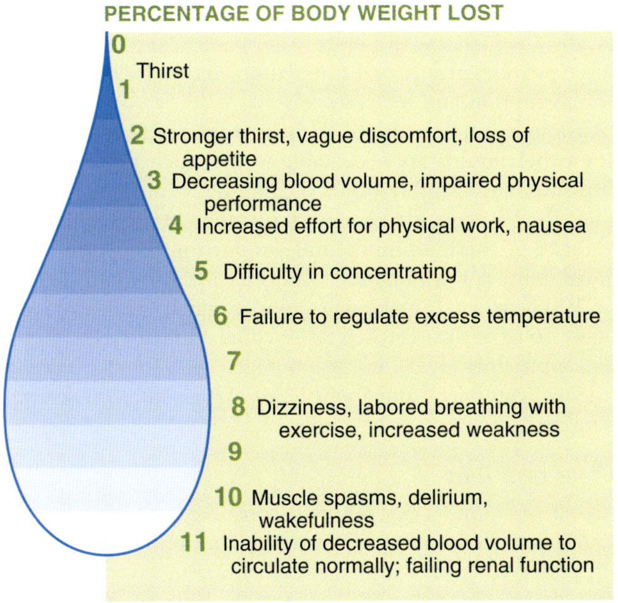

• **Figure 12.3** Percentage of body weight lost. Adverse effects of dehydration. (Reproduced with permission from Mahan LK, Raymond JL. *Krause's Food & the Nutrition Care Process.* 14th ed. St. Louis, MO: Elsevier, 2017.)

become disenchanted with tap water. Although not perfect, the United States has one of the safest public water supplies in the world. During the past century, many improvements in Americans' health can be attributed to improvements in drinking water, such as community fluoridation and infectious disease control. When groundwater becomes polluted, it is no longer safe to drink. Naturally occurring arsenic and radon in the environment and lead from corroded pipes can contaminate water, as occurred in Michigan in 2016. Other ways water can become contaminated are from use of fertilizers and pesticides, microbial contamination, and manufacturing processes.

Drugs have been detected in drinking water of several major metropolitan areas. This contamination could be from medications not absorbed by individuals and eliminated through physiologic discharges or numerous other reasons. Many pharmaceuticals pass through sewage and drinking-water treatment plants. Some gastrointestinal illnesses occur from small or individual water systems.

The Environmental Protection Agency (EPA) regulates levels of contaminants allowed in public drinking water; these amounts are provided to customers by water utility companies annually. Private well owners are responsible for ensuring that their water is safe from contaminants of high concern. Treated wastewater is not free of all drug residues and other contaminants. Although present in very low amounts, the effect of these drugs and contaminants on health is unknown.

Because of mistrust of the water supply, and a desire for a safer and more convenient form of fluid intake, consumers frequently choose bottled water. The bottled water market continues to increase but suffered a setback as a result of environmental concerns (energy required to produce plastic nonbiodegradable plastic bottles, bisphenol A BPA content of bottles, cost of marketing and shipping bottles of water) and the revelation that approximately 75% of reputable bottlers utilize groundwater (same source as the public water supply) or tap water. The letters P.W.S. on bottled water stands for "public water source." In 2016, Americans consumed more water than carbonated soft drinks (39.3 gallons of bottled water versus 38.5 gallons of soft drinks).[2] Bottled water, regulated by the U.S. Food and Drug Administration (FDA), is available with many labels: drinking water, sparkling water, mineral water, Artesian water, alkaline water, caffeinated water, oxygenated water, and purified water (distilled, demineralized, deionized, and reverse osmosis). Bottled water also includes flavored waters and

TABLE 12.2 Percentage of Water in Foods

Food Item	% Water
Beer and wine	90–95
Milk, fruit juice, fruit drinks	85–90
Cooked cereals	85–90
Fruits (strawberries, melons, grapefruit, peaches, pears, oranges, apples, grapes, cucumbers, tomatoes)	80–85
Vegetables (lettuce, celery, cabbage, broccoli, onions, carrots)	80–85
Cottage cheese and yogurt	75–80
Liquid drinks for weight loss, muscle gain, meal replacement	70–85
Fish and seafood	70–80
Vegetables (potatoes, corn)	70–75
Rice and pasta	65–80
Eggs	65–80
Stew, pasta and meat dishes, casseroles (with meat and meatless), meatloaf, tacos, enchiladas, macaroni and cheese	60–80
Sauces and gravies	50–85
Ice cream	50–60
Beef, chicken, lamb, pork, turkey, veal	45–65
Cheese	40–50
Breads, bagels, biscuits	30–45
Ready-to-eat breakfast cereals	2–5
Chips, pretzels, candies, crackers, dried fruit, popcorn	1–5

Adapted from Grandjean A, Campbell S. *Hydration: Fluids for Life.* Washington, DC: ILSI North America; 2004.

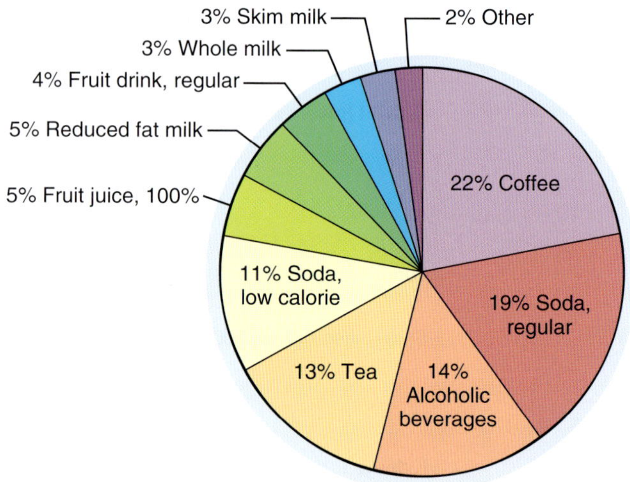

• **Figure 12.4** Distribution of intake (grams) across beverage types, U.S. adults (age 19+ years). Other beverages include fruit drink (low calorie), milk substitute/evaporated milk, and vegetable juice, each contributing less than 2%. Percentages do not add to 100% as a result of rounding. (Data source: NHANES 2005–2006. https://epi.grants.cancer.gov/diet/foodsources/beverages/figure4.html. Accessed January 7, 2017.)

nutrient-added water beverages. Broad claims for these various waters lack research to support them.

The FDA established maximum levels for contaminants and disinfection by-products (e.g., bromate, chlorite, and so on) and disinfectants (e.g., chlorine) in bottled water. This trend has resulted in increased water intake, but numerous problems are associated with this practice. Many consumers think bottled water is healthier, but most bottled waters do not contain fluoride. Fluoride does not have to be listed on the label unless it is added.

Many flavored beverages contain additional calories, which are consumed in excessive amounts by most Americans. The body does not treat calories from beverages differently from energy provided in foods. However, calories in beverages go down so smoothly that significant amounts can be consumed without realizing how much is being consumed. Water has been recommended for weight loss despite the fact that fluids satisfy thirst and not hunger. Based on a review of scientific evidence, a research team concluded that "increasing water intake to reduce energy consumption to promote weight loss" is only a presumption, not a fact.[3] Nevertheless, an increase of water intake by most people is beneficial. Water consumed with a meal does not affect caloric consumption at mealtime, but water incorporated into food (as in soup) increases satiety, ultimately leading to less caloric intake. Basically, foods that incorporate water tend to appear larger, more volume provides greater oral stimulation, and water bound to food slows absorption and increases satiety.

Although water is the only fluid truly needed by the body, many other liquids are acceptable; some, such as low-fat milk, contribute significant amounts of important nutrients. Fig. 12.4 depicts the beverage intake pattern of adults in the United States; beverages in these amounts and proportions represent almost 400 cal daily. A recommended healthier intake would include at least 100 fl oz total intake with approximately 50% from water, roughly 16 oz of unsweetened tea or coffee, at least 12 oz of low-fat milk, approximately 12 oz of beverages with some calories and nutrients (fruit juice), and about 12 oz of high-intensity sweetened beverages.

Coffees and Teas

Coffee is the number one beverage consumed at home. For many Americans, coffee tastes good and helps "jump start" the morning. Both coffee and tea, without added sugars or creamers, contain negligible calories, vitamins, or minerals. Both beverages contain caffeine, a compound that has received a lot of attention regarding its safety. In addition to contributing to fluid intake, both have some health benefits. In addition to caffeine, they both contain valuable polyphenols, antioxidants, and other bioactive compounds. These naturally present chemical compounds may be the reason numerous studies have discovered an inverse relationship between coffee consumption and chronic health conditions (Box 12.1).

Because of the addition of caffeine to many new products, the FDA continues to investigate the amount of caffeine that is safe (Table 12.3). Acute clinical toxicity begins at 1 g and 5 to 10 g of caffeine can be lethal. Coffee consumption has no detrimental effects on periodontal health.[4]

Most teas are benign, but the FDA has issued warnings regarding those that contain senna, aloe, buckthorn, and other plant-derived

• BOX 12.1 Caffeine Myths and Facts*

Caffeine occurs naturally in many plants, including coffee beans, tea leaves, kola nuts (used to flavor carbonated beverages), and cacao pods (used for chocolate products). Caffeine is sometimes added to medications and foods but is most frequently present in beverages. Most Americans consume about 300 mg/day. Despite the fact that other sources of caffeine are available, per capita of caffeine has remained stable.[1] Caffeine is a central nervous system stimulant, affecting the brain, spinal cord, and other nerves. The FDA considers caffeine both a drug and a food additive. Caffeine reaches a peak level in the blood within 1 hour after consumption and remains at these levels for 4 to 6 hours. High levels of caffeine intake have adverse effects, but little research has been conducted to validate benefits of excessively high caffeine intake.

Caffeine increases a person's metabolic rate and may be associated with increased wakefulness. Very high caffeine intake (> 500 mg/day) is associated with nervousness, restlessness, anxiety, insomnia, arrhythmia, gastrointestinal upset, tremors, and psychomotor agitation. Moderate amounts of caffeine (about 300 mg/day) do not cause these effects in most individuals.

1. Caffeine is not addictive. As a central nervous system stimulant, it can cause mild physical dependence, but it does not threaten physical, social, or economic health as addictive drugs do. Abruptly stopping caffeine may cause withdrawal symptoms such as headache, fatigue, anxiety, and depressed mood and concentration for a day or two.
2. Caffeine consumed within 6 hours of going to bed may cause insomnia. Caffeine is quickly absorbed but has a relatively short half-life. Drinking 1 or 2 cups of coffee in the morning will not interfere with nighttime sleep for most people.
3. Moderate amounts of caffeine do not increase risk for osteoporosis. High levels (more than 700 mg/day) do not increase risk for bone loss if adequate amounts of calcium are consumed. (The addition of 2 tbsp of milk in a cup of coffee can offset calcium loss.) However, older adults may be more sensitive to the effects of caffeine on calcium metabolism and, to be cautious, postmenopausal women should limit caffeine intake to less than 300 mg per day.
4. Low amounts of caffeine (less than 200 mg caffeine/day) have not been found to interfere with the ability to get pregnant or cause miscarriages, birth defects, premature birth, or low birth rate. One cup of coffee (containing approximately 200 mg caffeine) is considered safe during pregnancy.
5. Caffeine is not dehydrating. Caffeine acts as a mild diuretic, but fluid in caffeinated beverages offsets the effect of fluid loss and does not cause dehydration.
6. Caffeine has been linked to a number of harmful health effects in children, including effects on the developing neurologic and cardiovascular systems. The position of the American Academy of Pediatrics (AAP) is that "stimulant-containing energy drinks have no place in the diets of children and adolescents."[2] The AAP recommends that children avoid caffeine-containing beverages, including carbonated beverages, and that adolescents limit caffeine to less than 100 mg caffeine daily.[3] Health Canada has issued the following maximum levels of intake: 4 to 6 year olds, 45 mg/day; 7 to 9 year olds, 62.5 mg/day; 10 to 12 year olds, 85 mg; adolescents 13 and older, no more than 2.5 mg/kg; healthy adults, 400 mg; pregnant or breastfeeding women, 300 mg.[4] Popular drinks (carbonated beverages, energy drinks, and sweetened teas) put children at higher risk for obesity due to the empty calories and dental caries because of their low pH.
7. Caffeine has no effect in helping people under the influence of alcohol to sober up. Reaction time and judgment are still impaired.

Caffeine has some health benefits: improved alertness, concentration, and energy, slower decline in cognitive ability, possible improvement in immune function, and relief from allergic reactions. The International Agency for Research on Cancer (IARC), part of the World Health Organization, found no evidence of coffee drinking causing human cancer, and it helps to reduce the risk of several forms of human cancer. Coffee consumption may reduce the risk of liver diseases, diabetes mellitus, and high blood pressure.[5–7] Evidence indicates that it is not harmful and may be beneficial in helping prevent CVD, congestive heart failure, heart arrhythmias, and stroke.[8–11] A growing body of research suggests that moderate coffee drinkers are less likely to have Parkinson and Alzheimer disease, dementia, and may contribute to longevity.[12–14] However, coffee has not been shown to prevent these conditions, and whether the health benefits are causal or associative findings is unknown. Scientists are unsure which element in coffee and tea contribute to these health benefits, but they agree it is not the caffeine.

Energy drinks and soft drinks may contain sugar and/or caffeine. In general, soft drinks contain less caffeine than energy drinks per ounce. Caffeine content of many beverages, candies, over-the-counter medications, and energy drinks are listed in Table 12.3.

References

1. Fulgoni VL, Keast DR, Lieberman HR. Trends in intake and sources of caffeine in the diets of US adults: 2001–2010. *Am J Clin Nutr.* 2015;101(5): 1081–1087.
2. Branum AM, Rossen LM, Schoendorf KC. Trends in caffeine intake among US children and adolescents. *Pediatrics.* 2014;133(3):386–393.
3. American Academy of Pediatrics. Kids should not consume energy drinks, and rarely need sports drinks, says AAP. May 30, 2011. https://www.aap.org/en-us/about-the-aap/aap-press-room/pages/Kids-Should-Not-Consume-Energy-Drinks,-and-Rarely-Need-Sports-Drinks,-Says-AAP.aspx. Accessed January 6, 2017.
4. Health Canada reminds Canadians to manage their caffeine consumption. June 11, 2013. http://222.healthycanadians.gc.ca/recall-alert-rappel-avis/hc-sc/2013/34021a-eng.php. Accessed January 6, 2017.
5. Santos RM, Lima DR. Coffee consumption, obesity and type 2 diabetes: a mini-review. *Eur J Nutr.* 2016;55(4):1345–1358.
6. Saab S, Mallam D, Cox GA 2nd, et al. Impact of coffee on liver diseases: a systematic review. *Liver Int.* 2014;34(4):495–504.
7. Furman D, Chang J, Lartigue L, et al. Expression of specific inflammasome gene modules stratifies older individuals into two extreme clinical and immunological states. *Nat Med.* 2017;23:174–184.
8. Lee J, Lee JE, Kim Y. Relationship between coffee consumption and stroke risk in Korean population: the Health Examinees (HEXA) Study. *Nutr J.* 2017;16(1):7.
9. Grosso G, Micek A, Godos J, et al. Coffee consumption and risk of all-cause, cardiovascular, and cancer mortality in smokers and non-smokers: a dose–response meta-analysis. *Eur J Epidemiol.* 2016;31(12):1191–1205.
10. Larsson SC. Coffee, tea, and cocoa and risk of stroke. *Stroke.* 2014;45(1):309–314.
11. Cheng M, Hu Z, Lu X, et al. Caffeine intake and atrial fibrillation incidence: dose response meta-analysis of prospective cohort studies. *Can J Cardiol.* 2014;30(4):448–454.
12. Loftfield E, Freedman ND, Graubard BI, et al. Association of coffee consumption with overall and cause-specific mortality in a large US prospective cohort study. *Am J Epidemiol.* 2015;182(12):1010–1022.
13. Ding M, Satija A, Bhupathiraju SN, et al. Association of coffee consumption with total and cause-specific mortality in 3 large prospective cohorts. *Circulation.* 2015;132(24):2305–2315.
14. Carman AJ, Dacks PA, Lane RF, et al. Current evidence for the use of coffee and caffeine to prevent age-related cognitive decline and Alzheimer's disease. *J Nutr Health Aging.* 2014;18(4):383–392.

Adapted from Ratini M. Caffeine myths and facts. 2017 WebMD, LLC. April 30, 2017. Accessed October 19, 2017. www.webmd.com/diet/caffeine-myths-and-facts#3.

TABLE 12.3 Caffeine Content of Beverages and Other Products*

Beverage or Product	Portion or Size	Caffeine Content (mg)
Coffee		
Coffee, brewed, single-serve	8 oz	75–150
Latte or mocha	8 oz	63–175
Espresso, restaurant-style	1 oz	47–75
Coffee, instant		27–173
Coffee, decaffeinated, brewed or instant	8 oz	2–12
Espresso, decaffeinated	1 oz	0–15
Tea		
Green tea, brewed	8 oz	24–45
Black tea, brewed	8 oz	14–70
Iced tea, instant	8 oz	11–47
Tea, bottled, ready-to-drink	8 oz	5–40
Black tea, brewed, decaffeinated	8 oz	0–12
Soft Drinks		
Mountain Dew, regular and diet	12 oz	42–55
Dr. Pepper, regular and diet	12 oz	36–42
Pepsi	12 oz	32–39
Diet Pepsi	12 oz	27–39
Diet Coke	12 oz	23–47
Coca-Cola	12 oz	23–35
Barq's Root Beer	12 oz	16–18
A&W Root Beer; 7-Up; Sierra Mist, regular and diet; Sprite, regular and diet	12 oz	0
Energy Drinks		
5-Hour Energy	2 oz	200–207
Rockstar, regular or sugar free	8 oz	79–80
Red Bull, regular or sugar free	8.4 oz	75–80
Amp, regular or sugar free	8 oz	71–74
Full Throttle, regular or sugar free	8 oz	70–100
Over-the-Counter Medications		
NoDoz Max Strength	1 tablet	200
Excedrin Extra Strength	1 tablet	65

*Data adapted from Mayo Clinic Staff. Caffeine content for coffee, tea, soda, and more. http://www.mayoclinic.org/healthy-lifestyle/nutrition-and-healthy-eating/in-depth/caffeine/art-20049372. Accessed January 6, 2017.

laxatives. The FDA has granted permission for unauthorized health claims for some teas and requested that some manufacturers remove health claims on their labels.

Soft Drinks

Sugar-sweetened beverages constitute 47% of added sugar intake, with soft drinks being the highest contributor (see Fig. 12.4).[5] In 2012, the Center for Disease Control and Prevention's Behavioral Risk Factor Surveillance System found that 17% of respondents reported consuming regular sugar-sweetened beverages at least once daily.[6] A typical 20-oz soft drink contains 15 to 18 tsp of sugar or approximately 240 calories. In 2015, per capita consumption of carbonated soft drinks, including diet soft drinks, was at its lowest level since 1985.[7] The declining soft drink consumption is being replaced with liquids such as bottled water, sports drinks, and teas.

Approximately half of the increase in energy intake occurring over the past 20 years is attributed to sweetened beverages. Most people are unaware of how many calories are in their beverages, but these calories may be a contributor to the alarming increase in obesity and other chronic conditions. In a voluntary effort to control obesity and decrease added sugars in diets, the beverage industry is working to cut calories and sugar from beverages. Lower calories and smaller-size beverage portions are being marketed to determine acceptability.[8]

Energy Drinks

Energy drinks were introduced in the United States in 1997. Sales of energy drinks and shots have more than doubled in the past 5 years; they are especially appealing to teenagers and young adults, especially young men. Sales in the United States increased to almost $12.5 billion in 2012 and are predicted to be $21.5 billion in 2017.[9] Energy drinks are marketed as an **ergogenic** (enhance physical performance, stamina, or recovery) to delay fatigue and increase alertness. They promise to make a person feel more awake and boost attention span.

Energy drinks contain ingredients acting as stimulants, such as caffeine, **guarana** (a seed containing four times as much caffeine as coffee beans), and **taurine** (an amino acid with antioxidant properties). Guarana is one of the stimulants in the National Collegiate Athletic Association's (NCAA) 2016 banned drugs list. Although marketed to delay fatigue and increase alertness, research on these beverages supporting this claim is scant and results are equivocal.[10] Scientific evidence does not support the use of these supplements for performance enhancement.[11] Energy shots (approximately 2 oz) contain the same stimulants as energy drinks but are more concentrated. Decaffeinated energy drinks have eliminated caffeine but are packed with B vitamins and **quercetin** (bioflavonoid reported to energize muscles). Energy drinks containing "natural" ingredients, such as ginkgo or guarana, are considered a dietary supplement rather than a food or medication by the FDA. Contrary to what commercial advertisements would lead one to believe, vitamins only help the body use energy from foods; extra B vitamins do not provide additional energy bursts. These vitamins and amino acids are present in larger quantities than found naturally occurring in foods and plants; their combined effect combined with caffeine may be enhanced. Almost all Americans get adequate amounts of B vitamins in their diets, yet marketers would lead people to believe that a megadose of B vitamin will energize. Energy drinks usually contain 140 cal per 8-oz serving from carbohydrates. These beverages may include some nutrients but lack principal nutrients deficient in Americans' diets. Protein in energy drinks has not been shown to improve athletic performance, but protein enhances muscle recovery when ingested promptly after exercise.

Several energy drinks have been linked to unexpected deaths in apparently healthy adults and children, leading to closer scrutiny and regulation by the FDA.[12] Energy drinks have contributed to increases in emergency department visits resulting from excessive caffeine intake, especially when these drinks are combined with alcohol.[13] Many in the medical community are concerned about potential negative problems associated with stimulants in beverages and lack of disclosure about the amount of stimulants in the product, especially when consumed by children.[14] Energy drinks may increase risk for caffeine overdose in caffeine abstainers as well as in habitual consumers of caffeinated coffee, soft drinks, and tea.

The amount of caffeine in a product is not required on labels because it is not a nutrient.

Sports Drinks

Recent emphasis on Americans increasing their physical activity appears to have sparked an interest in supplemental products by sports enthusiasts and people who are attempting to maintain their health. The availability of sports nutrition products is ubiquitous.

Sports drinks and energy drinks are significantly different products, but the terms are confusing and used interchangeably by many consumers. Sports drinks (e.g., Gatorade and Powerade), popular among children and sports enthusiasts, are designed to restore fluid balance, to replace fluid and electrolytes lost in sweat during physical activity, and, ultimately, to optimize athletic performance. Sports drinks often contain carbohydrates (a source of calories), minerals (e.g., calcium and magnesium), electrolytes (e.g., sodium and potassium), and sometimes vitamins or other nutrients, such as protein and/or amino acids. Adulteration and contamination of some sports supplements have led the FDA and some consumers to question the safety of these products. There is no advantage to consuming vitamins and/or the minerals calcium and magnesium in sports drinks; these are readily available in a well-balanced diet.

Most sports products are designed for highly trained endurance athletes who exercise at high intensity for long periods. This type of athlete can benefit from a sports beverage that contains carbohydrates and electrolytes, and sometimes protein. Sports nutrition products are sometimes recommended to recreational athletes who have very different reasons for exercising and therefore different nutritional needs than endurance athletes.

For most people engaged in routine physical activity, sports drinks offer little to no advantage over plain water. Sports drinks can be helpful for young athletes engaged in prolonged (>1 hour) vigorous physical activities; they are probably unnecessary during school physical education or in the school lunchroom. Sports drinks containing 6% to 8% carbohydrate are recommended when exercise is longer than 1 hour. These drinks can easily meet carbohydrate and fluid needs as well as sodium and potassium lost in sweat.

Scientific studies do not support claims of improved performance and recovery for many sports drinks and protein shakes, making it is virtually impossible for the public to make informed choices about the benefits and harms of advertised sports products.

Dental Erosion

Most sports and energy drinks have a pH in the acidic range (pH 3–4), which is associated with enamel demineralization. The increase in use of sports and energy drinks by children and adolescents causes irreversible damage to teeth because high acidity levels (citric acid) in drinks erode tooth enamel. Damage to tooth enamel is evident after just 5 days of exposure to sports or energy drinks. Energy drinks cause twice as much damage to teeth as sports drinks. Calcium added to sports drinks lessens the erosive potential to teeth. Beverages with a low pH but containing high levels of fluoride promote some remineralization while beverages without fluoride roughen enamel surfaces. Hot coffee also causes some dental erosion.[15] Research suggests that enamel erosion with various beverages occurs in the following order (from greatest to least): energy drinks, sports drinks, regular soda, and diet soda.

DENTAL CONSIDERATIONS

- Individuals who do not ordinarily consume caffeine are not encouraged to change this habit.
- Small to moderate amounts of caffeine are not a concern for most individuals, but excessive consumption can cause insomnia, headaches, irritability, and nervousness.
- If caffeine is added to a food product, it must be included in the ingredients food label. However, the amount does not have to be disclosed.

NUTRITIONAL DIRECTIONS

- With regard to hydration and fluid intake, water is the gold standard. Water should be served with most meals. Starting the day by drinking 2 glasses of water is a great way to begin the day well hydrated.
- Milk and milk-based beverages (including chocolate milk) can be more effective than traditional sports drinks for rehydration following physical activity.[16]
- The *Dietary Guidelines* suggest choosing beverages with no added sugars (such as water), reducing portion sizes of sugar-sweetened beverages and choosing those beverages less often, and selecting beverages low in added sugars or with high-intensity sweeteners (saccharin, aspartame, acesulfame K, and sucralose).
- Habitual intake of caffeinated beverages (coffee, tea, soft drinks, and other caffeinated beverages) contributes to the daily total water intake similar to that contributed by noncaffeinated beverages. The health benefits for drinking coffee and tea clearly outweigh the risks of not drinking adequate fluids.
- Drinking coffee and tea cannot substitute for an overall healthy lifestyle and eating patterns. The quality of food habits is always the sum of its parts.
- Be aware of caffeine consumption from all sources.
- Energy drinks can potentially be dangerous for individuals under 18, women who are pregnant, have a caffeine sensitivity or do not consume caffeine regularly or are taking certain medications such as Adderall (for attention deficit disorder).
- Beverages are important to satisfy nutritional and hydration needs and fluid preferences.
- Energy drinks containing caffeine are inappropriate for children and athletic activities.
- The FDA, Health Canada, and the European Union have recommended limiting caffeine intake to 400 mg per day (4 to 5 cups of coffee), except for pregnant women, who should limit caffeine intake to 200 to 300 mg.
- Increase fluid intake and salivary production by chewing sugarless gum, preferably gum containing xylitol.
- High-protein diets, such as diets in which fruit and vegetable intake is minimal, require larger fluid requirements to eliminate higher levels of urinary waste products.
- Drink fluids during exercise to replace fluid loss through perspiration. (Loss of 1 lb of body weight during exercise means at least 2 cups of water have been lost.) In most cases, water is the most appropriate choice.
- To make wise beverage choices, read labels on bottled waters to see what ingredients they contain.
- Most tap water is safe and economical.
- Beverages with no or few calories should take precedence over consumption of beverages with more calories.
- Make water more exciting by adding slices of lemon, lime, cucumber, or watermelon, or add a splash of 100% juice to plain sparkling water.
- When selecting a sugar-sweetened beverage, choose a smaller size (6–8 oz).

Hyper States and Hypo States

Regulation of fluid intake and excretion by the kidneys usually maintain fluid balance in the body despite a wide range of intake. Imbalances may occur, however. **Fluid volume excess (FVE)** is the relatively equal gain of water and sodium in relation to their losses; **fluid volume deficit (FVD)** results from relatively equal losses of sodium and water.

Fluid Volume Excess

FVE mainly occurs in ECF compartments secondary to an increase in total body sodium content (Fig. 12.5C). Because water follows sodium, an excess leads to an increase in total body water. Excess fluid moves into interstitial compartments, located between cells and in body cavities such as joints, pleura, and the gastrointestinal tract, causing edema.

Congestive heart failure, chronic renal failure, chronic liver disease, and high levels of steroids may predispose an individual to FVE because of sodium retention. Conditions causing a loss of protein and reduced serum albumin levels (e.g., malnutrition and renal diseases) may contribute to FVE resulting from osmotic forces ordinarily exhibited by proteins and albumin. Common manifestations of FVE include rapid weight gain, puffy eyelids, distended neck veins, and elevated blood pressure. **Peripheral edema** is commonly observed in the legs and feet. Treatment involves correction of underlying problems or therapy for the specific disease; fluid or sodium may be restricted (or both) or diuretics prescribed.

Fluid Volume Deficit

In FVD (see Fig. 12.5A), the sodium-to-water ratio remains relatively equal; ADH and aldosterone secretions are not activated. Prolonged inadequate fluid intake can result in FVD. However, FVD is usually associated with excessive loss of fluids from the gastrointestinal tract (vomiting, diarrhea, or drainage tubes), urinary tract (diuretics, polyuria, or excessive urination), or skin (profuse sweating). Medications such as diuretics and laxatives may also increase risk of dehydration and heat-related illness in hot weather. Fever increases the need for electrolytes, increases fluid losses in dehumidified air, and causes excessive sweating.

Dehydration temporarily leads to weight loss but, more important, adversely influences cognitive function and motor control (see Fig. 12.3). Decreased food and fluid intake can result from illness, dementia, anorexia, nausea, or fatigue. Other less obvious reasons are an inability to (a) obtain water, such as with impaired movement; (b) activate the thirst mechanism, as in **hypodipsia** (diminished thirst); or (c) swallow, as in neuromuscular problems or unconsciousness. Excessive fluid losses occasionally occur with prolonged exercise.

Common characteristics of FVD include weight loss, confusion and fatigue, sunken eyes, hypotension, and orthostatic hypotension. Classic signs are dry tongue with **longitudinal fissures** (slits or wrinkles that extend lengthwise on the tongue; Fig. 12.6), xerostomia, shrinkage of oral mucous membranes, decreased skin turgor, dry skin, and decreased urinary output. A diminished salivary flow is associated with inadequate fluid intake. Treatment involves replacing lost fluid. If FVD is mild, oral fluids are likely to be sufficient; intravenous solutions are needed with significant FVD.

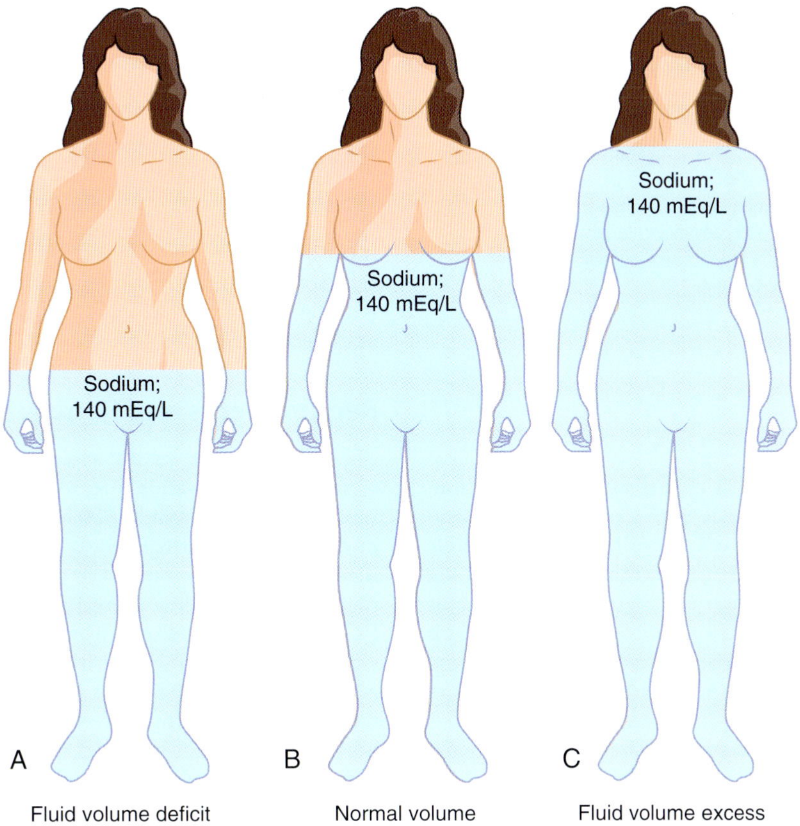

• **Figure 12.5** Fluid-volume disturbances. Compared with normal body fluids (B), in FVD (A), equal percentages of water and sodium losses occur, producing an isotonic depletion. In FVE (C), water and sodium are retained, producing an isotonic expansion. (Adapted from Davis JR, Sherer K. *Applied Nutrition and Diet Therapy for Nurses*. 2nd ed. Philadelphia, PA: Saunders Elsevier; 1994.)

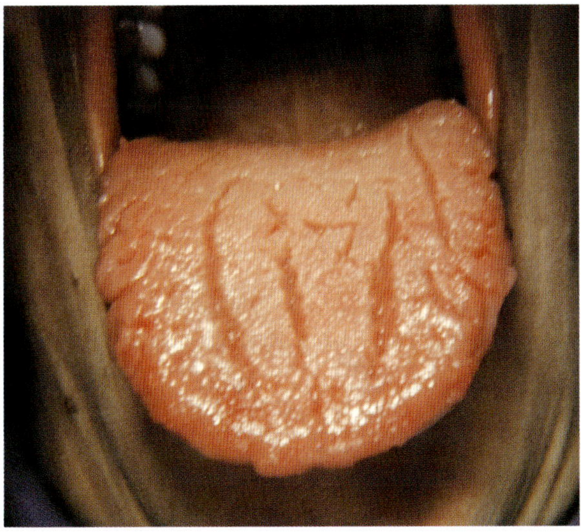

• **Figure 12.6** Fissured tongue. (Reproduced with permission from Ibsen OAC, Phelan JA. *Oral Pathology for the Dental Hygienist*. 6th ed. St. Louis, MO: Saunders Elsevier; 2014.)

DENTAL CONSIDERATIONS

- To help with conversion of total water intake: 1 L = 33.8 fluid oz and 1 cup = 8 fluid oz.
- Direct measurement of the total amount of body water is impossible. Evaluation of physical signs of fluid deficit or excess is vital to diagnosis and treatment.
- Assess patients for puffy eyelids or distended neck veins; inquire about recent unintentional weight changes, check blood pressure, and refer to a health care provider if necessary. A rapid weight loss or gain of 3% or greater of total body weight is significant.
- Observe for dry tongue with longitudinal fissures, xerostomia, or shrinkage of oral mucous membranes; adequacy of salivary flow; decreased skin turgor; and dry skin. Inquire about frequency and amount of urine output and fluid intake.
- Salivary flow measurements may be indicated for patients who present with FVD.
- Several physiologic and social factors prevalent in older patients place them at risk for dehydration (see Chapter 15). In addition, this population may drink less fluid because of dementia, immobility, or fear of incontinence.
- The oral mucosa is especially sensitive to the body's fluid volume; increases and decreases in body fluid affect the fit of a denture. FVD generates a loose-fitting prosthesis, whereas FVE may create a tight-fitting prosthesis. Patients may present with ulcerations in each situation and find the prosthesis uncomfortable to wear.

NUTRITIONAL DIRECTIONS

- Rapid weight changes generally indicate loss or gain of water rather than fatty tissue; a loss or gain of 480 mL (2 cups) of fluid is equivalent to a loss or gain of 1 lb.
- Monitor infants and children closely; their larger surface area-to-body mass ratio places them at risk for FVD.
- Pale yellow or almost colorless urine indicates adequate hydration. Dark-yellow urine with a strong odor, advancing to painful urination, and (eventually) cessation of urine output are progressive signs of inadequate water intake and dehydration.

Electrolytes

Electrolytes are compounds or ions that dissociate in solution; they are also known as **cations** if they have a positive charge and **anions** if they have a negative charge. Cations in the body include sodium, potassium, calcium, and magnesium; anions include chloride, bicarbonate, and phosphate. The body's hydration status depends on an electrolyte balance of equal concentrations of cations to anions. Because the electrolyte concentration in plasma is so low, it is expressed as milliequivalents per liter (mEq/L). Electrolytes are important in water balance and acid–base (pH) balance.

Electrolyte distribution is different in ICF and ECF compartments. The principal cation in plasma and interstitial fluid is sodium; the principal anion is chloride. The principal cation in ICF is potassium; the principal anion is phosphate. The major difference between intravascular fluid and interstitial fluid is the large amount of protein in the former. Because sodium and potassium are the major cations, these are discussed in more detail.

Sodium

Physiologic Roles

The important physiologic roles of sodium include (a) maintaining normal ECF concentration by affecting the concentration, excretion, and absorption of potassium and chloride, and water distribution; (b) regulating acid–base balance; and (c) facilitating impulse transmission in nerve and muscle fibers. Sodium is present in calcified structures; its function in bones and teeth is unclear. It is also present in saliva. Sodium concentration in saliva determines one's recognition of salt in food.

Requirements and Regulation

Because sodium is readily available in foods, no RDA has been established. The National Academy of Medicine estimates a safe minimum intake might be 500 mg per day. This amount is increased in the face of abnormal losses. Sodium regulation involves several mechanisms. To keep the ECF concentration normal, the sodium–potassium pump is constantly moving sodium from the cell to ECF. Aldosterone released by the adrenal cortex results in sodium reabsorption or excretion by the kidneys depending on the body's need (Fig. 12.7). The kidneys can adjust sodium excretion to match sodium intake despite large variations in intake. If serum sodium is high, aldosterone is inhibited, and sodium is excreted; the opposite is true for depressed serum sodium levels.

For most adults, the AI for sodium is 1500 mg per day; the *Dietary Guidelines* recommendation is consistent with the UL, 2300 mg per day (Table 12.4). This AI does not apply to highly active individuals, such as endurance athletes, who lose large amounts of sodium through sweat.

TABLE 12.4 National Academy of Medicine Recommendations for Sodium and Chloride

	AI[a] FOR SODIUM		UL[b] FOR SODIUM		AI FOR CHLORIDE		UL FOR CHLORIDE	
Life Stage	Male (g/day)	Female (g/day)	Male (g/day)	Female (g/day)	Male (g/day)	Female (g/day)	Male (g/day)	Female (g/day)
0–6 months	–	0.12	ND[c]	ND[c]	0.18	0.18	ND[c]	ND[c]
7–12 months	0.37	0.37	ND[c]	ND[c]	0.57	0.57	ND[c]	ND[c]
1–3 years	1	1	1.5	1.5	1.5	1.5	2.3	2.3
4–8 years	1.2	1.2	1.9	1.9	1.9	1.9	2.9	2.9
9–13 years	1.5	1.5	2.2	2.2	2.3	2.3	3.4	3.4
14–50 years	1.5	1.5	2.3	2.3	2.3	2.3	3.6	3.6
51–70 years	1.3	1.3	2.3	2.3	2	2	2.3	2.3
> 70 years	1.2	1.2	2.3	2.3	1.8	1.8	2.3	2.3
Pregnancy								
14–50 years		1.5		2.3		2.3		3.6
Lactation								
14–50 years		1.5		2.3		2.3		3.6

[a]AI (Adequate Intake) *The AI is not equivalent to a Recommended Dietary Allowance.*
[b]UL (Tolerable Upper Intake Level).
[c]ND (Not Determinable).
Data from Institute of Medicine (IOM), Food and Nutrition Board: *Dietary Reference Intakes for Water, Potassium, Sodium, Chloride, Chloride, and Sulfate.* Washington, DC: National Academies Press; 2005.

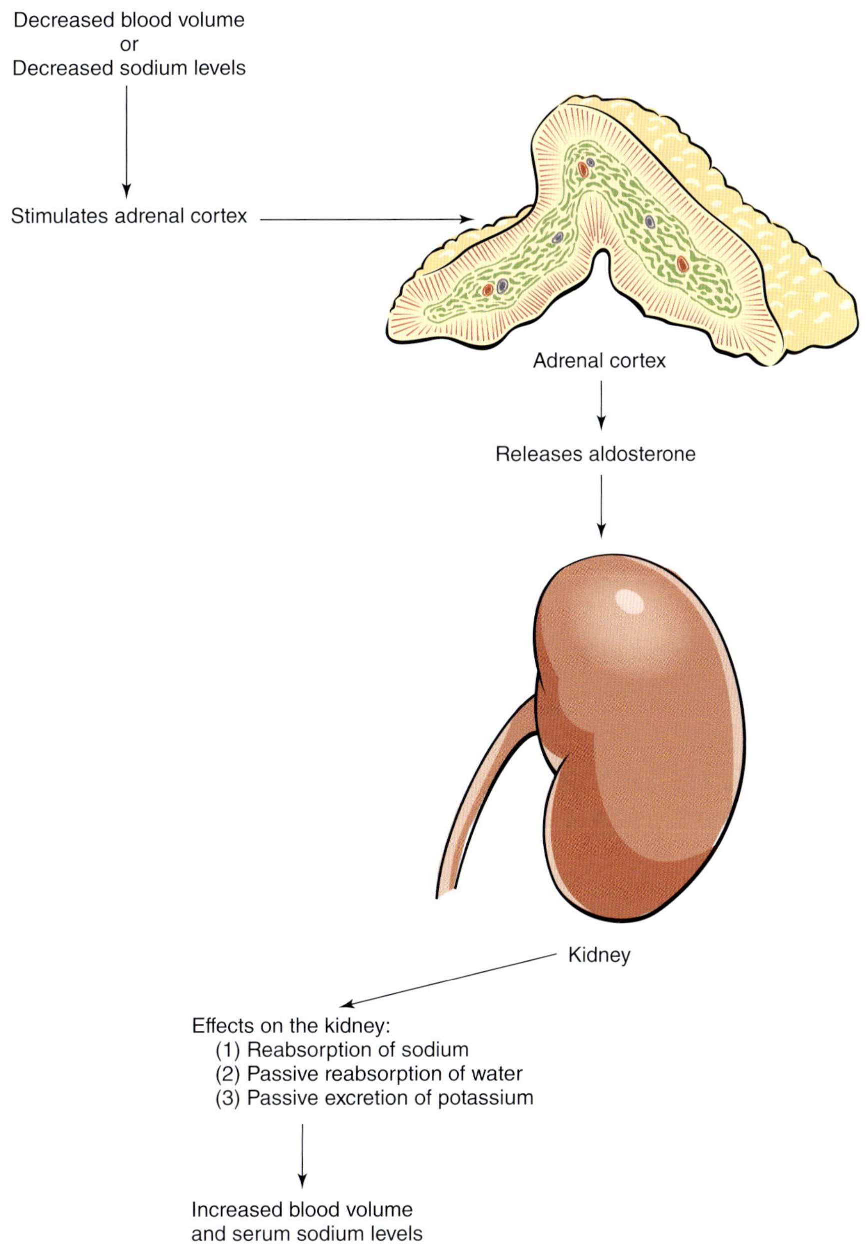

• **Figure 12.7** Effects of aldosterone on sodium levels. (Adapted from Davis JR, Sherer K. *Applied Nutrition and Diet Therapy for Nurses*. 2nd ed. Philadelphia, PA: Saunders Elsevier; 1994.)

Average daily consumption of salt is 3400 mg, considerably above the 2300 mg per day *Dietary Guidelines* recommendation. Adults with hypertension and prehypertension would benefit from reducing sodium intake to 1500 mg per day. Approximately 90% of adults exceed the recommendation of consuming more than 2300 mg of sodium per day. Approximately one-third of Americans have hypertension; daily sodium intake increased among people with hypertension by more than 14% from 1999 to 2012.[17] In comparison with sodium intakes in 1988 to 1994, average intake in 2009 to 2012 has not changed significantly. The World Health Organization recommends a maximum daily intake of 2000 mg for adults.[18]

Scientific studies irrefutably agree that reducing salt intake reduces blood pressure in individuals with hypertension. However, numerous well-designed studies and even systematic reviews of studies indicate conflicting outcomes as to whether or not lower sodium intake will prevent blood pressure–related cardiovascular events. While there is scientific uncertainty that reducing sodium intake for individuals with normal blood pressure will be beneficial for all, the current public health recommendation in many countries is to reduce salt intake by about half. Many randomized controlled trials and evidence-based medicine do not support benefits of reducing sodium to 2300 mg per day by normotensive individuals.[19-23]

Sources

Approximately 10% of the sodium consumed comes from natural content of foods and fluids regularly ingested. Sodium is a natural constituent of most foods (Table 12.5) and all food groups (except for minimal amounts from fruits); thus, lowering intake requires careful choices from all food groups. Animal foods such as meat, saltwater fish, eggs, dairy products, and some vegetables (beets, carrots, celery, spinach, and other dark green leafy vegetables) contain measurable amounts of sodium. Bread and rolls are the number

TABLE 12.5 Where's the Sodium?

Food Groups	Sodium (mg)
Whole and Other Grains and Grain Products[a]	
Cooked cereal, rice, pasta, unsalted, ½ cup	0–5
Ready-to-eat cereal, 1 cup	0–360
Bread, 1 slice	110–175
Vegetables	
Fresh or frozen, cooked without salt, ½ cup	1–70
Canned or frozen with sauce, ½ cup	140–460
Tomato juice, canned, ½ cup	330
Fruit	
Fresh, frozen, canned, ½ cup	0–5
Low-Fat or Fat-Free Milk or Milk Products	
Milk, 1 cup	107
Yogurt, 1 cup	175
Natural cheeses, 1½ oz	110–450
Processed cheeses, 2 oz	600
Nuts, Seeds, and Legumes	
Peanuts, salted, ⅓ cup	120
Peanuts, unsalted, ⅓ cup	0–5
Beans, cooked from dried or frozen, without salt, ½ cup	0–5
Beans, canned, ½ cup	400
Lean Meats, Fish, and Poultry	
Fresh meat, fish, poultry, 3 oz	30–90
Tuna canned, water pack, no salt added, 3 oz	35–45
Tuna canned, water pack, 3 oz	230–350
Ham, lean, roasted, 3 oz	1,020

[a]Whole grains are recommended for most grain servings.
From U.S. Department of Health and Human Services, National Institutes of Health. *Your Guide to Lowering Your Blood Pressure with Dash.* NIH Publication No. 06-4082. Revised April 2006. http://www.nhlbi.nih.gov/health/public/heart/hbp/dash/new_dash.pdf. Accessed January 6, 2017.

one source of sodium in the American diet. The large quantity of bread products consumed accounts for more than twice as much sodium as snack foods such as potato chips and pretzels.[24]

Most consumers believe regular salt contains more sodium than sea salt, which has been marketed as containing "natural" nutrients and more minerals than table salt. Trace elements in sea salt are minuscule and meaningless, with no known health benefits. Far more relevant is the fact that, unlike table salt, sea salt is not fortified with iodine, which is important for thyroid health, especially during pregnancy.

Approximately 75% to 80% of the sodium consumed is added to processed foods and foods prepared in restaurants and fast food establishments (Fig. 12.8). Processed, cured, canned, pickled, convenience, and fast foods, as well as condiments, are significant sources of sodium (Box 12.2). "Hidden" sources include softened

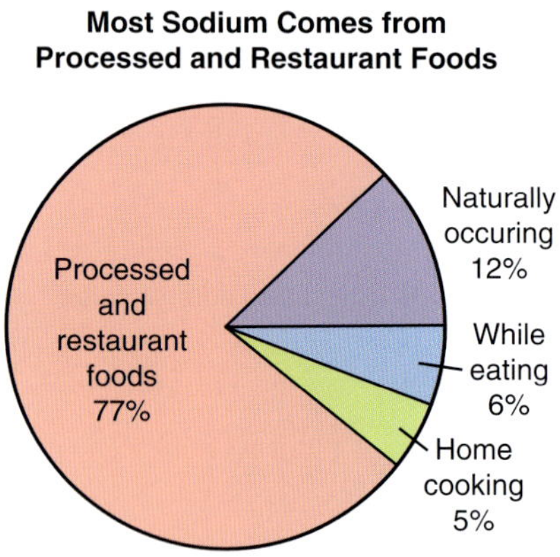

• Figure 12.8 Most of the sodium that Americans eat comes from packaged, processed, store-bought, and restaurant foods. Only a small amount comes from salt added during cooking or at the table. In fact, most Americans already get more daily sodium than recommended before using a salt shaker. Increasing access to lower-sodium food options and giving the power of choice to the consumer could help prevent millions of cases of high blood pressure and save billions of health care dollars. (From Centers for Disease Control and Prevention (CDC). Salt—Sodium and food sources. Last updated February 29, 2016. https://www.cdc.gov/salt/food.htm. Accessed January 7, 2017.)

• BOX 12.2 Implementing the *Dietary Guidelines* for Americans for Sodium Intake (2400 mg)

- Avoid foods with concentrated sources of sodium and do not add salt to foods.
- Avoid adding salt to food at the table or in recipes. Flavor foods with herbs, spices, wine, lemon, lime, or vinegar (see Table 12.6 for additional ideas).
- Salt substitutes can contain sodium, potassium, and other minerals. Salt substitutes should not be used unless approved by a health care provider or RDN.
- Sodium is found naturally in most foods. Animal products such as meat, fish, poultry, milk, and eggs are naturally higher in sodium than fruits and vegetables.
- Restaurant meals should be selected carefully because of their high sodium content.
- Limit the following high-sodium processed foods:
  Meats: Smoked, cured, salted, or canned meats, fish, or poultry, including bacon, cold cuts, ham, frankfurters, and sausages; sardines, anchovies, and marinated herring; pickled meats or pickled eggs
  Dairy products: Processed cheese, blue cheese, buttermilk
  Vegetables: Sauerkraut, pickled vegetables prepared in brine, commercially frozen vegetable mixes with sauces
  Breads and cereals: Breads, rolls, and crackers with salted tops
  Soups: Canned soups, dried soup mixes, broth, bouillon (except salt-free)
  Fats: Salad dressings containing bacon bits, salt pork, dips made with instant soup mixes or processed cheese
  Beverages: Commercially softened water, cocoa mixes, club soda, sports drinks, tomato or vegetable juice
  Miscellaneous: Casserole and pasta mixes; salted chips, popcorn, and nuts; olives; commercial stuffing; gravy mixes; seasoning salts (garlic, celery, onion), light salt, monosodium glutamate (MSG); meat tenderizer; catsup, prepared mustard, prepared horseradish, soy sauce
- Read food labels. Compare the sodium content of products.
- Use reduced sodium or no-salt-added products. Read the ingredient list on food labels to identify and avoid sources of sodium additives such as salt, sodium chloride (NaCl), sodium caseinate, MSG, trisodium phosphate, sodium ascorbate, and sodium bicarbonate.
- Foods making nutrient claims must meet certain labeling guides (see Chapter 1, Box 1.4.

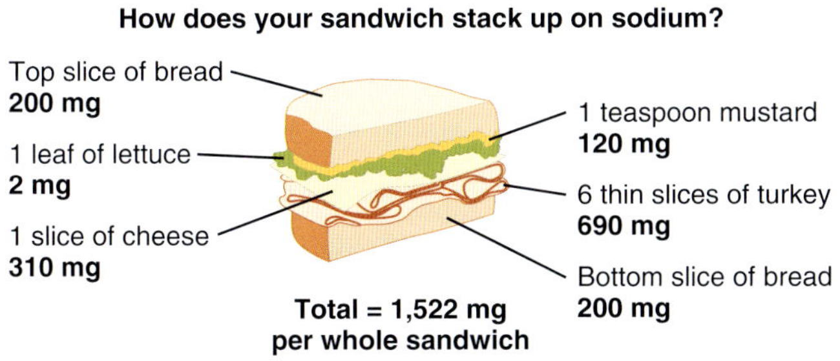

• **Figure 12.9** How does your sandwich stack up on sodium? Total = 1,522 mg per whole sandwich. (From Centers for Disease Control and Prevention (CDC). Sodium and Food Sources, Top 10 Sources of Sodium. Last updated, February 29, 2016. https://www.cdc.gov/salt/sources.htm. Accessed January 7, 2017.)

and bottled water, baking powder, baking soda, dentifrices (including toothpastes containing baking soda or sodium fluoride), antibiotics, chewing tobacco, and over-the-counter medications (e.g., antacids, cough medicines, and laxatives). Many foods such as bread and salsa do not taste salty. As shown in Fig. 12.9, a sandwich, a staple in the American diet, may provide over 1500 mg sodium (more than 60% of the recommended *Dietary Guidelines* amount). Sodium can be replaced in foods with spices, as noted in Table 12.6, to enhance taste appeal. Recommendations for implementing the *Dietary Guideline* to reduce sodium intake are provided in Box 12.2.

Because people have acquired a taste for high levels of salt in their food, food products with less sodium are not as palatable; thus, these products are not competitive with higher-sodium products on the market. The flavor of a food is the major determinant of food choices, overriding other factors, such as healthy choices. Reducing sodium added to foods by food manufacturers and restaurants is fundamental to lowering sodium intake to levels consistent with the *Dietary Guidelines*. The U.S. government and numerous other governments are working with food manufacturers to reduce sodium content of products. The goal is to slowly, and without loss of consumers' acceptance, achieve safer levels of sodium that are consistent with public health recommendations. Between 2000 and 2014, sodium content decreased significantly for packaged foods overall and top food sources of sodium. Despite this reduction, 98% of households purchase foods with sodium density exceeding optimal levels.[25] Reformulation by the food industry is the most cost-effective strategy for salt reduction.

TABLE 12.6 Herbs and Spices to Complement Foods

Food	Herbs/Spices
Beef	Onion, bay, chives, cloves, cumin, garlic, pepper, marjoram, rosemary, thyme, ginger, tumeric
Bread	Caraway, marjoram, oregano, poppy seed, rosemary, thyme
Carrots	Cinnamon, cloves, nutmeg, marjoram, sage
Cheese	Basil, chives, curry, dill, fennel, garlic, marjoram, oregano, parsley, sage, thyme
Fish	Dill, curry powder, paprika, fennel, tarragon, garlic, parsley, thyme
Fruit	Cinnamon, coriander, cloves, ginger, mint
Green beans	Dill, oregano, tarragon, thyme
Lamb	Garlic, marjoram, oregano, rosemary, thyme
Other vegetables	Basil, chives, dill, tarragon, marjoram, mint, parsley, pepper, thyme, tumeric
Pork	Onion, coriander, cumin, garlic, ginger, hot pepper, pepper, sage, thyme, ginger
Potatoes, rutabaga	Dill, garlic, paprika, parsley, sage, tumeric
Poultry	Garlic, ginger, oregano, rosemary, sage, tarragon
Salads	Basil, chives, French tarragon, garlic, parsley, arugula, sorrel (best if fresh or added to salad dressing, or use herbs and vinegars for extra flavor), tumeric
Soups	Bay, tarragon, marjoram, parsley, rosemary, tumeric
Winter squash/ sweet potatoes	Cloves, nutmeg, cinnamon, ginger

Hyper States and Hypo States

Serum sodium concentration is an index of water deficit or excess, not an index of total sodium levels in the body. Sodium levels in the blood are significantly higher than potassium levels because sodium is the major cation in intravascular fluid. **Hypernatremia** (elevated serum sodium level) and **hyponatremia** (low serum sodium level) are usually a result of hormonal imbalances or increased fluid loss or retention. "True" hypernatremia or hyponatremia, or imbalances caused by too much or too little sodium intake, rarely occurs in adults. If renal and hormonal mechanisms for sodium retention and excretion function efficiently, and water intake is adequate, the amount of dietary sodium causes little change in total body sodium. Sodium fluctuations do affect plasma volume.

Because water and sodium are closely related, a change in one causes a change in the other. Hypernatremia can be associated with FVD or FVE. A very high sodium intake can be toxic, especially if intake is insufficient.

Water deprivation (as occurs in unconscious, debilitated individuals or infants), insensible water loss (as a result of exposure to dry heat, sweating, or hyperventilation), and watery diarrhea lead to a loss of water in excess of sodium. Infants are more prone to watery diarrhea, whereas older patients are susceptible to water deprivation. If polyuria is not balanced with increased water intake, hypernatremia may occur.

Symptoms of hypernatremia are a result of fluid moving from the ICF to the ECF in an attempt to equalize sodium and water balance. This movement of fluid causes atrophy of tissue cells. Cells in the central nervous system shrink, producing hallucinations, disorientation, lethargy, and possibly coma. Other signs are extreme thirst; dry, "sticky" tongue and oral mucous membranes; fever; and convulsions. A sticky tongue can be identified by slowly rolling a tongue depressor over the lateral side of the tongue; tacky filiform papillae stick to the tongue depressor and rise up.

Hyponatremia, a potentially life-threatning condition, may develop when sodium losses exceed water losses, or when fluids are retained, leading to a greater concentration of water than sodium. The resulting changes in sodium–water movement to rebalance equilibrium leads to cellular edema. Problems are especially evident in the cranium, where there is no room for expansion. Sodium deficiency may lead to a decrease in salivary flow or a decrease in sodium concentration of saliva. Water intoxication or hyponatremia can occur when individuals drink too much water (several liters a day). The blood sodium level decreases to a dangerously low level, causing headaches, blurred vision, cramps, swelling of the brain, coma, and possibly death.

Heat exhaustion in unacclimated individuals may result in a sodium deficit. Hyponatremia also may occur in individuals who drink excessive quantities of water as part of a psychiatric disorder or when excessive amounts of diuretics are given. Excessive vomiting and diarrhea, especially in infants, can also lead to a sodium deficit.

Early symptoms of hyponatremia are fatigue, nausea, headache, and abdominal cramps. Other symptoms—headache, confusion, lethargy, and coma—are the result of cellular edema. Even though there is cellular edema, peripheral edema is not present. This is because water is primarily retained within cells rather than in the interstitial compartment. Chronic hyponatremia is usually well tolerated. It may or may not be treated, depending on the precipitating cause and severity.

DENTAL CONSIDERATIONS

- The salt recognition threshold is determined by sodium concentration of saliva (i.e., the lower the level of sodium in saliva, the easier it is to detect a small amount of salt in food).
- A low salt recognition threshold is desirable for patients who should curtail salt intake for health reasons; however, in a hyponatremic patient, diminished salt consumption could contribute further to sodium depletion.
- Sodium deficiency may lead to a decreased salivary flow rate.
- Assess patients for signs and symptoms of hypernatremia (thirst; dry, sticky tongue; xerostomia) and hyponatremia.
- Patients with hypertension need to consume 1500 mg or less of sodium daily. Refer patients who would benefit by reducing sodium intake to 1500 mg per day to a registered dietitian nutritionist (RDN).
- Encourage patients to use herbs and spices to flavor food instead of high-sodium seasonings (see Table 12.6).
- High levels of sodium (> 2 g/day) cause calcium loss in the urine.
- Identify "hidden" sources of sodium in a patient's diet. Discuss ways to reduce sodium.
- To convert milligrams of sodium to milliequivalents, divide the number by 23 (the atomic weight of sodium). For example, 1000 mg of sodium ÷ 23 = 43 mEq of sodium.
- Table salt contains sodium and chloride (40% sodium and 60% chloride); 1 tsp of salt is equivalent to 2000 mg of sodium.

NUTRITIONAL DIRECTIONS

- Use the Nutrition Facts label to choose foods lower in sodium.
- Prepare more meals at home, choosing fresh or frozen products.
- Purchase fewer processed and deli meats and sausage; opt for fresh options, such as seafood and lean meats and poultry.
- Be aware of various sources of sodium in your food and beverage choices and maintain as low sodium intake as possible or as recommended by the health care provider.
- Dietary sodium restriction is rarely the cause of hyponatremia. Sodium depletion may occur in combination with excessive losses as a result of vomiting, diarrhea, surgery, or profuse perspiration from exercise or fever.
- Sea salt is not a viable sodium reduction strategy.
- Many low-sodium or reduced-sodium foods are available as alternatives to processed foods made with higher salt content. Compare labels for their sodium content to find the lowest amount.
- The water supply and use of water softeners are "hidden" sources of sodium.

Chloride

Physiologic Roles

Chlorine is the primary anion connected with sodium in ECF to help maintain ECF balance, osmotic equilibrium, and electrolyte balance. Large concentrations of chloride are present in gastric secretions, which are important for protein digestion and creating an acidic environment to inhibit bacterial growth and enhance iron, calcium, and vitamin B_{12} absorption.

Requirements and Regulation

The AI for chloride has been established by the National Academy of Medicine at 2300 mg per day (see Table 12.4). Chloride intake and losses parallel those of sodium.

Sources

Most chloride intake is from salt (sodium chloride). Sources of chloride are the same as those for sodium, including processed foods. Water is an additional source of chloride.

Hyper States and Hypo States

Toxicity from chloride can be caused by excessive intakes of salt, dehydration, renal failure, diarrhea, and Cushing syndrome. Conditions associated with sodium depletion, such as persistent heavy sweating, chronic diarrhea, vomiting, or chronic renal failure, may precipitate hypochloremia and an electrolyte imbalance.

Potassium

Physiologic Roles

Potassium has the following important physiologic roles: (a) maintains cellular (ICF) concentration, (b) directly affects muscle contraction (especially cardiac) and electrical conductivity of the heart, (c) facilitates transmission of nerve impulses, and (d) regulates acid–base balance. Potassium is important to maintain good muscle function for physically active individuals.

Requirements and Regulation

Potassium is one of the nutrients mentioned in the *Dietary Guidelines* with consumption levels below the AI level. Similar to sodium, there is no RDA for potassium. As shown in Table 12.7, the AI for potassium has been established by the National Academy of Medicine at 4700 mg per day for all adults. This is equivalent to approximately 10 servings of fruits and vegetables (but potassium is present in all food groups). No UL has been established for healthy adults.

Fruits and vegetables are among the richest sources of potassium; low potassium intake is the result of low intakes of fruits and vegetables. High intake of meats and other animal proteins cause further depletion of this mineral. Average potassium intake of the U.S. population has declined; the average dietary potassium intake was 2640 mg per day in 2009 to 2010.[26] Low potassium consumption can cause sensitivity to salt, further increasing risk of hypertension.

The sodium–potassium pump regulates potassium levels. Depending on cellular needs, potassium is constantly moving

TABLE 12.7 National Academy of Medicine Recommendations for Potassium

	AI[a]	
Life Stage	**Male (g/day)**	**Female (g/day)**
0–6 months	0.4	0.4
7–12 months	0.7	0.7
1–3 years	3	3
4–8 years	3.8	3.8
9–13 years	4.5	4.5
≥ 14 years	4.7	4.7
Pregnancy		
≥ 18 years		4.7
Lactation		
≥ 18 years		5.1

[a]AI (Adequate Intake): *The AI is not equivalent to a Recommended Dietary Allowance.*
Data from Institute of Medicine (IOM), Food and Nutrition Board. *Dietary Reference Intakes for Water, Potassium, Sodium, Chloride, Chloride, and Sulfate.* Washington, DC: National Academies Press; 2005.

TABLE 12.8 Potassium Content of Selected Foods

Food	Portion	Potassium (mg)
Beet greens, cooked	1 cup	1309
Beans, mature, white, boiled	1 cup	1004
Lima beans, cooked	1 cup	969
Potato, baked with skin	1 med	941
Pinto beans	1 cup	746
Sweet potato with skin, baked	1 med	542
Beets, cooked	1 cup	518
Tomato juice	1 cup	527
Orange juice	1 cup	496
Tomato, fresh, chopped	1 cup	427
Cantaloupe	1 cup	417–427
Banana, small	1 med	422
Milk, 1%	1 cup	366
Sirloin steak, broiled	3 oz	334
Raisins	1 small box	322
Yogurt, nonfat, plain	8 oz	320–345
Spinach, cooked from frozen	1 cup	287
Salmon, canned	3 oz	292
Carrots, baby, raw	10	24
Orange	1 med	238
Gatorade sports beverage	8 oz	31

U.S. Department of Agriculture (USDA), Agricultural Research Service, Nutrient Data Laboratory. *USDA National Nutrient Database for Standard Reference, Release 28.* Version Current: September 2015, slightly revised May 2016. http://nea/bhnrc/ndl. Accessed January 6, 2017.

either into or out of cells. Aldosterone indirectly affects serum potassium levels. If aldosterone is released, sodium is reabsorbed, but potassium is excreted. Subsequently, if aldosterone is inhibited, potassium is retained (see Fig. 12.7). Approximately 92% of ingested potassium is excreted in urine, but a small amount is lost through feces or sweat.

Sources

Potassium is naturally available from foods and fluids regularly consumed (Table 12.8). Dairy, meat, and grains contribute 31% of total dietary potassium. Fruits and vegetables contribute 20% of total dietary potassium. Milk is the number one single food source of potassium for all age groups in the United States. Processed foods usually contain less potassium than fresh products. Potassium supplements and salt substitutes are another source; salt substitutes (potassium chloride [KCl]) often replace sodium with potassium.

Hyper States and Hypo States

Minor deviations in serum potassium levels can be life-threatening. Abnormal levels are referred to as either **hyperkalemia** (elevated serum potassium level) or **hypokalemia** (low serum potassium level).

Hyperkalemia has three causes: (a) impaired renal excretion, (b) increased shift of potassium out of cells, and (c) increased potassium intake. Most potassium is excreted through the kidneys. Acute or chronic renal failure impairs potassium excretion, resulting in potassium being retained. Increased serum potassium levels can result from an increased dietary intake, excessive administration of potassium supplements orally or intravenously, or excessive use of potassium-containing salt substitutes. In catabolic situations (burns, trauma, and so on) large amounts of potassium are released; a healthy kidney will increase potassium excretion.

Hyperkalemia is life-threatening because cardiac arrest may occur. Elevated potassium levels are irritating to the body; symptoms include muscle weakness (the first sign), tingling and numbness in the extremities, diarrhea, bradycardia, abdominal cramps, confusion, and electrocardiographic changes. Treatment for hyperkalemia involves potassium restriction or using medications to remove potassium.

Potential consequences of chronic potassium deficiency are often unrecognized. Problems include hypertension, heart attacks, strokes, kidney stones, and a loss of bone minerals that can lead to osteoporosis. Potassium deficiency can cause individuals to feel tired, weak, and irritable while unable to pinpoint a cause.

Excessive loss or inadequate intake of potassium can result in hypokalemia. Potassium loss occurs through the gastrointestinal and renal tracts and by excessive sweating. Because potassium is contained in gastric and intestinal secretions, vomiting and diarrhea may cause hypokalemia. Some potassium is lost through sweat; excessive perspiration can lead to hypokalemia. Drugs, such as diuretics (e.g., furosemide and hydrochlorothiazide) and antibiotics (e.g., carbenicillin and amphotericin B), are major offenders. Cushing syndrome, hyperaldosteronism, an excess of insulin, hypomagnesemia, alcoholism, and alkalosis also cause hypokalemia.

Potassium is the major ICF cation; deficits can affect every body system. Death from cardiac or respiratory arrest can occur. Clinical manifestations are anorexia, absence of bowel sounds, muscle weakness in the legs, leg cramps, and electrocardiographic changes.

DENTAL CONSIDERATIONS

- Be aware of factors that can cause potassium to increase or decrease. Refer the patient to the health care provider or RDN as needed.

NUTRITIONAL DIRECTIONS

- Choose at least 2 servings of fruit and 3 to 4 servings of vegetables daily in addition to recommended amounts of milk to obtain adequate amounts of potassium.
- Read labels; salt substitutes may be high in potassium. Consult a health care provider or RDN before using potassium-containing salt substitutes.
- If a potassium-wasting diuretic has been prescribed, consume high-potassium foods or take a potassium supplement.
- Medical conditions that can interfere with excretion of potassium include diabetes, renal failure, severe heart events, and adrenal insufficiency.
- Medications that can interfere with excretion of potassium are angiotensin-converting enzyme inhibitors, angiotensin receptor blockers, and potassium-sparing diuretics.

Iron

Physiologic Roles

Every cell contains iron; approximately 4 g (less than 1 tsp) is present in the entire body. Iron is a major component of hemoglobin, which transports oxygen from the lungs to the tissues, including both oral soft and hard tissues. It also catalyzes many oxidative reactions within cells and participates in the final steps of energy metabolism. Other roles include (a) conversion of beta-carotene to vitamin A, (b) synthesis of collagen, (c) formation of purines as part of nucleic acid, (d) removal of lipids from the blood, (e) detoxification of drugs in the liver, and (f) production of antibodies. Lactoferrin, a salivary glycoprotein, is capable of binding iron. It has an antibacterial action by competing with iron-requiring organisms in the mouth for limited amounts of available iron.

Requirements

The National Academy of Medicine recommends 18 mg daily for women 19 to 50 years old, 8 mg per day for women 51 years old and older, and 8 mg per day for men 19 years old and older (Table 12.9). The RDA is higher for premenopausal women than for men or postmenopausal women because of blood loss during menstruation. During the reproductive phase of a woman's life, iron loss is at least twice that of a man or of a postmenopausal woman. Although premenopausal women need more iron, they tend to consume less than men. Iron requirements also increase during times of impaired absorption (e.g., diarrhea), periods of

TABLE 12.9 National Academy of Medicine Recommendations for Iron

Life Stage	EAR (mg/day)[a]		RDA (mg/day)[b]		AI (mg/day)[c]		UL (mg/day)[d]
	Male	Female	Male	Female	Male	Female	
0–6 months					0.27	0.27	40
7–12 months	6.9	6.9	11	11			40
1–3 years	3	3	7	7			40
4–8 years	4.1	4.1	10	10			40
9–13 years	5.9	5.7	8	8			40
14–18 years	7.7	7.9	11	15			45
19–50 years	6	8.1	8	18			45
≥ 51 years	6	5	8	8			45
Pregnancy							
14–18 years		23		27			45
19–50 years		22		27			45
Lactation							
14–18 years		7		10			45
19–50 years		6.5		9			45

[a]EAR (Estimated Average Requirement). [b]RDA (Recommended Dietary Allowance). [c]AI (Adequate Intake). For healthy human milk–fed infants, the AI is the mean intake. *The AI is not equivalent to an RDA.* [d]UL (Tolerable Upper Intake Level). Data from Institute of Medicine (IOM), Food and Nutrition Board. *Dietary Reference Intakes For Vitamin A, Vitamin K, Arsenic, Boron, Chromium, Copper, Iodine, Iron, Manganese, Molybdenum, Nickel, Silicon, Vanadium, and Zinc.* Washington, DC: National Academy Press; 2001.

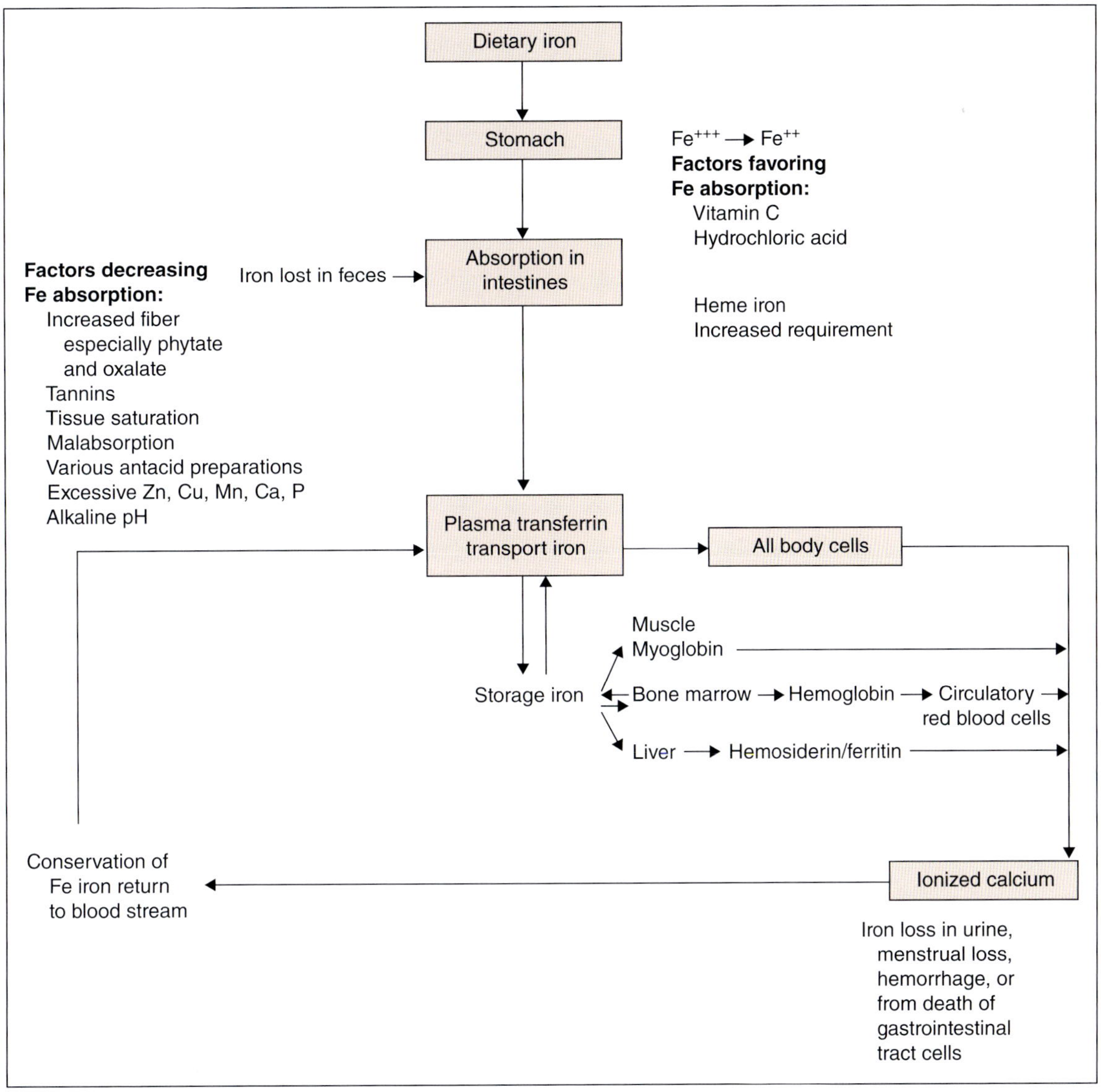

• **Figure 12.10** Iron absorption and use. (Adapted from Davis JR, Sherer K. *Applied Nutrition and Diet Therapy for Nurses*. 2nd ed. Philadelphia, PA: Saunders Elsevier; 1994.)

rapid growth, and heavy physical activity because of the increased need for oxygen transport and energy production.

The RDA is based on the approximation that 10% of dietary iron is absorbed. The demand for iron replenishment is constant because cells are continually being replaced; the life of a red blood cell is 120 days. When a cell dies, iron is recycled, being released and transported to various storage sites to be used again. A UL for iron was established at 45 mg per day for adults.

Absorption and Excretion

Similar to calcium, iron is poorly absorbed. Most of the iron in food is in the oxidized form of ferric iron (Fe^{3+}). Gastric acid in the stomach helps promote iron absorption. By binding to the serum protein **transferrin**, iron is continuously transported through the body because transferrin functions to recycle iron.

Absorption of **heme iron** parallels the body's need; absorption of **nonheme iron** depends on intraluminal and meal composition and physiologic need. Heme iron is provided by meat sources containing hemoglobin from red blood cells and myoglobin from muscle cells. The RDA is based on consumption of at least 75% of iron intake from heme sources. Nonheme iron is present in eggs, milk, and plants. Acidic conditions enhance iron absorption, but calcium and manganese interfere with its absorption. Fig. 12.10 lists factors affecting iron absorption. Combinations of food can enhance iron absorption; a meal of roast beef (rich in iron) with potatoes (rich in vitamin C) increases iron absorption.

Sources

Iron is probably the most difficult mineral to obtain in adequate amounts in the American diet. Although liver is often considered the best source of iron, meats (especially beef), egg yolk, dark-green vegetables, and enriched breads and cereals all contribute significant amounts (Table 12.10). Iron supplements come in two forms; the ferrous form is absorbed better than the ferric form. Even though iron can be considered toxic because of the body's inability to excrete excess amounts, supplementation is a safe and effective treatment for iron-deficiency anemia.

TABLE 12.10 **Iron Content of Selected Foods**

Food	Portion	Iron (mg)
Total cereal, whole-grain	1 cup	24.0[a]
Multi-Wheat Chex cereal	1 cup	19.2[a]
Chicken liver, braised	3 oz	11.6[b]
Raisin Bran	1 cup	10.8[a]
Oatmeal, instant, fortified, prepared with water	1 packet	10.6[a]
Lentils, boiled	1 cup	6.6[a]
Beef liver, pan-fried	3 oz	6.5[b]
Oysters, canned	3 oz	4.6
Lima beans, mature, boiled	1 cup	4.5[a]
Spinach, frozen, boiled	1 cup	4.3[a]
Kidney beans, mature, boiled	1 cup	3.6[a]
Pinto beans, mature, boiled	1 cup	3.6[a]
Beef, chuck roast, lean only, cooked	3 oz	2.1[b]
Beef, ground, 85% lean, broiled	3 oz	2.2[b]
Turkey, dark meat, roasted	3 oz	0.9[b]
Molasses, blackstrap	1 tbsp	0.9[a]
Raisins, seedless	¼ cup	0.8[a]
Turkey, light meat, roasted	3 oz	0.7[b]

[a]Nonheme iron.
[b]Heme iron.
U.S. Department of Agriculture (USDA), Agricultural Research Service, Nutrient Data Laboratory. *USDA National Nutrient Database for Standard Reference*, Release 28. Version Current: September 2015, slightly revised May 2016. http://nea/bhnrc/ndl. Accessed January 6, 2017.

Hyper States and Hypo States

The body cannot easily eliminate excess iron; this may explain why iron absorption rates are poor. The body seldom overcomes its regulation of intestinal absorption. Iron overload may occur, however, if ingestion of iron is extremely elevated. **Hemochromatosis** is an uncommon disorder in which iron is absorbed at a high rate despite elevated iron stores in the liver. Accumulation of iron throughout the body may develop with excessive iron intake or multiple blood transfusions. Inexpensive red wines contain wide variations in iron content (10–350 mg/L) and have been associated with hemochromatosis. Initially, it is difficult to diagnose because of its resemblance to other conditions in which fatigue and general weakness are symptoms. Elevated iron stores have been associated with increased risk of cardiovascular disease (CVD) and liver disease. Iron supplements should not be taken indiscriminately and without a comprehensive laboratory workup.

Inadequate dietary iron intake, chronic and acute inflammatory conditions, and obesity are individually associated with iron-deficiency anemia. As the leading nutrient deficiency in both developed and developing countries, iron-deficiency anemia continues to be a global health issue. Anemia has been linked to unfavorable outcomes of pregnancy resulting in a high risk of preterm delivery and subsequent low birth weight and possibly poor neonatal health. A deficiency can lead to various symptoms, such as microcytic anemia, fatigue, faulty digestion, blue sclerae, pale conjunctivae, and tachycardia. Iron-deficiency anemia may be caused by inadequate dietary intake; accelerated demand or losses; and inadequate absorption secondary to diarrhea, decreased acid secretions, or antacid therapy. Iron deficiency is frequently the result of postnatal feeding practices and has a serious impact on growth and mental and psychomotor development in infants and children.

The most prominent oral signs of iron deficiency include pallor of the lips and oral mucosa, angular cheilitis, atrophy of filiform papillae, and glossitis (see Chapter 17, Figs. 17.1 and 17.2). Oral candidiasis and a reduced resistance to infection are frequently associated with iron deficiency.

DENTAL CONSIDERATIONS

- Despite the prevalence of iron-deficiency anemia, supplements are not recommended without laboratory testing to indicate a deficiency.
- The most prominent sign of iron deficiency in the oral cavity is pallor and swelling of the tongue. The patient also may complain of soreness and a "burning" tongue. Atrophic changes progress from a patchy denudation of papillae to a smooth, reddened tongue.
- Hemochromatosis is common among chronic alcoholics, usually men, who may drink more than 1 L of inexpensive wine daily. Do not recommend iron-rich and iron-fortified foods to patients with this condition.
- Iron-containing supplements are one of the leading causes of poisoning deaths in children younger than 6 years old in the United States. Encourage storing iron supplements in a place inaccessible to children.
- Assess food intake of patients with renal failure, individuals experiencing periods of rapid growth (e.g., pregnant women, infants, toddlers, and teenage girls), and vegans for consumption of iron-rich foods.
- Encourage good oral hygiene practices when iron supplements are taken to prevent extrinsic staining of teeth. The abrasive effect of baking soda can help reduce staining. Liquid forms of iron can be taken through a straw.
- Because older adults may have a reduced production of gastric acid, this can interfere with iron absorption, increasing the risk of an iron deficiency. Referral to the health care provider may be necessary.
- Do not encourage patients with iron-deficiency anemia to consume tea with meals or an iron supplement.

NUTRITIONAL DIRECTIONS

- A food rich in vitamin C with supplements or meals increases iron absorption, especially nonheme iron. Take iron with orange juice, tomato juice, or vitamin C–enriched juices, such as apple juice.
- If nonheme-containing grains or vegetables are consumed with small amounts of heme iron, absorption of the nonheme iron doubles.
- Because iron provided in a vegan diet is the nonheme form, iron absorption is lower than for individuals consuming animal foods. Iron requirements may double for vegans.
- Polyphenols (not caffeine) in tea and coffee decrease iron absorption. No decrease in iron absorption occurs when tea or coffee is drunk 1 hour before or 2 hours after a meal.
- Vitamin A deficiency can cause iron deficiency because vitamin A helps to transport iron from the storage sites.
- Taking iron supplements with food and in divided doses reduces gastrointestinal symptoms associated with these supplements.
- A common treatment of hemochromatosis or iron overload is to donate blood regularly.
- For maximum absorption, avoid taking an iron supplement with a large calcium supplement (> 800 mg).

Zinc

Physiologic Roles

Zinc is a component in more than 300 enzymes that perform a variety of functions affecting cell growth and replication; sexual maturation, fertility, and reproduction; night vision; immune defenses; and taste, smell, and appetite. It is ubiquitous in the body–in organs, tissues, bones, fluids, and cells. Zinc is required for DNA, RNA, and protein synthesis. In this role, zinc is essential for bone growth and mineral metabolism. Zinc-containing enzymes are important in collagen synthesis and bone resorption and remodeling. Zinc might well be recognized as the most important essential trace mineral for humans.

Requirements

The National Academy of Medicine recommends a daily intake of 11 mg for men and 8 mg for women (Table 12.11). The RDA is based on the traditional American diet in which most people consume meat. Vegans absorb less zinc than individuals who consume animal products. The zinc requirement for vegans is definitely higher, and may be twice the RDA for individuals consuming meats. Although some concerns have been expressed about marginal intakes, zinc deficiencies have not been reported in Americans consuming a variety of foods, but it affects one-third of the world's population. The UL for zinc is 40 mg per day.

Absorption and Excretion

Bioavailability of zinc varies widely; approximately 25% to 40% of dietary zinc is absorbed. Absorption depends on several factors, including body size; total dietary zinc; and the presence of other potentially interfering substances, such as calcium, fiber, and phosphate salts. Higher-quality protein improves zinc absorption. Many substances in plant products (e.g., fiber and phytate) interfere with zinc absorption. Zinc is lost in the feces; abnormal losses from diarrhea increase zinc requirements.

Sources

Protein-rich foods are good sources of zinc. Lamb, beef, crustaceans (especially oysters), eggs, and peanuts contain significant amounts of zinc (Table 12.12).

Hyper States and Hypo States

Consumption of high levels of zinc normally causes vomiting and diarrhea, epigastric pain, lethargy, and fatigue, and can result in renal damage, pancreatitis, and death. Supplementation is recommended only under medical supervision.

In developing countries, severe zinc deprivation has been related to excessive consumption of inhibitors, which adversely affect zinc absorption, rather than inadequate zinc intake. Individuals at particular risk of zinc deficiency include those whose zinc requirements are high (e.g., during periods of rapid growth and during pregnancy and lactation), alcoholics, total vegetarians whose

TABLE 12.11 National Academy of Medicine Recommendations for Zinc

	EAR (mg/day)[a]		RDA (mg/day)[b]		AI (mg/day)[c]		
Life Stage	Male	Female	Male	Female	Male	Female	UL (mg/day)[d]
0–6 months					2	2	4
7–12 months	2.5	2.5	3	3			5
1–3 years	2.5	2.5	3	3			7
4–8 years	4	4	5	5			12
9–13 years	7	7	8	8			23
14–18 years	8.5	7.5	11	9			34
≥ 19 years	9.4	6.8	11	8			40
Pregnancy							
14–18 years		10		12			34
19–50 years		9.5		11			40
Lactation							
14–18 years		10.9		13			34
19–50 years		10.4		12			40

[a]EAR (Estimated Average Requirement). [b]RDA (Recommended Dietary Allowance). [c]AI (Adequate Intake). *The AI is not equivalent to an RDA.*
[d]UL (Tolerable Upper Intake Level). Data from Institute of Medicine (IOM), Food and Nutrition Board. *Dietary Reference Intakes for Vitamin A, Vitamin K, Arsenic, Boron, Chromium, Copper, Iodine, Iron, Manganese, Molybdenum, Nickel, Silicon, Vanadium, and Zinc.* Washington, DC: National Academy Press; 2001.

TABLE 12.12 Zinc Content of Selected Foods

Food	Portion	Zinc (mg)
Oysters, canned	3 oz	77.3
Total cereal, whole-grain	1 cup	20.0
Baked beans, canned, plain or vegetarian	1 cup	5.8
Beef, chuck roast, braised	3 oz	56.6
Lobster, cooked	3 oz	6.2
Beef, hamburger, 85% lean, broiled	3 oz	5.4
Crab, canned	3 oz	3.2
Yogurt, plain, low fat	8 oz	2.0
Kidney beans, cooked, mature	1 cup	1.9
Cashews, dry roasted	1 oz	1.6
Cheese, Swiss	1 oz	1.2
Oatmeal, instant, plain prepared with water	1 packet	1.1
Peas, green, frozen, cooked	1 cup	1.1
Milk, low-fat or skim	1 cup	1.0
Almonds, dry roasted	1 oz	0.9
Chicken breast, roasted, skinless	3 oz	0.8
Flounder or sole, cooked	3 oz	0.3

U.S. Department of Agriculture (USDA), Agricultural Research Service, Nutrient Data Laboratory. *USDA National Nutrient Database for Standard Reference, Release 28.* Version Current: September 2015, slightly revised May 2016. http://nea/bhnrc/ndl. Accessed January 6, 2017.

diet consists primarily of cereal protein or is generally nutrient deficient, and individuals with severe malabsorption (ulcerative colitis, chronic diarrhea), sickle cell disease, or other chronic health problems.

Oral manifestations of zinc deficiency include changes in the epithelium of the tongue, such as thickening of epithelium; increased cell numbers; impaired keratinization of epithelial cells; increased susceptibility to periodontal disease; and flattened filiform papillae. Zinc deficiency in humans is associated with loss of taste and smell acuity, poor appetite, and impaired wound healing.

Decreased linear growth and hypogonadism in adolescent boys are principal manifestations of zinc deficiency. Zinc deficiency also results in congenital defects, such as skeletal abnormalities, especially cleft palate and lip. Collagen synthesis defects are seen in zinc-deficient animals. Even when adequate amounts of zinc are provided for an extended time, abnormalities in mineral metabolism are not completely reversed. When zinc deficiency is diagnosed, supplementation is vital.

DENTAL CONSIDERATIONS

- Patients with abnormalities of taste because of zinc deficiency may respond to supplementation, but additional zinc is ineffective in reversing abnormal taste acuity associated with other conditions.
- Supplementation in zinc-depleted patients is beneficial for wound healing, but unnecessary for healthy individuals.
- Zinc supplementation interferes with use of iron and copper and adversely affects high-density lipoprotein levels. Do not advocate indiscriminate use of zinc.
- Zinc lozenges and zinc supplements are marketed to treat cold symptoms. If taken at onset of cold symptoms, zinc may reduce the duration of a cold. However, notable side effects of of treating cold symptoms with zinc are bad taste and nausea. Currently, zinc formulations are not standardized and the best dosage is unknown.

NUTRITIONAL DIRECTIONS

- Small amounts of animal protein can significantly improve bioavailability of zinc from a legume-based meal.
- Fruits and vegetables are low in zinc, whereas peanuts and peanut butter have higher amounts.
- Meat, fish, and poultry are the preferred sources of zinc because of its bioavailability from plant foods.
- If a well-balanced diet is consumed, zinc supplements are rarely needed and may be harmful.
- Large amounts of iron can decrease zinc absorption from food. Iron supplements between meals allow greater zinc absorption from foods.

Iodine

Physiologic Role

Iodine is required for production of thyroxine, a hormone secreted by the thyroid gland. Thyroxine regulates the basal metabolic rate; an altered metabolic rate affects other nutrient requirements. Thyroid hormones are essential for normal brain development.

Requirements

The adult RDA for iodine is 150 μg daily. Because iodine is related to the metabolic rate, needs are increased during periods of accelerated growth, especially during pregnancy and lactation. As shown in Table 12.13, the RDA for pregnant and lactating women is higher because of critical needs of the fetus and infant during this period. The UL for iodine is 1100 μg/day.

Currently, iodine intake of the average American adult is adequate. However, iodine levels for pregnant and breastfeeding women are less than desirable—between 21% and 44% of third-trimester pregnant women in the United States may have inadequate levels of iodine.[27]

Sources

A major source of iodine is seafood (especially cod, shrimp, and tuna) and plants grown near the ocean. Other natural sources include seaweed, dairy products, grain products, and eggs. Breast milk contains iodine and is added to infant formulas. The iodine content of common foods varies significantly, ranging from as little as 10 μg/kg to 1 mg/kg dry weight. The iodine content of meat and animal products depends on iodine content of foods consumed by animals; iodine content of fruits and vegetables is

TABLE 12.13 National Academy of Medicine Recommendations for Iodine

	EAR (μg/day)[a]		RDA (μg/day)[b]		AI (μg/day)[c]		
Life Stage	**Male**	**Female**	**Male**	**Female**	**Male**	**Female**	**UL (μg/day)[d]**
0–6 months					110	110	ND[e]
7–12 months					130	130	ND[e]
1–3 years	65	65	90	90			200
4–8 years	65	65	90	90			300
9–13 years	73	73	120	120			600
14–18 years	95	95	150	150			900
≥19 years	95	95	150	150			1100
Pregnancy							
≥14 years		160		220			900
Lactation							
≥14 years		209		290			900

[a]EAR (Estimated Average Requirement). [b]RDA (Recommended Dietary Allowance). [c]AI (Adequate Intake). For healthy human milk–fed infants, the AI is the mean intake. *The AI is not equivalent to an RDA.* [d]UL (Tolerable Upper Intake Level). [e]ND (not Determinable). Data from Institute of Medicine (IOM), Food and Nutrition Board. *Dietary Reference Intakes for Vitamin A, Vitamin K, Arsenic, Boron, Chromium, Copper, Iodine, Iron, Manganese, Molybdenum, Nickel, Silicon, Vanadium, and Zinc*, Washington, DC: National Academy Press; 2001.

affected by the iodine content of soil and fertilizer and by irrigation practices. The iodine content of foods is not reflected on package labeling and is not available in the U.S. Department of Agriculture's Nutrient Database.

The best safeguard for acquiring an AI is the use of iodized salt. Until the 1920s, endemic iodine deficiency disorders were prevalent in the Great Lakes, Appalachian, and Northwestern regions of the United States. Iodized salt virtually eliminated endemic goiter and remains the mainstay of eradicating iodine deficiency in the United States and worldwide. Iodide in salt will remain stable for many months if kept dry, preferably in a cool place away from light.

Hyper States and Hypo States

Very high levels of iodine may cause adverse effects in some individuals. Excessive amounts of iodine can result in enlargement of the thyroid gland similar to the condition produced by deficiency. Thyroiditis, hypothyroidism, hyperthyroidism, **goiter** (enlargement of the thyroid gland), and sensitivity reactions have occurred in relation to excessive iodine intake through foods, dietary supplements, topical medications, and iodinated contrast media.

Iodine deficiency is a major public health problem internationally, especially for pregnant women. It is considered the most common cause of preventable intellectual impairment. With insufficient iodine intake, the thyroid cannot produce adequate amounts of thyroxine. The pituitary gland continues to secrete thyroid-stimulating hormone, resulting in further hypertrophy and engorgement of the thyroid gland. Goiter is usually associated with iodine deficiency but may be caused by excessively high intake of **goitrogens** contained in cabbage, cauliflower, brussels sprouts, broccoli, kale, raw turnips, and rutabagas.

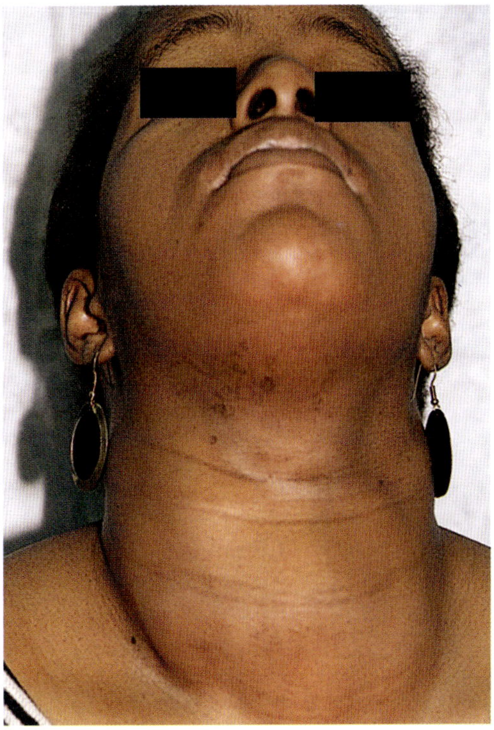

• **Figure 12.11** Goiter resulting from iodine deficiency. (Reproduced with permission from Swartz M. *Textbook of Physical Diagnosis: History and Examination*. 6th ed. St. Louis, MO: Saunders Elsevier; 2009.)

An iodine deficiency may cause profound metabolic and emotional disturbances ranging from a mild deceleration of catabolic functions, with sensitivity to cold, dry skin, and mildly elevated blood lipids, to mild depression of mental functions. Endemic goiter occurs where the soil or water is low in iodine content (Fig. 12.11).

Goiter is the main disorder resulting from low iodine intake. Other iodine-deficiency disorders include stillbirths, spontaneous abortions (i.e., miscarriages), and congenital anomalies; endemic **cretinism**, usually characterized by impaired mental development and deaf mutism related to fetal iodine deficiency; and impaired mental function. Children born to mothers with severe iodine deficiency have delayed eruption of primary and secondary teeth and an enlarged tongue. Craniofacial growth and development are altered; malocclusion is common.

A deficiency of iodine remains the most frequent cause worldwide, second only to starvation, of preventable mental retardation in children. Even a mild deficiency during pregnancy is related to mild and subclinical intellectual and psychomotor deficits in neonates, infants, and children. Severe iodine deficiency usually leads to infertility and increased risks for miscarriage or congenital anomalies. Further information regarding iodine deficiency in pregnancy is provided in Chapter 13.

DENTAL CONSIDERATIONS

- Assess patients for possible thyroid problems.
- Enlargement of the thyroid gland can indicate hyperthyroidism or hypothyroidism. Refer these patients to a health care provider.
- For women who are pregnant or breastfeeding, stress the importance of taking a prenatal multivitamin that contains at least 150 μg iodine.
- Severe hypothyroidism is termed **myxedema**; hyperthyroidism is also called Graves disease.

NUTRITIONAL DIRECTIONS

- Sea salt has been advocated by health food promoters, but its iodine content is negligible. Purchase salt that is fortified with iodine, as indicated on the label.
- Individuals consuming large amounts of seaweed, a rich source of iodine, may be at risk for iodine toxicity.

HEALTH APPLICATION 12

Hypertension

Of the more than 76 million Americans who have hypertension warranting some form of treatment, only 60% to 86% are aware of it, and 46% to 77% of hypertensive individuals receive treatment. Hypertension has been called mankind's most common disease. Approximately 1 in 3 adult Americans has hypertension.[28] Individuals who are of African American descent, are 60 years old and older, have a family history of hypertension, have sedentary lifestyles, consume a large amount of alcohol, have dyslipidemia and/or diabetes, and are obese are affected by it more often. Individuals who are normotensive at age 55 years have a 90% lifetime risk of developing hypertension.

Hypertension is defined as a persistent elevation of systolic blood pressure greater than 120 mm Hg and diastolic pressure greater than 80 mm Hg (Table 12.14). For patients with diabetes and chronic kidney disease, the goal is 130/80 mm Hg or less. For every increment of blood pressure above normal levels, there is a commensurate increase in risk of cardiovascular complications, stroke, peripheral vascular disease, and renal insufficiency. Hypertension may result in myocardial infarction, cerebrovascular accident, or heart failure. Uncontrolled hypertension can affect blood vessels in the eyes, kidneys, and nervous system. Hypertension cannot be cured, but it can be controlled. One of the goals of *Healthy People 2020* is to reduce the proportion of adults with hypertension from 29.9% to 26.9%.[29]

Causes

Several important causal factors for hypertension have been identified, including excess body weight, excess sodium intake, minimal physical activity, inadequate intake of fruits and vegetables and potassium, and excess alcohol intake. Body fat deposited in the trunk increases risk of developing essential hypertension independent of the overall level of obesity, whereas peripherally deposited fat does not. **Essential hypertension** is elevated blood pressure of unknown cause.

A weight loss of 10% is as effective at reducing blood pressure as pharmacologic treatment. Despite the fact that sodium restriction alone does not always result in lower blood pressure for all patients with hypertension, sodium reduction is effective in lowering mean blood pressure in salt-sensitive adults. There is no precise method of identifying salt sensitivity. Sodium restriction enhances effectiveness of diuretics and other pharmacologic treatments. The American Heart Association recommendations are consistent with the *Dietary Guidelines* in reducing sodium (see Box 12.2). Generally, when sodium must be restricted, hidden sources of sodium should be considered: (a) sodium bicarbonate and other sodium products used as leavening agents; (b) sodium benzoate, used as a preservative in margarine and relishes; (c) sodium citrate and monosodium glutamate, used to enhance flavors in gelatin desserts, beverages, and meats; (d) sodium bicarbonate or sodium fluoride added to dentifrices or used in place of commercial dentifrices and mouth rinses; (e) some medications, particularly when taken regularly and frequently, such as antacids, laxatives, and cough medicines; and (f) chewing tobacco.

High potassium intake has a protective effect against hypertension, has no adverse effect on blood lipids, and is associated with a lower risk of stroke.[30] Potassium increases urinary sodium excretion. A customary high sodium-to-low potassium ratio consumed when most foods are highly processed may be detrimental to normal blood pressure regulation. Increasing dietary potassium intake from natural foods is a factor in reducing blood pressure and development of CVD. Compared with carbohydrate, dietary protein intake is associated with a significantly lower blood pressure, regardless of the source of protein (vegetable or animal).[31] Overall, a diet rich in protein, potassium, magnesium, and calcium; whole grains; fruits and vegetables; and low-fat and nonfat foods, and low in sodium can lead to a 15% decrease in CVD and 27% fewer strokes.

Drug therapy is effective, but for prehypertensive and treated hypertensive individuals, lifestyle changes are also important. Dietary modifications reduce blood pressure for many individuals with mild to moderate hypertension. Health-promoting lifestyle modifications are recommended to prevent the progressive increase in blood pressure and CVD. Looking at the overall dietary pattern instead of one single nutrient is the key for assessing risk. Notable for the dental hygienist is that individuals with insufficient masticatory function, poor oral hygiene, and oral inflammation may be associated with hypertension; patients with these problems may need to be referred to a health care professional.[32] The dental hygienist can also help by monitoring blood pressure, and educating and

HEALTH APPLICATION 12

Hypertension—cont'd

supporting the patient's efforts toward reducing blood pressure values. The Dietary Approaches to Stop Hypertension (DASH) approach to prevention and treatment of hypertension combines all the dietary and lifestyle factors related to hypertension.

Dietary Approaches to Stop Hypertension (DASH)

The National High Blood Pressure Education Program recommends the DASH diet for preventing and managing hypertension. As recommended in the *Dietary Guidelines*, the DASH diet is a dietary pattern–based template for all healthy individuals to meet nutrient recommendations. Individuals following the DASH diet achieve at least two-thirds of the DRI recommendations for most nutrients despite reduced energy intake. The pattern offers individualization and flexibility in food choices.

By combining an eating plan with lifestyle modifications designed to prevent and treat hypertension, the DASH approach has been proven to be effective in reducing high blood pressure, and other chronic health conditions. DASH focuses on a dietary pattern instead of decreasing calories or restricting specific nutrients. It emphasizes fruits, vegetables, low-fat or nonfat dairy products, whole grains, nuts, fish, and poultry. In addition, it reduces and limits saturated fat, total fat, cholesterol, red meats, and sweets. The dietary pattern is rich in nutrients commonly lacking in American diets—fiber, potassium, magnesium, and calcium (Box 12.3 and Table 12.15). Participants with hypertension in the DASH study experience greater decreases in blood pressure than nonhypertensive participants. Blood pressure improvement occurred within 2 weeks after beginning the study. Adherence to the DASH diet is associated with reduced risks of strokes and other concerns linked to hypertension.

To reduce sodium intake, patients need to retrain their taste buds by gradually reducing salt intake. For example, patients should remove the salt shaker from the table and refrain from using the salt packet included with fast foods. Eventually, individuals will adjust to a 2300-mg sodium intake and find it acceptable.

Nonpharmacologic treatment of hypertension can work if supported by the health care provider and the patient is strongly motivated. When applied together, sodium restriction (less than 2300 g/day), moderate alcohol intake (less than two servings per day for men and less than one serving per day for women), weight loss for individuals whose body mass index is greater than 25, regular exercise, and following a DASH diet (providing > 3500 mg of potassium) can achieve decreases of approximately 10 to 15 mm Hg systolic blood pressure.

For many years, many health and wellness experts have named the DASH diet as the best for helping with weight loss and improvement of overall health. *US News and World Report* again rated the DASH diet as the best diet in their 2017 rankings for its nutritional completeness, safety, and its role in supporting heart health, describing it as a well-balanced, thorough approach to weight loss.[33] In addition to promoting lower blood pressure and cholesterol, research studies confirm that the DASH diet is beneficial in lowering risk of stroke, heart failure, osteoporosis, several types of cancer, kidney stones, type 2 diabetes, cognitive function and decline, and prevention and delay of disease progression in kidney disease.

TABLE 12.14 2017 High Blood Pressure (BP) Clinical Practice Guideline: Executive Summary *Categories of BP in Adults**

BP Category	Systolic Pressure (mm Hg)		Diastolic Pressure (mm Hg)
Normal	<120	and	<80
Elevated	120–129	and	<80
Hypertension			
Stage 1	130–139	or	80–89
Stage 2	≥140	or	≥90

*Individuals with systolic blood pressure and diastolic blood pressure in 2 categories should be designated to the higher BP category.
BP indicates blood pressure (based on an average of ≥2 carefull readings obtained on ≥2 occasions, as detailed in Section 4).
Data from Whelton PK, Carey RM, Aronow WS, et al. 2017 ACC/AHA/AAPA/ABC/ACPM/AGS/APhA/ASH/ASPC/NMA/PCNA Guideline for the Prevention, Detection, Evaluation, and Management of High Blood Pressure in Adults: A Report of the American College of Cardiology/American Heart Association Task Force on Clinical Practice Guidelines. *J Am Coll Cardiol.* 2017 Nov 7. pii: S0735-1097(17)41519-1. [Epub ahead of print].

• BOX 12.3 Tips for Implementing the DASH Eating Plan

Implement 1 or 2 of the following suggestions each week.

- Make gradual changes, such as adding a vegetable as a snack or choosing fruit as a dessert.
- Reduce total fat intake by using half the butter or margarine currently used. (Be sure it does not contain *trans* fats.)
- Reduce sodium intake by not adding salt at the table (for other suggestions, see Box 12.2).
- Maintain calcium intake using low-fat or nonfat dairy products. For lactose intolerance, try lactase enzyme pills or drops or buy lactose-free milk or milk with lactase enzyme added.
- Increase potassium intake by choosing more fresh fruits and vegetables.
- Consume rich sources of magnesium by selecting one serving of nuts as a snack, or dried beans or peas at mealtime.
- Increase dietary fiber by eating edible skins on fruits and/or vegetables.
- Get recommended amounts of minerals and fiber by choosing at least 1 whole-grain food (cereal or bread) daily.
- Treat meat as a part of the meal, instead of the focal point; try casseroles, pasta, and stir-fry dishes. Have at least one meatless meal a week; reduce the portion size of meat.
- Increase intake of omega-3 fatty acids by choosing at least one serving of fatty fish (e.g., mackerel, herring, salmon) weekly.
- Consume 3 smaller meals a day plus one or more snacks.

TABLE 12.15 The DASH Eating Plan[a]

Food Group	Daily Servings (Except as Noted)	Serving Sizes
Grains and grain products	7–8	1 slice bread 1 cup ready-to-eat cereal[b] ½ cup cooked rice, pasta, or cereal
Vegetables	4–5	1 cup raw leafy vegetable ½ cup cooked vegetable 6 oz vegetable juice
Fruits	4–5	1 medium fruit ¼ cup dried fruit ½ cup fresh, frozen, or canned fruit 6 oz fruit juice
Low-fat or fat-free dairy foods	2–3	8 oz milk 1 cup yogurt 1½ oz cheese
Lean meats, poultry, and fish	2 or fewer	3 oz cooked lean meat, skinless poultry, or fish
Nuts, seeds, and dry beans	4–5/week	⅓ cup or 1½ oz nuts 1 tbsp or ½ oz seeds ½ cup cooked dry beans
Fats and oils[c]	2–3	1 tsp soft margarine 1 tbsp low-fat mayonnaise 2 tbsp light salad dressing 1 tsp vegetable oil
Sweets	5/week	1 tbsp sugar 1 tbsp jelly or jam ½ oz jelly beans 8 oz lemonade

Nutrient Target Totals/2000-cal Dietary Pattern[d]

3932 mg potassium
450 mg magnesium
1131 mg calcium
18% protein
55% carbohydrates
28 g dietary fiber
27% fat
6% saturated fat
150 mg cholesterol

[a]The Dietary Approaches to Stop Hypertension (DASH) Eating Plan is based on 2000 cal per day. The number of daily servings per food group may vary depending on caloric needs. It closely follows the *Dietary Guidelines for Americans* and *MyPlate* with a few modifications.
[b]Serving sizes vary between ½ cup and 1¼ cups. Check the product's nutrition label.
[c]Fat content changes serving counts for fats and oils. For example, 1 tablespoon of regular salad dressing equals 1 serving, 1 tablespoon of low-fat salad dressing equals ½ serving, and 1 tablespoon of fat-free salad dressing equals 0 servings.
[d]Lin PH, Appel LJ, Funk K, et al. The PREMIER intervention helps participants follow the Dietary Approaches to Stop Hypertension dietary pattern and the current Dietary Reference Intakes recommendations. *J Am Diet Assoc.* 2007;107(9):1541–1551.
U.S. Department of Health and Human Services, National Institutes of Health. Your Guide to Lowering Blood Pressure. NIH Publication No. 03-5232, May 2003. http://www.nhlbi.nih.gov/files/docs/public/heart/hbp_low.pdf. Accessed January 6, 2017.

◆ CASE APPLICATION FOR THE DENTAL HYGIENIST

Your patient, an older gentleman, complains of a dry mouth and sore tongue. He states that he has not been thirsty and his intake of fluids has been poor for 4 days. His health care provider recently prescribed a diuretic for hypertension and told him to eliminate salt and add more fruits and vegetables to his diet. He complains that "nothing tastes good."

Nutritional Assessment

- Blood pressure value
- Oral mucous membranes, tongue characteristics
- Fluid likes and dislikes
- Mental changes

Nutritional Diagnosis

Fluid volume deficit related to diuretic and poor fluid or food intake.

Nutritional Goals

Patient will have good skin turgor, moist oral mucous membranes, and increase his intake of liquids and food.

Nutritional Implementation

Intervention: Explain the need for fluid intake.
Rationale: Knowledge and involvement in self-care increase compliance.
Intervention: Encourage the patient to drink his favorite fluids, preferably water, on a regular schedule.
Rationale: The patient is more apt to drink his favorite fluid, and, in doing so, he will replace fluids lost because of the diuretic.
Intervention: Identify methods to increase salivary flow and oral lubrication.
Rationale: The patient's degree of oral comfort will improve and soft tissue will heal.
Intervention: Explain the importance of oral hygiene and how to perform oral self-care procedures.
Rationale: Less saliva allows more food debris to remain on teeth, which may increase caries risk. Because oral mucosa and gingival tissues are more susceptible to trauma, an extra-soft bristle brush may be appropriate for plaque removal, and the patient should be cautioned against aggressive oral hygiene. Other oral physiotherapy aids may be warranted for optimal plaque biofilm removal.
Intervention: Explore challenges the patient will encounter with foods low in salt and discuss ways to enhance flavors of food without using sodium (see Box 12.2 and Tables 12.5 and 12.6). Explain that as his salt intake decreases, salt in the saliva will also decrease so that after about 3 months of moderately low intake, his preferred salt level in foods will decrease and his taste for food will gradually improve.

CASE APPLICATION FOR THE DENTAL HYGIENIST—cont'd

Rationale: Most Americans consume about four to seven times the recommended amount of sodium. Sodium concentration in saliva determines a patient's recognition of salt in food; higher levels of sodium in saliva means higher levels of sodium are needed for it to be detected.

Intervention: Discuss types of dentifrices consistent with the health care provider's order to eliminate salt.

Rationale: Sodium bicarbonate or sodium fluoride is added to some dentifrices and mouth rinses; these would increase his sodium intake, especially if oral hygiene is practiced several times a day and the patient ingests the dentifrice or mouth rinse.

Intervention: Have the patient record his dietary intake for 1 to 3 days. Compare this record with the Dietary Approaches to Stop Hypertension (DASH) diet (see Health Application 12).

Rationale: Suggestions can be tailored to the patient's needs. The patient can set a goal based on the information presented.

Evaluation

Desired outcomes include the patient's adequate consumption of preferred beverages each day, moist oral mucous membranes, and no dental caries.

Student Readiness

1. Define ICF and ECF. What are the principal electrolytes found in each?
2. Record your daily fluid intake. How does this record compare with the required intake? What percentage is water?
3. Fluid is essential for survival. Discuss advantages and disadvantages of water intake versus other fluids, such as milk, soft drinks, tea, and coffee.
4. List five clinical observations indicating FVD. What type of medication is frequently prescribed that affects hydration status?
5. What can cause hypernatremia? Hyponatremia? Why is altering salt intake of patients with these conditions not usually the mode of treatment?
6. What can cause FVD or FVE?
7. What is the general effect of food processing on sodium and potassium content of foods?
8. Explain the physiologic change that occurs when salt intake is decreased and why adding large amounts of salt to foods is unwise. Would you consider salt addictive?
9. Discuss dental hygiene interventions for iron-deficiency anemia. Discuss factors affecting iron absorption.
10. Which two nutrients discussed in this chapter are important for collagen formation?
11. Name the electrolyte(s) or mineral(s) discussed in this chapter associated with the following symptoms:
    - Shrinkage of mucous membranes
    - Thirst
    - Oral pallor
    - Taste abnormalities
    - Lethargy
    - Enlargement of thyroid
    - Poor wound healing
    - Swollen tongue
    - Loss of appetite
12. The *Dietary Guidelines* and the American Heart Association recommend restricting red meat. Their recommendations also include increasing fiber intake from cereal and vegetable sources to help reduce blood lipid levels. Discuss how these two recommendations affect the known deficiency of iron stores in the American population in general. Would you anticipate that long periods of compliance with lower saturated fat intake might necessitate use of iron supplements in affected individuals?
13. Identify guidelines in the DASH diet that would be beneficial to the older adult in the Case Application in this chapter.

CASE STUDY

A 17-year-old boy complains of a dry mouth; difficulty in swallowing food; dry, sticky tongue; and dry skin. The patient reports he has just recovered from the flu with fever, diarrhea, and vomiting. He also informs you he is currently training for an athletic competition and exercises 3 to 4 hours a day. A 24-hour diet recall reveals the patient's fluid intake includes 48 to 72 oz of caffeinated soft drinks without any other beverages and a high protein intake.

1. What other information should you obtain about the patient's dietary intake?
2. Could the patient's oral symptoms be attributed to his current fluid intake?
3. Is salivary analysis indicated for this patient?
4. What suggestions could you make that would decrease his symptoms of xerostomia? List suggestions to increase his fluid intake.
5. What oral self-care practices would you recommend to relieve his oral discomfort and facilitate swallowing?

CASE STUDY

A 15-year-old girl comes into the dental office reporting a history of iron-deficiency anemia. She has clinical symptoms typical of this anemia: glossitis; smooth, shiny, red tongue; and painful cracks at the corners of her mouth. Her health care provider has prescribed ferrous sulfate and zinc to correct this deficiency.

1. When evaluating dietary intake, what are some foods you would need to watch for to assess iron intake?
2. If the patient is having problems with the ferrous sulfate supplement (e.g., constipation or nausea), would it be advisable to resolve the anemia by just increasing dietary iron intake? Why or why not?
3. Why has the health care provider ordered zinc supplements?
4. What should you tell her about iron from plant or animal foods?
5. What can she do to help increase absorption of iron?

References

1. Rosinger A, Herrick K. Daily water intake among US men and women, 2009-2012. NCHS data brief, No. 242. Hyattsville, MD: National Center for Health Statistics, 2016.
2. CBS/AP. Bottled water sales outpace soda for first time in U.S. March 9, 2017. https://www.cbsnews.com/news/bottled-water-sales-outpace-soda-for-the-first-time/.
3. Casazza K, Brown A, Astrup A, et al. Weighing the evidence of common beliefs in obesity research. *Crit Rev Food Sci Nutr.* 2015;55(14):2014–2053.

4. Duarte PM, Reis AF. Coffee consumption has no deleterious effects on periodontal health but its benefits are uncertain. *J Evid Based Dent Pract*. 2015;15(2):77–79.
5. U.S. Department of Health and Human Services and U.S. Department of Agriculture. 2015–2020 Dietary Guidelines for Americans. 8th ed. December 2015. https://health.gov/dietaryguielines/2015/guidelines/. Accessed July 21, 2017.
6. Centers for Disease Control and Prevention. Sugar-sweetened beverage consumption among adults—18 states, 2012. *Morbidity and Mortality Weekly Report (MMWR)*. https://www.cdc.gov/mmwr/preview/mmwrhtml/mm6332a2.htm. Accessed January 3, 2017.
7. Kim S. US soda consumption at its lowest level in 30 years. March 30, 2016. http://abcnews.go.com/Business/us-soda-consumption-lowest-level-30-years/story?id=38036424. Accessed January 3, 2017.
8. FoodIngredientsFirst. US beverage initiative to cut calories targets soda guzzling communities. October 18, 2016. http://www.foodingredientsfirst.com/news/US-Beverage-Initiative-to-Cut-Calories-Targets-Soda-Guzzling-Communities.html. Accessed January 3, 2017.
9. Webb D. The truth about energy drinks. *Today's Dietitian*. 2013;15(10):62–67.
10. Rosenbloom C. Energy drinks, caffeine, and athletes. *Nutr Today*. 2014;49(2):49–54.
11. Mason BC, Lavallee ME. Emerging supplements in sports. *Sports Health*. 2012;4(2):142–146.
12. U.S. Food and Drug Administration. Energy "drinks" and supplements: investigation of adverse event reports. November 16, 2012. Last updated December 16, 2015. http://www.fda.gov/Food/RecallsOutbreaks Emergencies/SafetyAlertsAdvisories/ucm328536.htm. Accessed January 3, 2017.
13. Substance Abuse and Mental Health Services Administration, Center for Behavioral Health Statistics and Quality. The DAWN Report. Update on emergency department visits involving energy drinks: a continuing public health concern. Rockville, MD, January 10, 2013. https://www.samhsa.gov/data/sites/default/files/DAWN126/DAWN126/sr126-energy-drinks-use.pdf. Accessed January 3, 2017.
14. Visram S, Cheetham M, Riby DM, et al. Consumption of energy drinks by children and young people: a rapid review examining evidence of physical effects and consumer attitudes. *BMJ Open*. 2016;6(10):3010380.
15. Jameel RA, Khan SS, Abdul Rahim ZH, et al. Analysis of dental erosion induced by different beverages and validity of equipment for identifying early dental erosion, in vitro study. *J Pak Med Assoc*. 2016;66(7):843–848.
16. Desbrow B, Jansen S, Barrett A, et al. Comparing the rehydration potential of different milk-based drinks to a carbohydrate-electrolyte beverage. *Appl Physiol Nutr Metab*. 2014;39(12):1366–1372.
17. Bansilal S, Fonarow G, Heller S. Americans with high blood pressure still eating too much salt. HealthDay. 2017 Mar 8. https://consumer.healthday.com/vitamins-and-nutrition-information-27/salt-and-sodium-news-591/americans-with-high-blood-pressure-still-eating-too-much-salt-720479.html.
18. World Health Organization. WHO issues new guidance on dietary salt and potassium. http://www.who.int/mediacentre/news/notes/2013/salt_potassium_20130131/en/. Accessed January 7, 2017.
19. Expeimental Biology 2017. Low-sodium diet might not lower blood pressure: findings fro large, 16-year study contradict sodium limits in Dietary Guidelines for Americans. *Science Daily*. 2017;April. www.sciencedaily.com/releases/2017/04/170425124909.htm.
20. Mente A, O'Donnell M, Rangarajan S, et al. Associations of urinary sodium excretion with cardiovascular events in individuals with and without hypertension: a pooled analysis of data from four studies. *Lancet*. 2016;388(100433):465–475.
21. Trinquart L, Johns DM, Galea S. Why do we think we know what we know? A metaknowledge analysis of the salt controversy. *Int J Epidemiol*. 2016;45(1):251–260.
22. O'Brien E. Evidence-based policy for salt reduction is needed. *Lancet*. 2016;388(10043):439–440.
23. Heaney RP. Making sense of the science of sodium. *Nutr Today*. 2016;50(2):63–66.
24. Centers for Disease Control and Prevention (CDC). Top 10 sources of sodium. https://www.cdc.gov/salt/sources.htm. Accessed January 6, 2017.
25. Poti J, Dunford EK, Popkin BM. Sodium reduction in US households' packaged food and beverage purchases, 2000 to 2014. *JAMA Intern Med*. 2017;177(7):986–994.
26. Hoy MK, Goldman JD. Potassium intake of the US population: what we eat in America, NHANES 2009–2010. Food Surveys Research Group Dietary Data Brief No. 10. September 2012. https://www.ars.usda.gov/ARSUserFiles/80400530/pdf/DBrief/10_potassium_intake_0910.pdf. Accessed January 6, 2017.
27. Lumen A, George NI. Estimation of iodine nutrition and thyroid function status in late-gestation pregnant women in the United States: development and application of a population-based pregnancy model. *Toxicol Appl Pharmacol*. 2017;314:24–38.
28. Go AS, Mozaffarian D, Roger VL, et al. on behalf of the American Heart Association Statistics Committee and Stroke Statistics Subcommittee. Heart disease and stroke statistics—2013 update: a report from the American Heart Association. *Circulation*. 2013;127:e6–e245.
29. US Department of Health and Human Services. Progress toward Healthy People 2020 targets and objectives: heart disease and stroke. https://www.healthypeople.gov/2020/topics-objectives/topic/heart-disease-and-stroke/objectives. Accessed January 6, 2017.
30. Whelton SP, Blumenthal RS. Insights on potassium supplementation for the treatment of hypertension from the Canadian Hypertension Education Program Guidelines (CHEP). *Circulation*. 2017;135:3–4.
31. Buendia JR, Bradlee ML, Singer MR, et al. Diets higher in protein predict lower high blood pressure risk in Framingham Offspring Study adults. *Am J Hypertens*. 2015;28(3):372–379.
32. Darnaud C, Thomas F, Pannier B, et al. Oral health and blood pressure: the IPC Cohort. *Am J Hypertens*. 2015;28(10):1257–1261.
33. US News Staff. US News' 38 best diets overall. January 4, 2017. http://health.usnews.com/best-diet. Accessed January 6, 2017.

EVOLVE RESOURCES

Please visit http://evolve.elsevier.com/Stegeman/nutritional for additional practice and study support tools.

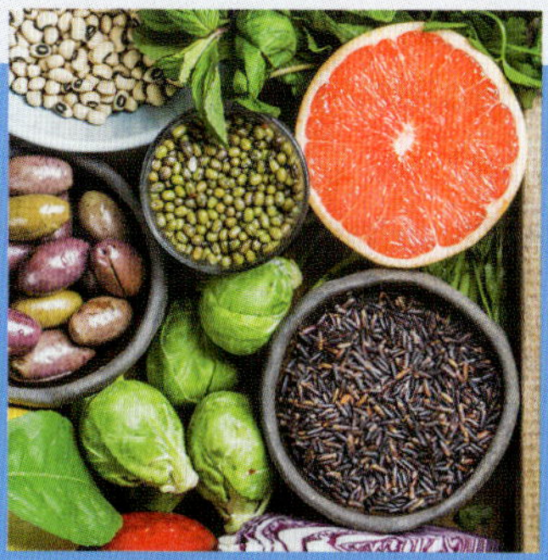

13 Nutritional Requirements Affecting Oral Health in Women

STUDENT LEARNING OUTCOMES

Upon completion of this chapter, the student will be able to achieve the following student learning outcomes:

1. Discuss the following related to factors affecting fetal development:
   - Explain the importance of prenatal weight and weight gain during pregnancy.
   - Advise prenatal patients who have unusual dietary patterns.
   - Discuss why good oral health is important before and during a pregnancy.
   - List foods pregnant women should avoid to decrease risk of foodborne illness.
2. Discuss factors affecting oral development.
3. Discuss nutritional requirements for pregnancy, including:
   - Name nutrients needed in larger amounts by pregnant women and explain why those increases are needed.
   - Identify nutrients frequently consumed in inadequate amounts by pregnant women and suggest ways to improve their intake.
   - Discuss nutrients commonly supplemented during pregnancy.
4. Discuss nutritional requirements for lactation, including:
   - Name nutrients needed in larger amounts by lactating women and explain why those increases are needed.
   - Identify nutrients frequently consumed in inadequate amounts by lactating women and suggest ways to improve their intake.
   - Discuss nutrients commonly supplemented during lactation.
5. List the nutrients affected by oral contraceptive agents (OCAs), as well as the increased risks associated with use of OCAs.
6. Describe the many hormonal changes that occur in a woman's body during menopause, as well as nutritional approaches that can be used to reduce menopausal symptoms.

KEY TERMS

Anencephaly
Atrophic gingivitis
Dysesthesia
Erythropoiesis
Gravidas
Hormone replacement therapy (HRT)
Listeriosis
Low birth weight (LBW)
Menopausal gingivostomatitis
Menopause
Nutritional insult
Perimenopause
Pica
Preeclampsia
Premature
Primigravida
Toxoplasmosis

TEST YOUR NQ

1. **T/F** All efforts should be made to satisfy a pregnant woman's food cravings because cravings reflect an innate need for certain nutrients.
2. **T/F** The fetus is nourished from the mother's nutrient stores.
3. **T/F** After pregnancy, most mothers have at least one carious lesion because calcium was pulled from teeth for the developing fetus.
4. **T/F** A woman should eat twice as much food when she is pregnant because she is eating for two.
5. **T/F** Most women should gain 25 to 35 lb during a pregnancy.
6. **T/F** Vitamin A is the only nutrient warranting global supplementation during pregnancy.
7. **T/F** Virtually all women can produce enough milk to support nutritional needs of the infant.
8. **T/F** Breast milk that is too thin must be nutritionally inadequate.
9. **T/F** If breast milk supply is inadequate, omit a feeding to have more milk available later.
10. **T/F** WIC is a governmental program that provides supplemental foods for women, infants, and children.

Healthy Pregnancy

Although there is no specific definition of a healthy pregnancy, the health of both mother and infant is important. A healthy baby begins with a healthy mother. In addition to continued preservation of the mother's physical health, her emotional and psychological well-being is important. Goals for the infant include being (a) full term (born between the 39th and 41st week of gestation) and (b) mature (weighing more than 6 lb). Infants with a **low birth weight** (**LBW**; weighing less than 5½ lb) or who are **premature** (gestational age less than 37 weeks, especially a gestational age of less than 32 weeks) have more long-term health and developmental problems, oral problems, and increased risk of early mortality. In 2014, approximately 34% of all infant deaths were born at less than 32 weeks gestation. The number of infants born prematurely dropped from 12.7% in 2007 to 9.54% in 2014.[1] Primary factors for a successful pregnancy are nutritional status before conception, appropriate weight gain, and adequate intake of essential nutrients during pregnancy. If the mother's nutritional status is poor, the placenta is unable to perform its function well.

The classic report published in 1970 by the National Academy of Sciences established a basis for increased nutritional requirements during pregnancy.[2] More recent workshops acknowledge that the report principally addressed undernutrition and inadequate weight gain, whereas current concern has shifted to focus on increased body weight of women in their childbearing years who are more likely to have chronic conditions such as hypertension or diabetes mellitus. Many health care providers and women of childbearing age are unaware of these guidelines for weight gain. Gaining either too little or too much weight during pregnancy can lead to poor outcomes of the mother and infant. With the exception of chromosomal issues, fetal health is determined by the mother's diet, exercise, and lifestyle choices. The quality of daily food choices is the most important and most ignored factor determining pregnancy outcomes (Fig. 13.1).

Factors Affecting Fetal Development

Preconceptional Nutritional Status

One of the most important times for "getting healthy" is prior to conception. Preconceptual obesity or underweight not only hampers fertility but also can set the stage for metabolic problems during pregnancy. Ideally, weight adjustments should be achieved before pregnancy begins. Because of the detrimental influence of maternal overweight and obesity on pregnancy outcomes, the Academy of Nutrition and Dietetics (AND) recommends counseling for all women of reproductive age (especially those who are overweight or obese) about maternal and fetal risks, addressing prepregnancy obesity, excessive weight gain, and postpartum weight retention, including benefits of lifestyle changes prior to a pregnancy.[3] Severe dietary restrictions are inappropriate when a woman is trying to conceive even though she is attempting to lose weight in anticipation of the pregnancy. Losing 15 to 20 lb before conception may be enough to avoid some weight-related pregnancy complications (e.g., preeclampsia, preterm birth, gestational diabetes, hypertension, assisted delivery, and large-for-gestational-age infants). **Preeclampsia** is a potentially serious complication of pregnancy involving high blood pressure that often leads to premature delivery.

Approximately half of all pregnancies are unplanned. By the time a woman has her first prenatal visit, fetal development has already progressed beyond a critical period during which a lack of folic acid or certain exposures may have already compromised the health and well-being of the mother and/or fetus. In addition to eating a well-balanced diet, prenatal vitamins are encouraged in anticipation of a pregnancy. Prenatal food choices may have enduring effects on the child's lifelong food preferences and negative metabolic outcomes.[4]

In pregnancies conceived less than 1 year after a previous pregnancy, maternal nutritional reserves may be inadequate, contributing to increased incidence of preterm births and fetal growth retardation. Risk of maternal mortality and morbidity is also higher. Body parts and organs develop rapidly during the first trimester; birth defects are likely to occur if usual dietary patterns are poor or if drugs are used during this critical period. With some nutrients, such as calcium and iron, higher requirements are met by increased maternal absorption, but for others, inadequate maternal intake may deplete the mother's stores (e.g., folic acid), potentially resulting in suboptimal infant stores at birth.

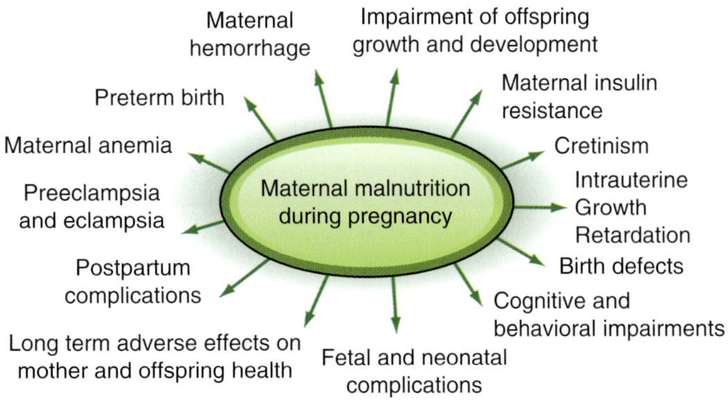

• **Figure 13.1** Major negative effects of maternal malnutrition (both undernutrition and overnutrition) on mother and infant. (Reproduced with permission from Mahan LK, Raymond JL. *Krause's Food and the Nutrition Care Process.* 14th ed. St. Louis, MO: Elsevier; 2016.)

Unusual Dietary Patterns

Pica, or an abnormal consumption of specific food and nonfood substances—such as dirt, clay, baking soda, paint chips, stones, cloth, baby powder, starch (laundry and corn), large quantities of ice/frost, or other inedible items—remains a millennia-old nutritional enigma. Women practicing pica behaviors are usually from lower socioeconomic groups or have less than a high school education; are in poor nutritional health; may be an adolescent having clinical problems; or are affected by behavioral/environmental factors, such as alcohol or substance abuse. Pica is more frequently practiced by African American women living in rural areas with a childhood and family history of pica. Micronutrient deficiencies, especially iron and zinc, may result from these abnormal behaviors. Additionally, pica may contribute to too little or too much weight gain.[5] Pica may result in lead poisoning and, depending on the nonfood item, the substance consumed can cause teeth to wear down quickly.

Personal beliefs about cravings and folklore influencing dietary selections are cultural and regional. Familiarity with local beliefs is beneficial in assessing how these practices affect nutritional status and advising a **gravida** (pregnant woman) about habits potentially detrimental to both her and the fetus. Patients are more receptive to changing their food habits when the dental hygienist provides unbiased guidance about desirable food choices.

Health Care

Availability and use of health care services are related to problems in pregnancy. Inadequate prenatal care leads to problems for both mother and fetus. Prenatal care is important to protect the embryo from effects of chronic health problems later in life.

Age

Maternal age can be a factor in the increased number of LBW infants among gravidas younger than 18 years old. Most adolescent girls do not complete linear growth and achieve gynecologic maturity until age 17 years. Nutritional requirements are quite high to meet growth needs for both adolescent and fetus. Additionally, many adolescents have an inadequate intake of numerous crucial nutrients (see Chapter 14). Approximately one of every three teenage mothers shows signs of significant bone loss after giving birth; greater calcium and vitamin D consumption during pregnancy may protect against bone loss.

Intake of calorie-dense foods and erratic eating may preclude adequate intake of required nutrients. Socioeconomic disadvantages of these young mothers may affect their diet as a result of the amount of food available and their uninformed selections. Ordinarily, caloric intake is more than adequate to meet increased energy requirements.

More women are choosing to become pregnant at an older age. A woman needs to be particularly aware of maintaining her nutritional health if a pregnancy after age 35 years is anticipated. Maternal risks involve chronic conditions, including overweight or obesity, and diabetes and hypertension. These conditions are closely supervised to lessen their impact on the fetus.

Weight Gain

Successful pregnancies depend on ideal preconceptional weight plus appropriate weight gain during gestation. One in four women (25%) are overweight prepregnancy, 20% to 22% are obese.[3] The goal for women who are overweight before pregnancy is to avoid excessive weight gain but to consume adequate calories to allow optimal fetal growth.

Current NAM recommendations take into consideration factors that affect pregnancy before conception and continue through the first year postpartum with regard to health of both infant and mother. These guidelines are based on body mass index (BMI) categories and include a relatively narrow range of recommended gain for obese women (to determine BMI, see page ix). The suggested range of weight gain accommodates differences such as age, race/ethnicity, and other factors that affect pregnancy outcomes. The guidelines are intended to be used along with good clinical judgment and a discussion between the woman and her health care provider about diet and exercise. Women whose prepregnancy weight is within a normal BMI should have a total weight gain of 25 to 35 lb, or 0.8 to 1 lb/week during the second and third trimesters (Table 13.1). More research is needed to determine appropriate weight gain for adolescents. Some women are concerned about gaining too much weight during pregnancy; others, recognizing the need to eat for two, consume excessive amounts of food. Excessive weight gain during pregnancy can increase maternal risk of gestational diabetes, pregnancy-induced high blood pressure, preeclampsia, assisted deliveries, postpartum hemorrhage, and weight retention.[6] Fetal risks include preterm delivery, increased mortality, large-for-gestational age, and congenital anomalies. Physical activity, such as walking briskly for 30 minutes a day, can help avoid adding many pounds during pregnancy. Among **primagravida** (first-time pregnancies) women, 66% experience gestational weight gain exceeding NAM recommendations.[7] Women who gain more than 22 lb during pregnancy are more likely to retain the weight and gain additional weight postpartum. Infants born to mothers who gain more than 50 lb during pregnancy are more likely to be heavier at birth and have a higher BMI later in life, but this may be more related to genes than the gravida's weight.[8] On the other hand, underweight women are at increased risk for spontaneous preterm birth and LBW, which is associated with health problems for the infant.

Oral Health

Only slightly more than half of pregnant women may receive dental care during their pregnancy.[9] Even when an oral problem exists, most women do not see their dentist. If they have not received routine dental care either before or during pregnancy, they are unaware of the importance of oral health care during this period. Even though a gravida may not have overt dental problems, maintaining proper oral hygiene care is important. Oral hygiene practices and dental service utilization are highly related to racial, ethnic, and economic disparities.

TABLE 13.1 Recommendation for Total and Rate of Weight Gain During Pregnancy by Prepregnancy Body Mass Index (BMI)

Prepregnancy BMI	BMI[a] (kg/m^2) (WHO)	Total Weight Gain Range (lb)	Rates of Weight Gain[b] Second and Third Trimester (Mean Range in lb/wks)
Underweight	< 18.5	28–40	1 (1–1.3)
Normal weight	18.5–24.9	25–35	1 (0.8–1)
Overweight	25.0–29.9	15–25	0.6 (0.5–0.7)
Obese (includes all classes)	≥ 30.0	11–20	0.5 (0.4–0.6)

[a]To determine BMI, go to https://www.nhlbi.nih.gov/health/educational/lose_wt/BMI/bmicalc.htm or use this formula: BMI = (weight in pounds/[height in inches × height in inches]) × 703
[b]Calculations assume a 0.5–2 kg (1.1–4.4 lb) weight gain in the first trimester.
Reprinted with permission from Institute of Medicine (IOM) and National Research Council (NRC): Weight Gain during Pregnancy: Reexamining the Guidelines, Washington, DC: National Academies Press: 2009. Web site. http://www.nationalacademies.org/hmd/Reports/2009/Weight-Gain-During-Pregnancy-Reexamining-the-Guidelines.aspx

Attitudes and behaviors about dental care during pregnancy may be influenced by fear of harm to the woman or fetus. Routine dental care (dental prophylaxis and tooth scaling) during pregnancy is not associated with an increased risk of serious medical events, preterm deliveries, spontaneous abortions, or fetal deaths or anomalies.

Hormonal changes (estrogen and progesterone) associated with pregnancy contribute to an increased susceptibility to pregnancy gingivitis and periodontitis. An intensive oral hygiene regimen may decrease gingivitis during pregnancy.[10] Pregnancy gingivitis (Fig. 13.2A) usually becomes evident in the second month of pregnancy. If plaque biofilm is allowed to accumulate and irritate the gingiva, gingivitis occurs and may result in large lumps called "pregnancy tumors" (Fig. 13.2B). Some studies indicate that periodontal disease during pregnancy is possibly a risk factor for adverse pregnancy outcomes such as preeclampsia, premature birth, and/or LBW infant.[11–13] However, treatment of periodontal disease during pregnancy does not appear to improve perinatal outcomes.[14–17] Currently, there is a lack of consensus among experts on the nature of periodontal disease and infant/maternal outcomes, so health care providers and the public may be confused by how to interpret the numerous conflicting reports. The etiology of preterm birth and/or LBW is multifactorial, involving consumption habits and socioeconomic and health factors. Periodontal disease is more prevalent in populations at highest risk of adverse pregnancy outcomes; whether or not periodontal disease increases the risk for adverse pregnancy outcomes, use of dental services for pregnant women needs to be encouraged.

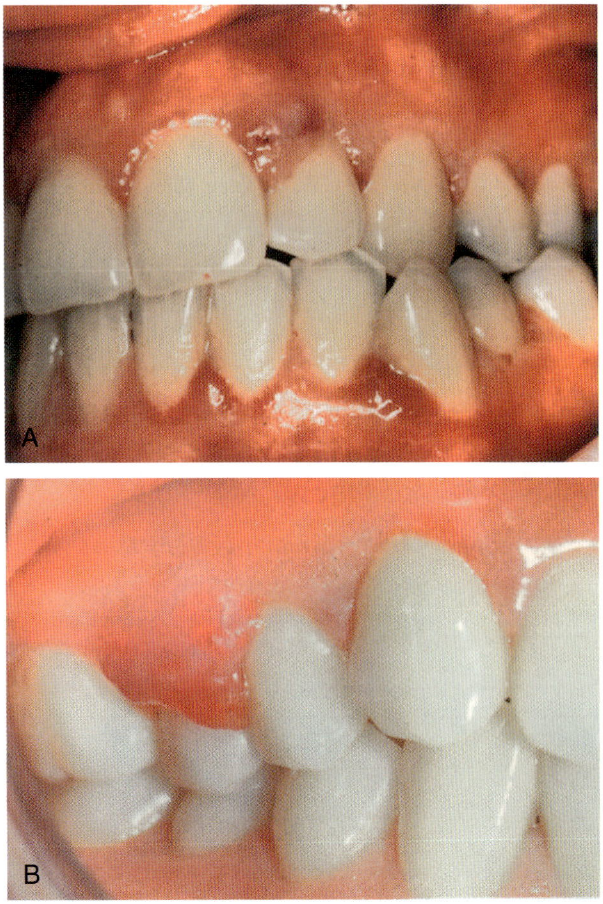

• **Figure 13.2** (A) Pregnancy gingivitis. (B) Pregnancy tumor. (Reproduced with permission from Perry DA, Beemsterboer PL. *Periodontology for the Dental Hygienist*. 4th ed. St. Louis, MO: Saunders; 2014.)

Nausea is common during pregnancy; recurring vomiting increases oral exposure to gastric acid secretions, which may erode tooth enamel. In addition to nausea and vomiting, gastroesophageal reflux disease occurs frequently during pregnancy because of normal physiologic changes that affect the lower esophageal sphincter. Evidence shows a strong association between gastroesophageal reflux disease and dental erosion. Acidity from repeated regurgitation should be treated by rubbing the teeth with a paste of baking soda and water to neutralize oral pH, rinsing after 30 seconds, then brushing and flossing.

Drugs and Medications

Use of tobacco, alcohol, caffeine, some medications, megadoses of nutrients, and illegal drugs can harm the fetus. Caffeine, a stimulant and a diuretic, crosses the placenta. Epidemiologic studies have shown inconsistent conclusions about the effect of caffeine intake during pregnancy on the risk of LBW or preterm birth.[18,19] However, the current recommendation is to eliminate caffeine or limit it to less than 200 mg/day.[20] Brewed coffee, for example, can contain 150 to 500 mg caffeine per 16-oz cup. Considering the popularity of coffee, sodas, and energy drinks, minimizing caffeine intake may be challenging for some pregnant women (see Chapter 12).

Alcohol is a folic acid antagonist and can cross the placenta. For decades, doctors and researchers have known that alcohol intake during pregnancy may cause birth defects, especially fetal alcohol syndrome (discussed in *Health Application 13*). The effects of a small amount of alcohol on the fetus are not well understood. Prenatal exposure to alcohol can harm the fetus and is the leading preventable cause of birth defects and intellectual and neurodevelopmental disabilities. Alcohol-related birth defects and developmental disabilities are completely preventable when women abstain from alcohol. During pregnancy, no amount of alcohol intake is considered safe; all forms of alcohol (beer, wine, liquor) pose similar risks.[21]

Artificial Sweeteners

Nonnutritive sweeteners, while classified as generally safe, have received little attention regarding their safety during pregnancy. The U.S. Food and Drug Administration (FDA) has approved aspartame, acesulfame-K, rebaudioside (Stevia), and sucralose for moderate consumption during pregnancy. Saccharin crosses the placenta; thus, its use is questionable during pregnancy. Pregnant women with the genetic disorder phenylketonuria should not use aspartame throughout their life span.

Food Safety

During pregnancy, women are at high risk for foodborne illness because of physiologic changes that may increase exposure of the gravida and fetus to hazardous substances. Pregnant and breastfeeding women, in particular, should heed food-handling precautions discussed in Chapter 16 in addition to other precautions discussed here.

The U.S. Department of Agriculture advises pregnant women to avoid unpasteurized (raw) milk and cheese and juices; raw or undercooked animal foods such as seafood, meat, poultry, and eggs; and raw sprouts because of high risk of foodborne illness.[22] Certain foodborne illnesses can be especially dangerous; for example, listeriosis can cause miscarriage, premature birth, stillbirth, or acute illness in newborns. **Listeriosis** is a disease usually caused by food contaminated with the bacterium *Listeria monocytogenes,* which principally affects infants and adults with weakened immune systems. These harmful bacteria grow slowly at refrigerated temperatures. The disease caused by *Listeria* can be transmitted to the fetus even if the mother does not show signs of illness. Symptoms include gastrointestinal problems followed by fever and muscle aches. To reduce risk of listeriosis, pregnant women should heat leftovers and ready-to-eat foods (e.g., deli meats, hot dogs, and luncheon meats) until steaming (165°F); and avoid unpasteurized (raw) milk, soft cheeses (Brie, feta, blue-veined, Camembert, and queso blanco, queso fresco) and homemade cheese if prepared with unpasteurized milk; smoked fish and pâtés; meat spreads from a meat counter or refrigerated section of the store; and store-prepared salads such as ham, chicken, egg, tuna, and seafood salads.

Toxoplasmosis, caused by a parasite, is a leading cause of death related to foodborne illness in the United States. The gravida may be symptom free because the immune system prevents the parasite from causing illness, but the infection is passed on to the fetus. In addition to observing safe food handling precautions listed in Box 16.3, gravidas should be especially mindful of cooking meat, poultry, and seafood to safe minimum internal temperatures; washing all cutting boards and knives with hot soapy water after use; avoiding drinking untreated water; washing hands with soap and water after touching soil, sand, cat litter, raw meat, or unwashed vegetables; and wearing gloves when gardening or handling sand, or cleaning cat litter boxes.[23]

Pregnant women are encouraged to consume at least 8 oz (2–3 servings) of cooked seafood weekly (especially salmon, herring, mussels, trout, sardines, and pollock, which are rich in omega-3 fatty acids) but limit total intake of acceptable fish, including shrimp and catfish, to 12 oz/week. Raw fish should be avoided. Mercury can affect the developing nervous system in a fetus or young baby. Therefore, as shown in Fig. 13.3, the FDA and the Environmental Protection Agency have provided advice about best or good choices and fish to avoid while ensuring 2 to 3 servings of fish weekly to prevent ingesting dangerous levels of mercury. State and local health departments have information relevant to fish caught locally or sold in a particular location. If the information is unavailable, pregnant women should limit consumption of fish from local water to 6 oz per week.[24]

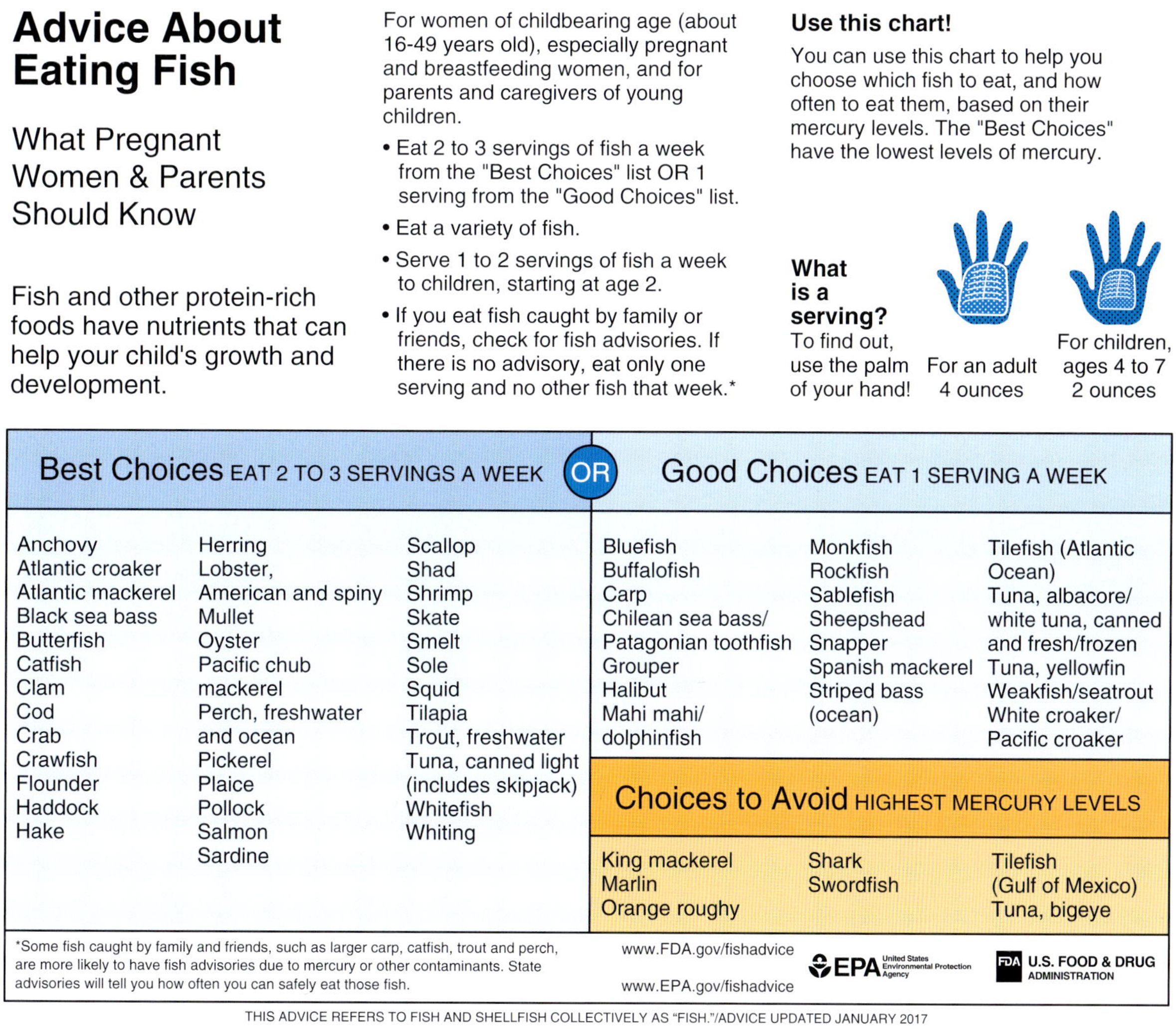
Advice About Eating Fish
What Pregnant Women & Parents Should Know
Fish and other protein-rich foods have nutrients that can help your child's growth and development.
For women of childbearing age (about 16-49 years old), especially pregnant and breastfeeding women, and for parents and caregivers of young children.
• Eat 2 to 3 servings of fish a week from the "Best Choices" list OR 1 serving from the "Good Choices" list.
• Eat a variety of fish.
• Serve 1 to 2 servings of fish a week to children, starting at age 2.
• If you eat fish caught by family or friends, check for fish advisories. If there is no advisory, eat only one serving and no other fish that week.*
Use this chart!
You can use this chart to help you choose which fish to eat, and how often to eat them, based on their mercury levels. The "Best Choices" have the lowest levels of mercury.
What is a serving?
To find out, use the palm of your hand!
For an adult 4 ounces
For children, ages 4 to 7 2 ounces
Best Choices EAT 2 TO 3 SERVINGS A WEEK
OR
Good Choices EAT 1 SERVING A WEEK
Anchovy
Atlantic croaker
Atlantic mackerel
Black sea bass
Butterfish
Catfish
Clam
Cod
Crab
Crawfish
Flounder
Haddock
Hake
Herring
Lobster, American and spiny
Mullet
Oyster
Pacific chub mackerel
Perch, freshwater and ocean
Pickerel
Plaice
Pollock
Salmon
Sardine
Scallop
Shad
Shrimp
Skate
Smelt
Sole
Squid
Tilapia
Trout, freshwater
Tuna, canned light (includes skipjack)
Whitefish
Whiting
Bluefish
Buffalofish
Carp
Chilean sea bass/ Patagonian toothfish
Grouper
Halibut
Mahi mahi/ dolphinfish
Monkfish
Rockfish
Sablefish
Sheepshead
Snapper
Spanish mackerel
Striped bass (ocean)
Tilefish (Atlantic Ocean)
Tuna, albacore/ white tuna, canned and fresh/frozen
Tuna, yellowfin
Weakfish/seatrout
White croaker/ Pacific croaker
Choices to Avoid HIGHEST MERCURY LEVELS
King mackerel
Marlin
Orange roughy
Shark
Swordfish
Tilefish (Gulf of Mexico)
Tuna, bigeye
*Some fish caught by family and friends, such as larger carp, catfish, trout and perch, are more likely to have fish advisories due to mercury or other contaminants. State advisories will tell you how often you can safely eat those fish.
www.FDA.gov/fishadvice
www.EPA.gov/fishadvice
EPA United States Environmental Protection Agency
FDA U.S. FOOD & DRUG ADMINISTRATION
THIS ADVICE REFERS TO FISH AND SHELLFISH COLLECTIVELY AS "FISH."/ADVICE UPDATED JANUARY 2017

• **Figure 13.3** Advice about eating fish. (From U.S. Environmental Protection Agency and U.S. Food and Drug Administration. Updated January 2017. http://www.fda.gov/Food/FoodborneIllnessContaminants/Metals/ucm393070.htm?source=govdelivery&utm_medium=email&utm_source=govdelivery.)

Lead, present in tap water leached from plumbing and in dust from deteriorating lead-based paint, can negatively affect socialization and behaviors. Absorbed lead accumulates; maternal bones can release stored lead into the bloodstream. Regardless of the source, lead is absorbed by fetal brain cells in place of calcium needed for thought processes. This results in lifelong developmental problems, such as reduced attention span, increased impulsive behavior, and lower intelligence.

Other chemicals, or pesticides in the food supply may pass through the placenta. As a prudent measure, encourage pregnant women to wash all produce thoroughly, or purchase organic fruits and vegetables most likely to contain pesticides (Box 16.4).

Factors Affecting Oral Development

In general, potential arrangement of teeth, their eruption time, and pits and fissures on enamel are attributed to heredity. However, availability of nutrients in utero is closely associated with whether teeth achieve their optimum genetic potential.

Critical periods for various stages of tooth development occur at different times. Nutrients supplied by the mother must be available when needed for development of pre-eruptive teeth and soft tissues. All primary teeth and many permanent teeth are at various stages of development at birth.

Tooth development begins by the sixth week of gestation. Calcification of deciduous teeth begins about the fourth month; development of more than 60% of the 52 deciduous and permanent teeth is initiated during gestation (Table 13.2). By the fourth month of pregnancy, the mandible is calcified.

Severe and irreversible damage results if **nutritional insult** (deficiency or excessive amounts of specific nutrients) or infection occurs during critical stages, especially in dentin or enamel formation (Table 13.3). After eruption, the tooth has no mechanism to repair itself. Severe nutrient deficiencies can result in malformations such as cleft palate, cleft lip, and shortened mandible. Less-severe nutrient deficiencies can reduce the size of the tooth, interfere with tooth formation, delay time of tooth eruption, and increase susceptibility of teeth to caries. Most nutrient deficiencies that occur in utero affecting developing teeth increase the child's susceptibility to dental caries. When an infection in a gravida causes a fever, the resultant calcium and phosphorus imbalance disrupts developing fetal tooth structure, which continues until the body regains calcium–phosphorus equilibrium.

TABLE 13.2 Chronology of Development of the Human Dentition

Tooth	Hard Tissue Formation Begins	Amount of Enamel Formed at Birth	Enamel Completed	Eruption	Root Completed
Primary Dentition					
Maxillary					
Central incisor	4 months in utero	Five-sixths	1½ months	7½ months	1½ years
Lateral incisor	4½ months in utero	Two-thirds	2½ months	9 months	2 years
Canine	5 months in utero	One-third	9 months	18 months	3¼ years
First molar	5 months in utero	Cusps united	6 months	14 months	2½ years
Second molar	6 months in utero	Cusp tips still isolated	11 months	24 months	3 years
Mandibular					
Central incisor	4½ months in utero	Three-fifths	1½ months	6 months	1½ years
Lateral incisor	1½ months in utero	Three-fifths	3 months	7 months	1½ years
Canine	5 months in utero	One-third	9 months	16 months	3¼ years
First molar	5 months in utero	Cusps united	5½ months	12 months	2¼ years
Second molar	6 months in utero	Cusp tips still isolated	10 months	20 months	3 years
Permanent Dentition					
Maxillary					
Central incisor	3–4 months	—	4–5 years	7–8 years	10 years
Lateral incisor	10–12 months	—	4–5 years	8–9 years	11 years
Canine	4–5 months	—	6–7 years	11–12 years	13–15 years
First premolar	1½–1¾ years	—	5–6 years	10–11 years	12–13 years
Second premolar	2–2¼ years	—	6–7 years	10–12 years	12–14 years
First molar	At birth	Sometimes a trace	2½–3 years	6–7 years	9–10 years
Second molar	2½–3 years	—	7–8 years	12–13 years	14–16 years

TABLE 13.2 Chronology of Development of the Human Dentition—cont'd

Tooth	Hard Tissue Formation Begins	Amount of Enamel Formed at Birth	Enamel Completed	Eruption	Root Completed
Mandibular					
Central incisor	3–4 months	—	4–5 years	6–7 years	9 years
Lateral incisor	3–4 months	—	4–5 years	7–8 years	10 years
Canine	4–5 months	—	6–7 years	9–10 years	12–14 years
First premolar	1¾–2 years	—	5–6 years	10–12 years	12–13 years
Second premolar	2–2¼ years	—	6–7 years	11–12 years	13–14 years
First molar	At birth	Sometimes a trace	2½–3 years	6–7 years	9–10 years
Second molar	2½–3 years	—	7–8 years	11–13 years	14–15 years

Adapted and slightly modified by Massler and Shour from Logan WAG, Kronfeld R. Development of the human jaws and surrounding structures from birth to the age of fifteen years. *J Am Dent Assoc* 1933;20:379–428; From Touger-Decker R, Radler DR, Depaola DP. Nutrition and dental medicine. In: Ross AC, Caballero B, Cousins, RJ, et al. (eds). *Modern Nutrition in Health and Disease.* 11th ed. Philadelphia, PA: Wolters Kluwer Health/Lippincott Williams & Wilkins; 2014:1016–1040.

TABLE 13.3 Nutrient Deficiencies and Tooth Development

Nutrient	Effect on Tissue
Protein	Delayed tooth eruption; increased caries susceptibility; dysfunctional salivary glands
Vitamin A	Disturbed keratin matrix of enamel; increased enamel hypoplasia; increased caries susceptibility; decreased epithelial tissue development; dysfunction of tooth morphogenesis
Vitamin D	Poor calcification; pitting
Calcium/phosphorus	Decreased calcium concentration; hypomineralization (hypoplastic defects)
Ascorbic acid	Disturbed collagen matrix of dentin; alterations of dental pulp
Fluoride/iron/zinc	Increased caries susceptibility
Iodine	Delayed tooth eruption
Magnesium	Hypoplasia of enamel

Compiled from information in Touger-Decker R, Radler DR, Depaola DP. Nutrition and dental medicine. In: Ross AC, Caballero B, Cousins RJ, et al. (eds.). *Modern Nutrition in Health and Disease.* 11th ed. Philadelphia, PA: Wolters Kluwer Health/Lippincott Williams & Wilkins; 2014:1016–1040; Nizel AE. Preventing dental caries: the nutritional factors. *Pediatr Clin North Am* 1977;24:144–155; and Shaw JH, Sweeney EA. Oral health. In: Schneider HA, Anderson CD, Coursin DB, et al. (eds.). *Nutritional Support of Medical Practice*, Philadelphia, PA: Harper & Row; 1983:517–540.

Dentin and enamel depend on many nutrients: vitamin C for formation of collagen matrix; and calcium, magnesium, phosphorus, and vitamin D for mineralization. An inadequate amount of any of these nutrients during tooth development results in an imperfect matrix, with subsequent imperfection of mineralization (see Table 13.3). Infants whose mothers have low levels of vitamin D during pregnancy may be at increased risk for tooth enamel defects and early childhood tooth decay.[25] Keratin in enamel depends on vitamin A for its synthesis. Folate deficiency, known to cause neural tube defects, can result in incomplete formation of cranial bones.

Benefits of fluoride supplements during pregnancy in preventing infant dental caries are uncertain. Small amounts of fluoride are allowed to pass through the placenta, which are incorporated into fetal bones and teeth. Although fluoride supplements are considered safe for the mother and fetus, oral fluoride supplements during pregnancy seem to have minimal benefits on the developing fetus and are not recommended. Use of fluoridated products, such as toothpaste and mouth rinses, and fluoridated water are encouraged.

Nutritional Requirements for Pregnancy

Dietary Reference Intakes (DRIs) for pregnancy indicate advisable nutrient intake for optimal health of both mother and fetus. Accelerated growth and metabolism increases most nutrient requirements to some extent. Each vitamin and mineral is not separately discussed in this chapter; Table 13.4 shows the increased amounts recommended for each of the nutrients. The following mean nutrient intakes are commonly below the Recommended Dietary Allowances (RDAs) for pregnant women: fiber, vitamin D, folate, iron, and polyunsaturated fatty acids (PUFA). In addition to low intake of these nutrients, gravidas on vegan diets frequently consume inadequate amounts of vitamin B_{12} and are at increased risk of an inadequate intake of iron and vitamin D. Adolescent females with childbearing potential frequently have inadequate intakes of nutrients, potentially affecting pregnancy outcomes.[26]

Energy and Calories

During pregnancy, calorie requirements increase slightly to ensure nutrient and energy needs. The estimated energy requirement does not increase during the first trimester of pregnancy, allows an additional 340 cal per day during the second, and allows an additional 452 cal during the third trimester. This additional energy is needed to (a) build new tissues, including added maternal tissues and growth of the fetus and placenta; (b) support increased

TABLE 13.4 **Vitamin and Mineral Recommended Dietary Allowances**

			PREGNANT (19–30 YEARS OLD)			LACTATING (19–30 YEARS OLD)	
Nutrient	Nonpregnant Women (19–30 Years Old)	Pregnant (14–18 Years Old)	Amount of Nutrient	Percent Increase[a]	Lactating (14–18 Years Old)	Amount of Nutrient	Percent Increase[a]
Vitamin A	**700 μg**	**750 μg RE**	**770 μg RE**	10	**1200 μg RE**	**1300 μg RE**	71
Vitamin D	**15 μg**	**15 μg**	**15 μg**	0	**15 μg**	**15 μg**	0
Vitamin E	**15 α–TE**	**15 α–TE**	**15 α–TE**	0	**19 α–TE**	**19 α–TE**	27
Vitamin K	90 μg*	75 μg*	90 μg*	0	75 μg*	90 μg*	0
Vitamin C	**75 mg**	**85 mg**	**85 mg**	13	**115 mg**	**120 mg**	60
Thiamin	**1.1 mg**	**1.4 mg**	**1.4 mg**	27	**1.4 mg**	**1.4 mg**	27
Riboflavin	**1.1 mg**	**1.4 mg**	**1.4 mg**	27	**1.4 mg**	**1.6 mg**	45
Niacin	**14 mg NE**	**18 mg NE**	**18 mg NE**	28	**17 mg NE**	**17 mg NE**	21
Vitamin B_6	**1.3 mg**	**1.9 mg**	**1.9 mg**	46	**2.0 mg**	**2 mg**	54
Folate	**400 μg**	**600 μg**	**600 μg**	50	**500 μg**	**500 μg**	25
Vitamin B_{12}	**2.4 μg**	**2.6 μg**	**2.6 μg**	8	**2.8 μg**	**2.8 μg**	17
Calcium	**1000 mg**	**1300 mg**	**1000 mg**	0	**1300 mg**	**1000 mg**	0
Phosphorus	**700 mg**	**1350 mg**	**700 mg**	0	**1250 mg**	**700 mg**	0
Magnesium	**310 mg**	**400 mg**	**350 mg** **360 mg**[¶]	9	**360 mg**	**310 mg**	0
Fluoride	3 mg*	3 mg*	3 mg*	0	3 mg*	3 mg*	0
Iron	**18 mg**	**27 mg**	**27 mg**	50	**10 mg**	**9 mg**	[–50%]
Zinc	**8 mg**	**12 mg**	**11 mg**	38	**13 mg**	**12 mg**	50
Iodine	**150 μg**	**220 μg**	**220 μg**	47	**290 μg**	**290 μg**	93
Selenium	**55 μg**	**60 μg**	**60 μg**	9	**70 μg**	**70 μg**	27
Copper	**900 μg**	**1000 μg**	**1000 μg**	11	**1300 μg**	**1300 μg**	44

[a]Percent increase for pregnant women above nonpregnancy recommendation.
[¶]Ages 31–50 years old.
Data from National Research Council. *The Guide to Nutrient Requirements.* Washington, DC: National Academies Press; 2006 and National Research Council. *Dietary Reference Intakes for Calcium and Vitamin D.* Washington, DC: National Academies Press; 2011. *Note:* This table presents Recommended Dietary Allowances (RDAs) in **bold type** and adequate intakes (AIs) in regular type followed by an asterisk (*).

metabolic expenditure; and (c) enable physical movement of additional weight. Appropriate weight gain reflects adequacy of energy intake and influences birth weight. When caloric intake is slightly inadequate, physiologic adaptations spare energy for fetal growth.

Gestational weight gain within the recommended range produces optimal pregnancy outcomes; many women exceed the guidelines. Increasing energy intake as recommended may encourage excessive weight gain.[27] Clearly, the key to adhering to the NAM guidelines for weight gain is to limit energy intake while increasing nutrient density and maintaining levels of physical activity.[28] Focusing on portion size may be a valuable tool to help prevent excess weight gain.[29]

Dieting for weight loss is not recommended during pregnancy even though studies indicate that interventions can improve some outcomes for the mother and baby. Dietary interventions are effective to control the amount of weight gain since most women tend to gain too much weight. Avoidance of carbohydrate-rich foods—such as enriched breads and cereals—to reduce calories, either preconceptionally or during pregnancy, negatively affects folic acid intake; this situation may be detrimental to the fetus. Moreover, added sugars and excess saturated fat should be avoided in favor of nutrient-dense foods (Fig. 13.4).

A gravida who is significantly underweight before conception may need additional calories during the first trimester. Because requirements for many nutrients are increased, it is more important that foods be chosen wisely, principally using nutrient-dense foods.

Fat

Vitamin and mineral requirements during pregnancy increase proportionately higher than caloric needs. Saturated fats should be limited because of their minimal nutrient contribution, but

Breakfast

1½ c Frosted Mini-Wheat cereal
2 c skim milk
12 oz decaffeinated coffee, black

Mid-morning snack

12 oz water
1 oz (22) dry roasted almonds, unsalted
1 medium orange

Lunch

Sandwich with:
1 c tuna salad with egg, low-calorie mayonnaise
¼ c thin sliced cucumber
3 thin slices tomato
2 lettuce leaves
2 thin slices 100% wheat bread
8 raw baby carrots
1 medium applesauce cookie
1 c grapes
12 oz herbal tea with low calorie sweetener

Mid-afternoon snack

6 oz vanilla yogurt, low fat
1 oz single-serve bag unsalted pretzels
8 oz herbal tea with low calorie sweetener

Dinner

4 oz pot roast beef, braised, lean only with ½ c sauteed mushrooms
1 c white and wild rice blend, cooked with margarine and ¼ c low sodium vegetable juice
2 c garden salad with avocado, lettuce, tomato, carrots
¼ c shredded low-fat Muenster cheese
2 tbsp vinaigrette salad dressing
1 medium roll, enriched
2 tsp soft margarine
⅛ medium cantaloupe
12 oz water

Evening snack

3 c low-fat microwave popcorn
12 oz water

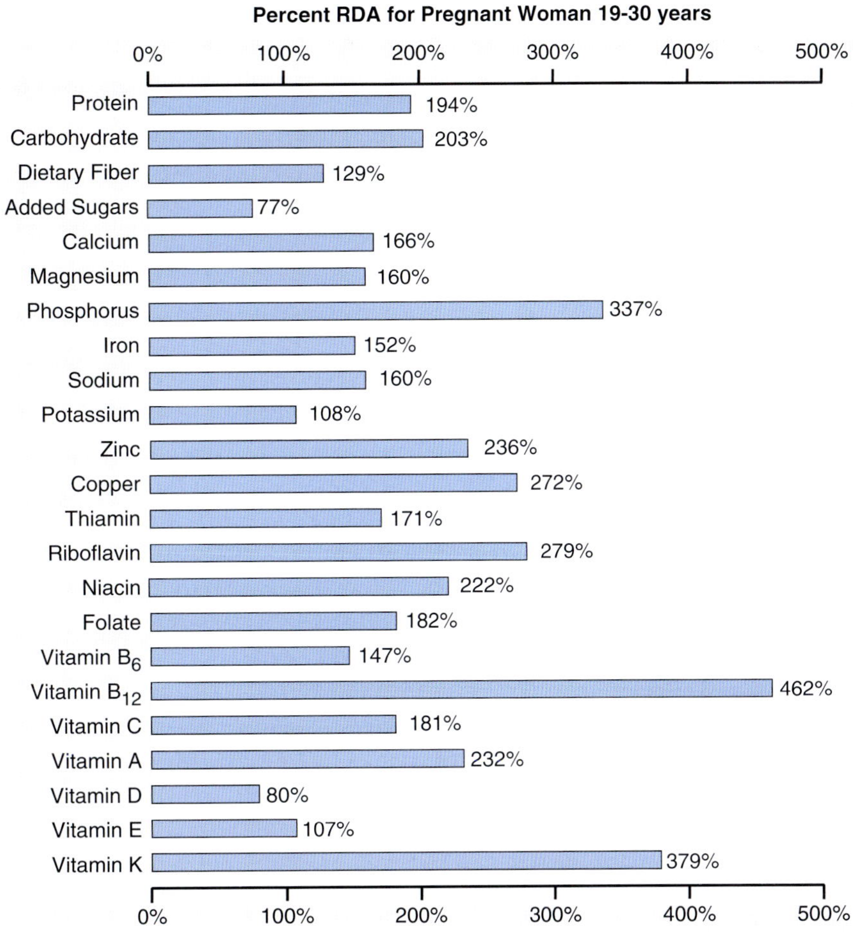

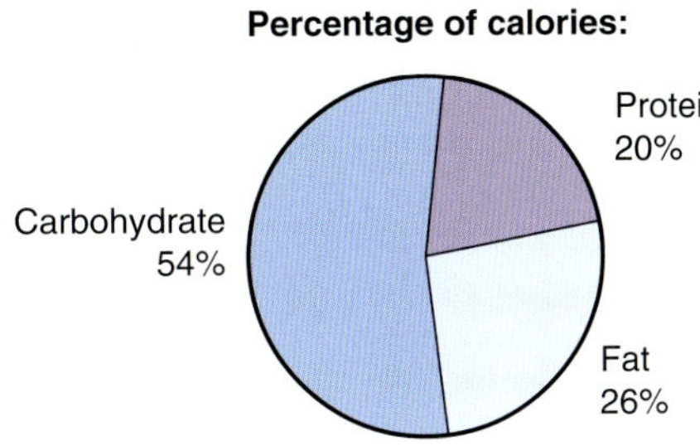

	Target	Eaten
Grains	9 oz	9½ oz
Whole grains	≥4½ oz	5 oz
Refined grains	≤4½ oz	4½ oz
Vegetables	3½ c	4 c
Fruits	2 c	2¼ c
Dairy	3 c	3¼ c
Protein Foods	6½ oz	9½ oz

• **Figure 13.4** Sample menu for pregnancy based on information provided by the mother: pregnant in the second trimester; age 28 years; height 5 ft, 7 in; prepregnancy weight 140 lb; and moderately active (30–60 minutes of physical activity 5 days a week).

PUFAs are needed to reduce serum lipids and for adequate fetal central nervous system development. Hormonal changes result in significant elevations of serum cholesterol and triglycerides during the second trimester of pregnancy.

More important during pregnancy (and lactation) is the fact that maternal intake of omega-3 fatty acids has a positive impact on maternal, infant, and child health.[30] Requirements for omega-3 fatty acids (docosahexaenoic acid/DHA) have not been established, but some experts have recommended at least 200 mg per day of DHA during pregnancy.[31] Omega-3 fatty acids are crucial for infant brain and visual development, especially during the latter part of gestation and early postnatal life. Maternal fish intake, but not dietary supplements, is associated with improved outcomes. Prenatal consumption of two servings weekly corresponds to

200 to 2400 mg omega-3 fatty acids/day, depending on the fish chosen. Two servings per week of low-mercury fish appear to be a safe level.[32]

Protein

Protein is the basic nutrient for growth; an additional 21 g of protein, or a total of 67 g daily, is recommended. This can be accomplished with an additional 3 oz of meat or meat substitute (21 g protein) or by adding 2 oz of meat and 8 oz of milk (24 g protein; see Fig. 13.4). Because Americans normally consume more than 65 g of protein daily, additional amounts may not be needed.

Calcium and Vitamin D

Calcium and vitamin D work together in the formation of skeletal tissue and teeth. During pregnancy, hormonal and physiologic adjustments promote increased calcium absorption and retention; thus, the DRI is the same as that of nonpregnant women of the same age. This extra calcium is thought to be stored in maternal bone for fetal availability in the third trimester, when fetal bone growth is rapid. If calcium intake meets the DRI, additional calcium supplementation is believed to be unnecessary.

The recommended 1000 mg per day of calcium for women older than 19 years of age can be met by three servings of milk or dairy products. Pregnant women younger than 19 years of age may need 4 cups of milk to provide the necessary 1300 mg per day. Dairy products may be incorporated into cooking or eaten in different forms—such as cheese, ice cream, or yogurt—for variety (see Table 9.2 and Box 9.2). A commonly reiterated erroneous myth is that a fetus removes calcium from the mother's teeth. If the gravida has sufficient calcium intake, problems do not develop. A calcium deficit ensures that fetal requirements are met first with resorption of calcium from the gravida's bones, not from her teeth.

Vitamin D intake during pregnancy has traditionally been associated with infant growth, bone ossification, tooth enamel formation, and neonatal calcium homeostasis, but the function of vitamin D during pregnancy is uncertain. The NAM established 600 IU per day for pregnant women; current Tolerable Upper Intake Level is 4000 IU (100 μg). Most American and Canadian women consume less than the recommended amount. Suboptimal vitamin D status has been documented in many urban populations, including those with adequate sunlight, which suggests that maternal vitamin D insufficiency during pregnancy is common. The American College of Obstetrics and Gynecology and the NAM currently recommend 600 IU (15 μg) daily vitamin D supplementation during pregnancy to support maternal and fetal bone metabolism.[33]

Clinical studies have established relationships between vitamin D levels and adverse pregnancy outcomes. Vitamin D supplements improve serum levels, but the needs, safety, and effectiveness of supplementation during pregnancy remain controversial. Screening for pregnant women thought to be at increased risk of vitamin D deficiency should be considered; if justified, 1000 to 2000 IU per day of vitamin D is considered safe.[33]

B Vitamins

Several of the B-vitamin requirements are based on energy or caloric intake; usually, their intake increases automatically with intake of additional calories. However, adequate intake of some B vitamins is difficult to achieve without careful selection of foods or supplementation.

The RDA for folate (600 μg) during pregnancy is significantly more than for the nonpregnant woman (400 μg). The role of folate as a coenzyme is essential for nucleic acid synthesis. Folate is also required for increased red blood cell formation. Folate deficiency impairing cell growth and replication may cause fetal anomalies. Orofacial clefts and neural tube defects, such as spina bifida and **anencephaly** (absence of a major portion of the brain and skull), are attributed to inadequate folate intake before conception and during the first trimester. Ideally, attention is focused on folate intake when a woman is capable of becoming pregnant because 50% to 70% of neural tube defects can be prevented if sufficient amounts of folic acid are consumed before conception and throughout the first trimester.[34] The U.S. Preventive Services Task Force recently reviewed its 2009 recommendation on folic acid supplementation in women of childbearing age, examining the effectiveness of supplementation and new evidence on the benefits and harms of supplements, and reaffirmed its previous recommendation.[35]

Because of crucial effects on a pregnancy, the FDA requires supplementation of all enriched grain products with specific amounts of folic acid. Since implementation of folic acid fortification in the United States in 1996, neural tube defects have fallen almost 35%.[35] Even with folic acid fortification, nearly 25% of reproductive-age women, especially Hispanic women, fail to get enough of the B vitamin. In 2016, the FDA approved folic acid fortification of corn masa flour, allowing manufacturers to voluntarily add folic acid in amounts consistent with levels of other enriched cereal grains.[36] The seal "Folic Acid for a Healthy Pregnancy" was developed to help women quickly and easily identify products fortified with folic acid.

Meeting the gravida's requirement for folate solely from food intake is difficult for most women. Education promoting consumption of folic acid from folate-rich foods, supplements, and foods fortified with folic acid can help prevent neural tube defects. Conscientious daily selections of raw fruits and vegetables, especially green leafy vegetables, can help ensure adequate intake. Folic acid–fortified breads and cereals also contribute significant amounts (see Tables 1.5 and 11.12). Every woman of reproductive age should be encouraged to consume a daily supplement containing 400 μg folic acid; absorption from supplements is better than from natural folate in foods. The March of Dimes indicates only 33% of women take a multivitamin supplement containing folic acid.[34]

Although folate intake is essential, some women take excessive amounts (up to eight times the RDA), which may adversely affect vitamin B_{12} levels (see Chapter 11).

Iron

A common problem among nonpregnant women is iron-deficiency anemia; many women begin pregnancy with diminished iron stores. Increased iron during gestation is needed for production of red blood cells and the placenta, and to compensate for cord and blood loss at delivery.

The fetus acts as a parasite in that fetal **erythropoiesis** (the formation of red blood cells) occurs at the expense of maternal iron stores. Iron-deficiency anemia is seldom seen in full-term infants. During the last half of pregnancy, iron absorption increases from the normal 10% to 20% to approximately 25% if it is available. Fetal accumulation of iron occurs principally in the last trimester. Premature infants, having a shortened gestation, have insufficient time to acquire adequate iron and may be born with iron-deficiency anemia; however, premature infants absorb iron very efficiently.

Approximately 27 mg of iron is needed daily during pregnancy. Because the average American diet does not provide this amount within normal caloric requirements, daily iron supplements (30 mg elemental iron) are usually recommended. Initiation of supplements before gestational week 24 prevents iron deficiency. Low-dose iron supplementation during pregnancy, even if the gravida is not anemic, improves the woman's iron status and seems to protect the infant from iron-deficiency anemia. Infant iron status has been associated with cognitive and neurobehavioral outcomes, indicating the importance of optimal iron status at birth.

Iron supplements frequently cause nausea and constipation, and occasionally high hemoglobin levels. Iron supplements taken one to three times weekly on nonconsecutive days reduces side effects and increases acceptance and adherence while maintaining safe hemoglobin levels. If iron supplements are not provided, it may take 2 years after delivery for maternal serum iron levels to return to normal.

High hemoglobin levels have been associated with an increased risk of LBW and premature births; thus, levels should be routinely monitored.

Zinc

Zinc is crucial early in pregnancy during the formation of fetal organs, but requirements are highest in late pregnancy for fetal growth and development. The RDA for zinc is 12 mg during pregnancy. An increase in high-protein foods, especially meats, improves zinc intake.

Iodine

Dietary iodine requirements are higher during pregnancy as a result of increased maternal thyroid hormone production and fetal iodine requirements. Iodine nutritional status has declined among United States women of childbearing age over the last three decades; between 21% and 44% of third-trimester pregnant women may have inadequate levels of iodine.[37] Adherence to the *Dietary Guidelines* recommendation to decrease use of salt (usually iodized), increased use of processed foods (not iodized), and increased popularity of sea salt (contains no iodine), may be affecting iodine intake. Adverse effects of iodine deficiency in pregnancy include maternal and fetal goiter; cretinism; fetal brain development and intellectual impairments; neonatal hypothyroidism; and infant mortality. Iodine deficiency is a significant global public health problem.

The NAM recommends a daily iodine intake of 220 μg during pregnancy. Because many women of reproductive age in the United States are marginally deficient in iodine, the American Thyroid Association, Teratology Society, and the American Academy of Pediatrics recommend a supplement containing adequate iodide during pregnancy and lactation.[38,39] The American Thyroid Association has stressed that adequate maternal iodine is necessary to ensure the health of the mother and infant; the addition of 150 μg of potassium iodide in prenatal vitamins would be effective. Nonprescription and prescription prenatal multivitamins in the United States contain a mean level of 119 μg iodine per daily dose despite the amount indicated on the label.[40]

Although an infrequent occurrence, congenital hypothyroidism may also result from excess prenatal intake of iodine supplements. The NAM has not determined a safe upper limit for iodine during pregnancy and lactation.

Vitamin-Mineral Supplements

Keeping vitamin and nutrient levels up during pregnancy is essential for a healthy baby. In the United States, vitamin and mineral supplementation is commonly recommended during pregnancy. The specific nutrient amounts for a daily multivitamin-mineral supplement appropriate for gravidas of any age are shown in Table 13.5.

TABLE 13.5 Nutrient Supplementation During Pregnancy

Nutrient	Amount of Supplement Recommended
Vitamin C	50 mg
Vitamin B_6	2 mg
Folate	300 μg
Iron	30 mg
Zinc	15 mg
Copper	2 mg

Data from Institute of Medicine, Food and Nutrition Board: *Nutrition during Pregnancy.* Washington, DC: National Academy Press; 1990.

Supplementation should be based on an identified nutritional need, evidence of a benefit, and lack of harmful effects. Multivitamins seem to improve brain development and cognitive abilities with long-term benefits.[41] Food is considered to be the optimal vehicle for providing nutrients, but supplements may be warranted during this period because many women fail to meet their prenatal nutrient requirements through diet alone. Excessive amounts of many nutrients may have detrimental effects on the fetus (Table 13.6). A supplement should not reduce the woman's motivation to maintain or improve the quality of her diet because, in most instances, nutrients in foods are better absorbed than those available in pills (except for folic acid).

The NAM subcommittee concluded that iron is the only known nutrient warranting global supplementation during pregnancy. A goal for *Healthy People 2020* is to reduce iron-deficiency anemia among pregnant females. Approximately 16% of pregnant females may be iron deficient.[42] Consequently, 30 mg of ferrous iron is recommended to provide adequate amounts of iron during the second and third trimesters of pregnancy.

Dietary folate intake does not usually meet the RDA, but since folate enrichment of cereal products began in 1998, maternal folate status has improved significantly. Whole-grain products do not contain as much folate (and are not absorbed as well) as enriched grains and cereals; therefore, only one-half of the gravida's grain selections should be whole grains. A supplement containing folate may be prudent if intake is questionable. It should be initiated before conception because birth defects from inadequate folate intake may occur before the gravida realizes the pregnancy. A multivitamin supplement containing folic acid is recommended for all young women 15 to 24 years old because of the number of unintentional pregnancies in that age group.

As a result of several studies showing a relationship between high doses of vitamin A supplements and birth defects, the FDA provided recommendations for women of childbearing age. Ordinary multivitamins typically contain 5000 IU of vitamin A, but some brands can contain much more—sometimes 25,000 IU. Excess vitamin A (10,000 IU of vitamin A preformed from animal sources) during the first trimester can result in severe craniofacial and oral clefts and limb defects. Intake of preformed vitamin A should be limited to approximately 100% of the Daily Value (5000 IU). Liver and other animal products and

TABLE 13.6 Nutrient Supplementation Associated With Deleterious Fetal Outcomes

Nutrient	Effects on Fetus
Vitamin A	Pharmacologic use of vitamin A analogs has resulted in major congenital defects (malformation of cranium, face, heart, thymus, and central nervous system) and spontaneous abortion, especially during first trimester.
Vitamin D	Excessive intake of vitamin D can result in hyperabsorption of calcium, hypercalcemia, calcification of soft tissues, and mental retardation.
Vitamin E	Excessive intake of vitamin E is associated with higher incidence of spontaneous abortions.
Vitamin K	Menadione administered parenterally has been associated with hemolytic anemia, hyperbilirubinemia, and kernicterus in the newborn.
Vitamin C	Megadoses of vitamin C have been reported to cause vitamin C dependency, with symptoms of conditional scurvy observed postpartum.
Iodine	Large amounts of iodides have resulted in infants with congenital goiter, hypothyroidism, and mental retardation.
Zinc	Large amounts of zinc supplements during the third trimester were implicated in premature delivery and stillbirth.
Fluoride	Well water containing 12 to 18 parts/million (ppm) fluoride produced offspring with significant mottling of deciduous teeth.

Data from Worthington-Roberts B. Nutrition deficiencies and excesses: impact on pregnancy, part 2. *J Perinatol* 1985;5(4):12. Reprinted by permission from Macmillan Publishers Ltd.

fortified foods and vitamin supplements listing retinyl palmitate and retinyl acetate as ingredients contain preformed vitamin A. Beta-carotene, which the body converts to vitamin A, is much less toxic. Fortified foods containing beta-carotene and fruits and vegetables that contain natural beta-carotene should be chosen whenever possible.

Nutritional supplementation may be warranted in high-risk pregnancies, including adolescent pregnancies; multiple gestations (carrying more than one fetus); and pregnancies in women who use cigarettes, alcohol, or other drugs. Women who are younger than 25 years of age—or who do not routinely consume milk, dairy products, or foods fortified with calcium and vitamin D—should take a calcium supplement. Vitamin D supplementation may be beneficial for some women living in northern latitudes with limited exposure to sunlight; more study is needed to determine the most effective dosage. Iron supplements containing more than 30 mg of iron necessitate supplemental amounts of zinc and copper.

Compliance with taking a nutrition supplement is poor; only about half of the vitamins are taken. Many women do not take the supplement because of nausea and vomiting or previous adverse effects, whereas others indicate the size of the pill is a factor. Patients should be encouraged to take the prescribed supplement and informed of the importance and reasons why it is needed. Compliance with use of prenatal supplements is enhanced by convenient supply, affordability, and reinforcement by health care providers.

Dietary Intake and Education

Prenatal nutritional care improves outcome by saving lives, averting LBW, and decreasing costs of care that are consequences of LBW. Nutrient intake warrants more attention than weight gain. Although adequate weight gain is the most reliable measurable tool for assessing adequacy of energy intake, food choices can provide adequate calories yet may be deficient in vital nutrients. For this reason, the NAM subcommittee recommends routine assessment of dietary practices for all gravidas in the United States to determine the need for improved diet or vitamin-mineral supplementation. Most women are highly motivated to make dietary changes during their pregnancy.

Because maternal nutrition has profound effects on infant health, the *MyPlate* website (https://www.choosemyplate.gov/moms-pregnancy-breastfeeding) has links that provide a myriad of information for pregnant and breastfeeding mothers, including calculations for a healthy weight gain and other tips for making healthy food choices. Dental hygienists can use these tools to discuss nutritional requirements and shortages in patients' diets. *SuperTracker* can be used to personalize a food plan based on age, height, prepregnancy weight, and physical activity level. Other topics for the gravida covered through links on the *MyPlate* website include dietary supplements, food safety, and special health needs.

Some pregnant women may have little or no nutritional knowledge. Although knowledge is the key to wise food choices, nutrition counseling is often unavailable or ignored during pregnancy. The AND recommends that women receive nutritional counseling during pregnancy for optimal outcomes.[31] Interventions prior to conception, as well as during pregnancy, improve fetal development and long-term health. Low-income expectant mothers have more opportunities to receive nutritional information through established programs such as the Supplemental Nutrition Program for Women, Infants, and Children (WIC) than more affluent women receive through the private sector.

Identification of poor and desirable food habits and dietary patterns can serve as the foundation for appropriate nutrition education and intervention. Identified nutritional problems, such as pica or fad dieting, or risk factors, such as alcohol abuse, may require special attention. Most important, the gravida should understand what foods she should be eating and the importance of choosing nutrient-dense foods. Breastfeeding should also be promoted during pregnancy.

DENTAL CONSIDERATIONS

Assessments

- *Physical:* Level of education, income status, culture, religion, prenatal health care, medical history (including drugs taken), dental history, oral examination, feelings about weight gain.
- *Dietary:* Health and nutritional knowledge and skills; adequacy of intake based on a well-balanced diet using a variety of foods, including enriched grain products; vegetarianism; food budget; food cravings and aversions; fad diets; beliefs about nutrition during pregnancy; pica; alcohol use; and caffeine intake.

Interventions

- Become familiar with local nutritional practices and beliefs about pregnancy; these beliefs are regional and may be affected by cultural beliefs.
- During routine dental recare for women of childbearing age, discuss the importance of maintaining oral health and dental appointments during pregnancy.
- Refer patients at risk of inadequate intakes of specific nutrients to a registered dietitian nutritionist (RDN) or health care provider.
- Emphasize consumption of a well-balanced diet, with three to six meals throughout the day to ensure optimal intake of nutrients. Discuss the importance of consuming 2 servings of low-mercury fish per week, focusing on the benefits of consumption and not just the risks by providing a broad range of fish that are low in mercury and high in omega-3 fatty acids.
- Patients who might become pregnant should have a high folate intake. If a woman of childbearing age is not taking a multivitamin supplement and is following a carbohydrate-restricted diet, refer her to a health care provider or an RDN.
- Ask pregnant patients whether they are taking a prenatal supplement. If not, refer them to a health care provider.
- Seize pregnancy as the ideal opportunity to discuss good nutritional and oral hygiene habits needed during this period and for the newborn infant. Proper oral tissue development of the fetus depends on adequate maternal nutrition.
- Encourage foods high in calcium. Low calcium intake may impair bone–mineral deposition, especially in women younger than 25 years of age. Consuming the recommended 1300 mg of calcium daily is particularly important for pregnant teens to meet calcium demands. The use of dietary calcium is preferred because these foods also provide other valuable nutrients—protein, riboflavin, and vitamin D and other components that enhance calcium absorption.
- Snacking is acceptable for pregnant women. Provide information on avoidance of acid attacks and resultant tooth decay by recommending appropriate oral hygiene techniques after snacking and encouraging foods such as nuts, raw vegetables, yogurt, and popcorn.
- If the mother has a strong preference for sweets, the infant's diet is also likely to be high in sugar. Review the gravida's diet for the form and frequency of sugar-containing foods, and suggest modifications or substitutions as indicated. This could create a healthier pattern for the patient and alleviate potential dental problems for the infant.
- Discuss the risk of early childhood caries with all pregnant women (see Chapter 14).
- Encourage pregnant patients to use iodized salt, and choose good dietary sources of iodine (e.g., milk and dairy products and fish). Avoid kelp supplements because of excessive levels of iodine.
- Because of potentially increased risk of preterm or LBW infants associated with pregnancy gingivitis and other periodontal issues, encourage excellent oral hygiene habits throughout the day.
- Encourage sexually active women of childbearing age who drink alcohol to use reliable methods to prevent pregnancy, plan their pregnancies, and stop drinking before becoming pregnant.
- Stress the importance of enrolling in educational breastfeeding classes that address benefits, techniques, common problems, myths, and skills training.

NUTRITIONAL DIRECTIONS

- Pregnant women should consult their health care provider before taking any drug, including nonprescription drugs and herbal products.
- Preventive oral care, including limiting frequency of fermentable carbohydrate intake and adequate oral hygiene care (brush the teeth at least 2 times a day, floss daily, and use an antibacterial mouthwash), is important for both mother and fetus.
- Nutrient needs must be met by deliberate preplanning and informed food choices.
- Low-fat or skim milk may be used to control weight, decrease saturated fat intake, and provide equivalent nutrients.
- Although the pregnant patient is "eating for two," energy requirements are not double.
- Moderate increases in whole grains, milk, and legumes can provide additional protein and other important nutrients.
- Calcium, vitamin D, and vitamin B_{12} supplements are advisable for vegans because they exclude all animal products. Pregnant vegans should be referred to an RDN.
- Vitamin D may be a special concern for women with minimal exposure to sunlight or routine use of sunscreens. Regular exposure to sunlight and foods fortified with vitamin D (e.g., milk and cheese) are recommended.
- Powdered milk (⅓ cup) can be added to soups, cooked cereals, mashed potatoes, or casseroles if the gravida has an aversion to drinking milk.
- Adverse symptoms, such as nausea or constipation, frequently occur from iron supplementation. Rather than discontinuing the supplement, take it with meals, or consult the health care provider about possibly decreasing the dosage or taking it three to four times a week.
- Absorption of iron from supplements or foods is enhanced if taken between meals with vitamin C–rich foods, such as orange juice, while avoiding milk or tea.
- Moderately intense exercise during pregnancy (such as 30-minute brisk walks) is beneficial if medical reasons do not prevent it. Exercise enhances blood flow, which delivers nutrients to the fetus, improves mood and energy level, and increases cardiovascular fitness and endurance.

Lactation

Exclusive breastfeeding for 4 to 6 months and continuing until 12 months is the ideal method of feeding infants. Complementary foods should begin at least by 6 months. United States health authorities began to promote breastfeeding about 25 years ago, a healthy practice that has been slowly gaining in popularity. In 2016, approximately 81.1% of mothers breastfed newborns, with 51.8% still breastfeeding 6 months later, and 30.7% at 12 months.[43] The target for breastfeeding established in *Healthy People 2020* is 81.9% at birth, 60.6% at 6 months, and 34.1% at 1 year.[44] Breastfeeding rates vary by race/ethnicity, participation in the WIC supplemental nutrition program, mother's age and education, and geography. Despite increases in the prevalence of infants initially being breastfed, the prevalence of breastfeeding among African American infants remains below that for whites and Hispanics. In 2008, 58.9% of African American mothers, and 80% of Hispanic mothers initiated breastfeeding.[45] This increase in breastfeeding rates shows outstanding gains, particularly for groups less likely to breastfeed—women who are African American, are younger than 20 years of age, have less than a high school education, are in their first pregnancy, and are employed. Numerous breastfeeding initiatives have been launched to increase breastfeeding rates: the Baby-Friendly Hospital Initiative, *Ten Steps to Successful Breastfeeding*,

• BOX 13.1 Advantages of Breastfeeding

For the Mother

- Maternal hormones produced as a result of lactation facilitate contractions of the uterus and control postpartum bleeding.
- Prepregnancy weight is achieved sooner because breastfeeding burns calories.
- Breastfeeding is less expensive than formula feeding.
- Mother–infant bonding is enhanced with breastfeeding.
- Breastfeeding saves time because there are no bottles to clean, prepare, warm, or sterilize.
- Working mothers who breastfeed miss less work because of a sick infant.
- Prolactin, the hormone that helps the milk "let down," relaxes the mother.
- The mother is at reduced risk of premenopausal breast and ovarian cancer.
- Breastfeeding is associated with reduced visceral adiposity, leading to lower risk of type 2 diabetes and hyperlipidemia.

For the Infant

- Human milk is nutritionally balanced with maximum bioavailability for infants. It is easy for the infant to digest.
- Breast milk has immunologic properties that help reduce infant morbidity (especially certain infectious gastrointestinal and respiratory diseases, and earaches) and mortality. Within 4 hours after exposure to germs, antibodies in the milk change to meet the needs of the infant.
- Breast milk constantly changes in composition to meet the changing needs of the infant, especially a premature infant.
- Human milk reduces the risk of food allergies and asthma (wheezing) and prevents or delays the occurrence of atopic dermatitis in early childhood.
- Breastfeeding promotes infant oral–motor and structural development; this can mean fewer dental bills or a decreased need for orthodontic work.
- Incidence of thumb sucking and tongue thrusting is lower in breastfed infants.
- Breastfed infants are exposed to a variety of tastes through the mother's milk.
- Breast milk reduces a child's risk for diabetes.
- Breast milk provides better brain development. Longer periods of exclusive breastfeeding during an infant's first year increase some measures of a child's cognitive development; this may lead to a smarter child and adult.
- Prolonged breastfeeding may reduce the risk of overweight in childhood. Breastfeeding has an indirect influence on body fat accumulation and selectively protects against extremes in body size and fat deposition.
- Breastfeeding longer than 6 months provides health benefits well beyond the breastfeeding period. A quantitative review of the evidence indicates that exclusively breastfed infants may have lower blood cholesterol concentrations in later life.
- Breastfeeding is associated with a reduction in risk for postneonatal death.

and numerous initiatives by state health departments and state and local WIC agencies designed to raise awareness of the importance and benefits of breastfeeding infants. In 2016, the U.S. Preventive Services Task Force recommended providing supportive interventions during pregnancy and after birth to support breastfeeding.[46]

Despite extensive evidence for short-term and long-term health benefits from breastfeeding for both mother and baby, and practical benefits, such as lower cost (Box 13.1), many women choose to bottle feed. Personal and social biases (such as attitudes of family and close friends, and problems with breastfeeding in public and employment practices) are principal factors in this decision. A mother's decision to breastfeed can be positively influenced by health education and peer support; her success is greatly improved through active support from her family, friends, communities, clinicians, health care providers, employers, and policymakers. Peer counseling, lactation consultation, and formal breastfeeding education during pregnancy appear to increase both initiation and duration of breastfeeding. The breastfeeding food package for mothers who breastfed was enhanced by providing mothers with more food, and the amount of formula allowed for formula-fed infants was decreased, but this effort yielded less than the desired results.

Virtually all women are able to produce enough breast milk providing essential nutrients to support infant growth and health. Breastfeeding has many advantages for the infant and mother (see Box 13.1). Further discussion regarding infant feeding is provided in Chapter 14.

Breast milk provides all the infant needs for about the first 6 months of life to support optimal growth and development, with rare exceptions. Principal reasons given by mothers for stopping breastfeeding is that they perceive the infant is not satisfied by breast milk alone, pain associated with breastfeeding, and returning to work. Breastfeeding continues to meet important nutritional needs and provides protection from illness and infection beyond the first 6 months of life. Mothers are encouraged to continue breastfeeding beyond the minimum of 6 months. Prolonged breast feeding (>2 years) may increase the risk for dental caries.[47]

Nutritional Recommendations for Breastfeeding

For most nutrients, recommendations for lactating women are similar to those for pregnant women. Energy requirements are proportional to the quantity of milk produced. Approximately 85 cal are needed for every 100 mL of milk produced, requiring approximately a 500-cal daily increase. Although this increase may not be fully adequate to cover the needs for milk production, the 2 to 4 kg of fat accumulated during pregnancy is available to supply additional calories. Return to prepregnancy weight is accelerated. The major determinant of milk production is the infant's demand for milk, not maternal energy intake. Weight loss during lactation has no apparent deleterious effects on milk production.

Carbohydrate intake from whole grains, dairy, fruits, and vegetables is important for maintaining lactose synthesis and milk volume. The amount of protein recommended is slightly higher than for pregnancy—an additional 25 g or a total of 70 g daily. Breastfeeding is positively related to mental development of the infant but may be influenced by maternal education, social class, a nurturing environment, and intelligence of the parents than diet. Long-chain PUFAs, especially DHA, seem to play a beneficial role in children's mental development and possibly immune response; thus, a prenatal omega-3 fatty acid supplement should be considered. Other nutrients needed in larger quantities during pregnancy include vitamins A, E, C, riboflavin, B_6, and B_{12}, along with the minerals copper, zinc, iodine, and selenium. Maternal vitamin B_6 status affects amounts found in breast milk, and, thus, infant growth. A source of vitamin B_{12} intake, from either foods or supplements, is crucial for optimal infant nutriture. Neurologic impairments have occurred in children of breastfeeding vegan mothers who were eating no or very limited foods of animal origin, the source of vitamin B_{12}. A lactating woman also requires additional fluids to replace those secreted in the milk. An additional 1000 mL per day (4 cups) of fluids is needed.

Dietary Patterns for Lactating Women

The dietary pattern of a lactating woman is similar to that of a pregnant woman (Fig. 13.5). Consumption of 3 cups of milk or dairy products fortified with vitamin D daily provides approximately

Breakfast

1¾ c Frosted Mini-Wheat cereal
2 c skim milk
12 oz decaffeinated coffee, black

Mid-morning snack

12 oz water
1 oz (22) dry roasted almonds, unsalted
1 medium orange

Lunch

Sandwich with:
1 c tuna salad with egg, low-calorie mayonnaise
¼ c thin sliced cucumber
3 thin slices tomato
2 lettuce leaves
2 thin slices 100% wheat bread
8 raw baby carrots
1 medium applesauce cookie
1 c grapes
12 oz herbal tea with low calorie sweetener

Mid-afternoon snack

6 oz vanilla yogurt, low fat
1 oz single-serve bag unsalted pretzels
8 oz herbal tea with low calorie sweetener

Dinner

3 oz pot roast beef, braised, lean only with ½ c sauteed mushrooms
1 c white and wild rice blend, cooked with margarine and ¼ c low sodium vegetable juice
2 c garden salad with avocado, lettuce, tomato, carrots
¼ c shredded low-fat Muenster cheese
2 tbsp vinaigrette salad dressing
1 medium roll, enriched
1 T soft margarine
⅛ medium cantaloupe
12 oz water

Evening snack

3 c low-fat microwave popcorn
12 oz water

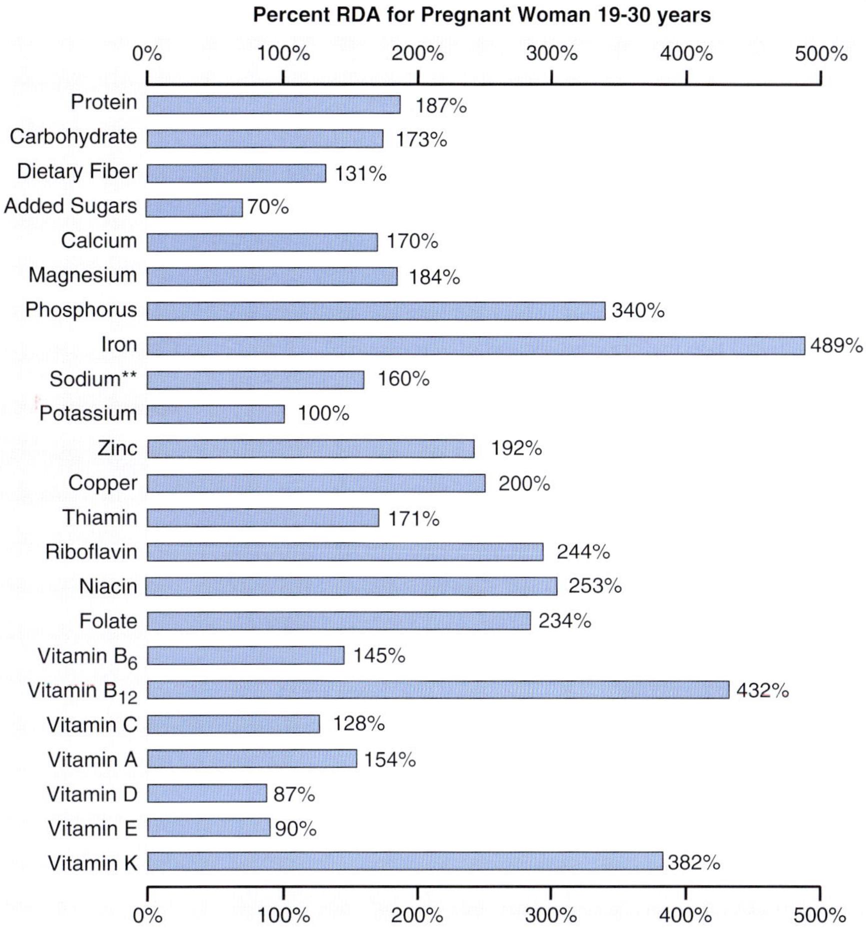

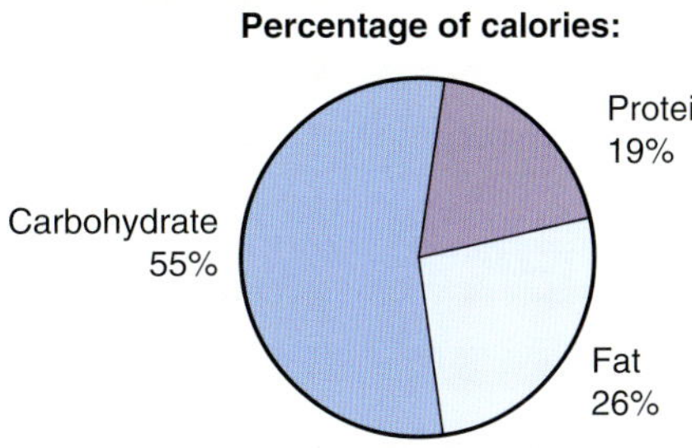

	Target	Eaten
Grains	9 oz	10 oz
Whole grains	≥4½ oz	5½ oz
Refined grains	≤4½ oz	5 oz
Vegetables	3½ c	4 c
Fruits	2 c	2¼ c
Dairy	3 c	3¼ c
Protein Foods	6½ oz	9 oz

• **Figure 13.5** Sample menu for lactation based on information provided by the mother: 100% breast-feeding 3-month-old infant; age 29 years; height 5 ft, 7 in; weight 150 lb; and moderately active (30–60 minutes of physical activity 5 days a week).

1000 mg of calcium and 300 IU of vitamin D, which are adequate amounts for women older than 19 years. Much higher doses of vitamin D are needed to achieve adequate concentrations in exclusively breastfed infants; thus, vitamin D supplementation for these infants is recommended.[48] Other high-calcium foods may also be used. High-protein foods may include 6 to 8 oz of meat daily, depending on the quantity of milk consumed. Adequate servings of fresh fruits, vegetables, and whole-grain products help provide the additional calories.

Low iron stores has a deleterious effect on the mother; a prenatal vitamin is encouraged for postpartum women to provide adequate iron and folate to replenish stores. Women who have mild iron deficiency are less sensitive to their infants' cues and have more difficulty bonding with their infants. Women who are anemic are more likely to experience postpartum depression.

Many substances consumed by the mother may affect breast milk. Certain foods, especially strongly flavored foods such as raw onion, garlic, curry, chili peppers, and chocolate, may cause gastrointestinal distress, rash, or irritability in the infant. These foods only need to be omitted if they affect the infant.

Many nonnutritive substances and drugs may be secreted in breast milk. Alcohol may impair milk flow and is transmitted in breast milk in approximately the same proportions as in the mother's blood. Intake should be limited to less than 0.5 g/kg daily. Large amounts of coffee and tea intake may adversely affect the iron content of human milk. Caffeine can be transferred to the infant in breast milk; therefore, caffeine intake should be moderate (300 mg).

Because of the risk of medications being passed into breast milk, all drugs, including over-the-counter medications and herbal remedies, should be used cautiously and only if essential. Medications less likely to be secreted into the milk can be prescribed by the health care provider.

MyPlate (https://www.choosemyplate.gov/moms-pregnancy-breastfeeding.gov) provides a plethora of health and nutrition information for breastfeeding women. Individualized nutrition guidance is available on the Internet consistent with the *Dietary Guidelines* to assist breastfeeding mothers (see Fig. 13.6). Nutrition information is provided for exclusively breastfeeding and partially breastfeeding mothers. Tips are available for eating a balanced diet, healthy weight maintenance or weight loss, physical activity, and use of dietary supplements.

Dietary assessment of routine food intake by an RDN is suggested, followed by nutrition counseling regarding foods rich in nutrients deficient in the diet. Continued use of the prenatal vitamin or a multivitamin supplement is recommended to ensure an adequate supply of folate if the woman may become pregnant again.

DENTAL CONSIDERATIONS

Assessments

- *Physical:* Socioeconomic status, types of drugs, over-the-counter medications, supplements, and herbals used.
- *Dietary:* Adequacy of calories, nutrients, and fluid intake; alcohol and caffeine intake.

Interventions

- For a postpartum patient, encourage gradual return to prepregnancy weight (maximum weight loss of 4 lb/month for lactating women) through a balanced diet and moderate exercise.
- Encourage lactating women to obtain their nutrients from a well-balanced diet.
- Stress the importance of choosing a well-balanced diet utilizing fruits and vegetables, enriched and whole-grain breads and cereals, calcium-rich dairy products, and protein-rich and carbohydrate-rich foods to provide required nutrients.
- Encourage intake of at least 10 to 12 cups of fluid each day.
- Discuss increasing intake of nutrient-dense foods to achieve a caloric intake of at least 1800 cal daily.
- Discourage the use of strict weight loss diets and appetite suppressants.
- Emphasize the importance of reduced-fat milk, cheese, or other calcium-rich dairy products.
- Encourage intake of vitamin D–fortified foods, such as fortified milk or cereal, for women with limited exposure to ultraviolet light.
- To support women during lactation, use the Internet to access *MyPlate* (www.choosemyplate.gov/moms-pregnancy-breastfeeding) to provide nutrition education.
- For vegans who are breastfeeding, stress the importance of a balanced diet with appropriate supplements, especially vitamin B_{12}, in sufficient quantities. Offer a referral to an RDN.

NUTRITIONAL DIRECTIONS

- Breastfeeding helps with weight loss.
- Limit intake of coffee (regular and decaffeinated), other caffeine-containing beverages, and medications. Choose fluids such as juice, milk, and water.
- The *SuperTracker* can be an effective tool for improving dietary intake and promoting weight loss during lactation.

Oral Contraceptive Agents

Many nutrients (especially folate, vitamins B_6 [pyridoxine], B_{12} [cobalamine], C, and E, zinc, magnesium, and selenium) are affected by oral contraceptive agents (OCAs),[49] but vitamin deficiencies have been identified with marginal diets only. Low-estrogen preparations currently on the market do not adversely affect the woman's vitamin levels as much as earlier preparations. Lower levels of water-soluble vitamins are a result of decreased intestinal absorption and increased metabolism. Low body reserves of B_6 may put women at risk for vitamin B_6 inadequacy during pregnancy upon cessation of OCAs.[50]

Increased amounts of pyridoxine may be indicated because estrogen increases the production of tryptophan, which uses pyridoxine in its metabolism. Supplements are appropriate if a deficiency is diagnosed by laboratory evaluation; increasing intake of vitamin B_6-rich foods is appropriate to avoid side effects of excessive amounts. Depression and impaired glucose tolerance attributed to OCAs may be alleviated with pyridoxine supplementation. Since nutrient intake of many women taking OCAs may not be adequate, or they may have an unhealthy lifestyle or poor nutrient absorption, to reduce side effects of OCAs and prevent vitamin and mineral deficiencies, a multivitamin–mineral supplement may be advisable.[49,51] Progestins can cause weight gain related to increased appetite and altered carbohydrate metabolism. Estrogens may lead to an increase in subcutaneous fat and fluid retention.

Use of OCAs is associated with increased risk of cardiovascular disease (CVD) related to changes in serum lipids. Progestin may cause elevation of low-density lipoprotein, total cholesterol, and triglyceride levels (discussed in Chapter 6). The net effect on serum lipids depends on the amount and ratio of progestin and estrogens.

Menopause

During different stages of life, hormonal changes have many repercussions on general health. Female hormonal changes may be related to increased incidence of osteoporosis, which may be accompanied by some oral conditions, CVD, and certain cancers that occur later in life.

Genetics, general health, and the age of menarche influence when perimenopause and menopause actually begin (usually in the late 40s). For several years before menopause, a range of symptoms may be experienced, including changes in menstruation, fatigue, night sweats, hot flashes, insomnia, loss of bone density, and mood swings. This cluster of symptoms is called **perimenopause**. **Menopause** (decreased production of estrogen and progesterone by the ovaries, resulting in termination of menses) occurs between the ages of 35 and 58 years. Estrogen production decreases approximately 60%. Loss of beneficial effects of estrogen causes health and nutrition issues.

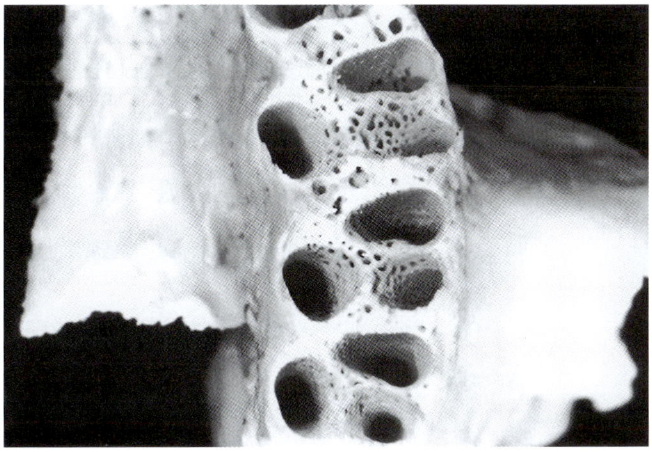

• **Figure 13.6** Alveoli of the molar area. Note the thinness of the buccal plates over the first molar roots compared with those of the second and third maxillary molars. The third molar alveoli are rarely separated as distinctly as in this specimen. (Nelson SJ. *Wheeler's Dental Anatomy, Physiology, and Occlusion.* 10th ed. St. Louis, MO: Elsevier Saunders; 2015.)

Lower estrogen levels affect the natural process of bone turnover, resulting in a decrease of bone mass. Estrogen receptors on the bone-resorbing osteoclasts increase activity in response to the estrogen level, whereas estrogen receptors on the bone-forming osteoblasts decrease their activity. Bone resorption exceeds bone formation, with significant trabecular and cortical bone loss. Rate of bone loss is rapid in early menopause, then slows and gradually decreases for 8 to 10 years after menstruation ceases. This bone loss may result in osteopenia or osteoporosis (discussed in *Health Application 9* in Chapter 9). The alveolar bone provides a potential labile source of calcium; changes in the alveolar process may signify potential diagnosis of osteoporosis (Fig. 13.6). A referral to the health care provider should be offered.

Reduced salivary gland secretion is a possible cause for increased dental caries and may lead to increased prevalence of oral **dysesthesia** (impairment of the sense of touch) and taste alterations. Senile **atrophic gingivitis** (abnormally pale gingival tissues) may develop concurrently. **Menopausal gingivostomatitis** (dry and shiny gingivae and edematous mucosa) results in easily bleeding gingiva that may be abnormally pale to quite erythematous. Postmenopausal women with osteoporosis exhibit an exaggerated response to dental plaque biofilm, including increased bleeding on probing, loss of dentoalveolar bone height, and decreased bone mineral density of the alveolar crestal and subcrestal bone. Uncontrolled osteoporosis may lead to edentulism; markedly resorbed residual alveolar ridges may be unsuitable for conventional dentures (see Fig. 13.6).

Declines in estrogen and progesterone production are accompanied by unfavorable changes in body composition (increased abdominal fat and decreased lean tissue). Weight gain is a major health concern of postmenopausal women. Weight loss becomes more difficult because body metabolism is lower and physical activity may be reduced. Weight loss during this stage of life requires greater focus on dietary monitoring, home-prepared meals, and increasing physical activity. Weight loss has been associated with bone mineral density loss and increased fracture risk that may not recover with weight regain.[52–54] Following intentional weight loss, weight gain frequently follows; even partial weight regain is associated with increased cardiometabolic risk.[55] Despite the possible need to lose weight, maintaining lean muscle mass is more important to prevent age-related functional and mental declines. Higher levels of protein consumption (up to 2.02 g/kg body weight) along with physical activity are positively associated with maintaining lean muscle mass.[56]

Medically, symptoms of perimenopause and menopause may be treated with **hormone replacement therapy (HRT)**, which consists of low levels of estrogen and progesterone. This treatment is controversial, but when HRT treatment is initiated at the onset of menopause, increased osteoblastic activity may reduce risk of osteoporosis and promote oral health by inhibiting gingival inflammation, periodontitis, and consequent loss of teeth. If symptoms significantly affect quality of life, decisions regarding HRT should involve the woman's genetic and medical history. Plant-based foods, such as legumes and soybeans, provide phytoestrogens and soluble fiber that may potentially reduce menopausal symptoms (i.e., hot flashes and night sweats) and may regulate blood cholesterol levels. Foods containing phytoestrogens include soy products or isoflavone extracts. Herbal supplements also used to decrease menopausal symptoms include Ginkgo biloba, black cohosh, and flaxseed. Studies acknowledge that soy isoflavone supplements containing a sufficient amount of genistein, derived by extraction or chemical synthesis, alleviate hot flashes and are safe. Approximately 40 to 50 mg per day may be necessary, but further studies are needed to confirm dose, isoflavone form, and treatment duration.[57,58]

Nutritional approaches to reducing menopausal symptoms continue to focus on quality of dietary choices and healthy weight maintenance. Adequate amounts of calcium, vitamins D and K, and magnesium are important for protecting bone health. Intake of adequate amounts of fruits, vegetables, and grains, following the *Dietary Guidelines*, are effective in possibly reducing risk of cancer and CVD. Although a reduction in total energy consumption is necessary to prevent weight gain, adequate protein intake is important—at least three servings of iron-rich foods daily. Physical exercise, including aerobic activity and resistance and weight-bearing exercise, is beneficial for bone and cardiovascular health and weight control.

DENTAL CONSIDERATIONS

Assessments

- *Physical:* Age, medical history (including drugs taken), dental history, oral examination, physical activity, oral radiographic findings.
- *Dietary:* Health and nutritional knowledge and skills, adequacy of calcium and vitamin D intake from food and supplements, caffeine intake.

Interventions

- Maintain meticulous daily oral self-care to reduce the risk for periodontal disease resulting from an exaggerated response to plaque biofilm.
- For xerostomia, provide information on preventive strategies, such as home and therapeutic fluoride applications; use of xylitol gum or mints; and minimizing choices of cariogenic snacks and beverages to reduce caries risk (see Chapter 20).
- Patients not prescribed HRT or other medications to deter progressive bone loss may exhibit increased alveolar bone loss; their periodontal condition should be carefully monitored at regular intervals with the use of oral radiographs.

NUTRITIONAL DIRECTIONS

- Encourage a minimum of three servings of low-fat dairy products or foods fortified with calcium and vitamin D to maintain bone mass. Consumption of greater than 90 mg per day of isoflavones in soy products may be effective in increasing bone mass of menopausal women.
- Calcium and vitamin D supplementation beyond the UL is not advisable unless recommended by a health care provider.
- Encourage good sources of lean protein and regular exercise to maintain muscle mass.
- Choose whole grains, vegetables, fruit, low-fat dairy products, and lean meat or soy substitutes to minimize risk of CVD and to maximize bone health.
- If xerostomia is present, recommend avoidance of alcohol and alcohol-containing products to minimize burning and discomfort in the oral tissues.
- Provide nutritional advice about noncariogenic snack choices.

HEALTH APPLICATION 13

Fetal Alcohol Spectrum Disorder

The Centers for Disease Control and Prevention, American College of Obstetricians and Gynecologists, American Academy of Pediatrics, and March of Dimes all recommend total abstinence from alcohol intake during pregnancy. No prenatal period has proven to be safe from the deleterious effects of alcohol. Consumption of alcohol during pregnancy is the leading cause of preventable birth defects and intellectual and neurodevelopmental disabilities.[22]

Fetal alcohol syndrome (FAS) is a cluster of birth defects resulting from prenatal alcohol exposure. An infant with FAS exhibits full effects of the alcohol (Box 13.2), characterized by a pattern of minor facial anomalies, prenatal and postnatal growth retardation, and functional or structural central nervous system abnormalities. Fetal alcohol spectrum disorder (FASD) is a combination of irreversible birth defects and behavioral challenges in infants and children whose mothers consumed alcohol during pregnancy. Approximately 2% to 5% of school-age children show signs of prenatal alcohol exposure.[59] Worldwide, about 119,000 infants are born each year with fetal alcohol syndrome; approximately 15 per 10,000 people have fetal alcohol syndrome.[60] Small amounts of alcohol consumption may be associated with adverse effects, such as spontaneous abortion, growth retardation, cleft palate, or some of the neurologic and behavioral effects of FASD without physical abnormalities. Prenatal alcohol exposure can cause damage to the brain, resulting in significant problems with regulating behavior and optimal thinking and learning. This condition, called fetal alcohol effects, is difficult to diagnose.

A group of experts on FASDs proposed clinical guidelines for diagnosing FASD in 2016.[59] These new guidelines clarify and expand previous guidelines to help clinicians distinguish among the four distinct subtypes of FASD (see Box 13.3), to evaluate facial and physical deformities characteristic of FASD and information about cognitive and/or behavioral impairments seen in different FASD subtypes.

The first trimester, especially the first month, is the most vulnerable time for the fetus because the woman may not even be aware of the pregnancy. Four to five drinks a day, or at least 45 drinks per month, can produce the full FAS (see Box 13.2). The FAS child has specific physiologic deformities (Fig. 13.7), but how alcohol affects the fetus is not fully understood. Accumulation of toxic levels of alcohol may interfere with cell formation. Several nutrients—especially folic acid, magnesium, and zinc—may be involved. The mental and physical abnormalities cannot be reversed.

Even with adequate nutrition, normal development of fetal organs is jeopardized. Other habits that usually accompany alcohol consumption (e.g., smoking, excessive amounts of coffee the “morning after,” poor eating habits with little attention to needed nutrients, and perhaps use of tranquilizers) may also adversely affect the unborn child. Ethanol is a source of energy; chronic alcoholics may have a relatively low intake of protein, essential fats, vitamins, and minerals. Alcohol may impair placental transport of amino acids, calcium, and some vitamins.

Because the brain has a special affinity for alcohol, it is one of the first organs affected. Intellectual impairment is frequently reported in children with FAS. Even at birth, the circumference of the head is small (microcephaly), indicating abnormal brain capacity (i.e., weight of 140 g in an infant with FAS compared with a normal brain weighing 400 g). Fewer brain cells exist, with damaged cells preventing normal functioning; fewer neurons result in disorganized thought. The thinking ability of the brain is permanently disturbed. The average IQ is 68; maladaptive behaviors are common. Additionally, as a result of fewer total body cells, abnormal weight gain affects normal cell development and growth.

Because of global adverse effects of alcohol intake, health care providers should advise pregnant women and women who might become pregnant to abstain from alcohol. Nutritional information and other efforts to improve food intake, such as referral to a social worker for food or monetary resources, are warranted. The NAM subcommittee recommended multivitamin–mineral supplements for heavy substance abusers who have difficulty changing their habits to improve nutrient intake.

BOX 13.2 Signs of Fetal Alcohol Syndrome

Fetal alcohol syndrome is a cluster or pattern of related problems, not just a single birth defect. The severity of symptoms varies, but the symptoms are irreversible. Facial features are more difficult to identify in preschool-age children. Signs of fetal alcohol syndrome may include the following:

- Small head circumference and brain size (microcephaly)
- Distinctive facial features: small eyelid openings; eyes close together; a sunken nasal bridge; a short, upturned, undefined nose; an exceptionally thin upper lip; and a smooth skin surface between the nose and upper lip
- Oral cavity: small teeth with faulty enamel, prominent ridges in palate, cleft lip or palate, and small jaws
- Ears poorly formed and incorrectly positioned
- Heart defects
- Deformities of joints, limbs, and fingers
- Weak skeletal muscles (hypotonia) and poor coordination
- Slow physical growth before and after birth
- Vision difficulties, including nearsightedness (myopia)
- Intellectual disabilities and delayed development
- Abnormal behavior such as poor judgment, distractibility and short attention span, hyperactivity, poor impulse control, extreme nervousness and anxiety, and social interaction problems

• BOX 13.3 Subtypes of Fetal Alcohol Syndrome

- Fetal alcohol syndrome (FAS)—most profoundly affected
- Partial fetal alcohol syndrome (PFAS)—display some but not all physical/neurodevelopmental characteristics of FAS
- Alcohol-related neurodevelopmental disorder (ARND)—demonstrate cognitive or behavior impairment with characteristic physical features
- Alcohol-related birth defects (ARBD)—physical malformations linked to maternal drinking with no other symptoms.

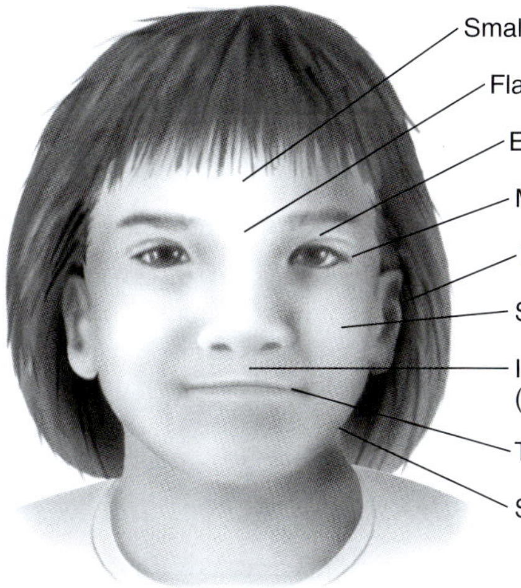

• **Figure 13.7** Fetal alcohol syndrome. (Reproduced with permission from Moore M. *Pocket Guide to Nutritional Assessment and Care.* 6th ed. St. Louis, MO: Mosby; 2009.)

◆ CASE APPLICATION FOR THE DENTAL HYGIENIST

Your regular patient, Betty, a 16-year-old, confides to you on her 6-month recare appointment that she is 3 months pregnant. Even though she and her parents have decided to keep the infant, she has not seen a health care provider yet. Betty indicates that her mother lost a tooth with each child; thus, she expects the same thing will happen to her.

Nutritional Assessment

- Knowledge about nutrition during pregnancy
- Special dietary restrictions; food fad practices; ethnic, cultural, or religious customs
- Adequacy of diet, especially calories, protein, calcium, vitamin D, iron, and folate
- Medications (including vitamin supplements), drug, and tobacco use
- Support of parents, living arrangements, and social support
- Psychological status and feelings about the reality of becoming a mother at such a young age

Nutritional Diagnosis

Altered nutrition: less than body requirements related to lack of nutritional information and weight concerns.

Nutritional Goals

The patient will consume a well-balanced diet (based on *MyPlate* website for pregnant and breastfeeding women, https://www.choosemyplate.gov/moms-pregnancy-breastfeeding) with additional calories during the second and third trimesters, and will verbalize ways to increase protein, iron, calcium, and folate intake.

Nutritional Implementation

Intervention: Encourage Betty to visit a health care provider as soon as possible.

Rationale: Fetal outcome is affected by nutrient intake during pregnancy; birth defects are likely to occur if dietary habits are poor, or if drug use occurs early in the pregnancy. Inadequate prenatal care leads to poor outcomes for the mother and fetus.

Intervention: Clarify nutritional misconceptions by providing written material and discussing the principal nutrients that need to be increased. Provide the name of an RDN with whom she can discuss these concerns.

Rationale: Nutritional requirements are quite high to meet the growth needs of the adolescent and fetus because Betty is still growing and storing nutrients in her own body.

Intervention: Teach Betty about the importance of consuming enough calcium and vitamin D during the pregnancy.

Rationale: Calcium and vitamin D are important in formation of skeletal tissue and teeth.

Intervention: Discuss fermentable carbohydrates, and determine how frequently Betty consumes them.

Rationale: Fermentable carbohydrates, especially soft foods, stick to teeth, enhance plaque formation, and increase severity of periodontal issues. Parental food selections reflect foods that a child is exposed to and accepts.

Intervention: Talk to Betty about gingivitis during pregnancy, why it occurs, and risks associated with it.

Rationale: Hormonal changes during pregnancy lead to an increased risk of oral problems affecting pregnancy outcome.

Intervention: Discuss increased nutrients requirement during pregnancy. Provide snack ideas (cheese, nuts, yogurt, milkshakes, popcorn, raw vegetables, and fruits) that contain these nutrients.

Rationale: Most teenagers have an inadequate intake of calcium, iron, and vitamins A and D. Adequate intake of calories, protein, calcium, iron, B vitamins, and zinc is essential for a healthy infant and to protect maternal stores.

Intervention: Explain the effects of her nutritional status on oral development of her infant.

Rationale: Nutrition can determine whether teeth achieve their optimum genetic potential.

Intervention: Explain why she should limit intake of coffee, tea, and especially carbonated beverages containing caffeine. Explain why she should abstain from alcohol use.

Rationale: Large amounts of caffeine could be responsible for malformations and increased susceptibility to decay of the primary first molars. Alcohol consumption may cause fetal alcohol spectrum disorder (FASD).

Evaluation

Betty should improve eating habits to consume at least the number of food groups recommended in *MyPlate* for pregnant and breastfeeding women. Other behaviors, such as decreasing sugar intake, consuming milk and dairy products (for calcium and vitamin D intake), and consuming raw fruits and green leafy vegetables (for folate intake), will increase intake of nutrients needed during pregnancy. Betty has been taking appropriate action toward oral hygiene self-care to prevent or minimize periodontal problems.

Student Readiness

1. Plan food intake for 1 day with two snacks for a gravida who has four new carious lesions. What reasons would you give her for restricting sugar intake?
2. Explain what pica is, and the type of individuals who may be practicing this behavior.
3. Why is it undesirable to lose weight during pregnancy?
4. List five effects on oral development of the fetus when maternal nutrient intake is inadequate.
5. Why is oral health care especially important during pregnancy?
6. Which nutrients may be needed if dietary assessment indicates deficient intake that cannot be corrected by changing eating habits?
7. List advantages of breastfeeding, especially on oral–motor development.

CASE STUDY

A 32-year-old mother of two children (3 years and 6 months old) who is breastfeeding complains of bleeding and sore gums and tongue. She has not visited her health care provider since the birth of her younger child because of lack of time. She has returned to her job as a clerk at a local department store. When questioned about her diet, she reports drinking a cup of coffee on her way to work; she usually takes a peanut butter and jelly sandwich and soft drink for lunch; and during the evening, she grabs something fast and easy to eat such as hot dogs, canned soup, crackers, cookies, chips, or soft drinks. She complains of being tired and irritable and feels this is because of the stress imposed on her by the two children and her work.

1. List probable causes of the mother's symptoms.
2. Discuss the added stress of pregnancy and lactation on her nutritional needs.
3. Determine other foods that should be readily available for her, such as cottage cheese, yogurt, nuts, fresh fruit, and raw vegetables.
4. Discuss possible nutrition-related causes of the "bleeding and sore gums and tongue."
5. As a dental hygienist, outline the steps to take to reach your recommendations.

References

1. Ferré C, Callaghan W, Olson C, et al. Effects of maternal age and age-specific preterm birth rates on overall preterm birth rates—United States, 2007 and 2014. *MMWR Morb Mortal Wkly Rep*. 2016;65(43):1181–1184.
2. Board on Children, Youth and Families, Food and Nutrition Board. Influence of Pregnancy Weight on Maternal and Child Health: Workshop Report. Washington, DC: National Academies Press; 2007.
3. Stang J, Huffman LG. Position of the Academy of Nutrition and Dietetics. Obesity, reproduction, and pregnancy outcomes. *J Acad Nutr Diet*. 2016;116(4):677–691.
4. Gugusheff JR, Ong ZA, Muhlhausier BS. The early origins of food preferences: targeting the critical windows of development. *FASEB J*. 2015;29(2):365–373.
5. Corbett RW, Kolasa KM. Pica and weight gain in pregnancy. *Nutr Today*. 2014;49(3):101–108.
6. Hung TH, Chen SF, Hsu JJ, et al. Gestational weight gain and risks for adverse perinatal outcomes: A retrospective cohort study based on the 2009 Institute of Medicine guidelines. *Taiwan J Obstet Gynecol*. 2015;54(4):421–425.
7. Haugen M, Brantsaeter AL, Winkvist A, et al. Associations of pre-pregnancy body mass index and gestational weight gain with pregnancy outcome and postpartum weight retention: a prospective observational cohort study. *BMC Pregnancy Childbirth*. 2014;14:201.
8. Richmond RC, Timpson NJ, Felix JF, et al. Using genetic variation to explore the causal effect of maternal pregnancy adiposity on future offspring adiposity: a Mendelian randomisation study. *PLoS Med*. 2017;14(1):e1002221.
9. Azofeifa A, Yeung LF, Alverson CJ, et al. Dental caries and periodontal disease among U.S. pregnant women and nonpregnant women of reproductive age, National Health and Nutrition Examination Survey, 1999–2004. *J Public Health Dent*. 2016;76(4):320–329.
10. Geisinger ML, Geurs NC, Bain JL, et al. Oral health education and therapy reduces gingivitis during pregnancy. *J Clin Periodontol*. 2014;41(2):141–148.
11. Poza E, Mesa F, Ikram MH, et al. Preterm birth and/or low birth weight are associated with periodontal disease and the increased placental immunohistochemical expression of inflammatory markers. *Histol Histopathol*. 2016;31(2):231–237.
12. Soroye AM, Ayanbadejo P, Savage K, et al. Association between periodontal disease and pregnancy outcomes. *Odontostomatol Trop*. 2015;38(152):5–16.
13. Hickman MA, Boggess KA, Moss KL, et al. Maternal periodontal disease is associated with oxidative stress during pregnancy. *Am J Perinatol*. 2011;28(3):247–252.
14. Srinivas SK, Parry S. Periodontal disease and pregnancy outcomes: time to move on? *J Womens Health (Larchmt)*. 2012;21(2):121–125.
15. Fogacci MF, Vettore MV, Leão AT. The effect of periodontal therapy on preterm low birth weight: a meta-analysis. *Obstet Gynecol*. 2011;117(1):153–165.
16. Uppal A, Uppal S, Pinto A, et al. The effectiveness of periodontal disease treatment during pregnancy in reducing the risk of experiencing preterm birth and low birth weight: a meta-analysis. *J Am Dent Assoc*. 2010;141(12):1423–1434.
17. Polyzos NP, Polyzos IP, Zavos A, et al. Obstetric outcomes after treatment of periodontal disease during pregnancy: systematic review and meta-analysis. *BMJ*. 2010;341:c7017.
18. Rhee J, Kim R, Kim Y, et al. Maternal caffeine consumption during pregnancy and risk of low birth weight: a dose–response meta-analysis of observational studies. *PLoS ONE*. 2015;10(7):30132334.
19. Jahanfar S, Jaafar SH. Effects of restricted caffeine intake by mother on fetal neonatal and pregnancy outcomes. *Cochrane Database Syst Rev*. 2015;(6):CD006965.
20. March of Dimes. Caffeine in pregnancy. Last reviewed October 2015. http://www.marchofdimes.org/pregnancy/caffeine-in-pregnancy.aspx. Accessed January 17, 2017.
21. Williams JF, Smith VC. Committee on Substance Abuse. Fetal alcohol spectrum disorders. *Pediatrics*. 2015;136(5):e1395–e1406.
22. U.S. Department of Agriculture (USDA). Keep yourself and your baby safe from listeriosis. Updated July 2, 2015. https://www.choosemyplate.gov/moms-food-safety-listeriosis. Accessed January 17, 2017.
23. U.S. Department of Agriculture (USDA). Keep yourself and your baby safe from toxoplasmosis. Updated July 2, 2015. https://www.choosemyplate.gov/moms-food-safety-toxoplasmosis. Accessed January 17, 2017.
24. U.S. Food and Drug Administration (FDA). Fish: what pregnant women and parents should know. Draft updated advice by FDA and EPA, June 2014. http://www.fda.gov/Food/FoodborneIllnessContaminants/Metals/ucm393070.htm. Accessed January 17, 2017.
25. Schroth RJ, Lavelle C, Tate R, et al. Prenatal vitamin D and dental caries in infants. *Pediatrics*. 2014;133(5):e1277–e1284.
26. Banfield EC, Liu Y, Davis JS, et al. Poor adherence to US *Dietary Guidelines* for children and adolescents in the National Health and Nutrition Examination Survey population. *J Acad Nutr Diet*. 2016;116(1):21–27.

27. Jebeile H, Mijatovic J, Louie JC, et al. A systematic review and metaanalysis of energy intake and weight gain in pregnancy. *Am J Obstet Gynecol.* 2016;214(4):465–483.
28. Gilmore LA, Butte NF, Ravussin E, et al. Energy intake and energy expenditure for determining excess weight gain in pregnant women. *Obstet Gynecol.* 2016;127(5):884–892.
29. Blumfield ML, Schreurs M, Rollo ME, et al. The association between portion size, nutrient intake and gestational weight gain: a secondary analysis in the WATCH study 2006/7. *J Hum Nutr Diet.* 2016;29(3):271–280.
30. Jia X, Pakseresht M, Wattar N, et al. Women who take n-3 long-chain polyunsaturated fatty acid supplements during pregnancy and lactation meet the recommended intake. *Appl Physiol Nutr Metab.* 2015;40(5):474–481.
31. Kaiser LL, Campbell CG. Practice paper of the Academy of Nutrition and Dietetics: Nutrition and lifestyle for a healthy pregnancy outcome. *J Acad Nutr Diet.* 2014;114(7):1099–1103.
32. Cusack KL, Smit E, Kile ML, et al. Regional and temporal trends in blood mercury concentrations and fish consumption in women of child bearing age in the United States using NHANES data from 1999-2010. *Environ Health.* 2017;16(1):10.
33. American College of Obstetrics and Gynecology (ACOG) Committee on Obstetric Practice. Opinion No. 495: Vitamin D: Screening and supplementation during pregnancy. *Obstet Gynecol.* 2011;118(1):197–198. Reaffirmed 2015. http://www.acog.org/Resources-And-Publications/Committee-Opinions/Committee-on-Obstetric-Practice/Vitamin-D-Screening-and-Supplementation-During-Pregnancy. Accessed January 18, 2017.
34. Women falling short on birth defect prevention. MedlinePlus. October 13, 2017. http://www.health.com/healthday/women-falling-short-birth-defect-prevention. Accessed October 24, 2017.
35. U.S. Preventive Services Task Force (USPSTF). Recommendation Statement. Folic acid supplementation for the prevention of neural tube defects. *JAMA.* 2017;317(2):183–189.
36. U.S. Food and Drug Administration New Release. FDA approves folic acid fortification of corn masa flour. April 14, 2016. http://www.fda.gov/NewsEvents/Newsroom/PressAnnouncements/ucm496104.htm. Accessed January 18, 2017.
37. Lemen A, George NI. Estimation of iodine nutrition and thyroid function status in late-gestation pregnant women in the United States: development and application of a population-based pregnancy model. *Toxicol Appl Pharmacol.* 2017;314:24–38.
38. De Leo S, Pearce EN, Braverman LE. Iodine supplementation in women during preconception, pregnancy, and lactation: current clinical practice by US Obstetricians and Midwives. *Thyroid.* 2017;27(3):434–439.
39. Council on Environmental Health, Rogan WJ, Paulson JA, et al. Iodine deficiency, pollutant chemicals, and the thyroid: new information on an old problem. *Pediatrics.* 2014;133(6):1163–1166.
40. Leung AM, Pearce EN, Braverman LE. Iodine content of prenatal multivitamins in the United States. *N Engl J Med.* 2009;360(9):939–990.
41. Prado EL, Sebayang SK, Apriatni M, et al. Maternal multiple micronutrient supplementation and other biomedical and socioenvironmental influences on children's cognition at age 9–12 years in Indonesia: follow-up of the SUMMIT randomised trial. *Lancet Glob Health.* 2017;5(2):3217.
42. United States Department of Health and Human Services (USDHHS). Healthy People 2020: Reduce iron deficiency among pregnant females, NWS-22. https://www.healthypeople.gov/2020/topics-objectives/topic/nutrition-and-weight-status/objectives?topicId=29. Accessed January 18, 2017.
43. Centers for Disease Control and Prevention (CDC). Breastfeeding rates continue to rise in the US. https://www.cdc.gov/breastfeeding/data/breastfeeding-report-card-2016.html. Accessed January 18, 2017.
44. Centers for Disease Control and Prevention (CDC). Healthy People 2020 Objectives for the Nation. Healthy People 2020 Breastfeeding Objectives. https://www.cdc.gov/breastfeeding/policy/hp2020.htm. Accessed on January 18, 2017.
45. Centers for Disease Control and Prevention (CDC). Progress in increasing breastfeeding and reducing racial/ethnic differences—United States, 2000–2008 Births. *MMWR Morb Mortal Wkly Rep.* 2013;62(05):77–80.
46. U.S. Preventive Services Task Force, Bibbins-Domingo K, Grossman DC, et al. Primary care interventions to support breastfeeding: US Preventive Services Task Force Recommendation Statement. *JAMA.* 2016;316(16):1688–1693.
47. Peres KG, Nascimento GG, Peres MA, et al. Impact of prolonged breastfeeding on dental caries: a population-based birth cohort study. *Pediatrics.* 2017;140(1):e20162943. doi:10.1542/peds.2016-2943.
48. Bagnoli F, Casucci M, Toti S, et al. Is vitamin D supplementation necessary in healthy full-term breastfed infants? A follow-up study of bone mineralization in healthy full-term infants with and without supplemental vitamin D. *Minerva Pediatr.* 2013;65(3):253–260.
49. Palmery M, Saraceno A, Vaiarelli A, et al. Oral contraceptives and changes in nutritional requirements. *Eur Rev Med Pharmacol Sci.* 2013;17(13):1804–1813.
50. Wilson SM, Bivins BN, Russell KA, et al. Oral contraceptive use: impact on folate, vitamin B_6, and vitamin B_{12} status. *Nutr Rev.* 2011;69(10):572–583.
51. Mohammad-Alizadeh-Charandabi S, Mirghafourvand M, Froghy L, et al. The effect of multivitamin supplement on continuation rate and side effects of combined oral contraceptives: a randomised controlled trial. *Eur J Contracept Reprod Health Care.* 2015;20(5):361–371.
52. Compston JE, Wyman A, FitzGerald G, et al. Increase in fracture risk following unintentional weight loss in postmenopausal women: the global longitudinal study of osteoporosis in women. *J Bone Miner Res.* 2016;31(7):1466–1472.
53. Von Thun NL, Sukumar D, Heymsfield SB, et al. Does bone loss begin after weight loss ends? Results 2 years after weight loss or regain in postmenopausal women. *Menopause.* 2014;21(5):501–508.
54. Villalon KL, Gozansky WS, Van Pelt RE, et al. A losing battle: weight regain does not restore weight loss-induced bone loss in postmenopausal women. *Obesity (Silver Spring).* 2011;19(12):2345–2350.
55. Beavers DP, Beavers KM, Lyles MF, et al. Cardiometabolic risk after weight loss and subsequent weight regain in overweight and obese postmenopausal women. *J Gerontol A Biol Sci Med Sci.* 2013;68(6):691–698.
56. Martinez JA, Wertheim BC, Thomson CA, et al. Physical activity modifies the association between dietary protein and lean mass of postmenopausal women. *J Acad Nutr Diet.* 2017;117(2):192–203.
57. Thomas AJ, Ismail R, Taylor-Swanson L, et al. Effects of isoflavones and amino acid therapies for hot flashes and co-occurring symptoms during the menopausal transition and early postmenopause: a systematic review. *Maturitas.* 2014;78(4):263–276.
58. Messina M. Soybean isoflavones warrant greater consideration as a treatment for the alleviation of menopausal hot flashes. *Womens Health (Lond).* 2014;10(6):549–553.
59. Hoyme HE, Kalberg WO, Elliott AJ, et al. Updated clinical guidelines for diagnosing fetal alcohol spectrum disorders. *Pediatrics.* 2016;138(2):pii: e20154256.
60. Popova S, Lange S, Probst C, et al. Estimation of national, regional, and global prevalence of alcohol use during pregnancy and fetal alcohol syndrome: a systematic review and meta-analysis. *Lancet Glob Health.* 2017;5(3):e290–e299.

EVOLVE RESOURCES

Please visit http://evolve.elsevier.com/Stegeman/nutritional for additional practice and study support tools.

14

Nutritional Requirements During Growth and Development and Eating Habits Affecting Oral Health

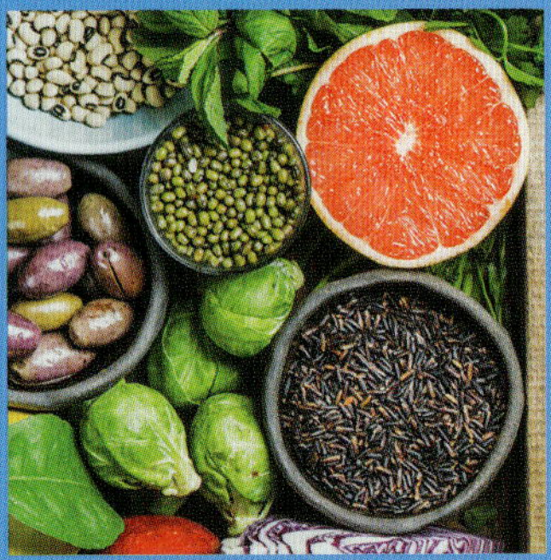

STUDENT LEARNING OUTCOMES

Upon completion of this chapter, the student will be able to achieve the following student learning outcomes:

1. The following are related to the growth and development of infants:
   - Discuss the growth and nutritional requirements of infants.
   - Describe how breast milk and artificial milk affect the oral health of infants.
   - Outline the timetable for introducing complementary foods and list reasons for their introduction.
   - Discuss ways to handle typical feeding problems that occur in infants.
   - Discuss oral health concerns and physiologic changes that alter the nutritional status of infants.
2. Discuss dietary recommendations for children older than 2 years of age as described in the *Dietary Guidelines*, *Healthy People 2020*, and *MyPlate*.
3. With regard to growth and development of toddlers and preschool children:
   - Discuss the growth and nutritional requirements of toddlers and preschool children.
   - Describe feeding patterns of toddlers and preschool children and how they relate to oral health.
4. Describe various theories behind the root cause of attention-deficit/hyperactivity disorder (ADHD), as well as oral hygiene implications related to children who have various special needs.
5. Discuss the dental caries and food habits of school-age children.
6. Discuss growth and nutrient requirements of adolescents, as well as influential factors that may affect food choices in an adolescent, and how to give nutritional advice to an adolescent.

KEY TERMS

Bruxism
Cleft lip
Cleft palate
Complementary feeding period
Early childhood caries (ECC)
Food jags
Hydrolyzed protein
Innate
Necrotizing enterocolitis
Nonnutritive sucking
Overjet
Retrognathic
Sealants
Suckling

TEST YOUR NQ

1. **T/F** Commercial infant formulas are standard in their nutrient content.
2. **T/F** Fluoride should be provided to all infants from birth if the water supply is not fluoridated.
3. **T/F** Solid foods should be introduced at 6 weeks of age.
4. **T/F** Peanuts and peanut butter should not be given to infants before age 2 to avoid peanut allergy.
5. **T/F** More nutrients are required during adolescence than during any other stage of life.
6. **T/F** Toddlers may refuse to eat anything except one food for several days.
7. **T/F** Breastfed infants do not need any supplements during the first 4 months.
8. **T/F** Bottle-fed infants are less likely to develop malocclusion.
9. **T/F** Children outgrow their need for milk.
10. **T/F** To reduce risk of plaque biofilm, toddlers and children should not be given snacks.

Proper nutrition during the first 1000 days is a critical period, having a profound impact on an infant's ability to grow, learn, and thrive. The first 1000 days includes nutrition of the mother during pregnancy until the infant reaches age 2 years. During this period, optimal nutrition builds the foundation for brain structure and capacity, lifelong health, and well-being. Achievement of goals established in *Healthy People 2020* will benefit the health of infants and children in the United States, affecting their long-term health status and lifespan.

Infants

An infant's health status, beginning at conception and affecting lifelong well-being, depends on feeding and nurturing the newborn by the mother or caretaker. Infancy is a time of rapid transition from virtually nothing but milk to a varied diet consisting of selections from all the food groups being consumed daily. The infant is normally able to thrive on human milk or commercially available, artificial infant milk, but many physiologic systems are immature at birth. Because of limited stomach capacity, frequent feedings are needed.

Pregnant patients expect the dental hygienist to provide information concerning infant feeding methods affecting the oral cavity. Practitioners should be prepared to address these issues basing their advice on scientific evidence. Feeding patterns present during the child's first 2 years create an environment for optimal development of genetically determined factors contributing to orofacial development and swallowing patterns.

Growth

Growth is the definitive test of health and is used as the most sensitive and specific indicator of nutritional status. Increased size results in greater nutritional requirements, but the need for calories per kilogram decreases as one grows. Dental hygienists working with new parents, infants, and children should be familiar with normal growth and developmental patterns that reflect adequacy of nutritional intake. The birthweight of an infant doubles in 4 months (from 7.5–15 lb) and usually triples by 1 year of age. Length or height increases 50% by 1 year of age. Charts developed by Centers for Disease Control and Prevention (CDC) for determining appropriate growth rates are available on the Evolve website.

Nutritional Requirements

Adequate nutrition is more important during infancy and childhood than during any other stage of the life cycle. As might be expected from the rapid growth rate, energy requirements are much higher per pound or kilogram of weight than for an adult: 95 to 83 cal/kg per day between 3 and 12 months of age (energy needs per kg decrease from birth to 12 months) versus 29 to 37 cal/kg per day for adults. Infants have a higher resting metabolic rate and intestinal absorption is relatively inefficient.

Adequate Intake (AI) for protein is 1.52 g/kg daily from birth to 6 months of age, and the Recommended Dietary Allowance (RDA) for older infants is 1.2 g/kg; this translates to about 9.1 to 13 g per day (Table 14.1). Recommended protein intakes are

TABLE 14.1 Dietary Reference Intakes (DRI) for Infants Compared With Nutrient Content of Human Breast Milk, Cow's Milk, and Artificial Breast Milk

	DIETARY REFERENCE INTAKE[a]				
Nutrient	**0–6 Months Old**	**7–12 Months Old**	**Human Breast Milk (Per Liter)**	**Cow's Milk[b] (Per Liter)**	**Average Artificial Breast Milk (Per Liter)[c]**
Calorie	95 cal/kg (3 months)*[d] 85 cal/kg (6 months)*[d]	83 cal/kg[c]	670 cal	563 cal	660 cal
Protein	9.1 g/day*	**13.5 g/day**	13 g	29 g	13–15 g
Fat	31 g/day*	30 g/day*	40–45 g	30 g	36 g
Cholesterol	ND	ND	100–200 mg	92 mg	10–30 mg
Calcium	200 mg/day*	260 mg/day*	350 mg	1043 mg	510–520 mg
Phosphorus	100 mg/day*	275 mg/day*	121–150 mg	776 mg	280–300 mg
Iron	0.27 mg/day*	**11 mg/day**	0.76 mg	0.27 mg	12 mg
Sodium	120 mg/day*	370 mg/day*	150–170 mg	397 mg	160–180 mg
Potassium	400 mg/day*	700 mg/day*	530 mg	1162 mg	690–720 mg
Renal solute load (mOsm/L)	N/A	N/A	91.1	221	126–136

Note: Recommended Dietary Allowances (RDAs) are presented in **bold type** and Adequate Intakes (AIs) are followed by an asterisk (*).
N/A, Not applicable; ND, not determined.
[a]Data from National Research Council: *The Guide to Nutrient Requirements.* Washington, DC: National Academies Press; 2006, and National Research Council: *Dietary Reference Intakes For Calcium and Vitamin D.* Washington, DC: National Academies Press; 2011.
[b]Whole milk (3.5% fat content). U.S. Department of Agriculture, Agricultural Research Service, Nutrient Data Laboratory. USDA National Nutrient Database for Standard Reference, Release 28. Version Current: September 2015. https://ndb.nal.usda.gov/ndb/search/list Accessed February 14, 2017.
[c]Standard infant formulas–Enfamil with iron, Similac with iron. US Department of Agriculture, Agricultural Research Service, Nutrient Data Laboratory. USDA National Nutrient Database for Standard Reference, Release 28. Version Current: September 2015. https://ndb.nal.usda.gov/ndb/search/list. Accessed February 14, 2017.
[d]Total energy expenditure.

based on mean protein intake of breastfed infants. At birth, renal functions are immature; total protein should not exceed 20% of the calories. Breast milk and artificial breast milk (commercial formula) provide approximately 50% of calories from fat to supply the high-energy needs.

Breast Milk

Human milk, nature's superfood for infants, is the optimal source of appropriate amounts of nutrients to help infants reach their maximum potential (Fig. 14.1). Human milk is very complex, and its exact chemical makeup is unknown. It contains living cells, hormones, active enzymes, and antibodies. Specific protein fractions synthesized in breast tissue promote colonies of healthy bacteria in the gastrointestinal tract that aid nutrient absorption and help protect infants from infections and illness. This is especially advantageous because the infant's immune system is not fully developed. Exclusive breastfeeding for at least 4 months is strongly recommended by numerous organizations in the United States and worldwide to reduce the incidence of gastrointestinal and respiratory infections, ear infections, and eczema; and to reduce long-term incidence of obesity and other chronic health conditions. The availability of required nutrients promotes optimal brain development.[1] Regardless of the mother's nutritional status, overall breast milk composition is constant, yet changing to meet the infant's nutritional needs.

Breast milk is normally thin, with a slightly bluish color. Breast milk contains substantial amounts of long-chain fatty acids (arachidonic acid [ARA] and docosahexaenoic acid [DHA]), which are important in brain and retinal tissue development. Human milk is relatively high in cholesterol. Lipase enzyme inherent in breast milk improves fat digestion. The low mineral and relatively low protein content of human milk is ideal for the infant's immature kidneys. Inherent compounds in human milk promote efficient iron utilization. Iron deficiency in exclusively breastfed infants is rare despite the low iron content of breast milk. Additional sources of iron are unnecessary during the first 4 to 6 months for breastfed infants. Supplemental foods during that time may reduce iron absorption.

Breast milk is least likely to trigger an allergic reaction; therefore, breastfeeding is highly recommended, especially for infants at risk for developing food allergies. Breastfeeding for at least 4 months may potentially prevent allergies (especially asthma and eczema), but its role in preventing allergies is controversial.[2–5] Some studies fail to confirm conventional wisdom that breastfeeding is protective against allergy and asthma.

Breast milk provides approximately 0.01 mg per day of fluoride, regardless of drinking water and maternal plasma levels. Despite the low fluoride levels, infants who are breastfed up to 12 months are not at risk of dental caries.[6] As shown in Table 14.2, the American Dental Association and American Academy of Pediatric Dentistry (AAPD) recommend delaying fluoride supplements for all infants until 6 months of age.

Artificial Infant Milk

Although nutrients differ slightly for various brands, all commercial formulas comply with standards set by the Infant Formula Act established in 1980 (see Table 14.1). The U.S. Food and Drug Administration requires that these products meet strict standards. Artificial infant milk formulas duplicate breast milk as closely as technology allows, but the exact composition of breast milk cannot be reproduced and artificial infant milk cannot match the benefits of breast milk. Artificial infant formulas are continually being modified to ensure growth and performance of formula-fed infants matches that of breastfed infants. Adequate nutrients (except for fluoride) are provided in 150 to 180 ml/kg per day commercial formula with iron or an appropriate caloric concentration (about

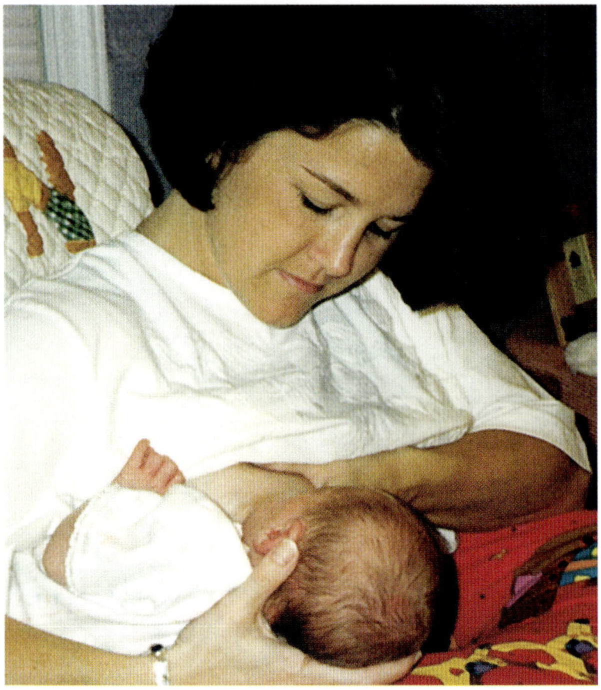

• **Figure 14.1** Breastfeeding promotes a special bonding between mother and infant. (Reprinted with permission from Lowdermilk DL, Perry SE. *Maternity Nursing*. 8th ed. St. Louis, MO: Mosby Elsevier; 2011.)

TABLE 14.2 Fluoride Supplementation[a]

Age	Fluoride Ion Level in Drinking Water (PPM)[a] <0.3	0.3-0.6	>0.6
Birth–6 months	None	None	None
6 months–3 years	0.25 mg/day[b]	None	None
3–6 years	0.50 mg/day	0.25 mg/day	None
6–16 years	1.0 mg/day	0.50 mg/day	None

Fluoride Supplement Dosage Schedule—2010
Approved by the American Dental Association Council on Scientific Affairs
[a]1.0 part per million (ppm) = 1 mg per liter (mg/L)
[b]2.2 mg sodium fluoride contains 1 mg fluoride ion.
American Dental Association. Oral Health Topics: Fluoride Supplements. Facts about Fluoride. http://www.ada.org/en/member-center/oral-health-topics/fluoride-supplements#dosage. Accessed January 30, 2017; and American Academy of Pediatric Dentistry (AAPD). *Clinical Practice Guidelines Reference Manual.* Revised 2014. http://www.aapd.org/media/Policies_Guidelines/G_FluorideTherapy.pdf. Accessed January 30, 2017.
From R. Gary Rozier, Steven Adair, et al. Evidence-Based Clinical Recommendations on the Prescription of Dietary Fluoride Supplements for Caries Prevention: A report of the American Dental Association Council on Scientific Affairs; The Journal of the American Dental Association;141(12), Dec 2010, Pages 1480-1489.

20 cal/oz) until the infant is 4 to 6 months old. Infants given artificial infant milk tend to weigh more than breastfed infants, a negative factor that may put them at greater risk for obesity as adults. However, more research is needed to confirm this association. Breastfed infants develop better control of their milk intake than bottle-fed infants.

Numerous commercial formulas are available to meet different needs and conditions. A health care provider should be consulted regarding any perceived intolerance to artificial breast milk. Almost all are available in different forms; the choice of powdered, concentrate, or ready-to-use is determined by the parent's preference and lifestyle. Some of the types of formulas available include: (1) standard cow's milk with and without iron, (2) soy based, (3) hypoallergenic (**hydrolyzed protein** [protein broken down into amino acids]), (4) reduced lactose or lactose free, (5) elemental formulas, and (6) specialized formulas for special metabolic problems. Other ingredients added to formulas based on new information available include DHA and ARA (natural ingredients of breast milk), added rice (for acid reflux), prebiotics and probiotics, antioxidants, and organic ingredients. When determining which formula to use, parents should discuss any problems or concerns with their health care provider. Formula manufacturers promote products that have no proven benefit; increased regulation of marketing claims by manufacturers is needed to protect consumers and ensure that they make wise decisions.[7]

Fluorosis has been associated with fluoride intake during enamel development; the severity is dependent on dose, duration, and timing of intake. Because of reported cases of fluorosis, no fluoride is added to artificial infant milk, but a small amount is inherently present as a result of some of the ingredients and processing. After 6 months of age, all infants need fluoride supplementation if local drinking water or bottled water contains less than 0.3 parts per million (ppm) of fluoride. Infants receiving breast milk or formula do not need additional water. Most bottled water does not contain fluoride. If bottled water is used for formula dilution, water specially marketed for babies (sometimes called "nursery water") contains appropriate amounts of fluoride. If local water contains too much fluoride, water that contains no or minimal amounts of fluoride—purified, demineralized, deionized, distilled, or reverse osmosis filtered water—are readily available in local stores.

Commercial artificial infant milk is more appropriate for infants than cow's or goat's milk. Malnutrition has been reported in infants fed home-recipe formulas. This may be related to variations in nutrient composition or unsanitary handling practices that may result in frequent infections or gastrointestinal disorders. In other countries, infants become malnourished and die when food manufacturers fail to include required nutrients or prevent contaminants, or when water mixed with the formula is dirty or contaminated.

Infant formulas should be discontinued by 12 to 14 months of age, and vitamin D–fortified whole milk should be provided until age 2. Low-fat milk is not recommended for children before the age of 2. Special toddler formulas are nutritionally safe and do not need refrigeration, but they are unnecessary.

Feeding Practices

Although rigid feeding schedules were employed in the past, infants today are generally fed on demand (when they are hungry). A pattern usually develops within about 2 weeks, with the infant eating six times daily at 4-hour intervals. This feeding pattern gradually evolves, eventually allowing the infant and parents to sleep through the night. Touching helps to strengthen feelings of love, security, and trust; this is as important as nutrients. An infant should never be left alone with a bottle propped during feedings.

Oral and Neuromuscular Development

Sucking is more difficult from the breast than from a bottle. Breastfeeding requires the infant to open the mouth wide, move the jaws back and forth, and squeeze with the gingiva to extract the milk, a process called **suckling**. Suckling encourages mandibular development by strengthening the jaw muscle, thus promoting maximum development of the genetically defined jaw and chin.[8] Breastfed infants are less likely to develop malocclusion—high premaxilla, abnormal alveolar ridges, and palate and posterior crossbite. Early weaning may interrupt oral motor development leading to malocclusion and oral breathing, and negatively affect swallowing, breathing, and speaking.[9–11] Infants breastfed for 1 year require 40% less orthodontia than bottle-fed infants. The fatty acid profile of human milk may confer a measure of protection against persistent stuttering.[12] Sucking from a bottle may result in narrower upper and lower dental arches. When the bottle presses against the soft bones of the palate, narrow or V-shaped palates may occur; this may be predictive of snoring and sleep apnea.[13]

Nonnutritive sucking (sucking on thumb, fingers, or a pacifier), which begins in utero, is normal, giving the child a feeling of relaxation. It is also important in development of self-regulation and ability to control emotions. Exclusive breastfeeding appears to diminish the risk of acquiring nonnutritive sucking habits.[14] Nonnutritive sucking is more prevalent in infants who were breastfed less than 6 months versus those exclusively breastfed longer than 6 months.[15,16] Use of a pacifier does not seem to interfere with successful breastfeeding if introduced after breastfeeding is established.

The effects of nonnutritive sucking on developing dentition are minor in a child under 3 years. However, if it continues after this age, dental-maxillary anomalies may occur: open-bite, narrow maxilla with upper protrusion, cross-bite; and possibly retrognathic mandible.[17–19] **Retrognathic** is the condition of a mandible posterior to its normal relationship with other facial positions. Prolonged digit-sucking increases the probability of an anterior open bite, while a pacifier-sucking habit increases problems with tooth alignment and jaw development, excessive **overjet** (horizontal projection of upper teeth beyond the lower teeth) and absence of lower arch developmental space.[18] Prolonged habits altering dento-skeletal development may lead to orthodontic problems and persist into the permanent dentition.[20] Eating is not instinctive but rather a combination of behaviors that develops during the first month, followed by primitive motor reflexes and learned behaviors. Eating is the most complex physical task humans do—using all the body's organ systems and requiring simultaneous coordination of all the sensory systems.

A successful feeding regimen (which foods or texture of food) is based on developmental stage of the infant or toddler. Nutrition is related to neuromuscular maturation, especially for infants. Suckling is replaced with sucking by 4 months of age, when orofacial muscles are used with the mouth more pursed, and the tongue moving back and forth. A forward motion of the tongue and dropping the mandible is typical during the first 3 months. If semisolid foods are offered at this time, the tongue may force food out; no discriminating taste is occurring, just reflex action.

The sucking motion becomes developed enough for the infant to eat and handle semisolid foods from a spoon around 4 to 6 months of age. Development of fine, gross, and oral motor skills to consume foods correlates with demands for additional calories and nutrients. If foods are not added by 6 months of age, growth may fall below normal growth curves.

At about 6 to 8 months old, infants develop the ability to receive food and pass it to the gingiva in a chewing motion. Eight teeth normally erupt between 6 and 12 months of age. When the infant can chew, pureed foods are not required; some variety of texture is mandatory if infants are going to accept unfamiliar foods later. Unless textured foods are offered, the development of oral musculature may be slow or delayed, affecting the child's speech.

Introduction of Foods

Good nutrition is essential for rapid growth and development that occurs during an infant's first year. As foods are added to the infant's selections to include more food groups, timing of the transition, how the infant is fed, and quality of foods offered can have important health implications.

Table 14.3 lists recommendations from Health Canada for feeding infants from birth to 24 months, indicating timing of introduction of supplements and types of appropriate complementary foods. The **complementary feeding period**, also called the sensitive period or critical window, occurs at about 4 months of age (but not before this time) when neither breast milk nor formula adequately meets all the nutrient requirements to promote growth and development.[21] Complementary foods begin the infant's education for developing a broad repertoire of food preferences. Complementary feeding begins when infants are mature enough to start eating from a spoon, to hold their necks steady and sit with support, draw in their lower lip as a spoon is removed from the mouth, and retain and swallow food. At 4 to 6 months of age, infants are usually developmentally ready to eat semisolid foods. The goal for introducing complementary foods is to promote a pattern of food consumption that matches the child's energy and nutrient needs for ideal growth and development but does not increase risk for becoming overweight.[22]

Numerous false assumptions are associated with introduction of solid foods. Despite the fact that many parents introduce solid foods, especially cereals, during the first month, this practice has no nutritional advantage and may be detrimental. The most common reason for early feeding is to help the infant sleep through the night. Infants will begin sleeping through the night between 1 and 3 months of age; this developmental milestone is not related to feedings.

Foods should be presented to the infant with a spoon, never in a bottle. Disadvantages in starting semisolid foods too early are (a) unnecessary costs, (b) high probability of overfeeding, (c) effects on the immature digestive system, (d) reduction of milk intake in lieu of a less nutritionally complete food, and (e) decreased iron absorption. After introduction of foods at 4 to 6 months, formula intake should remain around 32 oz daily.

There is no nutritional advantage to providing fruit juice for infants younger than 6 months; in 2017 the American Academy of Pediatrics (AAP) issued new guidelines regarding fruit juices:[23] (1) juice not be introduced to infants before 12 months of age; (2) between age 1 year and 3 years of age, 4 oz per day; and (3) increase to 4 to 6 oz per day for children 4 through 6 years of age. Their rationale for this recommendation is that juice (1) could interfere with infants consuming the amount of milk or formula needed; (2) lacks the fiber of whole fruit; (3) is easily overconsumed, possibly contributing to weight concerns; and (4) can increase the risk of tooth decay. For infants and toddlers, fruit juice can be diluted with equal portions of water in a cup, but dilution with water does not reduce the cariogenicity of the juice. To decrease risk of dental caries, fruit juice should not be given in bottles or sippy cups because these allow babies to drink easily throughout the day. Too much fruit juice—including apple, pear, and

TABLE 14.3 Key Recommendations of the Joint Statement by Health Canada on Feeding of Infants From Birth to 24 Months

Birth to 6 Months	
1	Exclusive breastfeeding for the first 6 months.
2	Supplemental vitamin D for breastfed infants.
3	Cow milk-based, commercial infant formula is the alternative when not breastfeeding. Homemade formula is not an appropriate choice. Need careful preparation and storage of the formula to reduce the risks of bacteria-related illness.
4	Feeding changes are unnecessary for most common health conditions in infancy (e.g., colic, constipation, reflux, acute gastroenteritis/diarrhea).
6–24 Months	
1	Introduction to solid foods at 6 mo when signs of physiologic and developmental readiness are observed.
2	First complementary foods should be iron-rich meat, meat alternatives, and iron-fortified cereal.
3	Offer a variety of nutritious foods from the family meals, providing a range of textures with a gradual progression.
4	Unless there is a family history of food allergy, common allergenic foods can be introduced at 6 months (consult health care provider).
5	Responsive feeding to promote the development of healthy eating skills.
6	Infant food should be prepared, served, and stored safely.

Adapted from Critch JN, Canadian Paediatric Society and Nutrition and Gastroenterology Committee. Nutrition for healthy term infants, six to 24 months: an overview. *Paediatr Child Health.* 2014;19(10):547–549. From Perreault M, Mikail S, Atkinson SA. New Health Canada Nutrition recommendations for infants birth to 24 months address the importance of early nutrition. *Nutr Today.* 2016;51(4):186–191.

prune—can cause diarrhea and decreases intake of other foods containing essential nutrients for infants and toddlers.

One of the most important factors in determining what foods to provide is to ensure that a balanced diet is offered. Providing the essential vitamins, minerals, and nutrients as needed during critical developmental stages is important. Iron-rich foods or a daily low-dose oral iron supplement should be initiated at 4 to 6 months. Table 14.4 indicates the role in growth and development for required nutrients, consequences of deficiency, critical time periods needed, and dietary sources. Age-appropriate foods of the correct consistency using an appropriate method are important for developmental and nutritional reasons.

According to the Food Allergy Research and Education organization, 8% of children have a documented food allergy. Between 1997 and 2011, food allergies increased approximately 50% in children.[24] Infants are at increased risk of developing allergies if they have at least one first-degree relative (parent or sibling) with allergies and are not exclusively breastfed for 4 to 6 months.

TABLE 14.4 The ABCs of Nutrition–Key Nutrients in the First 1000 Days

Nutrient	Role in the Body	Consequences of Deficiency	Vital Time Periods During the First 1000 Days	Dietary Sources*
Vitamin A	Critical for vision, supports cell growth and differentiation, playing a key role in the normal formation and maintenance of the heart, lungs, kidneys and other organs, immune function	Damage to the eyes, poor growth, loss of appetite, susceptibility to infections. Vitamin A deficiency is rare in the United States.	Pregnancy, infancy, early childhood	Egg yolks, liver, yellow and dark-green leafy vegetables and fruits such as spinach, kale, broccoli, sweet potatoes, pumpkin
Vitamin B6	Essential for normal brain development and function, development of neurotransmitters, chemicals that carry signals from one nerve cell to another, helps the body make the hormones serotonin and norepinephrine, which influence mood, and melatonin, which regulates the body clock.	Muscle weakness, irritability, depression, difficulty concentrating	Pregnancy, infancy, early childhood	Meat, liver, fish, chicken, potatoes and other starchy vegetables, bananas
Vitamin B12	Essential for cell health; aids in the production of DNA, the genetic material in all cells; together with folic acid, helps make red blood cells and helps iron work better in the body	Increased risk of birth defects such as neural tube defects, may contribute to preterm delivery, increased risk of poor cognitive function, failure to thrive	Pregnancy, infancy, early childhood	Meat, fish, poultry, eggs, milk and cheese
Calcium	Bone growth and health, tooth development and function, blood clotting, maintenance of healthy nerves and muscles	Greater risk of rickets, a disease characterized by swollen joints and poor growth, increased risk of bone fractures, increased vulnerability to the adverse effects of lead	Pregnancy, infancy, early childhood	Milk, cheese, yogurt and other dairy products, salmon, calcium-fortified foods

Continued

TABLE 14.4 The ABCs of Nutrition–Key Nutrients in the First 1000 Days—cont'd

Role in the Body | Consequences of Deficiency | Vital Time Periods During the First 1000 Days | Dietary Sources*

Choline

Category	Description
Role in the Body	A critical component of the cell membrane, choline is necessary for the normal function of all cells, critical during pregnancy for the development of the brain, where it can impact neural tube closure and lifelong memory and learning functions
Consequences of Deficiency	Reduced blood vessel growth in baby's brain in utero, increased risk for brain and spinal-cord defects, nerve and muscle problems, may make folate deficiency more likely
Vital Time Periods	Pregnancy, infancy
Dietary Sources	Meat, seafood, liver, egg yolks, broccoli and brussels sprouts, breast milk also has high concentrations of choline

Vitamin C

Category	Description
Role in the Body	Essential to forming collagen, a protein that gives structure to bones, muscle and other connective tissue; plays an important role in immune function and body's ability to resist infections; enhances the absorption of iron
Consequences of Deficiency	Can lead to scurvy, a serious disease which in infants can cause poor bone growth, bleeding, and anemia, bleeding gums
Vital Time Periods	Pregnancy, infancy, early childhood
Dietary Sources	Citrus fruits, tomatoes, red and green peppers, broccoli, potatoes

Vitamin D

Category	Description
Role in the Body	Critical to bone growth and health, key to a healthy immune system and immune response, promotes calcium absorption
Consequences of Deficiency	Bones can become thin, brittle or misshapen; causes rickets in children, a disease characterized by swollen joints and poor growth
Vital Time Periods	Pregnancy, infancy, early childhood
Dietary Sources	Vitamin D is produced by the skin when exposed to sunlight. Food sources of vitamin D include: fortified milk, fish, liver, egg yolks. Breast milk typically contains little vitamin D, and it is recommended that either breastfeeding mothers or breastfeeding infants take a vitamin D supplement.

Folate

Category	Description
Role in the Body	Essential for the proper development of a baby's brain and spinal cord; required for cell division, growth, and the development of healthy blood cells
Consequences of Deficiency	Greater risk of neural tube defect—a birth defect in which spinal cord does not close properly, leading to learning disability, paralysis, and babies being born with little to no brain
Vital Time Periods	Before pregnancy, pregnancy
Dietary Sources	Green leafy vegetables such as spinach and broccoli, beans, certain fruits such as bananas and melons, beef liver, fortified breads and cereals. In 1998, the U.S. Food and Drug Administration (FDA) began requiring manufacturers to add folic acid to breads, cereals, flours, cornmeals, pastas, rice, and other grain products.

Iron

Category	Description
Role in the Body	Critical for the proper brain development and function in young children, delivers oxygen to tissues, contributes to regulation of immune function and metabolism
Consequences of Deficiency	Extreme fatigue and depression, impaired cognitive development, reduced resistance to infection
Vital Time Periods	Pregnancy, infancy, early childhood
Dietary Sources	Eggs and meat, dark leafy vegetables such as spinach, legumes (e.g., beans, lentils), whole grains, fortified breads and cereals. Full-term, healthy babies typically receive enough iron from their mothers in the third trimester of pregnancy to last for the first four months of life. Exclusively breastfed babies may need to receive an iron supplement starting at four months.

TABLE 14.4 The ABCs of Nutrition–Key Nutrients in the First 1000 Days—cont'd

Role in the Body / Consequences of Deficiency / Vital Time Periods During the First 1000 Days / Dietary Sources*	
Vitamin K	
Role in the Body	Plays a key role in helping the blood clot, preventing excessive bleeding
Consequences of Deficiency	Increases the risk of uncontrolled bleeding, vitamin K deficiency bleeding can potentially result in gross motor skill deficits; long-term neurologic, cognitive, or developmental problems; organ failure or death.
Vital Time Periods	Newborn, early infancy
Dietary Sources	Because all babies are born vitamin K-deficient, a single injection of vitamin K administered at birth is standard practice in the U.S.
Long-Chain Polyunsaturated Fatty Acids (LC-PUFAs)	
Role in the Body	These fats, particularly DHA, play a major role in brain development and health. DHA is a major component of retinal and brain tissues, necessary for the formation of healthy cell membranes and support growth and immunity.
Consequences of Deficiency	Poor weight gain, lowered immunity, poor attention span, hyperactivity, or irritability, problems learning
Vital Time Periods	Pregnancy, infancy
Dietary Sources	Fresh fish and fish oils are ideal sources of LC-PUFAs. Cold water/oily fish such as salmon, mackerel, herring, tuna, sardines, anchovies are high in LC-PUFAs; as well as some seeds and nuts such as flax seeds and walnuts. Breast milk contains small but significant amounts of LC-PUFAs that are necessary for optimal development of the brain, the retina and other infant tissues.
Protein	
Role in the Body	Essential component of all cells in the body, muscle tissue, organs, and neurotransmitters in the brain, critical for proper brain development, regulates metabolism
Consequences of Deficiency	Fatigue, increased infections, muscle weakness, failure to thrive
Vital Time Periods	Pregnancy, infancy, early childhood
Dietary Sources	Eggs, meat, poultry, fish, legumes (e.g., dry beans, peas, nuts), milk and dairy products
Zinc	
Role in the Body	Essential for cell growth and metabolism, supports healthy growth and brain function, immune system, bone growth
Consequences of Deficiency	Decreased fetal movement and heart rate variability during pregnancy, possible increased risk of preterm birth, increased risk of infection, poor growth in children
Vital Time Periods	Pregnancy, infancy, early childhood
Dietary Sources	Red meat, poultry, whole grains, milk and dairy products, oysters

*In general, healthy, full-term breastfed infants receive an adequate amount of all of these nutrients with the possible exceptions of vitamin d and iron.

Courtesy of 1,000 days, 1020 19th Street NW, Suite 250, Washington, DC 20036. From *The First 1,000 Days: Nourishing America's Future.* Web site. www.thousanddays.org/resource/nourishing-americas-future.

From World Health Organization And Food and Agriculture Organization, Vitamin and Mineral Requirements in Human Nutrition, 2004;National Institutes of Health (NIH), Pediatric Nutrition Handbook, AAP 2009.

Parents report more infant adverse reactions to food than are confirmed clinically.

Because of the possibility of a food allergy, only one new food should be introduced at a time. Iron-fortified infant cereal—such as rice, oat, or barley cereal mixed with breast milk or artificial formula—may be introduced at 4 months without increasing the risk of developing an allergy to wheat. After introducing a new food, a waiting period of 2 to 3 days is recommended before introducing another new food to observe for allergic reactions. Foods most commonly causing allergies are cow's milk (including ice cream), eggs, peanuts, tree nuts (e.g., walnuts, almonds, cashews, pistachios, pecans), wheat, soy, fish, and shellfish. Infants with allergies to milk, egg, wheat, and soy may outgrow their allergy by age 5 years. Peanuts, tree nuts, fish, or shellfish allergies are generally lifelong.

The previous recommendation to withhold foods that most commonly cause allergies until after 12 months of age is outdated. Based on new evidence, the European Academy of Allergy and Clinical Immunology Taskforce on Prevention concluded that there is no reason to either postpone or encourage exposure to highly allergenic foods after 4 months once weaning has commenced, irrespective of atopic heredity.[25] Based on a recent landmark clinical trial and other research, the American Academy of Allergy, Asthma, and Immunology endorsed new guidelines recommending introduction of high allergenic foods (including peanuts) between 4 and 6 months of age along with introduction of other solid foods. Three separate guidelines and recommendations developed for health care providers describe infants based on risk of having or developing peanut allergy.[26] Introduction of these foods should be initiated at home rather than at a restaurant or day care center.

The recommended order of introduction for complementary foods (vegetables, meats, and fruits) varies among pediatricians. Some advise introduction of vegetables after cereals, then meats followed by fruits. Meats should be introduced early, especially for breastfed infants, to provide essential nutrients, such as iron and zinc.

Preference for sweet, salty, and unami flavors is an **innate** (inborn) preference over bitter or sour flavors. Because sweet flavors are well accepted, other foods (meats or vegetables) are offered first. Complementary foods without added sugars and salt and introducing a variety of flavors, including bitter green vegetables early, may influence later food preferences. Infants of weaning age may learn to like vegetables more quickly and sometimes with just one exposure to the food. Infants introduced exclusively to vegetables for the first two weeks of the complementary feeding period are much more likely to consume more vegetables at 1 year.[27] A mother's food choices, particularly for fruit and vegetables, influence later preferences and food behaviors. An infant's grimace when offered a new food is innate, not a sign of dislike. When the spoon is offered again, it is very likely to be accepted.

Commercial infant food may be used, but foods from the family menu can be pureed or finely chopped. When semisolid foods are introduced, the goal should be to include all food groups as soon as possible to ensure a well-balanced diet. Recommendations for feeding infants to provide a balance of nutrients are similar to the *Dietary Guidelines* except that fats are not limited.

Supplements

The American Academy of Pediatrics (AAP) and Health Canada recommend that exclusively breastfed infants and all nonbreastfed infants consuming less than 1000 mL of formula each day receive 400 IU (10 μg) vitamin D supplementation beginning during the first 2 months to prevent rickets and continuing until infants are weaned and are consuming 1000 mL/day or more of vitamin D–fortified formula or whole milk.[28,29] Artificial formulas marketed in the United States provide 400 IU or more of vitamin D per 1000 mL. Vitamin D supplements marketed for infants supply 400 IU/day. Despite recommendations, most American and Canadian infants do not consume adequate amounts of vitamin D.

Healthy, full-term infants require minimal amounts of iron during the first 6 months and more significant amounts after 6 months of age. If iron-fortified formula is not used, iron supplementation is recommended for infants after 4 months of age, breastfed infants at 4 to 6 months of age, and preterm infants after 2 months of age. Iron supplementation (usually ferrous sulfate or ferric ammonium citrate) is ordinarily given as liquid drops. Iron drops can cause staining on erupting teeth; this can be reduced by putting the drops in water.

Fluoride supplementation is recommended for infants older than 6 months and children to increase the strength and acid resistance of developing tooth enamel. Before fluoride supplementation is prescribed, however, the AAPD recommends a caries risk assessment along with an evaluation of dietary sources of fluoride (e.g., fluoridated water).[30] Vitamin supplements containing fluoride may be prescribed by a health care provider or dentist (see Table 14.2).

DENTAL CONSIDERATIONS

Assessment

- *Physical:* Infant's developmental stage, neuromuscular development, age, lip biting, thumb sucking, tongue thrusting, pacifier use.
- *Dietary:* Parent's knowledge of bottle-feeding, feeding of solid foods, necessity of providing oral care for the infant, source of iron, fluoride (drinking water from home, day care, and school; beverages such as soda, juice, and artificial infant milk; prepared food, and toothpaste), and use of other supplements.

Interventions

- Avoid recommending sugar-free foods, especially those containing sorbitol, which may cause diarrhea in infants and children.
- Inform parents that supplements containing fluoride should never be added to milk; fluoride binds with milk and soy proteins, decreasing availability of fluoride significantly.
- Exposure to too much fluoride before enamel maturation may alter the structure and cause fluorosis.
- Nonfluoridated or minimally fluoridated water is recommended for reconstituting powdered formulas to reduce risk of fluorosis.

NUTRITIONAL DIRECTIONS

- All water (tap or bottled, mixed with artificial infant milk or given plain) given to infants younger than 3 months old first should be boiled for 1 to 2 minutes.
- For the first 4 months of life, 32 oz of formula daily satisfies and provides all the nutrients needed for full-term infants.
- The rate of growth is faster during infancy than at any other stage of life. Fats, a concentrated source of energy, are needed to support growth (40%–50% of the total calories is recommended). Reduced-fat milk is inappropriate for children younger than 2 years.
- Children older than 1½ years of age who are still taking a bottle containing milk or sweetened liquids are more likely to be overweight and to develop anemia because of low iron intake. In addition they will have an increased risk of tooth decay.
- Despite growing concerns over cardiovascular disease (CVD), cholesterol intake is important during early developmental stages of infancy. Recommending changes in fat intake before age 2 years could be detrimental.
- Store all vitamin–mineral supplements in a place that is protected from children; many children die each year from accidental iron overdose.
- Children younger than 2 years should not consume foods or beverages with added sugars.
- Honey is inappropriate for children younger than 1 year of age because of the risk of botulism.

NUTRITIONAL DIRECTIONS—cont'd

- Toddlers learn about food by touching and playing with it. Encourage this by offering finger foods when the child can sit alone and pick up items.
- During the first year, habits and preferences are beginning to form. Fostering healthy eating habits early will promote healthful lifelong eating patterns.
- After solid foods are introduced, the goal is to gradually include a variety of vegetables and fruits on a daily basis. Offer dark green, leafy, and deep-yellow vegetables and colorful fruits frequently.
- Nutritious foods give children a healthy head start.

Oral Health Concerns in Early Childhood

Tooth formation begins before birth and is not completed until about 12 years of age; the structure of the tooth is affected by food intake during this time. A clear relationship has been shown between nutritional deficiency during tooth development and tooth size, tooth formation, time of tooth eruption, and susceptibility to caries. One occurrence of mild to moderate malnutrition during the first year of life is associated with increased caries in primary and permanent teeth later in life. Calcium and vitamin D must be present for proper calcification of dentin and normal enamel. Vitamin D is crucial to tooth development; later deficiency may promote tooth decay.[31]

Dental caries are largely preventable, but they remain the number one chronic disease of children and adolescents. Based on the mid-course review of *Healthy People 2020*,[32] 27.9% of U.S. children ages 3 to 5 years had dental caries in their primary teeth; 11.7% of children in this age group have untreated dental caries. As shown in Table 14.5, 29.2% of Hispanic and 24.2% African American children have untreated dental caries; 26.1% of 2 to 5 year olds in households below 100% of poverty level have untreated dental caries.[31] Dental caries in young children are significantly associated with lower parental education level, living at or below poverty level, no breastfeeding, skipping breakfast, low fruit and vegetable intake, no annual dental visit, and amount and frequency of sugar-sweetened beverages.

TABLE 14.5 Untreated Dental Caries (Cavities) in Children Ages 2 to 19, by Sex, Race, and Hispanic Origin, and Percent of Poverty Level, United States

	1971–1974	2001–2004
2–5 years		
Male	26.4%	20.0%
Female	23.6%	19.1%
6–19 years		
Male	54.9%	23.9%
Female	54.5%	22.0%
Race and Hispanic Origin		
2–5 years		
Not Hispanic or Latino		
White only	23.7%	14.5%
Black or African American	29.0%	24.2%
Mexican	—	29.2%
6–19 years		
Not Hispanic or Latino		
White only	51.6%	19.4%
Black or African American	71.0%	28.1%
Mexican	—	30.6%
Percent of Poverty Level		
2–5 years		
Below 100% of poverty level	32.0%	26.1%
100%–less than 200%	29.9%	25.4%
200% or more	17.8%	12.1%
6–19 years		
Below 100% of poverty level	68.0%	31.5%
100%–less than 200%	60.3%	32.7%
200% or more	46.2%	14.7%

Modified from Centers for Disease Control and Prevention (CDC). Untreated dental caries (cavities in children ages 2–19, United States. https://www.cdc.gov/Features/dsUntreated-CavitiesKids/. Accessed February 1, 2017.)

Infant Oral Care

Dental problems can begin early. Children who have caries as infants or toddlers have a much greater probability of subsequent caries in primary and permanent teeth.

Good dental care starts in infancy, before the first tooth emerges. Decay and early loss can damage permanent teeth before they erupt. The infant's gingiva should be cleaned daily with gauze, with a soft infant toothbrush and water, or with an infant tooth cleaner to remove plaque biofilm.

When teeth begin erupting, parents should continue brushing the teeth with a soft infant toothbrush using no more than a smear or rice-size amount of fluoride toothpaste twice daily for children under 3 years. The AAPD recommends a visit to the dentist following eruption of the first tooth, typically around 6 months of age, but no later than 1 year.[33] The earlier the dental visit, the better the chances of preventing dental problems. When the child is able to expectorate (usually around 3 years old), a pea-sized amount of fluoride toothpaste can be used. Because the child does not have the dexterity to brush the teeth thoroughly, the parent should continue brushing the child's teeth as long as needed.

After the first baby teeth begin to erupt, at-will nighttime feedings should be avoided. Infants and toddlers should never be given a bottle or sippy cup of milk or juice in bed. If the infant is given a bottle in bed, it should contain only water. Children should be weaned from the bottle by 14 months of age. When children are allowed to take the bottle longer, numerous problems can develop, including speech problems, tooth erosion and deformation, and more difficulty in weaning.

Children should be offered a cup as soon as they can hold it in their hands. Between meals, the sippy cup should contain only water. Prolonged use of sugary drinks in sippy cups is a leading cause of pediatric tooth decay.

Early Childhood Caries

Early childhood caries (ECC) is the presence of one or more decayed, missing (as a result of caries), or filled tooth surfaces in any primary tooth in a child younger than 6 years old. ECC is a leading oral health problem among children younger than age 3

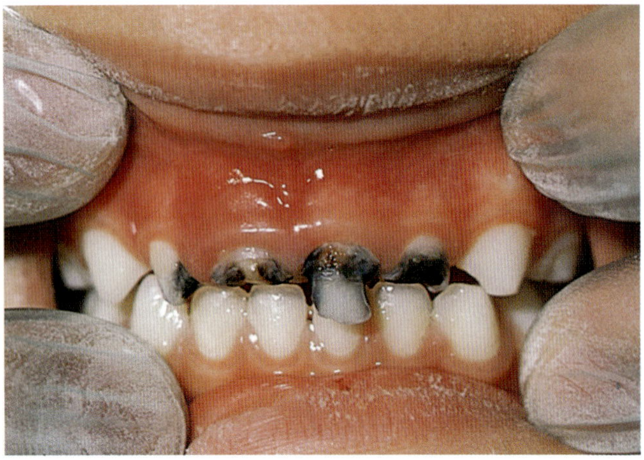

• **Figure 14.2** Early childhood caries. (Reprinted with permission from Swartz MH. *Textbook of Physical Diagnosis, History, and Examination.* 7th ed. St. Louis, MO: Saunders Elsevier; 2014.)

years. ECC, the term currently used, replaces the terms *severe early childhood caries, nursing bottle caries,* and *baby bottle tooth decay* and is characterized by early rampant decay associated with inappropriate feeding practices (Fig. 14.2). Any sign of smooth surface caries in children younger than age 3 years is indicative of ECC, which is a serious public health problem, especially prevalent in lower socioeconomic groups. Growth of infants with ECC may be inhibited because of pain associated with eating. Baby teeth are the pattern for the bite for permanent teeth.

Treatment of ECC is costly, requiring extensive extractions or restorations or both, and causing serious future oral health problems and unnecessary suffering. Severe cases are treated under general anesthesia in a hospital. Because it is preventable, health care professionals and caregivers need to watch for early warning signs to detect the disease.

Contributing Factors

Diet is the primary etiologic factor in the caries process. Unfortunately, to advise parents to "avoid sugar or sweets" is meaningless because the dietary factors involved in the caries process are more complex than simply avoiding sweets. The primary contributing factor to ECC is infection with *Streptococcus mutans* (cariogenic bacterium). Colonization of *S. mutans* occurs only after the infant's teeth erupt. Infection with the pathogen *S. mutans* is transmitted from the caregiver to the infant. Kissing and sharing utensils or other objects contaminated with saliva are contributing factors. The infant is more likely to be infected if the caregiver has a high level of *S. mutans*. The addition of frequent or prolonged exposure to a fermentable carbohydrate feeds *S. mutans*, allowing it to proliferate and produce cariogenic acid. Destruction of the tooth surface begins and can ultimately progress to rampant caries and abscesses.

Dental caries occur when a sweet liquid (e.g., juice or milk) pools around the lingual surfaces of the teeth for extended periods in the presence of caries-producing bacteria within plaque biofilm (Box 14.1). Acid produced by bacteria leads to demineralization of enamel. Allowing an infant to go to bed at night or at naptime with a bottle, frequent daytime bottles, and habitual use of a no-spill training cup are risk factors for ECC. Breast milk and artificial infant milk are equally cariogenic.

• BOX 14.1 Sources of Fermentable Carbohydrates for Infants

Liquids

- Cow's milk, plain and flavored
- Breast milk
- Artificial infant milk
- Unsweetened fruit juice
- Sweetened fruit juice and fruit drinks
- Syrup added to water
- Sweetened soft drinks
- Any sugar-sweetened beverages

Other Sources

- Some infant foods
- Medication
- Use of sweets to comfort or reward infant or relieve constipation, such as a pacifier dipped in honey or corn syrup
- Infant cereals, teething biscuits, crackers
- Dry cereals
- Arrowroot biscuits and other cookies, pretzels
- Fruits

As the child sleeps, cleansing action of saliva is diminished because of reduced salivary flow. The ultimate effect is poor clearance of the drink pooled in the mouth. Also, the natural or artificial nipple rests on the palate during sucking, allowing the liquid to pool around the maxillary incisors. The position of the tongue covers and protects the mandibular incisors. Because the disease state follows the eruption pattern, maxillary incisors are affected, followed by first molars and then canines.

Nutritional Advice

Parents must understand their role in preventing childhood dental disease. Begin dietary advice as soon as the dental team is apprised of the pregnancy. During the initial visit with the child, an assessment can be made to determine the level of fluoride intake and risk of oral problems. Recommendations to parents about controlling oral bacteria and appropriate infant and preschool feeding practices are important. Obtain diet histories of both parents, especially focusing on the primary caregiver to reveal cariogenic eating patterns that may be transferred to the infant. Critically analyze the frequency of fermentable carbohydrate intake and oral hygiene habits to alert parents to potential problems (see Chapter 18). Intercepting and modifying damaging health practices before birth can prevent ECC and decrease the likelihood of rampant caries.

DENTAL CONSIDERATIONS

Assessment

- *Physical:* Cursory oral examination to detect decalcification or carious lesions in teeth; frequency of daily cleaning; destructive habits such as lip biting, thumb sucking, tongue thrusting, or pacifier use.
- *Dietary:* Parental knowledge of ECC and what causes it; parental preferences for sweets; sharing of utensils contaminated with saliva; use of bottle propping, especially at night, or continual availability of a sippy cup throughout the day; use of corn syrup in the bottle; dipping the bottle nipple or pacifier in honey or molasses; continued use of the bottle after age 1 year; and appropriate fluoride consumption.

DENTAL CONSIDERATIONS—cont'd

Interventions

- Recommend routine dental visits and provide guidance to parents on feeding practices and nutritional needs.
- Teach parents to clean the infant's gingiva after feedings with a clean cloth. A soft infant toothbrush and water can be used when the infant has several teeth.
- If the water supply is optimally fluoridated, encourage using a smear or rice-sized amount of toothpaste until the child learns to expectorate.
- Discuss possible future problems of rampant decay in an infant (discomfort, dental phobia, infection, cost, tongue-thrust habit).
- Educate all expectant parents and parents of infants about techniques for avoiding ECC: when feeding an infant, hold the infant and bottle; avoid bottle propping or using the bottle or sippy cup as a pacifier at bedtime or throughout the day. Use other methods instead of a bottle at bedtime and naptime to quiet and relax the child, such as rubbing the child's back, rocking in a chair, singing to the child, or providing a stuffed toy.
- Parents should be advised to avoid saliva-sharing practices, such as sharing a spoon when tasting food, to prevent transmission of caries-causing bacteria (*S. mutans*) to the infant.
- Educate parents about ECC when (a) carious lesions are initially noted in a young child, (b) either parent has active caries or dentures, or (c) sweets are used to comfort or reward the infant.
- Explain the importance of primary teeth (appearance, speech, ability to eat). Patients may be under the false impression that because primary teeth fall out anyway, they serve no purpose.
- Discuss the role of carbohydrates (including those present in fruit juice and milk) in the decay process.

NUTRITIONAL DIRECTIONS

- Do not let the infant suck the bottle unattended.
- Avoid putting fruit juice or other carbohydrate-containing beverages in a bottle. Offer juice in a cup.
- If a fluoride supplement is recommended, tablets should be thoroughly chewed and swished between the teeth before swallowing. The child should not eat or drink for 30 minutes after taking the supplement and should avoid milk products for 1 hour because calcium may interfere with bioavailability of fluoride.
- Limit the child's access to a bottle or sippy cup containing milk or juice.
- Home filtration systems may remove fluoride; thus, filtered and treated water should be tested to measure fluoride content. Most state health departments assess the fluoride content of water for a minimal fee.
- During the first year, foods that require chewing should be added based on the number of erupted teeth.
- Wean infants from the bottle soon after the first birthday or fill the bottle with water.

Cleft Palate and Cleft Lip

One of the most common birth defects in the United States is **cleft lip** or **cleft palate**, or cleft lip/palate, a malformation in which parts of the upper lip or palate fail to grow together. National data for the prevalence of cleft lip or palate is incomprehensive as data is only available from 11 states. Based on this limited data, approximately 1 of 1000 live births is born with cleft lip with or without cleft palate.[34] Scientists believe numerous factors, including drugs, heredity, and folic acid deficiency, may cause this malformation.

When feeding the infant with a cleft palate, with or without a cleft lip, the main priority is to ensure adequate nutrition in spite of unique problems. Because of the opening between the roof of the mouth and floor of the nasal cavity, negative pressure needed for sucking cannot be created (see Figs. 14.3 and 14.4A). However, breastfeeding sometimes can be successful; the infant adapts by squeezing or chewing the nipple. Breastfeeding may promote better growth than spoon-feeding following surgery for cleft palate.[35]

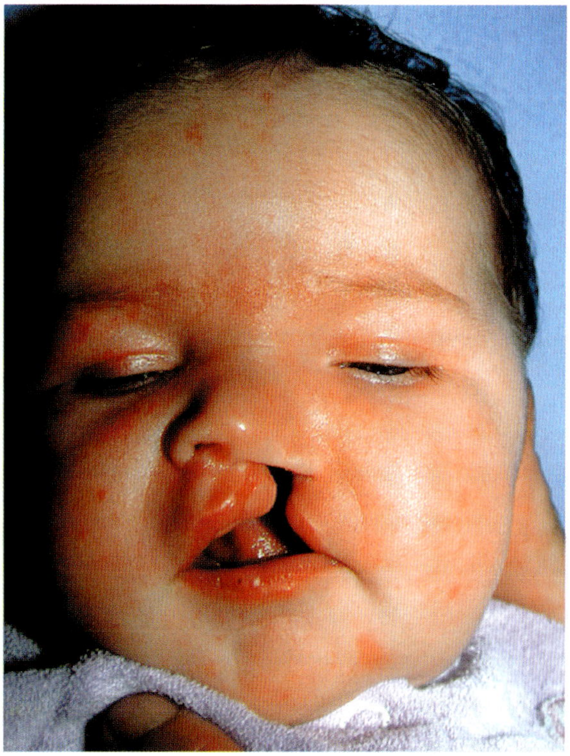

• **Figure 14.3** Cleft lip/palate. (Reprinted with permission from Kaban L, Troulis M. *Pediatric Oral and Maxillofacial Surgery*. Philadelphia, PA: Saunders Elsevier; 2004.)

The infant is held in a semi-upright position to prevent formula from entering the nose. Squeezable bottles appear easier to use than rigid feeding bottles.[35] Other feeding difficulties include nasal regurgitation, excessive air intake, and frequent burping. As soon as possible, spoon feeding is introduced. In severe cases, a prosthesis is made when the child is older (see Fig. 14.4B). Length of time needed for feedings to provide adequate nutrients can be exhaustive for both mother and infant. Special feeding devices available are recommended when lengthy feedings are necessary (see guidelines in Box 14.2).

Babies born with cleft lip, with or without cleft palate, have no greater risk for health problems and death than infants born with no disability, but they have increased rates of dental abnormalities, including supernumerary, missing, or malformed teeth.[36]

DENTAL CONSIDERATIONS

Assessment

- *Physical:* Cleft palate/lip, aspiration.
- *Dietary:* Feeding technique and past experiences in feeding infants.

Interventions

- Explain that the principal problem is a lack of normal suction and, by modifying feeding techniques, the infant can obtain adequate nutrients.
- Feed the infant slowly at a 60- to 80-degree angle to provide nutrients while minimizing risks.

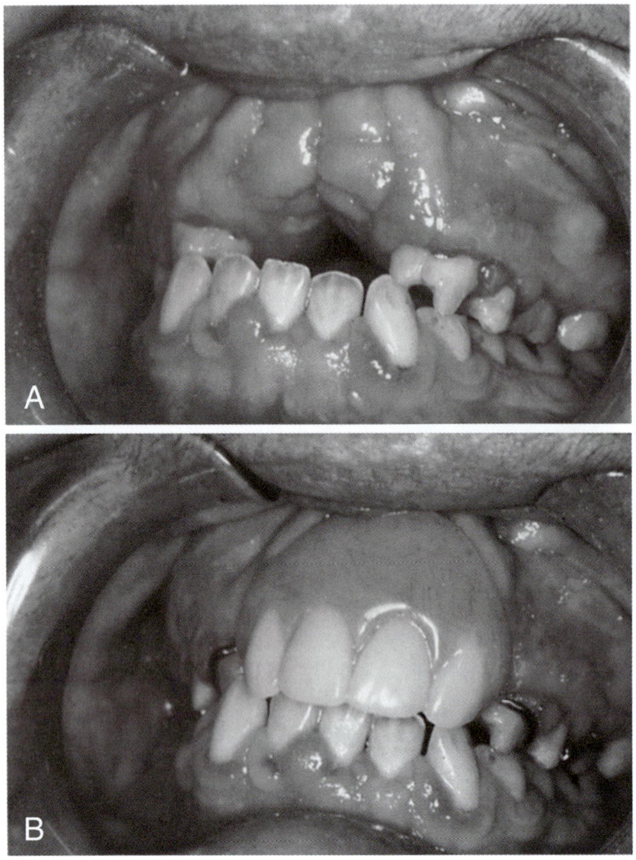

• **Figure 14.4** (A) Cleft palate. (B) Cleft palate with removable prosthesis. (Courtesy of Kathleen B. Muzzin, Texas A&M University College of Dentistry, Dallas, TX.)

NUTRITIONAL DIRECTIONS

- Introduce spoon feeding as soon as possible.
- Oral skills develop after surgery to correct the problem.
- Acidic and spicy foods may irritate delicate tissue in the cleft area.
- Young children with cleft palate are at increased risk for choking on foods that may slip into the trachea.
- Because of increased incidence of enamel hypoplasia, encourage meticulous oral hygiene practices and limited cariogenic food or liquids to avoid carious lesions at these sites.
- Refer parents to local support groups and to the American Cleft Palate Association for literature and suport.

• BOX 14.2 Suggestions for Feeding an Infant With Cleft Palate

- The infant should consume a specific amount in a feeding that takes no more than 30 minutes.
- Enlarge the hole in the bottle's nipple or use a special feeding device that enables the infant to get milk more easily.
- Boil new nipples before use to soften them.
- Mix pureed foods (fruits, vegetables, meats) with milk or broth for a thin consistency to flow from a bottle with an enlarged hole in the nipple.
- Burp frequently to aid in releasing excessive air intake.
- To prevent regurgitation, teach an older child to eat slowly and take small bites.
- Some children take liquids more easily by using a straw.
- Feeding a child with cleft palate takes longer than feeding a normal child; the mother needs to allow the necessary time. Fatigue on the part of the parent may interfere with the child's receiving adequate nourishment.
- Use saline drops before and after feeding to help clear any food or liquid that is in the nasal passage secondary to the cleft palate.
- After repair, recommend foods requiring that the patient uses the tongue and muscles for mastication.

Children Older Than 2 Years of Age: *Dietary Guidelines* 2015–2020 and *Healthy People 2020*

Healthy eating and physical activity patterns optimize normal growth and development, promote cognitive development, and reduce risk for future health problems. Consuming appropriate amounts of nutrients can best be achieved by considering the child's whole diet pattern, using principally nutrient-dense food from each of the main food groups. The AAP recommends a five-step approach to choosing foods for meals, including school or packed lunches, snacks, and social events[37]: (1) select a mix of foods from the five food groups—vegetables, fruits, grains, low-fat dairy, and quality protein sources, including lean meats, fish, nuts, seeds, and eggs; (2) offer a variety of food experiences; (3) avoid highly processed foods; (4) use small amounts of sugar, salt, fats, and oils with highly nutritious foods to enhance enjoyment and consumption; and (5) offer appropriate portions.

The general consensus is that most children's diets "need improvement" or are "poor" and are below the recommendations indicated in the Dietary Reference Intakes; (DRIs Table 14.6). For children ages 2 to 17 years, the Healthy Eating Index–2010 scores ranged from 47% to 50% out of an ideal score of 100% in 2007 to 2008. The Healthy Eating Index measures the quality of diets based on the *Dietary Guidelines*. Dairy and protein food groups scored highest (approximately 85%). Foods needing the most improvement are intake of vegetables (especially dark greens and beans), replacing refined grains with whole grains, and substituting seafood for some meat and poultry.[38] Prevalent and persistent childhood nutritional concerns include energy balance, excessive intakes of saturated fats, added sugar, and sodium. Physical activity decreases for most children after age 7 years, partially due to more nonacademic screen time, while calorie intake for children ages 2 to 6 years increased slightly more than 100 calories daily from 1994 to 1998 and 2003 to 2004.[39,40] Underconsumed nutrients of public health concern include calcium, potassium, magnesium, dietary fiber, and vitamin D (nutrients contributed from dairy foods, vegetables, fruits, seafood, and whole grains).[41] Intake of many of these nutrients decreases with age; intake of teenagers, especially girls, is notably lower than intake of younger children. Also of concern are excessive amounts of several nutrients; sodium, total and saturated fat, added sugars, and total caloric intake are significantly above amounts recommended in the *Dietary Guidelines* and the Acceptable Macronutrient Distribution (AMDR) (Box 14.3). The rationale behind the AAP recommendations to limit fruit juice consumption to 8 oz per day for children 7 to 18 years of age is to encourage whole fruit consumption for the benefit of fiber intake and because of the longer time to consume the same amount of calories as opposed to juice consumption.[23]

TABLE 14.6 Daily Nutritional Goals for Vitamins and Minerals Based on Dietary Reference Intakes for Age-Sex Groups

	Source of Goal	Female 4–8	Male 4–8	Female 9–13	Male 9–13	Female 14–18	Male 14–18
Calorie Level(s) Assessed		1200	1400–1600	1600	1800	1800	2200, 2800, 3200
Minerals							
Calcium, mg	RDA	1000	1000	1300	1300	1300	1300
Iron, mg	RDA	10	10	8	8	15	11
Magnesium, mg	RDA	130	130	240	240	360	410
Phosphorus, mg	RDA	500	500	1200	1250	1250	1250
Potassium, mg	AI*	3800	3800	4500	4500	4700	4700
Sodium, mg	UL	1900	1900	2200	2200	2300	2300
Zinc, mg	RDA	5	5	8	8	9	11
Copper, mcg	RDA	440	440	700	700	890	890
Manganese, mg	AI*	1.5	1.5	1.6	1.9	1.6	2.2
Selenium, mcg	RDA	30	30	40	40	55	55
Vitamins							
Vitamin A, mg RAE	RDA	400	400	600	600	700	900
Vitamin E, mg AT	RDA	7	7	11	11	15	15
Vitamin D, IU	RDA	600	600	600	600	600	600
Vitamin C, mg	RDA	25	25	45	45	65	75
Thiamin, mg	RDA	0.6	0.6	0.9	0.9	1.0	1.2
Riboflavin, mg	RDA	0.6	0.6	0.9	0.9	1.0	1.3
Niacin, mg	RDA	8	8	12	12	14	16
Vitamin B_6, mg	RDA	0.6	0.6	1.0	1.0	1.2	1.3
Vitamin B_{12}, mcg	RDA	1.2	1.2	1.8	1.8	12.4	2.4
Choline, mg	AI*	250	250	375	375	400	550
Vitamin K, mcg	AI*	55	55	60	60	75	75
Folate, mcg DFE	RDA	200	200	300	300	400	400

*AI, Adequate Intake; AT, α-Tocopherol; DFE, Dietary Folate Equivalents***; RAE, Retinol Activity Equivalents***; RDA, Recommended Dietary Allowance; UL, Tolerable Upper Intake Level.

Sources: Institute of Medicine. *Dietary Reference Intakes: The Essential Guide to Nutrient Requirements.* Washington, DC: National Academies Press; 2006. Institute of Medicine. *Dietary Reference Intakes for Calcium and Vitamin D.* Washington, DC: National Academies Press; 2010. U.S. Department of Health and Human Services and U.S. Department of Agriculture. *2015–2020 Dietary Guidelines for Americans.* 8th ed. Washington, DC. https://health.gov/dietaryguidelines/2015/guidelines/. Accessed February 6, 2017.

Nutrient inadequacies and excesses are more prevalent in children from households with lower incomes. Higher food security is associated with higher consumption of fruit and vegetables, consumption of unhealthy foods, and sedentary behavior.[42]

Healthy People 2020 objectives directly linked to weight and food and nutrition consumption for children age 2 years through adolescence are shown in Table 14.7. These established objectives were monitored for changes from 2005 to 2008 and 2008 to 2012.[43] Improvements in consumption (increased or decreased toward more desirable) have been documented for most of the objectives. Progress in some of these areas was very small, but at least indicated some positive trends toward the goals.

The key message of *Dietary Guidelines* (variety, moderation, and balance in food choices) applies to childhood nutrition. Between ages 2 and 5 years, children should adopt a diet consistent with the *Dietary Guidelines.* The main concerns with providing dietary recommendations and guidelines for children older than 2 years are to (a) provide adequate calories and nutrients to support growth and development and ensure genetic potential, and (b) reduce risk of diet-related chronic diseases later in life. Children's diets containing adequate energy and 25% to 35% of total energy from fat have positive effects on health later in life.

Most children are born with ideal cardiovascular health. The AAP Committee on Nutrition recommends universal serum lipid

• BOX 14.3 Acceptable Macronutrient Distribution Ranges for Children and Adolescents

Acceptable macronutrient distribution ranges (AMDRs) as a percent of energy intake for carbohydrates, fat, and protein are as follows:

- Carbohydrates—45% to 65% of total calories for ages 1 to 18 years
- Fat—30% to 40% of calories for ages 1 to 3 years, and 25% to 35% of calories for ages 4 to 18 years
- Protein—5% to 20% for ages 1 to 3 years, and 10% to 30% for ages 4 to 18 years

Added sugars should not exceed 25% of total calories (to ensure sufficient intake of essential micronutrients). This is a maximum suggested intake and not the amount recommended for achieving a healthful diet.

Consumption of saturated fat, *trans* fatty acids, and cholesterol should be as low as possible, while maintaining a nutritionally adequate diet.

Adequate Intake (AI) for total fiber is as follows:

- Children ages 1 to 3 years: 19 g per day
- Children ages 4 to 8 years: 25 g per day
- Boys ages 9 to 13 years: 31 g per day
- Girls ages 9 to 13 years: 26 g per day

Data adapted from A Report of the Panel on Macronutrients, Subcommittees on Upper Reference Levels of Nutrients and Interpretation and Uses of Dietary Reference Intakes, Standing Committee on the Scientific Evaluation of Dietary Reference Intakes. Dietary Reference Intakes for Energy, Carbohydrate, Fiber, Fat, Fatty Acids, Cholesterol, Protein, and Amino Acids (Macronutrients). Washington, DC: National Academies Press; 2005 and U.S. Department of Agriculture and U.S. Department of Health and Human Services: Dietary Guidelines for Americans. 7th ed. Washington, DC: U.S. Government Printing Office; December 2010.

• BOX 14.4 American Heart Association's Components of the Healthy Diet Score

Fruits and vegetables: ≥ 4.5 cups per day
Fish: ≥ two 3.5-oz servings per week (preferably oily fish)
Fiber-rich whole grains (≥ 1.1 g of fiber per 10 g of carbohydrate): ≥ three 1-oz equivalent servings per day
Sodium: ≤ 1500 mg per day
Added sugars: < 6 tsp per day
Sugar-sweetened beverages: ≤ 450 cal (36 oz) per week
Nuts, legumes, and seeds: ≥ 4 servings per week
Processed meats: none or ≤ 2 servings per week
Saturated fat: ≤ 7% of total energy intake

Reproduced with permission from Lloyd-Jones DM, Hong Y, Labarthe D, Mozaffarian D, et al. Defining and setting national goals for cardiovascular health promotion and disease reduction: the American Heart Association's Strategic Impact Goal through 2020 and beyond. Circulation. *2010;121(4):586-613.*

TABLE 14.7 *Healthy People 2020* Objectives for Children Over Age 2 Years

Objective	Progress (☺☹)
Reduce the proportion of children and adolescents who are considered obese.	☹
Increase contribution of intake from	
• fruits	☺
• total vegetables	☺
• dark-green vegetables, red and orange vegetables, beans and peas	☹
• whole grains	☺
Increase calcium intake.	☺
Reduce consumption of calories from	
• solid fats	☺
• saturated fat	☺
• added sugars	☺
• sodium	☺

(From *Healthy People 2020. National Health Promotion and Disease Prevention Objectives.* https://www.healthypeople.gov/2020/topics-objectives/topic/nutrition-and-weight-status/objectives. Washington, DC: U.S. Department of Health and Human Services. Accessed February 20, 2017.

screening for children between ages 9 and 11 years and again between ages 17 and 21 years; screening is recommended for children ages 2 to 8 years and 12 to 16 years who have cardiovascular risk factors such as hypertension, obesity, or a family history of premature CVD.[44] The American Heart Association advocates total cholesterol levels for children 6 to 19 years of age to be less than 170 mg/dl. By age 11 years, children in the United States do not meet ideal criteria in four cardiovascular categories—blood pressure, weight, diet, and total cholesterol. Rates of ideal cardiovascular health decline further during the first and second decades of life, indicating that the seeds of CVD accelerate in childhood primarily in conjunction with weight gain and obesity. The criterion established for ideal cardiovascular health is a body mass index (BMI) of less than the 85th percentile. Between 40% and 48% of teens have a BMI above this level. Approximately 90% of U.S. children are classified as having a poor heart-healthy diet score, 9% as having an intermediate diet score and less than 0.5% as having an ideal diet score. The percentage of children having a poor diet quality is higher than for adults. Fortunately, dietary intake of children has been slowly improving. Avoiding obesity by balancing energy intake in children is key. Measured physical activity shows less than 50% of school-age boys and 33% of girls meet the goal of 60 or more minutes/day of moderate to vigorous-intensity physical activity at least 3 days per week.[45]

The diet recommended by the American Heart Association is consistent with the *Dietary Guidelines* and the Dietary Approaches to Stop Hypertension (DASH)–type eating plan, curtailing intake of total fat, saturated and *trans* fat (Box 14.4). The amount of total fat should be 30% or less of daily total calories with saturated fat less than 10% and avoidance of *trans* fat. By using fat-free or low-fat or equivalent milk products instead of reduced-fat products or whole milk (for children older than age 2 years), lean meats in place of higher-fat meats, or lower fat products rather than high-fat products, energy and nutrient requirements can be achieved.

Serving a variety of foods is important to provide all the nutrients that children need. Another essential way to provide nutrients is to replace processed meats and other highly processed foods with unsalted nuts, seeds, legumes, and vegetable sources of protein and unsaturated fats. Although there are no studies showing long-term safety or effectiveness of nutritional modifications, lifestyle changes, or medications to prevent development of CVD, the safety and efficacy of these modifications appear to be similar to effects in adults. If more dietary restrictions are needed than the *Dietary Guidelines* (for children in the high-risk group), a registered dietitian nutritionist (RDN) can help families make appropriate changes without compromising good nutrition. Children can learn how to read food labels and determine which foods are healthier selections. The entire family usually benefits from implementing these guidelines.

The *Dietary Guidelines* recommend less than 10% of total energy intake from added sugars, which would mean between 120 and 200 cal or 30 to 40 g of sugar daily. As shown in Fig. 14.5, almost two-thirds of U.S. youth consumed at least one sugar-sweetened beverage on a given day. Children ages 2 to 19 years are consuming a little over 7% of their total energy requirements in sugar-sweetened beverages.[46] More than this amount of sugar prohibits adequate intake of required nutrients without exceeding energy needs. Energy needs of children and adolescents are high to support growth and development, but energy intake must be balanced with physical activity and/or other genetic and environmental factors.

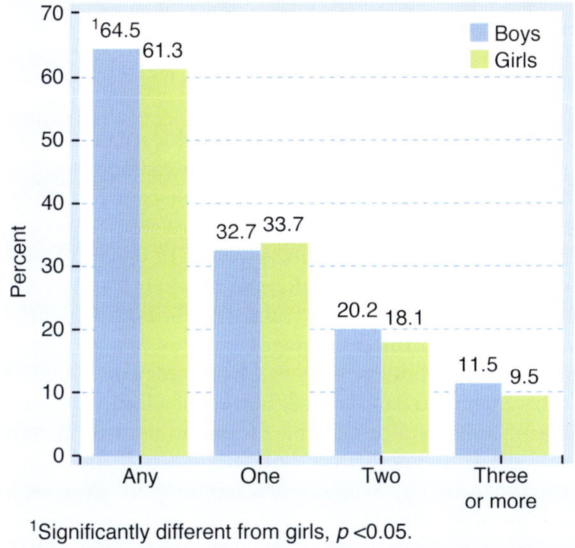

• **Figure 14.5** Percentage of youth aged 2 to 19 years who consumed sugar-sweetened beverages on a given day, by number of beverages and sex: United States, 2011–2014.

The most powerful predictor for how much children eat is the quantity of food put on their plate. Sections on the *MyPlate* for children are the same as for adults, but serving sizes differ; thus, smaller-sized plates are advantageous. Portion sizes and numbers of servings increase when children reach puberty, and needs are greater because of accelerated growth rate and increased size, but a principle concern is inappropriate portions contributing to the prevalence of overweight. One of the keys to the cause and prevention of overweight is the caregiver's knowledge. When parents assume control of food portions or coerce children to eat rather than allowing them to focus on internal cues of hunger, children's ability to regulate their own meal size is diminished.

Large portions of snacks and choice of restaurants, including fast food establishments, parallel dramatic increases in childhood obesity. Extra-large portions of single-serving items on kids' menus may contain more than 600 calories, the maximum amount recommended for a total meal.[47] Table 14.8 indicates recommended levels for kids' menu items of nutrients traditionally overconsumed as determined by the National Restaurant Association's Kids LiveWell Program; Table 14.9 itemizes single food items from kids' meals that exceed recommended calories and portions.[48]

Physical activity is important for bone mineralization, growth, and cardiovascular health. Parents should encourage individual physical activities and model them for the children (Fig. 14.6). Children should be given the opportunity to participate in a variety of activities, from walking to jumping rope to competitive sports. In reality, children will not be physically active unless they are having fun. Activity is important in helping control weight and reducing the risk for CVD, diabetes, and high blood pressure.

The National Academy of Medicine (formerly the Institute of Medicine) recommends that childcare providers give toddlers and

TABLE 14.8 National Restaurant Association Kids LiveWell Program[a]

Full Kid's Meals (Entree, Side Option, and Beverage)	Side Items
600 calories or less	200 calories or less
≤ 35% of calories from total fat	≤ 35% of calories from total fat
≤ 10% of calories from saturated fat	≤ 10% of calories from saturated fat
≤ 0.5 g *trans* fat (artificial *trans* fat only)	≤ 0.5 g artificial *trans* fat
≤ 35% of calories from total sugars (added and naturally occurring)	≤ 35% of calories from total sugars (added and naturally occurring)
≤ 770 mg of sodium	≤ 250 mg of sodium
2 or more food groups (of 5 listed in the legend)†	1 food group (of 5 listed in the legend)†; 100% fruit, vegetables, or juice; and low-fat (1%) and skim milks are permitted

[a]National Restaurant Association. Kids LiveWell. 2012. http://www.restaurant.org/foodhealthyliving/kidslivewell/about. Accessed February 6, 2017.
†(1) Fruit: > ½ cup (includes 100% juice); (2) Vegetable: > ½ cup; (3) Whole grains: contains whole grains; (4) Lean protein (skinless white meat poultry, fish/seafood, beef, pork, tofu, beans, egg): > 2 ounces meat, 1 egg or egg equivalent, 1 oz nuts/seeds/dry bean/peas (lean as defined by USDA); (5) Lower-fat dairy (1% or skim milk and dairy): > ½ cup (while not considered low-fat, 2% milk is allowed if included in the meal and the meal still fits the full meal criteria)

TABLE 14.9 Percentage of Single Food Items that Exceed Recommended Portion Sizes and the 600-Calorie Maximum for an Entire Kid's Meal[a]

	% Not Meeting Single Food Item Guidelines	% Exceeding 600 Calories for a Single Food Item
Beverages (milk)	97[b]	2
Fries	97	0
Burgers	78	17
Chicken nuggets	60	21
Pizza	85	37
Mac and cheese	71	23
Soups	57	0
Sandwiches	59	11
Fruit	4	0
Desserts	84	10

[a]Reproduced with permission from Cohen DA, Lesser LI, Wright C, et al. Kid's menu portion sizes. *Nutr Today.* 2016;51(6):273-280.
[b]Either not milk, or calories are greater than 130.

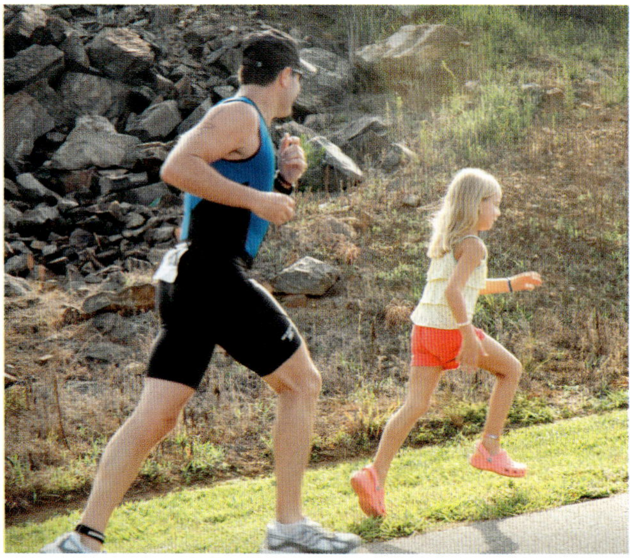

• **Figure 14.6** Parents should encourage individual physical activities and model these behaviors. (Photo courtesy of Sara Birkemeier, Raleigh, NC.)

preschool children "opportunities for light, moderate, and vigorous physical activity for at least 15 minutes per hour while children are in care." This translates to 3 hours daily for children in daycare for 12 hours, consistent with Australia and Great Britain recommendations. The Physical Activity Guidelines for Americans advocates 1 hour or more of physical activity daily for children 6 to 17 years old. The 60 or more minutes of physical activity should include each of the following at least 3 days a week: (1) either moderate- or vigorous-intensity aerobic activity, (2) muscle-strengthening activity, and (3) bone-strengthening activities.[49]

A reasonable goal for dietary fiber intake during childhood and adolescence is approximately equivalent to the age of the child plus 5 g per day. This formula represents a level that would provide health benefits, such as normal laxation, without compromising mineral balance or caloric intake in children older than 2 years. Based on this formula, the daily minimal dietary fiber intake would be 8 g per day for a 3-year-old, and would gradually increase to 20 g for a 15-year-old. The gradual increases are consistent with current guidelines for adult dietary fiber intake (25–35 g/day). Average dietary fiber intake among children 2 to 5 years old is 11 to 12 g; 14 g for children 6 to 11 years old; and 13 to 16 g for 12- to 19-year-olds, significantly lower than the recommendation.[50] By ensuring at least half of the grain servings are whole grains, as recommended in the *Dietary Guidelines*, fiber and other nutrient guidelines can be met. The *Dietary Guidelines* and *MyPlate* promote increasing fruit and vegetable consumption to five or more servings daily. To increase fiber intake, fresh fruits are recommended over fruit juice.

Because of the high calcium requirement to increase bone mineral density in children, milk and dairy products are essential components. Calcium levels were established for achievement of optimal bone mineral health to decrease the risk of osteoporosis later in life. Inadequate amounts of calcium and vitamin D during the toddler years could cause rickets when infants are weaned to diets with minimal dairy content. Adolescents (12–19 years old) typically consume about 1 cup of milk daily, and children (2–11 years old) consume about 1⅓ cup. Calcium intake can be favorably increased by using calcium-fortified beverages, such as orange juice with calcium, or milk products, such as low-fat yogurt. Some school districts have removed flavored milk because of added sugar content; a Canadian study revealed that this restriction resulted in children consuming half as much milk.[51] Lower-sugar formulations of chocolate milk may be a better option to ensure intake of essential nutrients contributed by milk—calcium, phosphorus, magnesium, and potassium.

Utilizing the ChooseMyPlate Website

The *MyPlate* website (http://www.ChooseMyPlate.gov) for preschoolers (ages 2–5 years) and children (ages 6–11 years) provides guidance for healthy food choices and an active, healthy lifestyle. The website is designed for parents, providing information to help children make wise food choices. As discussed in Chapter 1, and depicted in Fig. 1.4, the plate divides foods into five major food groups: grains, vegetables, fruits, dairy, and proteins. As children grow, needs may differ from those in the *MyPlate* guide. A doctor, nurse, or RDN should be consulted about a child's nutritional needs and how to best meet them if problems are observed, such as lethargy, undernutrition, excess weight gain, or symptoms of any chronic disease.

ChooseMyPlate.gov (https://www.choosemyplate.gov/children) provides guidelines, tips, and encouragements for preschoolers, kids, and students to help improve health and well-being. For preschoolers, links provide further information to help children (a) grow up healthy, (b) develop positive eating habits, (c) try new foods, (d) play actively every day, and (e) follow food safety rules. This website provides information about appropriate foods and portion sizes and suggestions for meal patterns or snacks. After creating a profile in *SuperTracker*, menus can be analyzed for adequacy, and *Food-A-Pedia* can help determine nutritional information for specific foods. Additionally, age-appropriate activities for preschoolers and school-age children include cooking skills, games, activity sheets, videos, and songs. Getting children involved in food preparation and cooking early increases their kitchen responsibilities.

These activities help children become more aware of the connection between their food choices and feeling healthy and their ability to participate in physical activities, thus providing a fun way to learn about nutritional needs. The website can also be helpful for teachers to plan activities and classroom materials. The *Physical Activity* link on the *MyPlate* website provides information and encourages physical activities for balancing energy intake. *SuperTracker* (https://health.gov/paguidelines/guidelines/children.aspx) can be used to record time spent in various activities to determine calories expended.

Toddler and Preschool Children

Growth

After the child reaches 1 year of age, the growth spurt slows down. A toddler gains approximately 4 to 6 lb until 2 years old, and height doubles by age 4 years. In a normally growing child, height increases parallel that of weight. Children grow approximately 2 to 3 inches a year and gain around 5 lb a year. One-half of adult height is achieved by 2½ to 3 years of age.

Nutrient Requirements

During the past 30 years, the nutritional status of children in the United States has improved, with few nutrient deficiencies observed. As previously discussed, poor nutritional status of children (as measured by growth rate and biochemical indices) is generally more prevalent in lower socioeconomic groups, for whom the amounts and variety of foods may be limited.

Anemia remains a public health concern among young (less than 2 years old) low-income children. Approximately 10% of all children, regardless of socioeconomic background, may be iron deficient. The incidence of anemia usually declines with age and is observed more often in African American children than in white, Asian, Native American, or Hispanic children. Iron-rich foods, such as meat, and fresh fruits and vegetables that contain vitamin C, which enhance iron absorption, are expensive compared with calorically dense foods such as chips or candy. Milk is a poor source of iron and large amounts of milk deter iron absorption. Iron deficiency during infancy results in lower cognitive abilities and motor skills that continue throughout childhood and adolescence.

As mentioned earlier, research studies note that ensuring vitamin D sufficiency throughout childhood and during the time of maximal bone mineral accrual seems particularly warranted. Depending on vitamin D intake and amount of sun exposure, a supplement may be needed.

Because of high activity level, basal metabolic rate, and growth, the caloric requirement for children is relatively high, roughly 1000 calories plus 100 calories per year of life. Younger children need to eat foods with high nutrient and energy density because they are unable to eat large quantities of food at any particular time. Healthy snacks can contribute vital nutrients, but snacks are frequently energy-dense foods and beverages. The extra nutrient needs for growth and development result in dietary deficiencies occurring more quickly and with more severe consequences than in adults. Interventions are needed to improve the nutritional quality of snacks consumed by children.[52]

However, overweight is pandemic (see *Health Application 14*), and eating patterns established at this age may be problematic for lifelong health. Energy intake of preschool children was significantly higher in 2009 to 2010 than in 1989 to 1991, especially in families of Hispanic origin, with low income and low educational levels.[53] By striving toward healthy eating and physically active habits, children may achieve healthful weights, possibly preventing lifetime risks of chronic health problems.

Food-Related Behaviors

Lifelong habits and food attitudes are formed during preschool years that, to some extent, affect health throughout life. A variety of foods should be available that provide the needed nutrients. Basic understanding of nutrient content of foods, the role of foods in health, and food-related behaviors for these age groups is important for parents to promote food habits conducive to adequate nutrient intake. Healthful eating produces benefits in cognitive and physical performance, fitness, psychological well-being, and energy level.

Parental attitudes and food preferences, eating habits, and food choices are influential factors in the child's food preferences. Being healthy role models by eating a variety of foods is more effective than telling them what to eat. Foods disliked by one or both parents are not served often or may not be served at all; children tend to enjoy foods preferred by their parents. When parents eat more fruits and vegetables, so do their children. Providing fruits for snacks and serving vegetables at mealtime affect a preschooler's eating patterns for life.

When planning menus, parents must consider the child's food preferences, but parents still must maintain control over the options. Without appropriate guidance, young children do not independently make healthy food choices; the parents' role is to offer nutritious foods. Children can choose how much or even whether they will eat the food provided. Feeding problems can result when either the parent or child crosses this line of responsibility (i.e., the parent bribes or forces the child to eat, or the child is allowed to tell the parent what to prepare). Family mealtime is essential for children's nutrition, health, and overall well-being. More food is eaten by the child when the family eats together rather than just offering food for the child to eat alone.

Toddlers (1 to 3 Years Old)

By the age of 2 to 3 years, the child will have acquired the type of stable eating habits and food preferences in a routine that tends to persist over time. During the second year of life, toddlers develop fine motor skills while learning to feed themselves, but skills and capabilities do not occur at exactly the same time for every child. Although this is a messy learning process, this transitional period stabilizes by age 2. Finger feeding may be preferred to spoon feeding; some finger foods should be provided at every meal. A toddler can manipulate a cup by about 18 months of age. Rotary chewing skills develop in the second year. Until then, finely chopped meats are accepted more readily and minimize the risk of choking.

Toddlers prefer regularity; thus, eating at the same time each day is desirable and helps control appetite. Regular meals also help to avoid fatigue, which can lead to an overly emotional situation that interferes with appetite. Tired children eat poorly. If the child has been very active, a short rest period before the meal improves intake.

Small amounts of food should be offered several times a day. Serving sizes should be based on appetite, but initially about 1 tbsp can be offered for each year of age. When children serve themselves from family-size bowls, they choose smaller portions and are less likely to overeat. The amount of liquids consumed can result in a poor appetite for foods or more food is consumed in addition to the calories provided in liquid form.

Food jags (refusing to eat anything except one food for several days) in toddlers and children are common and are a way to assert independence. This typical developmental stage is temporary, used frequently to attract attention. Overreaction by parents may prolong rather than correct such behaviors. Appetites, which are erratic and unpredictable, are a strong reflection of the current growth rate. Parents should not force children to eat when they are not hungry. When well-balanced meals are provided, caloric intake at any given meal varies greatly, but compensation at subsequent meals results in little variability in total energy intake. If sufficient amounts are not eaten at the meal, parents may limit snacking or provide nutrient-dense snacks. Snacks can contribute significantly to adequate nutrient intake (Box 14.5).

Until age 4 years, children are at risk for choking on food that gets caught in the airway. Food is not chewed thoroughly until the molars erupt. To prevent choking, closely supervise children while eating and do not allow walking, playing, talking, laughing, crying, or lying down while they are eating. Additionally, avoid foods most likely to cause choking: (a) small nuts and seeds; (b) round, firm, smooth foods such as grapes, hard candy, hot dogs, and round candies; (c) dry or hard foods, such as raw carrots, cookies, pieces of pretzels, potato chips, and popcorn; and (d) sticky or tough foods such as peanut butter, raisins, tough meat, and caramel candy.

Children under age 6 years are very susceptible to caffeine. United States poison control centers report that serious cardiac and neurologic symptoms occur frequently as a result of high-energy drink consumption. Of 5156 reported cases of energy drink exposure, 40% were unintentional exposures by young children.[54]

Preschool Children (4–6 Years Old)

Preschoolers are relatively independent at the table and can feed themselves. Mealtimes should be a pleasant occurrence rather than an ordeal. By allowing children to eat with adults, they imitate adults in manners and food habits. Parental insistence on proper utensil usage, manners, and other demands is inappropriate for this age group and may result in less food intake. Parents need to ignore some inappropriate mealtime behaviors and focus on positive nonmealtime activities. Conversation and role modeling can reinforce appropriate eating behavior and promote food intake.

Strong-flavored vegetables (overcooked cabbage and onions) are generally disliked by children, but are more popular if served raw. Crisp, raw vegetables are well accepted. Because preschool children still enjoy eating with their fingers, cutting fruits and vegetables into small pieces increases their acceptance. Preschoolers generally prefer their foods separate; casseroles and stews may not be well accepted. Foods that can be easily chewed are more readily accepted. Snacks are still important for adequate nutrient intake (see Box 14.5). The body uses food more effectively and energy levels are more consistent when children "refuel" every 2 to 4 hours. The number of snacks varies, depending on the family schedule and the child's activity and hunger levels. Preschoolers are likely to be suspicious of any new foods introduced. Eight to 15 exposures to a new food may be needed to achieve acceptance. Even after they have accepted a food, preschool children may not eat it every time it is served. Rather than bargaining with a child who does not want what is on the menu or becoming a short-order cook, it is better to give the child the option to eat or not. Children eventually eat more of what they should eat if they are not forced into it.

• BOX 14.5 Healthy Snack Choices

- Cut-up fresh vegetables with low-fat dip or salad dressing
- Air-popped popcorn with a sprinkle of parmesan cheese
- Fresh fruit[a]
- Frozen fruit (grapes, bananas)[a]
- Nuts
- Low-fat cheese (sticks, strings, cubes, or slices)
- Low-fat cottage cheese or yogurt
- Peanut butter on apple slices[a] or celery sticks
- Pretzels[a]
- Baked chips[a]
- Hard-boiled eggs
- Animal crackers[a]
- Graham crackers[a]
- Sliced turkey or chicken
- Dry, low-sugar cereal[a]
- Rice cakes[a]
- Low-fat pudding[a]
- Sugar-free gelatin with fruit
- Mini bagels[a]
- Pickles
- Frozen juice bars[a]

[a]*Cariogenic potential. Encourage tooth-brushing after snacks.*

DENTAL CONSIDERATIONS

Assessment

- *Physical:* Socioeconomic level, child's age, and child's developmental level.
- *Dietary:* Eating environment, frequency of meals and snacks, quantity of foods consumed, adequacy of intake, parental beliefs and food preferences.

Interventions

- Encourage eating meals at regular times. Serve food shortly after being seated to avoid restless behavior.
- Evaluate and assess children's diets at regular intervals.
- Growth charts are available on the *MyPlate* and Evolve websites for children that can be used by parents to ensure appropriate growth rates.
- Stress the importance of providing adequate amounts of protein; vitamins A, C, and D; calcium; phosphorus; and fluoride during formation and calcification of teeth.
- If sufficient amounts are not eaten, limit snacking or provide nutrient-dense snacks, as shown in Box 14.5.
- Consider the parents' attitudes, cultures, beliefs, fears, and educational levels when developing and providing oral health education.
- Help parents clarify any misconceptions interfering with a child's ability to consume foods to meet their nutrient needs for growth and development, such as "healthy foods do not taste good" or "healthful eating means eliminating all high-fat foods."
- Recommendations for fluoride usage should be determined by need, based on risk indicators.
- Encourage the use of fluoridated toothpastes for children older than 2 to 3 years.
- Encourage parents to assume responsibility for the child's oral health care and model good oral health behaviors.
- Refer low-income patients to any government or local social programs (Women, Infants, and Children [WIC] program, Supplemental Nutrition Assistance Program [SNAP]) for which they may be eligible.

NUTRITIONAL DIRECTIONS

- Eating habits developed during the preschool years track into adulthood.
- The goal for parents is to prevent caries and plaque biofilm formation.
- The child is expected to taste each new food prepared and served, but the "bite" may be very small.
- Risk of heart disease begins in childhood; a reduction of dietary fats (especially saturated) after the second birthday is recommended to reduce the risk of CVD. However, undue restriction of fat intake could compromise a child's growth and development and potentially lead to eating disorders or unhealthy attitudes about food.
- Until age 6 years, a good rule of thumb for a serving size is one-half an adult portion. Food, especially sweet foods, should not be used as a bribe or reward.
- Teach children to recognize and honor their hunger and satiety cues rather than cleaning their plates. Children who are told to "clean your plate" may have a more negative response, consuming less food.
- Diet and lifestyle choices during early childhood affect lifelong eating patterns and impact later disease risk. Accelerated weight and fat mass gain seem to predict adult disease conditions.
- Present disliked foods in a matter-of-fact manner, serving small portions (1–2 tbsp); discard without comment if the child does not eat them.
- Successful childhood feeding may be best accomplished by providing a variety of healthful foods and allowing children to eat without coercion.
- Provide healthy snacks, but prevent the child from grazing throughout the day to ensure a good appetite at meal time.
- Children who avoid drinking milk are at increased risk for prepubertal fractures.
- Children generally eat better when the family or at least one adult sits at the table and eats with them.
- Provide a wide variety of vegetables and fruits daily, especially dark-green, leafy, and deep yellow vegetables and colorful fruits.
- Purchase only 100% juice (not fruit drinks with added sugar or other sweeteners).
- Food children willingly eat, parents purchase, and industry produces often contain added sugars. Sweetness enhances food acceptance for young children. Parents expecting their child to "just eat" because the food is healthful may conflict with the realities of getting children to eat.[55]
- Water is the ideal beverage between meals; omitting sugar-sweetened beverages (sodas and fruit juice) helps prevent risk of excess weight gain by limiting extra calories and dental caries by lowering the frequency of tooth exposure to sugar.
- By offering a wide variety of foods to toddlers who are healthy and growing appropriately, parents need not be overly concerned about risk of nutrient deficiency.
- Teach the child to use an age-appropriate rice-size smear or pea-size amount of toothpaste to limit the amount accidentally swallowed.
- Ensure that the child receives a dental examination every 6 to 12 months; topical fluoride may be applied if the water supply is not fluoridated. The dental team determines an appropriate fluoride regimen for each child.
- Offer children whole fruits rather than fruit juices or fruit drinks.
- Good oral health is directly correlated to dietary habits that promote daily breakfast consumption and fruit and vegetable intake in conjunction with fluoridation.

Attention-Deficit/Hyperactivity Disorder

Attention-deficit/hyperactivity disorder (ADHD) is the most common neurologic disorder of childhood, but symptoms may persist into adulthood. Hyperactivity is characterized by chronic age-inappropriate behaviors, including inattention, impulsiveness, hyperactivity, restlessness, and problems in social interaction and academic performance. Many theories have been proposed on the causes of hyperactivity, but none has been proven conclusively. Inherited genetic factors affecting the function of chemicals in the brain that help regulate attention and activity may be responsible.

A common misconception is that sugar causes hyperactivity, or ADHD, in children, but controlled research studies fail to support this belief.[56,57] The origin of the idea that sugar is responsible for hyperactivity seems to be purely based on the fact that sugar is a source of energy, as are other carbohydrates. External cues, such as parties or celebrations, usually associated with a higher sugar intake, may cause hyperactivity, not the amount of sugar intake.

Some studies suggest that several food additives (e.g., artificial food colorings, flavorings, and sodium benzoate, a preservative) may be associated with these behaviors in children. Restriction of synthetic food color additives for children with ADHD has been beneficial for some children but appears to be more effective in individuals with food sensitivities. More research is needed to determine the effects of ingredients present in the food supply.

For children exhibiting behavior problems such as hyperactivity, the use of dietary manipulation tends to be a more acceptable approach to treatment than use of drugs, but evidence of an association between diet and behaviors is considered weak and limited. The use of dietary treatments alone is unlikely to be sufficient treatment for many children with ADHD. A nutritionally well-balanced, high-protein diet that limits added sugars and highly processed foods is encouraged. Inappropriate dietary treatment without scientific support could (a) detract from efforts to identify effective treatment and prevention of delinquent behavior; (b) lead to nutritional deficiencies or excesses; and (c) provide offenders with a dietary excuse for their behavior, rather than assuming responsibility for their own behavior. Data supporting new treatments for ADHD should be scrutinized for scientific study design, clinical safety, and scientific validity before recommending them as modes of therapy.

Children With Special Needs

Health conditions, such as mental retardation of unknown origin, cerebral palsy, Down syndrome, infantile autism, and muscular dystrophy, have significant oral health and oral hygiene implications. Mastication and swallowing problems occur in all of these conditions except Down syndrome. Some children with oral–motor problems can improve; others cannot. Gum disease is frequently observed in children with Down syndrome.

Children with cerebral palsy and Down syndrome may practice bruxism. **Bruxism** is involuntary grinding or clenching of teeth, which results in abnormal wear patterns on teeth and joint or neuromuscular problems. Loosened teeth interfere with eating chewy foods, such as meats. Children with cerebral palsy, Down syndrome, and intellectual disabilities are likely to have abnormal sensory input and muscle tone. Difficulties with sucking, swallowing, spoon-feeding skills, chewing development, and independent feeding are common. Tongue thrust associated with many of these conditions results in significant food waste and may jeopardize nutritional status. Dental problems may become exaggerated in the child as a result of difficulty in maintaining good oral hygiene, the child's unique dietary habits and patterns, and the effect of prescribed medications. Such problems include oral infections, dental caries, and periodontal disease.

Treatment by a team of health care providers, including a dental hygienist, is individualized depending on the child's potential capabilities and skills. Nutritional intervention for feeding-skill difficulties involves assistance in planning a diet easiest for the child to eat and meets nutritional needs.

DENTAL CONSIDERATIONS

Assessment

- *Physical:* Condition of the oral cavity, presence of dental caries, plaque biofilm, abnormal oral–motor habits, such as tongue thrust, bruxism, oral–motor development, medications.
- *Dietary:* Intake of fermentable carbohydrates, frequency of snacking, calcium and vitamin D intake, source of fluoride, pica.

Interventions

- Behaviors that are rewarded will increase in frequency. Provide reinforcement throughout the dental procedure by verbally praising desirable behavior, tangible rewards (stickers, tattoos, baseball cards) or a behavioral contract. Provide appropriate recommendations or referrals.
- These children are less likely to maintain good oral hygiene; schedule more frequent recare appointments.

NUTRITIONAL DIRECTIONS

- Provide nutritious snacks, such as cheese cubes or raw vegetables. Fibrous foods promote salivary flow, increasing the buffering capacity of saliva.
- Vitamin D–fortified milk and cheeses not only provide nutrients needed for healthy teeth but also are cariostatic.
- Provide an opportunity to brush the teeth after eating; if brushing is impossible, rinse with water.
- Inappropriate dietary habits and unhealthy food preferences developed during childhood have lifelong implications.
- Limit sticky carbohydrate foods—such as candies, cookies, crackers, pastries, and raisins—between meals. Frequently choosing these at snacktime may contribute to dental caries risk.

School-Age Children (7–12 Years Old)

The middle childhood years continues to be an important period for formation of eating habits. Habits established during this time will shape food-related perceptions and behaviors and contribute to lifelong healthy eating patterns. Reserves provide stores for upcoming rapid adolescent growth. New activities and friends begin to influence choices and broaden the child's horizon. Students who consume an adequate amount of fruit, vegetables, milk, protein, fiber, and other components of a healthy diet are more likely to perform better in school and maintain good nutrition practices that affect lifelong health. The child exposed to different foods and food patterns usually enjoys more foods. New ideas experienced with friends and at school may affect food choices at home.

Almost all foods are liked by school-age children. Vegetables are the least favorite, with only 22% of all children consuming three servings daily. Planning menus around food groups is important to include all the necessary nutrients. Foods containing sugars or fats need not be eliminated, but should be limited to less than 10% of the calories needed. The important fact is that foods with a high sugar content or refined grains should not replace recommended amounts from the food groups.

The appetite in this age group is usually good; but food habits and intake may suffer because children do not take time for meals (15–20 minutes). Enforcement of a specific amount of time to eat may prevent the child from forming the habit of eating too fast. Poor appetite may be caused by stresses, such as schoolwork and emotional difficulties. Nutrients available from family dinner meals are significantly associated with the child's overall dietary intake.[58] Overall dietary quality of students participating in the National School Lunch Program is better than when students bring food from home.[59]

Students are ravenous after school. Although bakery products, soft drinks, candy, and chips are favorites, nutritious snacks are preferable. More access to money and the influence of peers and mass media may result in expenditures at fast food restaurants and from vending machines, increasing the potential for choosing foods high in saturated fat, salt, and sugar.

Dental Caries in School-Age Children

According to the CDC, trends in prevalence of untreated tooth caries in the permanent teeth of children has improved, but more than 55% of children aged 6 to 15 have dental caries, and 21.5% ages 6 to 9 years and 11.4% of children 13 to 15 have untreated cavities. The increment of dental caries is slightly higher between the ages of 6 and 12 years than between 12 and 18 years. Black and Hispanic children and children in families below 100% of the poverty level have a significantly higher percentage of untreated cavities than white, non-Hispanic children (see Table 14.5). Only 35% of low-income children and adolescents received preventive dental service in 2012.[32] Untreated dental disease can lead to pain, infection, school absences, and poor academic performance. In addition, children could experience feelings of embarrassment, withdrawal, and anxiety.

This age range generally marks exfoliation of all or most of the primary teeth and the eruption of most permanent teeth. Systemic fluoride is effective before eruption and during the mineralization phase of erupting teeth. When 1 ppm of fluoride in drinking water is present during tooth formation, the caries rate is reduced 60% along with reduction in prevalence of plaque biofilm and remineralization of teeth. To provide maximum protection, systemic fluoride is recommended through age 16 years for children in nonfluoridated or inadequately fluoridated areas. Even cessation of water fluoridation for short periods, as has occurred in numerous communities, adversely affected the rate of children's dental caries.[60] Application of topical fluoride (professionally applied and self-applied) becomes as effective as systemic fluoride for school-age children. Topical administration of fluoride (dentifrices, rinses, gels, fluoride supplements, varnishes, and fluoridated water) can help in reduction of tooth decay.

Application of **sealants** (a clear or shaded plastic material applied to occlusal surfaces of permanent teeth) acts as a barrier protecting decay-prone areas of teeth from plaque biofilm and acid. However, even the combined use of a toothbrush, dental floss, fluoride toothpaste, and sealants cannot completely control caries formation.

Another factor in caries formation is food selection and patterns of consumption. Cariogenicity of food is influenced by the presence of fermentable carbohydrates, physical properties, and frequency of consumption (see Chapter 18). The use of products (e.g., chewing gum, candy, topical oral syrup) containing xylitol can be effective in preventing tooth decay by reducing levels of harmful *S. mutans* bacteria in plaque biofilm.

DENTAL CONSIDERATIONS

Assessment

- *Physical:* Schoolwork or emotional difficulties, activity level, sports interests.
- *Dietary:* Nutrient and fluid intake, appetite, food preferences and eating patterns, child's and parent's beliefs about nutrition.

Interventions

- Evaluate sources of fluoride to ensure optimal intake to protect erupting and newly erupted teeth while minimizing excessive intake and risk for fluorosis.
- Provide motivating education (explain, demonstrate, encourage, and reinforce) for children and parents to instill proper oral hygiene habits for caries prevention.
- Antimicrobial agents, such as chlorhexidine, can be used to control existing plaque biofilm and formation of new plaque biofilm by controlling bacteria and limiting acid production.
- Ask low-income parents about the child's participation in governmental child nutrition programs (National School Lunch, School Breakfast, Summer Food Service, and Special Milk).

NUTRITIONAL DIRECTIONS

- Cutting foods into shapes (smiley faces, stars, or animals) often creates interest in the food or snack.
- Children involved in meal preparation are more likely to eat the food they prepare and to be aware of what is in the food.
- Have nutritious foods available for snacks (see Box 14.5).
- As children grow older, they consume larger quantities of food, but food choices deviate more from the *Dietary Guidelines*.
- Encourage appropriate oral hygiene techniques.

Adolescents

Growth and Nutrient Requirements

Major biological, social, psychological, and cognitive changes occur during adolescence. Because of these changes and rapid growth rates, American teenagers are considered to be at nutritional risk, consuming inadequate amounts of nutrients and placing them at risk for developing chronic diseases later in life. Healthy eating helps reduce one's risk for becoming obese or developing osteoporosis, iron-deficiency anemia, and dental caries. Girls ages 9 to 18 years are getting between two-thirds and three-fourths of their RDAs from foods and supplements.[61]

Poor food choice is a result of noncompliance with *MyPlate* and the *Dietary Guidelines*. Numerous organizations are concerned that poor cardiovascular health behaviors, especially physical activity and dietary intake, will contribute to a worsening prevalence of obesity, hypertension, hypercholesterolemia, and diabetes as adolescents reach adulthood. Declining fitness levels are another contributing factor for weight gain.

The slow childhood growth rate accelerates with pubescence until the rate is as rapid as that of early infancy. Growth of long bones, secondary sexual maturation, and fat and muscle deposition create increased nutrient requirements. The end of this adolescent growth spurt is signaled by a deceleration of growth, completion of sexual maturation, and closure of the epiphyses of long bones.

Although the Dietary Reference Intakes (DRIs) provide nutrient recommendations based on chronological age, nutrient needs closely parallel physical development. Adolescent girls need to increase their energy intake sooner and decrease it more quickly than boys because of earlier onset of puberty and lower total body weight after adulthood is reached. Adolescent boys have greater nutritional needs than adolescent girls because of growth rates and body composition changes (see Table 14.6). A very active 18-year-old boy requires approximately 3800 cal compared with almost 2900 cal for an 18-year-old girl. Most adolescents need and are able to eat large quantities of food many times a day. However, teens need to be careful of amounts and frequency of eating when their rapid growth rate levels off.

Average protein intake is well above recommendations but may fall below required amounts due to weight-loss diets or chronic illness, or becoming a vegan/strict vegetarian. Dietary protein may be used to meet energy needs and would not be available for needed growth and repair.

The need for calcium, vitamin D, and iron is of particular importance throughout childhood. Adolescents are particularly vulnerable to an insult to their bones. A lack of calcium or vitamin D can have profound implications for future skeletal health because a mild deficiency of either can be unrecognized until severe skeletal damage has occurred. During adolescence, 45% of adult skeletal mass is formed; calcium needs are greater than at any other time of life. Building good bone mass during adolescence is thought to be the best way to prevent osteoporosis in old age. Health care providers should talk with teenagers about the importance of bone health, achieving maximum bone density, and maintaining strong bones. Daily calcium intake of 1300 mg in addition to exercise during adolescence promotes calcium retention and bone mineral density. Milk intakes generally decline in the teen years. American children have low levels of vitamin D and naturally occurring sources are not popular. Calcium–vitamin D supplements may be the best solution currently available to lessen risks of later osteoporosis.[61]

Increased iron is required because of the expansion of blood volume, increase in red blood cell mass and muscle mass, and the need to replace iron losses associated with menstruation in girls. Concern is especially warranted for adolescent girls because depletion of iron stores in women starts during adolescence with the onset of menstruation; over 10% of babies each year are born to adolescent girls between the ages of 15 and 19 years.[62] Participation in sports activities leads to red blood cell destruction. Iron supplementation among adolescents can significantly decrease the prevalence of anemia in this age group.[63]

Influential Factors on Eating Habits

Eating is an important part of socialization and exerting one's independence. Food choices are influenced by complex external factors, such as family, peers, mass media, economic and sociocultural factors, and internal factors, such as physiologic needs, body image, self-concept, food preferences, and personal values and beliefs about health and nutrition. Probably the strongest influential factor among teenagers is peer pressure.

Most adolescents are stressed because of continual changes. Sexuality, body image, scholastic and athletic pressures, relationships with friends and relatives, finances, career plans, and ideological beliefs may cause conflicts as adolescents try to establish and understand their identity. Stress can decrease utilization of several nutrients, particularly vitamin C and calcium.

Increasing numbers of children and adolescents are overweight (see *Health Application 14*). Adolescents, especially girls, are often obsessed about their body image and a desire to be thin. They are eager to try fad diets and other unsafe weight-loss methods, which may affect their ability to reach their growth potential. Dieting is not recommended for adolescents because nutrients during this period are necessary to build and strengthen their bodies to last a lifetime. Obesity, anorexia nervosa, and bulimia are serious health concerns amenable to early treatment. Extreme weight control behaviors during adolescence increase the risk for anorexia and bulimia 10 years later in life. Intervention for individuals in preadolescence and adolescence is most appropriate to prevent weight concerns from becoming life-threatening conditions, as experienced with anorexia nervosa. A discussion of problems associated with eating disorders is presented in Chapter 17.

Between 2004 and 2010, energy intake declined, with subsequent decreases in intake of sugar-sweetened beverages, pizza, pasta dishes, breads and rolls, and savory snacks while fruit intake increased.[53] Adolescents have increased their snacking in recent years, consuming an average of more than 500 calories, but snacking frequency is not associated with higher BMI.

Adolescents consume more added sugars than younger children. In 2011 to 2012, children 2 to 18 years old consumed 325 cal/day, or 14% of their total energy intake, from added sugars.[64] Surprisingly, 59% of the added sugar came from foods and 41% from beverages. More added sugars were consumed at home than away from home.

Adolescents consume more sugar-sweetened beverages than adults, contributing to their higher sugar intake. The recommendation by numerous organizations to eliminate the sale of soft drinks, sports drinks, and energy drinks in schools may have had some positive effects. Current data indicate that the percentage of children age 6 to 17 years who drink sugar-sweetened beverages is significantly less now than it was between 2001 and 2006. In 2011 to 2014, 64.5% of boys and 61.2% of girls consumed at least one sugar-sweetened beverage daily, and an average of 143 cal or 7.3% of total energy intake.[53] When cups are provided near water fountains at school, the percentage of students choosing plain water with fewer sugary drinks more than doubles.[65] Increasing fluid intake with a low-energy drink, such as skim milk or water, replacing sugar-sweetened beverages appears advantageous for weight maintenance.[66,67] Potential health problems are likely to occur as a result of high intake of sweetened-sweetened beverages: (a) overweight attributable to additional caloric intake; (b) displacement of milk consumption, resulting in calcium and other nutrient deficiencies; and (c) dental caries and potential enamel erosion.

High-intensity sweetened (nonnutritive, diet or low-calorie) beverages have gained popularity among children and adolescents, probably replacing sugar-sweetened beverages. Approximately 25% of children report consuming nonnutritive sweeteners at least once daily.[68] Changing to nonnutritive sodas is not especially helpful in regard to oral health because the phosphoric and citrus acids in all soft drinks can cause tooth enamel erosion.

Additionally, health care providers and parents are urged to monitor inappropriate use of sports drinks and energy drinks because large amounts of caffeine and other stimulant substances present are not advisable for children and adolescents. The AAP maintains that stimulant-containing energy drinks have no place in the diets of children and adolescents. Overall caffeine intake of children has actually slightly decreased in recent years because of less caffeinated soft drinks, but energy drink and coffee intake has increased.[69]

Adolescents have more access to food outside the home. Foods readily available from fast food outlets, vending machines, convenience stores, restaurants, and schools fit perfectly into adolescents' busy, active lifestyles. These foods increase daily caloric intake by more than 100 calories and lower diet quality because of increased amounts of saturated fat, sugar, and sodium compared with food prepared at home. A recent study indicated that the percentage of children consuming fast foods dropped from 38.8% in 2003 to 2004 to 32.6% in 2009 to 2010, resulting in a significant reduction in energy intake from burgers, pizza, and chicken from fast food establishments.[70] Average sodium intake among adolescents is between 2919 and 3565 mg. Foods obtained from stores contributed 58% of sodium intake, fast-food/pizza restaurants contributed 16%, and school cafeterias, 10%.[71] Fast foods are acceptable nutritionally when consumed in moderation as a part of a well-balanced diet. Lower-calorie items and a wider variety of menu selections, such as salads and low-fat milkshakes, can contribute to nutrient requirements without providing excessive calories.

Adolescents are notorious for skipping breakfast. Despite the availability of school breakfasts, omission of this meal is more prevalent with children from lower socioeconomic levels. A high-protein breakfast may reduce daily food intake and improve weight management and body fat gain, which is especially important in adolescents from lower socioeconomic levels who have higher rates of overweight and obesity. Short-term effects of breakfast positively affect cognitive functioning and alertness; the effect of skipping breakfast on mental stability and academic performance is stronger for boys than girls.

Nutritional Advice

Despite adolescents being knowledgeable about healthful eating and wise food options, they frequently make injudicious choices. Promoting change is more important than providing information. Factors negatively affecting food choices are time, availability of healthy foods, and lack of concern about healthy eating. Listening to adolescents' feelings followed by sound advice works well for those who are willing to listen and make changes. Adolescents can frequently be motivated by responsibility, collaboration, fear of failure, and respect for the health care provider. Techniques such as negotiation and reflective listening can enhance their critical thinking skills (see Chapter 21).

Effective tactics for providing adolescent nutritional advice are to appeal to their physical image or their muscular development and competitiveness for sports and to praise better food choices, ignore choices that are neutral, and discourage harmful choices. By presenting nutrition and health information in terms relevant to adolescent lifestyles and personal interests, dental professionals can help teenagers understand how current eating and exercise habits affect their current and future health.

DENTAL CONSIDERATIONS

Assessment

- *Physical:* Activity level, growth spurt, use of illicit drugs, use of tobacco products, body image, self-efficacy, influence of peer pressure, stress level.
- *Dietary:* Adequacy of nutrient intake based on *MyPlate;* amount and frequency of sodas and energy drinks; use of fast foods, convenience foods, or vending machine foods; food preferences and personal values and beliefs about health and nutrition; dietary and nutritional supplements; breakfast; and alcohol intake.

Interventions

- Encourage use of calcium-rich and vitamin D–rich foods.
- Praise good eating patterns; collaboratively work with adolescents to modify food choices and suggest substitutions.
- Determine the frequency, quantity, and form of cariogenic foods.
- Encourage a smoking cessation program for adolescents who smoke (see Chapter 19, *Health Application 19*).
- Provide knowledge to teens regarding risks of using smokeless tobacco and other tobacco products.
- Encourage parents to promote healthy dietary behavior and provide healthy choices that can contribute to oral health and appropriate weight gain.

NUTRITIONAL DIRECTIONS

- Teenagers should be knowledgeable of long-term risks and benefits of good nutrition, but the best approach is to focus on short-term benefits of eating well.
- Restriction of calorie intake during rapid growth periods compromises lean body mass accumulation despite a seemingly adequate protein intake.
- Intense physical activity can cause increased urinary loss of calcium and red blood cell destruction. Referral to an RDN may be needed to ensure adequate nutritional intake.
- Snacking can have a positive influence on overall nutritional and health status of the teenager. Kitchens should be stocked with nutritious snack foods (see Box 14.5) to encourage good eating habits.
- Water and low-fat or fat-free milk are the most healthful beverages; moderate use of 100% fruit juice has health benefits as well.
- Routine ingestion of sports drinks and soda (with sugar or nonnutritive sweeteners) can lead to dental caries.
- Use of dietary supplements by most adolescents is not needed.
- An inadequate intake of calcium and vitamin D during childhood or adolescence may fall short of achieving the genetically predetermined peak height and bone mass.
- Children and adolescents who skip breakfast miss the opportunity to consume a nutrient-rich meal; unhealthful dietary behaviors may have an adverse effect on body weight.
- An adolescent with light skin needs to spend about 5 to 10 minutes in the sun with only part of the body exposed (arms or legs) two or three times a week to produce enough vitamin D; an African American needs to spend 15 to 30 minutes. Additionally, calcium intake should be adequate (3 cups of milk or equivalent milk products).

HEALTH APPLICATION 14

Childhood and Adolescent Obesity

Childhood obesity is the greatest challenge to child health in the 21st century, and children born since 1980 may be the first generation in America to have shorter life expectancy than their parents as a direct consequence of the obesity epidemic.[72] Childhood obesity, similar to adult obesity, is a complex disease caused by an imbalance between calorie intake and output. The rate of childhood obesity tripled in the 1980s, yet the fact that no statistically significant changes occurred from 1999 to 2000 and 2001 to 2014 is encouraging. The prevalence of obesity is about the same in both boys and girls.[73] Childhood obesity is more prevalent in families from lower socioeconomic groups. This is probably related to a number of factors: prepregnancy and current maternal weight, lower household education, lack of knowledge, and lack of availability of nutrient-dense foods.

The Centers for Disease Control and Prevention recommends that World Health Organization growth standards be used to monitor growth for infants and children from birth to age 2 years. BMI charts are appropriate for boys and girls older than 2 years of age (see Evolve website). Because children grow in spurts and frequently grow in height for a while, followed by an increase in muscle mass and adiposity before growing taller again, the BMI is a screening tool used to detect potential weight problems. The BMI correctly identifies most children who are overweight or obese and is a reasonably good, simple diagnostic test for identifying childhood obesity and adiposity.[74] Overweight has been defined as a BMI that is greater than or equal to the 85th but less than or equal to the 95th percentiles for age and sex. Obesity is greater than or equal to the 95th percentile and extremely obese is a BMI of greater than or equal to 120%. Children with a high BMI do not necessarily manifest clinical complications or health risks related to increased body fat. A high BMI is a clue necessitating more in-depth assessment of the individual child to ascertain health status but is more sensitive and easier than other tests.

Obesity in children can potentially cause significant physiologic and psychosocial complications leading to negative health consequences. Health problems associated with childhood obesity include diabetes; high cholesterol and blood pressure levels, which are risk factors for CVD; sleep apnea (interrupted breathing while sleeping); orthopedic problems; liver disease; and asthma. While one would hope a child's obesity resolves over time, the bulk of scientific research demonstrates that childhood overweight and obesity adversely affect adult morbidity and mortality. The U.S. Preventive Services Task Force regards the prevalence and problems of obesity in childhood as being so serious, they recomend that all health care providers screen children over 6 years old and adolescents and refer them to comprehensive, intensive behavioral interventions to promote improvements in weight status.[75] Identifying young and preteen children at highest risk for sustained obesity with focus on both primary prevention and early intervention may be the only way to curtail the obesity trend.

Obesity is an important issue for all health care professionals to discuss with their patients. Obesity is a systemic problem, not isolated from oral health. The topic is a difficult subject to discuss even in a clinical setting because of current societal culture and values. To many mothers, a little "fluff" on their child looks healthy, and they do not recognize and accept the fact that their child is overweight. They may become defensive when the issue is mentioned or take offense at comments. Individuals from low-income groups frequently possess different perceptions of weight than the health care provider and may be unconcerned about the child's weight. Furthermore, they lack the skills and knowledge to change behaviors.

Continued

HEALTH APPLICATION 14

Childhood and Adolescent Obesity—cont'd

Treatment of obesity for any child or adolescent requires the expertise of many health care disciplines.

Perhaps more devastating to an overweight child is social discrimination. Overweight children often experience psychological stress, poor body image, low self-esteem, and depression. Children are more concerned about their current appearance and athletic performance than the long-term effects of weight on their mental and physical capacities and shortened lifespan.

Despite these distressing effects on American youth, the consensus seems to be that the environment, especially a sedentary lifestyle, supports a genetic predisposition to gain excessive weight. A recent study found 35 to 40% of a chil'd BMI is inherited from the parents.[76] The cycle of obesity and disease seems to begin before birth: women who are overweight are more likely to give birth to larger infants, who are more likely to become obese adults.[77] At-risk children begin gaining inordinate amounts during preschool years. Preschool children who are modestly overweight often continue to gain weight during their school years, making later weight loss even tougher. Assisting an overweight toddler or school-age child is easier than assisting a teenager because parents have a greater control over food choices inside and outside the home. Weight maintenance in a growing child or adolescent is as effective as weight loss in an adult.[78]

Although the cause of the childhood obesity epidemic is multifaceted, factors driving this phenomenon include rapid changes in modern food selections and activity levels of children superimposed onto genetic and metabolic predispositions for weight gain. The problems of American children eating too many high-calorie fast foods and snacks along with being inactive are well recognized as contributing factors. The problem will not be resolved by any single action; rather, concerted action is needed across many disciplines, sectors, and settings, such as childcare facilities, communities, health care professionals, and schools.

Weight loss or gain reflects inadequate or excessive intake, which should be balanced with an appropriate amount of physical activity. This simple equation is confounded by complex social factors influencing children's eating habits, exercise, and play.

It remains very difficult for overweight children and adolescents to lose weight and even more tedious to sustain that weight loss. The ultimate goal is prevention of overweight in children and adolescents. Prevention is important for numerous reasons: (a) obesity is very expensive to treat; (b) an older child regains most of the weight after an obesity management program; (c) success rates for long-term treatment of morbidly overweight teens is extremely low; and (d) access to an effective weight-loss program is limited for high-risk children. Treatment requires a motivated child and parent, and indeed the whole family.

The goal for obese children has been weight maintenance or reduction in the rate of weight gain while height increases. By "growing into their weight," body fat decreases without compromising lean body mass and growth. Many experts believe that overweight children should not be restricted because of the importance of providing adequate nutrients to promote optimal linear growth, but rather should focus on nutrient-dense foods and portion control. Although an ideal BMI goal is established for these children, this goal should be secondary to healthy eating and activity.

Beneficial effects of child obesity prevention programs exist, especially if the target audience is between 6 and 12 years of age. Favorable outcomes are more likely to occur when these components are included: (a) school curriculum that includes healthy eating, physical activity, and body image; (b) increased sessions for physical activity and development of fundamental movement skills throughout the school week; (c) improvements in nutritional quality of the food supply in schools; (d) environments and cultural practices that support children eating healthier foods and being active throughout each day; (e) support for teachers and other staff to implement health promotion strategies and activities (e.g., professional development, capacity-building activities); and (f) parental support and home activities that encourage children to be more active, eat more nutritious foods, and spend less time on screen-based activities. A key parenting practice is to create a protective home environment, substituting nutritious foods for unhealthful ones and facilitating physical activities instead of sedentary pursuits.

Interventions to reduce BMI are aimed at changing lifestyle behaviors—including physical activity and healthy dietary habits that prevent pediatric obesity. The multifaceted topic of food consumption includes types of food consumed, location, food preparation, and eating habits of other household members. Food choices of children and adolescents are usually dictated by the mother (or other primary caregiver), which is influenced by her heritage and level of education. The first step in addressing this epidemic is to teach parents of young children how to provide and encourage healthful choices. Nutritional imprinting starts early; thus, early childhood is the ideal time to start discussing proper feeding practices.

Nutrition education for the child and both parents is needed to provide a well-balanced diet with some caloric restriction. It is questionable whether children should be required to eat food that is different than the rest of the family; only food portions should be different. A limited amount of juice is natural and healthy, but fresh fruits are preferable. When parents change how the whole family eats and offer children wholesome rewards for not being sedentary, obese children begin to shed pounds. Instead of rewarding children with snacks, alternative ways of spending quality time with them is recommended. Environmental change is fostered by restructuring family mealtimes and leisure-time activities, and reinforcing appropriate eating cues (Box 14.6).

Technology has increased the use of media devices such as televisions, video game devices, smartphones, and other interactive portable devices. These electronic advancements expose children to advertisements that influence their perceptions of foods. "Inactive entertainment" or noneducational screen time has paralleled the disturbing increase in obese and overweight children.

Necessary lifestyle changes, although challenging to the child and family, are effective in improving weight. Physical activity should be encouraged with consideration of the child's interests and preferences. The whole family should engage in some form of physical activity on a routine basis.

Behavioral treatment of obesity may be more effective for children than adults. A family-based, multifactor intervention can be implemented by a multidisciplinary team after a comprehensive, in-depth assessment when obesity is diagnosed. Effective behavioral programs are labor intensive and require intensive parental involvement but can be successful. Changes such as taking time to chew food, minimizing sugar-laden beverages, eating more vegetables, and walking for exercise can be effective in gaining control of the weight problem.

The goal is to establish an environment that supports behavior changes while minimizing any perceptions of restrictions or limitations on the child. Successful programs focus on encouragement and "small victories" to sustain involvement in improving fitness levels. Parents need help in communicating about eating and exercise habits with their children in positive and encouraging ways.

Because of the lack of success in weight loss and maintenance programs for severely obese children and adolescents, even with intensive behavioral treatment, clinicians have begun resorting to medication therapy and bariatric surgery to ameliorate pediatric obesity. Comprehensive weight-management programs that incorporate counseling and behavioral management techniques targeting diet and physical activity are the most effective. Medication or surgical treatment should not be offered to overweight or obese children until more modest measures—including intensive dietary, behavioral, and activity-related lifestyle changes—are attempted.[78] Only adolescents who have not lost weight through lifestyle modifications should be considered for medication or gastric surgery and even then only when other comorbidities exist and the individual continues to adhere to previously implemented diet and exercise interventions.

• BOX 14.6 Help Children Maintain a Healthy Body Weight

- Be supportive. Children know if they are overweight, and do not need to be reminded or singled out. They need acceptance, encouragement, and love.
- Be a positive role model. Note lifestyle habits contributing to overeating and inactivity and help them avoid the situation.
- Start the day off on the right foot. Breakfast helps spread the calories throughout the day and helps avoid mid-morning unhealthy snacks.
- Set guidelines for the amount of time that children spend watching television, playing video games, or playing on the computer.
- Set goals for physical activity; plan family activities involving physical activity. Instead of watching TV, go hiking or biking, wash the car, or walk around a mall. Offer choices and let children decide.
- Be sensitive. Find activities children will enjoy that are not difficult or could cause embarrassment.
- Eat meals together as a family and eat at the table, not in front of a television. Eat slowly and enjoy the food. Eating at home with family often translates into a healthier diet.
- Avoid using food as a reward or punishment. Spend some quality time together; take a walk or go on a long bike ride.
- Focus on positive goals. Allow children to determine goals they want to achieve, such as being able to swim five laps in a specified time. Focusing on positive goals is better than focusing on weight loss.
- Do not be too restrictive; focus on moderation. Children should not be placed on restrictive diets unless ordered by a pediatrician (for medical reasons). Encourage kid-sized portions. Sweets and fast foods should be curtailed, but they can be used sparingly.
- Children need food for growth, development, and energy, but if they are forced to clean their plates, they are doing their bodies a disservice.
- Make eating a family activity. Involve children in meal planning, grocery shopping, and meal preparation. This helps them learn about healthy eating and gives them a role in decision making.
- Keep healthy snacks on hand. Good options include fresh, frozen, or canned fruits and vegetables; low-fat cheese, yogurt, or ice cream; frozen fruit juice bars; and cookies, such as fig bars, graham crackers, gingersnaps, and vanilla wafers.
- Monitor what children drink. High-energy drinks provide a lot of sugar with little health benefit.
- Stock the refrigerator and pantry with nutrient-dense healthy foods; do not purchase foods they should not eat.
- Make small changes as a family. Menu changes should be implemented for all family members. Begin parking the car a little farther away or eating fast food less often.
- Focus on small, gradual changes in eating and activity patterns. This helps form habits that can last a lifetime.
- Get active. Plan activities involving the whole family, such as skating, hiking, or biking. Make an after-dinner walk a regular part of the family's evening.

◆ CASE APPLICATION FOR THE DENTAL HYGIENIST

A mother brings her 3-year-old son in because of the need for a routine oral examination required by the Head Start program he is attending. She knows he has some white spots on his front teeth, but he will not allow her to brush his teeth and she does not routinely ensure that he brushes his teeth. He is still using a sippy cup but gave up the bottle at age 18 months.

Nutritional Assessment

- Willingness to seek nutritional information
- Desire for increased knowledge of nutritional health habits
- Knowledge of community resources
- Cultural or religious influences
- Knowledge regarding the *Dietary Guidelines,* Nutrient Facts, and *MyPlate*

Nutritional Diagnosis

Health-seeking behaviors related to lack of knowledge concerning optimal nutrition practices in relation to dental health.

Nutritional Goals

The parent verbalizes correct information concerning the importance of oral hygiene and foods and beverages affecting the oral cavity; is aware of snacks that do not promote dental caries; is able to read food labels; and can name the food groups in *MyPlate*, the number of servings needed for the child, and portion sizes from each group.

Nutritional Implementation

Intervention: Ask the parent to write down everything the child ate yesterday and from the time he got up this morning until the office visit. Also ask the parent to document everything she ate.

Rationale: This will help tailor the information provided to the needs of the patient. You especially need to know the child's access to the sippy cup during the day, what beverage is in the cup, and whether he goes to bed with it. The parent's diet recall reflects the primary caregiver's preferences and habits. Any changes in her diet ultimately help the child.

Intervention: (a) Encourage variety of food intake, using *MyPlate.* Review the number of servings needed and what consists of a serving size. (b) Recommend substituting fresh fruit for juices and limiting fruit juice to 4 to 6 oz daily. (c) Instruct her to avoid products that contain fermentable carbohydrates, such as cookies, crackers, or cereal, between meals.

Rationale: It is the total balance of diet that matters, and the best balance incorporates variety to promote optimal nutrition. Providing the minimal number of servings prevents nutritional deficiencies in healthy individuals. Certain foods, although they may be wholesome and nutritious, may not be advisable for oral health.

Intervention: (a) Explain how to read labels for carbohydrate content. The name of most sugars ends in *"-ose."* (b) Emphasize moderation of sugar intake. (c) Explain that "dietetic" and "sugar free" do not mean that the product is low in calories or low in cariogenic potential. (d) Explain the relationship between carbohydrate and the caries process; emphasize the importance of proper oral hygiene after its use.

Rationale: Refined sugar contains calories and no other nutrients but is acceptable when used in items that contain appreciable amounts of other nutrients (e.g., a pudding would provide more nutrients than a gelatin dessert or carbonated beverage).

Intervention: (a) Review an entire label with the mother to help her understand how to use it, (b) determine a serving size, and (c) explain the types of carbohydrates.

Rationale: Knowledge increases compliance and allows the mom to make informed choices regarding food selections.

Intervention: Discuss the importance of three regular mealtimes and three healthy snacks and avoidance of grazing.

Rationale: Adequate nutrients are important for growth and health of the child; snacking is needed for a 3-year-old to obtain adequate nutrients. Assist the child in tooth brushing after meals and snacks.

Intervention: Ask the mother how she feels about being able to implement the changes.

Continued

CASE APPLICATION FOR THE DENTAL HYGIENIST—cont'd

Rationale: This will give you the opportunity to empathize with her about the difficulties of changing food habits and perhaps make further suggestions for implementing changes.

Intervention: Refer the patient to governmental programs for which she may be eligible—WIC, food stamps, or expanded nutrition programs.

Rationale: These agencies may help in providing healthful foods and provide practical guidelines via newsletters, workshops, and written materials to improve health.

Evaluation

To determine effectiveness of care, have the parent read labels; have the parent state the number of servings and portion sizes needed for her son. Additionally, the parent should be able to plan a menu using foods recommended and to state how to obtain or use community information and support. The parent should be able to indicate how changes in food choices will not only improve overall health but also maintain health of the oral cavity and ensure optimal growth of her son with minimal or no problems in the oral cavity.

Student Readiness

1. Plan meals for 1 day for a family with a 2-year-old toddler, a 10-year-old boy, and a 15-year-old girl.
2. Discuss feeding an infant from birth to 12 months.
3. What is considered normal weight for a newborn?
4. Create an outline for discussing ECC with an expectant parent.
5. A mother wants to know why snacks are needed and which ones to give her preschooler to lessen the risk of developing dental caries. What would you tell her? Provide a list of specific suggestions and food choices for the mother.
6. A mother states that because her child is hyperactive, she is going to eliminate all sugar. What is a good response to this statement?
7. List barriers for not being able to decrease use of fast food restaurants. List healthier choices available at favorite fast food restaurants.

CASE STUDY

Mrs. C. is at her 6-month recall visit and talks about her 6-month-old daughter, Jennifer. Jennifer weighed 7 lb at birth and now weighs 15 lb. She was bottle fed from birth. At 3 months, Mrs. C. introduced cereals, but Jennifer has resisted all attempts to increase her solid food intake. She is allowed to go to sleep with a bottle propped in her crib at the daycare center.

1. What additional assessment data do you need?
2. Is Jennifer's weight gain within the expected range?
3. How much should she gain in the next 6 months?
4. What tentative dental diagnosis could you derive?
5. The dental hygienist encourages Jennifer's mother to discontinue the habit of putting her in bed with a bottle and to request that the daycare center do the same. Why?
6. The health care provider recommends solid foods be introduced gradually to Jennifer. What foods should be introduced first?
7. When will Jennifer be old enough for finger foods?
8. Why should honey be withheld until 1 year of age?
9. Why would the dental hygienist want to assess Mrs. C's dietary intake?

CASE STUDY

R.J. is a large 16-year-old boy (6 feet, 4 inches, 190 lb) who has complained to you about pain from dental caries. He is active in athletics in school and has a part-time job. You determine from his dietary history that his appetite is very good, and his nutrient intake is adequate except for vegetables. Snacking, principally soft drinks, candy, and cookies, constitutes almost 50% of his total caloric intake.

1. How would you advise R.J.? What motivational factors would you consider for him?
2. What are some dental nutritional diagnoses and goals and interventions for Raymond?
3. What further data are needed for a complete assessment?
4. When having R.J. choose better snack options, what are some that you would recommend?
5. How do you think R.J. will feel about your suggestions?

CASE STUDY

Norma returns for a 6-month recall visit. Since her last checkup, this 17-year-old girl has developed 12 new dental caries in the mandibular anterior teeth. Norma's parents are in their 50s. Her father has lost numerous teeth as a result of periodontal disease, and her mother is completely edentulous. Norma has no medical problems other than rhinitis (inflammation of the nasal mucous membranes secondary to allergies), which causes her to breathe through her mouth much of the time. The oral examination showed normal color and tone of the oral mucosa, tongue, and gingiva. Her decayed, missing, filled rate was 17. She reports eating a varied, well-balanced diet, except for fruit and vegetable intake. Because of the dryness in her mouth, she relies heavily on cough drops and chewing gum.

1. What is a possible cause of these new dental caries?
2. What suggestions would you give her to relieve mouth dryness?
3. Based on her dietary habits, what nutrient(s) may be inadequate?

References

1. Cusick SE, Georgieff MK. The role of nutrition in brain development: the golden opportunity of the "first 1000 days". *J Pediatr*. 2016;175:16–21.
2. Jelding-Dannemand E, Malby Schoos AM, Bisgaard H. Breast-feeding does not protect against allergic sensitization in early childhood and allergy-associated disease at age 7 years. *J Allergy Clin Immunol*. 2015;136(5):1302–1308.
3. Lodge CJ, Tan DJ, Lau MX, et al. Breastfeeding and asthma and allergies: a systematic review and meta-analysis. *Acta Paediatr*. 2015;104(467):38–53.
4. Luccioli S, Zhang Y, Verrill L, et al. Infant feeding practices and reported food allergies at 6 years of age. *Pediatr*. 2014;134(1):S21–S28.
5. Hong S, Choi WJ, Kwon HJ, et al. Effect of prolonged breast-feeding on risk of atopic dermatitis in early childhood. *Allergy Asthma Proc*. 2014;35(1):66–70.
6. Richards D. Breastfeeding up to 12 months of age not associated with increased risk of caries. *Evid Based Dent*. 2016;17(3):75–76.
7. Belamarich PF, Bochner RE, Racine AD. A critical review of the marketing claims of infant formula products in the United States. *Clin Pediatr (Phila)*. 2016;55(5):437–442.
8. Picard PJ. Bottle feeding: a preventive orthodontic. *J Calif State Dent Assoc*. 1995;35:90–95.
9. Sum FH, Zhang L, Ling HT, et al. Association of breastfeeding and three-dimensional dental arch relationships in primary dentition. *BMC Oral Health*. 2015;15:30.
10. Galán-Gónzalez AF, Aznar-Martin T, Cabrera-Dominguez ME, et al. Do breastfeeding and bottle feeding influence occlusal parameters? *Breastfeed Med*. 2014;9(1):24028.
11. Thomaz EB, Cangussu MC, Assis AM. Maternal breastfeeding, parafunctional oral habits and malocclusion in adolescents: a multivariate analysis. *Int J Pediatr Otorhinolaryngol*. 2012;76(4):500–506.
12. Mahurin-Smith J, Ambrose NG. Breastfeeding may protect against persistent stuttering. *J Commun Disord*. 2013;46(4):351–360.
13. Brew BK, Marks GB, Almqvist C, et al. Breastfeeding and snoring: a birth cohort study. *PLoS ONE*. 2014;9(1):e84956.
14. Lopes-Freire GM, Cárdenas AB, Suarez de Deza JE, et al. Exploring the association between feeding habits, non-nutritive sucking habits, and malocclusions in the deciduous dentition. *Prog Orthod*. 2015;16:43.
15. Agarwal SS, Nehra K, Sharma M, et al. Association between breastfeeding duration, non-nutritive sucking habits and dental arch dimensions in deciduous dentition: a cross-sectional study. *Prog Orthod*. 2014;15:59.
16. Lopes TS, Moura Lde F, Lima MC. Breastfeeding and sucking habits in children enrolled in a mother-child health program. *BMC Res Notes*. 2014;7:362.
17. Lopes-Freire GM, Espasa Suarez de Deza JE, Rodrigues da Silva IC, et al. Non-nutritive sucking habits and their effects on the occlusion in the deciduous dentition in children. *Eur J Paediatr Dent*. 2016;17(4):301–306.
18. Chen X, Xia B, Ge L. Effects of breast-feeding duration, bottle-feeding duration and non-nutritive sucking habits on the occlusal characteristics of primary dentition. *BMC Pediatr*. 2015;15:46.
19. Festilă D, Ghergie M, Muntean A, et al. Suckling and non-nutritive sucking habit: what should we know? *Clujul Med*. 2014;87(1):11–14.
20. Silva M, Manton D. Oral habits–part 1: the dental effects and management of nutritive and non-nutritive sucking. *J Dent Child (Chic)*. 2014;81(3):133–139.
21. Fewtrell M, Bronsky J, Campoy C, et al. Complementary feeding: a position paper by the European Society for Paediatric Gastroenterology, Hepatology, and Nutrition (ESPGHAN) Committee on Nutrition. *J Pediatr Gastroenterol Nutr*. 2017;64(1):119–132.
22. Murray RD. Influences on the initil dietary pattern among children from birth to 24 months. *Nutr Today*. 2017;52(25):S25–S29.
23. Heyman MB, Abrams SA, Section on Gastroenterology, Hepatology, and Nutrition; Committee on Nutrition. Fruit juice in infants, children and adolescents: current recommendations. *Pediatrics*. 2017;139(6). pii: e20170967. doi:10.1542/peds.2017-0967.
24. Food Allergy Research and Education. Food allergy facts and statistics for the US. https://www.foodallergy.org/facts-and-stats. Accessed January 31, 2017.
25. Muraro A, Halken S, Arshad SH, et al. EAACI food allergy and anaphylaxis guidelines. Primary prevention of food allergy. *Allergy*. 2014;69(5):590–601.
26. Togias A, Cooper SF, Acebal ML, et al. Addendum guidelines for the prevention of peanut allergy in the United States: Report of the National Institute of Allergy and Infectious Diseases–sponsored expert panel. *J Allergy Clin Immunol*. 2017;139(1):29–44.
27. Barends C, de Vries JH, Mojet J, et al. Effects of starting weaning exclusively with vegetables on vegetable intake at the age of 12 and 23 months. *Appetite*. 2014;81:193–199.
28. American Academy of Pediatrics (AAP). Vitamin D supplementation for infants. https://www.aap.org/en-us/about-the-aap/aap-press-room/Pages/Vitamin-D-Supplementation-for-Infants.aspx. Accessed January 31, 2017.
29. Perreault M, Mikail S, Atkinson SA. New Health Canada Nutrition Recommendations for infants birth to 24 months address the importance of early nutrition. *Nutr Today*. 2016;51(4):186–190.
30. American Academy of Pediatric Dentistry (AAPD). Recommendations for pediatric oral health assessment, preventive services and anticipatory guidance/counseling. https://www.aap.org/en-us/about-the-aap/aap-press-room/Pages/Vitamin-D-Supplementation-for-Infants.aspx. Accessed January 31, 2017.
31. Schroth RJ, Rabbani R, Loewen G, et al. Vitamin D and dental caries in children. *J Dent Res*. 2016;95(2):173–179.
32. National Center for Health Statistics. Chapter 32: Oral Health. Healthy People 2020 Midcourse Review. Hyattsville, MD, 2016. https://www.cdc.gov/nchs/data/hpdata2020/HP2020MCR-C32-OH.pdf. Accessed August 23, 2017.
33. American Academy of Pediatric Dentistry (AAPD). Recommendations for pediatric oral health assessment, preventive services and anticipatory guidance/counseling. https://www.aap.org/en-us/about-the-aap/aap-press-room/Pages/Vitamin-D-Supplementation-for-Infants.aspx. Accessed January 31, 2017.
34. National Institute of Dental and Craniofacial Research (NIDCR). Craniofacial Birth Defects. https://www.nidcr.nih.gov/DataStatistics/FindDataByTopic/CraniofacialBirthDefects/. Accessed August 1, 2017.
35. Bessell A, Hooper L, Shaw WC, et al. Feeding interventions for growth and development in infants with cleft lip, cleft palate or cleft lip and palate. *Cochrane Database Syst Rev*. 2011;(2):CD003315.
36. Berg E, Haaland ØA, Feragen KB, et al. Health status among adults born with an oral cleft in Norway. *JAMA Pediatr*. 2016;170(11):1063–1070.
37. Hassink SG, American Academy of Pediatrics. AAP recommends whole-diet approach to children's nutrition. Healthy Children. Back to School. https://www.healthychildren.org/English/tips-tools/e-magazine/Documents/HC_Emagazine_2015_BacktoSchool.pdf. Accessed February 13, 2017.
38. Hiza HAB, Guenther PM, Rihane CI. Diet quality of children age 2-17 years as measured by the Healthy Eating Index–2010. Nutrition Insight 52. July 2013. USDA Center for Nutrition Policy and Promotion, Alexandria VA.
39. Farooq MA, Parkinson KN, Adamson AJ, et al. Timing of the decline in physical activity in childhood and adolescence: Gateshead Millennium Cohort Study. *Br J Sports Med*. 2017;119(8):926–933.
40. Ford CN, Slining MM, Popkin BM. Trends in dietary intake among US 2- to 6-year-old children, 1989-2008. *J Acad Nutr Diet*. 2013;113(1):35–42.
41. US Department of Health and Human Services and US Department of Agriculture. 2015-2020 Dietary Guidelines for Americans. 8th ed. December 2015. http://health.gov/dietaryguidelines/2015/guidelines/.

42. Asfour L, Natale R, Uhlhorn S, et al. Ethnicity, household food security, and nutrition and activity patterns in families with preschool children. *J Nutr Educ Behav*. 2015;47(6):498–505.
43. Healthy People 2020. National health promotion and disease prevention objectives. https://www.healthypeople.gov/2020/topics-objectives/topic/nutrition-and-weight-status/objectives. Washington, DC: US Department of Health and Human Services. Accessed February 8, 2017.
44. Howard T, Grosel J. Updated guidelines for lipid screening in children and adolescents. *JAAPA*. 2015;28(3):30–36.
45. Steinberger J, Daniels SR, Hagberg N, et al. Cardiovascular health promotion in children: challenges and opportunities for 2020 and beyond: a scientific statement from the American Heart Association. *Circulation*. 2016;134(12):e236–e255.
46. Rosinger A, Herrick K, Gahche J, et al. Sugar-sweetened beverage consumption among U.S. youth, 2011-2014. NCHS data brief, no 271. Hyattsville, MD: National Center for Health Statistics; 2017.
47. Cohen DA, Lesser LI, Wright C, et al. Kid's menu portion sizes. *Nutr Today*. 2016;51(6):273–280.
48. National Restaurant Association. Kids LiveWell. 2012. http://www.restaurant.org/foodhealthyliving/kidslivewell/about. Accessed February 6, 2017.
49. Office of Disease Prevention & Health Promotion (ODPHP). Physical Activity Guidelines: Children and Adolescents. https://health.gov/paguidelines/guidelines/children.aspx. Accessed February 8, 2017.
50. Hoy MK, Goldman JD. Fiber intake of the U.S. population. What We Eat in America, NHANES 2009-2010. Food Surveys Research Group Dietary Data Brief No. 12. September 2014.
51. Henry C, Whiting SJ, Finch SL, et al. Impact of replacing regular chocolate milk with the reduced-sugar option on milk consumption in elementary schools in Saskatoon, Canada. *Appl Physiol Nutr Metab*. 2016;41(5):511–515.
52. Shriver LH, Marriage BJ, Bloch TD, et al. Contribution of snacks to dietary intakes of young children in the United States. Matern Child Nutr. 2017 Mar 23. doi:10.1111/mcn.12454. [Epub ahead of print].
53. Slining MM, Mathias KC, Popkin BM. Trends in food and beverage sources among US children and adolescents: 1989-2010. *J Acad Nutr Diet*. 2013;113(12):1683–1694.
54. American Heart Association News. Poison control data show energy drinks and young kids don't mix. November 16, 2014. http://news.heart.org/poison-control-data-show-energy-drinks-young-kids-dont-mix/. Accessed February 7, 2017.
55. Johnson SL, Hayes JE. Developmental readiness, caregiver and child feeding behaviors, and sensory science as a framework for feeding young children. *Nutr Today*. 2017;52(25):S30–S40.
56. Fitch C, Keim KS, Academy of Nutrition and Dietetics. Position of the Academy of Nutrition and Dietetics: use of nutritive and non-nutritive sweeteners. *J Acad Nutr Diet*. 2012;112(5):739–758.
57. Wolraich ML, Wilson DB, White JW. The effects of sugar on behavior or cognition in children. a meta-analysis. *JAMA*. 1995;274(20):1617–1621.
58. Trofholz AC, Tate AD, Draxten ML, et al. What's being served for dinner? An exploratory investigation of the associations between the healthfulness of family meals and child dietary intake. *J Acad Nutr Diet*. 2017;117(1):102–109.
59. Au LE, Rosen NJ, Fenton K, et al. Eating school lunch is associated with higher diet quality among elementary school students. *J Acad Nutr Diet*. 2016;116(11):1817–1824.
60. McLaren L, Pattenson S, Thawer S, et al. Measuring the short-term impact of fluoridation cessation on dental caries in Grade 2 children using tooth surface indices. *Community Dent Oral Epidemiol*. 2016;44(3):274–282.
61. Altschwager DK, Dwyer JT. Making micronutrient adequacy of American children a reality. *Nutr Today*. 2017;52(1):26–40.
62. World Health Organization. *Adolescent Pregnancy*. Geneva: WHO; 2012.
63. Salam RA, Hooda M, Das JK, et al. Interventions to improve adolescent nutrition: a systematic review and meta-analysis. *J Adolesc Health*. 2016;59(4S):S29–S39.
64. Powell ES, Smith-Taille LP, Popkin BM. Added sugars intake across the distribution of US children and adult consumers: 1977-2012. *J Acad Nutr Diet*. 2016;116(10):1543–1550.
65. Kenney EL, Gortmaker SL, Carter JE, et al. Grab a cup, fill it up! an intervention to promote the convenience of drinking water and increase student water consumption during school lunch. *Am J Public Health*. 2015;105(9):1777–1783.
66. Andersen LB, Arnberg K, Trolle E, et al. The effects of water and dairy drinks on dietary patterns in overweight adolescents. *Int J Food Sci Nutr*. 2016;67(3):314–324.
67. Schwartz AE, Leardo M, Siddhartha A. Effect of a school-based water intervention on child body mass index and obesity. *JAMA Pediatr*. 2016;170(3):220–226.
68. Sylvetsky AC, Jin Y, Clark EJ, et al. Consumption of low-calorie sweeteners among children and adults in the United States. *J Acad Nutr Diet*. 2017;117(3):441–448.
69. Tran NL, Barraj LM, Bi X, et al. Trends and patterns of caffeine consumption among US teenagers and young adults, NHANES 2003-2012. *Food Chem Toxicol*. 2016;94:227–242.
70. Rehm CD, Drewnowski A. Trends in energy intakes by type of fast food restaurant among US children from 2003 to 2010. *JAMA Pediatr*. 2015;169(5):502–504.
71. Quader ZS, Gillespie C, Silva SA, et al. Sodium intake among US school-aged children: National Health and Nutrition Examination Survey, 2011-2012. *J Acad Nutr Diet*. 2017;117(1):39–47.
72. American Heart Association. Statement from CEO Nancy Brown on Dec. 2016 NCHS Mortality Data Report. December 8, 2016. http://newsroom.heart.org/news/american-heart-association-statement-from-ceo-nancy-brown-on-dec-2016-nchs-mortality-data-report. Accessed February 13, 2017.
73. Centers for Disease Control and Prevention (CDC). Childhood Obesity Facts. Prevalence of Childhood Obesity in the United States, 2011-2014. Last updated December 22, 2016. https://www.cdc.gov/obesity/data/childhood.html. Accessed February 13, 2017.
74. Simmonds M, Llewellyn A, Owen CG, et al. Diagnosis of childhood obesity using BMI: potential ethicolegal implications and downstream effects: a response. *Obes Rev*. 2017;18(3):382–383.
75. US Preventive Services Task Force, Grossman DC, Bibbins-Domingo K, et al. Screening for obesity in children and adolescents: US Preventive Services Task Force Recommendation Statement. *JAMA*. 2017;317(23):2417–2426.
76. Dolton P, Xiao M. The intergenerational transmission of body mass index across countries. *Econ Hum Biol*. 2017;24:140–152.
77. Richmond RC, Timpson NJ, Felix JF, et al. Using genetic variation to explore the causal effect of maternal pregnancy adiposity on future offspring adiposity: a Mendelian randomisation study. *PLoS Med*. 2017;14(1):e1002221.
78. Styne DM, Arslanian SA, Connor EL, et al. Pediatric obesity—assessment, treatment, and prevention: an Endocrine Society Clinical Practice Guideline. *J Clin Endocrinol Metab*. 2017;102(3):1–49.

EVOLVE RESOURCES

Please visit http://evolve.elsevier.com/Stegeman/nutritional for additional practice and study support tools.

15

Nutritional Requirements for Older Adults and Eating Habits Affecting Oral Health

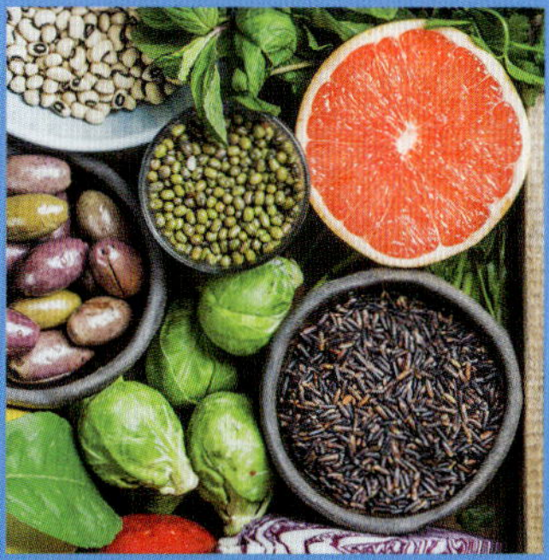

STUDENT LEARNING OUTCOMES

Upon completion of this chapter, the student will be able to achieve the following student learning outcomes:

1. Identify oral nutritional problems typically observed in older adults.
2. Predict physiologic changes that may alter an older individual's nutritional status.
3. Name socioeconomic and psychological factors influencing food intake of older patients.
4. Explain why nutrient requirements of older patients differ from younger patients.
5. Describe typical eating patterns of older adults, relate *Dietary Guidelines* and *MyPlate* to the diet of an older adult, and suggest implementation of dietary changes to provide optimum nutrient intake for older patients.

KEY TERMS

Age-related macular degeneration
Alternative medicine
Atrophic gastritis
Botanical
Complementary medicine
Denture stomatitis
Dysphagia
Genomics
Herb
Homeopathy
Homeostatic mechanisms
Hypogeusia
Incontinence
Naturopathy
Nocturia
Polypharmacy
Quality of life
Sarcopenia
Spices

TEST YOUR NQ

1. **T/F** Normal physiologic changes occurring in older adults do not affect nutritional requirements.
2. **T/F** Nutritional requirements for a 50-year-old patient are different from those for an 81-year-old patient.
3. **T/F** Food selection is highly correlated with dentition.
4. **T/F** Edentulous patients should puree their food.
5. **T/F** Dehydration is seldom observed in older adults.
6. **T/F** Older adults need more vitamins D and B_{12} than individuals younger than 51 years of age.
7. **T/F** Healthy older women require increased amounts of iron.
8. **T/F** Energy requirements decrease with age.
9. **T/F** Self-medication with vitamins is a healthy practice for older adults.
10. **T/F** Exercise is of no benefit to older adults.

Major shifts in the age of the United States population are affecting health care needs. Compared with 2000, when more than 35 million people were age 65 years and older (13% of the population), this group is expected to increase to approximately 74 million by 2030 (21% of the population). The 85-years-and-older group is the fastest growing segment of the older population (Fig. 15.1), and this group is projected to increase from 6 million in 2014 to 20 million in 2020.[1] U.S. life expectancy may rise to over 80 by 2030.

Genetics accounts for about 20% to 30% of an individual's lifespan, with the rest attributed to diet and lifestyle choices. Individual healthy lifestyle choices (never smoking, moderate alcohol consumption, physical activity, and regularly choosing a healthy diet) are moderately associated with successful aging; their combined impact is substantial. Improved medical care from infancy has improved Americans' lifespan, but it is important to increase the

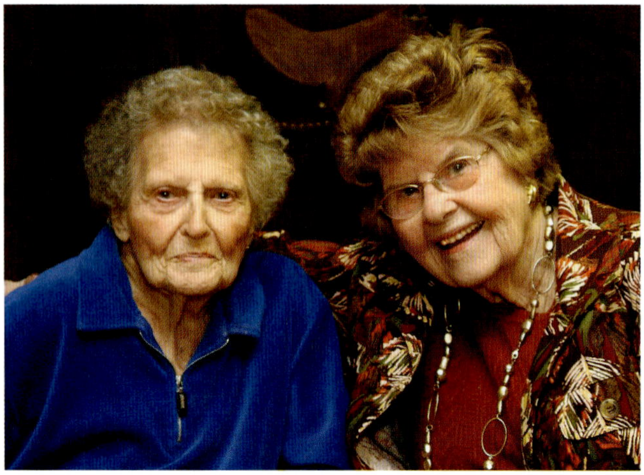

• **Figure 15.1** Relatives celebrating their 100th (*left*) and 90th (*right*) birthdays. Life expectancy is higher for baby boomers than for the current older population. (Reproduced with permission of D2 Studios, www.d2studios.net.)

quality of the older years by adopting healthy lifestyles and consistently choosing nutrient-dense foods.

Quality of life is defined by the World Health Organization as individuals' perception of their position in life in the context of the culture and value systems in which they live and in relation to their goals, expectations, standards, and concerns.[2] Oral health impacts systemic health. Therefore, oral care is an important consideration in maintaining quality of life. Whereas people were once disabled by conditions such as poor vision and cardiovascular disease (CVD), which are now more treatable, currently degenerative conditions, such as Alzheimer disease and dementia, are plaguing older individuals. By age 85 years, 50% of older adults will have dementia, which may impact function and nutritional status.

The *Dietary Guidelines* recognize that the health and nutritional status of people older than 50 years needs special consideration; changes in food habits are needed to adjust to physical and metabolic changes that occur with aging. It is never too late to make lifestyle changes to improve one's health, longevity, and quality of life.

General Health Status

The most common nutritional disorder in older individuals is obesity. The prevalence of obesity increases progressively from 20 to 60 years of age and decreases after age 60. Between 2003 to 2004 and 2011 to 2012, the percentage of people older than age 60 years who were obese increased from 31.5% to 35.4%. More men than women are overweight, but more women than men are obese. Obesity is more common among African Americans and slightly higher among Mexican Americans than among non-Hispanic whites.[1]

Obesity causes serious medical complications, impairing quality of life by exacerbating the age-related decline in physical function and cognitive disability. Approximately 80% of older Americans have at least one noncommunicable chronic disease, 68% have been diagnosed with two or more chronic conditions, and 36% have four or more chronic diseases.[3] Obesity contributes to some chronic conditions commonly seen in older adults, including CVD, diabetes, lung disease, arthritis, and Alzheimer disease. Most of these conditions increase the risk of poor nutritional status. Routine nutritional care for older adults can help prevent or manage chronic diseases.

Malnutrition is another nutrition-related problem diagnosed in older adults admitted to hospitals and long-term care facilities and in those with serious medical problems. Malnutrition is associated with impaired immune response, impaired muscle and respiratory function, delayed wound healing, overall increased complications, longer rehabilitation, longer hospitalizations, and increased mortality. Factors considered to be contributing causes of older individuals being at risk of malnutrition include less education and lower income; being housebound or unable to purchase food; multiple medications; physical disabilities, depression, and other mental challenges; recent drastic lifestyle changes, such as death of spouse; and lacking regularly cooked meals. An example of a nutritional assessment questionnaire is available on the Evolve website. Identifying individuals at nutritional risk is critical to cost-effectiveness for the health care system and to assist older patients in maintaining their independence and personal well-being. Food choices are also related to oral problems; thus, a dental assessment should include questions regarding food intake and oral problems affecting intake.

Dietary restrictions associated with management of chronic diseases, such as diabetes, renal disease, or CVD, can be confusing, especially if more than one condition exists. Improper food selection or fear of choosing unhealthy foods may be a factor for inadequate nutrition. The result of certain treatments can affect eating by creating loss of appetite, nausea and vomiting, diarrhea or constipation, xerostomia, or changes in the taste of food, for example, chemotherapy.

Prescription use, **polypharmacy** (use of at least five or prescriptions), and supplement use are prevalent. Approximately 36% of older adults take five or more prescriptions; 88% take at least one prescription medication; almost 64% are taking dietary supplements.[4] Some of these drugs depress appetite, interfere with nutrient absorption, and affect cognitive abilities. Classes of medications that place older adults at risk include (1) diuretics, (2) opioid painkillers, (3) tranquilizers, (4) antidepressants, (5) statins, (6) oral hypoglycemics, and (7) antacids and anticholinergics. Although drug–nutrient interactions can compromise anyone's nutritional status, these problems are amplified in older adults. Physiologic and pathophysiologic changes, such as decreased hepatic and renal clearance, result in greater variability and less predictability of a drug's effects.

Physiologic Factors Influencing Nutritional Needs and Status

Aging significantly impacts body composition. Many organ functions decline with age, some beginning as early as age 30 years. These physiologic changes can substantially influence nutritional requirements of older adults by affecting absorption, transportation, metabolism, and excretion of nutrients. With aging, the body is less able to correct nutrient imbalances, such as increasing absorption when intake is decreased. The precarious physiologic balance may be upset by disease; physical and mental challenges; and environmental, economic, and social disabilities. However, chronological age and functional capacity do not always correlate. Older individuals differ from one another in physiologic and health status more than any other age group, meaning that chronologic status is not useful in predicting physiologic abilities and health status.

Impairment of visual, auditory, and olfactory sensory organs is common. Poor vision makes food preparation difficult, even hazardous in some cases, and may be responsible for senior citizens not identifying contaminated foods, a potential cause of foodborne illness. Poor hearing increases isolation and decreases socialization.

Oral Cavity

Oral health problems (e.g., chewing, swallowing, compromised dentition) are indicators of nutritional risk and may be primary contributors to malnutrition. Persistent oral health problems are associated with impaired intake of certain foods and nutrients. A progressive decline in gustatory and olfactory sensitivity affects food choices and quantity because "nothing tastes good." Olfactory and taste receptors are affected by impaired chewing and swallowing.

Some conditions and certain medications also lead to deterioration of taste sensitivity. **Hypogeusia** (loss of taste) may be associated with certain disorders rather than being a normal component of the aging process. Older adults may confuse taste sensations, describing sour foods as metallic and salty foods as tasteless. Many people gradually begin to lose their sense of smell around age 50 years, a condition called anosmia. As a consequence of anosmia and hypogeusia, foods may be overly seasoned with salt or sugar. Losses in salt or sugar perception make it difficult to comply with low-sodium or diabetes guidelines. Other seasonings and spices can help replace the taste of salt or sugar.

Xerostomia, which affects half of all older adults, compromises oral processing of foods. Most individuals requiring polypharmacy report problems with xerostomia. A lack of saliva affects both the oral preparatory and oral phases of swallowing, thus leading to impaired bolus formation and oropharyngeal bolus transport. Xerostomia increases the risk for oral disease because antimicrobial components and minerals in saliva help rebuild tooth enamel after acid-producing, decay-causing bacterial attacks. Crunchy foods stimulate saliva flow, but foods such as raw vegetables and crispy fruits are more likely to be shunned. Dry foods, such as bread, and sticky foods, such as peanut butter, may also be avoided. Many patients may choose hard candy or gum to stimulate saliva flow and relieve the dryness. However, frequent exposure to fermentable carbohydrate promotes root caries and reduces intake of nutrient-dense foods (see Chapter 20 for further discussion of xerostomia).

Recession of gingival tissues exposes root surfaces of teeth to the oral environment; this process increases with aging. The lack of a protective enamel layer on the root, surface roughness of roots, and demineralization related to a lower pH, make the area highly susceptible to dental caries. The prevalence of root caries, further discussed in Chapter 20, is much higher in older adults than in younger individuals. In 1999 to 2004, almost 38% of adults age 75 years and older had root caries.[5] Root caries are more prevalent in men, usually with a history of tobacco use.

Osteoporosis and periodontitis are both diseases characterized by bone resorption. Periodontitis involves inflammatory bone loss in alveolar cortical bone supporting the teeth. A negative calcium balance results in calcium loss from the maxilla and mandible, which are primarily trabecular bone. Age-related bone loss affecting alveolar bone results in tooth loss and edentulism. Low bone mineral density and osteoporosis/osteopenia are both risk factors for tooth loss, especially prevalent in postmenopausal women.[6] Approximately two-thirds of individuals older than 65 years have periodontitis.[7] Periodontal disease increases the likelihood of weight loss in older adults; the more extensive and severe the disease, the greater the weight loss. This condition is partially responsible for loss of teeth; control of periodontal disease can significantly reduce tooth loss.

The prevalence of edentulism is nearly twice as high among people age 85 years and over (31%) as people ages 65 to 74 years (16%).[8] Edentulism is not inevitable with advancing age; its prevalence among adults older than age 50 has decreased significantly. Native Americans and African Americans have the highest rates of edentulism, possibly due to lack of receiving annual oral health services. More seniors with lower incomes are edentulous than those in higher income brackets.

The quality of chewing, or chewing ability, is affected by the number of teeth in functional occlusion. Tooth loss adversely affects chewing ability, causing difficulties in forming a bolus. A larger bolus size interferes with optimal swallowing, leading to additional swallowing abnormalities in the oral preparatory stage.[9,10] Patients with periodontal conditions, edentulous areas, and/or patients who wear dentures tend to alter food choices to reduce chewing or because of fear of choking. Many individuals in the United States older than age 60 only have 19 teeth. The function and position of the remaining teeth seem to indicate chewing ability more accurately than the total number of teeth present. Tooth loss may be an early indicator of accelerated aging. Weight changes can be a reason for an ill-fitting dental appliance. Weight gain (usually secondary to edema) results in a tight-fitting denture, which may cause ulcerations; weight loss causing loose-fitting dentures also can increase risk of ulcerations. Normally, alveolar bone is maintained in response to occlusal forces associated with chewing. If severe mandibular resorption occurs, it is very difficult to construct a well-fitting dental prosthesis. Many older individuals or their families do not believe the cost of a new or replaced appliance is warranted because of the patients' perceived life expectancy. Even if edentulous individuals own dentures, some may not wear them regularly, or they may be unable to chew because of a periodontal condition. Treatment with mandibular implant-supported dentures has a significant positive effect on both bite force and masticatory performance.[11]

Tooth loss, edentulous status, and conventional dentures reflect differences in healthy behaviors, attitudes toward oral health, and dental care. Nutrient intakes of patients with compromised dentition can fall below minimum requirements, increasing risk of malnutrition in older adults.[12,13] Even the loss of a few teeth affects nutrient quality of the diet; individuals have difficulty managing high-fiber fruits and vegetables, especially raw apples and carrots, tossed salads, and dietary fiber.

Compromised dental status also negatively affects animal protein intake. Nutrient intake decreases as the total number of teeth decreases, which may result in an inadequate amount of total protein, magnesium, zinc, vitamins B_1, B_6, and C, niacin, folate, pantothenic acid, and beta-carotene.

Denture stomatitis may affect over 75% of partial and complete denture wearers. **Dental stomatitis** is traumatization and chronic inflammation of mucus membranes supporting a removable denture. While many risk factors contribute to the etiology of denture stomatitis, *Candida albicans* is probably the main culprit. Any condition that allows proliferation of candida and possibly affects immune function of the host may result in irritation of the mucus membranes. A high sugar intake increases the risk of denture stomatitis as the sugar stimulates growth of *Candida*. This may be as significant as poor denture hygiene in the development of denture stomatitis. Other nutritional factors frequently implicated as increasing risk include dietary deficiencies (iron, folate, vitamin B_{12}) and xerostomia.[14]

Gastrointestinal Tract

Changes in esophageal motility and deterioration of nerve function may cause **dysphagia** (difficulty with swallowing). This frequently observed disorder increases risk of aspiration pneumonia and morbidity; individuals with swallowing problems eat slowly and may be unable to consume adequate amounts.

Atrophic gastritis, a chronic stomach inflammation with atrophy of the mucous membrane and glands and diminished hydrochloric acid production, is frequently observed in older patients. Diminished hydrochloric acid secretion may affect calcium, iron, and vitamin B_{12} absorption. Additionally, lack of acid permits overgrowth of bacteria that compromise vitamin B_{12} availability.

Constipation may be a consequence of altered gastrointestinal motility, loss of bowel muscle tone, medications, inadequate food and fluid intake, low-fiber diet, and inactivity. Additional causes include chronic laxative use and some medications, especially analgesics, antihypertensives, and narcotics. Problems with constipation may be averted by increasing fiber-containing foods, fluid intake, and activity level.

Hydration Status

Decreased thirst sensations are associated with aging; dehydration occurs more frequently in older adults. Fluid intake may not increase automatically to offset increased water losses from the compromised kidney. As a result of poor fluid intake, susceptibility to caries is increased.

Homeostatic mechanisms indicate the body's ability to correct imbalances, such as decreased nutrient intake accompanied by an increase in nutrient absorption or efficiency of use. Certain chronic illnesses (heart and kidney disease) lead to impairment of various homeostatic mechanisms controlling water balance. Fever, which can lead to mild dehydration in healthy individuals, may result in severe dehydration in older adults. Other seemingly mild stresses, such as the presence of infection or diarrhea or use of diuretics, can upset the normal homeostasis of an older individual.

Water is the single most important substance consumed. Regardless of the setting in which older adults are living, at home or in long-term care, dehydration or inadequate fluid intake is a common and costly disorder.[15] Dehydration is probably the primary cause of confusion in older patients and can occur because of the kidney's inability to concentrate urine, changes in thirst sensation, changes in functional status, side effects of medications, and lack of mobility. Dehydration can lead to loose-fitting dentures. The condition frequently results in hospitalization as a result of fecal impaction, cognitive impairment, and overall functional decline.

Musculoskeletal System

Two nutrition-related conditions encountered by older persons involving the musculoskeletal system are osteoporosis and sarcopenia; thus, maintaining bone health and muscle mass are primary concerns. As discussed in Chapter 9, *Health Application 9*, osteoporosis or shortening and outward bowing of the spine may develop. Bone resorption progresses rapidly in older patients. Trabecular bone loss may be associated with physical inactivity, unavailability of calcium (inadequate dietary intake, imbalance in calcium-to-phosphorus ratio, and decreased calcium absorption), changes in hormones affecting calcium metabolism, lack of vitamin D, or altered vitamin D metabolism associated with impaired renal function. Bone loss increases susceptibility to fractures, which can result in disability.

Sarcopenia is the loss of skeletal muscle mass (unintentional), strength (loss of muscle), and physical performance related to aging. The older person becomes weak and frail, creating functional problems that further contribute to sarcopenia. If enough muscle is lost, it can be debilitating. This complex multifaceted process also is observed in persons who have been physically inactive throughout their lives. Individuals with dependent ambulatory status experience a higher prevalence of sarcopenia compared with ambulatory patients.[16] Functional decline inevitably leads to frailty, reduced mobility, falls, fractures, and mortality. Hospital stays are longer and often functional recovery is incomplete even after rehabilitation.[17] Impaired dentition is significantly associated with sarcopenia.[18,19] As many as 30% of adults older than age 60 may have sarcopenia; prevalence increases to more than 50% of adults older than age 80 years.

Sarcopenia can even occur in an obese person (body mass index [BMI] > 27 kg/m^2; called sarcopenic obesity). A "fat frail" person suffers from the worst of both worlds, (decreased muscle strength expected to support increased body weight).[20] The prevalence of sarcopenic obesity differs substantially among studies because of the lack of a standard definition.

Inactivity is responsible for loss of muscle strength and balance. Physical activity can help ameliorate some chronic health problems, yet only 15% of people ages 65 to 74 years and 5% of those 85 years old and over meet the physical guidelines.[1] An active lifestyle also helps improve physiologic well-being, and relieves symptoms of depression and anxiety. Box 15.1 lists some benefits of physical activity. Many older adults can be motivated to make changes to prevent or delay a decline toward ill health and disability if information is presented with an understandable rationale.

The *Physical Activity Guidelines for Americans* (see Chapter 1) addressing older adults may help to deter sarcopenia.[21] Older adults unable to do 150 minutes of moderate-intensity aerobic activity a week because of chronic conditions should be as physically active as their abilities and conditions allow. Older adults with chronic conditions should understand whether and how their conditions affect their ability to safely participate in regular physical activities. Exercises that maintain or improve balance are recommended. Walking and other moderate exercise are linked to lower stroke and heart attack risk even for people in their 70s.[22] Physical activity (walking, swimming, or dancing) may improve quality of life for older adults by maintaining their independence longer, improving longevity, and increasing brain function and boosting memory.[23,24] Actually, the more physical activity older adults do, the greater the health benefit.[25] Optimizing physical activity should be encouraged for all adults—not just when symptoms of physical or cognitive decline appear.

Women have less muscle than men but lose it more slowly during aging. Because older women do not use protein as effectively as men, muscle that has been lost is harder to replace. Adequate amounts of protein are essential to replace muscle lost during the aging process.

With aging, intraabdominal fat increases more than subcutaneous or total body fat, and peripheral muscle declines more than central muscle mass. As musculature shrinks, fat tissue accumulates. When

• BOX 15.1 Health Benefits of Physical Activity

Strong Evidence

- Lower risk of early death
- Lower risk of cardiovascular disease (CVD)
- Lower risk of stroke
- Lower risk of adverse blood lipid profile
- Lower risk of type 2 diabetes
- Lower risk of metabolic syndrome
- Lower risk of colon cancer
- Lower risk of breast cancer
- Prevention of weight gain
- Weight loss, particularly when combined with reduced calorie intake
- Improved cardiorespiratory and muscular fitness
- Prevention of falls
- Reduced depression
- Better cognitive function (for older adults)

Moderate to Strong Evidence

- Better functional health (for older adults)
- Reduced abdominal obesity

Moderate Evidence

- Lower risk of hip fracture
- Lower risk of lung cancer
- Lower risk of endometrial cancer
- Weight maintenance after weight loss
- Increased bone density
- Improved sleep quality

Note: *The Advisory Committee rated the evidence of health benefits of physical activity as strong, moderate, or weak. To do so, the Committee considered the type, number, and quality of studies available, as well as consistency of findings across studies that addressed each outcome. The Committee also considered evidence for causality and* dose–response *in assigning the strength-of-evidence rating.*

Source: U.S. Department of Health and Human Services. 2008 Physical Activity Guidelines for Americans. *https://health.gov/PAGuidelines/pdf/paguide.pdf. Accessed February 26, 2017.*

older people reduce their food intake without exercising, they lose more lean muscle mass and less fat compared to those who exercise while dieting. A slightly higher BMI seems to be protective in maintaining immunity to diseases.

Even with no increase in weight, fat stores replace lean muscle mass. Low protein intake contributes to muscle loss and a negative nitrogen balance that evokes muscle breakdown. Maintaining muscle is essential to reduce the risk of falling.

Diminished sense of taste and smell, rapid satiety, poor oral health, decreased metabolism, gastrointestinal changes, and dementia—all increasingly common with aging—result in decreasing food intake and increased adiposity (caused by fatigue and lack of activity). This creates a vicious cycle that leads to more gain in fat and more muscle loss, eventually resulting in functional consequences (e.g., disability), reduced quality of life, and early death.

On the brighter side, sarcopenia is not inevitable with aging. High-protein foods stimulate muscle protein synthesis, even in older adults. Protein use may be impaired, but this can be overcome by consuming high-quality protein at each meal. Resistance exercise combined with adequate consumption of protein from animal sources elicits the greatest anabolic response and may help older individuals produce a "youthful" muscle protein synthesis response. The consensus is to ensure a high-protein diet with adequate amounts of fruits and vegetables to reduce risk of sarcopenia.[26,27]

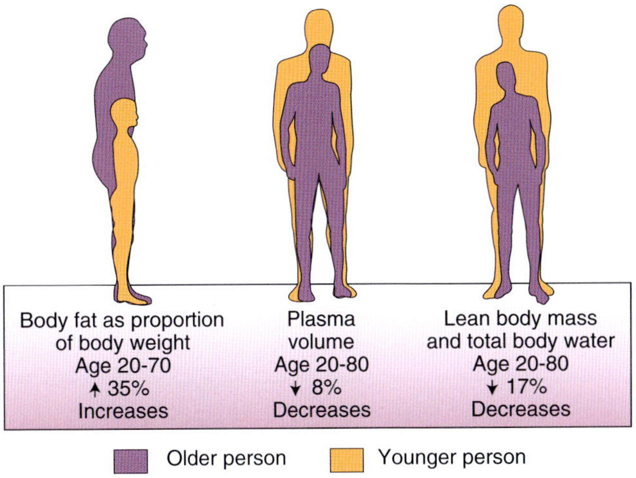

• Figure 15.2 Changes in the body with aging. Younger person, age 20 years. Older person, age 80 years. (Redrawn from Vestal RE. *Drugs and the Elderly*, NIH Publication No. 79-1449, Washington, DC: US Department of Health, Education, and Welfare, 1979.)

Protein supplementation has not consistently shown benefits on muscle mass and function. Maintaining appropriate blood levels of vitamin D may also aid in retaining muscle strength and physical performance.[28,29] Whether benefits of weight loss outweigh risks in individuals with sarcopenic obesity is unknown.[30] Muscle mass can be preserved by increasing physical activity. Less lean body mass results in a decreased basal metabolic rate (Fig. 15.2). In older individuals, the basal metabolic rate may be 10% to 12% below the level of 20-year-olds (see Fig. 7.5). In other words, the body burns fewer calories than during earlier years; thus, less food is needed to prevent weight gain. Less intake of vital proteins inhibits healing after a physiologic injury or insult and contributes to the declining function of many organ systems.

Socioeconomic and Psychological Factors

Many changes occur affecting food intake of older adults (Fig. 15.3). Most retired people live on fixed incomes significantly lower than when they were employed. In 2014, approximately 15.8% (10.2 million) older adults were faced with the threat of hunger; many have incomes above the poverty line and are white. Between 2001 to 2014, the fraction of older adults experiencing the threat of hunger increased by 47%.[31] Inflation, failing health, and medical bills (especially cost of medications) can have a devastating effect on fixed incomes. The food budget frequently is affected and is a risk factor for inadequate nutrition. Fresh fruit and vegetable choices may be curtailed because of their high cost and limited shelf life. Title III Nutrition Programs for the Elderly (congregate dining and Meals-on-Wheels) are available to improve nutritional and health status of older patients and possibly prevent or postpone more expensive services of long-term care institutions. Nutritious meals are furnished at a minimal charge to older adults or free for those who qualify. These programs have been proven to improve dietary intakes of recipients whose diets were previously below the Recommended Dietary Allowance (RDA).

An inability to drive or lack of access to transportation affects use of health services and availability of food. Approximately one-half

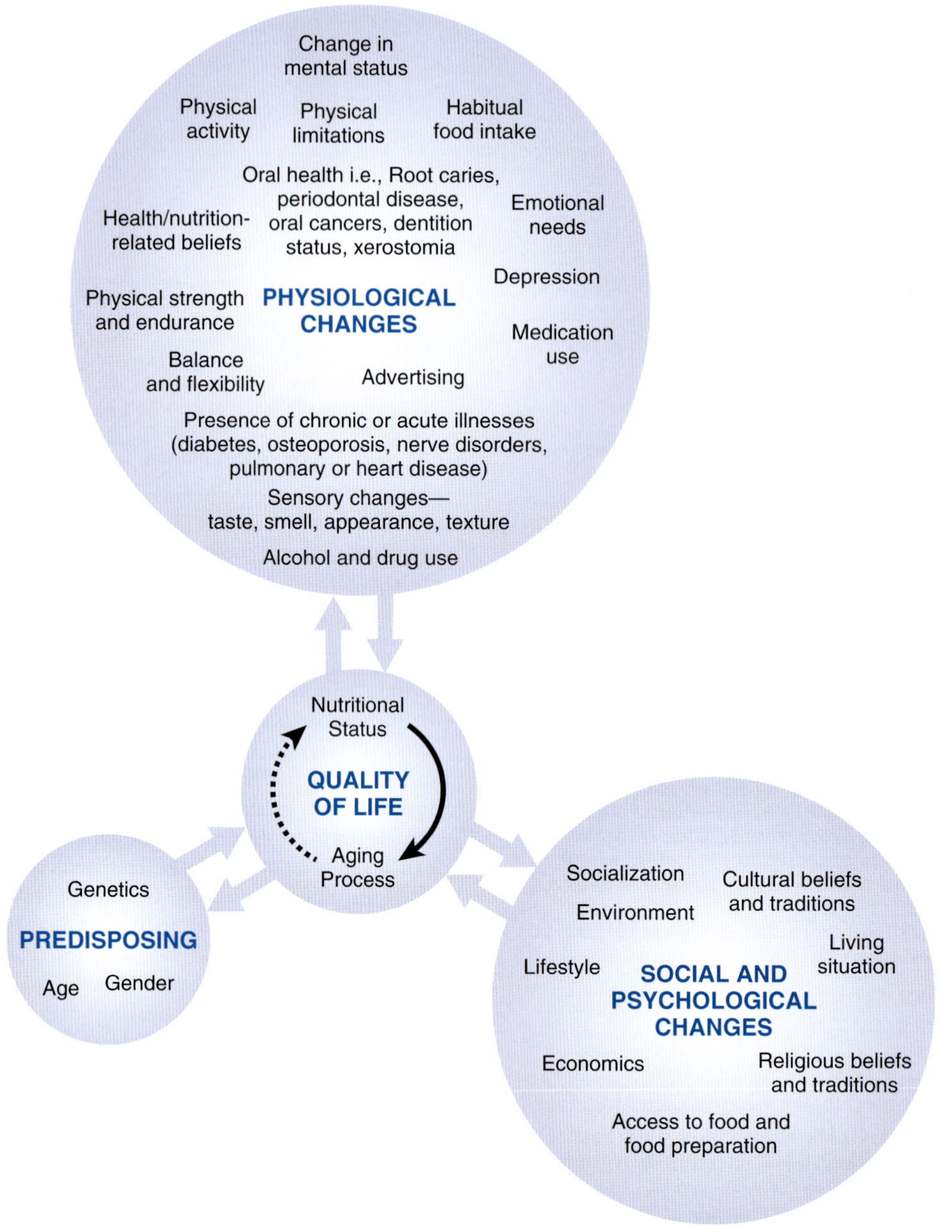

• **Figure 15.3** Multiple interrelated factors affecting nutritional status for older adults. (Reproduced with permission from the American Dietetic Association: Position of the American Dietetic Association: Nutrition, aging, and the continuum of care. *J Am Diet Assoc* 2000;100(5):580–594.)

of noninstitutionalized individuals older than age 65 years live alone.[31] Individuals who live with another person and are socially active tend to consume a larger variety of foods. An inactive person who lives alone may lack motivation to prepare well-balanced meals, especially if the appetite is poor.

Apathy and depression can predispose older individuals to decreased appetite and interest in food. Deterioration in oral health and oral health-related problems increase the risk of depressive symptoms among older adults, signifying the importance of maintaining good oral health as a determinant of subjective quality of life.[32] Depression is difficult to distinguish from symptoms related to stresses of later life, such as illness and changes in lifestyle. Some older individuals may consider depression as a natural, inevitable component of aging and may not seek treatment. Loneliness is related to dietary inadequacies.

DENTAL CONSIDERATIONS

Assessment

- *Physical:* Blood pressure; diagnosis of chronic disease, dentures, swallowing process, xerostomia, condition of oral cavity and gingiva; educational level; financial, socioeconomic, mental, and psychological status; types of drugs taken, including over-the-counter drugs, herbal supplements, and aspirin use.
- *Dietary:* Screen for nutritional health (see the assessment form available on the Evolve website); motivation to eat and drink; beliefs and attitudes about foods or products to delay the aging process.

Interventions

- Osteoporosis and periodontal disease both require interdisciplinary approaches for their prevention and management.

DENTAL CONSIDERATIONS—cont'd

- Encourage new denture wearers to swallow liquids with the dentures first, then to chew soft foods, and, last to bite and masticate regular foods. It is easier to master complex masticatory movements in this order, and the mouth is protected from becoming sore. New denture wearers need to eat slowly, chew food longer, and cut raw fibrous foods such as apples and carrots into bite-size pieces.
- Wearing dentures may promote positive calcium balance and decrease alveolar resorption. If calcium intake is poor, supplements containing both calcium and vitamin D may help promote positive calcium balance.
- For edentulous patients, inquire about the preferred texture of food. Do not assume that edentulous patients require pureed foods; because of lack of visual appeal and flavor, appetite may be affected if only pureed foods are offered.
- Sweet sensitivity declines with age, leading to a compensatory increase in desire to choose foods containing sugar and possibly other carbohydrate foods.
- Normal swallowing is closely associated with chewing ability and ample saliva secretion.
- Adequate oral care, provision of dentures, prevention of tooth loss, and swallowing training may have positive effects on general health in elderly adults.
- Without adequate oral care, general health, including swallowing, will steadily worsen.
- Improvement for problems associated with swallowing disorders related to xerostomia can be managed with oral moisturizers, lubricants, and careful use of fluids during mealtime.
- Tooth brushing may increase salivary flow for those with medication-induced dry mouth; mechanical stimulation of the salivary glands during tooth brushing may promote salivary flow.
- Well-fitted dentures are effective in increasing chewing ability and thus improve food intake and oral health–related quality of life.
- Teach older patients about appropriate oral hygiene techniques to minimize gingival recession, followed with a fluoride regimen.
- Assess the fit of a denture or any prosthesis. The dental team may need to make recommendations for adjusting the prosthesis for a better fit or refer the older patient to a health care provider for assessment and management of unintentional weight changes.
- Encourage older patients to eat slowly and chew their food well.
- Often, health care providers recommend lemon glycerin swabs to moisten oral tissues in patients with xerostomia. This may be detrimental to the mouth for two reasons: (a) because lemon is an acid, it may cause decalcification of the teeth, and (b) glycerin is a form of alcohol that can further dry oral tissues. A better alternative would be to moisten a swab with water and apply it to the dry mucosa.
- Avoidance of certain food categories (fresh fruit and vegetables and meats) because of masticatory difficulties may aggravate other nutrition-related problems; these foods are major sources of vitamins and minerals.

NUTRITIONAL DIRECTIONS

- Factors that slow the aging process include regular exercise, abstinence from smoking, and getting adequate sleep. Physical activity enhances muscle strength and preserves muscle mass.
- Preventing and controlling oral disease to achieve good oral health is essential to healthy aging.
- Less muscle tissue and a lower activity level result in a reduced caloric requirement.
- If xerostomia is present, use artificial saliva products (oral moisturizers), sugar-free gum or hard candies (preferably containing xylitol); practice frequent oral hygiene care; and drink adequate noncariogenic fluids.
- For compromised natural dentition or xerostomia, include fluids, sauces, or gravies with each meal to make chewing easier. However, beverage consumption should not interfere with food intake.
- Because of decreased stomach acid, older adults should take calcium citrate with vitamin D supplements between meals for optimal absorption or use calcium carbonate supplements with meals.
- Low calcium intake is related to increased risk of tooth loss.
- Moderate exercise, such as walking, is beneficial in reducing the risk of CVD in older adults.
- By exercising 45 minutes a day, significant improvements may be seen in muscle strength, preventing bone loss and reducing risks of many diseases associated with aging. Exercise may also improve balance and coordination to reduce the likelihood of falling. Physical activity should include moderate-intensity aerobic activity, muscle-strengthening activity, flexibility, and balance.

Nutrient Requirements

Dietary Reference Intakes (DRIs)

The revised DRIs added recommendations for individuals 51 to 70 years old and individuals older than 70 years. Metabolism to maintain body functions requires all the same nutrients, but the requirements for most micronutrients are increased because of the effects of aging on absorption, use, and excretion. With few exceptions, the recommended nutrient amounts for both groups are the same. Energy needs are lower for older individuals because of declining basal metabolism and activity level. Recommendations for several nutrients differ from those for adults 31 to 50 years old, including fiber, calcium, chromium, iron (for women), and vitamins D and B_6 (Table 15.1).

Fluids

In normal situations, at least eight glasses of fluids per day is recommended. Fluid intake is of particular concern because of susceptibility to fluid imbalances secondary to physiologic changes. An older patient may intentionally restrict fluids because of **nocturia** (excessive urination at night), **incontinence** (inability to control urinary excretion), pain associated with movement related to arthritis, or having to request assistance to go to the toilet.

Energy and Protein

Despite the fact that caloric requirements are less, energy balance is usually recommended for older adults. Clinical recommendation of weight loss remains controversial because of the potential for loss of lean muscle and physical function. If intentional caloric deficit to lose weight (and consequently fatty tissue) is accompanied by routine exercise to maintain physical fitness, mobility and walking speed can improve. While overweight and obesity are associated with a higher risk of CVD, and weight loss is normally recommended; physical activity may do more for cardiovascular health than losing weight does.[33] Weight loss, even with intentional caloric restriction and improved health indices, will not necessarily increase the lifespan in humans.

TABLE 15.1 **Dietary Reference Intakes (DRIs) for Selected Nutrients for Older Adults**

	AGE 51–70 YEARS		AGE OLDER THAN 70 YEARS	
Nutrients	**Men**	**Women**	**Men**	**Women**
Protein (g)	**56**	**46**	**56**	46
Carbohydrate (g)	**130**	**130**	**130**	130
Fiber (g)	30*	21*	30*	21*
Fat-Soluble Vitamins				
Vitamin A (μg)	**900**	**700**	**900**	**700**
Vitamin E (mg)	**15**	**15**	**15**	**15**
Vitamin D (μg/IU)[a]	**15/600**	**15/600**	**20/800**	**20/800**
Vitamin K (μg)	120*	120*	90*	90*
Water-Soluble Vitamins				
Ascorbic acid (mg)	**90**	**75**	**90**	**75**
Folate (μg)	**400**	**400**	**400**	**400**
Niacin (mg)	**16**	**14**	**16**	**14**
Riboflavin (mg)	**1.3**	**1.1**	**1.3**	**1.1**
Thiamin (mg)	**1.2**	**1.1**	**1.2**	**1.1**
Vitamin B_6 (mg)	**1.7**	**1.5**	**1.7**	**1.5**
Vitamin B_{12} (μg)[a]	**2.4**	**2.4**	**2.4**	**2.4**
Biotin (mg)	30*	30*	30*	30*
Choline (mg)	550*	550*	550*	550*
Minerals				
Calcium (mg)	**1000**	**1200**	**1200**	**1200**
Phosphorus (mg)	**700**	**700**	**700**	**700**
Iodine (μg)	**150**	**150**	**150**	**150**
Iron (mg)	**8**	**8**	**8**	**8**
Magnesium (mg)	**420**	**320**	**420**	**320**
Zinc (mg)	**11**	**8**	**11**	**8**
Selenium (μg)	**55**	**55**	**55**	**55**

Note: Recommended Dietary Allowances (RDAs) are presented in **bold type** and Adequate Intakes (AIs) are followed by an asterisk (*).

[a]1 μg cholecalciferol = 40 IU vitamin D.

Data from Institute of Medicine, Food and Nutrition Board: *Dietary Reference Intakes for Calcium and Vitamin D.* Washington, DC: National Academies Press; 2011. Institute of Medicine, Food and Nutrition Board: *Dietary Reference Intakes for Vitamin C, Vitamin E, Selenium, and Carotenoids.* Washington, DC: National Academies Press; 2000. Institute of Medicine, Food and Nutrition Board: *Dietary Reference Intakes for Calcium, Phosphorus, Magnesium, Vitamin D, and Fluoride.* Washington, DC: National Academies Press; 1997. Institute of Medicine, Food and Nutrition Board: *Dietary Reference Intakes for Vitamin A, Vitamin K, Arsenic, Boron, Chromium, Copper, Iodine, Iron, Manganese, Molybdenum, Nickel, Silicon, Vanadium, and Zinc.* Washington, DC: National Academies Press; 2001. Institute of Medicine, Food and Nutrition Board: *Dietary Reference Intakes for Carbohydrates, Fats, Protein, Fiber, and Physical Activity, Parts 1 and 2.* Washington, DC: National Academies Press; 2002.

Calorie needs decrease with age, but protein needs do not. Older adults tend to consume less protein than younger adults, primarily due to reduced energy needs. Protein intake may be compromised because of illness, debilitating injuries, depressed appetite, or difficulty eating. Approximately one-third of adults over age 50 fail to meet the RDA for protein; close to 10% of older women fail to meet even the Estimated Average Requirements (EAR) for protein (0.66 g protein/kg/day).[34] Despite what is indicated in the RDAs, protein needs are proportional to body weight, not energy intake. Essential amino acid requirement is increased for older adults to produce a positive response in muscle protein synthesis and metabolism and stimulate bone protein metabolism. Protein also plays a pivotal role in maintenance of bone health by increasing calcium absorption and muscle strength and mass, thereby benefiting the skeleton.

The percentage of protein from animal sources providing all the essential amino acids predicts the probability of meeting the RDA. Older persons who consume higher percentages of protein

• BOX 15.2 Recommended Protein Intakes

Routinely active adults: 1.2–2.0 g/kg[a]
Healthy older adults: 1.0–1.2 g/kg[b,c]
Older adults with acute or chronic disease: 1.2–1.5 g/kg[b]
Older adults with severe illness/marked malnutrition: up to 2 g/kg[b]

[a]Thomas DT, Erdman KA, Burke LM. Position of the Academy of Nutrition and Dietetics, Dietitians of Canada, and the American College of Sports Medicine. Nutrition and athletic performance. J Acad Nutr Diet. 2016;116(3):501–528.
[b]Bauer JM, Diekmann R. Protein and older persons. Clin Geriatr Med. 2015;31(3):327–338. Deutz NE, Bauer JM, Barazzoni R, et al. Protein intake and exercise for optimal muscle function with aging: recommendations from the ESPEN Expert Group. Clin Nutr. 2014;33(6):929–936.
[c]English KL, Paddon-Jones D. Protecting muscle mass and function in older adults during bed rest. Curr Opin Clin Nutr Metab Care. 2010;13(1):34–39.

can lose weight with less age-related reduction in lean tissue mass.[34] Exercise at any age increases the body's need for protein; thus, protein intake slightly above the RDA (1.0 g/day) may be needed for increasing bone-mineral density and muscle mass. Protein intakes above the RDAs have been supported by several expert groups (Box 15.2). Approximately 25 to 30 g (or slightly more than 3 oz of meat) of high-quality protein will maximize muscle protein synthesis, but this amount of protein is needed three times a day rather than consuming most of the protein at one meal.[35,36]

Vitamins and Minerals

Older patients (especially women) usually have a negative calcium balance and lose bone mass, leading to osteoporosis and spontaneous fractures. Inadequate calcium intake is one possible reason for this, but genetic, hormonal, and environmental factors are also important. Decreased physical activity contributes to calcium loss over the years. The RDA of 1200 mg of calcium for everyone older than age 70 years is higher than for younger adults so as to maintain bone mass and reduce risk of osteoporosis. Calcium supplements are largely ineffective for remodeling bone matrix unless adequate protein (at least 1.0 g/kg) is available. Calcium absorption, healthy bone density, and physical function all require adequate vitamin D levels.

To prevent problems with bone mineralization, the recommendation for vitamin D intake is higher for individuals over 70 years—20 μg/day (800 IU). It is important to ensure that patients receive adequate calcium in addition to vitamin D. Low vitamin D levels are linked to muscle weakness, loss of bone strength, and falls and fractures. Prevalence of vitamin D deficiency in Americans is a public health concern because of its effects on quality of life. Vitamin D insufficiency may occur in older adults because aging skin cannot synthesize vitamin D as efficiently, homebound or institutionalized individuals are less likely to spend much time outdoors, and vitamin D intakes may be inadequate. A deficiency may also be the result of reduced production of vitamin D_3 by the skin as a result of covering the skin and using sunscreen. Other causes of vitamin D deficiency include dietary insufficiency, malabsorption, kidney disease, and use of glucocorticoids.

As many as half of older adults in the United States could be vitamin D deficient as evidenced by the numbers of hip fractures. The RDAs may be adequate for most older individuals, but these amounts may not be adequate for high-risk seniors—those who are obese, have osteoporosis, have limited sun exposure, or experience malabsorption. For these individuals, the International Osteoporosis Foundation recommends providing supplementation based on measurement of serum 25-OHD (1,25-dihydroxyvitamin D3) level. In vitamin D insufficiency in older individuals, supplementation reduces bone loss. Supplementation with vitamin D reduces risk of falls only in older people whose serum vitamin D levels are low; higher levels of vitamin D seem to promote falls.[37,38] Muscle performance also is improved, which reduces the risk of falling and fracture risk.

Physiologic requirements for vitamins B_6 and B_{12} are increased to prevent a decline in cognitive function and physical mobility associated with aging and to reduce risk for CVD.[39] Economic factors and chewing problems may negatively affect meat consumption, thus negatively affecting vitamins B_6 and B_{12} intake. Edentulous men with inadequate natural masticatory function and no dentures could be at much greater risk of dementia than those with adequate natural chewing skills. Neurologic symptoms similar to dementia may result from deficiencies of vitamins B_6 and B_{12} when intake is reported to be marginal.

Cobalamin (vitamin B_{12}) may be less available in older adults because of atrophic gastritis and bacterial overgrowth. Approximately 10% to 30% of older adults have decreased absorption of vitamin B_{12} and many are at risk because of adverse effects of medications. Choosing foods fortified with vitamin B_{12} or taking a vitamin B_{12}-containing supplement is recommended to meet the DRIs. Symptoms such as cognitive decline, confusion, disorientation, and neurologic problems may improve in individuals treated with vitamin B_{12}.[40] Oral vitamin B_{12} rather than the painful and more expensive injections is effective in treating symptoms of depression in some older adults. Megaloblastic anemia occurs only in severely vitamin B_{12}–depleted individuals.

Whereas optimal folate levels help prevent damage to blood levels and atherosclerosis, higher folate levels may increase risk of cancer mortality. High folate levels can cause cognitive decline and impaired cognitive performance. Supplements may result in elevated folate concentrations, especially in nonsmokers.

Dietary mineral intake, especially sodium, may need to be adjusted based on the patient's physiologic status. Excess or even normal dietary levels can have deleterious consequences in certain diseases, particularly hypertension or congestive heart failure. Rigid and severe restrictions may seriously affect food acceptance. Individualization is crucial.

Aging may negatively affect absorption of magnesium from foods, and the kidneys may increase excretion. Some older adults need medications that interact with magnesium (especially diuretics and long-term prescriptions for proton-pump inhibitor drugs). Higher magnesium intake to offset aging physiologic changes may boost physical performance.[41] Dark green leafy greens and whole grains are good dietary sources.

Older adults generally have a weakened immune system, making them more susceptible to infection. Adequate amounts of zinc may play an important role in improving their immune system and susceptibility to infections, especially pneumonia.[42]

Eating Patterns

Deficiencies

Compared with younger age groups, the diets of Americans older than age 65 years rate better with regard to higher consumption of fruits and lower sodium and cholesterol intake (Fig. 15.4). As with most Americans, the prevalence of low-energy-dense diets are more likely to provide inadequate amounts of nutrients. Most older

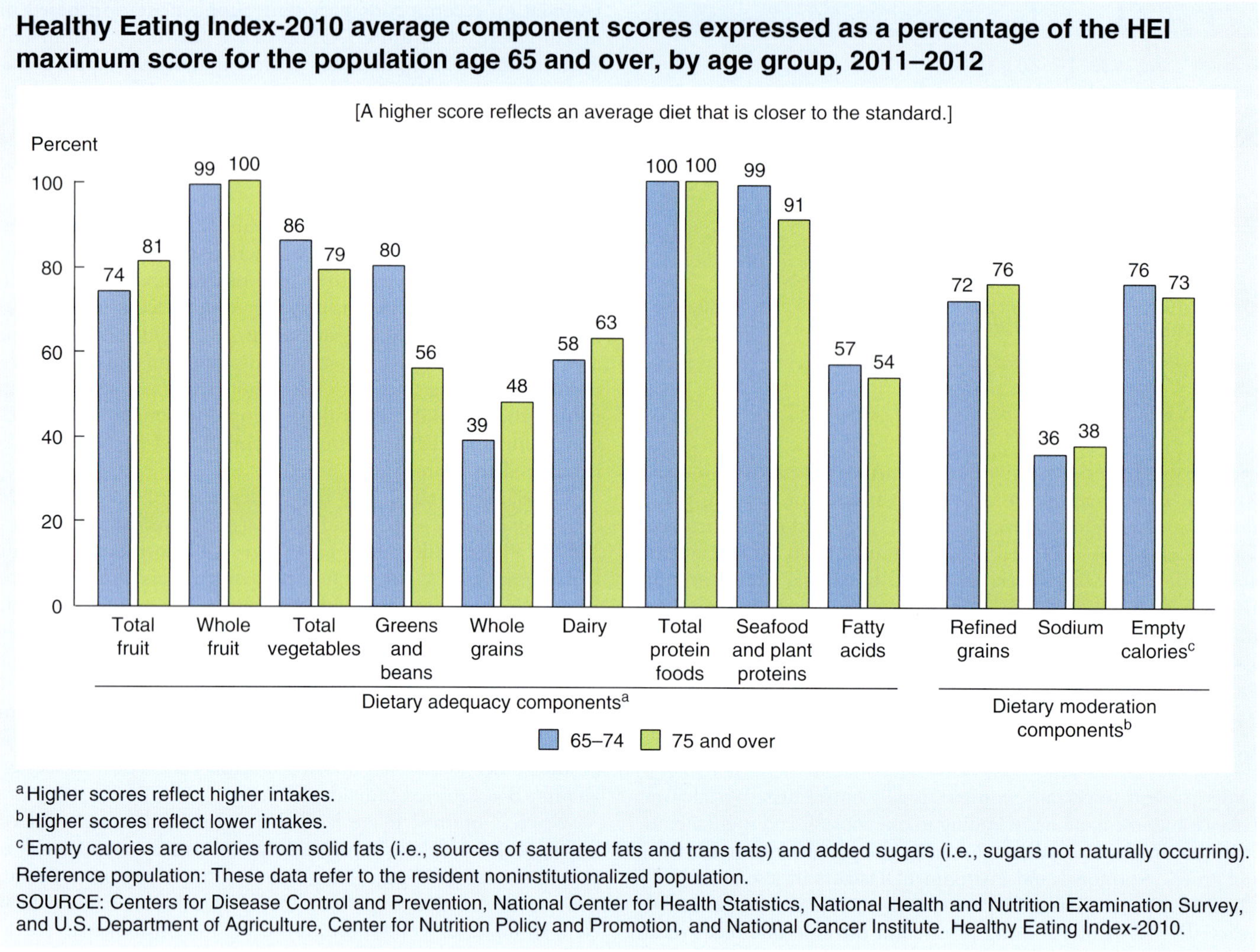

• **Figure 15.4** Healthy Eating Index–2010 average component scores.

individuals consume empty calories, exceeding the discretionary caloric allowances, and fail to meet the RDA for many nutrients. The choice of soft foods usually results in a decrease in protein and more simple carbohydrate intake. Inadequate monetary resources to purchase meat products may result in less protein consumption.

Dairy products, fruits, and vegetables are frequently lacking, especially for individuals living alone. Eating more fruits and vegetables can help ward off frailty. In a study of participants with ages ranging from 69 to 82 years, those who consumed three servings of fruit and two servings of vegetables daily were at 69% lower risk of developing frailty.[43] Older individuals at highest risk of consuming minimal amounts of fruits and vegetables are those who are socially isolated, are missing pairs of posterior teeth, have poor self-reported health, and are obese.

Milk is important for calcium needs, but daily consumption is difficult because of frequent trips needed to purchase it. Dry milk, although less palatable than regular milk, can be incorporated into many foods without deleterious effects on taste. Additionally, lactose intolerance may contribute to inadequate calcium intake (see Chapter 4, *Health Application 4*).

Snacks and Nutritional Supplements

For some older adults, energy intake declines. Snacking may ensure consumption of adequate amounts of calories and protein for those experiencing weight loss. Underweight is a recognized risk factor for disease and disability. Between-meal snacks can be used to offset some nutrient deficits.

Milk-based food supplements, such as an instant breakfast mix, are economical and can help prevent nutrient deficiencies. A tasty supplement can augment overall nutrient intake to maintain nutritional status. Commercial liquid nutrition supplements, such as Ensure (Abbott Nutrition) and Sustacal (Nestlè Lanka Group), are more convenient and may be preferred. These supplements, when used routinely, may produce a small but consistent weight gain, but there is no evidence that liquid supplements affect important clinical outcomes, such as quality of life, mood, functional status, or survival. These beverages are primarily "liquid candy" nutrition shakes, resembling a multivitamin in a bottle.[44] Oral nutritional supplements can be recommended for acutely ill patients who are malnourished. Referral to the health care provider or registered dietitian nutritionist (RDN) is appropriate for these patients.

Food Safety

Foodborne illness can be very serious for older patients. Many older adults are more susceptible to foodborne illness because of a compromised immune system (placing them at risk for infections), decreased secretion of gastric hydrochloric acid, and reduced smell and taste. Food poisoning (discussed more fully in Chapter 16) is caused by food contaminated with pathogenic bacteria, toxins, viruses, or parasites.

Dietary Guidelines and *MyPlate for Older Adults*

During 2011 to 2012, Americans age 75 years and over met the *Dietary Guidelines* for whole fruits; Americans between the age of 65 and 75 years met the recommendations for total protein foods (see Fig. 15.4). Older Americans need to better align with the *Dietary Guidelines* by increasing dietary intakes of whole grains, vegetables and legumes, fat-free or low-fat milk products, and foods and beverages lower in sodium and that have fewer calories from solid fats and added sugars. Fruits and vegetables are also smart choices for maintaining a healthy weight because they are nutrient-dense, containing fiber, vitamins, minerals and phytonutrients.[45] Incorporating colorful fruits and vegetables such as berries, peaches, and peppers into a diet helps combat gradual weight gain.

Dietary patterns, as exemplified in *MyPlate* and the Mediterranean diet (see Evolve website), higher in nutrient-rich, plant-based foods such as leafy green vegetables, berries and fruits, whole grains, nuts, olive oil, legumes and seafood while limiting red and/or processed meats, sugar-sweetened foods and drinks, refined grains, and added salt are generally associated with lower risk of age-related cognitive decline and dementia, muscle and physical deterioration and may improve quality of life and increase the lifespan.[46–51] Whereas only five servings of fruits and vegetables are recommended in the *Dietary Guidelines,* doubling that amount, or 10 servings of produce daily, may help increase the lifespan by preventing CVD, cancer, and premature mortality.[52]

The updated version of *MyPlate for Older Adults,* based on the *Dietary Guidelines* and *MyPlate,* focuses on the unique needs associated with the aging process (see Fig. 15.5). *MyPlate for Older Adults* emphasizes nutrient-dense food choices and the importance of fruits and vegetables, healthy oils, and herbs and spices to reduce the need for salt. Further guidelines for implementation and understanding are in Box 15.3. The groupings on this plate are slightly different than the USDA version: (a) icons of many bright-colored fruits and vegetables (fresh, frozen, dried, canned) occupy half of the plate; (b) whole, enriched, and fortified grains cover one-fourth of the plate; (c) protein sources, including nuts, beans, fish, lean meat, poultry cover one-fourth of the plate; and (d) fat-free and low-fat dairy products such as milk, cheese, and yogurts are on the top right side of the plate along with other beverages (e.g., water, coffee, tea, soup). In the center of the plate are icons depicting heart-healthy fats, for example, liquid vegetable oils and soft spreads. Figures below the plate are a reminder of the importance of staying active. The accompanying website spotlights herbs and spices as a replacement for salt to lower sodium intake.

Eating should be an enjoyable routine and, whenever possible, mealtimes should involve social interaction. Shifting toward healthier food choices can decrease risk for developing chronic diseases such as diabetes, hypertension and heart disease, neurodegenerative diseases, obesity, and early death. It is never too late to make changes in eating habits that will improve and extend peoples lives.[53]

• BOX 15.3 Strategies to Shift

Older adults can begin by making small shifts in food and beverage choices to improve their overall eating pattern, and then continue to build on them. Making small changes and sticking with them is the best approach to long-term improvements in eating habits. Before making major dietary changes, talk with a primary health care provider first.

When selecting foods:

- Buy a variety of fresh, frozen, or no-salt-added canned vegetables and fruit packed in its own juices so that they are readily available for eating as is or adding to sauces, soups, and salads.
- Choose reduced-sodium varieties of beans, salad dressings, and baked products, as available.
- If only varieties packed in sugary syrup or salty fluids are available, rinse them a before serving.
- Dried fruit and unsalted nuts make good portable snacks.
- When food is not prepared at home, try to identify, in advance, nearby restaurants and other food outlets that offer options consistent with healthy dietary patterns. When in doubt, ask the restaurant for information. Chain restaurants may post nutrition information on their website and sometimes have it available in the restaurant, and many restaurants allow some customization of entrées to better fit into a healthy dietary pattern.

Adapted from Updated nutrition for older adults. Tufts Health & Nutrition Letter. *2016;34(3):4–5.*

Vitamin–Mineral Supplements

Frequently food choices of older adults are not as well balanced as they should be or sometimes less food is consumed. Natural foods are the best source of vitamins and minerals; thus, if additional food is needed for adequacy, healthy snacks should be encouraged. Because of impaired absorption of nutrients and reduced food intake, daily multivitamin–mineral supplementation at 100% of the RDI levels may be helpful in protecting against a decline in immune response and preventing anemia. Because of increased need for calcium and vitamins D and B_{12}, accompanied by poor intake and decreased caloric requirements, a vitamin and/or mineral supplement may prevent deterioration of cognition and nutritional status.

A discussion with the health care provider about the need for nutritional supplements may be in order. The following recommendations about dietary supplements should be considered in concurrence with the individual's regular food intake with a goal of ensuring nutrients in the amounts listed in Table 15.1.

- Calcium: Calcium intake should be less than 2500 mg/day. For better absorption, supplements should be taken in two 600-mg doses. Calcium not only keeps bones healthy, but also helps muscles function properly and normalizes blood pressure.
- Vitamin D: Vitamin D supplements should be limited to less than 4000 IU each day. This should be taken in conjunction with calcium to increase calcium absorption. This amount should not be increased without a recommendation from the health care provider.
- Vitamin B_{12}: Because of poor absorption of vitamin B_{12}, increased amounts (above 2.4 μg) may be needed, which may help improve

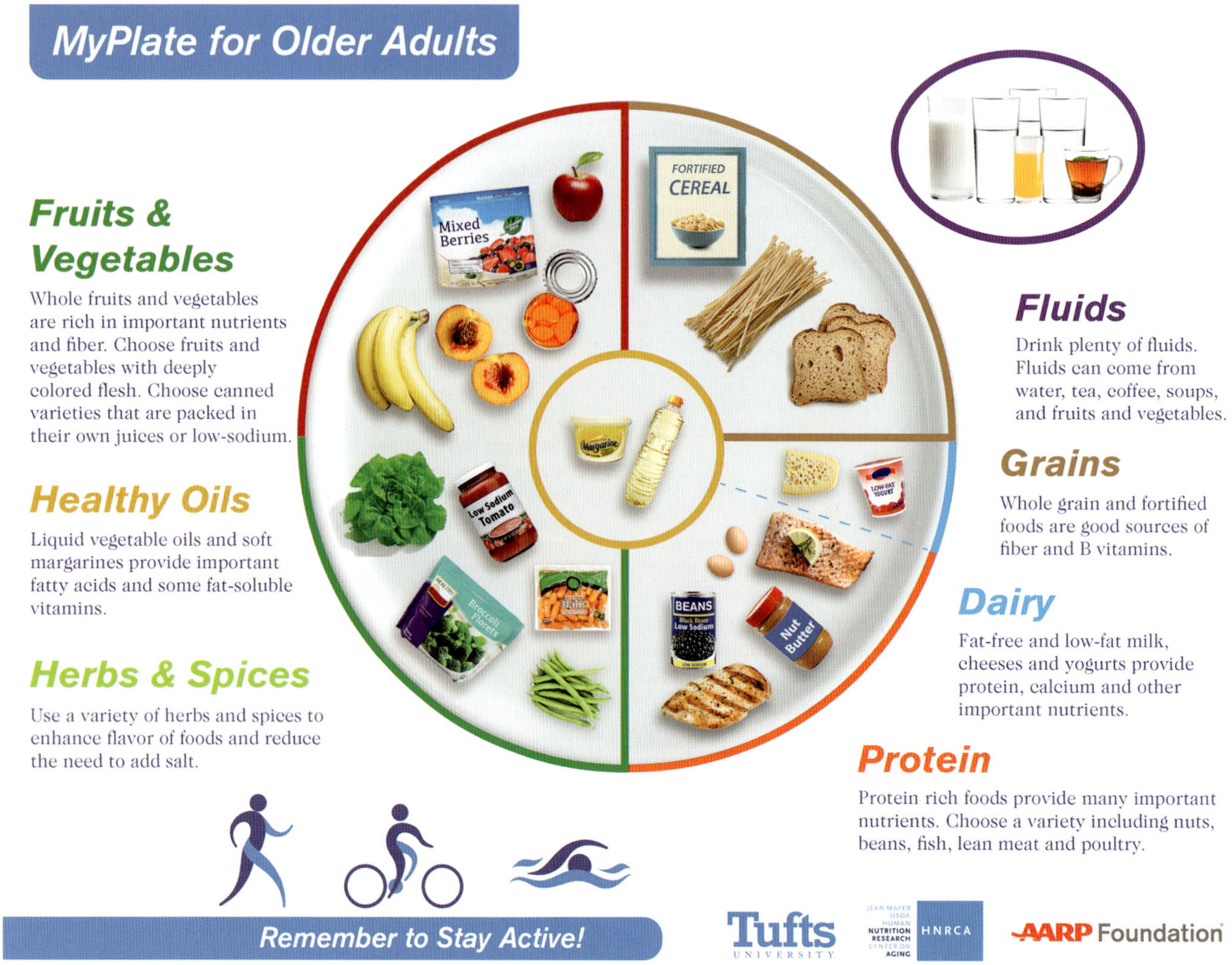

• **Figure 15.5** *MyPlate for Older Adults*. (Source: Tufts University copyright © 2017. Available at http://hnrca.tufts.edu/myplate/myplate-for-older-adults/download/.)

cognitive function and symptoms of depression and prevent pernicious anemia.

- Omega-3 fatty acids: People who do not eat fish at least weekly may benefit from a fish oil supplement (300 mg of omega-3 fatty acid).

As many as 70% of older adults take dietary (vitamin–mineral) supplements to maintain a healthy life or prevent a disease/medical problem because they know their eating patterns are not ideal or because a health care professional recommended them. Although many people choose to take dietary supplements, doing so frequently results in exceeding the upper limit for one or more nutrients.

Age-related macular degeneration is a deterioration in the central area of the retina (back of the eye) in which lesions lead to loss of central vision. Studies have found a lower risk of macular degeneration in people who consume a diet rich in lutein and zeaxanthin (carotenoid vitamins, related to beta-carotene and vitamin A) and diets rich in fatty fish, such as salmon. Researchers have reported that taking vitamin E, beta-carotene, or antioxidant supplements are unlikely to prevent age-related macular degeneration. Foods may contain something other than these nutrients that explains the lower risk of eye disease associated with eating them. These vitamin supplements are generally recognized as safe but could have harmful effects; clear evidence of benefit is needed before recommending them. Referral to the health care provider or an RDN is necessary to assess the need for supplements.

DENTAL CONSIDERATIONS

Assessment

- *Physical:* Visual appraisal of weight status; dry mucous membranes.
- *Dietary:* Adequacy of nutrients and fluid intake based on the *MyPlate for Older Adults*; multivitamin/mineral/herbal use.

Interventions

- To prevent dehydration, encourage older patients to use caffeine in moderation and to take medications with 8 oz of fluid. Encourage nutrient-dense foods, especially for older patients whose calorie expenditure is low.
- Discuss economical fruit, vegetable, and meat selections (see Chapter 16).
- Older patients who have had an unintentional weight change of 10% (loss or gain) in 6 months should be referred to a health care provider.
- Absorption of vitamin B_{12} from vitamin supplements or fortified foods is not affected by atrophic gastritis. Suggest enriched or fortified cereals to increase intake of iron and vitamin B_{12}.
- Encourage consumption of a vitamin C–rich food daily.
- Review economical sources of folate and cooking practices to retain folate.
- Vitamin supplements providing more than 100% of the RDI should be taken only in cases of specific need or if recommended by a health care provider.
- Encourage wise selections of convenience foods. Explain how to read food labels to make selections appropriate for restricted diets or to provide a well-balanced diet.

NUTRITIONAL DIRECTIONS

- Keep healthy snacks on hand, such as cheese, hard-boiled eggs, low-fat milk products, bananas, and canned fruit.
- A well-balanced diet following the *MyPlate for Older Adults* or the Mediterranean diet may delay symptoms of aging.
- Consume 2 to 4 oz of meat or other protein source at each meal.
- Adequate vitamin D levels in the blood are important; consult your health care provider before self-medicating with vitamin D.
- Lack of vitamin B_{12} can cause poor memory and impaired balance.
- Nutrition counseling by an RDN can provide information on consuming adequate amounts of high-quality protein on a limited budget and offer alternatives to eating problems.
- Nonfat or low-fat milk is the best source of calcium and vitamin D.
- Dietary intake should strive to optimize immune function and reduce risk of disease.
- Calcium supplements should also contain vitamin D to enhance calcium absorption.
- Adequate fluid intake is beneficial in preventing and treating constipation. Soups, juices, milk products, decaffeinated soft drinks, and decaffeinated tea and coffee can enhance fluid intake.
- The vitamin B_{12} present in breakfast cereals or supplements is better absorbed than the form present in animal foods.
- Consult your health care provider or RDN to find out whether supplements are needed.
- Contact your health care provider or an RDN when food choices are limited over a period of time because of illness, chewing problems, lack of appetite, or inability to shop for or prepare food.
- Use of vitamin–mineral supplements does not eliminate the need to consume a nutritionally balanced diet, and supplements do not protect against development of chronic diseases associated with inappropriate food intake.
- Excess supplementation of vitamins and minerals may cause more problems with hypervitaminosis and detrimental effects on other nutrients. Zinc supplements can result in copper imbalance and reduce high-density lipoprotein cholesterol levels. Consult your health care provider or RDN.
- Heed food safety guidelines to ensure that foods do not cause illness.

HEALTH APPLICATION 15

Complementary and Alternative Medicine (CAM) and Botanical Supplements

Complementary and alternative medicine (CAM) is using diverse medical and health care systems and products generally not considered part of conventional medicine. **Complementary medicine** utilizes CAM medicine together with conventional medicine, such as using acupuncture to alleviate pain. **Alternative medicine** pertains to use of CAM in place of conventional medicine. CAM practices often utilize herbal medicines and other "natural products." Many are available over the counter as dietary supplements. Interest in and use of CAM products have grown considerably in the past few decades. People have many reasons for turning to alternative medicine—failure of or dissatisfaction with mainstream medicine, scientific illiteracy, or possibly just having been swayed by media claims.

Medical systems that have evolved from different cultures apart from conventional or Western medicine include **homeopathy** (treatment of diseases with minute doses of drugs that cause symptoms of a disease in healthy people to cure similar symptoms in sick people) and **naturopathy** (support of the body's inherent ability to maintain and restore health, using noninvasive treatments with minimal use of surgery and drugs). Theoretically, if a certain substance causes a symptom in a healthy person, a very small amount of the same substance may cure the symptoms. The National Center for Complementary and Alternative Medicine (NCCAM), part of the National Institutes of Health (NIH), notes that most rigorous clinical trials and systematic analyses of research on homeopathy have concluded that "there is little evidence to support homeopathy as an effective treatment for any specific condition."[54] Some studies suggest that the results are similar to a placebo effect, whereas others have found positive effects not readily explained scientifically. In general, homeopathics are benign because, being so dilute, they are unlikely to cause harm if used properly.

As with any medical treatment, risks are associated with CAM therapies. Several general-principle precautions to help minimize risks are: (a) "natural" does not always mean "safe"; (b) herbal supplements may contain dozens of compounds and some active ingredients may not be known; (c) ingredients indicated on the label and actual ingredients in the product may be different; (d) some active ingredients may be lower or higher than indicated on the label; (e) the product may be contaminated with other herbs, pesticides, or metals; (f) some dietary supplements may interact with medications or nutrients, and may have their own side effects; and (g) inform all health care

Continued

HEALTH APPLICATION 15

Complementary and Alternative Medicine (CAM) and Botanical Supplements—cont'd

providers about use of any complementary and alternative practices. Most important, homeopathy should not be used as a replacement for proven conventional care or to postpone seeing a health care provider about a medical problem.

A **botanical** is a plant or plant part valued for its medicinal or therapeutic properties, flavor, and/or scent. **Herbs** are leafy green parts of a plant, whereas **spices** are from any other part of the plant that can be used for seasoning—seeds, fruits, flowers, bark, or roots. Herbs are a subset of botanicals. Botanical dietary supplements, also called herbal medicines or herbal supplements, have been used for centuries in attempts to maintain or improve health.

Many medications, prescription and over the counter, are actually based on naturally occurring active ingredients in plants. Until sometime in the 1970s, most medications were derived from herbs. These medications using natural substances have been thoroughly researched to verify benefits and adverse outcomes with standard quantities of active ingredients. Many natural plant materials are too toxic for human consumption.

In the 1990s, the German Commission E, generally acknowledged as Europe's leading regulatory authority for evaluating therapeutic activities of herbs and the equivalent of the U.S. Food and Drug Administration in the United States, published *The Complete German Commission E Monographs—Therapeutic Guide to Herbal Medicines.* In 1998, the National Center for Complementary and Alternative Medicine (NCCAM) already stated earlier in Health Application, was established to provide scientifically based information about CAM and herbs. About the same time, more publications focusing primarily on herbs popular in the United States were written to help health care professionals and consumers make informed decisions about herbal use and their interactions with medications.

Research-based information about specific CAM treatments and herbs is available on the NCCAM website: https://nccam.nih.gov/. NCCAM's Herbs at a Glance, a link on the same website, provides updated reliable information about more than 50 botanicals—research, potential side effects and cautions, and resources for more information. Box 15.4 shows the type of information found on the website for Ginkgo, a product that is used by many older adults. This herb is promoted to improve numerous conditions, but scientific evidence for efficacy for many of these uses is inconclusive.

Because herbs are not actual nutrients, when used for health benefits, they are considered CAMs or dietary supplements. The Dietary Supplement Health and Education Act (1994) discussed in *Health Application 11, Vitamin and Mineral Supplements* applies to herbal supplements. Herbs are not innocuous; most Americans are unaware of the potential toxicity of herbs. Consumers can purchase as much as they want of any of these products. Many people believe that "natural" products are safe and harmless.

Many botanicals provide a large array of phytochemicals, antioxidants, and biologically active compounds. Herbal supplements do not have to be tested for safety and effectiveness before they are marketed. Some botanicals have been evaluated in scientific studies, but the amount of scientific evidence supporting various botanical ingredients varies widely. In the amounts currently used, no negative side effects are expected. Some of the biologically active compounds have been identified and characterized, and many have unknown actions.

Herbal supplements are available in many forms—as fresh or dried products, liquid or solid extracts, tablets, capsules, powders, and teas. The form of the herb determines its potency. For instance, ginkgo seed and ginkgo leaves have different safety and clinical application profiles. Consumption of the seeds is associated with seizures and can be fatal; the active ingredient in *Ginkgo biloba* leaves (flavonoids) reduce clotting time and may be effective in improving cognitive disorders. The active compound is extracted from the plant by using a solvent such as water, fat, oil, or alcohol.

In the United States, dietary supplements are not required to be standardized. Standardization is a process manufacturers use to ensure that all batches are consistent with regard to specific chemicals. Standardization is a measure of quality control that is dependent on the manufacturer, supplier, and others in the production process. Herbs are living organisms comprised of thousands of ingredients, and the proportions may differ dramatically between two plants. Due to different growing conditions—such as the weather, amount of sun, level of soil acidity, and rainfall—known compounds present in herbs can vary significantly. The degree of accuracy between label statements and actual content is unreliable. Some products have been found to contain toxic substances.

Popular herbs do not contain any known, single active ingredients. Therefore, determining the effectiveness of a given herbal batch is almost impossible. Even names of botanicals can be confusing because of different names for the same herb—ginkgo (*Ginkgo biloba)* has a pharmacopeial name of ginkgo folium; other names include duck foot tree, maidenhair tree, and silver apricot.

Emerging evidence indicates that commonly used botanicals (herbs and spices) may help protect against certain chronic conditions, such as cancer, diabetes, and heart disease. Of particular concern is the fact that one-third of older adults use CAM, and 42% failed to discuss this practice with their primary care physicians,[55] thus putting as many as 15% of men and women ages 62 to 85 years at increased risk of drug–drug and drug–nutrient interactions.[5] The greatest health risk in use of CAM and botanical medicines is the potential of the product interacting with prescribed medications. It is very important for the health care provider to be aware of any use of CAM and/or botanical medicines.

• BOX 15.4 Ginkgo

This fact sheet provides basic information about ginkgo—common names, usefulness and safety, and resources for more information.

Common Names: ginkgo, *Ginkgo biloba*, fossil tree, maidenhair tree, Japanese silver apricot, baiguo, yinhsing

Latin Name: *Ginkgo biloba*

Background

- Ginkgo, one of the oldest living tree species in the world, has a long history in traditional Chinese medicine. Members of the royal court were given ginkgo nuts for senility. Other historical uses for gingko were for asthma, bronchitis, and kidney and bladder disorders.
- Today, the extract from ginkgo leaves is used as a dietary supplement for many conditions, including dementia, eye problems, intermittent claudication (leg pain caused by narrowing arteries), tinnitus, and other health problems.
- Ginkgo is made into tablets, capsules, extracts, tea, and cosmetics.

How Much Do We Know?

- There have been a lot of studies on the possible health effects and risks of people using ginkgo.

• BOX 15.4 Ginkgo—cont'd

What Have We Learned?

- There is no conclusive evidence that ginkgo is helpful for any health condition.
- Ginkgo does not help prevent or slow dementia or cognitive decline according to studies, including the long-term Ginkgo Evaluation Memory Study, which enrolled more than 3000 older adults and was funded in part by the National Center for Complementary and Integrative Health (NCCIH).
- There is no strong evidence that ginkgo helps with memory enhancement in healthy people, blood pressure, intermittent claudication, tinnitus, age-related macular degeneration, the risk of having a heart attack or stroke, or with other conditions.
- Ongoing NCCIH-funded research is looking at whether a compound in ginkgo may help with diabetes.

What Do We Know About Safety?

- For many healthy adults, ginkgo appears to be safe when taken by mouth in moderate amounts.
- Side effects of ginkgo may include headache, stomach upset, and allergic skin reactions. If you are older, have a known bleeding risk, or are pregnant, you should be cautious about ginkgo possibly increasing your risk of bleeding.
- In a 2013 research study, rodents given ginkgo had an increased risk of developing liver and thyroid cancer at the end of the 2-year tests.
- Ginkgo may interact with some conventional medications, including anticoagulants (blood thinners), research reviews show.
- Eating fresh (raw) or roasted ginkgo seeds can be poisonous and have serious side effects.

Keep in Mind

- Tell all your health care providers about any complementary or integrative health approaches you use. Give them a full picture of what you do to manage your health. This will help ensure coordinated and safe care.

For More Information

- Using Dietary Supplements Wisely (https://nccih.nih.gov/health/supplements/wiseuse.htm)
- *Ginkgo* (https://www.niehs.nih.gov/health/assets/docs_f_o/ntp_ginkgo_508.pdf)
- Know the Science: How Medications and Supplements Can Interact (https://nccih.nih.gov/health/know-science/how-medications-supplements-interact)
- Know the Science: 9 Questions To Help You Make Sense of Health Research (https://nccih.nih.gov/health/know-science/make-sense-health-research)

Source: National Center for Complementary and Integrative Health, National Institutes of Health. Ginkgo. https://nccih.nih.gov/health/ginkgo/ataglance.htm. Accessed February 28, 2017.

CASE APPLICATION FOR THE DENTAL HYGIENIST

A 75-year-old edentulous patient is not eating because he states he has difficulty chewing and food does not taste good. He reports he dislikes a lot of red meat and milk. He has lost 14 lb since his last recare appointment (usual weight 170 lb).

Nutritional Assessment

- Height; weight; appropriateness of BMI; significant weight changes, especially loss
- Nutrient and fluid intake in relation to DRIs
- Medications
- Alterations in taste, smell, or vision
- Support group, significant others, living arrangements, social support
- Psychological status

Nutritional Diagnosis

Altered nutrition: less than body requirements related to taste changes and chewing difficulty.

Nutritional Goals

The patient will consume a well-balanced diet (based on the *MyPlate for Older Adults*) and verbalize ways to increase protein and calcium intake and exercise.

Nutritional Implementation

Intervention: Encourage small, frequent meals.
Rationale: This helps the older patient consume adequate amounts of nutrients by decreasing fatigue and feelings of fullness that may occur with larger meals.
Intervention: Suggest use of spices such as pepper, thyme, and basil.
Rationale: These spices may improve the taste of foods because the older patient's ability to detect tastes is altered.
Intervention: Encourage fluids with meals.
Rationale: Drinking fluids with meals makes chewing and swallowing easier.
Intervention: Examine and question about the fit of the prosthesis. Clinically, conduct an intraoral and extraoral examination, especially noting any deviations from normal of the underlying tissue.
Rationale: The weight change may have created a loose-fitting denture and ultimately difficulty in chewing. An ill-fitting denture may also result in weight loss.
Intervention: Teach the patient to perform an oral self-examination.
Rationale: The patient also can identify oral problems earlier for more effective treatment.
Intervention: Emphasize use of eggs, turkey, chicken, fish, tenderized meat in marinades (e.g., wine or vinegar), and soy products, such as tofu.
Rationale: Because he does not like red meats, the patient may obtain needed protein in a more acceptable manner with these options.
Intervention: Emphasize the use of low-fat or nonfat dairy products, such as yogurt, cream cheese, cheese, or frozen yogurt.
Rationale: His dislike of milk lessens the likelihood of his choosing milk; these foods are alternatives to supply the needed calcium.
Intervention: Encourage adding powdered milk to soups, sauces, cereals, and casseroles.
Rationale: These are methods to increase protein and calcium consumption.
Intervention: Encourage the patient to walk outdoors for 10 to 20 minutes daily and eat foods that require more chewing, such as lettuce salads, raw carrots, cabbage, and apples.
Rationale: Exercise is important to maintain bone density in the mandible and throughout the body. Available dietary calcium is better absorbed because it is dependent on vitamin D, which can be obtained through sunshine.
Intervention: Suggest mixing meat with vegetables.
Rationale: Because he enjoys vegetables, this form may be more palatable for him and would enhance protein intake.
Intervention: Refer the patient to Meals-on-Wheels or another federally funded program (e.g., food stamps), community meals centers, or church-sponsored centers.
Rationale: Anorexia may be a result of a lack of socialization during mealtimes.

Evaluation

The patient should be eating at least 75% of the number of food servings from *MyPlate for Older Adults* and steadily gaining weight until desired body weight is achieved. Other behaviors, such as consuming yogurt, eggs, fish, and dry milk in foods, will increase calcium and protein intake.

Student Readiness

1. Plan a day's menus for an older edentulous patient.
2. What are some vitamin and mineral deficiencies that might influence mental attitudes of older patients?
3. Discuss reasons older patients might not eat adequately.
4. Visit a group meal program. Review the menu with an RDN and discuss beneficial effects of the program's various activities.
5. List nutritional interventions to help a healthy older patient with full dentures to eat a well-balanced diet.
6. Observe the staff at an long-term care facility, and note positive activities related to maintaining good oral health and activities that can be improved.
7. Why are older individuals prone to dehydration? How can dehydration affect oral status?
8. Describe procedures for encouraging adequate food intake for new denture wearers.
9. What are some suggestions you could make for a patient experiencing xerostomia?
10. Name three differences in *MyPlate* and *MyPlate for Older Adults*.

CASE STUDY

A 75-year-old man widowed for 2 years is seen in the health care clinic for decreased intake and a weight loss of 6 lbs in the past year. He states nothing tastes good. He is on a fixed income from Social Security. His current weight is 130 lb, and his height is 5 feet, 7 inches. He is edentulous and refuses to get dentures because he feels he is "too old."

He fixes a bologna sandwich occasionally, but mostly eats frozen food dinners. He thinks meats and fruits are too expensive to buy and states, "They spoil before I can eat them." He eats overcooked vegetables in the summer because a neighbor shares fresh produce from his garden. He does not want to use any community resources because he objects to "a handout."

1. Explain why "food does not taste good."
2. What psychological and social factors may influence his dietary patterns?
3. What are some practical ways to increase protein and calcium in his diet?
4. How could you address his attitude of not wanting to accept "a handout"?
5. What medical and dental information should you assess on this man to determine nutritional status?
6. What are the strengths and weaknesses of his diet?
7. What behaviors would indicate this patient is meeting his nutritional needs?

References

1. Federal Interagency Forum on Aging-Related Statistics. *Older Americans 2016: Key Indicators of Well-Being*. Federal Interagency Forum on Aging-Related Statistics. Washington, DC: U.S. Government Printing Office; 2016.
2. World Health Organization Quality of Life Group (WHOQOL). *WHOQOL Measuring Quality of Life*. Geneva, Switzerland: World Health Organization; 1997. http://www.who.int/mental_health/media/68.pdf. Accessed February 21, 2017.
3. National Council on Aging. Chronic Disease Management. https://www.ncoa.org/healthyaging/chronic-disease/. Accessed February 21, 2017.
4. Qato DM, Wilder J, Schumm LP, et al. Changes in prescription and over-the-counter medication and dietary supplement use among older adults in the United States, 2005 vs. 2011. *JAMA Intern Med*. 2016;176(4):473–482.
5. U.S. Department of Health and Human Services. Healthy People 2020. Oral Health. https://www.healthypeople.gov/2020/topics-objectives/national-snapshot/untreated-dental-decay-adults-1999%E2%80%932004-and-2011%E2%80%9312. Accessed February 21, 2017.
6. Kim CS, Kim EK, Lee KS, et al. Relationship between bone mineral density, its associated physiological factors, and tooth loss in postmenopausal Korean women. *BMC Womens Health*. 2015;15:65.
7. Eke PI, Wei L, Borgnakke WS, et al. Periodontitis prevalence in adults ≥ 65 years of age, in the USA. *Periodontol 2000*. 2016;72(1):76–95.
8. Federal Interagency Forum on Aging-Related Statistics. *Older Americans 2016: Key Indicators of Well-Being*. Federal Interagency Forum on Aging-Related Statistics. Washington, DC: U.S. Government Printing Office; 2016.
9. Okamoto N, Morikawa M, Yanagi M, et al. Association of tooth loss with development of swallowing problems in community-dwelling independent elderly population: the Fujiwara-kyo Study. *J Gerontol A Biol Sci Med Sci*. 2015;70(12):1548–1554.
10. Furuta M, Yamashita Y. Oral health and swallowing problems. *Curr Phys Med Rehabil Rep*. 2013;1:216–222.
11. van der Bilt A. Assessment of mastication with implications for oral rehabilitation: a review. *J Oral Rehabil*. 2011;38(10):754–780.
12. Felton DA. Complete edentulism and comorbid diseases: an update. *J Prosthodont*. 2016;25(1):5–20.
13. Andreas ZA, Rammelsberg P, Cabrera T, et al. Prosthetic rehabilitation of edentulism prevents malnutrition in nursing home residents. *Int J Prosthodont*. 2015;28(2):198–200.
14. Puryer J. Denture stomatitis—a clinical update. *Dent Update*. 2016;43(6):529–535.
15. Marra MV, Simmons SF, Shotwell MS, et al. Elevated serum osmolality and total water deficit indicate impaired hydration status in residents of long-term care facilities regardless of low or high body mass index. *J Acad Nutr Diet*. 2016;116(5):828–836.
16. Maeda K, Shamoto H, Wakabayashi H, et al. Sarcopenia is highly prevalent in older medical patients with mobility limitation. *Nutr Clin Pract*. 2017;32(1):110–115.
17. Landi F, Calvani R, Ortolani E, et al. The association between sarcopenia and functional outcomes among older patients with hip fracture undergoing in-hospital rehabilitation. *Osteoporos Int*. 2017;28(5):1569–1576.
18. Watanabe Y, Hirano H, Arai H, et al. Relationship between frailty and oral function in community-dwelling elderly adults. *J Am Geriatr Soc*. 2017;65(1):66–76.
19. Iwasaki M, Kimura Y, Ogawa H, et al. The association between dentition status and sarcopenia in Japanese adults aged ≥75 years. *J Oral Rehabil*. 2017;44(1):51–58.
20. Shao A, Campbell WW, Chen C-Y Oliver, et al. The emerging global phenomenon of sarcopenic obesity: role of functional foods; a conference report. *J Func Foods*. 2017;33:244–250.
21. U.S. Department of Health and Human Services. 2008 Physical Activity Guidelines for Americans. https://health.gov/paguidelines/pdf/paguide.pdf. Accessed February 22, 2017.
22. Soares-Miranda L, Siscovick DS, Psaty BM. Physical activity and risk of coronary heart disease and stroke in older adults: The Cardiovascular Health Study. *Circulation*. 2016;133(2):147–155.
23. Hayes SM, Hayes JP, Williams VJ, et al. FMRI activity during associative encoding is correlated with cardiorespiratory fitness and source memory performance in older adults. *Cortex*. 2017;pii: S0010-9452(17)30005-9.
24. Holme I, Anderssen SA. Increases in physical activity is as important as smoking cessation for reduction in total mortality in elderly men: 12 years of follow-up of the Oslo II study. *Br J Sports Med*. 2015;49(11):743–748.

25. Hupin D, Roche F, Oriol M. Physical activity for older adults: even a little is good! *Ann Phys Rehabil Med*. 2016;59S:e58.
26. Liao CD, Tsauo JY, Wu YT, et al. Effects of protein supplementation combined with resistance exercise on body composition and physical function in older adults: a systematic review and meta-analysis. *Am J Clin Nutr*. 2017;106(4):1078–1091.
27. Muscariello E, Nasti G, Siervo M, et al. Dietary protein intake in sarcopenic obese older women. *Clin Interv Aging*. 2016;11:133–140.
28. Verlaan S, Maier AB, Bauer JM, et al. Sufficient levels of 25-hydroxyvitamin D and protein intake required to increase muscle mass in sarcopenic older adults—The PROVIDE study. *Clin Nutr*. 2017;pii: S0261-5614(17)30010-9. [Epub ahead of print].
29. Bhattoa HP, Konstantynowicz J, Laszcz N, et al. Vitamin D: musculoskeletal health. *Rev Endocr Metab Disord*. 2017;18(3):363–371.
30. Yanai H. Nutrition for sarcopenia. *J Clin Med Res*. 2015;7(12):926–931.
31. Ziliak JP, Gundersen C. The State of Senior Hunger in American 2014: An Annual Report. June 2016. http://www.nfesh.org/wp-content/uploads/2016/05/State-of-Senior-Hunger-in-America-2014.pdf. Accessed February 22, 2017.
32. Rouxel P, Tsakos G, Chandola T, et al. Oral health—a neglected aspect of subjective well-being in later life. *J Gerontol B Psychol Sci Soc Sci*. 2016;gbw024, doi:10.1093/geronb/gbw024.
33. Koolhaas CM, Dhana K, Schoufour JD, et al. Impact of physical activity on the association of overweight and obesity with cardiovascular disease: the Rotterdam Study. *Eur J Prev Cardiol*. 2017;24(9):934–941.
34. Paddon-Jones D, Campbell WW, Jacques PF, et al. Protein and healthy aging. *Am J Clin Nutr*. 2015;101(6):1339S–1345S.
35. Porter Starr KN, Pieper CF, Orenduff MC, et al. Improved function with enhanced protein intake per meal: a pilot study of weight reduction in frail, obese older adults. *J Gerontol A Biol Sci Med Sci*. 2016;71(10):1369–1375.
36. Bauer JM, Diekmann R. Protein and older persons. *Clin Geriatr Med*. 2015;31(3):327–338.
37. Bischoff-Ferrari HA, Dawson-Hughes B, Orav EJ, et al. Monthly high-dose vitamin D treatment for the prevention of functional decline: a randomized clinical trial. *JAMA Intern Med*. 2016;176(2): 175–183.
38. Hansen KE, Johnson MG. An update on vitamin D for clinicians. *Curr Opin Endocrinol Diabetes Obes*. 2016;23(6):440–444.
39. Struijk EA, Lana A, Guallar-Castillon P, et al. Intake of B vitamins and impairment in physical function in older adults. *Clin Nutr*. 2017;pii:SO261-5614(17)30177-2, doi:10.1016/j.clnu.2017.05.016. [Epub ahead of print].
40. Barnes JL, Tian M, Edens NK, et al. Consideration of nutrient levels in studies of cognitive decline. *Nutr Rev*. 2014;72(11):707–719.
41. Veronese N, Berton L, Carraro S, et al. Effect of oral magnesium supplementation on physical performance in healthy elderly women involved in a weekly exercise program: a randomized controlled trial. *Am J Clin Nutr*. 2014;100(3):974–981.
42. Barnett JB, Dao MC, Hamer DH, et al. Effect of zinc supplementation on serum zinc concentration and T cell proliferation in nursing home elderly: a randomized, double-blind, placebo-controlled trial. *Am J Clin Nutr*. 2016;103(3):942–951.
43. García-Esquinas E, Rahi B, Peres K, et al. Consumption of fruit and vegetables and risk of frailty: a dose–response analysis of 3 prospective cohorts of community-dwelling older adults. *Am J Clin Nutr*. 2016;104(1):132–142.
44. AGS Choosing Wisely Workgroup. American Geriatrics Society identifies five things that healthcare providers and patients should question. *J Am Geriatr Soc*. 2013;61(4):622–631.
45. Bertoia ML, Rimm EB, Mukamal KJ, et al. Dietary flavonoid intake and weight maintenance: three prospective cohorts of 124,086 US men and women followed for up to 24 years. *BMJ*. 2016; 352:i17.
46. Masana MF, Koyanagi A, Haro JM, et al. N-3 fatty acids, Mediterranean diet and cognitive function in normal aging: a systematic review. *Exp Gerontol*. 2017;91:39–50.
47. Yannakoulia M, Ntanasi E, Anastasiou CA, et al. Frailty and nutrition: from epidemiological and clinical evidence to potential mechanisms. *Metabolism*. 2017;68:64–76.
48. Shlisky J, Bloom DE, Beaudreault AR, et al. Nutritional considerations for healthy aging and reduction in age-related chronic disease. *Adv Nutr*. 2017;8(1):17–26.
49. Anderson JJ, Nieman DC. Diet quality—the Greeks had it right! *Nutrients*. 2016;8(10):pii:E636.
50. Miller MG, Thangthaeng N, Poulose SM, et al. Role of fruits, nuts, and vegetables in maintaining cognitive health. *Exp Gerontol*. 2017;94:24–28.
51. Knight A, Bryan J, Wilson C, et al. The Mediterranean Diet and cognitive function among healthy older adults in a 6-month randomised controlled trial: The MedLey study. *Nutrients*. 2016;8(9):pii: E579.
52. Aune D, Giovannucci E, Boffetta P, et al. Fruit and vegetable intake and the risk of cardiovascular disease, total cancer and all-cause mortality—a systematic review and dose–response meta-analysis of prospective studies. *Int J Epidemiol*. 2017;46(3):1029–1056.
53. Sotos-Prieto M, Bhupathiraju SN, Mattei J, et al. Association of changes in diet quality with total and cause-specific mortality. *N Engl J Med*. 2017;377:143–153.
54. National Institutes of Health (NIH), National Center for Complementary and Integrative Health (NCCIH). Homeopathy. https://nccih.nih.gov/health/homeopathy. Accessed February 28, 2017.
55. Johnson PJ, Jou J, Rhee TG, et al. Complementary health approaches for health and wellness in midlife and older US adults. *Maturitas*. 2016;89:36–42.

EVOLVE RESOURCES

Please visit http://evolve.elsevier.com/Stegeman/nutritional for additional practice and study support tools.

16

Food Factors Affecting Health

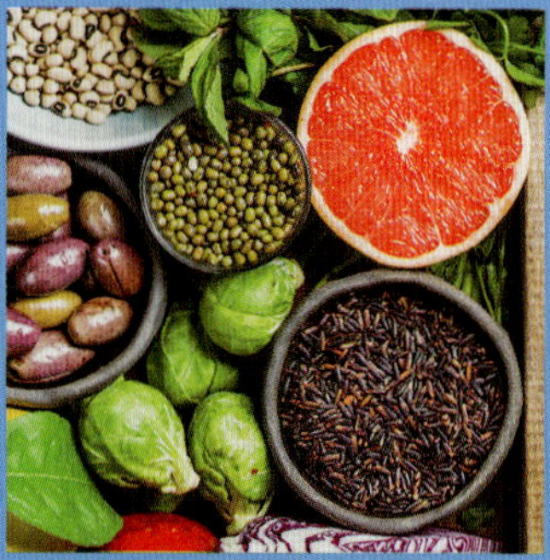

STUDENT LEARNING OUTCOMES

Upon completion of this chapter, the student will be able to achieve the following student learning outcomes:

1. Discuss health care disparities and how they relate to oral health.
2. Regarding (or With regard to) food patterns:
   - Explain how a patient can obtain adequate nutrients from different cultural food patterns.
   - Identify reasons for food patterns.
   - Respect cultural and religious food patterns while providing nutritional recommendations for patients.
3. Pertaining to food budgets:
   - Explain to a patient how to prepare and store food to retain nutrient value.
   - Inform patients of ways to make economical food purchases.
   - Explain to a patient how food processing, convenience foods, and fast foods affect overall intake.
   - Discuss reasons why food additives are used.
4. Describe food fads, and list reasons why health quackery can be dangerous. Also, identify common themes of health quackery and why they are contrary to evidence-based research.
5. Provide referrals for nutritional resources, and describe the role of dental hygienists in combating nutrition fads and misinformation.

KEY TERMS

Chelation therapy
Colonics
Detoxification
Dietary acculturation
Evidence-based
Food deserts
Food fad
Food insecurity
Food patterns
Food quackery
Hunger
Irradiated foods
Meta-analysis
Observational studies
Organic
Stable nutrients
Systematic reviews
Very low food security

TEST YOUR NQ

1. **T/F** Religion can affect food patterns.
2. **T/F** Adults usually avoid the foods they ate during childhood.
3. **T/F** The nutritional content of food is the most important reason for an individual's food choices.
4. **T/F** Most consumers spend about 25% of their income on food.
5. **T/F** Fad diets are usually well balanced and nutritious.
6. **T/F** Organic foods are more nutritious.
7. **T/F** All food processing is detrimental to the nutritional quality of foods.
8. **T/F** Fast foods are usually a good source of protein.
9. **T/F** Food additives improve the nutritional value of foods.
10. **T/F** Individual food preferences do not ordinarily influence nutritional adequacy of the diet.

Health Care Disparities

Health care disparities are a serious problem in the United States for the underprivileged of all ages, especially for ethnic minorities and low-income groups. The Centers for Disease Control and Prevention (CDC) reports that quality of health care in the United States varies according to the patient's race and ethnicity, resulting in health care disparities.[1] By 2060, 56.4% of the American population may consist of ethnic minorities in contrast to 37.8% in 2014.[2] Not all ethnic minorities are disadvantaged, but many come from different cultural backgrounds with dissimilar beliefs and expectations, are not cognizant of American health care systems and policies, and may experience communication problems as a result of language barriers. The health status of many underprivileged and racial and ethnic minority groups is poor.

Patients who speak, understand, or read only a language other than English, have different levels of acculturation and socioeconomic status, understand illness uniquely, or have a different perspective on health care are challenging to health care workers educated in the American mainstream system. Health professionals need to be able to provide health care to accommodate different cultural attitudes. Cultural competence of health care providers contributes substantively in reducing racial and ethnic disparities in health and health care that pervade the U.S. health care system. Cultural competency requires a dedication of dental professionals to understand and serve others and be responsive to a variety of attitudes, perspectives, values, verbal cues, and body language. Additionally, they should be familiar with health problems common among the ethnic groups served most frequently in their locale, whether they be African Americans, Asians, Hispanics/Latinos, Native American/Alaskan Natives, Pacific Islanders, or poorly educated and impoverished Americans. The CDC identified these specific oral health disparities in *Healthy People 2020*[2]:

- Lack of annual preventive dental services for children and adolescents from families at or below 200% of the federal poverty level.
- More untreated dental caries in children age 3 to 9 years from families with incomes less than 100% of the federal poverty level.
- Fewer dental sealants in African American adolescents.
- Fewer African American adults between 45 and 64 years of age and persons with activity limitations having a full set of permanent teeth (excluding third molars).
- Fewer Hispanic adults received needed dental care (because of cost).
- More edentulous older adults age 65 to 74 years who have less than a high school education.

Food Patterns

In terms of food choices, people are creatures of habit. Patterns throughout societies are quite evident; however, the term "habit" connotes inflexibility. People change their food habits for numerous reasons; thus, the term "food pattern" is more descriptive of food choices. Many factors are associated with formation of food patterns and preferences. **Food patterns** are generally developed during childhood and reflect the family's lifestyle and its ethnic or cultural, social, religious, geographical, economic, and psychological components. All of these influence one's attitudes, feelings, and beliefs about food. However, cultural and economic factors typically have the greatest influence on food choices.

No culture has ever been known to make food choices solely on the basis of nutritional and health values of food. Nutritional value is secondary, especially if a food has established social, religious, or economic status. For example, kale is one of the most nutritious vegetables (based on nutrient density) available in the United States but is a less-popular vegetable. On the other hand, the tomato, the most commonly eaten vegetable, rates comparatively low as a source of vitamins and minerals. A raw carrot is more nutrient dense than a candy bar because the carrot contains more nutrients per calorie.

Cultural Influences

The United States is more culturally diverse today than at any time in its history. The immigrant population has changed dramatically. Dietary needs unique to foreign-born individuals have a direct impact on the national health of the United States. One of the most interesting and visible ways that cultural identity is expressed is through an individual's food choices. Although milk is the only food used worldwide, many cultures consider it appropriate only for infants and children.

Children of different cultures accept as the norm what adults in their family eat. Cultural food patterns establish the foundation for a child's lifelong eating patterns regarding meal times and frequency of eating, foods acceptable for specific meals, preparation methods, likes and dislikes, foods suitable for specific members of a group or specific time of day, table manners, the social role of foods and eating, and attitudes toward eating and health (Fig. 16.1).

Many ethnic groups have brought a rich heritage of various food patterns to the United States, resulting in distinct and discrete patterns of food consumption. American diets have become more homogeneous because of transportation, advertising, mobility, new methods of production, changes in income distribution, and appreciation of one another's heritage. Food preferences are influenced by the influx of immigrants, yet some regional food patterns are still evident—few people in northern states would routinely choose grits and many Southerners would not recognize lentils. Individual food preferences do not influence nutritional adequacy of the diet.

Status and Symbolic Influences

Two cultures often regard a food differently. For example, beef is regarded as a high-status food among some people in the United States, but some Hindus from India consider cows sacred and do not eat beef. The choice of different foods is influenced by religious beliefs, availability, cost, cultural values, and traditions or even the endorsement or condemnation of a highly respected person.

Because of symbolic meanings of food, eating becomes associated with sentiments and assumptions about oneself and the world. Foods sometimes become symbolic because of religious connotations and use as rewards. After a child has fallen, a mother may give

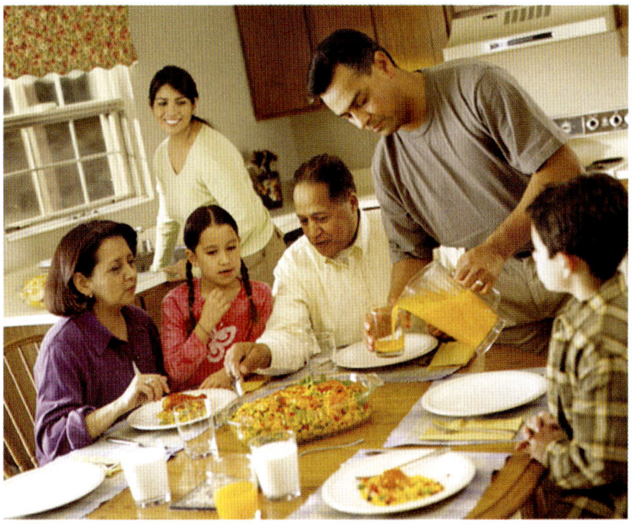

• **Figure 16.1** An extended family eating a dinner together. (From Food and Nutrition Service, U.S. Department of Agriculture and Food and Nutrition Information Center, National Agricultural Library: SNAP-Ed Connections: photo gallery. Beltsville, MD. https://snaped.fns.usda.gov/extended-family-eating-dinner-together. Accessed April 11, 2017.)

the child ice cream or candy to help forget the pain and stop crying. Food is also withheld for bad behavior.

Working With Patients With Different Food Patterns

Respect for Other Eating Patterns

Dental hygienists must be prepared for the unexpected. People are partial to their own food pattern; however, too many people, including dental professionals, are convinced their own beliefs, attitudes, and practices are best and assume that everyone should follow them. Multicultural competence is the ability to discover each patient's cultural and ethnic preferences and effectively adapt interventions.

Even when the facts are known, an analysis of the situation may be clouded because of unique individual habits. Information should be obtained regarding food habits using open-ended questions, rather than questions that put words into a patient's mouth. For example, "Tell me everything you had to eat this morning" might elicit a different response than the open-ended question, "What did you have for breakfast this morning?"

Effecting Change

Knowledge of food preferences and attitudes is important for recognizing and respecting differences to effect change if needed. An empathetic, observant dental hygienist understands and is aware of unique characteristics of local cultures and treats each patient with respect while attempting to promote sound nutritional practices.

Cultural food patterns have contributed to survival of the group in a particular environment. People have a remarkable ability to obtain a nutritious diet out of available foodstuffs. Some eating patterns that seem strange may actually be adaptive by enhancing or preserving nutritional value.

Food patterns of other countries are in some instances nutritionally superior or at least comparable to "ordinary" American traditions. When people relocate, they retain their traditional food patterns only if their native foods are available in a new location at an affordable price. Finding native foods that were the basis of their family traditional food pattern may be a challenge.

Problems arising within various cultural groups are generally economic rather than faults of traditional food patterns. Foods from the country of origin, which were cheapest at "home," may be very expensive or possibly unavailable in the new location. Immigrants may find their culturally preferred foods easily in urban areas because many Americans are interested in exotic and ethnic cuisines, increasing availability of ethnic foods in supermarkets and ethnic restaurants. If the location is a rural, less populated area, finding native foods may be more difficult.

Each food, food-related behavior, and tradition can be categorized as beneficial, neutral, or potentially harmful. A food that is beneficial promotes health by contributing necessary nutrients. Neutral foods are not especially beneficial but are not harmful to health. Foods are not usually harmful, but customs affecting nutritional content of the food may be potentially harmful. Efforts should be made to alter only patterns undesirably affecting nutritional value or health. For example, because many water-soluble vitamins are destroyed by heat, the practice of cooking foods (especially vegetables) for long periods is discouraged unless the liquids are consumed or iron cookware is used.

Food patterns are generally deeply ingrained, contribute to psychological stability, and are hard to change. If dietary changes are indicated for health or dental reasons, suggest minimal alterations in the patient's normal patterns and, if possible, present the information with options. Rather than indicating that a patient needs to stop eating a food that is a part of the cultural heritage, talk about portion control of the food. Health care workers who do not address individual patient needs are ineffective, and patients feeling uncomfortable with the information will not use it.

Cultural patterns tend to be used more consistently by older family members. First-generation immigrants are still rooted in their homeland and usually prefer at least one native meal a day. Dental professionals should learn about ethnic foods for immigrants in the area so they can assist in suggesting alternatives or similar types of foods. Gradually, the diet conforms to food resources of the new location, a process called **dietary acculturation**. Second-generation Americans are raised without that direct native connection, and their parents, often struggling with new foods themselves, may not have the knowledge to educate their children about healthy American foods.

It is impossible to cover the dietary practices of all cultures and religions in this text. Fig. 16.2 is a food guide for Mexico. The Canadian Food Guide was presented in Chapter 1 (see Fig. 1.7). Additional food guides can be found in the back of the book and on the Evolve website. A list of different cultural and regional foods with brief descriptions is available on the Evolve website.

Religious Food Restrictions

Religious beliefs affect eating patterns, attaching symbolic meanings to food and drink. Some examples are the bread and wine served during Christian communion service and Hindu reverence for the cow. Many Seventh Day Adventists are vegetarians; some are vegans. These patterns do not usually result in any nutritional problems but could affect one's food patterns and require consideration before making dietary recommendations.

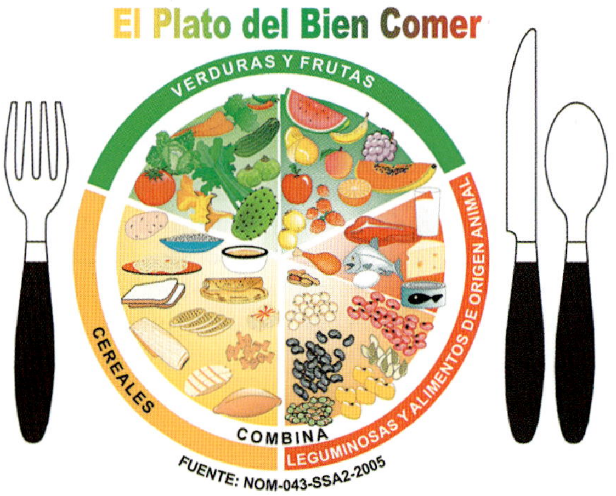

• **Figure 16.2** Mexican food guide. (Reproduced with permission from Mahan LK, Escott-Stump S, Raymond JL: *Krause's Food and the Nutrition Care Process*. 13th ed. St Louis, MO: Saunders; 2012.)

DENTAL CONSIDERATIONS

- Patients sometimes refuse to eat a particular food or comply with recommended changes because of cultural or religious beliefs.
- Advice that takes into consideration a patient's needs and food preferences is more likely to be followed.
- The increasing ethnic and cultural diversity of the United States presents new challenges to health professionals in offering culturally sensitive interventions to improve the health of their patients.
- When working with patients who have strong cultural ties, maintain a sensitive, nonjudgmental, and respectful perspective of their preferences.
- A heavy accent or lack of English proficiency is not indicative of educational level or intelligence.
- Patients are more likely to disclose crucial information to an open-minded dental hygienist who avoids cultural biases.
- Be tactful and allow longer response times for patients from different cultures.
- Patients are more receptive to minor changes in the diet pattern. The key is to ease patients into change.
- Identify advantages and faults for each cultural food pattern in your area.
- Use an understanding of ethnic food habits to encourage or incorporate beneficial practices into the patient's diet.
- Compliance is improved when a patient has input into changes in food choices, understands why changes are indicated, and feels responsible for following any suggestions.
- Individuals from all cultures have unique tastes and preferences; stereotyping members of cultural groups should be avoided.
- In many cases, American food practices adopted by immigrants have been deleterious to their health by contributing to the same chronic diseases typical in the United States.

NUTRITIONAL DIRECTIONS

- Patterns and attitudes internalized during childhood promote a sense of stability and security for adults.
- Insufficient quantities of any food group (milk, fruits, vegetables, cereals, and meats) have the greatest effect on nutritional adequacy rather than specific aversions, such as a dislike of turnips or rye bread.
- An adequate diet can be planned incorporating most cultural and religious beliefs.

Food Budgets

Foods available in the home are primarily the result of food shopping behaviors. If nutrient-dense healthful foods are not purchased, they cannot be consumed. Likewise, if more energy-dense foods are purchased, they compete with more healthful choices even if more nutritious foods are available. Despite increasing interest in optimal nutrition, many Americans are anxious about food prices and constantly attempt to conserve their food dollars. In 2016, retail food prices decreased by 1.3%—the first time in almost 50 years that grocery store prices did not increase.[3] Fluctuating prices from year to year reflect supply and demand both within the United States and internationally, with supply being affected significantly by weather conditions. Evidence that poor or fair health status and malnutrition increase as income level decreases is discussed in *Health Application 16*.

The average American family spends approximately 10% to 15% of its income on food; families at the poverty level may spend 33%.[4] American families report spending anywhere from $50 per week to $300 per week, with an average expenditure of $151 weekly.[5] Based on U.S. Department of Agriculture (USDA) food plans for 2012, the weekly cost of food for a family of 4 ranges between $128 and $294 (based on all meals and snacks being prepared at home).[6]

In 2014, Americans spent more on food away from home ($0.33 of every dollar or 50% of total food expenditures) than for foods purchased for the home.[7] In general, a large proportion of the food dollar is spent on processed foods. A general awareness of food costs can be used to assist patients in stretching their food dollar (Box 16.1). The amount of money a household spends on food provides insight into how adequately nutritional needs are being met. Households with better financial management skills are better equipped to provide enough food for the household. Palatable, healthful foods can be provided economically.

Consumers sometimes believe that healthy food must be more expensive than less expensive foods and that higher-priced food is healthier.[8] Most people believe that healthful foods (such as fruits and vegetables) are more expensive than calorie-dense foods (e.g., foods high in sodium, added sugars, or saturated fats). The USDA's Economic Research Service concluded that following *Dietary Guidelines* recommendations were not more expensive; most people simply need to reallocate their food budget.[9] Approximately 35% of grocery store purchases includes "miscellaneous foods"—soft drinks and other sugar-sweetened beverages, frozen meals, snacks, canned and packaged soups, salad dressings, candy, condiments, gourmet and specialty items, and seasonings.

Cheap foods that provide few nutrients may actually be "expensive" from a nutritional economic perspective, whereas a food with a higher retail price providing large quantities of nutrients may actually be quite cheap. By shifting the amount spent on fruits and vegetables from 26% to 40% of the budget, the family can buy the quantity and variety of produce needed. Reducing the amount spent on meat proteins and incorporating more plant protein meals frees up about $20 per week. The greatest cost savings and dietary improvements are from substituting a table-service meal with one prepared at home and changing from fast food to home cooking.[10] "Eating out" accounts for 43% of the annual food expenditures for the average family.[11] Additionally, most restaurant menus provide too much saturated fats, calories, and added sugar, and more alcohol may be consumed. Only about one in five meals consumed outside the home meets the *Dietary Guidelines* recommendations and costs almost $100 more monthly.[12] Consumers can save money and eat healthier by reducing portion sizes, especially of energy-dense foods, and buying fewer calorie-dense foods.

Based on the *Dietary Guidelines*, food choices of low-income households are generally less desirable than those of higher-income households. Compliance with recommendations for fruits and vegetables is the biggest concern. Low-income households earning below 130% of the poverty line are more likely to spend less on all categories of foods except for eggs. This suggests that low-income households may consume less food and/or lower-quality foods. More food can be purchased with less money by choosing lower-priced foods, by selecting less-expensive meats and fresh fruits and vegetables, and by reducing the amount of energy-dense foods. As a rule, small increases in income result in increased expenditures on more expensive foods, such as beef and frozen prepared foods, rather than increasing variety and quality of foods. A systematic review of studies concluded that subsidizing healthful foods to lower their cost significantly increased consumption of produce,

• BOX 16.1 Basic Principles for Economical Food Purchases

1. Take inventory before going to the supermarket.
2. Plan weekly menus using *MyPlate* as a guideline. Prepare a shopping list and stick to it.
3. Plan menus around seasonal foods or weekly specials.
4. Never shop when hungry.
5. Purchase the least-expensive items in each food group that you will eat.
6. Rely on minimal servings of meats. On the average, purchase 1 lb ground beef or turkey for 4 people. When purchasing steaks, check the weight; most would serve at least 2 people.
7. Use meat substitutes (e.g., legumes, nuts, peanut butter, and cheese) several times each week.
8. Serve adequate quantities of grains, cereals, and pasta products (6 to 11 servings per day), but be aware of portion sizes. For instance, one serving of pasta is ½ cup cooked, but pasta labels may identify 1 serving as 1 cup cooked.
9. Purchase smaller quantities of whole-grain products in place of a larger quantity of refined grains. The first ingredient in the bread should be 100% whole grain.
10. Prepare most foods from scratch rather than buying convenience items, such as frozen pizza.
11. Limit highly processed foods that are expensive or have low nutrient density (e.g., carbonated beverages and chips). Replace these foods with fresh fruits and vegetables.
12. Avoid impulse buying, and be prepared to make substitutions if a similar item is a better buy.
13. Purchase store brands, which are usually a wise choice. Store brands, often found on the lowest shelves, are equal in quality and taste to well-advertised national brands.
14. Read labels to determine nutritive value and compare with similar products.
15. Compare unit prices. If available, the price per unit (e.g., ounce) stated on the shelf below the grocery item facilitates comparing various sizes.
16. Buy larger sizes (which are usually cheaper per serving) if the food will be eaten before it spoils, but purchase individual serving sizes of products such as low-fat yogurt, if portion control is important.
17. Shop at large supermarkets rather than small stores or convenience stores for more economical purchases.
18. Avoid purchasing high-energy snack foods and breakfast cereals with a high sugar content.
19. Do most of your shopping around the perimeter of the store, where seasonal items and basic essentials such as fresh meat, milk, and eggs are located. Highly processed foods line the inner supermarket shelves.
20. Frozen meats are cheaper and as healthful as fresh meat.
21. Plan to use highly perishable items, such as fresh fish or strawberries, as soon as possible after purchasing.
22. Use convenience foods wisely. In general, the more someone else does in preparing food, the more the product will cost.
23. Use dating information on products to select the freshest foods. Do not let food in the pantry or refrigerator go to waste, but do not dispose of items just because they are past their "Best if used by" date without checking to see if the product is good.
24. Avoid purchasing bruised, moldy, and mushy produce.
25. Pay attention at the checkout counter to be sure the advertised price or the price indicated on the shelf is what is charged.
26. Plan to use leftovers for soups, salads, and sandwiches.

and taxation of unhealthful foods and beverages and fast food reduced their intake.[13]

On the basis of nutrient density, spinach, liver, turkey, canned tuna, lentils/beans, nonfat and low-fat milk, cottage cheese, tofu, eggs, and fresh carrots are usually the most economical. Some less-expensive fruits per serving size are bananas, watermelons, raisins, apples, grapefruit, grapes, and oranges; least-expensive vegetables include potatoes, carrots, cabbage, cucumbers, green beans, onions, mustard greens, kale, romaine and iceberg lettuce, bell peppers, tomatoes, and broccoli. Buying seasonal, homegrown fruits and vegetables is more economical. Generally, more of the food dollar should be spent for fruits, vegetables, whole grain products, low-fat milk, and dry beans; less is needed for meats and high-sugar, high-fat food items (e.g., candy, sugar-sweetened beverages, and chips).

People with limited financial resources are hampered by other constraints. **Food deserts** are located in lower-income inner-city and rural areas with few supermarkets; numerous small stores stock limited nutritious food items, particularly fruits and vegetables, at affordable prices. Low-income shoppers spend less on food purchases despite the fact that food prices are higher where they are compelled to shop. Without transportation, low-income consumers are often limited to shopping close to where they live or they must spend money for travel or delivery services. Lack of availability of a variety of produce and poor quality are deterrents to eating healthier for very-low-income consumers. Small, low-income-area grocery stores may inconsistently stock whole grains, low-fat cheeses, lean ground beef, and larger package sizes. Merely adding a supermarket in a food desert may not change people's habits of shopping and eating, however. The educational level of consumers is more predictive of food purchases.[14] Families on food stamps or on a very low food budget need to learn skills in buying and storing food.

Maintaining Optimal Nutrition During Food Preparation

From the time any produce is removed from the plant or a grain product is harvested, nutrient content begins to degrade. Harvesting, processing, and cooking food means nutrient losses are occurring, but good handling processes, such as chilling or freezing, minimize losses and bacterial growth.

Methods of Preparation

Many consumers would hope that all vitamins and minerals would be available and utilized by their bodies. In many instances, cooking enhances palatability, increases digestibility of food, and destroys pathogenic organisms. Cooking affects acceptability and nutritional value of food. Nutrients most susceptible to food preparation techniques are the water-soluble vitamins (C, thiamin, riboflavin, niacin, folate, B_6, and B_{12}). Minerals may also be affected but to a lesser degree than vitamins. Following a few guidelines can help preserve nutrients during cooking (Box 16.2).

Adding large amounts of fats during the cooking process, as in frying, is discouraged. Methods of preparing meats, such as broiling or cooking on a grill, are recommended to lessen natural fat content. Meats cooked to the well-done stage contain less fat. To remove fats during cooking, meats can be boiled, microwaved in a colander or on paper towels, or roasted or broiled on a rack. Absorption of fat-soluble vitamins requires availability of a small amount of fat; that is, absorption of vitamins A, D, E, and K from a vegetable salad is enhanced with a salad dressing (not fat-free) or cheese, or some other food containing fat.

Cooking increases digestibility of protein in meats. Cooking generally softens cellulose in fresh produce. Total volume and bulk of the food decrease; thus, a greater quantity of these low-calorie

• BOX 16.2 Guidelines for Preserving Nutrients During Preparation

1. Prepare fresh produce as near to serving time as possible to prevent deterioration of many nutrients when they are exposed to air. Refrigerate within 2 hours of cutting or peeling.
2. Do not soak fruits and vegetables that have been cut to prevent loss of water-soluble vitamins and some minerals (especially potassium) into the water. If cut-up fruits and vegetables are soaked in water, use the water in food preparation.
3. Scrub fruits and vegetables rather than pare them to increase fiber and nutrient intake. When necessary, pare as thinly as possible to maintain nutrients.
4. Boil nonconsumable parings and portions of vegetables in water and incorporate in soup stock or gravies. This is a very rich source of potassium and water-soluble vitamins.
5. Leave produce whole or in large pieces so that less surface area is available for oxidation of nutrients.
6. Carotenoids—such as beta-carotene, lycopene, and lutein—are more easily absorbed when vegetables are cooked than raw.
7. Store any fruits or vegetables that have been cut or otherwise processed, such as fruit juice, in airtight containers. Container size should be appropriate for the amount to be stored to prevent excessive oxidation from air inside the container.
8. Quick-cooking methods rather than extended cooking times are usually best to retain the B complex and C vitamins. Boiling leaches water-soluble vitamins; thus, quick steaming or sautéing is recommended to reduce loss into the cooking medium unless the liquid is also consumed (e.g., in soups or incorporated into a gravy).
9. A covered pan minimizes cooking time by increasing the temperature inside.
10. Use the least amount of liquid possible in cooking. Serve vegetables as soon as they are prepared.
11. Do not use baking soda when cooking vegetables.

foods can be eaten. Stir frying is an old Asian technique that is a highly recommended method, which has the added benefit of being quick. Bite-sized pieces of food are cooked very briefly over high heat with or without a small amount of vegetable oil. Vegetables retain their nutrient value, color, and crispness.

A microwave oven is another timesaver because of shorter cooking times. Vitamin content of foods cooked in a home microwave oven is about the same as foods prepared conventionally, especially if a minimal amount of water is added.

Greens, such as spinach, increase in folate, lutein, beta-carotene, and vitamins E and K content during exposure to light, even with continuous exposure to grocery store lighting.[16] The vitamin detrimentally affected most often is vitamin C. Apparently, as long as the plant is green, photosynthesis continues. Vitamin levels begin to degrade when wilting begins. Actually, baby greens are typically more nutritious than more mature greens—younger leaves have greater nutrient density than older leaves.[16]

Food Sanitation and Safety

Food carefully chosen for nutritional value may be adversely affected by handling techniques and preparation for consumption. Food-borne illness affects about 48 million people, contributing to 128 hospitalizations and 3000 deaths every year.[10] Of the 31 pathogens known to cause food-borne illness, six account for most of the illnesses, hospitalizations, and deaths annually—*Campylobacter*, *Escherichia coli* (*E. coli*), *Listeria monocytogenes*, *Salmonella*, *Vibrio*, and *Yersinia*. In recent years, progress has been made in significantly reducing food-borne infections caused by *E. coli*, *Listeria*, *Salmonella*, and *Campylobacter*; infections from *Campylobacter* and *Salmonella* caused the most illnesses. The official statistics are probably low, because many food-borne infections are not reported or are not identified.

In other words, despite the abundance of knowledge about food-borne illness, food safety is still a significant public health challenge and we are still "losing the battle" against food-borne illness.[17]

For most people, the illness resolves on its own, but these illnesses can be fatal for younger and older individuals and those with weakened immune systems. Illness caused by *Listeria* can result in miscarriage, fetal death, or severe illness or death of a newborn (see Chapter 13).

A food safety survey conducted in 2016 indicated most respondents thought that food poisoning was not common from food prepared at home; only 6% thought raw vegetables could have germs present.[18] Most food-borne illnesses can be prevented by following safe food-handling and preparation recommendations and by avoiding consumption of raw or undercooked foods of animal origin such as eggs, ground beef, and poultry; unpasteurized milk, cheese, and juices; and raw or undercooked oysters.

The *Dietary Guidelines* provide food safety principles and guidance in general terms to reduce the risk of foodborne illness: *Clean* (handwashing, food preparation surfaces, and food), *Separate* (to prevent cross-contamination), *Cook* (to recommended safe temperature), and *Chill* (maintain foods at a safe temperature). Edibles must be handled with care to prevent contamination with food-borne organisms, and some foods—especially meat, poultry, and eggs—must be cooked to sufficiently high temperatures to kill microorganisms naturally present. When foods remain in the "Danger Zone" (between 40°F and 140°F), bacteria can multiply rapidly, causing a single bacterium to multiply to 17 million in 12 hours. Box 16.3 lists some specific guidelines for handling food.

In recent years, nationwide recalls of tainted food products have included meats, peanut butter, vegetables, salad, snacks, fast foods, and dessert items, causing thousands of illnesses and even a few deaths. Many of these foods were imported, but some were domestic products grown in areas considered to be safe. New foods implicated—organically grown spinach, sprouts, and peanut butter—were perplexing problems. Increasing numbers of people consuming more fresh produce is good nutritionally, but harmful microbes on some fruits and vegetables have created problems. Contrary to popular opinion, pathogens that cause illness are odorless, colorless, and invisible. Therefore, smelling, tasting, or looking at food is not a good gauge of whether it may be contaminated. Spoilage bacteria evidenced by slimy films on lunch meat, soggy edges on vegetables, or sticky chicken are not as toxic as pathogens.

Concern has intensified over the possibility of contaminated food caused by terrorist acts. The U.S. Food and Drug Administration (FDA) is authorized in the Public Health Security and Bioterrorism Preparedness and Response Act of 2002 (Bioterrorism Act) to detain suspect food. The FDA Food Safety Modernization Act was signed into law in early 2010 and is slowly being implemented with regulations, processes, and systems developed based on science-based standards. These regulations encompassing growing, harvesting, and packing produce strengthen oversight of imported foods and require food producers to identify possible hazards and take steps to prevent outbreaks of food-borne illness. The Act

• BOX 16.3 Safe Sanitary Kitchen Guidelines

- Keep kitchen countertops, refrigerator, cookware, and cutlery clean. Disinfect countertops and sink with a weak chlorine (1 tsp household bleach in 1 gallon water) solution.
- Wash your hands before preparing meals and handling any foods.
- Purchase pasteurized juice to avoid harmful bacteria.
- Avoid cross-contamination by keeping fresh produce away from uncooked meats.
- Avoid washing fruits and vegetables until just before eating. Natural coatings keep moisture inside; washing makes them spoil sooner.
- Refrigerate fresh produce within 2 hours of cutting or peeling.
- Wash all prepackaged produce, even if the package says "prewashed."
- Refrigerate or freeze meat, poultry, eggs, and other perishables as soon as possible.
- Bacteria can live on the rinds or skins—clean the whole thing, even inedible parts. The knife cutting into the edible portion can transfer bacteria from the rind/peel.
- Gently rub fruits and vegetables under running water. Soaps, detergents, bleaches, or commercial sprays and washes will leave their own residue on the produce.
- Scrub firmer items such as apples and potatoes with a vegetable brush while rinsing with clean water to remove dirt and residues.
- Remove and discard the outer leaves of lettuce and cabbage heads; thoroughly rinse the rest of the leaves.
- Rinse berries and other small fruits thoroughly and allow them to drain in a colander.
- People with a compromised immune system should consider eating only cooked produce, especially sprouts, and well-cooked meats and fish.
- Never use the same utensils or cutting surfaces for preparing meats and vegetables. Use different cutting boards for fresh produce, dairy products, poultry, fish, and meats. Wash with a weak chlorine solution after using.
- Wash the tops of all cans, including pop-top beverages, before opening.
- Use an appliance thermometer to ensure that the refrigerator temperature is between 40°F and 32°F and freezer is 0°F or below. Use a food thermometer to ensure that meats are cooked to appropriate temperature—beef, pork, veal, and lamb at 160°F; turkey and chicken at 165°F; ham at 140°F; fish at 145°F; leftovers at 165°F.
- Refrigerate leftovers to 40°F or below within 2 hours of serving. Seal leftovers in an airtight, clean container labeled with the expiration date.
- Discard leftovers and other refrigerated foods as soon as possible after expiration date. Leftovers should be eaten within 2 days.
- Foods left unrefrigerated for more than 2 hours should be discarded.
- Wash reusable grocery bags.
- Defrost meats in the refrigerator or the microwave.

enables the FDA to better protect public health by focusing on preventing food safety problems rather than reacting to problems after they occur. Imported foods will have to comply with the same standards as domestic foods.

The FDA acknowledges that to progress in this battle against food-borne illness, reform of behaviors is needed. The FDA teamed with the Partnership for Food Safety Education to provide consumers and food safety educators information to implement safe food handling practices. The website for Fight Bac! (www.fightbac.org/) provides free resources regarding food safety basics, food poisoning, and food safety education to help prevent this unnecessary illness.

Most people feel that foods with a "sell by" or "use by" date somehow goes bad after that date. This may not be true. In addition to these phrases being confusing, these meaningless labels have led to disposal of millions of pounds of food that is wholesome and safe. Food Safety and Inspection Service (FSIS) has issued new guidance aimed at reducing food waste by encouraging food manufacturers and retailers to use a "Best if used by" date label. This terminology does not indicate a safety date but a guideline for enjoying the best flavor or quality.

Processed Foods

When the word "processed" is used, consumers often make the mistake of assuming that the food is automatically unhealthy and should be avoided. Actually, everything that is done to a food after harvesting to prepare for consumption is food processing, whether it occurs at home or by the food manufacturer. Food processing is a method used since ancient times to preserve and improve foods. Processed foods are not always unhealthy and may be beneficial, both nutritionally and for convenience. Active, mobile lifestyles and an increasing number of women working full-time or part-time outside the home have led to a continued increase in availability and consumption of processed foods. Although growing one's own food and making foods from "scratch" can give consumers control over how food is handled and what is added, this is not feasible for most Americans.

Effect of Processing on Nutrients

Many consumers have been misled in assuming that nutrient content of our food supply has deteriorated. Based on studies conducted by the USDA, nutrient changes are mixed—some nutrients have gone down whereas others have improved.

Nutrient content of foods can be affected by the way food is handled—that is, the type of processing to which the food is subjected (e.g., milling, cooking, freezing, canning, dehydration)—and how it is stored. In general, most minerals, carbohydrates, lipids, proteins, and vitamin K and niacin are **stable nutrients**. Nutrients are considered stable if at least 85% of the original level is retained during processing and storage. Thiamin, riboflavin, folate, and ascorbic acid are most likely to be seriously depleted by processing and storage and method of food preparation. The nutritional value of home-cooked foods is frequently about the same as processed foods.

Manufacturers involved in food processing attempt to maintain optimal qualities of taste, freshness, safety, cost, and value—five traits important in consumer choices. Not everything done to foods by food processors has been good; however, not all processing is detrimental. The milling process removes the bran coat of grains. Removal of the high lipid-containing bran produces a more stable grain, increasing its shelf life. Nutritionally, however, this results in a reduction of fiber and loss of 70% to 80% of thiamin, riboflavin, vitamin B_6, and other nutrients. Enrichment replaces some nutrients (thiamin, riboflavin, niacin, folic acid, and iron) lost in processing, but not all of them (see Chapter 1, Table 1.5). Without the enrichment and fortification processes, many American diets would be deficient in nutrient intake of vitamins A, C, and D and thiamin, iron, and folate.

Fresh fruits and vegetables have a higher nutritive value and better taste immediately after harvest but rapidly deteriorate if transported long distances or improperly stored. Frozen foods packed immediately after harvesting are frequently higher in nutritive value than their fresh counterparts available in the supermarket. Because canned vegetables have prolonged exposure to water, they usually lose more nutrients than frozen ones, but even canned vegetables are better than no vegetables at all. On the other hand, some canned foods, especially tomatoes, but also carrots, sweet potatoes, peaches, beans (legumes), tuna, and salmon, are cheaper and as nutritious as their counterpart fresh products.

The most negative effect of food processing has been the addition of ingredients that enhance taste and desirability of the product—sweeteners, salt, and artificial colors and flavors. Because of the way foods are processed quickly and transported rapidly, fresh produce is available year round, harmful microorganisms are reduced, maximum efficiency in production results in reduced costs, and foods are fortified or enriched with nutrients. Highly processed foods are usually less nutritious than the fresh form (i.e., potato chips are less nutritious than a baked potato; a handful of corn chips does not compare to a sweet ear of freshly picked corn). Consumers are free to choose foods that are minimally processed and thus healthier, or ready-to-eat foods that may contain less-desirable ingredients (Fig. 16.3). Reading nutrition and ingredient labels is important. Avoid processed foods that reduce a food's nutritional wealth or add ingredients that should be avoided—added sugar, sodium, or saturated or *trans* fats. Choose whole foods that have had a minimum amount of processing.

Convenience Foods

Convenience foods are usually popular because they save time in meal preparation, planning, purchasing, and cleanup. The variety of foods available has also expanded. Convenience foods prepared by food manufacturers may cost more because of extra handling and packaging (Table 16.1). Convenience foods also require more preservatives and may contain more sodium and fat than home-cooked products. On the positive side, foods that are convenient can actually increase the likelihood that the consumer will eat a healthier diet.

Irradiated Foods

Foods treated with controlled amounts of ionized radiation for a prescribed period to kill spoilage-causing and disease-causing bacteria and molds in meats and produce are known as **irradiated foods**.

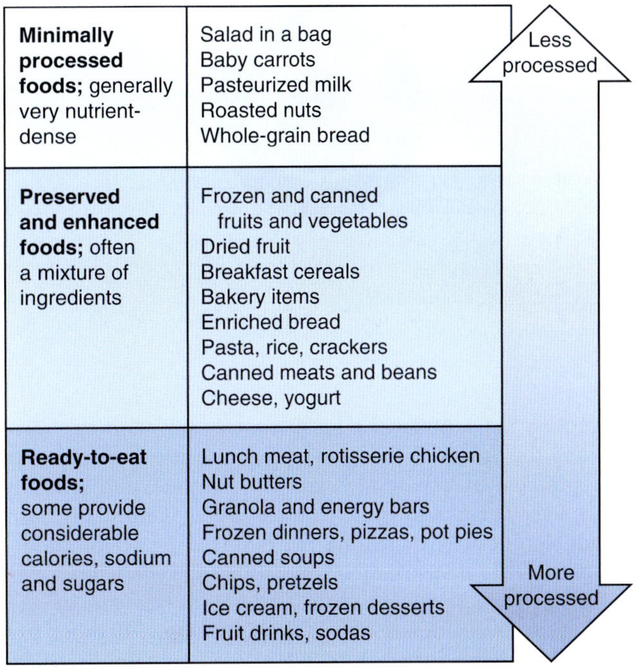
Minimally processed foods; generally very nutrient-dense
Salad in a bag
Baby carrots
Pasteurized milk
Roasted nuts
Whole-grain bread
Preserved and enhanced foods; often a mixture of ingredients
Frozen and canned fruits and vegetables
Dried fruit
Breakfast cereals
Bakery items
Enriched bread
Pasta, rice, crackers
Canned meats and beans
Cheese, yogurt
Ready-to-eat foods; some provide considerable calories, sodium and sugars
Lunch meat, rotisserie chicken
Nut butters
Granola and energy bars
Frozen dinners, pizzas, pot pies
Canned soups
Chips, pretzels
Ice cream, frozen desserts
Fruit drinks, sodas
Less processed
More processed

• **Figure 16.3** How do I make sure that I am eating "healthy" processed foods? The chart shows the range of processed foods available. Minimally processed foods are similar to, and sometimes even more nutritious than, the same foods in their unprocessed form. Although the ready-to-eat category contains some foods that are high in calories and nutrient poor, this category also includes convenient, ready-to-eat meals and snacks that provide a significant source of nutrients. (Reproduced with permission by the Dairy Council of California © 2013. Processed foods: a range, not a dichotomy. 2012. http://www.healthyeating.org/Portals/0/Documents/Health%20Wellness/White%20Papers/ProcessedFoods_72dpi.pdf.)

TABLE 16.1 Eating Healthy on a Budget

HIGHLY PROCESSED FOODS			MINIMALLY PROCESSED FOODS		
Food	Serving Size	Price/ Serving[a]	Food	Serving Size	Price/ Serving[a]
Chocolate milk	1 cup	0.40	Skim milk	1 cup	0.24
Brown rice, ready-to-serve	1 container	1.00	Brown rice, bulk, dry	⅓ cup	0.079
White bread	1 slice	0.07	Whole-grain bread	1 slice	0.19
Banana nut muffin	1 large	0.67	Banana nut muffin, mix	1 medium	0.25
Fruit Loops cereal	1 cup	0.56	Cheerios cereal	1 cup	0.39
Oatmeal, instant packaged	1 package (½ cup)	0.30	Old fashioned oats, dry	½ cup	0.27
Hamburger pattie (80/20)	4 oz	1.25	Hamburger meat, bulk (80/20)	4 oz	1.12
Fish sticks, frozen	5	0.83	Chunk light tuna in water	2 oz	0.55
Pinto beans, canned	½ cup	0.37	Dried pinto beans, cooked	½ cup	0.11
Tater tots	9 pieces	0.33	Potato, cooked	1 cup	0.20
Carrots, canned	½ cup	0.43	Carrots, raw	½ cup cooked	0.25

[a]Price per serving April 11, 2017 at Randalls grocery store in Lakeway, TX.

• **Figure 16.4** Official package label for irradiated foods. (From U.S. Food and Drug Administration [FDA]. https://www.fda.gov/Food/ResourcesForYou/Consumers/ucm261680.htm.)

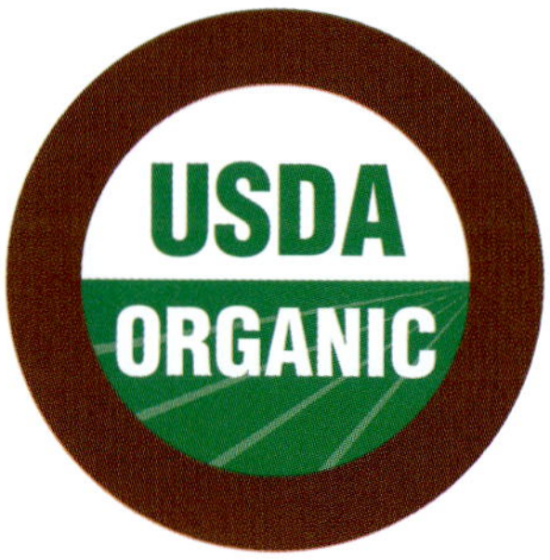

• **Figure 16.5** Official USDA organic seal. (From Agricultural Marketing Service, U.S. Department of Agriculture, Washington, DC. https://www.ams.usda.gov/sites/default/files/media/Organic4colorsealJPG.jpg.)

This process has stimulated a lot of controversy, with opponents criticizing the process as being a stopgap measure that ignores the bigger problem of how food is grown, processed, and sold. This process, which breaks down DNA molecules of harmful organisms without significantly increasing the temperature of the food, is often called "cold pasteurization." Irradiation can extend the period of ripeness of fruits and vegetables, prolong the freshness of many foods, and prevent certain food-borne illnesses. Washing fresh fruits and vegetables can reduce risk of food contamination, but irradiation kills bacteria that are beyond the reach of conventional chemical sanitizers, such as inside the leaves of curly spinach and lettuce. (Irradiated foods are not sterile.) At the low doses of radiation allowed, nutrient losses are either not measurable or are insignificant.[15] Foods have been safely irradiated in the United States for more than 50 years, and more than 40 other countries use the process. The process is carefully controlled and monitored by numerous government organizations; irradiated foods bear the label shown in Fig. 16.4.

Organic Foods

The sharp rise in consumer demand for organic food outpaces domestic supply. Organic sales account for over 5% of total U.S. food sales or an estimated $40 billion in 2015; sales are predicted to reach an estimated $320 billion by 2025.[19] The fastest-growing sector—the meat, fish, and poultry category—is still significantly less than fruit and vegetable sales. Organic foods receive significant price premiums over conventionally grown products. Average organic prices for 18 fruits and 19 vegetables were slightly less than 30% over conventionally produced products for over two-thirds of the items.[20]

This rapid growth may be driven by consumers' perception that organic foods are healthier, tastier, and contain fewer calories. Consumers who reported being more knowledgeable about organic food and choose it more frequently felt that processed organic foods were tastier and equally or more healthful than other foods.[21,22] Consumers indicate other good reasons for choosing organic foods: (a) organic farming tends to build topsoil; (b) environmental reasons, such as less use of fertilizer; (c) fresher; and (d) more humane treatment of animals and less antibiotic-resistant bacteria.

In 2002, the USDA passed regulations defining organic food and permitting use of a seal (Fig. 16.5) for foods meeting specific standards. Organic certification regulates how these foods are grown, handled, and processed. Foods labeled **organic** are grown without *synthetic* pesticides, growth hormones, antibiotics, or genetic engineering. Organic farmers are allowed to use pesticides approved by the National Organic Standards Board that are naturally occurring chemicals, principally animal and crop wastes; botanical, biologic, or nonsynthetic pest controls; or specific synthetic materials that quickly degrade when exposed to oxygen and sunlight. Contamination with the dangerous bacterium *E. coli* does not differ between organic and conventional produce.

Animals raised by organic producers cannot be given antibiotics to stimulate growth; thus, organic meats, poultry, milk, or eggs do not contain any residue of these drugs. New standards became effective in 2011 requiring that all organic animals have year-round outdoor access, ruminant animals must graze on pasture land during the entire grazing season, and at least 30% of their dry nutrition must be from the pasture while they are grazing. Beef and lamb must come from animals that were not confined during the finishing period (when animals are usually fattened on grain). The USDA states that organic agriculture is meant "to protect natural resources, conserve biodiversity, and use only approved substances," but the "organic" label does not have any bearing on the healthfulness of a product.[23]

Food manufacturers voluntarily provide information to the USDA about substances and practices used in food production, including how nonorganic and organic foods are kept separate. The USDA is responsible for inspecting the agricultural site annually and certifying a producer. Products labeled "Made with Organic Ingredients" must contain at least 70% organic ingredients. A product containing more than 5% of the allowable pesticide tolerance level established by the Environmental Protection Agency (EPA) cannot be labeled organic.

Whether organic foods are more nutritious than conventional foods has been a point of contention for years. Two systematic reviews, one analyzing more than 250 research studies and the other evaluating more than 160 studies published in the scientific literature over the past 50 years, found no overall difference in vitamin and mineral content between foods produced using organic and conventional methods.[24] After examining all available evidence, the American Association of Pediatricians concluded that organic foods (produce, meats, milk) do not have any meaningful nutritional benefits or deficits.[25] Numerous studies, however, indicate that organic produce contains more polyphenols or antioxidants having potential human health benefits.[24,26,27]

A study on organic versus conventional meat indicated that fatty acid content may be slightly more desirable in organic meat, but significant variations were influenced by animal species and meat cuts, and grazing/forage-based diets.[28] Organic whole milk also had a more desirable fatty acid composition and iron content than conventional milk but lower concentrations of iodine and selenium.[29] When it comes to nutritional benefits from organic foods, evidence is lacking that organic has any significant benefit—neither milk nor meat is a great source of omega-3 fatty acids and skim milk (recommended for everyone over 2 years of age) contains no fatty acids.

There are virtually no published studies from (1) long-term studies focusing on chronic disease (e.g., cardiovascular disease [CVD], diabetes, cancer, and neurodegenerative conditions) and (2) controlled human dietary intervention studies comparing effects of organic and conventional diets.[30] Eating a healthful, well-balanced diet incorporating a rainbow of vegetables and fruits plus adding nuts, fish, and eggs to the diet will more likely result in long-range health benefits.

The health risks of pesticides in humans are unclear; the amount and type of chemical pesticides permitted in agricultural use have been restricted since 1996. Pesticides in the U.S. food supply have decreased significantly; thus, approximately 99% of the products sampled in 2012 had residues below the EPA tolerances.[31] Although organic produce contains fewer pesticide residues than conventional produce, the difference is insignificant. Actual levels of pesticides in all foods grown in the United States are well below acceptable limits established by EPA. Pesticide chemical residues on foods are routinely tested since large intakes above established safe levels might possibly be toxic.

Organic produce can acquire synthetic pesticides from the environment (in the air) or in packing (from water or packing materials) or storage. Nonorganic produce is 30% more likely to have pesticides than organic fruits and vegetables.[24] Food surveys of conventional foods indicate that estimated exposures from 34 pesticides were less than 1% of the United Nations Food and Agriculture Organization/World Health Organization's Acceptable Daily Intake, and four other pesticides contributed 1% to 4.8% of the Acceptable Daily Intake. A typical human exposure at 1% of the acceptable daily intake represents an exposure 10,000 times lower than levels that do not cause toxicity in animals. Pesticides currently allowed metabolize quickly and are not stored in the body; a few days after ingesting a pesticide, it is completely absent from the body.

Several measures can be taken to ensure minimal intake of questionable chemicals other than purchasing only organic products, as described in Box 16.4. Blanching, boiling, canning, frying, juicing, peeling, and washing fruits and vegetables reduces pesticide residues. Even after washing fruits and vegetables, some foods still contain higher levels of pesticide residue than others. Annually, the Environmental Working Group (EWG) analyzes conventionally grown products for pesticide residue (see Box 16.4). Buying locally produced fresh vegetables and fruits in season is helpful because fewer pesticides are used when long storage periods and long-distance shipping are not required.

Beginning in January 2017, the FDA implemented voluntary guidelines that described policy direction regarding the judicious use of medically important antibiotics in animals. These new regulations (1) require that licensed veterinarians oversee the use of antibiotics on animals; (2) require a prescription or veterinary feed directive from a licensed veterinarian for the use of antibiotics in water and feed; and (3) prohibit the use of medically important antibiotics for anything other than treatment, control and prevention of disease. Nonorganic animals do not contain antibiotic residues because FDA regulations prohibit farmers from giving feed with antibiotics to conventionally raised animals during a "withdrawal time" before slaughter. This length of time is specific to the antibiotic used to ensure that the drug is not present in the animal's system before the meat or milk enters the food supply. Tests rarely detect traces of antibiotics or other drugs in conventionally produced meat, poultry, milk, or eggs. In both methods of farming, bacterial contamination of chicken and pork is common. Bacteria resistant to three or more antibiotics was higher in conventional than in organic chicken and pork.[24]

Organic food generally comes at a premium cost for many reasons, including higher production and labor costs, lower yields, and high demand. Also, profit margins are higher than those of conventional foods. Organic products cost approximately 10% to 50% more than conventional products. When deciding whether the additional cost for organic food is worth it, remember that eating a lot of fruits and vegetables with pesticides outweighs any possible risk from ingesting trace amounts of pesticides. Although organic foods have been on the market for many years, it is premature to say that either organic or conventional foods are superior with respect to safety or nutritional composition.

Organic farming is sustainable for a population of about 2 to 3 billion people, but not for the current worldwide population of more than 7 billion people. Available arable land is limited, prohibiting organic crop rotation to feed the world. Only drastically cutting consumption of poultry and meat could make the possibility of feeding everybody organic products conceivable.

The food industry has developed many new organic products that are not healthful choices. For instance, a jelly bean is all sugar and not a healthful food choice, whether it is 100% organic or not. To know whether a product is healthy, read food labels (nutrition and ingredient labels) to determine levels of calories, saturated fat, sugar, and sodium, as well as protein, fiber, and vitamins and minerals. An organic cracker may be made with wheat flour, but if whole grain is not the first ingredient, the cracker is inconsistent

• BOX 16.4 Facts About Pesticides

1. Both traditional and organic food production may use pesticides.
2. Pesticide residue levels on both traditional and organic produce are well below the limits established by the Environmental Protection Agency.
3. Washing fruits and vegetables prior to eating or cutting largely removes any remaining traces of pesticide residues.
4. The benefits of consuming fruits and vegetables far outweigh any risks from the amount of pesticide from these foods.
5. The presence of a pesticide residue cannot justify the recommendation to avoid conventional produce or consume only organic produce. Such a recommendation would only be appropriate after determining that exposure to the pesticide residue poses a risk to human health.[1]
6. To help avoid any possibility of consuming unhealthy amounts of pesticides, the Environmental Working Group (EWG) analyzes conventionally grown produce annually and has listed the following as the Dirty Dozen for 2017 (indicating that they tested positive for a number of pesticide residues and contained higher concentrations of pesticides than other produce)[2]:

   Strawberries, spinach, nectarines, apples, peaches, pears, cherries, grapes, celery, tomatoes, sweet bell peppers, potatoes, hot peppers.[15]
7. The EWG also lists the following as having the least amount of pesticide residue (relatively few pesticides detected on them, and low total concentrations of pesticide residues): sweet corn, avocado, pineapple, cabbage, onions, sweet peas (frozen), papaya, asparagus, mango, eggplant, honeydew, melon, kiwi, cantaloupe, cauliflower, grapefruit.[2]

[1] *International Food Information Council Foundation (IFIC). Facts & figures on pesticide safety & use in food production. (Updated).* Food Insight. *May 18, 2015. Last updated November 12, 2015. http://www.foodinsight.org/newsletters/facts-figures-pesticide-safety-use-food-production-updated. Accessed April 11, 2017.*

[2] *Environmental Working Group. Executive Summary: EWG's 2017 Shopper's Guide to Pesticides in Produce. https://www.ewg.org/foodnews/summary.php. Accessed April 3, 2017.*

with the *Dietary Guidelines*. Organic foods to avoid include sweetened beverages, crackers, candy, energy bars, and chips. These foods are high in calories and are not nutrient dense.

The term "natural" is popular on food packaging. Many consumers assume that a product labeled "natural" is healthier. "Natural" does not mean organic. The FDA has not established a standardized legal definition for this term, and use of this claim on food products is unregulated. The FDA does not allow foods to be labeled as "natural" if they contain added color, artificial flavors, or synthetic substances. "Natural" labels are meaningless and misleading for consumers.

Fast Foods and Other Food Establishments

Fast foods have become an integral part of the American fast-paced lifestyle. Spending for meals and snacks away from home has increased substantially since 1965 and accounts for more than double the amount spent on food eaten at home. Providing nutrition information at restaurants is one avenue for educating consumers about what they are eating. The Patient Protection and Affordable Care Act (2010) requires chain restaurants with 20 or more locations to post the number of calories and other nutritional information in each standard menu item. The FDA was authorized to establish uniform requirements affecting many chain restaurants, but implementation has been extremely slow. Restaurant owners must meet this federal requirement by May 2018. Nutrition information must be displayed prominently on menus and menu boards, including drive-through locations and next to self-service foods, such as items in a salad bar. In most cases, this regulation also applies to vending machines. Menu labeling will ensure that customers can process the calorie information when they are deciding what to eat at the point of purchase.

Although some people believe that fast food is junk food, this is not always true. Nutritional analyses by fast food chains and independent studies reveal that their menu items contain rich sources of protein: 30% to 50% of the Recommended Dietary Allowances (RDAs). Additionally, items are available that (if selected) provide 20% to 30% of the RDAs for thiamin, riboflavin, ascorbic acid, and calcium. When a hamburger or roast beef sandwich is selected, substantial amounts of iron are supplied. Most fast food menus lack a rich source of vitamin A. Consumer demand has resulted in salads and other healthier items being added to menus. Salads provide a source of vitamins A and C and dietary fiber; however, the cost may be two to seven times higher than the same foods purchased at supermarkets. Shortages of other nutrients—specifically biotin, folate, pantothenic acid, and copper—are also reported.

Several other problems with fast foods raise concern: (a) The calorie count of a large-sized bundled meal (cheeseburger, french fries, and regular sugar-sweetened beverage) represents 65% to 80% of a 2000 calories per day meal pattern; (b) sodium content 63% to 91% of the 2300 mg per day recommendation; and (c) more than 100% of the recommendation for added sugar per day. Cheeseburgers are the main contributor of saturated fat; on a positive note, saturated and *trans* fat content of a large order of french fries decreased between 2000 and 2013.[32] While sodium intake of fast food may be high, foods from fast food and pizza restaurants contributed only 16% of the sodium intake of school-aged children.[33] Based on NHANES studies, sharp declines of meals eaten by school-aged children from pizza and burger restaurants between 2003 and 2010 have been observed.[34]

The impact of fast foods on nutritional status depends on how frequently they are consumed, composition of each item selected, and other foods eaten during the day. Wise choices are possible when an individual's nutritional needs and nutrient content of menu items are known. New menu items and reduced-portion sizes by several fast food chains simplify decisions to choose healthier foods, but consumers need to comparison shop (Box 16.5). Nutritional analysis of menu items is available from most fast food chains; posted calorie content is the same as for other eating establishments.

While some consumers say labeling is helpful, others find it confusing or disregard the information. Numerous reviews have shown that menu labeling in restaurants and fast food establishments has had no significant impact on consumers' food choices.[35,36] Another possible advantage of labeling is that posting nutrition information may pressure chain restaurants to reformulate and make healthful changes in their products.

• BOX 16.5 Options for Healthful Eating Away From Home

Compare the nutrition numbers (calories, fat, and sodium) for your favorite items between fast-food chains. Be cognizant of new items on the menu that may appeal to you. Some simple switches that may be more healthful include:

- Instead of a quarter-pound cheeseburger, opt for a regular hamburger without cheese, potentially saving 280 calories, 9 g saturated fat, and 1.5 *trans* fat, and 630 mg sodium.
- Instead of a salad topped with crispy fried chicken, substitute with grilled chicken, potentially saving 160 calories, 2 g saturated fat, and 170 mg sodium.
- Instead of a fried-fish sandwich, order a veggie burger, potentially saving 110 calories, 2 g saturated fat, and 330 mg sodium.
- Instead of a sausage and cheese breakfast muffin, substitute oatmeal with maple and fruit, potentially saving 10 calories, 3.5 g saturated fat, and 590 mg sodium.
- Instead of a caramel mocha coffee drink, order a regular coffee (add nonnutritive sweetener and low-fat creamer if desired), potentially saving up to 320 calories, 7 g saturated fat, and 170 mg sodium.

Reproduced with permission from Tufts University. Fast food: why it pays to compare. Health & Nutrition Letter. *April 2015.*

Food Additives

The use of food additives is regulated by law. During the 1950s, the Delaney Committee investigated food additives. The Delaney Clause prohibits use of any food additive that is carcinogenic in humans or animals. Additives deemed to be harmless were labeled "generally recognized as safe." These substances met certain specifications of safety under what might be called a "grandfather clause"—in other words, they are generally recognized by experts as safe, based on their use in foods for years without any known occurrence of health problems.

In 1960, similar regulations were passed for color additives. Colors currently in use were required to undergo further testing to continue being marketed. Since then, approximately 90 of the original 200 color additives have been classified as safe and continue to be added to foods.

In 2016, the FDA issued regulations to strengthen oversight of substances added to human and animal food. Before a newly proposed additive can be marketed, it must undergo strict testing to establish its safety for the intended purpose; safe use of ingredients must be widely recognized by qualified experts. Safety levels of additives established by FDA limit the quantity and use of the additive. Currently, additives are specific, well-known substances meeting specifications for purity and have been shown as convincingly as possible to be free from harmful effects in amounts commonly used. All preservatives used in food products must be declared in the ingredient list on the food label. Preservatives cannot be used to conceal damage or inferiority, make the food appear better than it is, or adversely affect nutritive value of the food. "Safe" is defined as "a reasonable certainty" in the minds of competent scientists that the substance is not harmful under intended conditions of use.

Almost all food additives (99%) are derived from natural sources or are synthetically produced to be identical to the natural chemical substance. In many instances, effects of chemicals naturally present in a food are observed, and this chemical is added to other foods to achieve a similar effect. For instance, calcium propionate in Swiss cheese was observed to retard mold; therefore, it was added to bread to inhibit mold growth.

Currently, additives are as safe as science can make them. "Absolute safety" cannot be guaranteed for anything in life. They are designed not to be toxic, and most of them would have to be ingested in very large amounts to produce acute symptoms. Some people experience allergic reactions to food additives, just as allergies to natural foods can occur.

A few of the preservatives generally recognized as safe have been of concern. Meats processed using sodium nitrite/nitrate have been linked with an increased risk of colorectal cancer in studies when large amounts are eaten. Sodium benzoate is safe for most people, but sodium benzoate and some artificial food colorings may exacerbate hyperactivity in young children.

The use of food additives makes many foods more readily available by preventing spoilage and keeping food wholesome and appealing. Complicated chemical names found on labels can be intimidating. Many food manufacturers are abandoning artificial preservatives and chemical additives due to consumer concerns and attitudes. Consumers are more concerned about chemicals in foods than about avoiding added sugar and sodium and about limiting saturated fat. Even names of vitamins on labels (e.g., thiamin mononitrate or cyanocobalamin) can cause apprehension for consumers unfamiliar with the terms. Food additives have the following benefits (Table 16.2):

1. They improve nutritional value. Enrichment and fortification have helped reduce malnutrition in the United States. Nutrients added help ensure adequate intake of vitamins or minerals. All added nutrients must be listed on product labels.
2. They maintain wholesomeness and palatability of foods. Bacterial contamination can cause foodborne illnesses. Preservatives retard spoilage caused by mold, air, bacteria, fungi, or yeast and preserve natural color and flavor. Antioxidants prevent oxidation of fats and oils, fruits, and vegetables.
3. They maintain product consistency. Emulsifiers enable particles to mix and prevent separation. Stabilizers and thickeners contribute to a smooth, uniform texture.
4. They provide leavening or control pH. Leavening agents, such as yeast and baking powder, are used to make foods light in texture and to cause baked goods to rise.
5. They enhance flavor and appearance. These substances are the most widely used and the most controversial additives. Included in this category are coloring agents, natural and synthetic flavors, spices, flavor enhancers, and sweeteners. Sugar, corn syrup, and salt are used in the largest amounts. Without these additives, foods are less appealing, a factor that influences selection and nutrient intake.

DENTAL CONSIDERATIONS

- Stress following the recommendations on how to retain nutrients during preparation that are listed in Box 16.2.
- Clarify any misinformation about use of organic foods, but respect patients' beliefs and assist them in obtaining economical products that are acceptable to them.

NUTRITIONAL DIRECTIONS

- Products stored at room temperature should be kept in cool, dry areas in airtight containers.
- Regular ground beef is more economical than ground round, and total fat content can be significantly reduced by using a low-fat cooking method and rinsing crumbled ground beef after cooking.
- Organic foods cost more but are not more nutritious or significantly different in taste. Fresh, locally grown produce is ideal.
- Organic produce may not look as attractive and unblemished as traditionally grown produce; organically processed foods have a shorter shelf life than products containing preservatives.
- The terms "natural" and "organic" were used interchangeably in the past to describe food that was minimally processed and free of artificial additives or preservatives; however, consumers should be aware that only products with an organic label have met USDA standards. Legally, use of terms such as "natural" or "all-natural" can mean anything the manufacturer wants them to mean.
- Food additives are tested before they can be used. They are considered safe, but should be consumed in moderation. Cumulative amounts of additives such as added sweeteners or sodium (from many different sources) may be undesirable. Choosing fresh foods is usually the ideal situation; these foods usually have fewer additives.
- Populations consuming large amounts of fruits and vegetables, even with the use of fertilizers and pesticides, have a lower rate of cancer.
- Eat a wide variety of fruits and vegetables to limit exposure to any one type of pesticide residue.
- Purchase only fruits and vegetables subject to USDA regulations. Imported produce is not grown under the same regulations as those enforced by the USDA.
- Buying organic foods should be a personal choice, based on availability, price, appearance, and taste, as well as personal values of the consumer. The most important factor is eating a wide variety of fruits and vegetables.

Food Fads and Misinformation

Nutrition is a very popular subject, but even with all the current knowledge, it is no easier to understand today than it was in 1938:

> *More food notions flourish in the United States than in any other civilized country on earth, and most of them are wrong. They thrive in the minds of the same people who talk about their operations; and like all mythology, they are a blend of fear, coincidence, and advertising.*[37]

As consumers' interest in nutrition increases, myths surrounding the subject continue to confuse. Purveyors of nutritional misinformation capitalize on fears and hopes by exaggerating and oversimplifying health virtues or curative properties of foods. Too few consumers understand the effects of various nutrients on the body and how nutrients are used, opening the door to food faddism or nutrition quackery.

Food fad is a catchall term covering all aspects of nutritional nonsense, characterized by exaggerated beliefs about the value of nutrition in health and disease. A food fad may be based on a fact

TABLE 16.2 **Guide to Food Additives**

Type or Function	Commonly Used Additives	Food Usage
Vitamins and minerals improve nutritive value of foods.	Vitamin D; potassium iodide (iodine); thiamin mononitrate (vitamin B_1), riboflavin (vitamin B_2), niacin (vitamin B_3), folate and ferrous sulfate (iron); ascorbic acid/sodium ascorbate (vitamin C)	Milk, margarine; iodized salt; enriched or fortified breakfast cereals, macaroni, pastas, breads, flour; fruit juices and fruit drinks, cured meats, cereals
Preservatives maintain wholesomeness and palatability of foods.	Butylated hydroxyanisole (BHA); tocopherols (vitamin E)	Cereals, chewing gum, potato chips, vegetable oils
Antioxidants prevent unsaturated fats and oils, flavorings, and colorings from oxidation, which would result in rancidity, flavor changes, and loss of color.	Citric acid, ascorbic acid (vitamin C), propyl gallate, erythorbic acid	Instant potatoes, fruit drinks, sherbet, cured meats, vegetable oils, meat products
Other preservatives control growth of mold, bacteria, and yeast.	Sodium benzoate, calcium (or sodium) propionate and potassium sorbate, sulfites, sodium nitrite/nitrate, sorbic acid	Pickles, preserves, fruit juice; breads, rolls, pies, cakes; dried fruit, frozen potatoes, wines; bacon, ham, frankfurters, luncheon meats, smoked fish, cheese
Processing aids product consistency and texture; emulsifiers keep oil and water mixed together with uniform dispersion of tiny particles.	Monoglycerides and diglycerides, lecithin, polysorbate 60	Baked goods, margarine, candy, peanut butter; frozen desserts, imitation dairy products
Stabilizers (other processing aids) help maintain smooth texture and uniform color and flavor.	Alginate and propylene glycol alginate; carrageenan	Ice cream, cheese, yogurt; jelly, chocolate milk, artificial breast milk
Thickeners (more processing aids) provide desired thickness or gel.	Various gums (Arabic, guar, xanthan), casein/sodium caseinate, pectin, gelatin, starch/modified starch	Beverages, salad dressing, cottage cheese, frozen pudding; ice cream, sherbet, coffee creamers; jelly; powdered dessert mixes, yogurt, cheese spreads; soup, gravy, baby food
Acids and bases control the pH of many foods and may act as buffers or neutralizing agents or as leavening agents.	Citric acid and sodium citrate, fumaric acid, lactic acid, phosphoric acid, sodium bicarbonate	Frozen desserts, fruit drinks, carbonated beverages, candy; pudding, pie fillings, gelatin desserts; olives, cheese, powdered foods and drinks, instant potatoes, cured meats; breads, pastries, baked goods
Colorings, cosmetic additives in natural and synthetic forms, enhance the appearance of foods.	Beta carotene, caramel color, artificial colors, ferrous gluconate	Margarine, shortening, nondairy whiteners; carbonated beverages, candy; baked goods, cherries in fruit cocktail, gelatin desserts; sausage, black olives
Flavoring agents, cosmetic additives available in natural and synthetic forms, enhance flavors.	Artificial and natural flavoring, hydrolyzed vegetable protein (HVP), vanillin (substitute for vanilla), monosodium glutamate (MSG), quinine, salt (sodium chloride)	Carbonated beverages, candy, breakfast cereals, gelatin desserts; instant soups, frankfurters, sauce mixes, beef stew; ice cream, baked goods, chocolate; tonic water, bitter lemon; soup, potato chips, crackers
Sweeteners are cosmetic additives used to increase sweetness.	Dextrose (corn syrup, glucose), high-fructose corn syrup, invert sugar, sugar (sucrose), lactose	Candy, toppings, syrups, snack foods, imitation dairy foods; soft drinks, processed sweetened foods; whipped topping mix, breakfast pastry
Alternative sweeteners are cosmetic additives replacing sugar in products to reduce calories or to reduce risk of dental decay.	Acesulfame-K, aspartame, mannitol, saccharin, sorbitol, sucralose	Baked goods, chewing gum, gelatin desserts, soft drinks, drink mixes, frozen desserts, chewing gum, low-calorie foods; "diet" products; candy, shredded coconut
Other additives needed for processed foods to be prepared, stored, and shipped include anticaking agents; humectants; curing agents; sequestrants; and firming, bleaching, and maturing agents.	Calcium (or sodium) stearyl lactylate, ethylenediamine tetraacetic acid (EDTA), glycerin	Bread dough, cake fillings, processed egg whites; salad dressing, margarine, processed fruits and vegetables, canned shellfish; marshmallows, candy, fudge, baked goods

or fallacy. People often begin a diet or believe claims for specific foods or supplements on the basis of something they read or hear without investigating its validity or effectiveness. Some fad diets are nutritionally inadequate and can lead to serious deficiencies. A fad is sometimes harmful because a specific therapy is substituted for advice of a health care provider and consumers delay medical treatment.

Fad diets are prevalent in the United States as Americans continue to search for a magic formula to lose weight and defy the aging process. According to promoters of weight loss diets, specific foods or food combinations facilitate weight loss, implying that a specific food or combination of foods oxidizes body fat, increases metabolic rate, or inhibits voluntary food intake. These diets are frequently deficient in essential nutrients and can be dangerous. Other benefits, such as rapid weight loss, may not be long-lasting (see the Evolve website for information to evaluate popular diets).

Fad diets may promise to melt away fat with an immediate weight loss of several pounds, without exercise or limiting food intake. Miraculous promises are a good reason to run the other way. Diets that provide adequate nutrients and changes in lifestyle behaviors are desirable and more effective. Fads, whether for weight loss or other purposes, can be recognized instantly when they promise secret formulas to "cure all."

Food quackery is the promotion of nutrition-related products or services having questionable safety and/or effectiveness for claims made. These claims or promises may be due to ignorance, delusion, misconception, or deliberate deception. The question of why people turn to quackery instead of to legitimate health professionals cannot be understood in isolation. In some way the rational scientific approach fails to fulfill the desperate needs of suffering people; it is to these needs that quacks and cultists address themselves.[38] Americans spend more than $10 billion annually for cures that scientists deem to be quackery.

The unknowns of medicine and disagreement among reputable scientists regarding interpretation of research findings foster nutritional misinformation. Given the right circumstances, such as confronting a chronic or incurable disease, everyone is potentially capable of exchanging sound judgment and common sense for the promise of a miraculous cure.

Numerous unproven theories abound regarding food allergies and intolerances, ranging from illegitimate diagnostic testing to treatment with diets and supplements not proven effective in scientific studies.

Unconventional procedures for nutritional assessment are numerous. Hair analysis is used to recommend vitamin and mineral supplements. Hair analysis can indicate exposure to toxic heavy metals, but vitamins are not present in hair except in roots below the skin. Hair grows very slowly and does not reflect current body status. Hair mineral content can be affected by shampoos, bleach, dye, and many other factors, including environmental and geographical factors. Be cautious of recommendations for vitamin or mineral doses more than the RDAs or over the tolerable upper intake levels for the nutrient. Only certain conditions require doses beyond the RDAs, and a legitimate medical source should monitor the effects (see Chapter 11, *Health Application 11*).

Many theories have been proposed to delay the aging process and chronic diseases such as cancer, rheumatoid arthritis, multiple sclerosis, and migraine headaches. Nutritional manipulations are implemented based on theories to extend a person's life. To date, no proven methods exist to extend the lifespan.

Other than lead or arsenic toxicities, medical research has no proof of toxic levels from food; thus, little to no scientific support is available for detoxification methods. The American Academy of Nutrition and Dietetics defines **detoxification** as biochemical processes that transform non–water-soluble toxins and metabolites into water-soluble compounds excreted in urine, sweat, bile, or stool.[39] Doctors generally define toxins as something that enters the body having a damaging effect, such as lead or antifreeze, or in large quantities, such as alcohol or medication.

Alternative complementary medicine has been a promoter of detoxification. The media and popular culture advocate detoxification through diet, herbal supplements, fasts, juicing, cleanses, chelation therapy, purging products, and removal of mercury fillings. Many chemicals—especially heavy metals from food, water, and the environment —can be deposited in fat cells. The human body is an amazing machine, cleansing itself from the inside out; cells die and are removed naturally. Detoxification is what the body does naturally to neutralize, transform, or remove unwanted materials or toxins; the intestinal wall and liver are constantly neutralizing potentially toxic substances for elimination via the kidneys, colon, gallbladder, lungs, and skin. If one of these systems is not functioning properly or if the systems are overloaded with excess toxins, a state of toxicity could occur. Each chemical has a different level of toxicity.

During any of the detoxification diets, individuals may experience side effects of fatigue, malaise, aches and pains, emotional duress, headaches, and allergies. Despite the fact that detoxification diets are popular, they have not been proven to fulfill their claims. Research available on detoxification is largely testimonial—individual personal accounts of healing without controlled scientific experiments. Detoxification diets may be detrimental to people with diabetes; research has not shown that they improve blood pressure or cholesterol.

Detoxification diets may be high in fiber; vegetarian; low in fat, processed foods, alcohol, and caffeine; and utilize supplements with numerous vitamins, minerals, and antioxidants. A detoxification diet based on whole foods with fruits and vegetables, adequate fiber, and water may accelerate the body's detoxification pathways. Phytochemicals from numerous foods promote detoxification enzymes: cruciferous vegetables (broccoli, cabbage, Brussels sprouts, collard greens, kale, turnips, rutabaga, wasabi, etc), celery, herbs (cilantro, rosemary, turmeric, milk thistle, and curry), dark-green leafy vegetables, green and herbal teas, fibrous foods, probiotics, eggs, garlic, and onion. This diet can be well balanced and consistent with the *Dietary Guidelines*. The recommendation for using foods for detoxification is not endorsed by most science-based health care providers; claims are based on preliminary and questionable studies.

Juicing is the extraction of juice from fresh fruits or vegetables. This juice contains most of the vitamins, minerals, and phytonutrients found in the whole fruit; however, whole fruits and vegetables contain fiber lost in juicing. Whether juicing actually reduces risk of cancer, boosts the immune system, helps remove toxins, aids digestion, and helps with weight loss is unproven. Freshly squeezed juice can develop harmful bacteria unless consumed soon, and juices contain significant amounts of sugar that can lead to weight gain.

Herbal laxatives and high-fiber products, such as psyllium seeds, may be used to cleanse the digestive tract and promote elimination. The use of **colonics** to cleanse the lower intestines is based on the assumption that years of bad diet causes the colon to become caked with layers of accumulated toxins. This is a false assumption because colon examinations routinely performed on millions of people have not observed this even in people who routinely make poor food choices.

Chelation therapy uses specific chemicals to bind and eliminate heavy metals from the body. It has been proposed to rejuvenate the cardiovascular system, treat cancer and immune disorders, and retard aging. This treatment has caused kidney damage and may result in people not seeking competent medical treatment. Sweating therapies help release toxins stored in subcutaneous fat cells. In addition to saunas, therapeutic baths, and exercise, massage therapy and acupressure may be used.

The removal of mercury fillings is based on the concept that mercury in amalgam causes numerous health problems; thus, fillings are removed to prevent or treat disease. Although it is indisputable that mercury can be toxic, scientific evaluation generally indicates mercury levels in people with fillings are significantly below levels that cause toxic symptoms.

Because governmental organizations do not monitor the production and marketing of herbal supplements, numerous concerns are associated with their use. Herbal medicine should not be regarded as quackery but should be approached with caution. Herbs, including herbal teas and other plant-based formulations, are marketed as being the only natural method to prevent and cure numerous conditions. Herbal products available may be contaminated or contain alternative plant products not listed on the label. Deaths and severe health problems—including CVD, cirrhosis, and renal failure—have occurred from use of some herbal preparations in the United States.

Identifying Sources of Nutrition Misinformation

With the prolific amount of information broadcast in the news, it has become increasingly difficult to distinguish valid nutritional information on which to base one's decisions. Even within the medical and nutrition professions, recommendations have occasionally done an about face, causing confusion for consumers. Medical scientists and academics must publish their research to advance; medical organizations must release health recommendations to remain relevant.

News organizations feel they must report on new research and recommendations as they are released. The news media often have a poor understanding of research methods and statistics, seldom reporting the extent and limitations of information or important nuances of a research study. Frequently, reporters are anxious to publish before the competition and may jump the gun to get to press without fully checking out the story. They generally report medical findings as "facts." Many consumers become confused by listening to journalists presenting research studies that provide conflicting information. In the past, studies were read by other scientists, mulled over to assimilate with other known information, and only the most useful information was released to consumers.

Four valuable guidelines, published in the *New England Journal of Medicine* in 1994 to help prevent misinterpretation of scientific studies, remain valid[40]: (a) an association between two events is not the same as a cause and effect, (b) demonstrating one link in a postulated chain of events does not mean that the whole chain has been proven, (c) probabilities are not the same as certainties, and (d) the way that a scientific result is framed can greatly affect its impact. A single study seldom constitutes strong evidence of anything and is rarely a clinical game changer.

Sometimes it is hard to separate what is truly a medical certainty from what is merely solid scientific conjecture.[41] Current *Dietary Guidelines* have modified recommendations for fat, cholesterol, and added sugars. Why so much confusion among scientists and physicians? Recommendations are needed; sometimes a theory works for one group, so it is anticipated that it will work for other groups. Sometimes recommendations fail because high-quality research behind them is lacking. Observational trials or epidemiologic studies are not proof that a recommendation works for all. Sometimes, the downsides of recommendations are not considered until after the fallout. For instance, the recommendation to follow a low-fat diet resulted in more carbohydrate consumption, which may have led to increased obesity and triglyceride levels.

Very likely, some of the things in this text you have been taught may be contradictory to what you thought or were previously taught. Just remember, nutrition should be based on science, not opinions. Nutrition is a relatively young science (the word *vitamine* was first used in 1911). Nutrition is not a science of breakthroughs; it is evolution, not revolution. Confusion comes from constant evolving as new evidence adds to the existing body of research. In essence, the medical field agrees on and recommends the "boring and bland" facts that consumers need to implement basic simple lifestyle changes (exercise, do not smoke, do not drink too much, and so on) and to choose healthful foods in moderation—facts that they already know but continue searching for an instantaneous miracle easy solution.

The factors just mentioned cause confusion even within the health care field. Therefore, it is easy to understand how unscrupulous health promoters can get away with lies and fake products. Strict laws protect against false advertising and mislabeling.

The First Amendment to the United States Constitution protects free speech and free press; it also protects a person's right to dispense false, misleading, or deceptive health claims. If the label on a food product makes false or misleading claims, however, the FDA can take action because of mislabeling. Health-related claims are permitted on food labels if (a) it is well documented that a particular nutrient can reduce risk and (b) the benefits of this nutrient are not offset by another ingredient present. (For instance, a high-fiber cereal high in fat could not be touted as being healthful because of its fat content.) The Federal Trade Commission can take action if false claims are made in advertising; thus, claims made on labels or in promotions are not usually false. However, products can be legally promoted in the media and on the Internet because of protection under the First Amendment. Under the Food, Drug, and Cosmetic Act, a product is a drug if medical claims are made or if it affects body functions. All medical manufacturers who market products interstate must register and list the products with the FDA. The FDA prohibits introduction of any food, drug, device, or cosmetic not labeled correctly. Even though the FDA must approve products before they are marketed, the term *FDA* is not permitted in any claim suggesting approval. Consumers can request the firm's FDA registration letter, product's listing letter, or FDA marketing approval letter. The government actively pursues health swindlers, but enforcement agencies lack adequate staff and resources needed to handle all the problems reported.

Consumer interest in health and nutrition information is high as consumers are taking more responsibility for their own health care. The American culture is bombarded with nutrition information—television and radio talk shows, commercials, infomercials, magazines, newspapers, books, the Internet, family and friends, and health care providers. People are frequently influenced by testimonials. Celebrities, sports figures, fitness experts, and others without nutrition expertise frequently are featured in advertisements touting a nutritional product.

The Internet is an unregulated source of nutrition information, reaching millions of people with sales of fraudulent and illegal nutritional and medical products. The emergence of blogs and tweets on the Internet are other sources of information that need to be questioned for credibility. Information may be presented as fact, but the validity of information on websites, especially those with products to sell, should be verified before making a purchase. Therefore, the information is to be questioned regarding its scientific basis. Blogs and YouTube videos may contain personal testimonials from real people, but the conclusions drawn may not be related to any purported cause; that is, what works for one person may not work on anyone else.

A popular tactic is to discredit the interpretation of scientific research by the medical community and governmental agencies. Inaccurate information is based on misunderstanding and misrepresentation. Evaluating nutritional information for its legitimacy and validity can be tedious. Health care professionals, regardless of where the nutrition information is presented—on the Internet, on television, on podcasts, in print, or any other media—should evaluate the findings in light of well-established nutrition principles.

The best way to begin a search on the Internet is to go to credible websites of trusted health organizations with names you recognize, universities, and state and national government agencies and offices, and click on links provided on these websites. Reliable nutrition websites are given throughout this text and on the Evolve website. The Food and Nutrition Science Alliance is a partnership of several professional nutrition science associations, including the Academy of Nutrition and Dietetics, American College of Nutrition, American Society for Nutrition, and the Institute of Food Technologists who have combined their efforts to help debunk the junk advice. The information provided in Box 16.6 is helpful for evaluating oral or written claims.

Dental professionals and consumers can begin by checking credentials of the person making a questionable claim. Most articles appearing in established medical and scientific journals were submitted to a board of peer scientists for evaluation before publication. If peer reviewers consider conclusions to be well supported by the research, it is published for others to read. A single study never proves a theory; it may provide conclusive information but provoke more questions for further studies. A single study usually serves as another piece of the puzzle if it can be replicated.

When evaluating individual studies, consideration must be given to the number of participants and length of the study and other pertinent information, as described in Box 16.6. For instance, the Nurses' Health Study that began in 1976 has involved almost 122,000 women ages 30 to 55 years and is still ongoing. This study, funded by the National Institutes of Health to investigate potential long-term consequences of oral contraceptives, has limitations in its credibility because professionally trained health care workers may have different values and practices than a cross-cultural sample of women.

Many types of studies—epidemiologic, case control, placebo controlled, randomized, crossover design, double blind, clinical trials, or interventions—together help provide conclusive information. The gold standard for research studies is "**evidence-based**," a term used for medical practices that have been thoroughly evaluated using scientific methods. Interventions used in studies are evaluated based on risks and benefits revealed during clinical trials that are randomized and placebo controlled. Experts review data from numerous studies to determine whether treatment can be recognized as safe or effective. The Cochrane Collaboration is dedicated to creating systematic reviews of peer-reviewed studies. The Academy of Nutrition and Dietetics also maintains an evidenced-based library of nutrition-related studies.

Meta-analysis combines all relevant studies from independent sources using a statistical technique, most often used to assess clinical effectiveness of health care interventions. **Systematic reviews** also provide reliable information based on all relevant published and unpublished evidence, selecting studies for inclusion, assessing the quality of each study, then compiling the findings and interpreting them to present a balanced and impartial summary while defining limitations of the evidence. Meta-analysis studies and systematic reviews have been given a lot of prestige because they were considered a concise synopsis of multiple studies with reliable conclusions. However, they are currently being produced in massive amounts as a result of software that streamlines the process and may be biased with vested interests funding them. Instead of promoting evidence-based medicine and health care findings, they may be redundant and misleading, with methodological flaws.[42]

Observational studies are epidemiologic research studies with no type of intervention or experiment. These may be used to discover possible relationships between lifestyle and diseases. For instance, "people who love ice cream are obese" may survey thousands of participants, but does not clearly determine a cause.

DENTAL CONSIDERATIONS

- Assess patients' use of food fads, economic level, educational level, and the nutrient adequacy of any fad diet undertaken.
- If a patient restricts food choices because of a food fad or belief, ensuring nutrient adequacy is more difficult. A thorough assessment and evaluation by the dental hygienist may indicate risk for a nutritional insufficiency or deficiency. Referral to a registered dietitian nutritionist (RDN) may be needed.
- Encourage patients to choose a variety of foods to ensure a balanced intake and decrease amounts consumed of any particular food to minimize risk of excessive contaminants from any one source. For instance, consumption of fish is encouraged because of beneficial substances to prevent CVD. However, fish, especially large fish such as swordfish, shark, mackerel, tilefish, and tuna, contain methylmercury so that eating too much fish has the potential to cause neurologic problems.
- Provide patients with positive advice based on a broad knowledge base and understanding of nutritional concepts and current research findings.
- Answer any questions about therapies, products, or treatments that a patient may be contemplating or refer the patient to a reliable source.
- Speak out to protect the public from misinformation.
- Do not offer remedies unless they have been proven to be safe and effective.
- If a patient is using or contemplating using a food fad or diet you are unfamiliar with, do not hesitate to consult an RDN, home economist, or nutrition professor.

NUTRITIONAL DIRECTIONS

- Although some fads are physically harmless, they may create an economic hardship for individuals with limited income because the foods or supplements may be expensive.
- Results of fad diets can be devastating and have even led to death.
- The mainline medical community is divided on whether detoxification has any benefits.

• BOX 16.6 Debunk the Junk

The following are 10 red flags to help separate plausible but incorrect nutrition advice from the good stuff.

1. *Recommendations that promise a quick fix.* Ignore any product (sometimes foods, sometimes supplements or pills) that promises fast results. Scientific studies about the effectiveness of the product are usually conducted by the manufacturer; thus, the data is biased. Scientific literature does not use terms such as "amazing," "exclusive," "cure," or "long life." Quick-fix product claims are also peppered with medical jargon to further mislead the consumer. Serious medical problems cannot be cured with remedies marketed mail order, door to door, or on the Internet. In short, do not allow these companies to manipulate you.
2. *Dire warnings of danger from a single product or regimen.* One particular thing is not responsible for being overweight or unhealthy (fat makes you fat, carbohydrates are toxic, sugar is white death). Typically, it is a combination of factors and/or lack of exercise. Sometimes people swing from an all to nothing approach, swinging from paleo to vegan. Too much of any one thing in the diet is unhealthy, but it will not be the sole reason for weight gain.
3. *Claims that sound too good to be true.* Many consumers like it when the advice is consistent with what they want to do. Scrutinize the science behind the recommendation to determine whether the recommendation is worth following or just wishful thinking. Study the label on the product. (a) The instructions on the label should clarify the product's benefits. (b) Advertisements or promotional material should agree with the product label. Unsubstantiated false claims are usually found in books, television, brochures, infomercials, and promotional materials. Beware of "cures" for serious diseases and of products that claim to cure multiple health problems. Symptoms of many illnesses are similar, and a misdiagnosis can be hazardous if the condition is not being treated appropriately. A proper diagnosis requires an assessment, including a physical examination, by a health professional. Delaying treatment may allow progression of the disease beyond help.
4. *Simplistic conclusions drawn from a complex study.* Many consumers want a study to conclude with black-and-white answers but most science is very complicated, requiring analytical thinking and digging to understand it. A study will take into account previous research on the subject. Good scientific studies have limitations that scientists acknowledge, inviting further research to cover these areas. Anything that seems like it has the be-all-end-all simple answer probably is not trustworthy or may be flat out wrong in its conclusion.
5. *Recommendations based on a single study.* Be wary of any recommendations from a single study, especially if the conclusion is contrary to everything else that has been published. Be a skeptic; do not ignore studies that go against prevailing wisdom. Compare findings with all the published literature on the subject, not just the most recent.
6. *Statements refuted by reputable scientific organizations.* For a nutrition statement that seems too good to be true, too simplistic, or claims to be a quick fix, definitely verify what reputable scientific organizations have to say. If it sounds too good to be true, it probably is. A list of quality government agencies and nutrition organizations are listed along with their websites throughout this text and on the Evolve website.
7. *Lists of "good" and "bad" foods.* Lists are problematic because foods are not all good or all bad. Balance, variety, and moderation are all necessary. An occasional candy bar can be okay, and not every vegetable consumed has to be chock full of antioxidants and vitamins. The key, though, is restraint, moderation, and balance. Indulge on occasion, but ensure that you eat healthful well-balanced meals regularly. Attempting to use balance and moderation can be hard on consumers who are simultaneously barraged by food commercials and obesity issues. Specific direction is easy and mindless for some consumers; hence the appeal of the paleo diet or one with a set of rules. There are foods to avoid or eat in moderation, but no one food in reasonable amounts is going to be toxic.
8. *Recommendations made to help sell a product.* If the health article conveniently ends with a sales pitch for a supplement or if all the studies referenced at the end are by the author, the quackery alarm should sound. Due to government funding cuts for nutrition research, more studies funded by groups having a stake in the outcome are to be expected. This does not mean recommendations or studies are wrong, but be cautious and ensure that findings are not inconsistent with other studies. Investigate information based on testimonials or case histories or promoted by movie stars, sports figures, or any "big name" person. This is not scientific evidence. The FDA cannot regulate a testimonial about a product.
9. *Recommendations based on studies not peer reviewed.* Research published in a peer-reviewed journal mean that a group of outside reviewers have deemed the research well conducted, the results credible, and the findings significant. Peer review is necessary in science for reliability and accuracy.
10. *Recommendations from studies that ignore differences among individuals or groups.* Nutrition is not a "one size fits all" science. A study making blanket statements is likely not reliable. The results of a study on bone health conducted using teen-age athletes would not be applicable to older women experiencing osteoporosis.

Adapted from Food and Nutrition Science Alliance Gives 10 Bits of Advice on Junk Science. August 17, 2014. http://www.redorbit.com/news/health/1113214063/debunk-the-junk-science-in-nutrition-081714/. Accessed April 4, 2017; and Flaherty J. Debunk the Junk. TuftsNow. August 13, 2014. http://now.tufts.edu/articles/debunk-junk. Accessed August 6, 2017/

Referrals for Nutritional Resources

Frequently, patients need special assistance for nutritional and financial problems. At some point during 2015, approximately 25% of Americans participated in at least one of the USDA's 15 domestic food and nutrition assistance programs.[43] The number of people facing hunger in the U.S. declined 2.4% in 2016 to the lowest since 2007 as the unemployment rate fell.[44] A variety of governmental programs available may help financially, assist with food budgeting, teach basic nutrition and meal planning, or help clarify nutrition misconceptions. Local chapters of many health-related organizations, searchable on the Internet, furnish free or inexpensive literature, audiovisual material, and health-oriented programs on various topics. Dental hygienists can identify patients or families with nutritional needs, provide appropriate referrals, and help them participate in applicable programs (Table 16.3). RDNs and many nutritionists are trained to assist with nutritional or dietary problems.

One of the best sources is the city or county health department. State and local health departments usually have various programs to provide nutrition services, such as well-baby clinics and family health centers. Health departments and county hospitals are excellent resources for information about various programs available. The federal government administers several nutrition programs through the USDA and the U.S. Department of Health and Human Services. The Area Information Center (2-1-1) maintains comprehensive databases of resources, including federal, state, and local government agencies, and community-based and private nonprofit organizations.

TABLE 16.3 Referral Chart for Community Nutrition Resources

Population Group	Risk Factor	Referral Source[a]	Contact[b]
Pregnant and lactating women	Low income	Supplemental Nutrition Assistance Program (SNAP)	State food stamp hotline number available at https://www.fns.usda.gov/snap/state-informationhotline-numbers
	Anemia, inadequate weight gain, age-related risk factor, inadequate health care, or lack of food and nutrition information	Women, Infants and Children Program (WIC) Maternity and Infant Care Project Expanded Food and Nutrition Education Program (EFNEP)	City, county, or state health department State health department Land-grant universities Prenatal clinic or private health care team
Infants	Low-birth-weight, failure to thrive, or poor growth patterns	Prenatal education	City, county, or state health department
	Inadequate health care	WIC Program	State health department
Children	Poor growth patterns or overweight, inadequate diet, or anemia	WIC Program (up to 5 years old)	City, county, or state health department
	Low income	Children and Youth Project (up to 18 years old) Head Start (preschool) School lunch School breakfast	State health department Local community action project Board of education Local school district
Older adult	Low income	Supplemental Nutrition Assistance Program (SNAP)	State food stamp hotline number available at https://www.fns.usda.gov/snap/state-informationhotline-numbers
		Congregate meal sites	State and local agencies on aging
	Homebound	Meals on Wheels	Locations available at http://www.mealsonwheelsamerica.org/
General adult	Obesity	Weight Watchers International, Thin Within, Dieters Workshop, TOPS, and other weight reduction groups	Local chapters
	Hyperlipidemia, cardiovascular disease, or hypertension	American Heart Association	Local chapter
	Diabetes	American Diabetes Association	Local chapter
	Low income	SNAP	State food stamp hotline number available at https://www.fns.usda.gov/snap/state-informationhotline-numbers
	Reliable food and nutrition information	EFNEP	Land-grant universities
	General consumer information for all populations	Community nutrition groups and community cooperatives Academy of Nutrition and Dietetics (AND) Center for Science in the Public Interest U.S. Department of Health and Human Services Healthfinder WebMD	Local groups Available at www.eatright.org Available at http://www.cspinet.org Available at https://www.hhs.gov Available at https://healthfinder.gov Available at http://www.webmd.com

[a]This is only a partial listing. Programs may vary in different parts of the United States.
[b]Call 2-1-1 for free access to health and human services information and referrals in local communities.

Information and Referral Services is a national dialing code to link people in need of assistance with appropriate providers of services in their community.

The Supplemental Nutrition Assistance Program (SNAP; formerly the Food Stamp Program) is the cornerstone for nutrition safety in the United States. This federal assistance program is available to individuals with incomes up to 130% of the federal poverty level. The program, designed to help low-income households purchase nutritious food, is based on family income and household size. Local offices that administer the program are widely distributed throughout the United States. The program was initially designed to boost food consumption and energy intake. SNAP participants express frustration about the process of applying for and maintaining benefits related to communication problems and poor integration of services.[45]

In times of a declining and weak economy and high rates of unemployment or underemployment in the American workforce, increasing numbers of people need to rely on federal programs. The number of people on SNAP more than doubled between 2004 and 2013 (47 million persons or 23 million households) but dropped to 44 million persons/21 million households in 2016.[46] This decrease is partially related to the unemployment rate; additionally, more than one million people lost SNAP benefits in 2016 due to implementation of a three-month limit (in 21 states) on benefits for unemployed adults between the ages of 18 and 49 years who are not disabled or raising minor children. Currently, approximately 1 in 7 Americans receives SNAP benefits. According to the USDA, about 4.7 million SNAP recipients are deemed able-bodied adults without dependents, with only one in four having income from a job.[47] SNAP program benefits are critically important to help feed families in need. From October 2016 through September 2017, the maximum monthly allotment for a family of 4 with a net income of less than $2,025 was $632 per person and $347 for a family of 2.[46] Without good money management skills, the monthly food allowance runs out before the end of the month. The program is meant to supplement a household's food budget; it is not intended to be the total food budget. The SNAP benefit is a paltry amount for most Americans, but it can go far with careful planning and shopping. Eating healthy on the SNAP program is challenging but doable—a back-to-basics style of eating. Because most people who qualify for SNAP have less education, however, it is very difficult for them to keep healthful food on the table all month.

Because poor diets exert heavy costs in medical expenditures and lost productivity, measures for promoting healthful food choices could yield considerable benefits. State governments and health advocates recognize that additional modifications are needed to reinforce nutrition education, restrict foods allowed with food stamp benefits, and expand benefits to encourage purchases of more healthful foods, such as fruit and vegetables.

While the program is intended to improve the nutritional and health status of families needing help, consumers frequently do not use the funds to purchase foods wisely. Recipients can use the Electronic Benefit Card to buy any foods sold in participating grocery stores, with the exception of prepared hot foods. Billions of SNAP dollars purchase products inconsistent with the goal of helping improve health. A study conducted by Yale University's Rudd Center for Food Policy and Obesity estimated that, annually, at least $1.7 to $2.1 billion in SNAP benefits go toward sugar-sweetened beverages purchased in grocery stores.[48]

The Special Supplemental Food Program for Women, Infants, and Children (WIC) is designed to prevent nutritional problems in this high-risk, low-income group. The WIC program is available to pregnant and lactating women, infants, and children up to 5 years old who are considered to be at nutritional risk. Some of the criteria for nutritional risk are evidence of iron deficiency, inadequate weight gain during pregnancy, teenage pregnancy, failure to thrive, poor growth patterns, and inadequate dietary patterns. In addition to supplemental foods, nutrition education and referrals to health care sources are provided. Studies of the WIC program have shown positive effects on iron status, growth and development of infants and children, and breastfeeding rates. The program also saves millions of dollars by decreasing the rate of low-birth-weight infants; thus, funding has remained relatively stable.

In 2009, significant nutritionally beneficial changes were made in WIC food packages. The goals for changes were to better support breastfeeding and provide healthier foods more consistent with the *Dietary Guidelines*. Food packages for mothers and infants are financially equivalent in the costs of food provided, whether the mother is breastfeeding or not. For instance, since formula feeding is more expensive, breastfeeding mothers are allowed more foods equivalent to the cost received by the formula-fed infant. The full formula package provides less food for the mother and all food benefits for the mother stop when the formula-fed infant is 6 months old. Fresh fruits and vegetables are permitted, and only low-fat or skim milk is allowed for mothers and children older than 2 years of age. Foods allowed must meet strict nutritional standards by providing a specific amount of fiber, vitamin C, or vitamin D. These changes have resulted in food purchases more consistent with the *Dietary Guidelines.*

School breakfast and lunch programs provide nutritious meals for children at school. Nutritional standards for school lunch require that lunch provide at least one-third, and breakfast at least one-fourth, of the RDAs for children. Free and reduced-price meals are provided based on household income and size. School meals can account for approximately one-half of a child's daily caloric intake, with school lunches contributing up to 31% of daily calories and school breakfasts contributing up to 22%.[49] When elementary school students participate in school lunch, overall diet quality is higher than for children obtaining lunch from home.[50]

New guidelines for overhauling the school food program were implemented in 2012. These requirements are more consistent with the daily food group recommendations of the *Dietary Guidelines*; the new meal patterns provide fruit, more vegetables (with specific subgroups required each week) and whole grains, and minimum and maximum daily calorie level averages over a week.[51,52] Because of difficulties in meeting the lower sodium requirement, these targets will be gradually decreased through 2022. The standards for age-grade groups include more food groups and limiting calories. Milk must be fat free (plain or flavored) or plain low fat (1% milk fat). More whole fruit is required at both meals. Dark-green vegetables, red/orange vegetables, beans/peas (legumes), and starchy vegetables (1/2 cup equivalent) must be offered at least weekly. Fruits and vegetables are not interchangeable. All grains must be whole grain. Many students claimed the school lunch that met the guidelines did not provide enough calories and protein. The amount of fruits and vegetables wasted has been of concern; innovative strategies to improve consumption of these foods served in school meals are needed.[53]

The Nutrition Program for the Elderly (Title III) provides group and home-delivered meals. The purpose of this program is to improve nutritional and health status of older adults and offer participants opportunities to form new friendships and create informal support networks. The Elderly Nutrition Program provides a range of services (including social services) through approximately 4000 nutrition service providers. Of the participants served, 73% are at high nutritional risk, 25% at moderate risk; 25% reported they did not always have enough money or food stamps to purchase food. More than 3 million elderly participants receive an estimated 40% to 50% of required nutrients from meals provided by this program.[54]

The Expanded Food and Nutrition Education Program is designed to help lower socioeconomic groups with all aspects of nutrition. Low-income adults have varied levels of knowledge regarding nutrition and a healthy diet, cooking skills, and health overall. Thus, they would benefit from a more accurate understanding of nutrition and healthful eating to improve overall diet quality. The Expanded Food and Nutrition Education Program is available through county extension services of land-grant universities and assists with meal planning, budgeting, cooking, and other food-related and nutrition-related problems. Nutrition aides are low-income homemakers who are trained to visit homes of low-income families to assist in providing well-balanced meals. This program appears to be well suited for working with low-income families.[55]

Head Start is a preschool educational program for low-income families. Children are furnished breakfast, lunch, and snacks, and nutrition education is available for parents.

Locally funded food agencies providing assistance through food banks and food pantries have increased substantially. Food pantries, which usually do not base eligibility for benefits on income status, currently serve millions of Americans. The USDA reports that in 2014, 23 million American households receiving SNAP benefits had visited a food pantry in the previous month.[56]

DENTAL CONSIDERATIONS

- Identify patients needing food assistance and refer them to appropriate sources.
- If calories, sodium, and fat should be restricted, discourage patronage of fast food establishments or suggest appropriate fast food selections (e.g., salads or baked chicken).
- Low-income households must allocate a higher proportion of both their income and time to planning, purchasing, and preparing food if they wish to consume nutritious meals.
- When recommending foods to patients, consider the income level. Suggesting steak or lobster as a protein source for low-income patients is inappropriate.
- In addition to government health agencies already mentioned, numerous health and professional organizations listed on the Evolve website provide health information. Other organizations, such as the Better Business Bureau, may also be helpful.

NUTRITIONAL DIRECTIONS

- Protein sources are generally the most expensive budget items; however, it is unnecessary to buy choice quality grades of meat for good nutrition. ("Select" and "standard" are more economical grades of meat.)
- Discuss guidelines for economical food purchases (see Box 16.1) to help low-income patients modify food purchases.
- Health care professionals, including dental hygienists, can encourage communities and food banks to focus on more nutritious food, such as fresh fruits and vegetables.

Role of Dental Hygienists

What role can the dental hygienist play in combating nutrition fads and misinformation? Natalie Van Cleve stated in 1938, when times were different but widespread misinformation on diet was just as prevalent as today:[57]

> *It is the duty of all professions active in the field of food and nutrition to cooperate in clarifying any misconceptions of the laity. If the [health care providers] do not know their vitamins, the patients will find a radio announcer who does.*

Health care providers, dental hygienists, and even RDNs have sometimes promoted nutritional misinformation by failing to apply their knowledge, misunderstanding how nutrients are used, or searching for fame and fortune. The dental professional is in a unique position to understand the causes of food fads and to recognize their dangers. First, understanding patients and their love of "miracle" answers should help in recognizing the appeal of such misinformation. Second, a scientific background permits assessment of potential effects or uselessness of food fads. Dental hygienists can help patients understand the true essence of nutritional science—the process of nourishing or being nourished—rather than allowing them to trust in the polypharmacy of supernutrition. Many legitimate resources include governmental and professional organizations; these are referenced on the Evolve website to help evaluate the legitimacy of nutritional claims. Many legitimate medical journals are also available on the Internet, as listed on the Evolve website.

The dental professional can help by referring patients to appropriate resources and agencies or to a social worker for assistance in filling out forms. These embarrassing issues should be discussed in a matter-of-fact manner. Patients may benefit by ventilating feelings and beliefs about food "handouts." Information should be presented in a positive manner, stating how it would benefit the patient and family. Most parents desire the best for their children; it is important to stress benefits children would receive (e.g., increased growth, learning, productivity) by participating. Help patients recognize that having inadequate funds for food is not a sign of failure and that asking for help shows strength, courage, and wisdom. In due time, they may be able to help someone else. Dental professionals can also help by serving at community food resource centers or food donation drives. Some centers offer dental care using volunteer dental hygienists and dentists.

HEALTH APPLICATION 16

Food Insecurity in the United States

Food security—that is, access to enough food for an active, healthy life by all family members at all times—is a universal dimension of household and personal well-being and considered a fundamental requirement for a healthy, well-nourished population. However, food insecurity and hunger continue to exist in the United States. **Hunger**, or an uneasy or painful sensation caused by lack of food, typically precedes food insecurity. **Food insecurity** refers to the lack of access to enough food to meet basic needs fully at some time during the year because of insufficient funds or resources for food. Food insecurity means having to decide which bills to pay—food, housing, heat, electricity, water, transportation, childcare, or health care. Food insecurity remains a public health concern in the United States, particularly among low-income, urban, ethnically diverse families. Food insecurity is usually recurrent or transient but not chronic, and may involve a low-quality diet that is monotonous and lacking in nutrients. Approximately 12.7% of U.S. households were food insecure sometime during 2015. Prevalence of food insecurity in America increased and remained high between 2007 and 2014 when it finally decreased, but continues at higher rates than prior to 2007 (Fig. 16.6).

In 2015, the typical food-secure household spent 27% more on food than the typical food-insecure household of the same size and household composition. About 59% of food-insecure households participated in one or more of the three largest federal food and nutrition assistance programs during the month prior to the 2015 survey. In 2015, approximately 0.7% of households (7 million) experienced **very low food security** (at times during the year, food intake of household members was reduced and normal eating patterns disrupted because of insufficient funds or other resources to obtain food; Fig. 16.7).[47] Hunger rates decrease as income increases, but food insecurity is not exclusive to very-low-income families.

Rates of food insecurity are substantially higher than the national average for households with children headed by a single woman and in

Continued

HEALTH APPLICATION 16

Food Insecurity in the United States—cont'd

households with children (Fig. 16.8). African American and Hispanic households had rates of food insecurity more than twice those of non-Hispanic white households. Nearly half of American children live in homes that at some point receive governmental nutrition programs.[47]

A work-limiting disability substantially increases the risk of food insecurity for low-income families. In addition to the disabled individual being unable to work and incurring burdensome medical costs and other expenses, an adult caretaker may be restricted in work opportunities and hours. The homeless population makes up a large percentage of the hungry. Millions of people in the United States maintain a home and may even work full-time but live below the poverty level. (In 2017, the federal poverty guideline was an annual income less than $24,600 for a family of 4 in the 48 contiguous states.)

Several factors may account for food insecurity—the state of the American economy; unemployment rate; and the changing composition of the U.S. population, particularly households headed by single women. People who are unemployed for a long period deplete their assets, exhaust unemployment insurance, and turn to SNAP for help. Households attempt to avoid hunger by using various strategies, such as eating less-varied diets, skipping meals, participating in federal food assistance programs (57%), and/or getting emergency food from community food pantries.

Food pantries are now used to regularly supplement monthly shortfalls in contrast to earlier usage of food pantries for temporary acute food needs. A problem with food pantries is nutrient quality of the food, providing more energy-dense foods. Fresh produce may only be available intermittently. Foods available at food pantries provide inadequate amounts of vitamins A, C, D, and some B vitamins, and the minerals calcium, iron, magnesium, and zinc.[58] These facilities would like to improve the quality of foods that they provide but are dependent on donations of food or money. Emergency food providers serve a diverse population with different reasons for needing assistance. These providers are especially helpful for people during a short-term setback, such as an unexpected emergency medical bill; others need emergency kitchens to receive a hot meal or supplement food stamps. Two groups of low-income Americans frequently face problems, requiring more reliance on food banks—seniors and people enrolled in the SNAP program. Food insecurity may cause a variety of negative health outcomes for everyone affected, but younger populations are most at risk. In most households, older family members protect children, especially younger ones, from substantial reductions in food intake and ensuing hunger. Effects on health and behavior have been observed, especially with persistent or chronic food shortages. Insufficient food intake affects mental and physical health, having both acute and chronic effects. Food-insecure children younger than 3 years old are nearly twice as likely to be in "fair or poor" health, and a larger percentage of children are more likely to require hospitalization than food-secure children. Ensuring food security may reduce health problems and hospitalizations in children. Growth stunting without muscle wasting is characteristic of homeless children who experience moderate chronic nutritional stress. Hungry children are more likely to experience undesired weight loss, fatigue, irritability, concentration problems, and dizziness, frequent headaches, ear infections, and colds.

Cognitive and academic performance are also detrimentally affected. Missing a meal, particularly breakfast, can reduce a child's ability to respond to the environment, negatively affecting learning. Apathy, disinterest, irritability, and a low tolerance for frustration are common behaviors in hungry children who are unable to concentrate in school and are less likely to reach their potential to become fully productive adults. Additionally, psychosocial problems are observed more often: difficulty getting along with peers, suspension from school, and adolescent suicide. Having a healthy, balanced diet improves brain capacity, minimizes cognitive capabilities, and improves academic performance.[59]

Paradoxically, low-income individuals, especially women, with food insecurity have disproportionately higher rates of obesity than those with food security. A consensus of research indicates that participation in the program does not increase likelihood of being overweight or obese for men or children, but hunger along with food insecurity is related to greater body mass indexes.

Low-income people are subject to the same influences and problems as other Americans (e.g., more sedentary lifestyles, increased portion sizes), but they also face unique challenges in adopting healthful behaviors. Individuals who skip meals or postpone mealtimes are more likely to consume more calories when food is available. When adequate food supplies are not always available, people find themselves in a cycle of overeating followed by hunger when money or food stamps run out. Mothers, usually the food managers in the household, may take several actions to protect their children from hunger, including skipping meals and eating cheaper, less nutritious foods. Persistent household food insecurity without hunger is related to child obesity, but maternal weight is also an influential factor.

Overconsumption is even easier with more readily available cheap, energy-dense foods. In low-income neighborhoods, full-service grocery stores and farmers' markets are lacking, healthy food is more expensive or may not be available, and fast food establishments are plentiful. Households with very low food security tend to shop more frequently in stores that have less-healthful options such as convenience/dollar stores.[60] Lower-income neighborhoods provide fewer opportunities for physical activity (fewer parks, bike paths, and recreational facilities, unsafe playground equipment, more problems with crime and traffic, and fewer organized sports programs).

Nutritionally, adults and children from food-insufficient households are more likely to consume substantially less than recommended dietary allowances (RDAs) for certain food groups and nutrients. Unfortunately, SNAP participants have lower-quality diets than income-eligible nonparticipants. The food group first eliminated from an impoverished person's diet is produce. Over the long-term, these deficits increase the risk of developing chronic diseases, such as CVD and diabetes; more frequent and severe disease complications; and increased demands and costs for health care services. Diet-related disease is disproportionately higher in low-income communities, where produce consumption is very low.

Food insecurity represents a major public health and public policy challenge by causing health problems, increased education costs, and less than optimal productivity. Yet this serious health problem is treatable with a simple inexpensive cure: providing food. Proper nutrition can decrease money spent on health problems. SNAP participants choose how to spend their benefits. However, many lack money management skills, creating problems at the end of the month when benefits are depleted. They have no knowledge of which foods are the healthiest to purchase with their limited allotment. A brief waiting-room intervention with SNAP participants at a health center resulted in a nearly fourfold increase in produce consumption. Providing information about healthy food choices is a low-cost, easily implemented attempt to improve the quality of their diet and help with weight management.[61] A recent study revealed that the monetary amount of SNAP benefits may be insufficient to support the healthy diet recommended by the *Dietary Guidelines and MyPlate*.[62] The Academy of Nutrition and Dietetics (AND) advocates "systematic and sustained interventions to achieve food and nutrition security for everyone in the U.S.," recommending adequate funding for and increased use of food and assistance programs and innovative programs to promote and support economic self-sufficiency.[63]

Use of dietary supplements containing the recommended amounts of vitamins and minerals has been proposed because the average cost of one tablet is less than a dime. However, dietary supplements do not provide energy, which is especially important for children and older adults.

The goal of *Healthy People 2020* is to increase quality and years of healthy life and to eliminate health disparities; this requires improved food and nutrition security. The objective to eliminate very low food security among children showed some improvement—decreasing from 2.3% in 2009 to 1.1% in 2014; the objective to reduce household food insecurity and in doing so reduce hunger showed a slight decrease—from 14.6% in 2008 to 14% in 2014.[64] U.S. federal assistance programs discussed earlier in this chapter are available to address hunger. Full use of these programs—with increased availability and benefits and increased awareness of programs—is a good place to start.

Prevalence of food insecurity and very low food security in 2015 is down from 2014

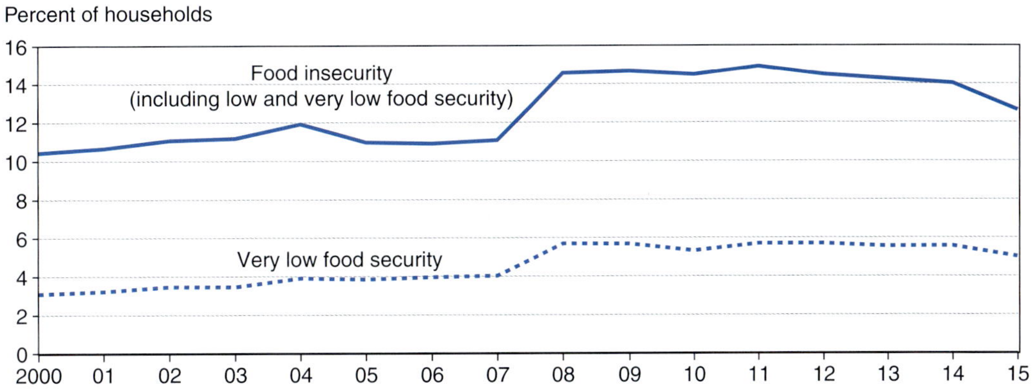

Source: USDA, Economic Research Service using data from U.S. Department of Commerce, U.S. Census Bureau, Current Population Survey Food Security Supplement.

• **Figure 16.6** Prevalence of food insecurity and very low food security in 2015 is down from 2014. (From Coleman-Jensen A, Rabbitt, Gregory CA, Singh A. Household food security in the United States in 2015. U.S. Department of Agriculture (USDA), Economic Research Service. Economic Research Report Number 215, September 2016. Source: U.S. Department of Agriculture, Economic Research Service using data from U.S. Department of Commerce, U.S. Census Bureau, Current Population Survey Food Security Supplement. https://www.ers.usda.gov/webdocs/publications/err215/err-215.pdf.)

U.S. households by food security status, 2015

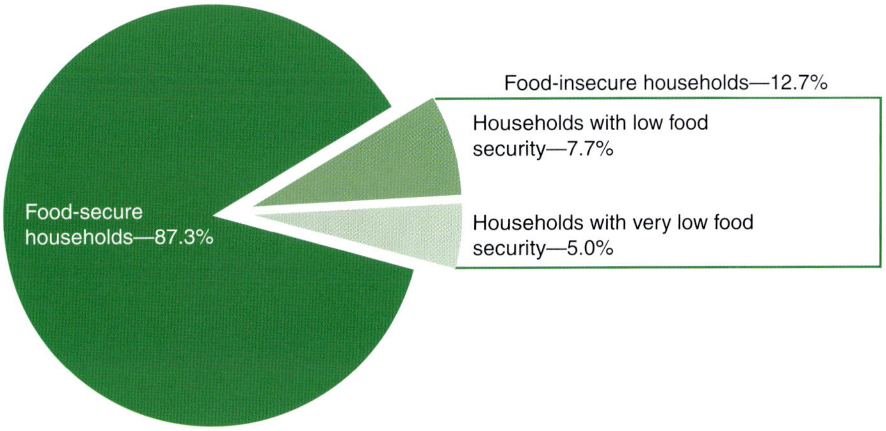

Source: USDA, Economic Research Service using data from U.S. Department of Commerce, U.S. Census Bureau, 2015 Current Population Survey Food Security Supplement.

• **Figure 16.7** U.S. households by food security status, 2015. (From Coleman-Jensen A, Rabbitt, Gregory CA, Singh A. Household food security in the United States in 2015. U.S. Department of Agriculture (USDA), Economic Research Service. Economic Research Report Number 215, September 2016. Source: USDA, Economic Research Service using data from U.S. Department of Commerce, U.S. Census Bureau, Current Population Survey Food Security Supplement. https://www.ers.usda.gov/webdocs/publications/err215/err-215.pdf.)

U.S. households with children by food security status of adults and children, 2015

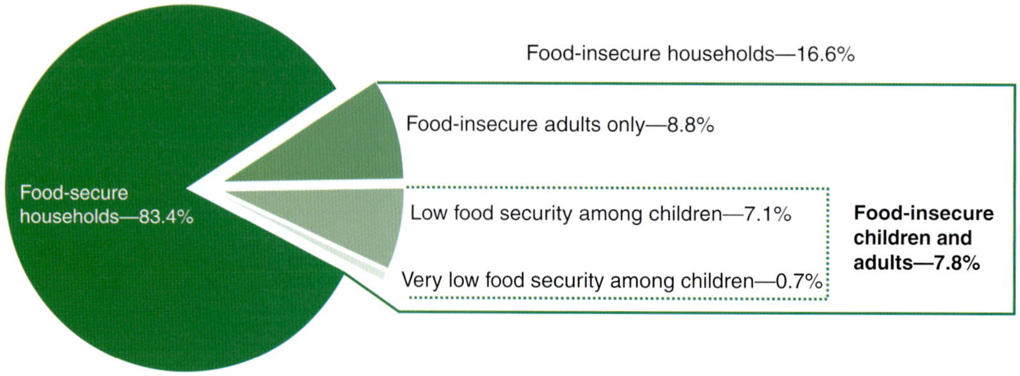

Source: USDA, Economic Research Service using data from U.S. Department of Commerce, U.S. Census Bureau, 2015 Current Population Survey Food Security Supplement.

• **Figure 16.8** U.S. households with children by food security status of adults and children, 2015. (From Coleman-Jensen A, Rabbitt, Gregory CA, Singh A. Household food security in the United States in 2015. U.S. Department of Agriculture (USDA), Economic Research Service. Economic Research Report Number 215, September 2016. Source: USDA, Economic Research Service using data from U.S. Department of Commerce, U.S. Census Bureau, Current Population Survey Food Security Supplement. https://www.ers.usda.gov/webdocs/publications/err215/err-215.pdf.)

CASE APPLICATION FOR THE DENTAL HYGIENIST

A patient reports he has found a miracle cure for his advanced periodontal disease. He plans to follow a diet and take recommended supplements "to strengthen my gums." This diet eliminates all foods from two food groups on *MyPlate*.

Nutritional Assessment

- Dietary intake, especially which of the food groups are omitted; nutrients most likely to be lacking
- Nutrition knowledge
- Supplements used and dosage
- Economic status
- Where most meals taken; food preparation

Nutritional Diagnosis

Knowledge deficit related to nutritional requirements.

Nutritional Goals

The patient will receive adequate nutrients to maintain oral health status by consuming a well-balanced diet.

Nutritional Implementation

Intervention: Discuss *MyPlate*—different groups, numbers of servings needed from each group, portion sizes, and nutrients provided from each group.

Rationale: Healthy oral structures depend on a variety of nutrients that can be obtained by following this guideline.

Intervention: Discuss nutrients that are deficient in his proposed diet and why those nutrients are important.

Rationale: When essential nutrients are omitted, the body cannot function effectively and its immune response is compromised.

Intervention: Discuss the importance of obtaining nutrients from foods rather than supplements.

Rationale: Foods are the natural way of obtaining nutrients; when supplements are used, many times they are in proportions that cannot be absorbed or they may interfere with absorption of other nutrients. Other components of food may affect use of the nutrient. In general, most supplements are not as effective as the food itself (see *Health Application 11* in Chapter 11).

Intervention: Discuss specific foods and oral care that would be helpful in preventing further deterioration.

Rationale: Adequate nutrition and oral self-care promote healing and repair of disease tissue. Maintaining a well-balanced diet provides the nutrients needed to support a healthy periodontium and resist disease activity.

Evaluation

The patient will practice effective oral care and consume a well-balanced diet; as a consequence, his periodontal health will improve.

Student Readiness

1. Which ethnic group is most prevalent in your area?
   - Identify at least one good thing about this ethnic group's food pattern.
   - List at least one potential dietary problem of this ethnic group and provide some suggestions for altering the diet.
   - Plan a 2-day menu that would fulfill the RDAs using many favorite foods or habits of the ethnic group.
   - Would a patient have any problem following that menu, such as economic hardship or the local availability of special foods?
   - Does this ethnic group have any predominant dental problems?
2. Think of two general statements that apply to all of your family/roommates (e.g., always eat breakfast, never drink milk, etc.). Discuss these statements with a group of your fellow students and see how many actually conform to your statements. Other than good foods to eat, what other lifelong eating customs are learned as a child?
3. State some reasons why people in the United States do not have similar eating patterns.
4. Plan an inexpensive menu for one day using low-cost foods.

5. A patient wants to know about convenience and fast foods. What would you tell the patient?
6. Study the meats at a grocery store. Categorize the types of meats that contain nitrate preservatives. Look at your own daily intake for three days and evaluate how frequently you are consuming nitrate-containing foods.
7. Some Americans are dependent on commercially prepared frozen foods or purchased foods outside the home. Look at the caloric density of foods consumed in commercial restaurants and the nature of the diseases that relate to obesity and cardiovascular health. What has consumer demand done to change selections offered in commercial food service establishments?
8. Prepare a rough budget showing how your personal funds are expended on a month-to-month basis. Evaluate the percentage of your own personal income that is earmarked for food prepared at home versus food prepared commercially in a restaurant or convenience items purchased in a grocery store. How well do you spend your own food dollar? Make some conclusions about how you could better use your dollar to provide nutrient-dense foods for you and your family.
9. Compare the cost of three foods from a health food store or health food section of a supermarket with the cost of similar items in a supermarket. Can you think of any reasons to justify the more expensive product?
10. Locate an advertisement in a popular magazine or newspaper for a health food product, and list merits of the product stated in the ad. List information about the product that might have been omitted or should be questioned.
11. Compare the cost of three organic foods with the same foods that are not labeled organic. Which would you choose to purchase and why?
12. Why are food faddism and quackery problems for medical professionals?
13. Discuss current food fads and how they may have adverse effects.
14. How can one spot a food quack?
15. Discuss the pros and cons of allowing nutritional claims on products.
16. A patient states, "I want to follow the _______ diet because _______ (popular actor) is advertising it." How would you respond?
17. Read a nutrition research article from a reputable journal. Using information provided in this chapter, point out some problems with the validity and applicability of the research. Does the article identify these as problem areas? Summarize the article in one page or less as if presenting to a patient.

◆ CASE STUDY

A young couple with 3 children—ages 3, 5, and 7 years—has been living on unemployment insurance payments for 9 months. The mother expresses concerns because of inadequate funds to feed the children. She is worried about their dental health.

1. Prepare a list of social services or federal service agencies in the community that should be contacted to determine potential sources of assistance to support recovery of this couple.
2. What are some nutritional concerns the dental hygienist could address with the patient?
3. What are some foods that are nutrient dense and economical purchases?
4. List some snack foods for the children that are nutritious, economical, and noncariogenic.
5. What methods of food preparation could be suggested to the mother that would preserve the nutritional quality of the food?

References

1. Centers for Disease Control and Prevention (CDC). Health disparities and inequalities report—United States, 2013. *MMWR.* 2013;62 (3 suppl):1–187. https://www.cdc.gov/mmwr/preview/ind2013_su.html#HealthDisparities2013. Accessed March 29, 2017.
2. Colby SL, Ortman JM. *Projections of the Size and Composition of the U.S. Population: 2014 to 2060.* Washington, DC: U.S. Census Bureau; 2014. Current Population Reports P25-1143.
3. Kuhns A, Levin D. Consumers paid less for grocery store foods in 2016 than in 2015. *Amber Waves.* 2017. https://www.ers.usda.gov/amber-waves/2017/march/consumers-paid-less-for-grocery-store-foods-in-2016.than-in-2015/. Accessed March 29, 2017.
4. Tuttle C, Kuhns A. Percent of income spent on food falls as income rises. *Amber Waves.* 2016. https://www.ers.usda.gov/amber-waves/2016/october/food-price-inflation-has-outpaced-economy-wide-inflation-in-recent-years/. Accessed March 29, 2017.
5. Mendes E. Americans spend $151 a week on food; the high-income, $180. August 2, 2012. http://www.gallup.com/poll/156416/americans-spend-151-week-food-high-income-180.aspx. Accessed March 29, 2017.
6. U.S. Department of Agriculture (USDA), Center for Nutrition Policy and Promotion (CNPP). Official USDA food plans. Cost of food at home at four levels, U.S. average, February 2017. https://www.cnpp.usda.gov/sites/default/files/CostofFoodFeb2017.pdf. Accessed March 29, 2017.
7. U.S. Department of Agriculture, Economic Research Service (ERS). Food expenditures. Last updated January 26, 2016. https://www.ers.usda.gov/data-products/food-expenditures.aspx. Accessed March 29, 2017.
8. Ohio State University. "The strange effects of thinking healthy food is costlier." *ScienceDaily.* December 19, 2016. http://www.sciencedaily.com/releases/2016/12/161219085423.htm.
9. U.S. Department of Health and Human Services and U.S. Department of Agriculture. 2015–2020 Dietary Guidelines for Americans. 8th ed. http://health.gov/dietaryguidelines/2015/guidelines/.
10. Carlson A, Frazão E. *Are Health Foods Really More Expensive? It Depends on How You Measure the Price. EIB-96.* Washington, DC: U.S. Department of Agriculture. Economic Research Service; 2012.
11. Morrell A, Gould S. A close look at Americans' food budget shows an obvious place to save money. *Business Insider.* February 17, 2017. http://www.businessinsider.com/americans-spending-food-bls-2017-2 Accessed March 29, 2017.
12. Tiwari A, Aggarwal A, Tang W, et al. Cooking at home: a strategy to comply with U.S. Dietary Guidelines at no extra cost. *Am J Prev Med.* 2017;doi:10.1016/j.amepre.2017.01.017. [Epub ahead of print]; pii: S0749-3797(17)30023-5.
13. Afshin A, Peñalvo J, Del Gobbo L et al. The prospective impact of food pricing on improving dietary consumption: A systematic review and meta-analysis. *PLoS ONE.* 2017;12(3):e0172277.
14. Handbury J, Rahkovsky I, Schnell M. Is the focus on food deserts fruitless? Retail access and food purchases across the socioeconomic spectrum. NBER Working Paper No. 21126. National Bureau of Economic Research. 2015.
15. Lester GE, Hallman GJ, Perez JA. Gamma irradiation dose: effects on spinach baby-leaf ascorbic acid, carotenoids, folate, alpha-tocopherol, and phylloquinone concentrations. *J Agric Food Chem.* 2010;58(8):4901–4906.
16. Sun J, Xiao Z, Lin LZ, et al. Profiling polyphenols in five Brassica species microgreens by UHPLC-PDA-ESI/HRMS(n.). *J Agric Food Chem.* 2013;61(46):10960–10970.
17. Crawford E. Four tools to help fight food borne illness and boost food safety efforts. Food Navigator-USA-com. January 30, 2017. http://www.foodnavigator-usa.com/content/view/print/1362296.
18. Lando A, Verrill L, Liu S, et al. *2016 FDA Food Safety Survey.* Center for Food Safety and Applied Nutrition, FDA. https://www.fda.gov/downloads/Food/FoodScienceResearch/ConsumerBehaviorResearch/UCM529453.pdf. Accessed March 29, 2017.

19. Research and Markets. Prediction: organic foods and beverages market to reach $320 billion by 2025. New Hope Network. June 12, 2017. http://www.newhope.com/news/prediction-organic-foods-and-beverages-market-reach-320-billion-2025. Accessed July 13, 2017.
20. U.S. Department of Agriculture, Economic Research Service (ERS). Organic market overview. https://www.ers.usda.gov/topics/natural-resources-environment/organic-agriculture/organic-market-overview.aspx. Accessed March 29, 2017.
21. Prada M, Garrido MV, Rodrigues D. Lost in processing? Perceived healthfulness, taste and caloric content of whole and processed organic food. *Appetite*. 2017;doi:10.1016/j.appet.2017.03.031. [Epub ahead of print]; pii:S0195-6663(16)30821-2.
22. Gwira Baumblatt JA, Carpenter LR, Wiedeman C, et al. Population survey of attitudes and beliefs regarding organic, genetically modified, and irradiated foods. *Nutr Health*. 2017;23(1):7–11.
23. U.S. Department of Agriculture, Agricultural Marketing Service (AMS). Organic Standards. https://www.ams.usda.gov/grades-standards/organic-standards. Accessed April 3, 2017.
24. Smith-Spangler C, Brandeau ML, Olkin I, et al. Are organic foods safer or healthier? *Ann Intern Med*. 2013;158(4):297–300.
25. Forman J, Silverstein J, Committee on Nutrition, Council on Environmental Health. Organic Foods. Health and Environmental Advantages and Disadvantages. *Pediatrics*. 2012;130(5):e1406–e1415.
26. Reganold JP, Andrews PK, Reeve JR, et al. Fruit and soil quality of organic and conventional strawberry agroecosystems. *PLoS ONE*. 2010;5(9):pii: e12346.
27. Dangour AD, Lock K, Hayter A, et al. Nutrition-related health effects of organic foods: a systematic review. *Am J Clin Nutr*. 2010;92(1):203–210.
28. Średnicka-Tober D, Barański M, Seal C, et al. Composition differences between organic and conventional meat: a systematic literature review and meta-analysis. *Br J Nutr*. 2016;115(6):994–1011.
29. Średnicka-Tober D, Barański M, Seal CJ, et al. Higher PUFA and n-3 PUFA, conjugated linoleic acid, α-tocopherol and iron, but lower iodine and selenium concentrations in organic milk: a systematic literature review and meta- and redundancy analyses. *Br J Nutr*. 2016;115(6):1043–1060.
30. Barański M, Rempelos L, Iversen PO, et al. Effects of organic food consumption on human health; the jury is still out! *Food Nutr Res*. 2017;61(1):1287333.
31. U.S. Department of Agriculture. USDA Releases 2014 Annual Summary for Pesticide Data Program. January 11, 2016. https://www.ams.usda.gov/press-release/usda-releases-2014-annual-summary-pesticide-data-program-report-confirms-pesticide. Accessed April 3, 2017.
32. Urban LE, Roberts SB, Fierstein JL, et al. Sodium, saturated fat, and trans fat content per 1,000 kilocalories: temporal trends in fast-food restaurants, United States, 2000–2013. *Prev Chronic Dis*. 2014;11:140335. https://www.cdc.gov/pcd/issues/2014/14_0335.htm. Accessed April 3, 2017.
33. Quader ZS, Gillespie C, Sliwa SA, et al. Sodium intake among US school-aged children: National Health and Nutrition Examination Survey, 2011–2012. *J Acad Nutr Diet*. 2017;117(1):39–47.e5.
34. Rehm CD, Drewnowski A. Trends in consumption of solid fats, added sugars, sodium, sugar-sweetened beverages, and fruit from fast food restaurants and by fast food restaurant type among US children, 2003–2010. *Nutrients*. 2016;8:12.
35. Platkin C, Yeh MC, Hirsch K, et al. The effect of menu labeling with calories and exercise equivalents on food selection and consumption. *BMC Obes*. 2014;1:21.
36. Ellison B, Lusk JL, Davis D. Looking at the label and beyond: the effects of calorie labels, health consciousness, and demographics on caloric intake in restaurants. *Int J Behav Nutr Phys Act*. 2013;10:21.
37. Anonymous. cited by Wilder RM. Fads, fancies, and fallacies in adult diets. *Sigma Xi O*. 1938;26:73.
38. Bruch H. The allure of food cults and nutrition quackery. *J Am Diet Assoc*. 1970;57(4):316–320.
39. Foroutan R. Defining detox. *Food Nutr*. 2012;1(3):13–15.
40. Angel M, Kassuer JP. Clinical research—what should the public believe? *N Engl J Med*. 1994;331(3):189–190.
41. Carroll AE. The whiplash from ever-changing medical advice. *The New York Times*, January 16, 2017.
42. Ioannidis JPA. The mass production of redundant, misleading, and conflicted systematic reviews and meta-analyses. *Milbank Q*. 2016;94(3):485–514.
43. Oliveira V. Food assistance landscape: FY 2016 annual report. United States Department of Agriculture, Economic Research Service. Economic Information Bulletin No. (EIB-169), March 2017. https://www.ers.usda.gov/webdocs/publications/eib169/eib169_summary.pdf?v=42823. Accessed April 5, 2017.
44. Bjerga A. Hunger in U.S. Drops to Lowest in a Decade as Economy Improves. September 7, 2017. https://www.bloombergquint.com/global-economics/2017/09/06/hunger-in-u-s-drops-to-lowest-in-a-decade-as-economy-improves. Accessed October 27, 2017.
45. Robbins S, Ettinger AK, Keefe C, et al. Low-income urban mothers' experiences with the supplemental Nutrition Assistance Program. *J Acad Nutr Diet*. 2017;[Epub ahead of print]; pii: S2212-2672(17)30030-8.
46. U.S. Department of Agriculture, Food and Nutrition Service (FNS). Supplemental Nutrition Assistance Program (SNAP). Last updated August 4, 2017. https://www.fns.usda.gov/pd/supplemental-nutrition-assistance-program-snap. Accessed August 4, 2017.
47. Coleman-Jensen A, Rabbitt MP, Gregory CA, et al. Household food security in the United States in 2015. U.S. Department of Agriculture, Economic Research Service. Economic Research Report Number 215. September 2016. https://www.ers.usda.gov/webdocs/publications/err215/err-215.pdf. Accessed April 5, 2017.
48. Andreyeva T, Luedicke J, Henderson KE, et al. Grocery store beverage choices by participants in federal food assistance and nutrition programs. *Am J Prev Med*. 2012;43(4):411–418.
49. Gordon AR, Cohen R, Crepinsek MK, et al. The third School Nutrition Dietary Assessment Study: background and study design. *J Am Diet Assoc*. 2009;109(2 suppl):S20–S30.
50. Au LE, Rosen NJ, Fenton K, et al. Eating school lunch is associated with higher diet quality among elementary school students. *J Acad Nutr Diet*. 2016;116(11):1817–1824.
51. U.S. Department of Agriculture, Food and Nutrition Service (FNS). Nutrition standards in the National School Lunch and School Breakfast Programs. GAO-12-458R. February 15, 2012. http://www.gao.gov/products/GAO-12-458R. Accessed April 5, 2017.
52. Government Accountability Office. *School Lunch: Implementing Nutrition Changes was Challenging and Clarification of Oversight Requirements is Needed*. Washington DC: US Government Accountability Office; 2014. http://www.gao.gov/products/GAO-14-104. Accessed April 5, 2017. GAO-14-104.
53. Cullen KW, Dave JM. The new Federal School Nutrition Standards and meal patterns: early evidence examining the influence on student dietary behavior and the school food environment. *J Acad Nutr Diet*. 2017;117(2):185–191.
54. Administration for Community Living, Administration on Aging. Elderly Nutrition Program. https://acl.gov/NewsRoom/Publications/docs/Elderly_Nutrition_Programs_1.pdf. Accessed April 5, 2017.
55. Murray EK, Baker S, Auld G. Nutrition recommendations from the US Dietary Guidelines critical to teach low-income adults: expert panel opinion. *J Acad Nutr Diet*. 2017;doi:10.1016/j.jand.2016.11.007. [Epub ahead of print]; pii: S2212-2672(16)31415-0.
56. Randall K. Nearly one-third of US food stamp recipients rely on food pantries. World Socialist Web site. March 9, 2016. Web site. https://www.wsws.org/en/articles/2016/03/09/food-m09.html. Accessed April 5, 2017.
57. Van Cleve N. Food: facts, fad, and fancy. *Am J Nurs*. 1938;38(3):285–287.
58. Simmet A, Depa J, Tinnemann P, et al. The dietary quality of food pantry users: a systematic review of existing literature. *J Acad Nutr Diet*. 2017;117(4):563–576.

59. Rausch R. Nutrition and academic performance in school-age children: the relation to obesity and food insufficiency. *Nutr Food Sci*. 2013; 3(2):190–192.
60. Ma X, Liese AD, Hibbert J, et al. The association between food security and store-specific and overall food shopping behaviors. *J Acad Nutr Diet*. 2017;doi:10.1016/j.jand.2017.02.007. [Epub ahead of print]; pii: S2212-2672(17)30119-3.
61. Cohen AJ, Richardson CR, Heisler M, et al. Increasing use of a healthy food incentive: a waiting room intervention among low-income patients. *Am J Prev Med*. 2017;52(2):154–162.
62. Mulik K, Haynes-Maslow L. The affordability of *MyPlate:* An analysis of SNAP benefits and the actual cost of eating according to the Dietary Guidelines. *J Nutr Educ Behav*. 2017;49:623–631.
63. Holben D. Position of the American Dietetic Association: Food insecurity in the United States. *J Am Diet Assoc*. 2010;110(9):1368–1377.
64. Center for Disease Control and Prevention, Office of Disease Prevention and Health Promotion. Healthy People 2020 Topics and Objectives. Nutrition and weight status. https://www.healthypeople.gov/node/3502/objectives#4936. Accessed April 5, 2017.

EVOLVE RESOURCES

Please visit http://evolve.elsevier.com/Stegeman/nutritional for additional practice and study support tools.

17

Effects of Systemic Disease on Nutritional Status and Oral Health

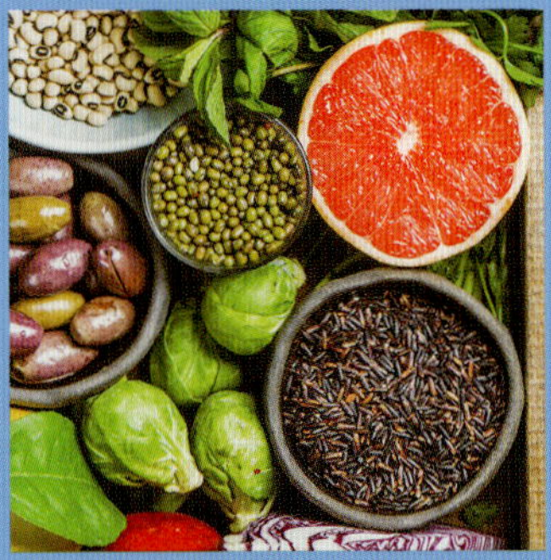

STUDENT LEARNING OUTCOMES

Upon completion of this chapter, the student will be able to achieve the following student learning outcomes:

1. Discuss the effects of anorexia, taste and smell disorders, and xerostomia on intake and oral health. Also, critically assess the implications of these chronic diseases, and plan appropriate dental interventions for patients with these disorders.
2. Describe the effects of various types of anemias, as well as neutropenia, on nutritional status and oral health. Also, critically assess the implications of these conditions, and plan appropriate dental interventions for patients with these symptoms.
3. Discuss the effects of various gastrointestinal and cardiovascular conditions on nutritional status and oral health. Also, critically assess the implications of these conditions, and plan appropriate dental interventions for patients who have these issues.
4. Discuss the effects of systemic bone disturbances, as well as metabolic problems, on nutritional status and oral health. Also, critically assess the implications of these conditions, and plan appropriate dental interventions for patients who have these issues.
5. Discuss the effects of neuromuscular problems, as well as neoplasia, on nutritional status and oral health. Also, critically assess the implications of these conditions, and plan appropriate dental interventions for patients who have these issues.
6. Discuss the effects of acquired immunodeficiency, as well as mental health problems, on nutritional status and oral health. Also, critically assess the implications of these conditions, and plan appropriate dental interventions for patients who have these symptoms.

KEY TERMS

Aneurysm
Anticholinergic
Atrophic glossitis
Binges
Bisphosphonates
Bradykinesia
Brown tumors
Chemotherapy
Dialysate
Epilepsy
Esophagitis
Gastroesophageal reflux disease
Gastrostomy
Glossodynia
Herpetic ulcerations
Hiatal hernia
Hirsutism
Human papillomavirus
Ischemia
Kaposi sarcoma
Leukemia
Leukoplakia
Lipodystrophy
Macroglossia
Materia alba
Micrognathia
Mucositis
Necrotizing ulcerative periodontitis
Neoplasia
Neutropenia
Odynophagia
Osteonecrosis
Osteosclerosis
Parkinson disease
Periapical
Pocketed foods
Purging
Renal osteodystrophy
Syrup of ipecac
Thrombus

TEST YOUR NQ

1. **T/F** Anorexia, associated with a chronic disease, can result in an increased susceptibility to infection.
2. **T/F** Antihypertensive, anticholinergic, and antidepressant drugs often cause a decrease in salivary flow.
3. **T/F** Iron supplements should be recommended to a patient who has anemia.
4. **T/F** It is within the scope of practice for a dental hygienist to provide nutritional advice to a patient recently diagnosed with diabetes.
5. **T/F** A patient with a hiatal hernia should be cautioned against eating before a dental appointment to prevent regurgitation while lying in a supine position.
6. **T/F** The health care provider should monitor protein intake closely in a patient with chronic renal failure.
7. **T/F** Kaposi sarcoma is a tumor that occurs frequently in patients with epilepsy.
8. **T/F** Phenytoin (Dilantin) can cause gingival hyperplasia and vitamin deficiencies.
9. **T/F** A dental hygienist should not confront a patient suspected to have an eating disorder but should casually refer the patient to a health care provider.
10. **T/F** Patients with bulimia generally have low body weight.

As you have already learned, nutritional deficiencies frequently are manifested in the oral and head and neck areas. Oral lesions can be a reflection of, or a marker for, disease elsewhere. The oral cavity cannot be isolated from, and is not immune to, what is occurring physiologically because oral tissues are nourished by the same blood supply providing oxygen and nutrients to cells throughout the entire body. Oral tissues may reflect changes in nutrient supply or other metabolic alterations. Oral manifestations are just a single part of the total systemic state.

Oral problems may develop as a result of disease processes or therapies or by nutritional deficiencies. Subsequent oral issues can cause inadequate intake. Systemic diseases or medications usually prescribed for these conditions may cause alterations in the oral cavity, such as oral lesions, xerostomia, or muscular weakness (Table 17.1). These oral alterations may lead to changes in eating patterns, which frequently have a general debilitating effect on the entire body. For example, food preferences are affected by an individual's ability to chew. Patients with reduced masticatory efficiency usually choose soft foods, which may not provide adequate amounts of essential nutrients. Dentate status, malocclusion, and ill-fitting dentures or partials increase risk of inadequate nutrient intake. The most common nutrients include protein, fiber, some B vitamins, vitamin D, iron, magnesium, and phosphorus. The body depends on nutrients from foods eaten to regenerate and repair diseased tissues; provisions must be made to provide these nutrients in adequate amounts on a regular basis.

All disease processes result from a combination of factors: the presence of an etiologic agent (e.g., plaque biofilm), the susceptibility or resistance of the host (or activation of immune response), and environmental factors. One of the most important factors in one's ability to combat hostile agents is availability of nutrients acquired from food. Infections can spread rapidly when the immune response is depressed.

Ramifications of a patient's systemic health are important to the dental hygienist because they provide cues to possible oral problems; may change treatment goals, priorities, or scheduling; or may influence dietary recommendations provided to the patient. Thus, the dental hygienist's dietary recommendations should take into consideration the systemic health of a patient and should not contradict dietary instructions provided by the patient's other health care providers. In other words, nutritional advice regarding oral health problems must be provided in the context of the whole patient.

More than one-third of the patients seen in a dental office do not frequently interact with a general health care provider.[1] Especially for these individuals, but often for other patients who visit their health care provider less frequently than they visit the dental office, dental hygienists are in a key position to assess and detect oral signs and symptoms of systemic health disorders. Clinical observations, radiographic findings, diet screening, and inquiries made while obtaining or updating the health history are used to detect signs and symptoms. They should be the basis for motivating the patient to visit a health care provider or registered dietitian nutritionist (RDN). This can potentially reduce health care costs.

This chapter presents oral problems frequently caused by systemic health conditions or their treatment because these problems typically affect eating patterns. No attempt is made to cover pathophysiology, and the information given should not be used to diagnose conditions. If the cause of oral signs and symptoms is unknown, refer the patient to a health care provider who can perform a thorough assessment, including diagnostic laboratory evaluation, for accurate diagnosis and treatment.

Effects of Chronic Disease on Intake

Anorexia and Appetite

The term *anorexia nervosa* refers to a disease associated with a distorted body image, but anorexia may also refer to a condition in which a patient has a poor appetite and/or decreased food intake for a variety of reasons (e.g., cancer treatment). Appetite is associated with enjoyment of food. Most healthy individuals have a good appetite with no problems eating adequate amounts. However, during illness, appetite may decrease because of pain, apathy, anorexia, drugs, inactivity, or many other reasons. Individuals may become depressed after the diagnosis of a chronic illness, causing mental stress about problems related to living with, or dying because of, the condition. A modified diet may be prescribed for a patient with a chronic illness, which may adversely affect intake. Poor food intake may further lessen the desire to eat. In some situations, it may be unknown whether anorexia is a cause of the illness or an effect of the illness. Malnutrition and other stresses—such as infection, surgery, and injuries resulting in anorexia—deplete body stores of calories, macronutrients (e.g., protein), and micronutrients (e.g., vitamin C) needed to regenerate and repair cells. In this situation, the body is more susceptible to bacterial or viral invasion.

Taste and Smell Disorders

The foods that people choose to eat are modulated by taste, smell, and oral textural perception. Taste and smell dramatically affect appetite and food intake. Various disease conditions (e.g., respiratory diseases and cancer), medications, smoking, and treatment for the conditions may result in chemosensory disorders (i.e., disorders of taste and smell). Taste perception declines during the normal

TABLE 17.1 Oral Problems Associated With Systemic Diseases

Condition	Xerostomia	Taste Alterations	Oral Lesions	Immune Response	Masticatory Efficiency	Delayed Wound Healing	Dysphagia	Sore Tongue	Risk of Bleeding	Dental Caries
Anemias										
Iron-deficiency	X	X	X	X		X		X		
Plummer-Vinson	X	X	X	X		X	X	X		
Megaloblastic		X	X	X				X		
Thalassemia					X					
Aplastic			X						X	
Other Hematologic Diseases										
Polycythemia									X	
Neutropenia			X	X						
Gastrointestinal Problems										
Medications for reflux	X							X		
Malabsorptive conditions		X	X			X				
Cardiovascular Conditions										
Cardiovascular accidents							X			
Antihypertensive medications	X									
Lipid-lowering medications		X							X	
Skeletal Anomalies										
Systemic bone disturbances					X					
Metabolic Problems										
Diabetes mellitus	X	X		X		X				X
Acromegaly					X					
Hypopituitarism					X					
Cushing syndrome					X			X		
Hypothyroidism					X					X
Hyperparathyroidism					X					
Renal Disease										
Diminished kidney function			X		X	X			X	
Neuromuscular Problems										
Parkinson disease	X				X		X			
Developmental disabilities					X		X			
Epilepsy	X									
Neoplasia										
Cancer		X								
Kaposi sarcoma			X							
Leukemia				X						
Acquired Immunodeficiency Syndrome										
AIDS	X		X	X						
Mental Health Problems										
Anorexia nervosa/bulimia				X						X
Medications for mental illness	X									

aging process. An aging adult loses salty and sweet tastes first, thereby requiring greater amounts of sodium and sugar to perceive these tastes.[2] Older adults have a tendency to dislike bitter and sour foods.[3] Reactions to loss of taste and smell vary. Patients with loss of smell eat less, use more spices, and eat and drink fewer sweets. Loss of saliva in disease and drug-induced xerostomia reduce solubility of flavors and the ability to taste. Many patients experiencing taste changes tend to have inadequate food intake and weight loss, resulting in malnutrition.[2,3]

Numerous drugs may adversely influence taste perception, either by decreasing function or producing perceptual distortions or **phantom taste** (lingering unpleasant taste even though nothing is in the mouth). Individuals taking three or more medications are likely to have less taste sensitivity.

Xerostomia

Saliva protects hard and soft oral tissues from mechanical, thermal, and chemical irritants in addition to its roles in buffering acids, antimicrobial activity, and remineralization. Medications (e.g., antidepressants, antihistamines, antihypertensives, diuretics, and gastrointestinal drugs), diseases or conditions (e.g., Sjögren disease), and therapies (e.g., radiation) may cause xerostomia. More than one-third of older adults experience xerostomia primarily as a result of **anticholinergic** (blockage of impulses through the parasympathetic nerves) medications.[4,5] Older individuals taking more than one medication are more likely to have xerostomia not caused by the aging process. Hyposalivation is a known risk factor for dental caries and periodontal disease but may also cause taste disturbances, swallowing problems, poor chewing ability, and malnutrition.

Xerostomia can affect nutritional status in several ways: (a) chewing is difficult because a bolus cannot be formed without additional moisture; (b) chewing is painful because the mouth is sore; (c) swallowing is difficult because of loss of lubrication from saliva; and (d) food intake may decrease because of changes in taste perception. Individuals with xerostomia tend to avoid dry, crunchy foods and sticky foods, which may result in malnutrition secondary to lower intake of calories and other essential nutrients.[6]

Anemias

Typical symptoms of all the anemias are pallor of the skin, oral mucosa, and conjunctival tissues, along with overall weakness as a result of inadequate oxygen-carrying power of the blood. The occurrence and severity of clinical symptoms depend on the degree of anemia and speed of onset. The type of anemia can be determined only after evaluation of blood tests.

Iron-Deficiency Anemia

Iron-deficiency anemia can be caused by a deficiency of dietary iron or by excessive bleeding. It is likely to occur during periods in which iron requirements are high, such as during infancy or pregnancy. Gradual depletion of iron stores may progress to iron-deficiency anemia, in which iron levels are inadequate for maintaining hemoglobin levels to provide cellular oxygen. Lethargy and fatigue—in addition to glossitis, aphthous ulcers, and xerostomia associated with iron-deficiency anemia—can lead to changes in appetite and food intake. Clinical symptoms in the oral cavity include gingival and mucosal pallor (Fig. 17.1), angular cheilosis, and atrophic glossitis. **Atrophic glossitis** is described as atrophy of the filiform and fungiform papillae beginning at the tip and lateral borders of the tongue and gradually spreading to the entire dorsum of the tongue. As the papillae gradually shrink in size, bald spots appear, and the tongue becomes smooth, shiny, and red (Fig. 17.2).

Iron-deficiency anemia affects the immune response and places a patient at increased risk for fungal infections, such as candidiasis. After iron supplementation is initiated, oral symptoms begin to resolve in 48 hours and filiform papillae regenerate in 3 to 4 weeks. Depending on the severity of iron-deficiency anemia, wound healing may be impaired in response to invasive dental treatments, such as tooth extraction, nonsurgical periodontal therapy, and periodontal surgery.

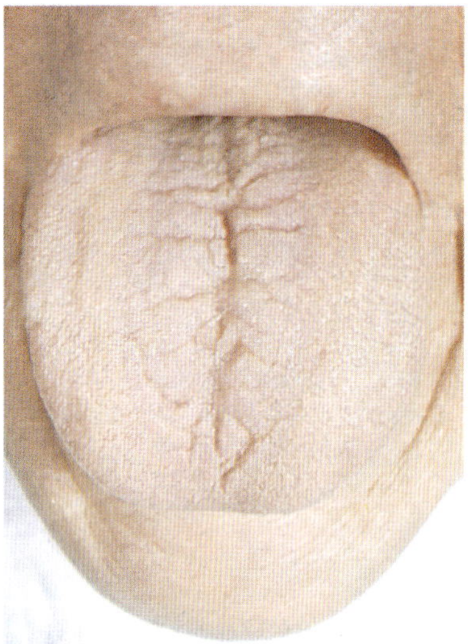

• **Figure 17.1** Clinical symptoms of iron-deficiency anemia include pallor of the gingiva, mucosa, and tongue. (Courtesy DW Beaven and SE Brooks. From McLaren DS. *A Colour Atlas and Text of Diet-Related Disorders*. 2nd ed. London: Mosby-Yearbook; 1992.)

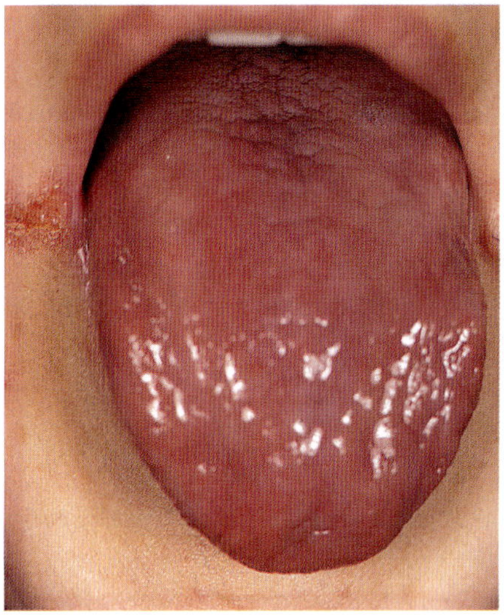

• **Figure 17.2** Iron-deficiency anemia. (Reproduced with permission from Cawson RA, Odell EW. *Cawson's Essentials of Oral Pathology and Oral Medicine*. 8th ed. Edinburgh: Churchill Livingstone; 2008.)

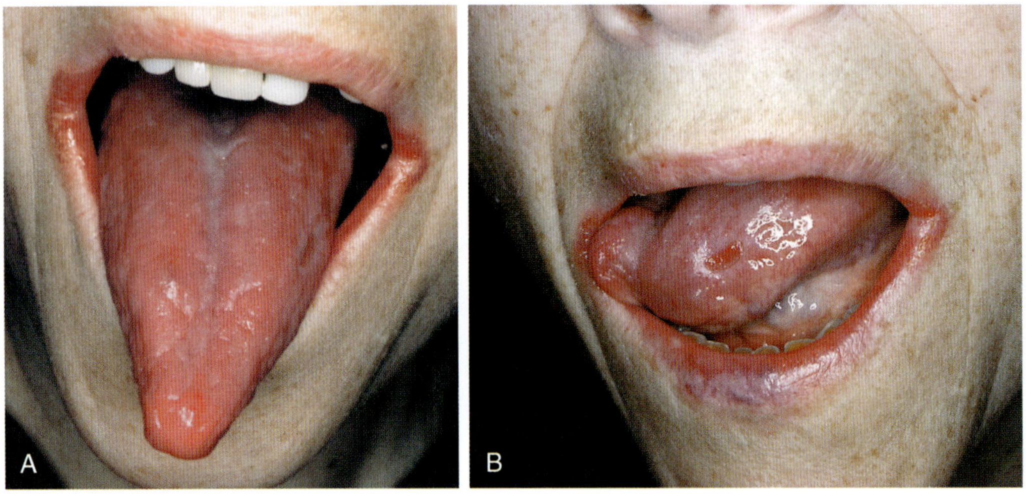

• **Figure 17.3** (A) and (B) Pernicious anemia. (Reproduced with permission from Ibsen OAC, Phelan JA. *Oral Pathology for the Dental Hygienist*. 6th ed. St Louis, MO: Saunders; 2014.)

DENTAL CONSIDERATIONS

Assessment

- *Physical:* Burning sensation of the tongue, xerostomia, gingival and mucosal pallor, atrophy of the filiform and fungiform papillae, atrophic glossitis, angular cheilosis, dysphagia, candidiasis.
- *Dietary:* Adequacy of dietary intake, especially red meats, dark-green vegetables, enriched cereals and bread; use of vitamin-mineral supplements.

Interventions

- Encourage iron-rich foods (see Table 12.9); if principally nonheme sources are consumed at a meal, a source of vitamin C enhances absorption of nonheme iron.
- If the iron supplement causes nausea, suggest that the patient take the supplement with food or discuss the problem with the health care provider rather than discontinue the supplement.

Evaluation

- Successful outcomes include the patient consuming iron-rich foods and taking the prescribed supplement.

NUTRITIONAL DIRECTIONS

- If the iron supplement is liquid, dilute with water or juice and drink with a straw to minimize tooth staining.
- Iron stores are replenished very slowly; therapy should be continued for at least 1 year.

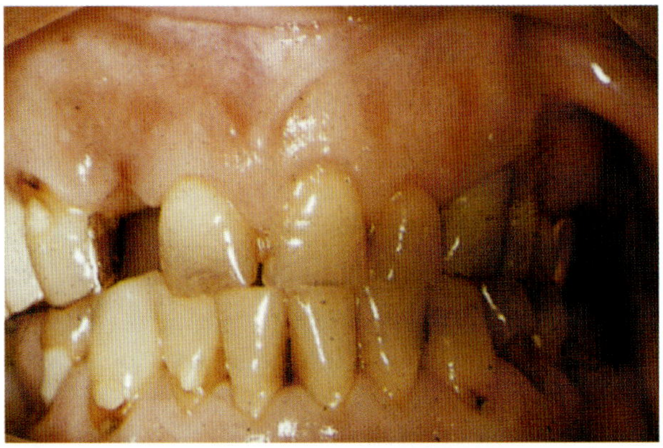

• **Figure 17.4** Gingival "appearance" owing to anemia. (Courtesy Dr. Edward V. Zegarelli. Reproduced with permission from Ibsen OAC, Phelan JA. *Oral Pathology for the Dental Hygienist*. 6th ed. St. Louis, MO: Saunders; 2014.)

Megaloblastic (Pernicious) Anemia

Vitamin B_{12} deficiency can result in a megaloblastic anemia (a small number of large red blood cells), also called pernicious anemia. This condition occurs when vitamin B_{12} is deficient in the diet, absorption is inadequate, or requirements are increased. With vitamin B_{12} malabsorption or no dietary source, normal body stores are usually sufficient for 3 to 4 years. Vitamin B_{12} deficiency is most common among vegans who consume no animal products.

Oral changes of vitamin B_{12} deficiency may be the only clinical evidence of the disease preceding significant anemia. Patients with pernicious anemia may initially present with angular cheilosis, recurrent aphthous ulcers (Fig. 17.3, A and B) and erythematous **mucositis** (inflamed, flat lesions with red borders on the mucous membrane and pale or yellowish oral mucosa (Fig. 17.4). Patients may also complain of a painful, sore, burning tongue with signs of atrophic glossitis associated with a beefy red color. Replacement therapy with vitamin B_{12} supplements or injections relieves symptoms within 36 to 48 hours, with evidence of regeneration of tongue papillae within 4 to 7 days, and the tongue may be normal in 3 to 4 weeks.

Another type of megaloblastic anemia, caused by folic acid deficiency, is frequently associated with poor diets or medications that interfere with folate absorption or metabolism, such as phenytoin (Dilantin) or methotrexate. Oral manifestations are similar to symptoms present in pernicious anemia: glossitis, atrophy of the papillae, ulcerations, and **glossodynia** (pain in the tongue). Angular cheilitis and fungal infections in the perioral area may also be observed.

Folate replacement is necessary because diet alone is inadequate to replace lost stores. Iron supplements may also be ordered because when folate is deficient, iron is usually low as well. Folate supplementation in a patient deficient in vitamin B_{12} may produce hematologic improvement, whereas neurologic damage from vitamin B_{12} deficiency continues to progress.

DENTAL CONSIDERATIONS

Assessment

- *Physical:* Sex; age; glazed, red, sore, or painful tongue; pale skin and oral mucous membranes; shortness of breath; malabsorption, previous gastrointestinal surgeries.
- *Dietary:* Dietary intake, especially dark-green leafy vegetables, animal products, whole-grain breads, and fortified foods; alcohol intake.

Interventions

- If the patient has megaloblastic anemia caused by folate deficiency, encourage rich sources of folate (especially grains fortified with folic acid) along with a supplement meeting the RDA for folate (400 µg; see Table 11.12).
- If the patient is not a vegan, encourage intake of foods from animal sources high in vitamin B_{12} for pernicious anemia. If the patient is a vegan, encourage fortified foods or supplementation. Dietary intake helps reestablish depleted stores.
- Refer the patient to an RDN; patients with megaloblastic anemia especially need nutritional counseling because of undesirable eating habits.

Evaluation

- Desired outcomes include the patient consuming a well-balanced diet and foods high in folate or vitamin B_{12} (as appropriate) and taking supplements to enhance the formation of red blood cells (erythropoiesis).

NUTRITIONAL DIRECTIONS

- Raw vegetables are a better source of folate than cooked vegetables; heat destroys folate.
- Daily intake of dietary folate is necessary.
- Patients with permanent gastric or ileal damage need monthly intramuscular or oral vitamin B_{12} supplementation for life.
- Vitamin B_{12} shots are not always indicated for "tired blood."
- When oral vitamin B_{12} or iron supplements are ordered, take with vitamin C–rich foods to enhance absorption.
- Large doses of folate can negate therapeutic effects of anticonvulsants; thus, consultation with the health care provider is recommended.

Other Hematologic Disorders

Neutropenia

Neutropenia is a diminished number of neutrophils, the most abundant type of white blood cells (WBCs) in the blood and may predispose an immunocompromised patient to life-threatening infections. The risk of infection is directly proportional to duration and severity of neutropenia. Neutropenia results from dysfunctional bone marrow: cancer (e.g., leukemia), drugs (e.g., chemotherapeutic agents or antibiotics), radiation therapy, autoimmune disease (e.g., rheumatoid arthritis or systemic lupus erythematosus), bone marrow transplant, nutritional deficiencies (e.g., severe vitamin B_{12} or folate deficiency), or certain bacterial or viral infections (e.g., human immunodeficiency virus [HIV], malaria, tuberculosis, or Epstein-Barr virus).

Mucositis and viral and fungal infections (e.g., candidiasis) are frequently occurring complications as a result of neutropenia. As the neutrophil count falls, incidence and severity of infection rise. Oral organisms from the dentition, **periapical** (area around the root apex), and periodontium can disseminate systemically, causing bacteremias and systemic infection. Mucositis may result in large ulcerative and necrotic lesions with extensive tissue destruction. Ideally, this condition is treated and managed before initiation of treatment that may result in neutropenia.[7] Meticulous oral hygiene is essential to prevent the progression of periodontal disease. When neutropenia is present, invasive dental treatment is usually contraindicated until WBC counts increase. If treatment is indicated, a consultation with the health care provider is necessary to determine if antibiotic prophylaxis is needed.

DENTAL CONSIDERATIONS

Assessment

- *Physical:* Painful oral mucosal ulcerations (mucositis), candidiasis.
- *Dietary:* Folate and vitamin B_{12} intake.

Interventions

- For neutropenia, encourage foods high in folate (see Table 11.12) and vitamin B_{12} (see Table 11.14) if the patient's intake is questionable.
- Stress the importance of frequent oral prophylaxis and meticulous oral self-care.
- Refer the patient to an RDN for nutritional counseling if eating habits are poor.

Evaluation

- Successful outcomes include patient adherence to a diet encompassing a variety of foods, concentrating on iron, vitamin B_{12}, or folate; use of supplementation as recommended by a health care provider or RDN; and frequent dental recare appointments and maintenance of good periodontal health.

NUTRITIONAL DIRECTIONS

- To ensure adequate iron intake, choose meat, fish, or poultry regularly.
- Choose a vitamin C–rich food with a meal or eat a small amount of meat with each meal to enhance iron absorption.

Gastrointestinal Problems

Gastroesophageal Reflux, Hiatal Hernia, and Esophagitis

Heartburn 30 minutes to 1 hour after eating is the most common symptom of **gastroesophageal reflux disease**, a return of gastric contents into the esophagus. This condition is commonly associated with **hiatal hernia** (partial protrusion of the stomach through the diaphragm; Fig. 17.5), pregnancy, and obesity. Normally, the lower esophageal sphincter prevents caustic gastric acid from refluxing into the esophagus. Acidity from the stomach, alkalinity, pepsin, or bile may damage the esophageal mucosa, and esophagitis may result if left untreated. **Esophagitis** is an inflammation of the lower esophagus and may cause discomfort when swallowing.

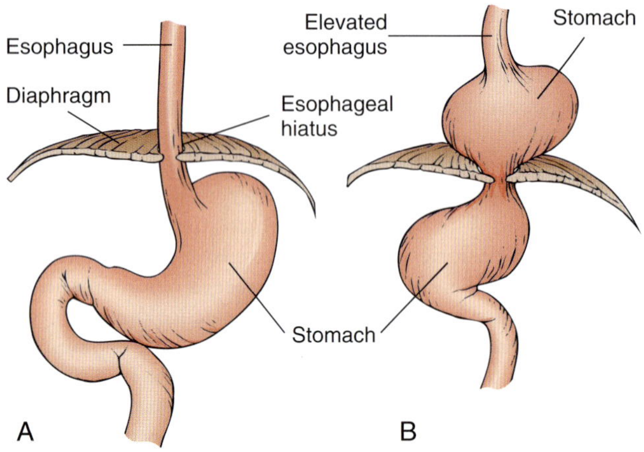

• **Figure 17.5** Gingival "appearance" owing to anemia. (Reproduced with permission from Grodner M, Escott-Stump S, Dorner S. *Nutritional Foundations and Clinical Applications: A Nursing Approach*, 6th ed. St. Louis, MO: Elsevier; 2016.)

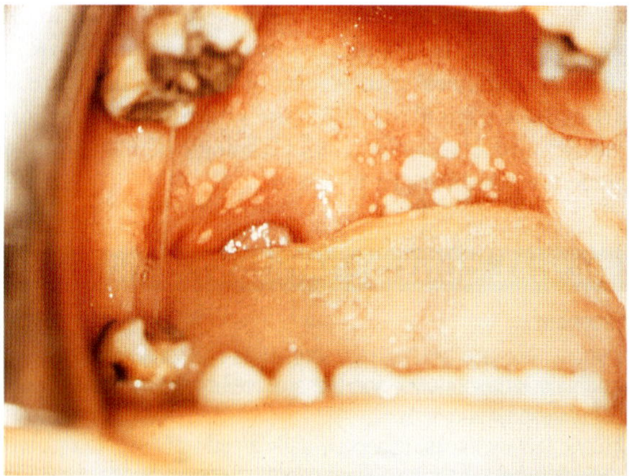

• **Figure 17.6** Oral ulcers "due to" ulcerative colitis. (Reproduced with permission from Ibsen OAC, Phelan JA. *Oral Pathology for the Dental Hygienist*. 6th ed. St. Louis, MO: Saunders; 2014.)

Patients are frequently advised to decrease their intake of foods that may precipitate reflux, such as fatty foods (e.g., gravy, pastries, chocolate, fatty meats, cheese, nuts, chips, salad dressing, and mayonnaise), peppermint, caffeinated foods (e.g., coffee, tea, chocolate, and some carbonated beverages), alcohol, and onions. Other foods to avoid are those directly irritating to the esophagus, such as citrus juices, tomato products, and red peppers. If appropriate, weight loss and/or tobacco cessation is recommended. Other suggestions to help reduce pain include eating small, frequent meals; using antacids to buffer gastric juices; wearing loose-fitting clothing; eating at least 2 to 3 hours before lying down; and sleeping with head and shoulders elevated 6 inches.

Anticholinergic medications prescribed for gastroesophageal reflux disease may interfere with absorption of vitamin B_{12} and folic acid. Observation for oral signs of vitamin deficiency is appropriate for patients taking these medications. Anticholinergic medications may also cause xerostomia.

DENTAL CONSIDERATIONS

Assessment

- *Physical:* Type of medications used, heartburn, bitter taste, visual appraisal of weight, enamel erosion, sensitivity of the dentin.
- *Diet:* Adequacy and frequency of intake; caffeine, fat, and alcohol intake; knowledge of foods that increase reflux or irritate the esophagus.

Interventions

- If weight loss is needed, refer to an RDN or a nationally recognized weight loss program, such as Weight Watchers, for a nutritionally sound reduction program.
- To reduce risk of regurgitation during dental treatment, the patient should be in semisupine position; the patient should not eat for 2 hours before the appointment; avoid the use of nitrous oxide because it may relax the lower esophageal sphincter.

Evaluation

- The patient plans frequent well-balanced meals, avoiding foods that cause reflux and irritate the esophagus.

NUTRITIONAL DIRECTIONS

- The effectiveness of avoiding or limiting foods that increase likelihood of reflux to prevent irritation of esophageal tissue varies among patients and is based on individual tolerances. General recommendations include limiting caffeine, chocolate, alcohol, mint, and carbonated beverages.
- If citrus fruits and tomato products are avoided or limited, other sources of vitamin C should be selected, including cantaloupe, potatoes, and strawberries.
- Heartburn is not caused by inadequate digestion; digestive enzyme tablets are inappropriate.
- Eat small meals, evenly distributed throughout the day.
- Reduce or eliminate cigarette smoking, which stimulates gastric acid secretion.

Malabsorptive Conditions

Many chronic diseases are associated with poor nutrient absorption, including Crohn disease, ulcerative colitis, cystic fibrosis, gluten-sensitive enteropathy (sprue or celiac disease), and AIDS. **Gluten** is a protein found mainly in wheat and to a lesser degree in rye, oat, and barley. Different parts of the gastrointestinal tract are affected in these disorders, and manifestations differ from one individual to another with the same condition (see Chapter 3, *Health Application 3*). Malabsorption may occur, affecting many macronutrients (e.g., gluten [protein], fat, and carbohydrates) and micronutrients (e.g., vitamin B_{12}).

Oral problems associated with Crohn disease and ulcerative colitis include swollen, bleeding, erythematous gingiva; diffuse pustular eruptions on the buccal gingiva; oral ulcerations (Fig. 17.6); swelling of the lips; and cobblestone-like, raised hypertrophic lesions. Additionally, taste alterations (metallic dysgeusia) and reduction in taste acuity may develop. Enamel defects and deep aphthous ulcerations may be a marker of Crohn disease, ulcerative colitis, or celiac disease, and precede gastrointestinal symptoms. These clinical signs appear when the disease is in the acute stage and disappear when it is inactive.

Diarrhea and malabsorption associated with these disease states create deficiencies of nutrients and trace elements. Nutritional requirements of these patients are usually increased; however, abdominal cramping precipitated by food intake and anorexia and intolerance to many different food components (gluten, fat, lactose, and fiber) inhibit intake. As a result, patients are finicky and apprehensive about eating; they may present with anemia, protein and energy malnutrition, poor wound healing, and suppressed immune response.

Different nutritional modalities are used with these conditions. A diet high in calories and protein with limited fat and fiber, and possible lactose or gluten restriction, may be recommended for patients by their health care provider or RDN. Small, frequent feedings are better tolerated and increase adequacy of intake. Irritating foods are excluded. Extremely hot and cold foods and high-fiber foods are avoided because they increase peristalsis.

DENTAL CONSIDERATIONS

Assessment

- *Physical:* Edema, anemia, weight loss, abdominal pain, diarrhea, fatigue, swollen and bleeding gingiva, enamel defects, aphthous ulcers (canker sores), and emotional stress.
- *Dietary:* Iron, folate, vitamin B_{12}, and adequate protein and calories.

Interventions

- Encourage the patient to eat a nutrient-rich, well-balanced diet. Reassess the diet as appropriate to monitor nutrient adequacy.
- The use of stress management techniques (e.g., the use of headphones with enjoyable music) during the appointment can prevent aggravating symptoms associated with the disease.
- Consult with the health care provider about the need for supplemental steroids and prophylactic antibiotics before the dental appointment. The health care provider or RDN may also recommend vitamin and mineral supplementation.

Evaluation

- Successful outcomes include the patient choosing foods that are well tolerated and promote weight gain or stability (as needed) and physical strength; also, minimal oral problems do not affect eating.

NUTRITIONAL DIRECTIONS

- Encourage the patient to use a food diary to note symptoms, specific foods, or dietary practices that cause problems.
- Adequate rest and a relaxed, calm day before the prophylaxis help to avoid aggravating symptoms.
- Probiotics may be beneficial (see Ch. 3, *Health Application 3*).[8]
- Multiple nutrient deficiencies are common and can interfere with effectiveness of the prescribed medication, compromising immune function.

Cardiovascular Conditions

Cardiovascular disease (CVD) encompasses numerous prevalent chronic heart problems, including hypertension, congestive heart failure, myocardial infarction, cerebrovascular accident, and arteriosclerosis. There may be a risk of CVD resulting from systemic exposure to periodontal pathogens. Periodontal interventions may reduce systemic inflammation and risk of CVD. However, meta-analyses and evidence-based research have revealed conflicting results regarding the association between periodontal disease and interventions to prevent or modify the outcomes of CVD. To date, randomized controlled trials evaluating the effect of periodontal treatment on CVD risk are lacking.[9–11]

In contrast to its many ill effects in other sites of the body, CVD produces few oral effects and usually does not have any oral manifestations that affect food intake. However, medications prescribed for cardiovascular conditions may have oral effects. Dietary adjustments recommended for these patients affect information that the dental hygienist provides.

Cerebrovascular Accident

A cerebrovascular accident (also known as a stroke) results if occlusion, or ischemia, occurs in an artery supplying the brain or if hemorrhaging in the brain occurs. **Ischemia** (inadequate blood flow and lack of oxygen because of constriction or obstruction of arteries) is caused by blockage of one of the arteries in a part of the body (cardiac ischemia, heart muscle). Most strokes are caused by ischemia. An artery may become blocked from atherosclerosis or a **thrombus** (blood clot). **Atherosclerosis** is caused by an accumulation of fatty materials (such as cholesterol) on smooth inner walls of arteries (see Fig. 6.3). As this plaque thickens, arteries become progressively narrow and rough, and blood flow carrying oxygen and nutrients may be disrupted. Hemorrhagic strokes may occur as a result of a bleeding **aneurysm** (weak or thin spot in an arterial wall). Occasionally, patients who have ministrokes do not seek medical care even though dysphagia can result. The patient may realize that things are not normal but may attribute these deficits to the aging process. A dental hygienist may suspect dysphagia in a patient who has facial muscle weakness (drooping mouth) or slurred speech; who has weak oral, neck, or tongue muscles; or who coughs or chokes frequently on foods, drinks, and secretions (e.g., saliva and mucus). Neurologically impaired patients may deny having swallowing problems. Patients suspected to have dysphagia should be referred to a health care provider. Normally, a speech-language pathologist and RDN work closely with these patients to ensure adequate fluid and nutrient intake. Severely impaired patients may receive their nutrition via **gastrostomy** (a tube that provides the feeding directly into the stomach) until the swallowing reflex improves.

Liquids are very difficult to control in the mouth, especially in the oral stage of the swallow. Because of this issue, use of water for rinsing or ultrasonic instrumentation may be contraindicated during dental care. The patient may be unable to lie in a supine position because of the potential for choking on saliva. Water should be used sparingly, and use of high-speed evacuation may help prevent aspiration.

Neurologic deficits may cause some patients to be unaware of the presence of food in the mouth. After meals, the mouth should be checked for any **pocketed foods** (foods retained in the mouth, especially in the vestibule) that should be removed to decrease risk of aspirating the food and developing dental caries.

Hypertension

Blood pressure consistently 140/90 mm Hg or higher is known as stage 1 hypertension. Patients with diagnosed hypertension or congestive heart failure may have been told to increase fruits and vegetables, use more low-fat or nonfat dairy products, limit sodium, limit intake of alcohol and caffeine, quit smoking, exercise, lose weight, and reduce stress (see Chapter 12, *Health Application 12*). When many older adults are told to limit salt in their diet because of high blood pressure, they may consume less food because it does not taste good and they may not adhere to the recommendations because of limited food choices and lack of palatability.

Diuretics are frequently prescribed for patients with congestive heart failure or hypertension to help eliminate excess fluid. These medications also negatively affect salivary flow, which causes xerostomia.

DENTAL CONSIDERATIONS

Assessment

- *Physical:* Slurred speech and inability to communicate effectively; unilateral weakness or paralysis; difficulty chewing and swallowing; loss of oral sensations; lack of tongue control (weak, flabby, and deviates to one side).
- *Dietary:* Chewing and swallowing difficulties, dietary inadequacies.

Interventions

- Monitor the patient's blood pressure at each dental visit.
- Refer to the RDN when dysphagia exists.
- Consult the health care provider before treatment to determine the need for antibiotic prophylaxis to prevent infective endocarditis and whether medications will have an anticoagulant effect.

Evaluation

- Desired outcomes include adequate nourishment using modifications according to the patient's disability, maintenance of good oral hygiene with formation of no new caries, and control of the periodontal condition.

NUTRITIONAL DIRECTIONS

- Encourage the patient or caregiver to maintain adequate oral hygiene, particularly because of limited self-cleansing action on the affected side of the oral cavity.

Hyperlipidemia

Patients with other types of heart disease involving elevated cholesterol levels or increased risk of atherosclerosis normally have a saturated, *trans* and total fat restriction as well as a calorically restriction (discussed in Chapter 6, *Health Application 6*). Low-fat diets can result in weight loss, which is beneficial to many. However, for patients who are trying to maintain their weight, snacks may be needed. Dental hygienists should recommend noncariogenic snacks relatively low in fat, such as low-fat or nonfat cheese or skim milk.

Long-term use of bile acid sequestrants (e.g., cholestyramine and colestipol), prescribed to reduce serum lipids, may cause malabsorption of fat-soluble vitamins and folic acid. Several bile acid sequestrants may cause gastrointestinal disturbances and affect overall food intake. Patients with heart disease may also be taking anticoagulants, such as warfarin (Coumadin), which may increase risk of bleeding and affect dietary intake because foods with vitamin K are limited.

DENTAL CONSIDERATIONS

Assessment

- *Physical:* Medications prescribed, xerostomia, blood pressure.
- *Dietary:* Dietary recommendations, adequacy of food intake.

Interventions

- Because stress is a negative risk factor for most patients with hypertension or heart conditions, minimize stress and consider effects of the disease on the proposed dental treatment. A shortened appointment and use of nitrous oxide may need to be considered.
- Generally, hypertension has no typical physiologic symptoms; monitoring blood pressure at each appointment is necessary.
- Refer the patient to the RDN for medical nutrition therapy.

Evaluation

- The patient's blood pressure is within a normal range; the patient takes prescribed medications and follows *MyPlate* guidelines.

NUTRITIONAL DIRECTIONS

- Most salt substitutes contain potassium and chloride. Remind patients to check with the health care provider or RDN for advice on the use of salt substitutes to minimize the intake of excessive dietary potassium.
- Assist the patient determine low-sodium, low-fat, and low-cholesterol foods feasible for individual lifestyle and food preferences.
- Antihypertensive drugs may be responsible for reduced salivary flow. Fluoride therapy may be necessary. Xylitol gum or mints also may be used to promote salivation and remineralization of early carious lesions.
- Calcium channel blockers can cause gingival hyperplasia. Encourage optimal oral hygiene.

Skeletal System

Systemic bone disturbances initially may be detected by the following changes in the maxilla or mandible during an oral examination: (a) significant increase in size or alteration in contour of the maxilla or mandible, (b) alteration in radiographic pattern, (c) mobility of individual teeth without significant periodontal disease, (d) pain or discomfort in the jaw without obvious dental pathology, (e) increased sensitivity of the teeth without obvious dental or periodontal disease, (f) changes in occlusion of the teeth, or (g) abnormal sequence of deciduous tooth loss or eruption of permanent molars in young patients. These changes may be caused by osteoporosis, metabolic disturbances such as hyperparathyroidism, or other conditions such as Paget disease or fibrous dysplasia. For denture-wearing patients with osteoporosis, rapid resorption of the alveolar ridges may lead to continuous loosening of the dentures with resultant oral lesions or the inability to consume foods that require chewing.

In addition to referring the patient to a health care provider for correct diagnosis and treatment, the dental hygienist needs to provide guidance to ensure adequate calcium and vitamin D for patients with missing teeth, sensitivity to hot or cold foods, or pain when eating hard foods.

Bisphosphonates are medications primarily prescribed for postmenopausal and glucocorticoid-induced osteoporosis and multiple myeloma; intravenous use is sometimes prescribed during chemotherapy for cancer. These drugs decrease bone turnover and

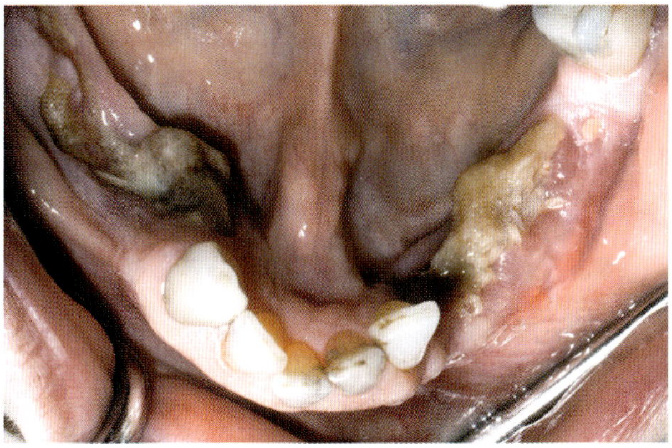

• **Figure 17.7** Bisphosphonate-associated osteonecrosis of mandibular arch. (Reproduced with permission from Damm DD, Bouquot JE, Neville BW, et al. *Oral and Maxillofacial Pathology*. 3rd ed. St. Louis, MO: Saunders; 2009.)

inhibit the bone's reparative ability. A growing concern for patients receiving bisphosphonates is the risk for **osteonecrosis** (destruction and death of bone tissue due to lack of blood flow to the area) after invasive dental procedures (Fig. 17.7). Patients at risk for osteonecrosis usually have a history of large doses of intravenous bisphosphonates (although patients taking oral bisphosphonates for long periods may also be at risk) with poor oral health requiring invasive dental procedures (e.g., extractions or dental surgery) or mechanical trauma.[12,13]

DENTAL CONSIDERATIONS

Assessment

- *Physical:* Postmenopausal changes involving bone; osteoporosis/osteopenia.
- *Dietary:* Variety and a well-balanced meal plan.

Interventions

- Encourage consultation with a health care provider to evaluate bone mineral density, possibly with dual-energy x-ray absorptiometry.
- As a part of the health care team, the dental professional can explain oral concerns related to bisphosphonate use and risk of osteonecrosis of the jaw.
- If necessary, chlorhexidine rinses, systemic antibiotics, and analgesics may be used for dental treatment.
- Resorption of the edentulous alveolar ridge requires frequent relining of the mandibular denture to avoid oral lesions and ensure the ability to masticate food.
- Provide counseling for tobacco cessation, if necessary (see Chapter 19, *Health Application 19*).

Evaluation

- The patient seeks medical guidance and adheres to prescribed recommendations.

NUTRITIONAL DIRECTIONS

- Dietary supplementation of calcium and vitamin D may slow bone loss or increase bone mass.
- Avoid excessive alcohol consumption.

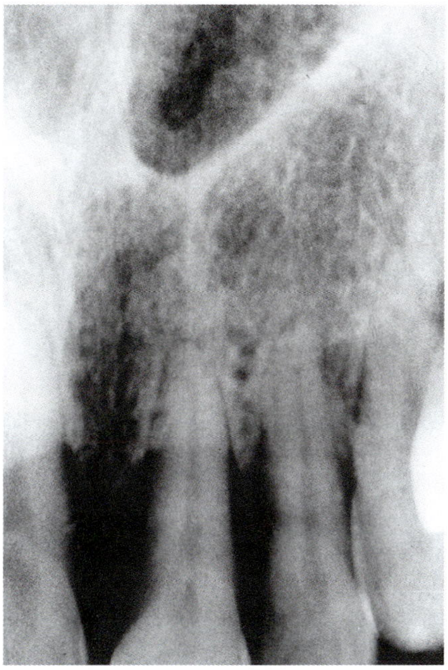

• **Figure 17.8** Alveolar bone loss in diabetes. (Reproduced with permission from Ibsen OAC, Phelan JA. *Oral Pathology for the Dental Hygienist*. 6th ed. St. Louis, MO: Saunders; 2014.)

• 3 Ps
• Polydipsia – ↑ thirst
• Polyphagia – ↑ hunger
• Polyuria – ↑ urination

Metabolic Problems

Diabetes Mellitus

Current evidence supports an interrelationship between diabetes and oral health problems. Type 2 diabetes and risk of periodontitis are correlated.[14] Periodontal disease is considered another long-term complication associated with diabetes, along with neuropathy and/or nephropathy. Studies are inconsistent in regard to the impact of periodontal treatment on improving glycemic control, but because periodontal disease is an infection, evidence indicates that periodontitis may be a risk factor for poor glycemic control.[14,15] Poorly controlled diabetes results in more severe periodontal disease and alveolar bone loss even in children and adolescents and may contribute to the progression of diabetes (Fig. 17.8).

Patients with uncontrolled or undiagnosed diabetes may have a characteristic fruity-smelling breath (more prevalent in type 1 diabetes), increased thirst, unexplained weight loss, or frequent urination. These symptoms are associated with elevated blood glucose levels. However, patients may be asymptomatic. Diabetes mellitus and nutrition recommendations are discussed in Chapter 7, *Health Application 7*.

Resistance to infections in these patients is lowered and the normal healing process is slow. In poorly controlled diabetes, minor trauma to the gingiva may result in extensive tissue necrosis with eventual denudation of the underlying bone and the possibility of osteonecrosis. Treatment of oral problems should be reserved until the diabetes is under good control.

Xerostomia is also prevalent and is partially responsible for altered taste, general tenderness or burning of the mucosa, and carious lesions, all of which may affect nutrient intake. Patients with longstanding, poorly controlled diabetes are at risk of developing oral candidiasis (Fig. 17.9), partly due to increased glucose levels in saliva, which provide a substrate for fungal growth.

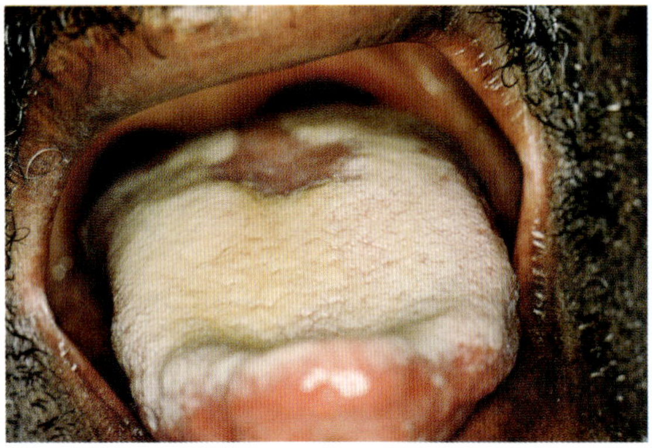

• **Figure 17.9** Oral candidiasis. (Reproduced with permission from Swartz MH. *Textbook of Physical Diagnosis: History and Examination*. 7th ed. Philadelphia, PA: Saunders: 2014.)

DENTAL CONSIDERATIONS

Assessment

- *Physical:* Polyuria, polydipsia, xerostomia, weight loss, weakness, ketosis, or asymptomatic.
- *Dietary:* Polyphagia (increased hunger); adherence to prescribed lifestyle modifications, particularly fruit and vegetable intake.

Interventions

- Dental professionals can have a significant, positive effect on the oral and general health of patients with diabetes mellitus.
- Educate patients with diabetes about oral manifestations (e.g., xerostomia) and complications (e.g., periodontitis and oral candidiasis) to promote proper oral health behaviors. Few dental and periodontal changes and no oral mucosal changes are observed in individuals with well-controlled diabetes.
- To prevent hypoglycemia during dental treatment, the patient at risk of low blood glucose levels must eat at the usual time and take prescribed medications.
- Patients taking insulin or an oral diabetes medication in which hypoglycemia can occur may require at least 15 g of a carbohydrate source to bring blood glucose levels to a normal range.
- Some oral diabetes medications (e.g., α-glucosidase inhibitor) do not cause hypoglycemia by themselves; however, they are often combined with an oral agent that does. In this scenario, the patient may require a glucose source. Have 3 to 4 glucose tablets available for such events.
- When working with individuals who have diabetes, watch for the following warning signs:
  - gingival bleeding when brushing, flossing or probing
  - red, swollen, or tender gingiva
  - oral candidiasis
  - xerostomia
  - suppuration
  - halitosis
  - recession
  - mobile teeth
  - malocclusion
  - changes in the fit of partial dentures or bridges
  - white or red patches on gingiva, tongue, cheeks, or roof of mouth
  - pain when chewing
  - sensitivity to cold, hot, or sweet
  - demineralized areas
- Periodontal infections may need to be managed with systemic antibiotic therapy and topical antimicrobials.
- Because of the risk of periodontal disease, meticulous daily oral self-care is imperative in conjunction with regular supportive periodontal therapy.
- Request patients bring their blood glucose monitor to appointments to check the blood glucose level. Before a dental procedure begins, the patient's blood glucose level should be between 70 and 200 mg/dL. Long and stressful appointments may require testing during the appointment. Testing at the end of the appointment is also suggested; individuals with blood glucose values of less than 70 mg/dL should be treated before leaving the dental office.

Evaluation

- The patient's fasting blood glucose levels are normal, and the glycated hemoglobin A1c is less than 7.0%, indicating that the diabetes is well controlled.[16]

NUTRITIONAL DIRECTIONS

- Read labels carefully for sources of carbohydrates and choose predominantly complex carbohydrates. Foods labeled "sugar free" may contain carbohydrates other than sucrose.

Hypopituitarism

The pituitary gland releases seven different hormones, including antidiuretic hormone, growth hormone, thyroid-stimulating hormone, and the sex hormones. Hypopituitarism may occur congenitally. In childhood hypopituitarism, decreased skeletal growth results in disproportionate retardation of mandibular growth. Prepubertal hypopituitarism, or decreased production of growth hormone, is usually caused by pressure from a cyst or tumor. Because of normal-size teeth erupting into the small mandible and maxilla, proper alignment is impossible. In addition to delayed eruption, malocclusion is the principal oral problem.

Hypopituitarism may also occur secondarily to a tumor, head trauma, stroke, radiation, or infections of the brain. Symptoms of hypopituitarism in adults include poor appetite, weight loss, low blood pressure, fatigue, headache, and visual disturbances.

Cushing Syndrome

Pharmacologic use of corticosteroids and endogenous secretion of excess cortisol, as seen in Cushing syndrome, results in a state of hypercortisolism. Physical signs of Cushing syndrome include upper body obesity; round face; increased neck size; relatively slender arms and legs; high blood pressure; glucose intolerance or diabetes; muscle weakness; thin, fragile skin that bruises easily; **hirsutism** (excessive hair growth); osteoporosis; and depression. Muscle weakness resulting from excess amounts of cortisol may affect muscles used for mastication and the tongue. The presence of diabetes and osteoporosis may affect management of periodontal disease and associated bone loss.

Hypothyroidism

Hypothyroidism may be related to (a) inadequate consumption of iodine, (b) an inborn error of metabolism, (c) high intake of goitrogens, (d) treatment of hyperthyroidism (surgical excision, irradiation, antithyroid drugs), (e) thyroid gland disorder, or (f) deficient secretion of thyrotropin (thyroid-stimulating hormone) by the pituitary gland. **Goitrogens** are chemicals present in broccoli, kale, kohlrabi, cabbage, rutabagas, turnips, cauliflower, Brussels sprouts, horseradish, and soybeans that inhibit thyroid uptake of iodine. When hypothyroidism occurs at birth or in young children,

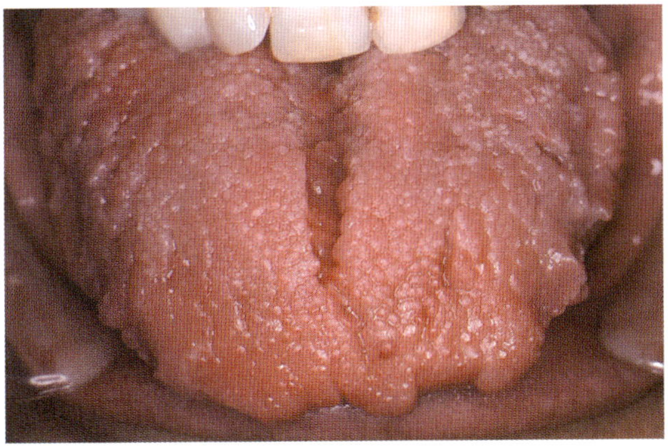

• **Figure 17.10** In hypothyroidism, the large tongue often protrudes from the mouth, showing indentation on the lateral borders caused by pressure from the teeth. (Reproduced with permission from Damm DD, Bouquot JE, Neville BW, et al. *Oral and Maxillofacial Pathology*. 3rd ed. St. Louis, MO: Saunders; 2009.)

the child is short in stature and has intellectual disabilities. Poor muscle tone results in a **macroglossia** (large, protruding) tongue, showing indentations on the lateral borders caused by pressure from the teeth (Fig. 17.10), and a tendency to choke. Eruption of the teeth is delayed, causing severe malocclusion, which makes proper oral hygiene difficult. Additionally, it places the patient at increased risk of dental caries and periodontal disease.

When hypothyroidism occurs in an adult, the tongue becomes enlarged and has decreased flexibility. Gingivitis and chronic periodontal disease may be a result of the patient's lack of oral hygiene care.

Hyperparathyroidism

Hyperparathyroidism results from hypersecretion of the parathyroid hormone, leading to alterations in calcium, phosphorus, and bone metabolism. Primary hyperthyroidism is seen more often in women older than 50 years of age. As a result of improved screening of serum calcium levels with routine laboratory tests, most cases of hyperparathyroidism are identified and treated before severe skeletal disease occurs. Clinical manifestations result from increased osteoclastic bone resorption, decreasing bone integrity. Systemic bone disturbances are reflected in the mouth by jaw enlargement and reduced bone density. In the terminal stage of the bone remodeling process, **brown tumors** (giant cell tumor replacement of bone as evidenced radiologically) may occur on the maxilla, palate, and mandible in addition to femur fractures.[17] These brown tumors may cause discomfort and may affect the patient's ability to consume an adequate diet but are normalized following treatment.

Renal Disease

The kidney is the primary organ that eliminates significant amounts of waste products; metabolic and endocrine functions are also affected by kidney disease. Progressive loss of nephrons in the kidney leads to chronic failure. When kidney function diminishes, complications arise as by-products accumulate from protein metabolism, and alterations occur in electrolyte levels and acid–base balance. Patients with renal disease may be on dialysis while awaiting a kidney transplant.

Because of calcium–phosphorus imbalances, various changes in bones are observed—a syndrome called **renal osteodystrophy**. This term describes various changes in bones associated with renal failure, such as classic hyperparathyroidism, osteomalacia, osteoporosis, and sometimes **osteosclerosis** (hardening or abnormal density of bone).

Manifestations occurring in the teeth and periodontium include delayed eruption, enamel hypoplasia, loss of the lamina dura, widening of the periodontal ligament, severe periodontal destruction, tooth mobility, drifting, petechiae of the oral mucosa, and pulp calcifications. Numerous manifestations are seen in the bone, such as bone radiolucent fibrocystic lesions, metastatic soft tissue calcifications, decreased trabeculation and thickness of cortical bone, jaw fracture after trauma or surgery, brown tumors, and abnormal bone healing after extraction.[18,19]

Nutritional care for these individuals is extremely complex. Anorexia is often present because of dietary restrictions, uremia, and bad taste experienced by many patients with chronic renal disease. High-quality, low protein intake is recommended to reduce nitrogen waste products (urea) and to minimize accumulation in the blood between dialysis treatments. In addition to protein, intake of minerals and electrolytes (e.g., sodium, potassium, and phosphorus) must be adjusted; adequate energy intake must be maintained; and potentially harmful intake of phosphorus, magnesium, aluminum, and some vitamins must be avoided. Fluid intake must be carefully monitored to prevent excess fluid buildup, which has a negative impact on blood pressure. For this reason, nutritional counseling should be left to an RDN who specializes in renal care.

The oral cavity reflects many signs of systemic involvement. Platelet abnormalities may result in gingival bleeding and bruising. Anemia is common; thus, gingival tissues may be pale in color. Other oral manifestations of chronic renal failure include complaints of a bad taste; malodor from urea buildup; xerostomia from fluid restriction; a variety of oral mucosal lesions (e.g., [inflammation of the mouth], lichen planus, oral hairy **leukoplakia** [an asymptomatic white, yellow, or gray patch or plaque on the oral mucosa that cannot be removed by scraping or rubbing]—Fig. 17.11); black hairy tongue, pyogenic granuloma, and nonspecific ulcerations); and oral infection (e.g., candidiasis and viral infections).[19] Periodontal disease is observed frequently in patients with poor oral hygiene habits leading to systemic problems (pneumonia) because of compromised immune status. Wound healing is slow because of general loss of tissue resistance and an inability to withstand normal traumatic insults. Evidence does not suggest an increased caries risk.

Many vitamin and mineral imbalances can develop in patients with renal disease, especially those on dialysis, due to poor appetite, depression, gastrointestinal symptoms, difficulty chewing and/or swallowing, and difficulty with grocery shopping and cooking. Also due to the dialysis process, the patient may have dietary restrictions, excretion alterations to maintain homeostasis, and **dialysate** (material that passes through the membrane during dialysis) contamination. Patients on dialysis are more likely to be deficient in water-soluble vitamins (B and C) and the minerals iron and zinc.

DENTAL CONSIDERATIONS

Assessment

- *Physical:* Oral manifestations and deteriorating physical status.
- *Dietary:* Appetite, prescribed diet, adequacy of oral intake.

Interventions

- Consult the health care provider before treatment because of a bleeding tendency as a result of platelet dysfunction and anticoagulant medication and to determine the necessity for antibiotic prophylaxis to

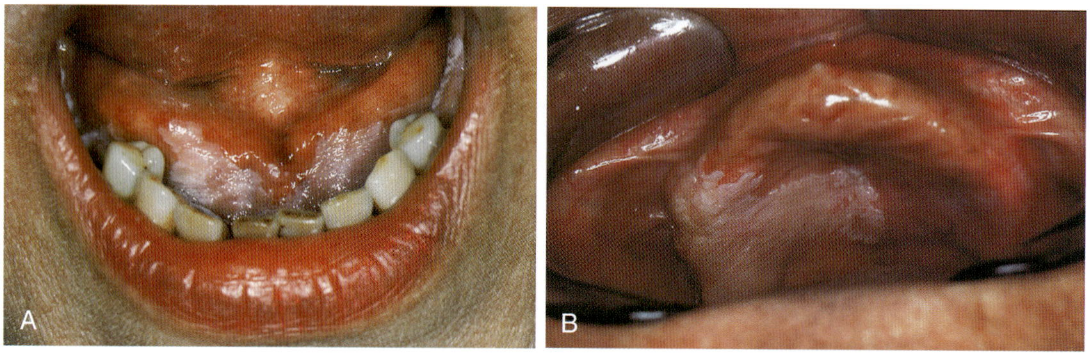

• **Figure 17.11** (A) Leukoplakia on the floor of the mouth. (B) Leukoplakia on the maxillary alveolar mucosa and palate. (Reproduced with permission from Ibsen OAC, Phelan JA. *Oral Pathology for the Dental Hygienist*. 6th ed. St. Louis, MO: Saunders; 2014.)

DENTAL CONSIDERATIONS—cont'd

prevent infective endocarditis or infection of the vascular access site for dialysis or both.

- Emphasize the importance of good oral hygiene and consequences of poor oral hygiene.
- Because of an increased occurrence of oral complications, perform a careful and thorough oral examination to detect problems early.
- Medical care becomes more complicated when systemic conditions (e.g., pneumonia and diabetes) occur secondary to oral infections.
- Because of fluid restrictions for patients on dialysis, minimize water used during treatment. Both amount of water generated when using ultrasonic and sonic instrumentation, it is essential to use high-speed evacuation.
- Patients normally require oral prophylaxis prior to being placed on the transplant waiting list.
- Consult with and refer to an RDN as needed.
- Schedule the dental appointment for a patient who is receiving dialysis the day after dialysis treatment.

Evaluation

- The patient is able to describe the relationship between the condition and effects of dietary intake on oral health.

NUTRITIONAL DIRECTIONS

- Meticulous oral hygiene and frequent recare appointments prevent or reduce oral infections commonly associated with metabolic problems that can lead to difficulties in eating certain foods.
- Antimicrobial mouth rinses are helpful to minimize possible bacterial and fungal infections.

Neuromuscular Problems

Parkinson Disease

Parkinson disease is a progressive neurologic condition characterized by involuntary muscle tremors, **bradykinesia** (slowness of movement), muscular weakness, rigidity, stooped posture, decreased fine motor coordination, masklike expression with absence of blinking, orthostatic hypotension, and a peculiar gait (rapid, short, shuffling steps with a loss of arm swing). It affects the oral cavity by causing an abnormal swallow pattern, with frequent drooling and tremor of the mandible, lips, and tongue (Fig. 17.12). Decreased voluntary muscle movement affects muscles used to masticate food. Patients with Parkinson disease may have many problems associated with feeding and receiving adequate nourishment: (a) mechanical difficulties may interfere with the transfer of food from the plate to the mouth, and (b) oral disturbances may alter normal chewing and swallowing mechanisms. These problems may necessitate a change in the form or consistency of food, or special eating utensils, or both.

Poor oral health of patients with Parkinson disease may be related to lack of muscular control both orally (affecting chewing and swallowing) and hand control (affecting use of toothbrush, toothpaste, and dental floss).

Dysphagia may affect the oral phase of swallow or the pharyngeal stage of swallow, thus causing problems such as pneumonia, dehydration, and malnutrition. The results include drooling of saliva, holding food in the mouth for extended periods, inability to tear food apart and mix it with saliva, food or liquid leaking from the nose, regurgitation, a gurgly voice, and food coating the tongue and palate after swallowing. Because of poor tongue control, a flowing, noncohesive bolus may spill over the base of the tongue before a swallow reflex is initiated, increasing risk for aspiration.

Another common oral implication of Parkinson disease is salivary dysfunction (xerostomia and drooling), leading to a disruption of microflora and increasing the risk of periodontal disease and caries. Unfortunately, the excess saliva does not relieve the symptoms of dry mouth. Dysphagia, burning mouth, changes in taste and smell, and increased plaque biofilm are also related to challenges with oral self-care.[20,21]

The Parkinson's Disease Foundation recommends eating a balanced diet to maintain a healthy weight, maintaining bone health, bowel regularity, and balancing medications and food. Frequently, patients with Parkinson disease lose weight during early stages of the disease related to avoidance of solid foods and a decrease in food intake because of eating difficulties. Attention to subtle cues can ensure that the patient does not lose a significant amount of weight and muscle mass. Nutritional supplements and high calorie foods can be encouraged.[22]

Medications are usually initiated when symptoms affect quality of life or affect work performance and disrupt an individual's daily activities. Recent research is working to find neuroprotective therapies to prevent the progression of disease since current medications only control symptoms.

The principle medication used for Parkinson disease is levodopa, which has drug–nutrient interactions with protein, reducing effectiveness of the drug. Despite these interactions, adequate protein intake is crucial. Xerostomia, nausea, and poor appetite resulting from medications can also negatively affect dietary intake. Challenges in maintaining body weight and health may necessitate consultation with an RDN to tailor a diet meeting the patient's needs.

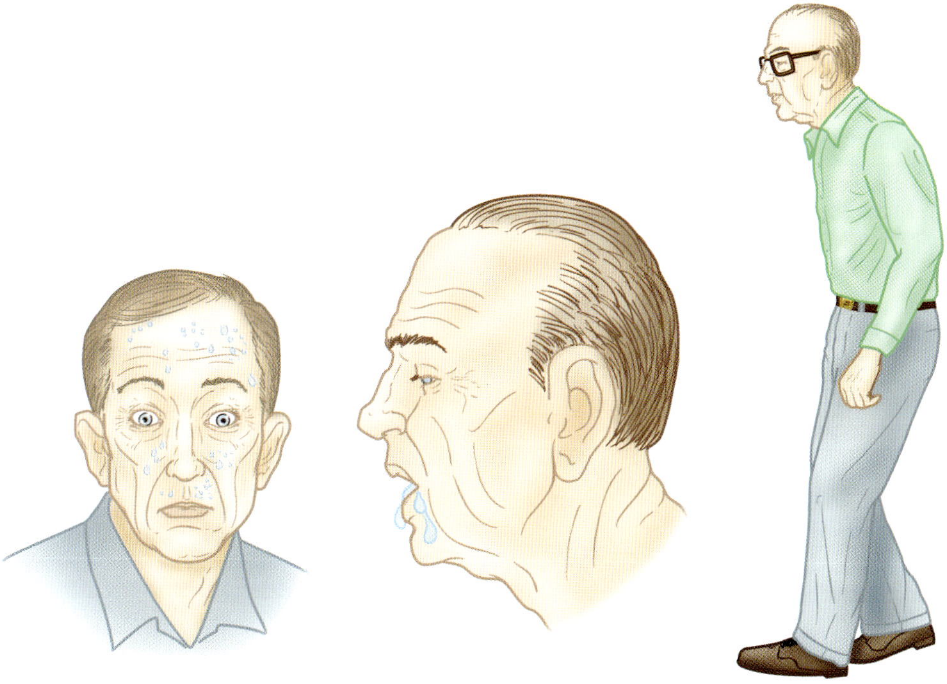

• **Figure 17.12** Characteristics of Parkinson disease. (A) Masklike appearance, stare and excessive sweating. (B) Drooling with excessive saliva. (C) Rapid, short and shuffling steps with low arm swinging. (Reproduced with permission from Seidel HM et al. Mosby's Guide to Physical Examination. 6th ed. St. Louis, MO: Mosby; 2011.)

Parkinson disease cannot be prevented. However, epidemiologic data suggest that dietary patterns with high intake of fruits, vegetables, legumes, whole grains, nuts, fish, and poultry; low intake of saturated fat; and moderate intake or abstinence of alcohol may protect against Parkinson disease. This is one more reason why dental hygienists need to encourage healthy eating.

Developmental Disabilities

Many disabilities may impair development of normal feeding reflexes (discussed in Chapter 14) and coordination of these reflexes with respiration. These feeding reflexes may be absent or weak and difficult to elicit. Abnormal oral–motor patterns and difficulties associated with feeding may result when structural malformations such as cleft palate, macroglossia, and **micrognathia** (abnormally small jaw) are present. Neuromuscular diseases, such as cerebral palsy, muscular dystrophy, and Down syndrome, may be associated with abnormal oral-motor development. The feeding experience, which is normally pleasurable, becomes a frustrating, time-consuming situation for everyone involved in the patient's care.

Oral–motor impairment may become evident during the spoon-feeding phase of feeding development. Tongue retraction, tonic bite reflex, tongue thrust, and persistence of a suckling pattern interfere with placing a spoon in the mouth and result in loss of food from the mouth (Table 17.2). A patient with tonic bite reflex may clamp down on a spoon inserted in the mouth and be unable to release the bite. Attempting to free the spoon by pulling is ineffective and may cause continued biting.

With tongue thrusting and tongue retraction, the tongue is unable to form a bolus and move it to the back of the mouth. Placing food in the mouth can be difficult with a severe tongue thrust, which also may affect the individual's ability to suck, chew, and swallow.

With lip retraction, lips may be unable to remove food from the spoon, and drinking or sucking may be impossible. Sensory defensiveness is associated with a strong emotional reaction to the unwanted tactile stimuli and can result in a severe food intake problem.

Inadequate chewing skills are associated with jaw and tongue thrusting, hyperactive or hypoactive gag reflex, abnormal intraoral sensation, and poor tongue lateralization. Oral–motor impairments make providing optimal nutritional care very difficult. Patients with an oral–motor problem or an inability to self-feed affecting food intake are at nutritional risk.

When oral–motor impairment is extremely severe, adequate nutrition cannot be provided with oral feedings, and nutrition may be provided via gastrostomy feedings. Treatment is facilitated using an interdisciplinary team to determine the best treatment promoting development of feeding skills and providing foods in a form that can be handled safely.

Epilepsy

Epilepsy, or psychomotor seizures, in itself does not usually result in any specific oral or feeding problems. However, a popular drug used for seizure control, phenytoin, can significantly cause bone loss within a year. Gingival hyperplasia is noted with long-term phenytoin use (Fig. 17.13). When good oral self-care techniques are routinely practiced, inflammation and gingival overgrowth are reduced.

TABLE 17.2 Feeding Problems

Condition	Description
Tonic bite reflex	Strong jaw closure when teeth or gingiva are stimulated
Tongue thrust	Forceful and often repetitive protrusion of an often bunched or thick tongue in response to oral stimulation
Jaw thrust	Forceful opening of the jaw to its maximal extent during eating, drinking, attempts to speak, or general excitement
Tongue retraction	Pulling back the tongue within the oral cavity at presentation of food, spoon, or cup
Lip retraction	Pulling back the lips in a very tight, smile-like pattern at the approach of food, spoon, or cup toward the face
Sensory defensiveness	A strong adverse reaction to sensory input (touch, sound, light)

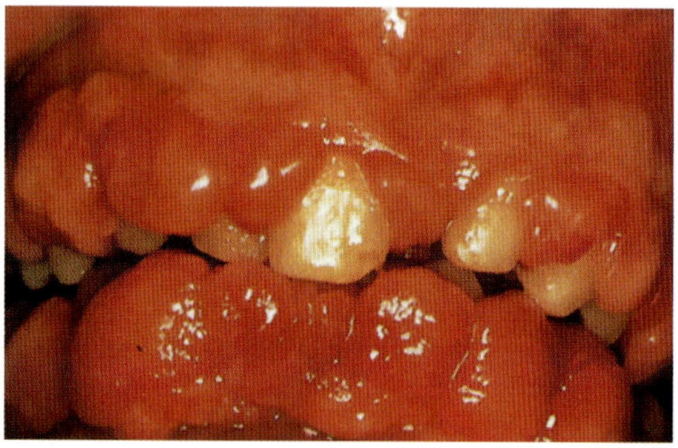

• **Figure 17.13** Hyperplasia associated with phenytoin use. (Courtesy of Barbara D. Altshuler, BSDH, MS, Clinical Assistant Professor, Texas A&M University College of Dentistry, Dallas, TX.)

Phenytoin also increases metabolism of vitamins D and K and folate, which may increase risk for loss of bone mineral density. Other dental considerations associated with phenytoin include increased incidence of infection, delayed healing, and gingival bleeding. Phenobarbital, which is also used to manage convulsions in epilepsy, may also affect bone health by increasing turnover of vitamins D and K. Despite increased need for these nutrients, supplementation of folate or vitamin B_6 may decrease bioavailability of phenytoin and must be carefully monitored by a health care provider.

DENTAL CONSIDERATIONS

Assessment

- *Physical:* Oral complications related to neuromuscular disorders; medications prescribed; nutrient supplements; orthostatic hypotension.
- *Dietary:* Adequacy of intake, signs of malnutrition.

Interventions

- Carefully assess oral status of patients taking anticonvulsants.
- To reduce stress and anxiety, keep appointments brief and relaxing.
- Encourage frequent recare visits.
- Assess saliva flow and provide tips for preventing xerostomia-associated oral problems (see Chapter 20).
- After supine positioning, have the patient with Parkinson disease sit upright for at least 2 minutes before standing to avoid orthostatic hypotension.
- Coping strategies for dysphagia, such as massaging the throat before beginning a feeding and reminding the patient to tilt the head forward before swallowing, aid swallowing problems, but become tedious and taxing for health care providers.
- For patients experiencing xerostomia, advise avoidance of alcohol, smoking, and caffeine.
- Instigate a rigorous preventive oral health regime tailored to the needs of individuals with neuromuscular problems.
- Schedule appointments at the individual's best time of day.
- Suggest dental gels, such as fluoride, and dentifrices for individuals with dysphagia rather than mouthrinses that may increase risk of aspiration.
- Refer the patient to the health care provider or RDN if nutrient supplementation is reported. Some nutrients may interfere with absorption of the prescribed medication.
- Suggest adaptations so that the patient can maintain independence for teeth or denture cleaning: for example, a mechanical toothbrush, toothbrush handle adaptations, or specialized toothbrushes, such as a Collis curve toothbrush (Fig. 17.14).

Evaluation

- The patient's dental health is maintained, and prescribed medications are taken.

NUTRITIONAL DIRECTIONS

- Check the fit of a dental prosthesis. An improper fit may impact nutritional status.
- Encourage small, frequent nutrient-dense meals and snacks for patients experiencing anorexia and weight loss. Refer to an RDN.
- Salivary substitutions and topical fluoride treatments may be recommended for patients experiencing xerostomia.
- Antimicrobial rinses are helpful to decrease the chance of bacterial and fungal infections.
- Patients with Parkinson disease are often at risk for osteoporosis. Foods high in or fortified with calcium, magnesium, and vitamins D and K may be suggested.
- Patients taking medications for Parkinson disease (e.g., levodopa or carbidopa) should take the medication at mealtime for best absorption and monitor foods high in vitamin B_6, protein and fat, as they may lengthen the time for the medication to take effect or decrease the effectiveness of the medication. Have the patient check with the health care provider on when to take the medication.
- Calcium supplements are not recommended for patients taking phenytoin and phenobarbital unless closely monitored by the health care provider because large amounts of calcium decrease bioavailability of both the drug and mineral.
- Pyridoxine and folate supplements may alter response of phenytoin and result in increased seizure activity.
- Carbamazepine (Tegretol), another popular anticonvulsant, causes xerostomia, altered taste, and oral sensitivity.

Neoplasia

Neoplasia (abnormal mass of tissue), more frequently referred to as tumors, causes problems not only in the primary site, but also in regional and remote areas. The manifestations at secondary sites away from the primary lesion may be the presenting feature in some cases. The mouth and jaw may be involved in generalized malignant disease.

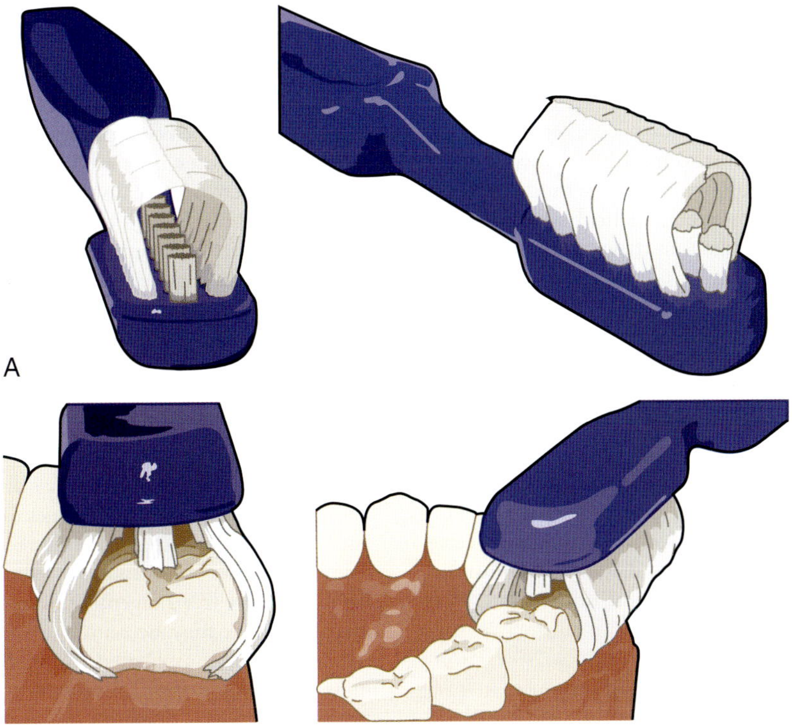

• **Figure 17.14** (A) Collis curve toothbrush. (B) Use of Collis curve toothbrush.

Nutritional requirements for patients with neoplasms are generally increased to maintain lean body mass and immune responses. Anorexia is an important symptom of an underlying neoplasm. Oral symptoms or signs may be secondary to malnutrition or nutrient deficiencies. Abnormalities in taste perception have been noted in some patients with cancer, such as an elevated threshold for sweets and a reduced threshold for bitter flavors. Altered taste sensations may be secondary to a deficiency of zinc. Hormonal factors affect the hypothalamic feeding center to reduce oral intake. Early satiety may be related to minimal digestive secretions or impaired gastric emptying.

The location of the tumor itself also may be a factor in reduced food intake, especially when the alimentary tract is affected. Intake is reduced in patients with cancer of the oral cavity, pharynx, or esophagus because of **odynophagia** (pain on swallowing) or dysphagia. Gastric cancer may lead to reduced gastric capacity or partial gastric outlet obstruction, resulting in early satiety, nausea, and vomiting.

Psychological factors undoubtedly affect appetite. Depression, grief, or anxiety resulting from the disease or its treatment may lead to poor appetite and abnormal eating behaviors.

Kaposi Sarcoma

Kaposi sarcoma is a highly malignant tumor of blood vessel origin that occurs on the skin and oral mucosa (Fig. 17.15). It is characterized by bluish-red cutaneous nodules, usually on the lower extremities, and occurs frequently in immunocompromised individuals. These lesions appear in many HIV-positive patients. Red-purple macular lesions in the mouth may progress to raised, indurated lesions with central areas of necrosis and ulceration. Lesions can cause obstruction of the esophagus, compromising food intake.

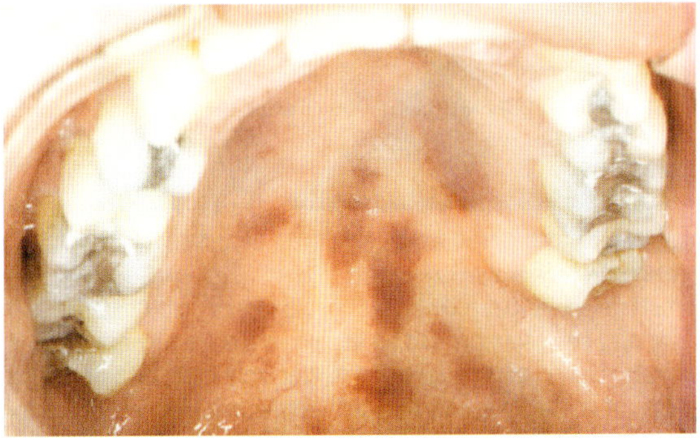

• **Figure 17.15** Kaposi sarcoma lesions on the hard palate. (Reproduced with permission from Silverman S Jr. *Color Atlas of Oral Manifestations of AIDS*. 5th ed. St. Louis, MO: Mosby; 1996.)

Leukemia

Leukemia is a generalized malignant disease characterized by distorted proliferation and development of WBCs. It is another neoplastic process with many oral manifestations that detrimentally affect food intake. Several types of **leukemia** are classified according to how quickly they progress (acute or chronic). Gingival tissues are especially susceptible to gingivitis because of an exaggerated inflammatory response to local etiologic factors: for example, calculus, plaque biofilm, and **materia alba** (soft white deposit around the necks of teeth). Rather than the normal response of chronic marginal gingivitis, the gingiva may become severely inflamed with tissue hyperplasia, areas of ulcerations, necrosis, and spontaneous bleeding. This is believed to be caused by the body's depressed immune response. Susceptibility to infection is increased and healing responses are delayed.

Cancer Treatments

Cancer treatment may include surgery, radiation therapy, chemotherapy, biologic therapy, or combinations of these modalities. **Chemotherapeutic** drugs are used to destroy malignant cells without loss of an excessive number of normal cells. Tumors involving the gastrointestinal tract affect the ability to ingest foods orally or digest and absorb nutrients adequately. Radical surgery in the oropharyngeal area may present problems in chewing and swallowing and alterations in taste sensations.

Radiation therapy significantly affects the alimentary tract. Early transient effects include general loss of appetite, nausea and vomiting, and diarrhea caused by malabsorption secondary to mucosal damage in the gastrointestinal tract. Food intake is affected because of loss of taste sensation, xerostomia, difficulty in swallowing, and a burning sensation in the mouth when the larynx or pharynx area is irradiated. A patient exposed to a food or beverage before radiation treatment or chemotherapy may associate the item with the therapy, resulting in an aversion to that particular food. Rampant caries and loss of teeth may complicate adequate dietary intake further.

Chemotherapy has more widespread effects on the body than either radiation or surgical treatment. Rapid cell turnover rate in the alimentary tract leads to stomatitis or mucositis, oral ulcerations, and decreased absorptive capacity. As a result, changes in taste sensation and learned food aversions occur.

DENTAL CONSIDERATIONS

Assessment

- *Physical:* Fatigue, caries, adequate weight, weight loss, oral ulcerations, medications.
- *Dietary:* Maintaining caloric intake, adequate fluids, food aversions (especially food groups), alterations in taste.

Interventions

- Use of an antimicrobial mouth rinse (i.e., alcohol-free chlorhexidine) may be indicated to reduce inflammation associated with cancer treatment.
- A mechanically altered (Box 19.3) or bland diet (see Chapter 19, Box 19.4) may be recommended as deemed necessary by oral conditions.
- Discuss the relationship between fermentable carbohydrate intake, effects of xerostomia, plaque biofilm formation, and caries. Caution against eating hard candy containing fermentable carbohydrates to relieve xerostomia.

Evaluation

- A dietary recall reveals adequate nutrients and calories with a minimum of fermentable carbohydrates.

NUTRITIONAL DIRECTIONS

- Small, frequent meals are appropriate to provide additional calories and to counteract nausea and vomiting.
- Meticulous oral hygiene, frequent recare appointments, and fluoride therapy are essential.
- Adequate food and fluid intake not only improve the physical response to cancer treatment but also create a more positive psychological outlook.
- Avoid foods that are hot, spicy, or acidic (e.g., citrus fruit and juices).
- Avoid alcohol-containing beverages and mouth rinses.
- Commonly used chemotherapeutic agents (bleomycin, cyclophosphamide, and methotrexate) generally cause complications such as stomatitis, nausea, vomiting, diarrhea, and anorexia.

Acquired Immunodeficiency Syndrome (AIDS)

HIV debilitates the body's immune system. Following identification of HIV antibodies in the blood, a positive diagnosis of HIV is made. This retrovirus causes a dysfunction in the genetic core of T lymphocytes or WBCs that normally function to resist infection. Retroviruses are characterized by the presence of reverse transcriptase, which interferes with production of DNA from RNA. Susceptibility to various opportunistic infections (especially *Pneumocystis carinii*, *Cryptosporidium*, *Candida*, *Mycobacterium*, and herpes simplex) and certain neoplasms (Kaposi sarcoma, non-Hodgkin lymphoma, and oral warts) is increased. These infections can appear in virtually every organ system. Because of the body's inability to fight infections, AIDS develops.

With the advent of highly active antiretroviral therapy (HAART), HIV-positive individuals no longer exhibit the classic gaunt appearance typical of wasting. Patients receiving HAART may still lose lean body mass, but because of a dramatic increase in fat cells and lipodystrophy (rearrangement of fat deposits that can be extremely disfiguring), it may be harder to diagnose. The course of HIV/AIDS is often complicated by weight loss, wasting of lean body mass, cachexia, opportunistic infections, malignancies, diarrhea, multiple nutrient deficiencies, and particularly protein-energy malnutrition. The cause of malnutrition is multifactorial and may involve inadequate intake, malabsorption, or hypermetabolism.

At present, nutritional status is not known to affect the length of time for HIV infections to progress to AIDS. Good nutrition does not cure AIDS, but malnutrition may hasten progression of the disease and affect outcome. Many oral problems in HIV-positive patients have predictive value for development of AIDS because of their effect on appetite and food intake. Adequate dietary intake can help maintain strength, comfort, and level of functioning. Providing optimal nutrition improves resistance to opportunistic infections. Good oral hygiene improves nutritional status by promoting a desirable environment that enhances food intake.

More than 30 different oral manifestations of HIV disease have been reported since the AIDS epidemic began in the 1980s. However, treatment of oral problems should not be avoided when a person is HIV positive. Individuals with a compromised immune system should practice preventive measures to avoid bacterial infections evidenced in dental caries and periodontal disease. A routine plan of care to prevent development of oral health problems is particularly important.

Anorexia may be attributed to respiratory and other infections, fever, dysgeusia, gastrointestinal complications, adverse effects of drugs, and depression. Specific nutritional deficiencies may depress appetite and exacerbate anorectic behavior. Oral and esophageal pain during eating also may decrease intake.

Several varieties of oral candidiasis are prevalent in HIV-positive individuals; *Candida* infection is a sign of immune dysfunction and should be reported to the health care provider. Oral candidiasis produces pain and inhibits production of saliva. Pharyngeal or esophageal lesions of Kaposi sarcoma may cause obstruction, whereas herpetic ulcerations or other ulcerations on the tongue or esophagus can cause difficulty in swallowing. Herpetic ulcerations are painful ulcerations of the oral mucosa with a red center and yellow border. The development of thrush may be attributed to herpes virus, candidiasis, chemotherapy, or drugs such as interferon.

Oral hairy leukoplakia (Fig. 17.16) is found predominantly on the lateral borders of the tongue or occasionally on the buccal or

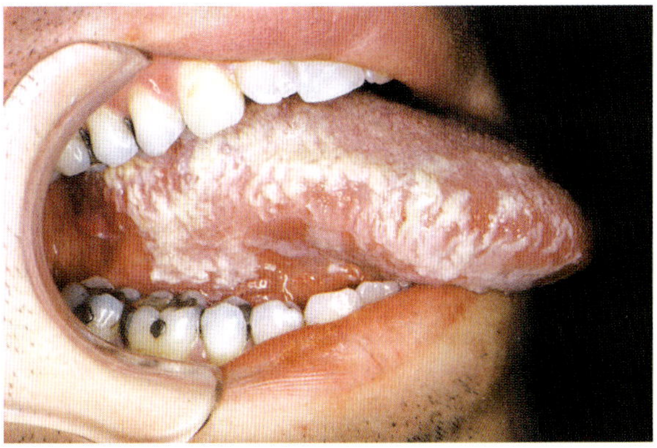

• **Figure 17.16** Hairy leukoplakia. (Reproduced with permission from Silverman S Jr. *Color Atlas of Oral Manifestations of AIDS*. 5th ed. St. Louis, MO: Mosby; 1996.)

labial mucosa in patients who are HIV positive. The white lesions or filamentous growth do not rub off. HIV-infected patients frequently have ulcerations that resemble aphthous ulcers that appear as well-circumscribed ulcers with an erythematous margin. These painful ulcers may become extremely large and necrotic; they may persist for several weeks.

The level of HIV control by HAART determines how the patient responds to periodontal therapy. Patients who are not well controlled may not respond normally to standard periodontal therapy; a mild case of gingivitis can progress to severe periodontitis in a few months, resulting in the need for extraction of affected teeth. Untreated periodontal disease can lead to necrotizing ulcerative periodontitis because of the compromised immune system. Necrotizing ulcerative periodontitis is a severe form of periodontal disease with rapid loss of soft tissue and bone (including exposure of the bone) and by rapid deterioration of tooth attachment and loss of surrounding teeth (see Chapter 19).

HIV-positive patients may have parotid gland swelling accompanied by xerostomia. Spontaneous oral bleeding may be associated with small purpuric lesions or ecchymoses or gingivitis.

DENTAL CONSIDERATIONS

Assessment

- *Physical:* Weight change, oral infections and malignancies, candidiasis, periodontitis, viral load.
- *Dietary:* Oral sensitivity, adequate levels of all nutrients.

Interventions

- Perform a careful intra- and extraoral examination to identify signs of HIV-infected patients so they can be treated appropriately.
- Individualize the care plan and treatment for each AIDS patient related to special needs.
- Systemic antibiotic therapy may be indicated for infections.
- Oral lesions will affect nutritional status because of discomfort in the mouth. Offer suggestions for palliative care (antimicrobial mouth rinse, antifungal lozenge or mouthwash; pain medication; and nonacidic foods) that will not exacerbate lesions.
- Consultation with the health care provider is necessary to gather information about laboratory values (e.g., platelet count, WBC count, and viral load), medications, and history of opportunistic infections, and to determine if antibiotic prophylaxis is needed.
- Encourage using a nonalcoholic antimicrobial rinse and antifungal and antiviral agents as prescribed by the dentist or health care provider.
- Encourage and try to motivate the patient to maintain the highest possible level of oral self-care and regular preventive dental care.
- Refer the patient to an RDN for medical nutrition therapy.
- Side effects of HAART include diarrhea, nausea, and vomiting. Frequent vomiting can cause enamel erosion. Preventive dental care and use of topical fluoride therapy at home is essential.

Evaluation

- The patient exhibits increased attention to oral hygiene care and is maintaining current weight.

NUTRITIONAL DIRECTIONS

- To promote healing and maintenance of oral tissues, encourage adequate nutrient intake. The *Dietary Guidelines* recommendation to decrease fat intake may be inappropriate for patients with HIV/AIDS.
- To add calories and protein, add nuts and dried fruits to hot and cold cereals; use cream instead of milk; add ground meat or poultry or grated cheese to soups, sauces, casseroles, and vegetable dishes; use peanut butter on fruit or crackers; dip vegetables in sour cream mixes; use nutritional supplements or instant breakfast drinks as snacks.
- Limit caffeine-containing and alcohol-containing beverages if xerostomia is present.

Mental Health Problems

Anorexia Nervosa, Bulimia Nervosa

More than 10 million Americans are affected by serious eating disorders. Although anorexia nervosa and bulimia nervosa are two different conditions, they are symptomatically related (Fig. 17.17). Anorexia nervosa is a disease primarily affecting adolescent girls and young women who have an exaggerated, intense fear of becoming fat. Zealous self-imposed restriction leads to extreme weight loss.

Individuals with anorexia nervosa may be described as achievement-oriented perfectionists who seek to rule their lives by refusing to eat in an effort to control their bodies. These young individuals are generally surrounded with all the evidences of success. Individuals with anorexia nervosa may become excellent gourmet cooks, spending hours planning menus, finding special recipes, and shopping for exotic ingredients. In-depth knowledge of nutritional and caloric value of foods is commonly exhibited by individuals with anorexia.

Diagnosis of anorexia nervosa includes weight loss equal to or exceeding 15% below expected or original body weight, rigid dieting, amenorrhea (for women), and an excessive desire for slimness with a distorted body image. Dental complications in advanced stages of malnutrition are generally observed in patients with anorexia nervosa.

Bulimia nervosa occurs more frequently than anorexia nervosa. Bulimia is an eating disorder that is not associated with significant weight loss. An individual with bulimia might even be normal weight or slightly overweight and appear healthy. Bulimia is characterized by intentional, although not necessarily controllable, secret **binges** (periods of overeating) usually followed by **purging** (a means of counteracting the effects of overindulgence).

Typically, bulimia and anorexia nervosa occur for the same reason: fear of becoming fat. However, individuals with bulimia try to control this fear by repeatedly restraining eating, but this backfires and leads to bingeing and purging. Individuals with

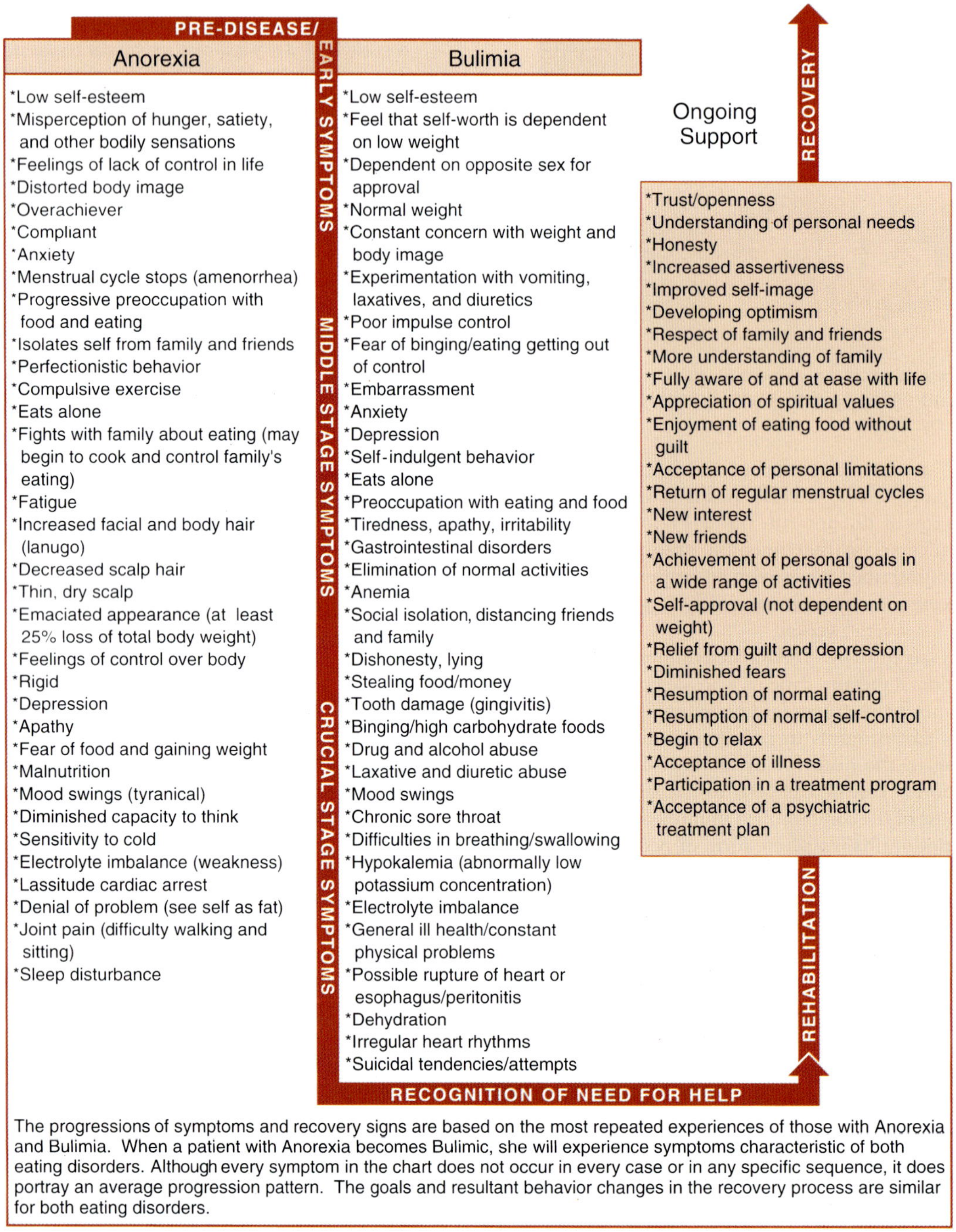
PRE-DISEASE/
EARLY SYMPTOMS
Anorexia
*Low self-esteem
*Misperception of hunger, satiety, and other bodily sensations
*Feelings of lack of control in life
*Distorted body image
*Overachiever
*Compliant
*Anxiety
*Menstrual cycle stops (amenorrhea)
*Progressive preoccupation with food and eating
*Isolates self from family and friends
*Perfectionistic behavior
*Compulsive exercise
*Eats alone
*Fights with family about eating (may begin to cook and control family's eating)
*Fatigue
*Increased facial and body hair (lanugo)
*Decreased scalp hair
*Thin, dry scalp
*Emaciated appearance (at least 25% loss of total body weight)
*Feelings of control over body
*Rigid
*Depression
*Apathy
*Fear of food and gaining weight
*Malnutrition
*Mood swings (tyranical)
*Diminished capacity to think
*Sensitivity to cold
*Electrolyte imbalance (weakness)
*Lassitude cardiac arrest
*Denial of problem (see self as fat)
*Joint pain (difficulty walking and sitting)
*Sleep disturbance
MIDDLE STAGE SYMPTOMS
CRUCIAL STAGE SYMPTOMS
Bulimia
*Low self-esteem
*Feel that self-worth is dependent on low weight
*Dependent on opposite sex for approval
*Normal weight
*Constant concern with weight and body image
*Experimentation with vomiting, laxatives, and diuretics
*Poor impulse control
*Fear of binging/eating getting out of control
*Embarrassment
*Anxiety
*Depression
*Self-indulgent behavior
*Eats alone
*Preoccupation with eating and food
*Tiredness, apathy, irritability
*Gastrointestinal disorders
*Elimination of normal activities
*Anemia
*Social isolation, distancing friends and family
*Dishonesty, lying
*Stealing food/money
*Tooth damage (gingivitis)
*Binging/high carbohydrate foods
*Drug and alcohol abuse
*Laxative and diuretic abuse
*Mood swings
*Chronic sore throat
*Difficulties in breathing/swallowing
*Hypokalemia (abnormally low potassium concentration)
*Electrolyte imbalance
*General ill health/constant physical problems
*Possible rupture of heart or esophagus/peritonitis
*Dehydration
*Irregular heart rhythms
*Suicidal tendencies/attempts
RECOGNITION OF NEED FOR HELP
REHABILITATION
RECOVERY
Ongoing Support
*Trust/openness
*Understanding of personal needs
*Honesty
*Increased assertiveness
*Improved self-image
*Developing optimism
*Respect of family and friends
*More understanding of family
*Fully aware of and at ease with life
*Appreciation of spiritual values
*Enjoyment of eating food without guilt
*Acceptance of personal limitations
*Return of regular menstrual cycles
*New interest
*New friends
*Achievement of personal goals in a wide range of activities
*Self-approval (not dependent on weight)
*Relief from guilt and depression
*Diminished fears
*Resumption of normal eating
*Resumption of normal self-control
*Begin to relax
*Acceptance of illness
*Participation in a treatment program
*Acceptance of a psychiatric treatment plan
The progressions of symptoms and recovery signs are based on the most repeated experiences of those with Anorexia and Bulimia. When a patient with Anorexia becomes Bulimic, she will experience symptoms characteristic of both eating disorders. Although every symptom in the chart does not occur in every case or in any specific sequence, it does portray an average progression pattern. The goals and resultant behavior changes in the recovery process are similar for both eating disorders.

• **Figure 17.17** Anorexia nervosa and bulimia: a multidimensional profile.

bulimia exhibit many of the same characteristics as individuals with anorexia, but those with bulimia are more sociable, while underneath they feel profoundly separated from other people. Usually, they appear very mature, but this is a defense mechanism to hide insecurities. Appearance is extremely important to them.

Individuals with bulimia acknowledge their eating behaviors are not normal. They have strong appetites and may binge several times a day, with intakes of 1200 cal or more per episode. Binges may last minutes to several hours and may be planned or spontaneous, but ordinarily are related to stress. Compulsive stealing of food and money to buy food is another common characteristic. Individuals binge on mainly high-carbohydrate, easily digested food.

These binges occur most often in the late afternoon or evening and end with purging. Self-induced vomiting is the main method of purging. Vomiting may be induced by sticking a finger or other object down the throat, applying external pressure to the neck, or drinking **syrup of ipecac** (emetic drug). Eventually, some individuals with bulimia can vomit by merely contracting their abdominal muscles.

In addition to poor overall health status, nutritional effects of bulimia stem from purging and the method employed for purging. Frequent episodes of self-induced vomiting can cause oral cavity trauma; bruises and irritations in the oral cavity may be observed. Frequent vomiting can cause erosion of tooth enamel (predominantly on the lingual surfaces of the maxillary teeth; Fig. 17.18), dentin

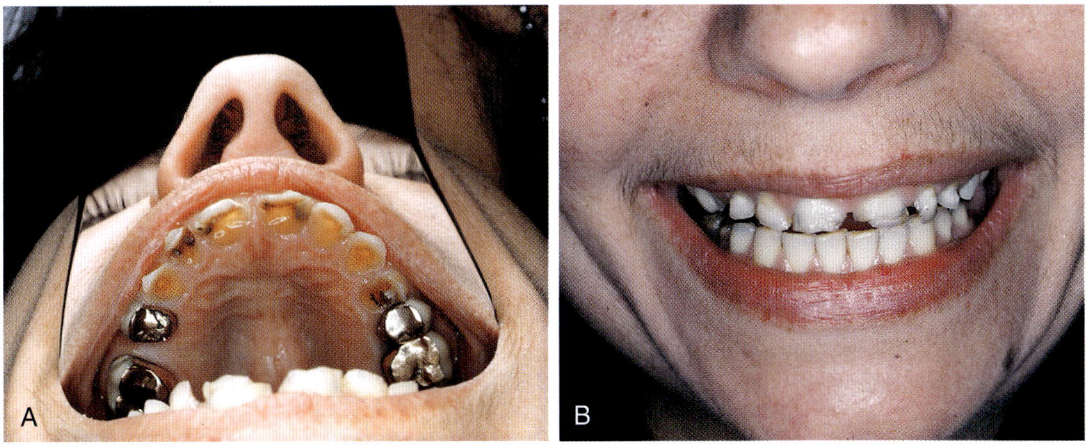

• **Figure 17.18** (A) and (B) Enamel erosion caused by bulimia nervosa. (Reproduced with permission from Ibsen OAC, Phelan JA. *Oral Pathology for the Dental Hygienist*. 6th ed. St. Louis, MO: Saunders; 2014.)

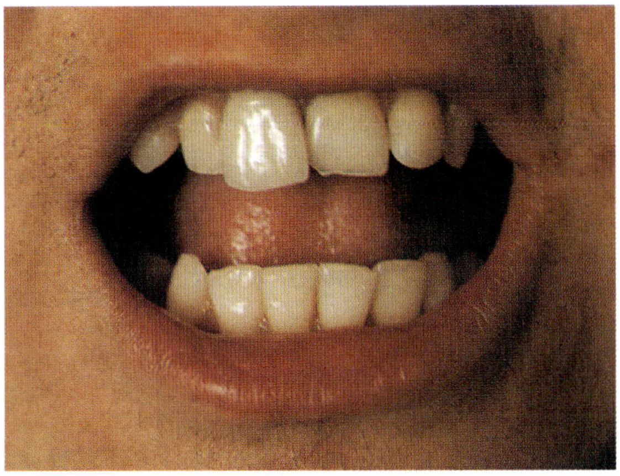

• **Figure 17.19** Bulimia nervosa. Incisor was capped because of dental caries. Continued vomiting has diminished the size of the surrounding teeth, while prosthesis remains unchanged. (Courtesy Dr. J. Treasure. From McLaren DS. *A Colour Atlas and Text of Diet-Related Disorders*. 2nd ed. London: Mosby-Yearbook; 1992.)

hypersensitivity, and enlargement of the parotid glands. Other signs can include lips that are red, dry, and cracked, and lesions on oral soft tissue that bleed easily. Erosion can occur in as short as 6 months after continued regurgitation (Fig. 17.19). An estimated 50% to 70% of those dealing with the challenges of frequent vomiting may experience erosion. A recent study suggested that minimal exposure to acid in some may cause erosion, while others may never develop dental erosions despite extensive exposure to acid.[23] Teeth may be sensitive to extreme temperatures. Signs of malnutrition may also be present and observed during an oral examination (e.g., dry brittle hair, spoon-shaped nails, and cheilosis). Dental hygienists should not falsely assume that oral problems result from poor dental hygiene practices; rather, these oral problems develop secondary to frequent vomiting. Another classic sign of bulimia associated with self-induced vomiting is the presence of abrasions and calluses on dorsal surfaces of fingers and hands secondary to friction of the teeth.

A third category of eating disorders is binge-eating disorder. It is defined as frequent episodes of eating significant quantities of food, even when not hungry. Accompanying feelings include lack of control, guilt, embarrassment, or disgust.[24]

Successful outcomes require comprehensive treatment by a multidisciplinary team that addresses individual psychosocial, nutritional, and medical problems. The team usually comprises a psychotherapist or psychiatrist, RDN, nurse, social worker, and health care provider. This pooling of specialties provides effective treatment for the patient and a support system for team members when difficult decisions are necessary or progress seems slow.

DENTAL CONSIDERATIONS

Assessment

- *Physical:* Signs of malnutrition (e.g., thinning hair, always cold, facial hair), fatigue, dehydration, trauma to the soft palate from fingernails or objects used to induce vomiting, location of enamel erosion, parotid enlargement, weight changes.
- *Dietary:* High-carbohydrate diet, very-low-caloric intake or other unusual dietary habits, obsession with diet or weight.

Interventions

- Goals of the dental hygiene treatment care plan for patients with psychiatric disorders are to realistically maintain oral health and to prevent and control oral disease.
- An increased caries rate can be indicative of high-carbohydrate bingeing, low pH of saliva from vomiting, and xerostomia. Office and home fluoride therapy should be recommended.
- Discuss specific characteristics observed in the dental assessment with the patient.
- Treatment of an eating disorder involves a multidisciplinary team of health care professionals, including the dental professional. It is the responsibility of the dental hygienist to recognize the signs and symptoms of a suspected eating disorder, refer patients to a health care provider or a local hospital or eating disorder facility for assessment and treatment, and document the findings and recommendations.
- Chronic use of syrup of ipecac can affect skeletal muscle and cardiac action, which can result in congestive heart failure, arrhythmia, and sudden death.
- Encourage meticulous oral hygiene.

Evaluation

- The patient is making realistic changes by protecting the hard and soft tissues, being plaque-free, and being treated by a multidisciplinary health care team.

NUTRITIONAL DIRECTIONS

- To prevent further damage to teeth, caution the patient against brushing immediately after vomiting; avoid use of hard toothbrushes, abrasive toothpaste, and a "scrubbing" toothbrush method; avoid rinsing with tap water because it reduces the protective effects of saliva; encourage use of a mouth guard during vomiting episodes; rinse with sodium bicarbonate to neutralize the oral environment; and encourage use of daily fluoride and dentinal hypersensitivity products.
- Inform the patient about various ways to relieve xerostomia and the effect of lack of saliva on hard and soft tissues.
- Nutritional advice provided should encourage health-centered behaviors rather than discussing caloric values or intake.

HEALTH APPLICATION 17

Human Papillomavirus

April is Oral Cancer Awareness Month. The American Dental Association recommends performing an oral cancer visual and tactile screening on a routine basis for early detection.[26] Several oral cancer screening technologies exist that may aid visual and tactile screening. Nearly 50,000 people in the United States will be diagnosed with oral or oropharyngeal cancer this year, 450,000 people worldwide. More disturbing is the fact that the survival rate after 5 years of diagnosis is only 57%.[27] Overall, cancer death rates are declining. However, oral cancer is on the rise. Dental professionals are well positioned to refer patients with lesions identified during an intra- and extraoral examination to the health care provider.

Human papillomavirus (HPV) is a common sexually transmitted infection that can also occur in the oral cavity, esophagus, and larynx. HPV is a risk factor for oral cancer (Box 17.1). These lesions can be recognized during an intraoral examination; however, HPV lesions vary in form (Fig. 17.20). More than 100 different types of HPV have been identified. Low-risk HPV strains can lead to the growth of a papilloma or wart. However, some high-risk strains have shown a strong association with cancer.[28] HPV strains are numbered; HPV-16 and HPV-18 have been identified as subtypes associated with risk factors for oral squamous cell carcinomas. Squamous cell carcinoma manifests as cancer in the head and neck area. Currently, two HPV vaccines, a series of three shots over 6 months, have received FDA approval for protection against HPV-16 and HPV-18.

HPV can be present and communicable even when lesions are not present. Salivary diagnostic testing is available to detect the presence of HPV.

Treatment regimens for cancer (surgery, chemotherapy, and/or radiation) vary according to the cancer site and stage. The treatments cause or exacerbate symptoms such as anorexia, alterations or loss of taste, xerostomia, mucositis, nausea, and vomiting, all of which have an impact on eating. Before, during, and after treatment, patients with oral cancer often experience complications related to these symptoms. Malnutrition, a frequent complication, has serious implications on the outcome and response to treatment.[29,30]

As the association between HPV and oral cancer strengthens, early detection and education is the emerging responsibility of dental professionals. Communicating the message on this sensitive topic may require additional training.

• BOX 17.1 Risk Factors for Oral Cancer

- Human papillomavirus
- Tobacco use
- Chewing betel quid (areca nut and lime wrapped in a betel leaf) and gutka (betel quid and tobacco)
- Heavy alcohol use
- Age
- Gender
- Family history
- Lichen planus
- Excessive exposure to sunlight
- Poor nutrition
- Weakened immune system
- Mouthwash[a]
- Irritation from dentures*

Data from American Cancer Society. What are the risk factors for oral cavity and oropharyngeal cancers? Last revised August 8, 2016. https://www.cancer.org/cancer/oral-cavity-and-oropharyngeal-cancer/causes-risks-prevention/risk-factors.html. Accessed April 15, 2017.
[a]Controversial

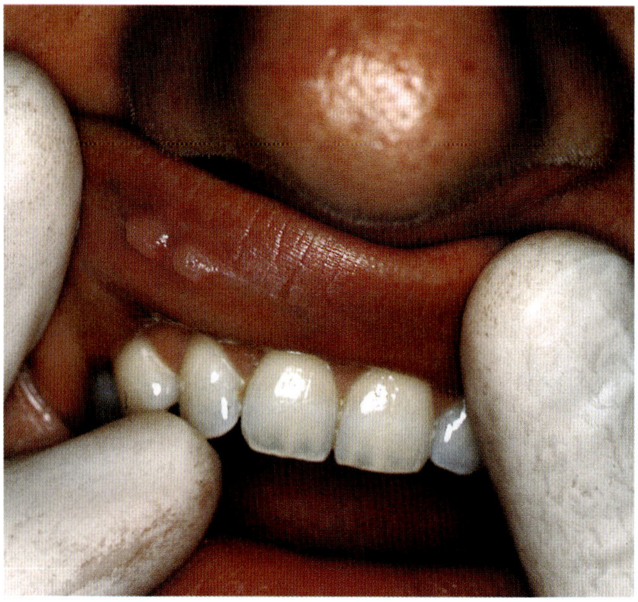

• Figure 17.20 Papillary lesion of the upper lip caused by human papilloma virus in a patient with human immunodeficiency virus infection. (Reproduced with permission from Ibsen OAC, Phelan JA. *Oral Pathology for the Dental Hygienist*. 6th ed. St. Louis, MO: Saunders; 2014.)

CASE APPLICATION FOR THE DENTAL HYGIENIST

Janie, a 17-year-old cheerleader in high school, came in for her 6-month recare appointment. She complained that "my teeth seem to be wearing down," and "I'm getting holes in my front teeth." Further questioning indicated frequent vomiting to control her weight because "everyone does it."

Nutritional Assessment

- Weight changes
- Oral assessment
- Food, nutrient, and calorie intake
- Awareness of the relationship between health and nutritional intake
- Dietary habits

Nutritional Diagnosis

Consumption of large amounts of high-carbohydrate, low-nutrient foods in a short time, several times a week, followed by regurgitation.

Nutritional Goals

Patient will limit fermentable carbohydrates to reduce the incidence of decay.

Nutritional Implementation

Intervention: Conduct an oral examination to note if any of the following complications are present: trauma to the soft palate, erythematous pharyngeal area, enamel erosion, angular cheilosis, salivary gland enlargement, and xerostomia.

Rationale: These self-inflicted oral complications can indicate to the dental professional the need to investigate further the possibility of an eating disorder in a patient who denies the problem.

Intervention: Discuss effects of frequent vomiting on the oral cavity and appropriate methods to prevent further damage.

Rationale: Not brushing immediately after purging, use of mouth guards during purging, and use of daily fluoride and desensitizing agents are practices Janie is encouraged to adopt to decrease further problems in the oral cavity. Providing such information may be a factor in reducing Janie's vomiting episodes.

Intervention: Become the dental liaison in the medical/psychological health care team for this patient.

Rationale: Because of complicated issues involved with an eating disorder, several health disciplines are required to treat patients. The dental hygienist plays a crucial role in overall care of these patients.

Intervention: Discuss specific foods that help to prevent further deterioration of the teeth.

Rationale: Adequate nutrition is essential to support a healthy periodontium and prevents destructive dental activities. Frequent intake of simple carbohydrate foods is a factor in the high caries rate.

Evaluation

The patient is actively seeking treatment for her eating disorder. She plans to achieve small goals as she works toward improving intake of all nutrients and decreasing episodes of bingeing and purging to improve her oral hygiene status.

Mental Illness

A few of the many different mental illnesses that occur include schizophrenia, depression, and bipolar disorder or mania. These disorders do not usually display any oral manifestations.[25] However, drugs frequently prescribed to treat the conditions may have side effects that affect oral status. Antipsychotics (e.g., haloperidol, thioridazine, fluoxetine, and thiothixene) used to treat schizophrenia frequently cause xerostomia. Anticholinergic properties of tricyclic antidepressants, monoamine oxidase inhibitors, and trazodone used to treat depression also cause xerostomia, dental caries, ulcerations, and periodontal disease. Trazodone can also cause an unpleasant taste in the mouth.

Student Readiness

1. List ways to make a low-sodium diet more appealing. Using favorite foods, create a low-sodium diet for yourself for one day.
2. Describe several oral manifestations seen in various systemic diseases that create a painful mouth, making eating difficult and less enjoyable.
3. Identify strategies for a patient who is experiencing (a) nausea and vomiting, (b) bitter or metallic taste in the mouth, (c) chewing and swallowing difficulties, (d) stomatitis, and (e) xerostomia.
4. What factors contribute to anorexia in a patient with HIV/AIDS?
5. What are some cancer treatments and what oral problems can result from these therapies?
6. Choose a systemic disease from this chapter. Search for a recent (within the past 3 years) systematic review and/or meta-analysis using the name of the disease, oral health, and nutrition as the key terms. Review the article and determine the outcomes. Present the outcomes to others in the course. Consider further researching and writing a journal article on the disease to submit to a dental hygiene journal for publication or present a poster at a dental hygiene association meeting.

CASE STUDY

A new patient is seen in the office with complaints of recurrent aphthous ulcers. These ulcers make it very difficult for him to eat, and he has lost about 8 lb. During an oral examination, candidiasis, hairy leukoplakia, and a flat, bluish, nonsymptomatic lesion on the palate, indicative of Kaposi sarcoma, are noted. HIV/AIDS may be a possible diagnosis.

1. What additional information would you like to obtain from this patient?
2. Would this patient benefit from nutrition information by the dental hygienist? If so, on what areas should the dental hygienist concentrate?
3. What dietary modifications and dental care instructions would you provide this patient?
4. Create a list of helpful additional resources, apps, and agencies for this patient.

References

1. Strauss S, Alfano MC, Shelley D, et al. Identifying unaddressed systemic health conditions at dental visits: patients who visited dental practices but not general health care providers in 2008. *Am J Pub Health*. 2012;102(2):253–254.
2. Landi F, Calvani R, Tosato M, et al. Anorexia of aging: risk factors, consequences, and potential treatments. *Nutrients*. 2016;8(2):http://www.mdpi.com/2072-6643/8/2/69/htm. Accessed March 29, 2017.
3. Sergi G, Bano G, Pizzato S, et al. Taste loss in the elderly: possible implications for dietary habits. *Crit RevFood SciNutr*. 2016;http://

www.tandfonline.com/doi/abs/10.1080/10408398.2016.1160208. Accessed March 29, 2017.
4. Desoutter A, Soudain-Pineau M, Munsch F, et al. Xerostomia and medication: a cross-sectional study in long-term geriatric wards. *J Nutr Health Aging*. 2012;16(6):575–579.
5. Shetty SR, Bhowmick S, Castelino R, et al. Drug induced xerostomia in elderly individuals: an institutional study. *Contemp Clin Dent*. 2012;3(2):173–175.
6. Nykänen I, Lönnroos E, Kautiainen H, et al. Nutritional screening in a population-based cohort of community-dwelling older people. *Eur J Public Health*. 2013;23(3):405–409.
7. National Cancer Institute, National Institutes of Health: Infection. Last modified December 16, 2016. http://www.cancer.gov/cancertopics/pdq/supportivecare/oralcomplications/HealthProfessional/page7. Accessed April 7, 2017.
8. Eales J, Gibson P, Whorwell P, et al. Systematic review and meta-analysis: the effects of fermented milk with Bifidobacterium lactis CNCMI-2494 and lactic acid bacteria on gastrointestinal discomfort in the general adult population. *Ther Adv Gastroenterol*. 2017; 101(1):74–88.
9. Lockhart PB, Bolger AF, Papapanou PN, et al. Periodontal disease and atherosclerotic vascular disease: does the evidence support an independent association?: a scientific statement from the American Heart Association. *Circulation*. 2012;125(20):2520–2544.
10. Berlin-Broner Y, Febbraio M, Levin L. Association between apical periodontitis and cardiovascular diseases: a systematic review of the literature. *Int Endod J*. 2016;http://aj2vr6xy7z.scholar.serialssolutions.com/?sid=google&auinit=Y&aulast=Berlin%E2%80%90Broner&atitle=Association+between+apical+periodontitis+and+cardiovascular+diseases:+a+systematic+review+of+the+literature&id=doi:10.1111/iej.12710. Accessed April 7, 2017.
11. Merchant AT, Virani SS. Evaluating periodontal treatment to prevent cardiovascular disease: challenges and possible solutions. *Curr Atheroscler Rep*. 2017;19(4):1–6.
12. Khan A, Morrison A, Cheung A, et al. Osteonecrosis of the jaw (ONJ): diagnosis and management in 2015. *Osteoporos Int*. 2016;27: 853–859.
13. Bagan J, Peydro A, Calvo J. Medication-related osteonecrosis of the jaw associated with bisphosphonates and denosumab in osteoporosis. *Oral Dis*. 2016;22:324–329.
14. Borgnakke WS, Ylostalo PV, Taylor GW, et al. Effect of periodontal disease on diabetes: systematic review of epidemiologic observational evidence. *J Clin Periodontol*. 2013;40(suppl 14):S135–S152.
15. Teshome A, Yitayeh A. The effect of periodontal therapy on glycemic control and fasting plasma glucose level in type 2 diabetic patients: systematic review and meta-analysis. *BMC Oral Health*. 2017; 17(31):1–11.
16. American Diabetes Association. Glycemic targets. *Diabetes Care*. 2017;40(suppl 1):S48–S56.
17. Brabyn P, Capote A, Belloti M, et al. Hyperparathyroidism diagnosed due to brown tumors of the jaw: a case report and literature review. *J Oral Maxillofac Surg*. 2017;http://aj2vr6xy7z.scholar.serialssolutions.com/?sid=google&auinit=P&aulast=Brabyn&atitle=Hyperparathyroidism+Diagnosed+Due+To+Brown+Tumors+Of+The+Jaw:+A+Case+Report+And+Literature+Review&id=doi:10.1016/j.joms.2017.03.013. Accessed April 10, 2017.
18. Dentistry iQ: Oral health and chronic kidney disease: building a bridge between the dental and renal communities. http://www.dentistryiq.com/articles/gr/print/volume-2/issue-3/original-article/oral-health-and-chronic-kidney-disease-building-a-bridge-between-the-dental-and-renal-communities.html. Accessed April 10, 2017.
19. Proctor R, Kumar N, Stein A, et al. Oral and dental aspects of chronic renal failure. *J Dent Res*. 2005;84(3):199–208.
20. Grover S, Rhodus NL. Dental management of Parkinson's disease. *Northwest Dent*. 2011;90(6):13–19.
21. Parkinson's Disease Foundation, Zwickey H Nutritional strategies for living with Parkinson's. News &Review, Winter 2016. http://www.pdf.org/winter16_nutrition. Accessed August 21, 2017.
22. Barbe AG, Bock N, Derman SHM, et al. Self-assessment of oral health, dental health care and oral health-related quality of life among Parkinson's disease patients. *Gerodontology*. 2017;34(1):135–143. http://www.pdf.org/parkinson_health_professionals_patienteducation. Accessed April 13, 2017.
23. Uhlen MM, Mulic A, Holme B, et al. The susceptibility to dental erosion differs among individuals. *Caries Res*. 2016;50(2):http://www.karger.com/Article/Abstract/444400#. Accessed April 15, 2017.
24. American Psychiatric Association. Feeding and eating disorders. http://www.dsm5.org/Documents/Eating%20Disorders%20Fact%20Sheet.pdf. Accessed April 15, 2017.
25. Araujo MM, Martins CC, Costa LCM, et al. Association between depression and periodontitis: a systematic review and meta-analysis. *J Clin Periodontol*. 2016;43:216–228.
26. Rethman MP, Carpenter W, Cohen E, et al. Evidence-based clinical recommendations regarding screening for oral squamous cell carcinomas. *J Am Dent Assoc*. 2010;141(5):509–520.
27. Oral Cancer Foundation: Oral cancer facts. http://oralcancerfoundation.org/facts/index.htm. Accessed April 15, 2017.
28. Li X, Gao L, Li H, et al. Human papillomavirus infection and laryngeal cancer risk: a systematic review and meta-analysis. *J Infect Diseases*. 2013;207(3):479–488.
29. Valentini V, Marazzi F, Bossola M, et al. Nutritional counseling and oral nutritional supplements in head and neck cancer patients undergoing chemoradiotherapy. *J Hum Nutr Diet*. 2012;25(3):201–208.
30. Kiss NK, Krishnasamy M, Loeliger J, et al. A dietitian-led clinic for patients receiving (chemo)radiotherapy for head and neck cancer. *Support Care Cancer*. 2012;20(9):2111–2120.

EVOLVE RESOURCES

Please visit http://evolve.elsevier.com/Stegeman/nutritional for additional practice and study support tools.

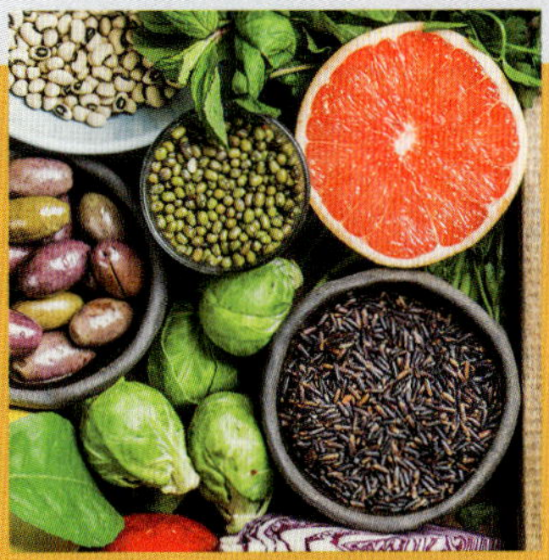

18 Nutritional Aspects of Dental Caries: Causes, Prevention, and Treatment

STUDENT LEARNING OUTCOMES

Upon completion of this chapter, the student will be able to achieve the following student learning outcomes:

1. Explain the role each of the following play in the caries process: tooth, saliva, food, and plaque biofilm.
2. Discuss the following related to cariogenic foods, as well as cariostatic and noncariogenic properties of food:
   - List cariogenic food and beverages.
   - List examples of fermentable carbohydrates potentially increasing risk to dental health.
   - Identify foods that stimulate salivary flow.
   - Suggest food and beverage choices and their timing to reduce the cariogenicity of a patient's diet.
   - Describe characteristics of foods having noncariogenic or cariostatic properties.
3. Provide nutrition education to a patient at risk for dental caries.

KEY TERMS

Acidogenic
Caries Management by Risk Assessment (CaMBRA)
Casein
Macrodontia
Noncariogenic
Silver diamine fluoride

TEST YOUR NQ

1. **T/F** Cariogenic carbohydrates are the only reason for development of carious lesions.
2. **T/F** Nutrients have a role in the composition and structure of teeth during development.
3. **T/F** Bicarbonates, phosphates, and proteins in saliva dilute and neutralize plaque acids in the mouth.
4. **T/F** Sucrose, fructose, glucose, and maltose have equal potential to cause dental caries.
5. **T/F** Most sugar alcohols—including sorbitol, mannitol, and xylitol—are cariogenic.
6. **T/F** For a tooth to demineralize, the plaque pH needs to be 6 or higher as a result of consuming cariogenic foods.
7. **T/F** The total quantity of sugar is of greatest importance when assessing the patient's diet.
8. **T/F** A fermentable carbohydrate consumed with a meal is less cariogenic than the same food consumed as a snack.
9. **T/F** The revised Recommended Dietary Allowances provide helpful nutrition information for patients trying to reduce dental caries.
10. **T/F** Providing patients with information about the caries process leads to desirable dietary and oral behavior changes.

Nutritional status and oral health have a strong interrelationship. Countless research studies have shown the importance of diet in the development, maintenance, and repair of hard and soft oral tissues. Dental caries is an oral infectious disease that is multifactorial, transmissible, and of bacterial origin (Fig. 18.1).

Diet and nutrients play a role in dental caries. Some foods exert a cariogenic effect, whereas others are cariostatic or anticariogenic and offer protection to reduce caries. Nutrients also have topical and systemic effects, which can be primary or secondary factors in the development of dental caries. However, many factors must be considered if the situation is to be defined as cariogenic. A list

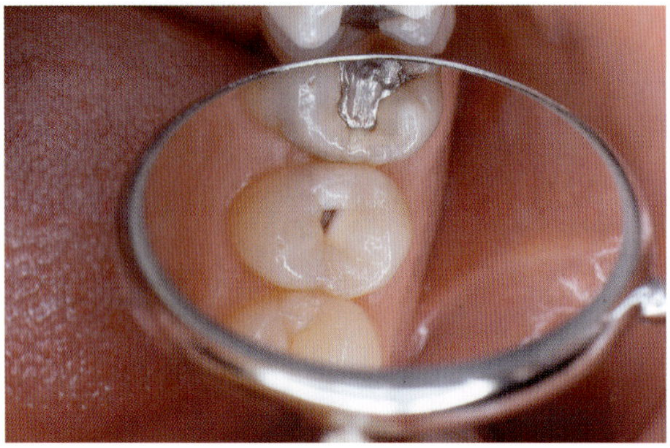

• **Figure 18.1** Dental caries. (Reproduced with permission from Iannucci JM, Howerton LJ. *Dental Radiography: Principles and Techniques*. 5th ed. St. Louis, MO: Elsevier; 2017.)

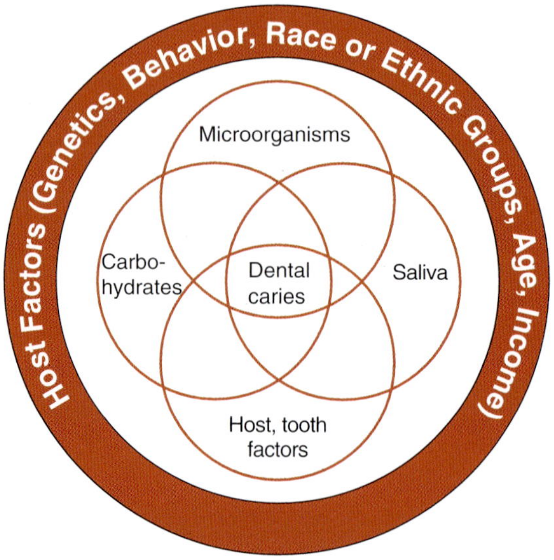

• **Figure 18.2** Major factors that interact in the dental caries process.

of cariogenic foods would be misleading because no food is cariogenic in all situations.

The primary oral health goals of *Healthy People 2020* are to reduce the number of caries in children and adolescents by 10% and to reduce untreated decay in this population group and adults by 10%.[1] Based on the mid-point review, 27% of preschool-age children 3 to 5 years and more than 57% of children ages 6 to 9 and adolescents have experienced decay. Regarding untreated decay, 11% of preschool-age children, 21.5% of children 6 to 9 years, 11.4% of adolescents, and 24.9% of adults up to age 44 years have at least one untreated area.[1]

Even with advancements in the quality of digital radiography, emerging technology for early detection of caries, improved restorative materials, multiple fluoride options, application of sealants, frequent dental care appointments, dental health education, and increased access to care, dental caries remain the most common chronic childhood disease. Although a remarkable reduction in caries has been observed in school-age children since the 1970s, certain racial, ethnic, and lower-income population groups continue to be problematic. *Healthy People 2020* estimates that only 44.5% of the U.S. population older than age 2 years have had a dental appointment within the past year.[1] Barriers to dental care include cost; lack of dental insurance, public programs, or providers for underserved groups; fear of dentistry; difficulties in accessing services; or poor awareness of the importance of oral health maintenance.

Major Factors in the Dental Caries Process

No single parameter is responsible for formation of a carious lesion (Fig. 18.2). A combination of factors is involved, including a susceptible host or tooth surface, a sufficient quantity of cariogenic microorganisms in the mouth, the presence of fermentable carbohydrates, and a particular composition or flow of saliva. All of these must be present simultaneously for an adequate time to allow decay to occur.

Tooth Structure

Increasing resistance of the tooth against demineralization begins in the pre-eruptive phase. An adequate intake of nutrients during growth and development of enamel and dentin is essential. The most influential nutrients include calcium; phosphorus; vitamins A, C, and D; fluoride; and protein. Indirectly, some fermentable carbohydrates play a role in the formation of caries before tooth eruption. Consider a child who snacks on cookies, candy, or ice cream throughout the day and is not hungry for meat, vegetables, fruit, and milk that may be offered at mealtime. A child's diet high in low-nutrient (or calorie-dense) carbohydrates may be deficient in required nutrients for optimal growth and development of the dentition. Other factors, such as genetic or metabolic disturbances, can be responsible for poor tooth formation. Dental anomalies include **macrodontia** (abnormally large teeth) and enamel hypoplasia.

After the tooth erupts, the depth of the natural anatomic pits and fissures and the position of the teeth are relevant factors in the development of dental caries. Deep pits and fissures increase susceptibility for dental caries because of the potential for plaque biofilm and food entrapment. Overlapping and crowding of teeth also offer areas for these materials to collect and ferment, compounded by difficulty keeping these areas clean.

Host Factors

Food selection, dietary patterns, oral hygiene habits, genetics, race or ethnicity, age, and income are factors that determine susceptibility to caries.

Saliva

Availability of essential nutrients during the development of salivary glands, which begins during the fourth week in utero, has a significant impact on the amount of saliva and its composition. Of particular importance are vitamin A, iron, and protein, which have a role in normal growth, development, and secretion of saliva.

The protection provided by an adequate salivary flow and buffering capacity of saliva ultimately reduce the destructive capabilities of fermentable carbohydrates on teeth. This fact is recognized in patients with xerostomia, who are at high risk for development of caries because of decreased salivary production.

Saliva provides protection against caries in several ways. First, saliva acts as a buffer by neutralizing much of the acid produced by plaque biofilm as a result of carbohydrate metabolism. Second, normal saliva contains bicarbonate, phosphate, and protein, which dilute and neutralize acids to maintain a neutral oral pH, which is around 7. After an acidic drink is consumed, the pH of the oral cavity is rapidly normalized by the components of saliva. However, if the frequency or duration of the acidic drink is extended, it becomes more difficult for saliva to buffer the continuous supply of acid and it loses its caries protection.

Particularly important to the prevention of dental caries is the flow of saliva. An adequate salivary flow enables rapid transport of foods from the mouth, decreasing the length of time harmful bacteria and food particles are able to attach to teeth and cause caries to develop. Consumption of citrus fruits (e.g., orange juice and lemonade) promotes saliva formation by means of their citric acid content; however, intake needs to be monitored because of the potential to cause enamel erosion.

Because saliva is saturated with calcium, phosphate, and fluoride ions, the potential for remineralization (restoration of damaged enamel) and resistance to enamel dissolution exists. Finally, antimicrobial elements in saliva, such as immunoglobulin A, either interfere with adherence of bacteria or compete with bacteria to attach to the tooth surface. An alkaline saliva offers protection, whereas an acidic saliva increases susceptibility to caries.

Plaque Biofilm and Its Bacterial Components

Plaque biofilm is a complex environment of bacteria, polysaccharides, proteins, and lipids. Plaque biofilm forms a local barrier on enamel and may interfere with demineralization. However, acids produced in plaque biofilm have harmful properties that offset the benefit of its barrier effect.

Composition of plaque biofilm is altered as it matures and is strongly influenced by diet. As a by-product of the metabolism of sucrose and glucose, bacteria produce acids that lower the pH, resulting in a more favorable environment for development of certain bacteria, such as *Streptococcus mutans*. *S. mutans,* a gram-positive, anaerobic, spherical bacterium, is widely implicated in initiation of dental caries. Other microorganisms, such as bacteria from other mutans streptococci and the *Lactobacillus* species, are capable of fermenting carbohydrates. They also thrive in an acidic environment.

When a carbohydrate has been ingested, its metabolism by salivary amylase begins within 2 to 3 minutes and can persist for hours. The metabolic products are acetic, butyric, formic, lactic, and propionic acids. Concentration of the acids escalates as carbohydrate intake continues, whereas the pH of the plaque decreases. Demineralization of enamel occurs when the "critical pH" of 5.5 is reached. The pH can increase to 6.7 for incipient demineralization of cementum and dentin to occur; this is a real concern for areas of gingival recession. In addition, demineralization is faster on root surfaces than on enamel because dentin contains less mineral content. In interproximal areas or in deep pits and fissures, the pH can decrease to 4 and remain at that pH for an hour. The pH of acids produced by bacteria in plaque biofilm is eventually neutralized after elimination of cariogenic foods as saliva exerts its protective action.

DENTAL CONSIDERATIONS

- Evaluate the patient for deep pits and fissures, amount of plaque biofilm in the oral cavity, and composition and flow of saliva. Encourage use of sealants in deep pits and fissures of young patients to prevent plaque biofilm accumulation.
- **Silver diamine fluoride** is a noninvasive and easily applied fluoride modality for caries management. The effectiveness of silver diamine fluoride can be a promising strategy for populations at risk for dental decay. Educating the patient on black staining of the arrested lesion is essential. Further studies are indicated.[2]
- Recommend a combination of fluoride sources for patients at high risk for caries. Fluoride in plaque biofilm and saliva inhibits demineralization and enhances remineralization of tooth surfaces.
- For patients with a high caries rate, the use of chlorhexidine or other antimicrobial agents may be beneficial due to their ability to disorganize dental biofilm. Educate the patient that this practice can suppress harmful plaque and organisms. Counsel the patient regarding the potential of chlorhexidine staining teeth. The research regarding the use of chlorhexidine for inhibiting caries formation is inconclusive. Further studies are indicated.[3]
- Encourage meticulous oral hygiene habits, including regular recare visits.
- Caution parents to avoid sharing utensils with children, a practice allowing transfer of the cariogenic microorganism *S. mutans*.

NUTRITIONAL DIRECTIONS

- Eating a variety of foods in moderation ensures adequate nutrient intake. Encouraging healthy eating habits is a factor in growth, development, and maintenance of teeth; prevention of dental caries; and general good health.
- Firm, fibrous foods (such as raw fruits and vegetables), chewing gum, sour foods, and citrus fruits stimulate salivary flow. An increase in the flow rate has a positive impact on resistance of teeth to caries.

Cariogenic Foods

Cariogenic foods and beverages are fermentable carbohydrates that can be metabolized by oral bacteria and reduce salivary pH below 5.5 (Fig. 18.3). As previously discussed, fermentable carbohydrates are a factor in the development of demineralization and dental caries. The average daily consumption from added sugars among 2- to 18-year-olds is 325 cals (over 80 g, or approximately 20 tsp).[4] The major sources of added sugars are sugar-sweetened beverages (e.g., sodas or fruit drinks), grain desserts (e.g., cookies or cakes), dairy desserts (e.g., ice cream), candy, and cold cereals.[5] Nondiet sports and energy drinks are fast-growing sugar-sweetened beverage choices. Almost 1 in 4 U.S. adults consumes sports and energy drinks at least one time per week.[6] A 16-oz bottle of a regular sports drink contains 33.6 g of added sugars, a 16-oz can of energy drink contains 54 g, and 16-oz sugar-sweetened soda may contain as much as 32.5 g of sugar.[7]

The small size of sugar molecules allows salivary amylase to split the molecules into components that can be easily metabolized by plaque bacteria. Sucrose is not the only culprit; other monosaccharides and disaccharides—such as fructose, glucose, and maltose—all produce similar amounts of substrate for metabolism by plaque bacteria to produce acid. Sucrose is used to produce glucans, facilitating the adherence of bacteria, such as *S. mutans,* to the dental pellicle. Glucose and other carbohydrates are also used to produce extracellular polysaccharides. Therefore, diets containing glucose, and the disaccharides can increase plaque biofilm mass and facilitate its retention and colonization. "Natural sugars"—such as honey (fructose and glucose), molasses (sucrose and invert sugar), and brown sugar (sugar and molasses)—have cariogenic potential similar to sucrose. Box 18.1 lists examples of fermentable carbohydrates potentially increasing risk to dental health.

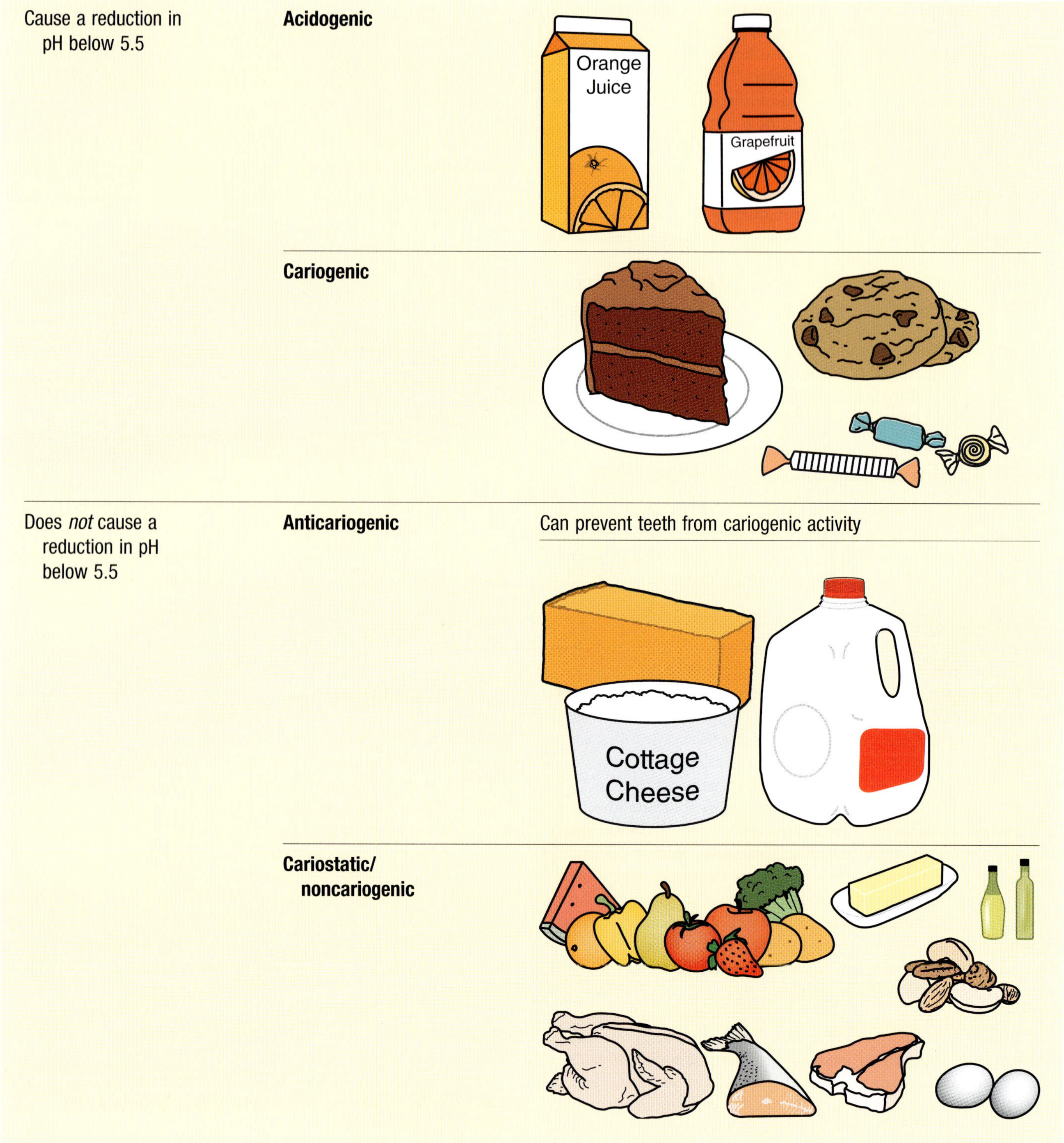

• **Figure 18.3** Cariogenicity of Foods and Beverages.

Polysaccharides—starchy foods such as rice, potatoes, and corn—are less cariogenic than monosaccharides and disaccharides. Physical and chemical properties of starches are very different from the properties of simple carbohydrates, and render complex carbohydrates less damaging to enamel. These unique properties prevent starch from providing a readily available energy source for cariogenic microflora, and it is less likely to produce caries than mono- or disaccharides. In contrast to sucrose, the large number of glucose units needed to form a starch make it almost insoluble. Because starch must be hydrolyzed (split into smaller glucose units) before acid can be produced, the time a starch is in the mouth is usually not long enough to be completely metabolized if oral self-care is completed promptly. Normal saliva flow readily neutralizes any acids produced by polysaccharides.

• BOX 18.1 Foods That Can Cause the pH of Plaque Biofilm to Fall Below 5.5

- Alcohol
- Bananas
- Beans, baked
- Bread
- Candy
- Cereals, non–presweetened, ready-to-eat
- Cereals, presweetened, ready-to-eat
- Chips
- Cookies
- Crackers
- Dill pickles
- Doughnuts, plain
- Energy drinks
- Flavored coffees and teas
- Fruit, dried
- Fruit drinks
- Fruit smoothies
- Gelatin, flavored
- Sugar-sweetened hard candy
- Honey
- Ice cream
- Jams and jellies
- Marshmallows
- Nondairy creamers
- Oatmeal, instant cooked
- Pasta
- Peanut butter
- Pretzels
- Rice, cooked
- Sauerkraut
- Snack cakes
- Soft drinks, regular and diet
- Sports drinks
- Tomato juice
- Yogurts

When starches and simple carbohydrates are combined (as in pastries or sugar-coated cereals), their potential to produce caries is equal to or greater than that of sucrose. Also, processed starches, as found in instant oatmeal, are often more fermentable than their nonprocessed counterparts because of partial hydrolysis or diminution of particle size. The cariogenic activity is also related to the form of starch.

Fresh fruit is another food group of low cariogenicity because of its low percentage of carbohydrate and high percentage of water. Firm fruits such as apples play a protective role by stimulating saliva flow. The high concentration of fructose found in juices is potentially a source of substrate for plaque bacteria that may influence caries risk. This is shown in early childhood caries, which occurs in children given unlimited amounts of fruit juice and other fermentable carbohydrate beverages. Citric fruits and juices are **acidogenic** and can reduce the salivary pH to less than 5.5. The sticky nature of dried fruit (e.g., raisins) also increases risk of decay. Each of these foods is important in its nutritional value, however, and should not be completely eliminated.

Cariostatic/Noncariogenic Properties of Food

Cariostatic or noncariogenic foods and beverages do not cause a reduction in salivary pH below 5.5 (see Fig. 18.3).

Nonnutritive Sweeteners

Aspartame, saccharin, sucralose, neotame, and acesulfame are a few examples of nonnutritive sweeteners. These sweeteners are not metabolized by microorganisms and do not promote dental caries. Foods made from these sweeteners are generally higher in cost, however, and may not be feasible for low-income patients. Other components of foods using these substitutes, such as raisins, may offset the benefits of using nonnutritive sweeteners to prevent dental caries.

Protein and Fat

Protein and fat are two nutrient classes that may be considered cariostatic because they do not lower plaque pH. Generally, protein may contribute to buffering effects of saliva. Consuming foods with fat and protein following a fermentable carbohydrate may increase plaque pH. Meat, seafood, poultry, eggs, nuts, seeds, margarine, and oils are examples of potentially cariostatic foods.

Anticariogenic Properties of Food

Anticariogenic foods or beverages do not cause a reduction in pH below 5.5 and may protect teeth from cariogenic activity (see Fig. 18.3).

Sugar Alcohols

Some food components can protect teeth by decreasing demineralization, enhancing remineralization, or increasing salivary flow, even in the presence of a fermentable carbohydrate. Sugar alcohols, such as mannitol and sorbitol, are often used as substitute sweeteners. They are viable alternatives to sugar because of their sweet taste but have the added benefit of being **noncariogenic**, a carbohydrate that does not increase salivary pH (see Table 4.1 in Chapter 4 and Fig. 18.3). Sugar alcohols ferment more slowly in the mouth than monosaccharides and disaccharides; buffering effects of saliva competently neutralize destructive acids produced by plaque bacteria.

Another sugar alcohol, xylitol, is found naturally in plants and is equal to or sweeter than sucrose. Xylitol may be classified as anticariogenic because oral flora may not contain enzymes to ferment it, and metabolizing microorganisms, such as *S. mutans,* are inhibited. Salivary pH does not drop below 5.5. Chewing gums, mints, and candies containing xylitol may inhibit enamel demineralization.[8] This inhibitory effect is enhanced by increased salivary flow, increased oral clearance, and greater buffering capabilities. Compounded by increased mastication, the outcome can be remineralization of incipient decay.

The U.S. Food and Drug Administration (FDA) recognizes sugar alcohols to be xylitol, sorbitol, mannitol, maltitol, isomalt, lactitol, hydrogenated starch hydrolysates, hydrogenated glucose syrups, and erythritol, or a combination of these. On food labels, products containing any of these sugar alcohols can state, "…the noncariogenic carbohydrate sweetener present in the food "does not promote," "may reduce the risk of," "useful [or is useful] in not promoting," or "expressly [or is expressly] for not promoting" dental caries.[9] The dental professional uses this information to educate the patient when choosing products containing sugar alcohols.

Phosphorus and Calcium

Phosphorus and calcium also provide qualities protecting against caries. Dispersion of these minerals throughout plaque biofilm may provide a buffering effect, increasing plaque pH. Ultimately, this action curtails demineralization of enamel.

Protein, especially the principal protein in milk, **casein**, and the minerals phosphorus and calcium are all ingredients of other anticariogenic—or even cariostatic—foods, such as cheese and milk. Despite the fact that lactose is cariogenic (although the least cariogenic of all mono-, di- and polysaccharides), these other elements in milk and dairy products decrease risk of dental caries. Cheese, produced from milk, contains several anticariogenic properties and has the potential to reduce demineralization (or enhance remineralization) of tooth enamel.

An increase of salivary flow occurs when chewing hard cheeses. This increased salivary flow provides a neutral environment and increases clearance of carbohydrates. Following the *MyPlate* recommendation for the milk and milk products group (using low-fat dairy products) is prudent advice for a dental patient. Eating these foods as snacks or at the end of a meal can provide anticariogenic effects.

Other Foods With Protective Factors

A constituent in chocolate, known as the cocoa factor, has shown anticariogenic properties. The classic Vipeholm study compared the caries rate of individuals consuming chocolate with the rate for individuals consuming other types of "nonchocolate" candies under similar circumstances. The results indicated a slightly lower caries incidence in individuals consuming chocolate.[10]

Glycyrrhiza, the active ingredient in licorice, can also be considered anticariogenic due to the potential to reduce *S. mutans* in saliva.[11] However, glycyrrhiza is contraindicated with some antihypertensive medications, has a staining capability, and can cause sodium retention and increased blood pressure. Grapefruit and other fruits containing citric acid can stimulate saliva production. However, they are generally considered acidogenic because of their ability to lower salivary pH and increase caries risk. Emerging research indicates that cranberries, tea, coffee, wine, and probiotics have properties that may interrupt caries formation.[12] Probiotics are live bacteria that are beneficial to the host (for more information see Chapter 3).

DENTAL CONSIDERATIONS

- Educate patients about the caries process and how to prevent demineralization of enamel, including the role that diet plays in initiation and progression of decay. Use terms that are appropriate and understandable for the patient.
- The dental hygienist should know which foods and situations have the potential to be cariogenic, create awareness of the potential harm, and offer suggestions for appropriate consumption of sweetened foods or alternative choices for sugar-containing foods (Box 18.1).
- Use of a variety of fluoride modalities, products containing appropriate levels of xylitol, and application of sealants increases protection of the tooth.
- Consider using an antimicrobial agent to control existing plaque biofilm, reduce the number of *S. mutans*, and prevent the formation of new plaque biofilm.
- Educate the patient regarding sports and energy drinks. Although these beverages are promoted to support intense physical activity since they contain electrolytes, vitamins, and minerals, remind patients that excessive consumption can lead to dental decay and in most cases are unnecessary.
- Exercise caution in recommending high-fat foods for their potential anticariogenic properties to patients with chronic diseases such as heart disease or diabetes mellitus because of their deleterious effects on these conditions.

NUTRITIONAL DIRECTIONS

- Using the *Dietary Guidelines* and *MyPlate*, evaluate the patient's diet for adequate nutritional intake and frequency of fermentable carbohydrate consumption.
- Substitute nonnutritive sweeteners for sucrose, if practical. Use a high-intensity sweetener NOTE–or you should list several, not just aspartame that many people distrust to sweeten coffee and tea instead of table sugar, especially if the beverage is consumed between meals.
- "Natural sugars," such as honey and molasses, are as cariogenic as refined carbohydrates.
- Encourage the consumption of healthy beverages, such as water, skim milk, and vegetable and 100% fruit juices.
- Food sources of probiotics include yogurt, kefir, buttermilk, tempeh, and miso.
- Energy drinks may contain vitamins and minerals, but the main ingredients are added sugars and stimulants (e.g., caffeine and guarana). The amount of caffeine varies widely among drinks but can be as high as 500 mg caffeine per can, which is comparable to approximately 14 cans of caffeinated soda. The consumption of energy drinks has been associated with insomnia, nervousness, and headache and can lead to tachycardia, seizures, and cardiac arrest.[6]
- Excessive intake of beverages or other products containing caffeine because of the potential interaction with certain drugs (e.g., bronchodilators, antibacterials, and antipsychotics).[6]
- Frequent use of medications containing fermentable carbohydrates, including antacids and cough drops.
- Increased use of products containing sugar alcohols (e.g., chewing gum, hard candy, dentifrices, and some medications) can cause gastrointestinal distress.
- Although sorbitol and mannitol ferment slowly in the mouth, which allows saliva to neutralize the acids produced, frequent use can potentially cause caries. This occurs especially in a patient with xerostomia using these products for relief of symptoms.
- Xylitol-containing chewing gums may inhibit growth of microorganisms, thereby reducing caries rate. Use of these gums after eating is recommended when proper oral care cannot be completed.
- High-sugar foods are generally high in fat as well. *MyPlate* recommends that intake of high-sugar and high-fat foods should be limited.
- The *Dietary Guidelines* and *MyPlate* recommend 10% of the total calories to be added sugar. The National Academy of Medicine (formerly the Institute of Medicine) recommends that added sugars should not exceed 25% of the total calories.[13]
- Popular sugar-sweetened beverages include sodas, fruit drinks, sports drinks, energy drinks, chocolate milk, and many vitamin waters.
- Compare some low-fat or nonfat foods that compensate for flavor by increasing sugar or sodium content (e.g., frozen dairy products).
- Because physical properties of milk are comparable to saliva, increasing low-fat milk intake as a saliva substitute may also offer protection against caries for a patient experiencing xerostomia.
- Encourage proper oral hygiene techniques to avoid complications associated with exposure to natural sugars (lactose in milk) and added sugars (some fruit juices).

Other Factors Influencing Cariogenicity

The amount and type of carbohydrates are not the only determinants of food intake that influence caries prevalence and severity. Other considerations include retentiveness of the carbohydrate, how often or how long teeth are exposed, sequence in which a carbohydrate is consumed, and whether food is eaten with a meal or as a snack. Some foods thought to have low cariogenic potential (e.g., cornflakes, crackers, or potato chips) may be more acidogenic than simple-carbohydrate foods because of their retentiveness in embrasures, pits, and fissures. Preventive practices, such as regular recare appointments, appropriate oral hygiene practices, sealants, xylitol, and fluoride use, should also be considered when discussing cariogenicity.

Physical Form

How quickly a cariogenic food is cleared from the mouth is a factor related to caries development. Ingestion of hard candy results in prolonged exposure. A sticky and retentive carbohydrate (e.g., chewy fruit snacks) remains in contact with the enamel surface for a longer period than sweetened fluids. Slow oral clearance of fermentable carbohydrate means longer exposure of the tooth to acid attack.

Fermentable carbohydrates that are chewy, such as caramels, adhere to teeth. However, the additional mastication required to process these foods stimulates saliva flow, making them less retentive and less damaging than dry, sticky foods, such as pretzels. Caramels are higher in sucrose than pretzels, supporting the concept of quantity of fermentable carbohydrates having a limited impact.

Frequency of Intake

Closely related to the physical form of a food in caries potential is frequency of fermentable carbohydrate intake. Longer periods of oral exposure to a fermentable carbohydrate lead to a greater risk of demineralization and less opportunity for teeth to remineralize. In comparing two individuals who eat equal amounts of fermentable carbohydrates, the one who eats more frequently throughout the day has the greatest potential for decay. With each exposure, a decrease in pH begins within 2 to 3 minutes; at a pH of 5.5 or less (the critical pH), enamel decalcification occurs. Within 40 minutes, the pH has increased to its initial value. The classic Stephan curve shows the pH changes of dental plaque after rinsing with a sugar solution (Fig. 18.4). Using a similar scenario, if a person eats a candy bar within a 5-minute period, the teeth would be exposed to a critical pH that lasts for approximately 40 minutes before the pH returns to the original level. If another person eats the same candy bar in five bites, but only takes a bite every hour, the total acid exposure would be approximately 200 minutes (5 bites × 40 minutes = 200 minutes of acid exposure).

Frequent consumption of soft drinks, sports drinks, energy drinks, and flavored coffees and teas compounded with a decline in dairy products can also influence caries risk and erosion despite the rapid oral clearance of these beverages (Fig. 18.5). The pH of diet and regular soft drinks, bottled iced teas, and sports drinks ranges from 2.5 to 3.5. Although these drinks are popular snacks, low-fat dairy products, 100% fruit juice, and water are preferable beverage alternatives. The American Academy of Pediatrics recommends infants under 6 months be fed only breastmilk or an infant formula; avoid fruit juice before 1 year of age Limit fruit juice to 4 oz per day for children 1 to 6 years old and 8 oz per day for children 7 to 18 years old.[14]

Timing and Sequence in a Meal

Another consideration is whether the cariogenic food is eaten with meals or snacks. Participants in the Vipeholm study who ate foods high in sugar between meals in addition to mealtime had a significantly higher decay rate than participants who consumed these foods at mealtime only.[10] Despite these results, recommendations to eliminate snacks are not always realistic. Children cannot eat enough food in three meals to get all the nutrients they need, and snacks are warranted. Foods chosen for snacks should produce little or no acid (Box 18.2), and oral self-care should follow a snack.

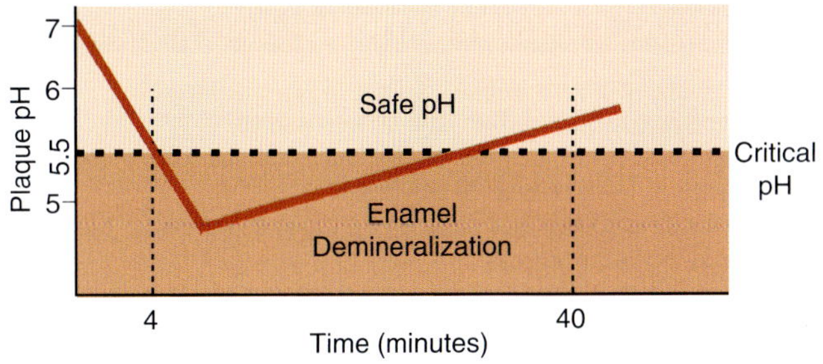

• **Figure 18.4** Stephan curve: time involvement of carbohydrate consumption and enamel demineralization.

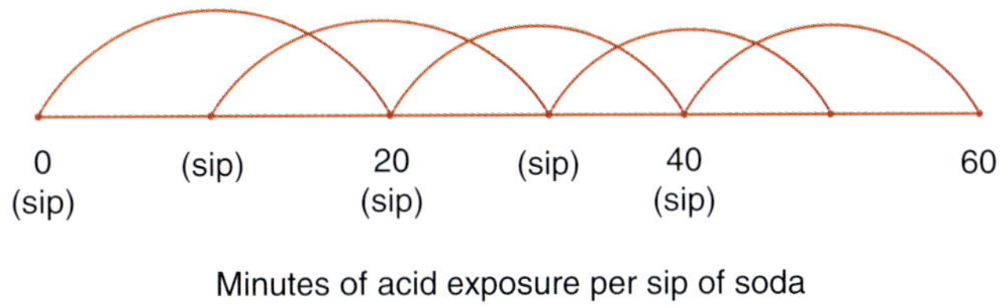

• **Figure 18.5** The increased consumption of soft drinks and sports drinks results in an enhanced caries risk. Although oral clearance is rapid, consuming such drinks over an extended time creates a cariogenic environment. If only soda is consumed, each sip results in at least 20 minutes of acid exposure. In this example, the patient took a sip at approximately 10-minute intervals and finished the drink in 5 sips for a total of 60 minutes of acid exposure.

• BOX 18.2 Snacks That May Produce Little or No Plaque Acid

- Cheeses[a]
  - American
  - Blue cheese
  - Brie
  - Cheddar
  - Cheese spread
  - Cream cheese
  - Gouda
  - Monterey jack
  - Mozzarella
  - Swiss
- Yogurt[b]
- Nuts
- Chewing gum with xylitol
- Cocoa products
- Protein food sources[c]
  - Meat
  - Seafood
  - Poultry
  - Eggs
- Fat food sources[c]
  - Margarine
  - Butter
  - Oils

[a]*These natural cheeses are high in fat. Reduced-fat or low-fat cheeses can be recommended.*
[b]*Encourage use of low-fat or skim versions, sugar free or plain.*
[c]*Follow* MyPlate *and* Dietary Guidelines *for serving sizes and low-fat choices and preparation methods.*

The location of an acidogenic food within a meal presents another consideration for caries potential. Drinking coffee with sugar after a meal has been determined to lower plaque pH, whereas consuming cheese after a fermentable carbohydrate within a meal prevents the decrease of plaque pH that would occur if this fermentable carbohydrate were eaten alone. Cariogenic foods create less risk of enamel demineralization if followed by a noncariogenic or cariostatic food.

DENTAL CONSIDERATIONS

- Review diet history for patterns of fermentable carbohydrate consumption, frequency, form, and time consumed.
- Further questioning can reveal dietary habits that the patient failed to recognize as being relevant to oral health.
- Fermentable carbohydrates alone do not cause dental decay. It is one factor in the decay process.

NUTRITIONAL DIRECTIONS

- Consume fermentable carbohydrates at mealtimes (when possible) to allow other foods to neutralize acids in saliva.
- Foods that require chewing (e.g., chewing gum, raw fruits, and vegetables) help increase salivary flow. This aids in providing additional buffering effects and accelerated removal of retentive foods.
- Noncariogenic snacks include raw fruits and vegetables, low-fat cheese, skim milk, low-fat yogurt, peanuts, popcorn, whole-grain bagels, seeds, pizza, and tacos.
- Cariogenic snacks before bedtime should be omitted or followed by careful oral hygiene. Salivary flow is reduced when sleeping; clearance of plaque acids is limited. Uninterrupted acid production for 2 hours can be harmful.
- Consume fermentable carbohydrates within a meal, or eat a noncariogenic food last.
- Carbohydrate foods that are retentive (e.g., graham crackers or potato chips) are retained in the mouth longer, creating a greater potential for decay.
- Use products made with a nonnutritive sweetener, such as aspartame or sucralose in moderation (two to three products per day). Some patients may not tolerate large amounts of aspartame or other nonnutritive sweetener, or choose not to use them. Choose alternative noncariogenic food items and practice oral self-care.
- Limit purchasing soft drinks and sports and energy drinks in large, resealable containers in an effort to decrease the frequency and duration of consumption.
- Athletes require fluid for hydration. In most events lasting less than 4 hours, water is the preferred source of hydration rather than high-carbohydrate sports drinks.

Dental Hygiene Care Plan

Providing nutrition information is an essential component of the preventive program. Although all patients benefit from nutrition education, certain populations (Box 18.3) require special attention by the dental hygienist. As mentioned, the quantity of fermentable carbohydrates consumed is of concern, especially nutritionally. However, the form of the carbohydrate, how often it is consumed, and whether it is eaten with meals or snacks are more important for oral health than the amount consumed.

Assessment

When a dental nutrition care plan is necessary, many factors must be considered. Anthropometric measures (i.e., height and weight), clinical signs, dental and dietary assessment, health and dental history, and laboratory data (if applicable) are addressed in Chapter 21. In addition, an assessment takes into account a patient's learning style, literacy level, cultural heritage, and socioeconomic status.

Caries Management by Risk Assessment (CaMBRA) is a popular tool used by dental professionals to identify risk of caries and to determine preventive and therapeutic goals for both children and adult patients. Figs. 18.6 and 18.7 show risk forms, approved by the American Dental Association and the American Academy of Pediatric Dentistry, differentiated by age. The patient or caregiver can answer the questions prior to the dental appointment or upon arrival at the dental office.

The first step is to identify disease indicators (e.g., low income), caries risk factors (e.g., frequent snacks), and caries protective factors (e.g., use of products with xylitol) along with the clinical evaluation (e.g., number of existing restorations). Note that the age 6-to-adult form (see Fig. 18.6) includes identification of medications associated with xerostomia while the 0-to-6-years form (see Fig. 18.7) highlights acid exposure associated with childhood caries, such as the availability of bottles or sippy cups between meals or in the bed. The second step is to create and implement a treatment plan of action based on the risk outcome. The risk form can be used as a pedagogical tool by the dental professional to educate the patient. Risk factors are color coded for ease in explanation. For example, green designates *low risk*. A risk score can be obtained and compared to future risk forms. Detailed instructions on use of the form and educating patients are available on the American Dental Association website. Accompanying patient education material and sources are also provided.

• BOX 18.3 Situations Presenting High Caries Risk and Educational Opportunities

Early Childhood Caries
- Parents before pregnancy
- Parents during pregnancy
- Parents of young children

Root Caries and Xerostomia
- Older adults
- Periodontal patients
- Chronic disease states, for example, diabetes mellitus, chronic renal disease
- Polypharmacy
- Radiation therapy
- Gingival recession

Habits
- Frequent use of hard candy or chewing gum, cough drops, chew tobacco, medication containing a fermentable carbohydrate source
- Frequent vomiting
- Poor oral hygiene
- Patients with orthodontic appliances
- Adolescents
- Patients with dexterity challenges

Dental Issues
- Intake of low-fluoridation or nonfluoridated water
- Unsealed deep pits and fissures
- Family history of high caries risk
- Levels of cariogenic bacteria

ADA American Dental Association®
America's leading advocate for oral health

Caries Risk Assessment Form (Age >6)

Patient Name:		
Birth Date:	Date:	
Age:	Initials:	

		Low Risk	Moderate Risk	High Risk
Contributing Conditions		**Check or Circle the conditions that apply**		
I.	**Fluoride Exposure** (through drinking water, supplements, professional applications, toothpaste)	☒ Yes	☐ No	
II.	**Sugary Foods or Drinks** (including juice, carbonated or non-carbonated soft drinks, energy drinks, medicinal syrups)	Primarily at mealtimes ☒		Frequent or prolonged between meal exposures/day ☐
III.	**Caries Experience of Mother, Caregiver and/or other Siblings** (for patients ages 6-14)	No carious lesions in last 24 months ☒	Carious lesions in last 7-23 months ☐	Carious lesions in last 6 months ☐
IV.	**Dental Home**: established patient of record, receiving regular dental care in a dental office	☒ Yes	☐ No	
General Health Conditions		**Check or Circle the conditions that apply**		
I.	**Special Health Care Needs** (developmental, physical, medical or mental disabilities that prevent or limit performance of adequate oral health care by themselves or caregivers)	☒ No	Yes (over age 14) ☐	Yes (ages 6-14) ☐
II.	**Chemo/Radiation Therapy**	☒ No		☐ Yes
III.	**Eating Disorders**	☒ No	☐ Yes	
IV.	**Medications that Reduce Salivary Flow**	☒ No	☐ Yes	
V.	**Drug/Alcohol Abuse**	☒ No	☐ Yes	
Clinical Conditions		**Check or Circle the conditions that apply**		
I.	**Cavitated or Non-Cavitated** (incipient) **Carious Lesions or Restorations** (visually or radiographically evident)	No new carious lesions or restorations in last 36 months ☒	1 or 2 new carious lesions or restorations in last 36 months ☐	3 or more carious lesions or restorations in last 36 months ☐
II.	**Teeth Missing Due to Caries in past 36 months**	☒ No		☐ Yes
III.	**Visible Plaque**	☒ No	☐ Yes	
IV.	**Unusual Tooth Morphology** that compromises oral hygiene	☒ No	☐ Yes	
V.	**Interproximal Restorations - 1 or more**	☒ No	☐ Yes	
VI.	**Exposed Root Surfaces** Present	☒ No	☐ Yes	
VII.	**Restorations with Overhangs** and/or **Open Margins; Open Contacts** with Food Impaction	☒ No	☐ Yes	
VIII.	**Dental/Orthodontic Appliances** (fixed or removable)	☐ No	☒ Yes	
IX.	**Severe Dry Mouth (Xerostomia)**	☒ No		☐ Yes

Overall assessment of dental caries risk: ☐ Low ☒ Moderate ☐ High

Patient Instructions:

• **Figure 18.6** Caries Risk Assessment form for ages 6 years to adult. (American Dental Association. http://www.ada.org/~/media/ADA/Science%20and%20Research/Files/topic_caries_over6.pdf?la.=en. Accessed May 15, 2017.)

Continued

ADA American Dental Association®
America's leading advocate for oral health

Caries Risk Assessment Form (Age >6)

Circle or check the boxes of the conditions that apply. Low Risk = only conditions in "Low Risk" column present; Moderate Risk = only conditions in "Low" and/or "Moderate Risk" columns present; High Risk = one or more conditions in the "High Risk" column present.

The clinical judgment of the dentist may justify a change of the patient's risk level (increased or decreased) based on review of this form and other pertinent information. For example, missing teeth may not be regarded as high risk for a follow up patient; or other risk factors not listed may be present.

The assessment cannot address every aspect of a patient's health, and should not be used as a replacement for the dentist's inquiry and judgment. Additional or more focused assessment may be appropriate for patients with specific health concerns. As with other forms, this assessment may be only a starting point for evaluating the patient's health status.

This is a tool provided for the use of ADA members. It is based on the opinion of experts who utilized the most up-to-date scientific information available. The ADA plans to periodically update this tool based on: 1) member feedback regarding its usefulness, and; 2) advances in science. ADA member-users are encouraged to share their opinions regarding this tool with the Council on Dental Practice.

• **Figure 18.6, cont'd**

Gathering information about the quality of the patient's meal pattern and eating habits is an important step in assessing the cariogenic potential of a diet. A food diary (Fig. 18.8), which provides food data for one day, can be obtained through an interview by the dental hygienist, or the patient can be asked to return the completed form at a recare appointment. This practical assessment tool is helpful in determining adequacy of the overall diet and habits related to carbohydrate intake. Several food records are available on the Internet. Choose one that meets the needs of the dental environment. Fig. 18.9 shows a second example of a food diary.

Using *MyPlate* as a guide, the dental hygienist can review adequacy of food intake with participation of the patient. Actively involving the patient in as many steps as possible enhances motivation and adherence. Ask the patient to highlight all fermentable carbohydrates on the food diary (see Figs. 18.8 and 18.9). Review the food diary and discuss any oversights with the patient as needed. Classify each fermentable carbohydrate as cariogenic or noncariogenic to assess caries potential (Fig. 18.10). This classification requires identifying the carbohydrate according to its form, frequency of consumption, and when it was eaten. More than two hours of acid exposure in one day is generally considered high.

Goals

When all the facts are gathered, help the patient develop realistic goals. These goals need to be flexible to meet the patient's needs, preferences, and lifestyle. Achievement of long-term goals is possible only if the patient is able and motivated to make behavioral changes, such as altering choices of cariogenic snacks or limiting frequency of cariogenic foods.

Education

Providing current information about detrimental dietary habits is instrumental in determining appropriate goals. Education alone does not guarantee behavioral change. For example, a patient may recite the process of decay and list components responsible for caries development, but if several areas of decay are evident at each 6-month recare visit, behavioral change has not occurred. Individualize dietary advice based on the patient's lifestyle, rather than requesting a change in lifestyle to accommodate recommendations. The patient's assessment and goals are the basis for any recommendations. The dental professional should attempt to dispel myths, redirect inappropriate habits, and provide new thoughts.

ADA American Dental Association®
America's leading advocate for oral health

Caries Risk Assessment Form (Age 0-6)

Patient Name:				
Birth Date:			**Date:**	
Age:			**Initials:**	
		Low Risk	Moderate Risk	High Risk
Contributing Conditions		Check or Circle the conditions that apply		
I.	**Fluoride Exposure** (through drinking water, supplements, professional applications, toothpaste)	☐Yes	☐No	
II.	**Sugary Foods or Drinks** (including juice, carbonated or non-carbonated soft drinks, energy drinks, medicinal syrups)	Primarily at mealtimes ☐	Frequent or prolonged between meal exposures/day ☐	Bottle or sippy cup with anything other than water at bed time ☐
III.	**Eligible for Government Programs** (WIC, Head Start, Medicaid or SCHIP)	☐No		☐Yes
IV.	**Caries Experience of Mother, Caregiver and/or other Siblings**	No carious lesions in last 24 months ☐	Carious lesions in last 7-23 months ☐	Carious lesions in last 6 months ☐
V.	**Dental Home**: established patient of record in a dental office	☐Yes	☐No	
General Health Conditions		Check or Circle the conditions that apply		
I.	**Special Health Care Needs** (developmental, physical, medical or mental disabilities that prevent or limit performance of adequate oral health care by themselves or caregivers)	☐No		☐Yes
Clinical Conditions		Check or Circle the conditions that apply		
I.	**Visual or Radiographically Evident Restorations/ Cavitated Carious Lesions**	No new carious lesions or restorations in last 24 months ☐		Carious lesions or restorations in last 24 months ☐
II.	**Non-cavitated** (incipient) **Carious Lesions**	No new lesions in last 24 months ☐		New lesions in last 24 months ☐
III.	**Teeth Missing Due to Caries**	☐No		☐Yes
IV.	**Visible Plaque**	☐No	☐Yes	
V.	**Dental/Orthodontic Appliances Present** (fixed or removable)	☐No	☐Yes	
VI.	**Salivary Flow**	Visually adequate ☐		Visually inadequate ☐

Overall assessment of dental caries risk: ☐ Low ☐ Moderate ☐ High

Instructions for Caregiver:

• **Figure 18.7** Caries Risk Assessment form for up to age 6 years. (American Dental Association. http://www.ada.org/~/media/ADA/Member%20Center/FIles/topics_caries_under6.pdf?la=en. Accessed May 15, 2017.)

Continued

ADA American Dental Association®
America's leading advocate for oral health

Caries Risk Assessment Form (Age 0-6)

Circle or check the boxes of the conditions that apply. Low Risk = only conditions in "Low Risk" column present; Moderate Risk = only conditions in "Low" and/or "Moderate Risk" columns present; High Risk = one or more conditions in the "High Risk" column present.

The clinical judgment of the dentist may justify a change of the patient's risk level (increased or decreased) based on review of this form and other pertinent information. For example, missing teeth may not be regarded as high risk for a follow up patient; or other risk factors not listed may be present.

The assessment cannot address every aspect of a patient's health, and should not be used as a replacement for the dentist's inquiry and judgment. Additional or more focused assessment may be appropriate for patients with specific health concerns. As with other forms, this assessment may be only a starting point for evaluating the patient's health status.

This is a tool provided for the use of ADA members. It is based on the opinion of experts who utilized the most up-to-date scientific information available. The ADA plans to periodically update this tool based on: 1) member feedback regarding its usefulness, and; 2) advances in science. ADA member-users are encouraged to share their opinions regarding this tool with the Council on Dental Practice.

• **Figure 18.7, cont'd**

Food Diary

Day ____________

Time	Place	Food Eaten	Amount Eaten	How Prepared
Example: 6:00 A.M.	Kitchen	Orange juice Whole wheat bread Diet margarine Egg	½ c 2 slices 1 tsp 1	Unsweetened Toasted Tub Fried in oil

Instructions:

1. List EVERYTHING you eat or drink on 3 consecutive, typical days.
2. Use 2 weekdays and 1 weekend day.
3. Include extras such as chewing gum, sugar and cream in coffee, or mustard on a sandwich.

• **Figure 18.8** Food diary. Typically used for 1 to 7 days. (A customizable version is available on Evolve.)

Daily Food and Activity Diary

	Monday	Tuesday	Wednesday	Thursday	Friday	Saturday	Sunday
Breakfast							
Lunch							
Dinner							
Activity							

GOALS: DIET	PHYSICAL ACTIVITY
BEHAVIOR	

• **Figure 18.9** Another example of a food diary. (U.S. Department of Health and Human Services. National Heart, Lung and Blood Institute. Available at: https://www.nhlbi.nih.gov/health/educational/lose_wt/eat/diary.pdf. Accessed May 15, 2017.)

Carbohydrate Intake Analysis Worksheet

Fermentable CHO	Cariogenic?	Reason	Period of Exposure to Enamel
Banana and coffee with sugar	Yes	2 carbohydrates eaten at the same time; banana is retentive.	40 minutes
Pizza and regular soda (consumed together)	No	If soda is consumed with meal, carbohydrates in pizza (crust, sauce) and soda will be neutralized by fat and protein of other components of pizza.	0 minutes
Pizza and regular soda (consumed separately)	Yes	If consumption of soda is continued after the meal, there are no components to neutralize the carbohydrates in the soda.	20 minutes

TOTAL EXPOSURE TIME: ____________

• **Figure 18.10** Example of a carbohydrate intake analysis. (A customizable version is available on Evolve.)

HEALTH APPLICATION 18

Genetically Modified Foods

Genetically modified organisms (GMOs) consist of taking genetic material (DNA) from one plant, animal, or microorganism and inserting it into the permanent genetic code of another. This technology is also referred to as "genetic engineering" and "biotechnology."

The first genetically modified (GM) food, introduced in the mid-1990s, was herbicide-resistant soybeans. Currently, more than 85% of corn, soybeans, cotton, and sugar beets in the United States are genetically engineered. Additionally, other GM plants include quinoa, canola (rapeseed), rice, potatoes, and bananas. While the United States is the leading producer of GM foods, developing countries are planting GM crops at a more rapid rate than rich countries. Currently, GM foods are mostly plants, but foods derived from GM microorganisms or GM animals may become available in the near future. Very few fresh fruits and vegetables are GM, but highly processed foods, such as vegetable oils or breakfast cereals, most likely contain some percentage of GM ingredients.

GM plants are modified in the laboratory and marketed because of a perceived advantage either to the farmer or consumer, such as lower price, improved durability, or nutritional value. The purposes of genetic engineering are to (a) speed growth, (b) resist disease, (c) repel insects, (d) withstand harsh growing conditions, and (e) improve nutritional quality. The world faces serious problems in feeding 9 billion people by 2050. Agriculture production must be increased and ecosystem services maintained at a time when conditions for growing crops are predicted to worsen in many parts of the world.[15]

Malnutrition in developing countries is a consequence of a dearth of certain vitamins in staple foods, losses during crop processing, and overreliance on a single primary food source. Golden Rice is a GM rice that provides vitamin A. The beta-carotene in this rice is effectively converted to vitamin A and can be used to improve the vitamin A status of young children in developing countries.[16]

Insect resistance is accomplished by incorporating the gene for a toxin from the bacterium *Bacillus thuringiensis*. This toxin, used as a conventional insecticide in agriculture, is safe for human consumption. Viral resistance makes plants less susceptible to diseases caused by viruses, resulting in higher crop production. The potential for GM seeds to result in bigger yields should lead to lower prices.

Altering the genetic makeup of plants and animals has been very controversial with concerns from many experts about the long-term effects on humans and the environment. Some of the concerns voiced include the potential for GM foods to cause (a) organ damage, (b) disrupt endocrine functions, (c) decrease fertility, (d) increase allergies, (e) increase pesticide resistance, (f) accelerate aging, and (g) promote immune system disorders. Indeed, no studies have tracked the long-term effect that GMOs may have on humans.

The main issues widely debated are the potential for GM foods to provoke allergic reaction, gene transfer, and cross-contamination. In response to the allegation that GM crops may increase allergenicity, foods that are considered highly allergenic are highly discouraged in producing GM products. When foods are digested and absorbed, a possibility exists that the genes can transfer through the digestive system, increasing antibiotic resistance and pesticide residues in the body. The World Health Organization indicates that the probability of transfer occurring is low, but using technology without antibiotic-resistant genes has been encouraged by an expert World Health Organization panel.[17] Some are fearful that modified plants or animals may have genetic changes that are unexpected and harmful. Some are concerned that the protein that was intended to be created during the manufacturing process may be different than what is actually created. Any minor error in a DNA sequence could cause various unintended effects and health issues.

A few of the concerns are legitimate. Whereas GM technology was supposed to decrease the need for pesticides to fight weeds and insects, herbicides in the production of two GM crops (soybeans and corn) have actually increased.[18] Resistant weeds have become a major problem for farmers using GM seeds. Genes from GM plants have cross-pollinated into conventional crops or related wild species as well as mixing with crops derived from conventional seeds with those grown using GM crops. This occurred when traces of maize approved for animals appeared in maize products produced for human consumption in the United States.[17]

The United States and Canada modified existing regulatory statutes to control GM foods. In the United States, three different government agencies have jurisdiction of GM foods. The U.S. Environmental Protection Agency (EPA) evaluates GM plants for environmental safety. The U.S. Department of Agriculture evaluates whether the plant is safe to grow; they are concerned with potential hazards of the plant itself. They ensure that the function of the introduced gene is known and the gene does not cause plant disease. The FDA evaluates whether the plant is safe to eat. The FDA has no control over the production of corn, but they regulate a box of cornflakes because it is a food product. To the FDA, GM foods are substantially equivalent to unmodified, "natural" foods, and are not subject to FDA regulations. Companies who create new GM foods are not required to consult the FDA nor are they required to follow any recommendations made by the FDA.

GM foods currently available have passed risk assessments and are not likely to present risks for human health. Conversely, there is little scientific data tracking the long-term effects that GMOs may have on humans, and the information available does not ensure complete safety. It is possible that GM foods may cause unexpected health consequences that will not be evident for years. Furthermore, it is impossible to design a long-term safety test in humans. Each new GM food should be assessed on an individual basis before being allowed on the market. General statements regarding the safety of all GM foods are inappropriate.

Most Americans would prefer that GM foods be labeled. Very low concentrations of GMOs in foods often cannot be detected. Proponents of labeling genetically engineered foods feel that consumers have a right to know where products come from when they are making food purchases. If all GM foods and food products are to be labeled, Congress must enact sweeping changes in the existing food labeling policy and establish acceptable limits of GM contamination in non-GM products. Labeling is mandatory in the European Union. Organic foods do not contain GM products.

There are many challenges for GM products in the areas of safety testing, regulation, international policy, and food labeling. This technology has enormous potential benefits, but caution is needed to avoid causing unintended harm to human health and the environment.

CASE APPLICATION FOR THE DENTAL HYGIENIST

At his 6-month recare visit, John S. presented with six new areas of decay: one occlusal area (class I carious lesion), two proximal surfaces of posterior teeth (class II), and three proximal surfaces of anterior teeth (class III). There is bleeding on probing, suggesting active periodontal disease. John admits that his busy schedule prevents him from flossing his teeth. He stopped smoking and replaced it with chewing gum and hard candy since his last appointment. When asked about work, John states he takes antacids to settle his stomach because of added pressures of his job.

Nutritional Assessment

- Food, nutrient, and caloric intake
- Frequency of eating between meals
- Eating habits
- Motivation level
- Knowledge level

Nutritional Diagnosis

Altered nutrition: frequent intake of chewing gum, hard candy, and antacids at various intervals throughout the day compounded by an increased plaque index, a measure of the quantity and location of plaque biofilm.

Nutritional Goals

The patient will improve his overall nutrient intake and make substitutions or modify the habits increasing his caries risk.

Nutritional Implementation

Intervention: Provide a food diary (see Figs. 18.8 and 18.9) with an explanation for its use and instructions emphasizing the importance of listing everything put into his mouth.

Rationale: The food record provides additional information about John's intake and reveals habits that he may have neglected to mention, thinking they were not relevant to his dental needs.

Intervention: Review the food record with John to identify health aspects and aspects needing revision. Allow John to make the necessary changes.

Rationale: The probability of a patient adhering to a recommended regimen is enhanced when the patient is actively involved in the decision-making process. The dental hygienist can suggest possible solutions and direct misguided changes. The patient ultimately makes required changes.

Intervention: Explain the caries process, factors involved, and that several of the carious lesions are in places usually unaffected.

Rationale: Understanding the total picture of his particular dental status can be motivating for John and may help him make needed changes.

Intervention: Stress that not only the quantity of fermentable carbohydrates in his diet but also spacing, duration, frequency, and form of intake lead to caries. Use the Carbohydrate Intake Analysis Worksheet (see Fig. 18.10) as an educational tool to enhance the explanation.

Rationale: Each time the patient consumes a fermentable carbohydrate, even if it is a small mint, he is decreasing the plaque pH to an acidic level for 40 minutes. By consuming sugar-containing mints six times throughout the day, the acid produced by plaque bacteria may be present for 4 hours.

Intervention: Educate John about the cariogenic potential of sugar-containing antacids and discuss options to avoid or reduce use of antacids. Another option may be to use sugar-free antacids, although his condition should be evaluated by his health care provider if it persists.

Rationale: Sugar-containing antacids contain simple carbohydrates and have cariogenic potential. Antacids are high in sodium and can interfere with absorption of many nutrients. Suggestions to decrease use of antacids include consuming small, frequent meals; eating slowly; avoiding excessive amounts of caffeine products and alcohol; and reducing stress. Referral to the health care provider is necessary for persistent heartburn to ensure diagnosis and management of gastroesophageal reflux, which may increase the risk for caries and dental erosion and esophageal cancer.

Intervention: Praise John for his ability to quit smoking (see Chapter 19, *Health Application 19*).

Rationale: Smoking is a very difficult habit to break; many who stop smoking will start again, especially in stressful situations.

Intervention: Recommend fluoride treatments in the office and at home; sealants, if applicable; an antimicrobial rinse; and optimum oral self-care practices.

Rationale: Omitting the carbohydrate source is not the only factor involved in the caries process. In John's situation, protecting susceptible tooth surfaces and removing plaque biofilm also help eliminate the potential for caries.

Evaluation

The patient returns for his 6-month recare appointment caries free with a reduction in gingival bleeding. He is still not smoking and uses a chewing gum and mints with xylitol. He has begun an exercise program, which is helping to relieve his stress, and he has decreased his use of antacids.

Student Readiness

1. Explain the role of firm, fibrous foods in protecting the tooth against caries.
2. List several noncariogenic substitutions for fermentable carbohydrate snacks.
3. What are the different roles that carbohydrates, protein, and fat play in the decay process?
4. Identify at least four nutritional foods contraindicated for a caries-active patient.
5. Complete a 1- to 3-day food diary (see Figs. 18.8 and 18.9). Assess for nutrient adequacy, comparing it with *MyPlate*. Highlight the fermentable carbohydrates.
6. Based on the food diary from Question 5, complete the example Carbohydrate Intake Analysis worksheet (see Fig. 18.10). Determine your cariogenic behaviors and the number of minutes of acid production. Based on this intake record, create a realistic and appropriate meal pattern. Discuss the rationale for modifications and substitutions.
7. Compare the pH, grams of sugar, and milligrams of caffeine for an 8-oz serving of 100% apple juice, skim milk, an energy drink, a sports drink, soda, a fruit drink, and water. Provide a conclusion based on your findings.

CASE STUDY

Carol is a 42-year-old married high school graduate with three teenage children. She is a homemaker and does all the cooking and grocery shopping. Each member of Carol's family continues to have new areas of decay at each recare visit. The dental hygienist decides to have Carol write down her food consumption from the previous day while waiting for her appointment. Her food record showed the following:

Breakfast: skipped
Morning snack: glazed doughnut, coffee with cream and sugar
Lunch: grilled cheese sandwich, taco chips, gelatin salad with fruit and whipped cream, coffee with cream and sugar
Afternoon snack: candy bar and two or three homemade cookies throughout the afternoon
Dinner: meat loaf, fried potatoes, buttered carrots, roll with margarine
Evening snack: chocolate chip ice cream

1. What other information needs to be obtained before starting to educate the patient?
2. What dental information does Carol need to have?
3. What dietary recommendations should a dental hygienist suggest? What are some specific substitutions and modifications that can be made?
4. Approximately how many minutes of acid production occurred on the enamel surfaces this day?

CASE STUDY

As a new mother, Barbara wanted to take precautionary measures to prevent her daughter from having rampant dental decay, like the neighborhood children. She breastfed the infant until 9 months of age and refused to allow any sugar-containing foods, including ice cream. The daughter was frequently observed carrying a box of crackers and her sippy cup around the house. By age 3 years, she has six carious lesions.

1. When should nutrition education have first been initiated for Barbara? Explain.
2. Describe the procedure that a dental professional would take to educate Barbara.
3. What suggestions would you recommend?

References

1. National Center for Health Statistics. Chapter 32: Oral Health. Healthy People 2020 Midcourse Review. Hyattsville, MD. 2016. https://www.cdc.gov/nchs/data/hpdata2020/HP2020MCR-C32-OH.pdf. Accessed August 23, 2017.
2. Gao SS, Zhao IS, Hiraishi N, et al. Clinical trials of silver diamine fluoride in arresting caries among children: a systematic review. *J Dent.* 2016;1(3):201–210.
3. Figuero E, Nobrega DF, Garcia-Gargallo M, et al. Mechanical and chemical plaque control in the simultaneous management of gingivitis and caries: a systematic review. *J Clin Periodontol.* 2017;44(suppl 18):S116–S134.
4. Powell ES, Smith-Taillie LP, Popkin BM. Added sugars intake across the distribution of US children and adult consumers: 1977-2012. *J Acad Nutr Diet.* 2016;116(10):1543–1550.
5. Kosova EC, Auinger P, Bremer AA. The relationships between sugar-sweetened beverage intake and cariometabolic markers in young children. *J Acad Nutr Diet.* 2013;113(2):219–227.
6. Park S, Onufrak S, Blanck HM, et al. Characteristics associated with consumption of sports and energy drinks among US adults: National Health Interview Survey, 2010. *J Acad Nutr Diet.* 2013;113(1): 112–119.
7. U.S. Department of Agriculture. Agricultural Research Service: USDA National Nutrient Database for Standard Reference, Release 28. 2016, Nutrient Data Laboratory. http://ndb.nal.usda.gov/. Accessed May 13, 2017.
8. Marghalani AA, Guinto E, Phan M, et al. Effectiveness of xylitol in reducing dental caries in children. *Pediatr Dent.* 2017;39(2): 103–110.
9. Food and Drug Administration. Code of Federal Regulations Title 21, Volume 2: Food labeling, specific requirements for health claims. Health claims: dietary noncariogenic carbohydrate sweeteners and dental caries. Updated 2016. https://www.accessdata.fda.gov/scripts/cdrh/cfdocs/cfcfr/CFRSearch.cfm?fr=101.80. Accessed May 15, 2017.
10. Gustaffson BE, Quensel CE, Lanke LS, et al. The Vipeholm dental caries study: the effect of different levels of carbohydrate intake on caries activity in 436 individuals observed for 5 years. *Acta Odontol Scand.* 1954;11:232–364.
11. Almaz ME, Sonmez IS, Okte Z, et al. Efficacy of a sugar-free herbal lollipop for reducing salivary *Streptococcus mutans* levels: a randomized controlled trial. *Clin Oral Invest.* 2017;21:839–845.
12. Van Loveren C, Broukal Z. Oganessian E. Functional foods/ingredients and dental caries. *Eur J Nutr.* 2012;52(suppl 2):S15–S25.
13. Institute of Medicine. *Dietary Reference Intakes for Energy, Carbohydrates, Fiber, Fat, Fatty Acids, Cholesterol, Protein, and Amino Acids (Macronutrients).* Washington, DC: National Academies Press; 2005.
14. Hayman MB, Abrams SA. Section on Gastroenterology, Hepatology and Nutrition and Committee on Nutrition. Fruit juice in infants, children, and adolescents: current recommendations. *Pediatrics.* 2017;139(6):e20170967.
15. Raybould A, Poppy GM. Commercializing genetically modified crops under EU regulations: objectives and barriers. *GM Crops Food.* 2012;3(1):9–20.
16. De Steur H, Demont M, Gellynck X, et al. The social and economic impact of biofortification through genetic modification. *Curr Opin Biotechnol.* 2017;44:161–168.
17. World Health Organization. Food safety—frequently asked questions on genetically modified foods. Updated May 2014. http://www.who.int/foodsafety/publications/biotech/20questions/en/. Accessed May 15, 2017.
18. Perry ED, Ciliberto F, Hennessy DA, et al. Genetically engineered crops and pesticide use in U.S. maize and soybeans. *Sci Adv.* 2016;2:e1600850.

EVOLVE RESOURCES

Please visit http://evolve.elsevier.com/Stegeman/nutritional for additional practice and study support tools.

19

Nutritional Aspects of Gingivitis and Periodontal Disease

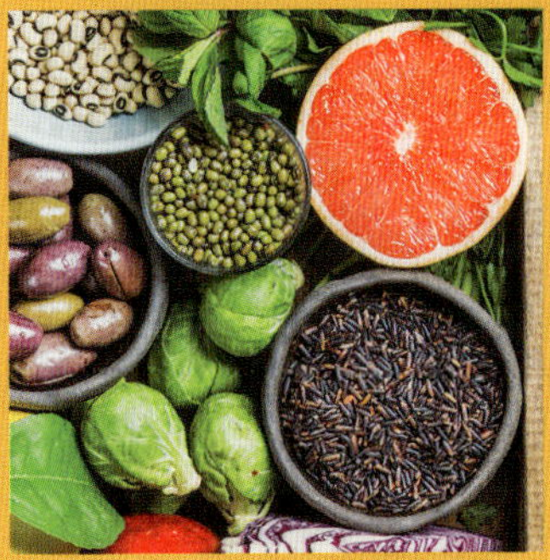

STUDENT LEARNING OUTCOMES

Upon completion of this chapter, the student will be able to achieve the following student learning outcomes:

1. Describe the role that nutrition plays in periodontal health and disease to a patient.
2. List the effects of food consistency and composition in periodontal disease.
3. Describe nutritional factors associated with gingivitis and periodontitis.
4. Discuss the following related to periodontal surgery and necrotizing periodontal disease:
   - Discuss components of nutritional education for a periodontal patient.
   - List major differences between full liquid, mechanically altered, bland, and regular diets.
   - Discuss nutrient deficiencies and oral health issues related to necrotizing periodontal disease.

KEY TERMS

Clinical attachment loss
Fibrotic
Full liquid diet
Mechanically altered diet
Purulent exudates
Suppuration

TEST YOUR NQ

1. **T/F** Vitamin-mineral supplementation beyond recommended levels is ineffective in controlling or preventing periodontal disease.
2. **T/F** Firm, fibrous foods physically remove plaque biofilm from the gingiva and tooth surface.
3. **T/F** A deficiency of vitamin C causes gingivitis.
4. **T/F** A bland, soft diet is commonly prescribed for a patient with necrotizing ulcerative gingivitis (NUG)/necrotizing ulcerative periodontitis (NUP).
5. **T/F** An appropriate instruction to a patient after periodontal surgery is, "Eat whatever foods you can manage."
6. **T/F** An individual with uncontrolled diabetes should be referred to a registered dietitian nutritionist for nutrition counseling if the diet needs to be modified because of oral discomfort, such as with NUG/NUP or after a periodontal procedure.
7. **T/F** Whole milk and milkshakes mixed with an instant breakfast mix are acceptable on a full liquid diet.
8. **T/F** A mechanically altered diet is similar to a regular diet except in consistency and texture.
9. **T/F** It is acceptable for a dental hygienist to recommend an instant breakfast drink or liquid supplement to a periodontal patient who is temporarily following a full liquid diet.
10. **T/F** The dental hygienist should complete the nutritional assessment and provide nutritional education immediately after periodontal surgery.

Gingivitis is characterized by inflammation, swelling, changes in contour or consistency, presence of plaque biofilm or calculus or both, no evidence of attachment loss, and bleeding on probing (Fig. 19.1A). Connective tissue and bone support are intact. Gingivitis is often reversible with appropriate oral hygiene techniques. If left untreated, gingivitis can progress to periodontal disease.

Periodontal disease is a chronic, inflammatory, and infectious disease (see Fig. 19.1B). It is the result of a loss of connective tissue and alveolar bone. Common findings are gingival bleeding, pain, infection, **suppuration** (formation or discharge of pus), tooth mobility, and tooth loss. Two targets for *Healthy People 2020* are (1) to reduce the prevalence of moderate and severe periodontitis from nearly 13% to 11% in people ages 45

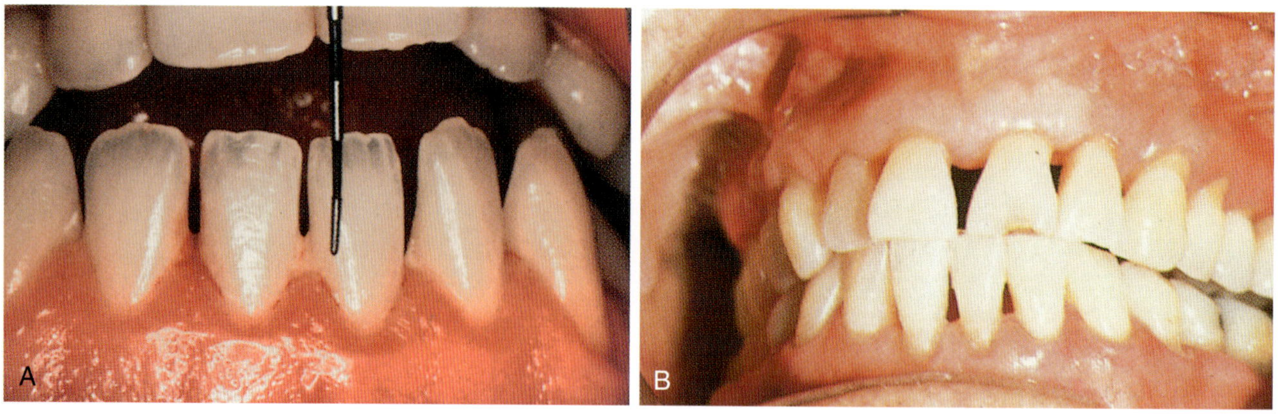

• **Figure 19.1** (A) Gingivitis. (B) Periodontal disease. (A reproduced with permission from Perry DA, Beemsterboer P, Essex G. *Periodontology for the Dental Hygienist*. 4th ed. St. Louis, MO: Saunders Elsevier; 2014. B courtesy of Barbara D. Altshuler, BSDH, MS, Clinical Assistant Professor, Caruth School of Dental Hygiene, The Texas A&M University System, Baylor College of Dentistry, Dallas, TX.)

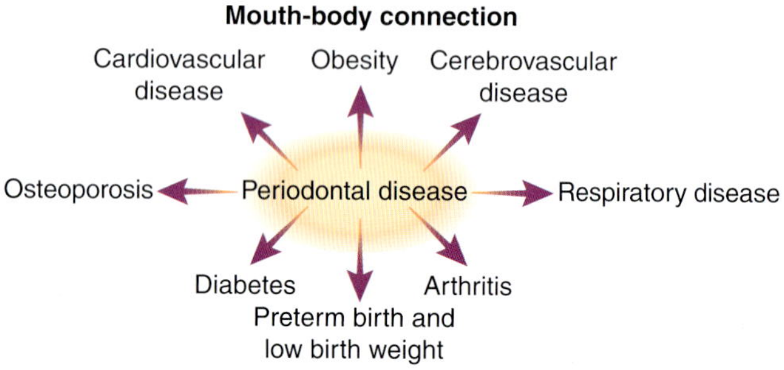

• **Figure 19.2** The possible connections between periodontal disease and other systemic diseases or conditions.

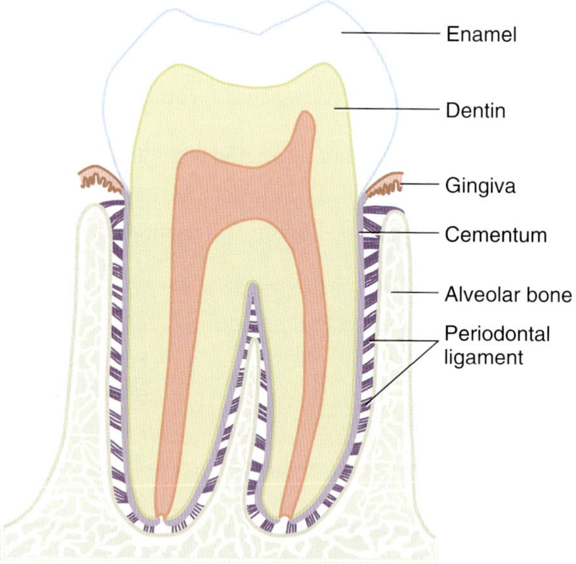

• **Figure 19.3** The periodontium consists of the gingiva, alveolar bone, cementum, and periodontal ligament. (Reproduced with permission from Fehrenbach MJ, Popowics T. *Illustrated Dental Embryology, Histology, and Anatomy*. 4th ed. St. Louis, MO: Saunders Elsevier; 2016.)

to 74 years and (2) to reduce the prevalence of tooth loss from periodontal involvement.[1]

The inflammatory process of gingivitis and periodontal disease is affected by the host's immune response—the body's ability to protect itself from destructive periodontal pathogens and infection. Nutritional deficiencies, which may occur from adolescence through adulthood, can modify the body's response to periodontal disease. Periodontal disease is the leading reason for tooth loss for individuals older than age 45 years. Bacteria associated with periodontal disease may increase the risk of systemic diseases or conditions such as cardiovascular disease, stroke, premature births, respiratory infections, and uncontrolled diabetes (Fig. 19.2).

The involvement of nutrition in periodontal disease is not as clear as it is for dental caries. Predisposing, etiologic, and contributing factors of periodontal disease are diverse; however, the primary initiating agent is plaque biofilm accumulation around teeth and gingiva. Nutrient deficiencies, excesses, or imbalances do not initiate periodontal disease, and megadoses of vitamin-mineral supplements do not cure or prevent periodontal disease. Indirectly, nutritional status may alter development, resistance, or repair of the periodontium (Fig. 19.3), which ultimately affects severity and extent of the disease. In addition, a patient's health, medications, and food choices influence the properties of plaque biofilm and saliva. The buffering and antimicrobial effects of saliva are significant factors in periodontal disease. A change in composition or amount of saliva can influence development and maturation of plaque biofilm (see discussion of xerostomia in Chapter 20).

Physical Effects of Food on Periodontal Health

Food Composition

The classes of macronutrients and micronutrients that have physiologic roles in growth, maintenance, and repair include carbohydrates, proteins, fats, vitamins, minerals, and water. At least 50 nutrients are provided by food, most of which are required for a healthy periodontium. An imbalance of one or more nutrients can be a factor in the disruption of tissue integrity and immune response. Consuming adequate amounts of each is the ultimate goal.

Normal growth and development of periodontal and oral mucosal tissues depend on sufficient intake of vitamin A (salivary glands, epithelial tissue), vitamin C (collagen, connective tissue), and

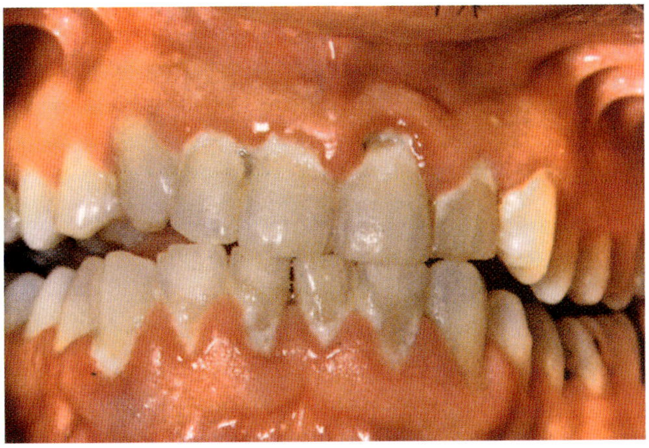

• **Figure 19.4** Gingivitis-related malnutrition. (Reproduced with permission from Perry DA, Beemsterboer P, Essex G. *Periodontology for the Dental Hygienist*. 4th ed. St. Louis, MO: Saunders Elsevier; 2014.)

vitamin B complex (epithelial and connective tissue). Calcification of the alveolus and cementum requires amino acids, calcium, phosphorus, vitamin D, and magnesium. Maintenance of oral tissues and integrity of the host's immune and repair responses requires sufficient amounts of vitamins A, C, D, and E; proteins; carbohydrates; fiber; calcium; iron; zinc; folic acid; and omega-3 fatty acids. Higher caloric ranges also are indicated for increased metabolic needs for individuals with periodontal disease.[2–4] (Refer to Chapters 4 through 12 for more descriptive information on the effects of specific nutrients on the periodontium.) Note the inflammation, bulbous tissue, edema, and suppuration in Fig. 19.4 depicting gingivitis-related malnutrition.

Supragingival plaque biofilm adhesion and formation is influenced by frequent dietary consumption of monosaccharides (e.g., glucose) and disaccharides, particularly sucrose. Subgingival plaque biofilm seems to be protected from local effects of sugars.

Nutritional intervention needs to be a component of the dental hygiene care plan for periodontal disease because poor nutrition affects the entire body, having an adverse effect on the periodontium. In combination with local irritating factors, such as plaque biofilm or tobacco use, systemic factors can increase risk or severity of periodontal disease of a patient but is not solely responsible for periodontal disease. A nutrition assessment by the dental hygienist can reveal dietary deficiencies that should be corrected for optimal healing. Referral to a registered dietitian nutritionist (RDN) may be indicated, particularly for compromised patients requiring medical nutrition therapy, such as patients with uncontrolled diabetes.

Food Consistency

Another factor affecting periodontal health is the texture of food. Chewing firm, coarse, and fibrous foods, such as raw fruits and vegetables, stimulates salivary flow. The increase in saliva enhances oral clearance of food, thereby reducing food retention. The less food debris that remains in the mouth, the less debris accumulates on the teeth. Plaque biofilm is not physically removed by eating firm foods, however. Soft, sticky foods increase accumulation of food, which enhances dental biofilm growth and retention.

• BOX 19.1 Nutritional Involvement in Periodontal Disease

A patient's dietary intake plays a role in periodontal health, directly and indirectly affecting:

- Growth and development, maintenance, and repair of the periodontium
- Amount and type of supragingival plaque biofilm
- Inflammation and immune response for optimal healing
- Amount and type of saliva
- Host resistance to decrease the susceptibility to infection

Nutritional Considerations for Periodontal Patients

Increased nutrients and energy are required by periodontal patients experiencing stress, tissue catabolism, or infection. A thorough assessment of the periodontal patient, as described in Chapter 21, provides valuable data needed to formulate a nutrition plan.

A medical and social history can indicate whether a patient is at risk of nutrient deficiencies because of alcoholism, anorexia, or other health problems. These patients would benefit from medical nutrition therapy by an RDN to normalize nutrient levels before treatment. Dietary education of all periodontal patients by the dental hygienist facilitates tissue repair and wound healing, improves resistance to infection, and reduces the number and severity of complications. Optimally, good nutritional status results in a shorter recovery and a more rapid return to health (Box 19.1).

Gingivitis

Gingivitis is a progressive inflammatory process beginning in the interdental papillae and advancing to the attached gingiva. The color of the gingiva varies from slight redness to a darker reddish blue. The gingiva bleeds easily and is either edematous and spongy or **fibrotic** (formation of fibrous tissue of the gingiva owing to chronic inflammation). The stippling of the gingiva disappears, and probing depths may increase without loss of attachment. Gingivitis is associated with a large accumulation of plaque biofilm and calculus on teeth (Fig. 19.5), which is exacerbated by frequent exposure to fermentable carbohydrates and retentive foods.

Gingival disease may be an indication of metabolic disease, such as diabetes mellitus. In combination with local factors, systemic factors, including an immunocompromised system (e.g., acquired immune deficiency syndrome [AIDS]); use of certain medications (e.g., antihistamines, antidepressants); hormonal changes (e.g., pregnancy, puberty); and a vitamin C deficiency can be elements in the development of gingivitis. Scurvy, a disease associated with vitamin C deficiency, is rarely seen in the United States because of the availability of fruits, vegetables, and foods fortified with vitamin C. Hemorrhage, bluish red gingiva, a widened periodontal ligament, and tooth mobility are characteristic oral symptoms of scurvy. Correcting the vitamin C deficiency through appropriate food choices, and sometimes supplementation, improves gingival health.

A lack of nutrients does not cause gingival inflammation but may be a predisposing factor by disrupting the process of tissue

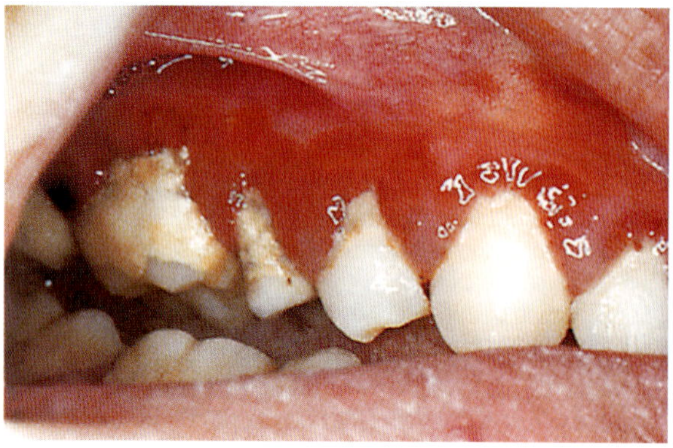

• **Figure 19.5** Gingivitis, with heavy calculus present. (Reproduced with permission from Darby ML, Walsh MM. *Dental Hygiene: Theory and Practice*. 4th ed. St. Louis, MO: Saunders Elsevier; 2015.)

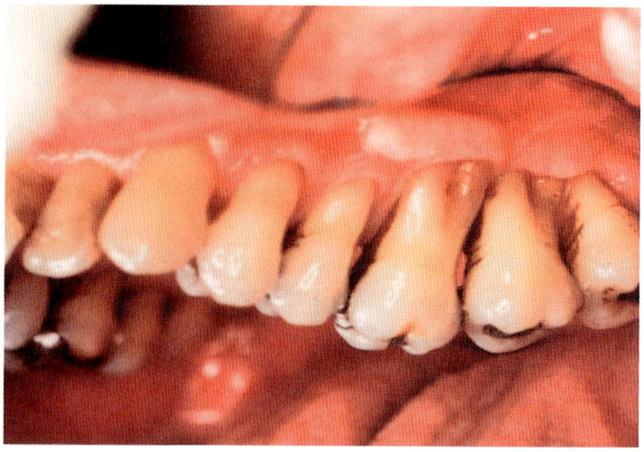

• **Figure 19.6** Clinical attachment loss. (Reproduced with permission from Perry DA, Beemsterboer P, Essex G. *Periodontology for the Dental Hygienist*. 4th ed. St. Louis, MO: Saunders Elsevier; 2014.)

repair. Adequate nutrients can hasten healing and repair processes. Controlling or modifying the etiologic factors can reverse clinical characteristics. Nutritional interventions for varying severities of gingivitis are the same as those for promoting overall health by encouraging adequate intake of all food groups and analyzing fermentable carbohydrate intake to determine potentially damaging habits that intensify the gingivitis.

DENTAL CONSIDERATIONS

Assessment

- *Physical:* Gingival tissue is red to reddish blue, or pink if fibrotic; interdental papillae are often bulbous; spontaneous bleeding on probing; the gingival margin is coronal to the cementoenamel junction; periodontal condition may be asymptomatic.
- *Dietary:* Adequate nutrient and calorie intake; frequency and amount of alcohol consumption.

Intervention

- Educate the patient that tissue damage associated with gingivitis is reversible.
- Encourage tailored oral self-care regimens.
- Provide oral prophylaxis, including biofilm and endotoxin debridement.

Evaluation

- Satisfactory response to therapy, resulting in healthy tissue; patient is able to demonstrate adequate oral hygiene techniques; adequate dietary intake.

NUTRITIONAL DIRECTIONS

- Optimal nutrient intake impacts the growth, development, maintenance, and repair of the periodontium throughout the life cycle.
- Encourage nutrient-dense foods that are not retentive. Soft foods are followed by appropriate oral hygiene.
- Encourage a variety of foods, including foods and beverages rich in vitamin C. Use the *Dietary Guidelines* and *MyPlate* as a guide.
- Poor nutrient intake is not the sole reason for periodontal disease. It is one risk factor that can affect the severity and extent of the disease.

Chronic Periodontitis

Periodontitis involves **clinical attachment loss** (Fig. 19.6), separation of collagen fibers from the cementum and apical movement of the junctional epithelium onto the root surface. Clinical attachment loss is a reliable method of determining disease activity, measuring from the cementoenamel junction to the bottom of the periodontal pocket. This destructive process results in bone loss. Inflammation is also present, affecting gingiva and other components of the periodontium. Severity of the gingival inflammation, recession, bone loss (Fig. 19.7), tooth mobility, and periodontal pocket formation varies according to duration of disease and the individual's resistance level or immune response. It can be localized or generalized in the mouth possibly with **purulent exudates** or drainage of fluids from the gingival sulcus.

Initiation and progression of periodontitis do not occur unless plaque biofilm and calculus are present. As with gingivitis, certain types of food (e.g., soft, retentive, or fermentable carbohydrate) can enhance food retention and severity of gingival inflammation. In addition to retentive carbohydrates, excess glucose and sucrose have been shown to increase rate of bacterial growth in the early stages of biofilm development. Biofilm development eventually reaches a steady state at this point, and the influence of diet is thought to be less important in the process of maturation of plaque biofilm.

Systemically, nutritional status determines immunocompetence of the periodontium. A deficiency of calcium, phosphorus, and vitamin D can contribute to severity of bone loss (although the deficiency is not the primary cause). Recovery from periodontitis also is enhanced by the positive effect of adequate nutrient reserves and intake on the immune system. Adequate vitamin C reserves can help ensure wound healing.[3–5] Nutrient intake exceeding the Recommended Dietary Allowance (RDA) may not improve or accelerate the healing process and can be detrimental because of interference with other nutrients or drugs. With assistance from the dental professional, the patient can make dietary adjustments necessary to meet the stresses and increased nutrient requirements of the disease and to ensure optimal wound healing.

Nutritional recommendations for a patient with gingivitis can be adapted to meet the needs of a patient with periodontitis. Importance is placed on maintaining a nutritionally adequate diet while avoiding retentive foods. The *Dietary Guidelines*

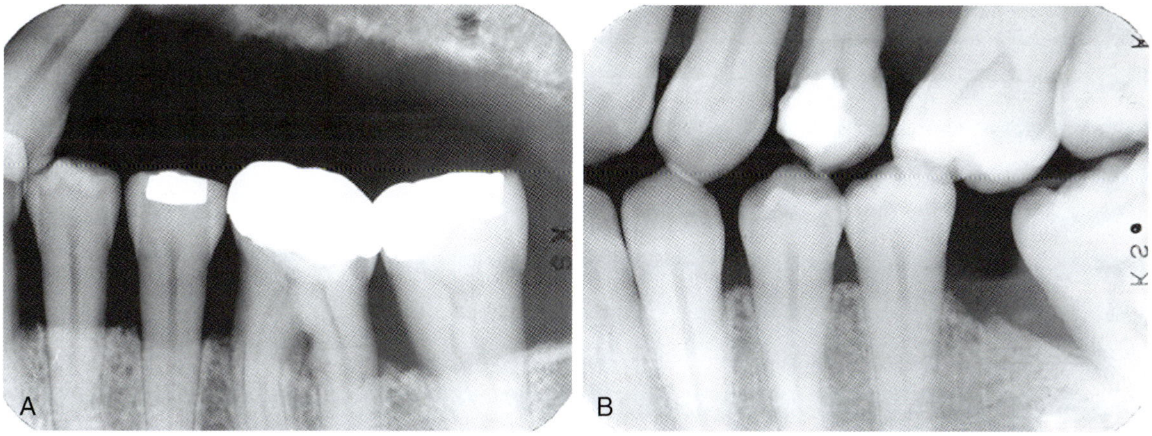

• **Figure 19.7** Horizontal (A) and vertical (B) bone loss. (Reproduced with permission from Iannucci JM, Howerton LJ. *Dental Radiography: Principles and Techniques*, 4th ed. St. Louis, MO: Saunders Elsevier; 2012.)

and *MyPlate* are valuable educational tools. The dental professional will analyze food intake for the amount and frequency of fermentable carbohydrate intake (see Fig. 18.9 in Chapter 18). By working toward improving or eliminating etiologic factors related to periodontitis, the healing process can minimize irreversible damage.

Periodontal Surgery

Preoperative

If periodontal surgery is indicated, the body's immunologic competency is important for optimal healing and preventing or minimizing infections. The dental hygienist should conduct a preliminary assessment of the patient for adequate nutrient reserves before the dental procedure. If the recommendations of the *Dietary Guidelines* and *MyPlate* are met, the patient's dietary intake is considered adequate. Generally, minor periodontal surgical procedures on a healthy patient with an adequate intake do not require special dietary modification. Surgery on a chronic alcoholic or a patient with an eating disorder could require preoperative replenishment of nutrient reserves. An elective surgery may need to be postponed for 1 or 2 weeks to allow improvement in nutritional status. A medically compromised patient is best served by an RDN who can appropriately assess and determine energy and other nutrient requirements.

Recommendation of a liquid nutritional supplement (e.g., instant breakfast) or multivitamin with minerals may be warranted. Coordinating efforts with an RDN provides the patient with continuity of care. To enhance compliance, the dental professional can provide a clear understanding of the relationship of nutrition to periodontal status.

Before surgery, the patient should be given a tailored meal plan listing nutrient-dense, fortified and enriched foods and beverages to consume during the recovery period. Milk and 100% fruit juices contain more nutrients than soft drinks, even if caloric value is similar. The dental hygienist should consider the extent of the surgery, its potential discomfort, and the patient's ability to eat after the periodontal procedure, and encourage food choices that avoid tissue trauma. The patient's food preferences and dislikes are other factors to be taken into consideration.

Postoperative

Because of blood loss, increased catabolism, tissue regeneration, and host defense activities after periodontal surgery, adequate nutrient intake is required. Meeting the requirements for calories, proteins, vitamins, minerals, and decaffeinated fluids (8–10 glasses a day) enhances recovery.

Dietary intake can be influenced by complications of anorexia, nausea, dysphagia, and oral discomfort. The texture of foods depends on extent of the surgery and symptoms of the patient. A full liquid diet may be required the first 1 to 3 days (Box 19.2). A **full liquid diet** provides food in a liquid form for patients who are unable to chew. It should consist of high-protein, high-calorie fluids and semisolid foods to promote optimal healing. Fluids can be drunk from a cup without the use of a spoon or straw. A full liquid diet is used only temporarily because nutrient and caloric value is usually inadequate. Any special diet modifications (e.g., low sodium, low fat) and patient preferences should be considered.

The full liquid diet can progress to a mechanically altered diet when tolerated. A **mechanically altered diet** (Box 19.3) is a regular diet altered in consistency and texture for ease in mastication when chewing may be compromised. This diet includes soft, ripened, chopped, ground, mashed, and pureed foods. Foods are generally moist. Most raw fruits (except bananas) and vegetables are avoided, as are any foods containing seeds or nuts. The mechanically altered diet is recommended for 3 to 7 days until the patient can tolerate regular foods. Consuming small, frequent meals (e.g., six small feedings one-half the size of a regular meal) may provide adequate intake and is easier for the patient. Bland foods (Box 19.4) may be necessary to avoid irritating sensitive tissue. A liquid nutritional supplement such as Carnation Instant Breakfast, Ensure (Abbot Nutrition), and Boost (Nestlē), a multivitamin with minerals, or both may be recommended to ensure adequate nutrients and accelerate recovery.

Periodontal dressing may be used to cover and protect the surgical site; shield the tissue from irritation; help control postoperative bleeding, edema, and infection; and prevent accumulation of food debris and bacteria. Also, encourage cool liquids and foods for the first 24 hours to allow the dressing to harden and prevent swelling. Discourage smoking and the use of straws because sucking pressure could dislodge a blood clot.

DENTAL CONSIDERATIONS

Assessment

- *Physical:* Pale-pink to purplish-red gingival tissue (firm to spongy); interdental papillae may not fill the interdental spaces; bleeding on probing and suppuration may occur; probing depths of 4 mm or more; tooth mobility, furcation involvement, and pain may be present.
- *Dietary:* Adequacy of dietary and fluid intake; avoidance of alcohol; use of vitamin-mineral supplements.

Interventions

- Oral prophylaxis to debride and deplaque teeth to eliminate or suppress infectious microorganisms.
- Recommend an antimicrobial (systemic or site specific).
- Instruct the patient to avoid hard, sticky, and brittle foods and to follow the guidelines for a mechanically altered diet for 1 to 2 days.
- Encourage appropriate techniques for optimal oral self-care.
- Provide smoking cessation counseling, if needed (see *Health Application 19* at the end of this chapter).
- Control any existing systemic disease, such as diabetes.
- Identify and recommend modification of open margins, overhangs, inadequate restorations.
- Recommend or provide fluoride therapy for desensitization, if needed.

Evaluation

- Absence of inflammation and other signs of periodontal issues, such as pain and ulcerations; adherence to an adequate diet; avoiding alcohol and smoking; maintaining regular recare appointments with a healthy periodontal clinical assessment.

NUTRITIONAL DIRECTIONS

- Postsurgical patients may require a full liquid or mechanically altered diet until the patient can chew comfortably.
- To meet energy and nutrient needs, postsurgical patients typically require small, frequent meals and nutrient-dense foods and beverages.
- A patient requiring a therapeutic meal plan, such as for diabetes, may need a referral to an RDN.
- Discuss with the patient how alcohol abuse may contribute to periodontal issues because of enhanced bleeding tendencies and a propensity toward malnutrition.
- There is emerging evidence that probiotics may inhibit growth of plaque biofilm and bacteria associated with periodontal disease (see Table 20.1 in Chapter 20). Probiotics vary in means of administration, including foods, tablets, chewing gums, and lozenges. Probiotics are live microorganisms differing in strains and strengths; therefore, selecting the correct strain for a specific oral issue is essential and complex (see Chapter 3). Other considerations for selecting a probiotic include mode and time of administration; health of the patient; and retention and exposure times in the oral cavity. Further rigorous research is needed in this area.[6–11]

BOX 19.2 Full Liquid Diet: Oral Surgery

Purpose

To provide a high-protein, high-calorie liquid diet to promote healing in cleft lip and cleft palate repair, oral surgery (when chewing is difficult), or mouth irritations when solid foods are not tolerated.

Adequacy

This diet meets the Dietary Reference Intakes for energy, carbohydrates, protein, fat, calcium, and vitamin C for children and adults. It may be inadequate in all other nutrients. Nutritional adequacy can be improved by the addition of a commercial nutritional supplement. For prolonged use, a multivitamin-mineral supplement should be considered.

Description

All foods are liquid or semisolid at room temperature. All foods are of a consistency that can be drunk from a cup without a spoon or straw (to avoid penetrating the repaired palatal tissue).

Guidelines

This is a transitional diet: it should be followed by the mechanically altered diet to a regular diet. Oral nutritional supplements are recommended after 48 hours. Refer to an RDN or a health care provider if the patient requires longer time on this diet. A multivitamin-mineral supplement may be needed. Six small meals are recommended.

Sample Menu for Full Liquid Diet for Oral Surgery Patients

Breakfast	Snack	Lunch	Snack	Dinner
½ cup apple juice	8 oz malted milk	½ cup cranberry juice	½ cup ice cream with chocolate syrup	½ cup grape juice
8 oz smoothie made with yogurt and fruit		8 oz strained cream of pea soup with pureed ham		½ cup gelatin
1 cup Cream of Wheat cereal with butter		12 oz milkshake mixed with instant breakfast powder		8 oz tomato soup made with milk and additional milk powder
1 cup whole milk		8 oz whole milk		8 oz vanilla yogurt
		½ cup custard		1 cup eggnog
				½ cup of pudding

Approximate Nutrient Composition for Sample Full Liquid Menu for Oral Surgery

Calories, 2649
Carbohydrate, 345 g
Protein, 102 g
Fat, 100 g
Cholesterol, 484 mg
Dietary fiber, 13 g
Sodium, 3622 mg
Potassium, 5191 mg
Calcium, 3019 mg
Iron, 18 mg
Vitamin A, 2086 μg RAE (retinol activity equivalents)
Vitamin C, 113 mg

Reproduced with permission of Texas Academy of Nutrition and Dietetics. Texas Academy of Nutrition and Dietetics MNT Manual. *Dallas, TX; 2013.*

• BOX 19.3 Mechanically Altered Diet

Purpose

To provide a well-balanced diet, soft in texture and consistency, for patients with chewing difficulties due to poor or missing dentition, oral surgery, or radiation of the head and neck area, which may make the mouth sore.

Adequacy

If a variety of foods are selected, this diet meets the Dietary Reference Intakes for nutrients for most adults.

Description

1. The diet consists of a regular diet with alterations in consistency and texture.
2. Foods are generally tender—finely chopped, ground, or pureed—although very soft whole foods may be eaten as tolerated.
3. Patient tolerance to food texture and consistency may vary; modifications should be made accordingly.

Mechanically Altered Diet Food List

Food	Allowed	Avoid
Soup	Broth or creamed soups made with allowed foods, or strained	Soup with large pieces of food or whole meats or crunchy vegetables
Meat and meat substitutes	Any chopped or ground meat or poultry, very tender, baked, broiled, creamed or stewed whole meat, fish, or poultry; bacon, cheese, and cottage cheese; eggs; smooth peanut butter; soft dried beans and peas; boiled, creamed, poached, scrambled, souffléd eggs; soft casseroles	Whole cuts of meat; fried meat, fish, poultry and eggs; hot dogs and other meat in casings; crunchy peanut butter; pizza with thick, tough crust
Potato and substitutes	Any white or sweet potatoes, mashed, baked, creamed, scalloped, or boiled; macaroni, noodles, rice, pasta	Fried potatoes, potato chips, potato skins; whole grain or brown rice
Vegetables	Vegetable juice; any well-cooked, soft vegetable without seeds or skins; peeled raw tomatoes	Corn and other raw vegetables, unless tolerated
Bread	Any enriched or whole grain breads, soft rolls, doughnuts, pancakes, crackers, and biscuits	Hard, crusty bread; bread containing nuts or dried fruit; bagels; taco shells; popcorn
Cereals	Cooked cereals, cereals that require minimal chewing	Cereals containing nuts, coconut, dried fruit; shredded wheat cereal; granola; cereals that remain crunchy in milk
Fats	Any	None
Fruits	Any fruit juice; all canned or cooked fruit, soft fresh fruit	All other raw fruits and fruits with skins, dried fruits
Milk	Any	None
Desserts	Any except those to "Avoid"	Desserts containing coconut, nuts, dried fruits; fried, tough, or chewy items
Beverages	Any	None
Miscellaneous	Honey, iodized salt, sugar, sugar substitutes, syrup, jelly, ketchup, mustard, pepper, herbs, ground spices, cream sauces and gravies, chocolate, vinegar, lemon juice, cranberry sauce	Whole spices, pickles, popcorn, nuts, coconut

Sample Menu for Mechanically Altered Diet

Breakfast	Lunch	Dinner	Snack
½ cup orange juice	3 oz ground beef	3 oz broiled salmon	1 tbsp smooth peanut butter
1 cup oatmeal with brown sugar	½ cup mashed potatoes with gravy	1 medium baked potato (no peel)	3 squares graham crackers
1 slice whole wheat toast	½ cup well-cooked green beans	½ cup well-cooked broccoli	½ cup apple juice
1 tsp margarine	2 slices peeled tomato	1 slice whole-wheat bread	
1 cup skim milk	1 ripe banana	1 tsp margarine	
	1 whole wheat bun	1 small brownie without nuts	
	1 tsp mayonnaise	1 cup chocolate skim milk	
	½ cup ice cream	½ cup vegetable juice	
	1 cup skim milk		

Approximate Nutrient Composition for Mechanically Altered Diet

Calories, 1898
Carbohydrate, 287 g
Protein, 154 g
Fat, 60 g
Cholesterol, 307 mg
Dietary fiber, 26 g
Sodium, 3114 mg
Potassium, 5700 mg
Calcium, 1587 mg
Iron, 16 mg
Vitamin A, 1199 μg RAE (retinol activity equivalents)
Vitamin C, 186 mg

Adapted from Texas Academy of Nutrition and Dietetics. Texas Academy of Nutrition and Dietetics MNT Manual. *Dallas, TX; 2013.*

• BOX 19.4 Bland Diet

Purpose

To provide a temporary well-balanced diet for dental patients with ulcerations.

Foods and Fluids to Avoid

- Caffeine-containing beverages (coffee, tea, cola, cocoa)
- Alcohol
- Peppermint
- Chocolate
- Black and red pepper
- Chili pepper
- Chili powder
- Acidic foods
- Citrus fruits

Intolerance to these and other foods varies. Foods that cause discomfort should be avoided.

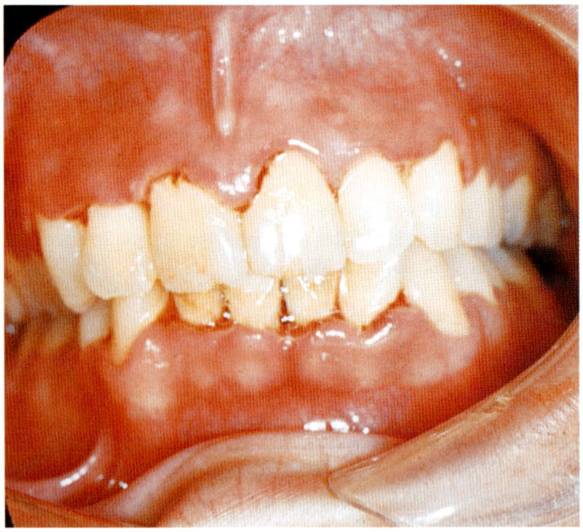

• **Figure 19.8** Necrotizing gingivitis. (Reproduced with permission from Ibsen OAC, Phelan JA. *Oral Pathology for the Dental Hygienist*. 6th ed. St. Louis, MO: Saunders Elsevier; 2014.)

Necrotizing Periodontal Diseases

Necrotizing Ulcerative Gingivitis and Necrotizing Ulcerative Periodontitis

Necrotizing ulcerative gingivitis (NUG) and necrotizing ulcerative periodontitis (NUP) are classified as acute periodontal diseases and are prevalent in young adults. NUG is characterized by red and shiny marginal labial and lingual gingivae that bleed when probed and by cratered interdental papillae, grayish sloughing of marginal gingiva, foul breath, metallic taste, occasional fever, and pain (Fig. 19.8). Common complaints include a burning mouth and anorexia. The etiology of NUG involves bacteria (e.g., *Borrelia vincentii*); systemic factors (e.g., increased susceptibility to infection, as in patients with diabetes or human immunodeficiency virus/AIDS); local factors (e.g., smoking, poor oral hygiene); and psychological factors (e.g., stress, fatigue) predisposing a patient to the disease.

Nutrient deficiencies, such as protein or vitamin C or B complex deficiency, are contributing factors to NUG because of lowered host resistance. These deficiencies commonly occur in young adults who have poor eating habits, consume primarily low nutrient-dense foods, and who rely primarily on convenience or fast food meals. Also, patients with NUG may lose the desire to eat because of pain or may choose soft foods that are easier to eat. Excessive alcohol intake and food impacted in the interproximal areas of open contacts are other possible factors related to the condition.

Tissue infection and destruction increase physiologic requirements for all nutrients. When fever is present, a 12% increase in total nutrient and energy intake is recommended for each degree above normal body temperature. Also, additional nutrients and energy are necessary for optimal tissue repair and healing. If left untreated, NUG can progress to NUP, in which attachment loss is present.

Obtaining the patient's health, dental, and social histories is the first step in nutritional management, followed by an extraoral and intraoral examination. In addition, a 24-hour food recall (see Chapter 18, Figs. 18.7 and 18.8) provides important insights into dietary practices and potential nutrient deficiencies. A 3- to 7-day food record may help provide a more accurate picture of food intake. Information gathered provides valuable clues regarding nutritional factors needing to be altered or eliminated. Dietary information allows the dental hygienist to make recommendations suited to the patient's eating patterns with consideration of the patient's food preferences and habits as well as financial resources. Maintaining food intake as closely as possible to the regular eating pattern generally results in greater compliance.

The severity of NUG determines initial dietary recommendations. The goal is to provide adequate nutrients and calories, avoid alcohol, and consume noncaffeinated fluids to maintain hydration. Based on the food record, a liquid nutritional supplement, or a multivitamin with mineral supplement may be suggested to ensure nutrient and caloric adequacy during acute periods of the disease. As soon as a nutritionally adequate diet is regularly consumed, any supplements recommended can be eliminated.

Lip and tongue ulcers, extremely painful inflamed gingival tissue, and possibly initial removal of calculus may warrant a full liquid diet for 1 to 3 days (see Box 19.2). As tolerated, the patient progresses to a mechanically altered diet (see Box 19.3). A patient's tolerance to consistency varies; the dental hygienist needs to tailor the dietary information to the patient. A patient with ulcerations may need to eliminate nuts and seeds that can lodge in the ulcer and cause further discomfort. Encourage fluids with meals to make chewing foods easier.

Provide examples of acceptable bland and soothing foods (e.g., gelatin, puddings), while recommending avoidance of spicy and acidic foods (e.g., citrus fruits and tomatoes), that can irritate the oral mucosa (see Box 19.4). Frequent small meals are beneficial for a patient who is having difficulty eating; choosing a variety of foods from each of the food groups is important. Additional protein intake (in the form of beans, low-fat cottage cheese, or skim milk) is effective in meeting the increased needs related to fever and infection. Adequate decaffeinated fluid intake is essential. When a regular diet can be reinstated, concentrate efforts on continuing to follow the *Dietary Guidelines* and *MyPlate*. Recurrence of NUG is possible, and preventive guidelines should be emphasized. Each episode of NUG increases the risk of progression to NUP.

DENTAL CONSIDERATIONS

Assessment

- *Physical:* Inflamed, hemorrhagic, and red labial and lingual gingivae; cratered interdental papillae; grayish sloughing of the marginal gingivae; metallic taste; foul odor; pain; fever; malaise.
- *Dietary:* Adequate nutrient, calorie, and fluid intake; amount and frequency of alcohol consumption.

Interventions

- Explain extrinsic and intrinsic etiologic factors associated with the type and severity of periodontal disease the patient is experiencing.
- Treatment includes debridement under anesthesia, pain control, and possibly antibiotics.
- Educate the patient on appropriate self-care procedures and recommend use of non–alcohol-containing antimicrobial mouth rinses.
- Explain how fermentable carbohydrates enhance plaque biofilm formation by providing substrates for bacterial growth and biofilm maturation. Also, explain how soft, retentive foods cling to the tooth, allowing adherence of plaque biofilm.
- When nutrient requirements are increased because of a periodontal condition and therapeutic treatment is needed, a multivitamin supplement may be recommended. Care should be taken to ensure that the nutrients in the supplement do not exceed 100% of the RDA unless recommended by an RDN.
- Many foods on a full liquid diet are milk based. Consider the needs of a patient who is lactose intolerant. A referral to an RDN may be needed.
- Ask the patient about any allergies to antibiotics.
- The methyl red sugar test can be incorporated into nutrition education as a practical motivational and educational tool. Its purpose is to determine a low pH (acid environment) in the oral cavity. Plaque is removed from the oral cavity and placed on a porcelain tile. Add a few drops of methyl red indicator to cover the plaque and sprinkle sugar on top. A change of color from red to yellow within 10 to 30 minutes indicates a decrease in the pH level. The patient should be taught not only about caries production but also how carbohydrates increase plaque biofilm adhesion and maturation.

Evaluation

- The patient improves nutritional adequacy of foods chosen; limits or avoids smoking and alcohol consumption; oral hygiene improves with each visit; and clinical signs and symptoms of NUP/NUG improve.

NUTRITIONAL DIRECTIONS

- Initially, a liquid diet may be needed; advancement to a mechanically altered diet is followed by a regular diet, depending on the patient's tolerance and comfort.
- Liquid nutrition supplements may be needed. Most of these products contain cariogenic sweeteners; these should be followed by appropriate oral hygiene care.
- Cooler-temperature foods are more soothing when ulcerations are present in the oral cavity.

HEALTH APPLICATION 19

Tobacco Cessation

Throughout this text, there are multiple references to the impact of smoking on health, including a negative influence on nutrient absorption. This health application focuses on one of the essential roles of dental professionals: implementing tobacco cessation protocols for dental patients.

Approximately 46.6 million U.S. adults smoke cigarettes, with cigarettes being responsible for 443,000 deaths each year. Furthermore, exposure to secondhand smoke affects 88 million nonsmoking Americans, 54% of whom are younger than age 11 years.[12] Cigarette smoke contains more than 4800 chemicals, 69 of which are known to cause cancer. Secondhand smoke is the number one cause of cancer in household pets. It is linked to premature births, low-birthweight babies, and cleft lip or palates in infants of women who smoke during pregnancy. Tobacco use is associated with cancer, coronary heart disease, stroke, respiratory diseases, and diabetes. In the oral cavity, tobacco use increases the risk of periodontal disease, oral cancers, leukoplakia, hairy tongue, delayed healing, failure of dental implants, loss of taste and smell, malodor, and extrinsic staining.

The addictive ingredient of tobacco is nicotine. Nicotine is a stimulant that increases the heart rate and blood pressure. All forms of tobacco have health consequences (Box 19.5). Because of the addictive nature of tobacco, an individual may attempt to quit on multiple occasions, requiring repeated intervention.

An established and frequently used protocol is the Five A's Approach: Ask, Advise, Assess, Assist, and Arrange.[13] *Ask* involves identifying and documenting tobacco use at every visit. Tobacco use should be a part of every health history. Fig. 19.9 provides an example of a tobacco use assessment form available for use with patients. The dental hygienist should determine if the patient is a current user, former user, or never used tobacco, as well as the form, frequency, and duration of tobacco use. Box 19.6 provides questions to aid the dental professional in starting and continuing this essential conversation.

Advise advocates all tobacco users to quit. The dental hygienist is to send a clear message about health risks at every appointment. It can be as simple as providing basic information about tobacco use. The message should be clear, nonjudgmental and tailored to the patient. A helpful statement may be, "I can't see what tobacco is doing to your heart, lungs, brain, and other organs, but I would like to show you some changes in your mouth." This opens opportunities to educate the patient on the importance of oral self-examinations in order to recognize abnormal situations.

Assess will focus on patients who report any type of tobacco use. The dental hygienist will assess the patient's willingness to quit. The response of the patient will determine the next step. Fig. 19.10 provides a flow chart on the process, including direction for when a patient is ready or not ready.

Assist is determined by the patient's willingness to quit. Whatever the response, the dental hygienist will provide information on the benefits of tobacco cessation. For those who are ready to quit, the dental hygienist will *elicit* information to enhance their motivation to quit; *provide* education (e.g., establish quit date, information on the available pharmacotherapy (Box 19.7); and refer the patient to support services. Popular resources include quitlines, online programs, pamphlets, or local smoking cessation programs. The final step within *Assist* is to *elicit* again by asking the patient to commit to an initial step in the action plan.

Continued

HEALTH APPLICATION 19

Tobacco Cessation—cont'd

Arrange is the final step, in which the dental professional will establish a follow-up contact (e.g., phone call, email, text), provide encouragement, answer questions, review information, and modify the plan as needed.

During the tobacco cessation process, the dental hygienist should encourage and praise the patient.

Tobacco quitlines are available in most states with a toll-free number. It is a free cessation service that includes coaching, self-help kits, cessation information, and referrals to local programs. The coaching is on an individual basis and anonymous. The ADHA quitline is a single access to the National Network of Tobacco Cessation quitlines: 1-800-QUIT-NOW. Online smoking cessation assistance is also anonymous, but group support is also available. A popular program is available at http://www.smokefree.gov/.

Except in the presence of contraindications, pharmacotherapy can be an effective support for patients going through smoking cessation (see Box 19.7). Medication can minimize the discomfort of nicotine withdrawal. A combination of tobacco cessation methods increases the likelihood for success.

Dental professionals are distinctively situated to provide tobacco education and promote abstinence or cessation. It is the responsibility and ethical obligation of all dental professionals to intervene and educate patients. The ADHA supports and encourages the dental hygienist to assess patients at each recare visit.

Tobacco Use Assessment Form

Name ______________________________

Date ____________

1. Do you use tobacco in any form? ☐ Yes ☐ No

1A. If no, have you ever used tobacco in the past? ☐ Yes ☐ No

How long did you use tobacco? _____ years _____ months

How long ago did you stop? _____ years _____ months

If you are not currently a tobacco user, no other questions should be answered. Thank you for completing this form.

Questions 2-10 are for current tobacco users only.

2. If you smoke, what type? (Check) How many? (Number)
☐ Cigarettes _____ Cigarettes per day
☐ Cigars _____ Cigars per day
☐ Pipe _____ Bowls per day

3. If you chew/use snuff, what type? How much?
☐ Snuff _____ Days a can lasts
☐ Chewing _____ Pouches per week
☐ Other (describe) ____________________
Amount __________ per ____________________

3A. How long do you keep a chew in your mouth?
________minutes

4. How many days of the week do you use tobacco?
7 6 5 4 3 2 1

5. How soon after you wake up do you first use tobacco?
☐ within 30 minutes ☐ more than 30 minutes

6. Does the person closest to you use tobacco?
☐ Yes ☐ No

7. How interested are you in stopping your use of tobacco?
☐ not at all ☐ a little ☐ somewhat ☐ yes ☐ very much

8. Have you tried to stop using tobacco before? ☐ Yes ☐ No

8A. How long ago was your last attempt to quit?
_____ years _____ months

9. Have you discussed stopping with another physician, dentist, or dental hygienist? ☐ Yes ☐ No

10. If you decided to stop using tobacco completely during the next two weeks, how confident are you that you would succeed?
☐ not at all ☐ a little ☐ somewhat ☐ very confident

Thank you for completing this form

Client Tobacco Use Assessment Form

Contact Record

Date client contacted	Client asked Y/N	Advice given Y/N	Assist describe service

• **Figure 19.9** Tobacco use assessment form. (Adapted from the U.S. Department of Health and Human Services: Tobacco effects in the mouth, National Institutes of Health Publication No. 94-3330, Bethesda, Md, 1992, U.S. Government Printing Office.)

• BOX 19.5 Tobacco Products

- Regular cigarettes
- Low-tar (light) cigarettes
- Smokeless tobacco
  - Spitless tobacco products
  - Moist snuff
  - Sticks
  - Orbs
  - Strips
- Cigars
- Pipes
- Electronic cigarettes
- Imported tobacco products
  - Hookah
  - Flavored tobacco

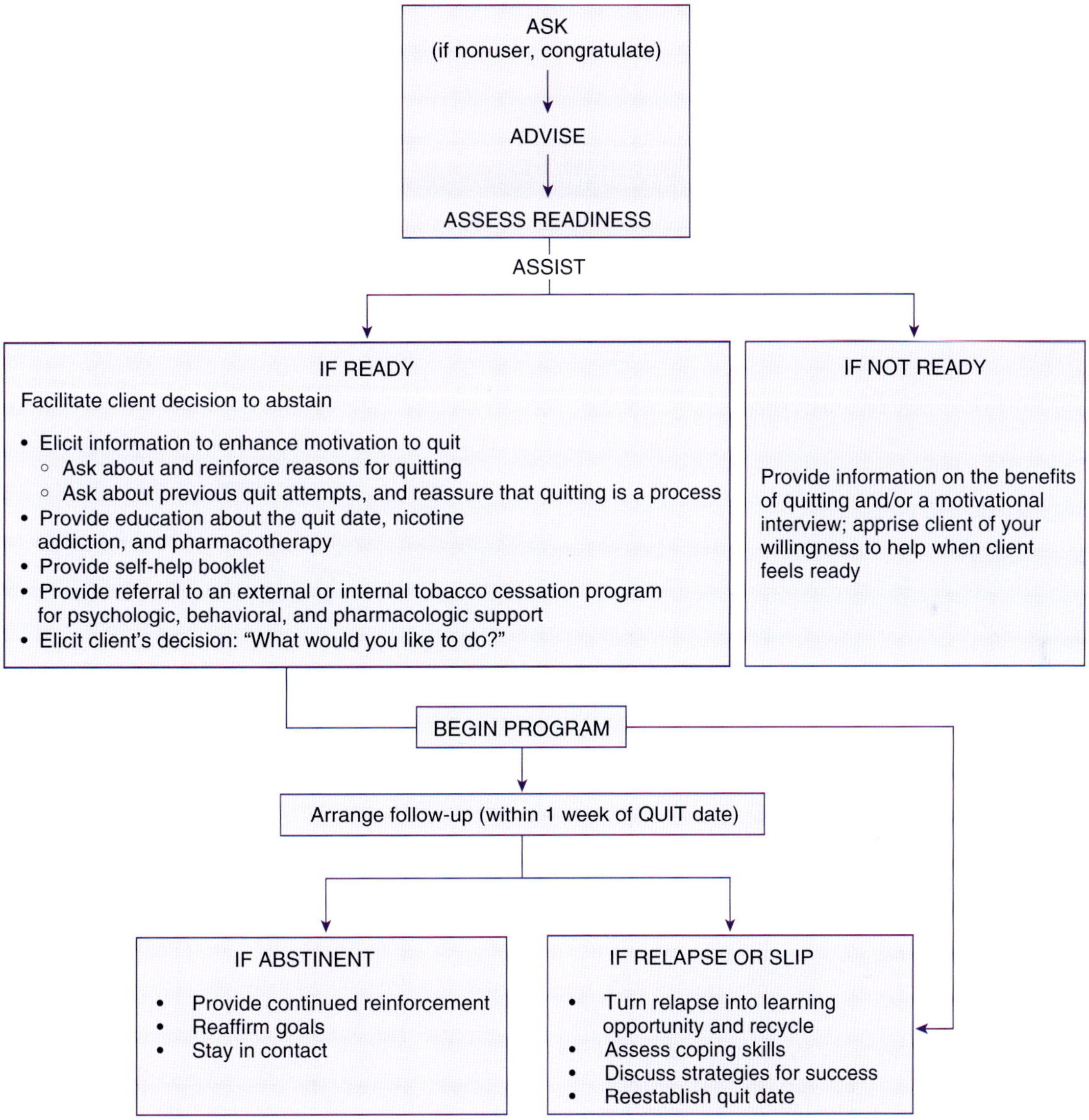
ASK
(if nonuser, congratulate)
ADVISE
ASSESS READINESS
ASSIST
IF READY
Facilitate client decision to abstain
• Elicit information to enhance motivation to quit
○ Ask about and reinforce reasons for quitting
○ Ask about previous quit attempts, and reassure that quitting is a process
• Provide education about the quit date, nicotine addiction, and pharmacotherapy
• Provide self-help booklet
• Provide referral to an external or internal tobacco cessation program for psychologic, behavioral, and pharmacologic support
• Elicit client's decision: "What would you like to do?"
IF NOT READY
Provide information on the benefits of quitting and/or a motivational interview; apprise client of your willingness to help when client feels ready
BEGIN PROGRAM
Arrange follow-up (within 1 week of QUIT date)
IF ABSTINENT
• Provide continued reinforcement
• Reaffirm goals
• Stay in contact
IF RELAPSE OR SLIP
• Turn relapse into learning opportunity and recycle
• Assess coping skills
• Discuss strategies for success
• Reestablish quit date

• **Figure 19.10** Tobacco intervention flow chart. (Reproduced with permission from Darby ML, Walsh MM. *Dental Hygiene: Theory and Practice*. 4th ed. St. Louis, MO: Saunders Elsevier; 2015.)

• BOX 19.6 Questions for Tobacco Cessation

- Do you use any tobacco products?
- Have you ever used tobacco in the past?
- How much do you smoke?
- What forms of tobacco do you use?
- How many cigarettes do you smoke each day?
- Why do you continue to smoke?
- How soon after you wake do you smoke your first cigarette?
- Do others in your household smoke?
- Do you smoke inside your home or car?
- Do you want to quit?
- Tell me about your last quit attempt(s).
  Did you use a smoking cessation medication?
  Did you receive any professional support?

• BOX 19.7 Pharmacotherapy for Tobacco Cessation

- Nicotine Replacement
  Gum
  Lozenges
  Patch
  Nasal spray
  Inhaler
- Nonnicotine Replacement
  Bupropion
  Clonidine
  Nortriptyline
  Varenicline
- Combination therapy

CASE APPLICATION FOR THE DENTAL HYGIENIST

Jenny is a 20-year-old college student. It has been 9 months since her last recare visit because of her busy school and work schedule. She continues to smoke despite the dental hygienist's encouragement to quit. An oral examination exhibits inflamed gingiva bleeding on touch and a grayish pseudomembrane covering the marginal gingiva. The dental hygienist also notices an unusual odor from the patient's mouth. A 24-hour dietary recall is as follows:

7:30 AM: large coffee with cream and sugar; pastry
10:00 AM: 12 oz cola; potato chips
2:30 PM: 3 slices pizza; 12 oz cola
7:30 PM: 12 oz can of ravioli; 8 oz milk
11:30 PM: hot chocolate; 8 sandwich cookies

Nutritional Assessment

- Food, nutrient, caloric intake
- Eating habits
- Social history
- Motivation level
- Knowledge level

Nutritional Diagnosis

Identify the patient's irregular eating patterns; choices of high-calorie, low nutrient-dense foods; stress from school and work; and smoking.

Nutritional Goals

Jenny will attempt to discontinue smoking or avoid smoking during periods of acute inflammation. With the help of the dental hygienist, she will review her busy schedule and prioritize events to incorporate a variety of foods, including some choices that are quickly prepared or more nutritious selections from vending machines.

Nutritional Implementation

Intervention: Question Jenny further on the level of oral discomfort she is experiencing. Determine whether a relationship exists between oral health and food choices. Depending on her response, a full liquid diet may initially be suggested, followed by a mechanically altered diet within 1 to 3 days, as tolerated.

Rationale: Oral conditions can interfere with chewing or swallowing. Jenny might be eating too little or omitting foods too painful to eat. Consequently, she may be experiencing a deteriorating nutritional status, which is negatively affecting her oral status. Altering the consistency of her diet can increase nutrient intake by minimizing the task of chewing and swallowing. Every patient's oral situation is unique and tolerance levels vary greatly. The dental hygienist should listen closely to Jenny's response to individualize recommendations to meet her needs.

Intervention: Encourage Jenny to eat a variety of foods, making choices as similar to her normal eating patterns as possible.

Rationale: Systemic factors, such as nutrient deficiencies, influence inflammatory response of the gingiva. The dental hygienist should explain the role of nutrients in maintaining a healthy periodontium, suggesting food choices that vary only slightly from Jenny's regular food intake to enhance compliance. Essential education tools include *MyPlate* and *Dietary Guidelines*. Temporary use of a multivitamin supplement may be recommended.

Intervention: Identify the frequency and form of fermentable carbohydrates in Jenny's diet, along with soft and sticky foods.

Rationale: Foods and drinks—such as coffee with sugar, pastries, potato chips, and cookies—influence formation of plaque. With Jenny's cooperation, practical and realistic modifications can be established in her diet that are compatible with the demands of her busy lifestyle. The dental hygienist should discuss use of dairy products (e.g., cheese on pizza and hot chocolate) in her diet.

Intervention: Continue efforts to eliminate smoking. Evaluate Jenny's readiness to quit tobacco use. Refer her to the National Network of Smoking Cessation quitlines at 1-800-QUIT-NOW, or www.smokefree.gov, or the state quitline.

Rationale: Smoking may promote plaque biofilm accumulation and inhibit the healing process. Heat, staining, and smoke from cigarettes can lead to unfavorable gingival changes. According to the American Dental Hygienists Association (ADHA), evidence suggests that quitlines are convenient, effective, and preferred by smokers.

Intervention: During an oral examination, note any areas of ulceration.

Rationale: Depending on the patient's tolerance, a bland diet may be recommended because discomfort may be experienced from highly seasoned or acidic foods. Nuts, popcorn hulls, and seeds are avoided because they can become lodged in an ulcerated area and become painful. Finally, cooler-temperature foods are more soothing.

Evaluation

The patient comes to each of her recare appointments, with improvement in oral health noted each time. At a 1-month reevaluation appointment, Jenny is (a) consuming a regular diet including a variety of foods; (b) eating fermentable carbohydrates only with meals; (c) choosing firm, fibrous foods more frequently; and (d) attending a smoking-cessation program. She is also able to verbalize reasons for these lifestyle changes.

Student Readiness

1. List at least four factors detrimentally affecting nutritional status in a periodontally involved patient. Why is it important to concentrate on nutrient intake?
2. Discuss the difference between a mechanically altered and a full liquid diet. What dental situations benefit from use of each of these diets?
3. Describe a periodontal situation in which small, frequent meals should be recommended. Explain the rationale to a patient.
4. What dietary strategies can be offered to a patient experiencing oral discomfort?
5. Conduct an Internet search for "supplements for periodontal disease" or "supplements for periodontal health." Choose one or two supplements identified to treat or prevent periodontal disease. Based on your knowledge of nutrition, dietary supplements, and periodontal disease, provide a rationale for suggesting or not suggesting the supplement(s).
6. If you are not in a "Tobacco-Free" work or school environment, investigate how you can begin this process. Find several tobacco-free policies at other schools of similar size to present to a professor or administrator or speak directly with the owner of your work environment. One person or a small group can make an impact.

CASE STUDY

A 43-year-old man comes to his recare appointment complaining of "sore and bleeding gums, especially after brushing." He is a busy executive and entertains his clients frequently. Consequently, he dines out often and averages two to three alcoholic drinks each day. His medical history is uneventful—no medications or health alerts. An oral examination reveals bleeding on probing with pocket depths generalized at 4 to 6 mm with moderate gingival inflammation.

The dental hygienist asks him to recall everything he has eaten on the previous day. His food consumption is high in fat, calories, and sodium because of heavy reliance on dining out. His diet also lacks variety and is low in nutrient value.

1. List several secondary factors precipitating the periodontal problem. What changes in his lifestyle could be suggested?
2. From the limited information presented, what additional data can the dental hygienist gather to help him modify his diet?
3. What vitamins and minerals might be deficient that could cause progression of his periodontal condition?
4. What diet should be suggested? What is the rationale? Provide a realistic menu for one day on the recommended diet.

References

1. U.S. Department of Health and Human Services: Healthy People 2020. https://www.healthypeople.gov/2020/topics-objectives/topic/oral-health. Accessed May 22, 2017.
2. Nielsen SJ, Trak-Fellermeier MA, Joshipura K, et al. Dietary fiber intake is inversely associated with periodontal disease among US adults. *J Nutr*. 2016;146:2530–2536.
3. Varela-Lopez A, Giampieri F, Bullon P, et al. A systematic review on the implication of minerals in the onset, severity and treatment of periodontal disease. *Molecules*. 2016;21:1183–1204.
4. Najeeb S, Zafar MS, Khurshid Z, et al. The role of nutrition in periodontal health: an update. *Nutrients*. 2016;8:530–568.
5. Chapple ILC, Bouchard P, Cagetti MG, et al. Interaction of lifestyle, behavior or systemic diseases with dental caries and periodontal diseases: consensus report of group 2 of the joint EFP/ORCA workshop on the boundaries between caries and periodontal diseases. *J Clin Periodontol*. 2017;44(suppl 18):S39–S51.
6. Martin-Cabezas R, Davideau J-L, Tenenbaum H, et al. Clinical efficacy of probiotics as an adjunctive therapy to non-surgical periodontal treatment of chronic periodontitis: a systematic review and meta-analysis. *J Clin Periodontol*. 2016;43:520–530.
7. Matsubara VH, Bandara HMHN, Ishikawa KH, et al. The role of probiotic bacteria in managing periodontal disease: a systematic review. *Expert Rev Anti Infect Ther*. 2016;14(7):643–655.
8. Koduganti RR, Sandeep N, Guduguntla S, et al. Probiotics and prebiotics in periodontal therapy. *Indian J Dent Res*. 2011;22(2):324–330.
9. Gupta G. Probiotics and periodontal health. *J Med Life*. 2011;4(4):387–394.
10. Chatterjee A, Bhattacharya H, Kandwal A. Probiotics in periodontal health and disease. *J Indian Soc Periodontol*. 2011;15(1):23–28.
11. Dhingra K. Methodological issues in randomized trials assessing probiotics for periodontal treatment. *J Periodontal Res*. 2012;47:15–26.
12. Centers for Disease Control and Prevention. Tobacco use: Targeting the nation's leading killer. https://stacks.cdc.gov/view/cdc/5527/. Accessed May 23, 2017.
13. Fiore MC, Jaen CR, Baker TB, et al. Treating tobacco use and dependence: 2008 update. Clinical Practice Guideline. Rockville, MD: U.S. Department of Health and Human Services. Public Health Service; 2008.

EVOLVE RESOURCES

Please visit http://evolve.elsevier.com/Stegeman/nutritional for additional practice and study support tools.

20 Nutritional Aspects of Alterations in the Oral Cavity

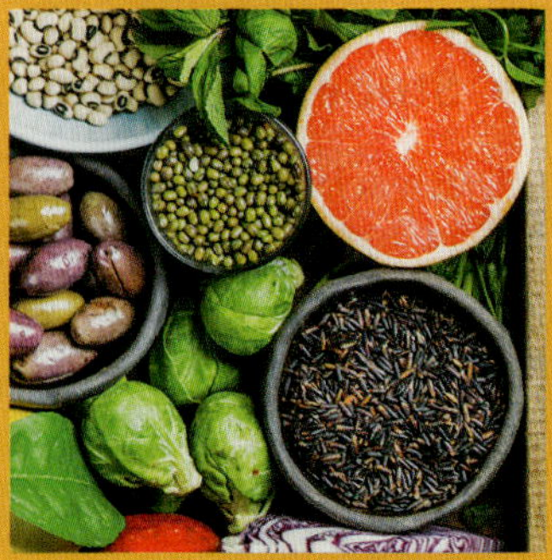

STUDENT LEARNING OUTCOMES

Upon completion of this chapter, the student will be able to achieve the following student learning outcomes:

1. Describe the common signs and symptoms of xerostomia. Also, synthesize appropriate dietary and oral hygiene recommendations for a patient with orthodontics, xerostomia, root caries, or dentin hypersensitivity.
2. Discuss normal dentition, and identify *Dietary Guidelines* appropriate for a patient undergoing oral surgery and a patient with a new denture, before and after insertion.
3. Describe the common signs and symptoms of glossitis. Also, synthesize appropriate dietary and oral hygiene recommendations for a patient with a loss of alveolar bone, glossitis, or temporomandibular disorder.

KEY TERMS

Abrasion
Benign migratory glossitis
Crepitus
Dentin hypersensitivity
Erosion
Functional food
Lichen planus
Temporomandibular disorder
Tinnitus

TEST YOUR NQ

1. **T/F** While charting for dental caries, the dental hygienist notes several root surface caries and documents xerostomia as the cause. This is a correct assessment.
2. **T/F** Xerostomia is a consequence of the aging process.
3. **T/F** Xerostomia can be a contributing factor to malnutrition in an older patient.
4. **T/F** Root caries are frequently seen in adolescents.
5. **T/F** The primary component of alveolar bone is compact cortical bone.
6. **T/F** Glossitis can be a symptom of a nutrient deficiency.
7. **T/F** Masticatory efficiency, or chewing, is a factor in providing a well-structured alveolar process.
8. **T/F** A relationship exists between nutritional status of a patient and tooth mobility, missing teeth, and denture performance.
9. **T/F** High fiber, nutrient-dense foods are recommended for the first few days after insertion of new dentures to promote healing and prevent loss of alveolar bone.
10. **T/F** To maintain a normal serum calcium level, calcium is obtained from the alveolar process when the patient is in negative calcium balance.

Instructing patients to follow the *Dietary Guidelines* and *MyPlate* is practical nutrition advice for optimum general and oral health. Various oral conditions can interfere with food intake and influence a patient's nutritional status. These situations require modifications of eating patterns based on individual needs. The oral health team is in an ideal position to provide dietary advice to a patient or to be a valuable member of a multidisciplinary team in complicated cases, such as patients with renal disease.

Orthodontics

Orthodontic treatment presents unique nutritional implications. Risk of decalcification, erosion, gingival inflammation, alveolar bone loss, and decline of the periodontal ligament are concerns that may compromise orthodontic outcomes and long-term oral health. Optimal nutrient intake is a factor that can minimize these negative oral health situations. The treatment time varies widely and is dependent on the complexity of the situation and patient compliance. The level of comfort and duration of discomfort also varies, with common complaints of pain localized to the teeth, soft tissues, and tongue, particularly in the first days after placement or adjustment. Pain can last from 1 day to 2 weeks.[1] These symptoms impact food choices, quantity of foods, and food preparation. Eating foods that require biting and chewing may be difficult.

Chaotic meal patterns and snack habits typical of many adolescents create an additional challenge during orthodontic treatment. Health and science courses at school provide adolescents with sufficient knowledge to make better choices, but this information is often ignored. Choosing snacks or meals from vending machines, convenience stores, or fast food restaurants is commonplace. Fortunately, many schools are opting to have nutrient-dense snack or meals in on-site vending machines. In addition, fast food restaurants and convenience stores are offering progressively more nutrient-dense options to consumers.

DENTAL CONSIDERATIONS

Assessment

- *Physical:* Gingival inflammation, dental caries, decalcification of teeth, soft tissue lesions from sharp appliances, erosion, root resorption, and accumulation of food debris around brackets.
- *Dietary:* Frequency and times fermentable carbohydrates are consumed, form of food chosen.

Interventions

- Individualize nutrition education to motivate adolescents to improve their eating and oral hygiene habits. For any plan to succeed, the adolescent must be willing to change. Remind adolescents that this procedure is to help improve their appearance.
- After initial placement, adjustments or repairs in orthodontic care may require a full liquid (see Box 19.2 in Chapter 19) or mechanically altered (see Box 19.3 in Chapter 19) diet for 1 to 2 days.
- Emphasize the importance of oral self-care, daily fluoride use, and possibly an alcohol-free antimicrobial rinse.
- Because fermentable carbohydrates are a factor in demineralization and plaque biofilm formation, conduct a carbohydrate analysis using a 3- to 7-day food diary (see Figs. 18.7, 18.8, and 18.9 in Chapter 18). Based on this assessment, counsel the orthodontic patient to use caution, including recommendations to modify the frequency of consuming fermentable carbohydrates.
- Remind the patient that appliances can be damaged with sticky, hard, or firm foods, or chewing ice.
- Soft tissue trauma caused by sharp appliances can lead to discomfort and avoidance of certain foods. Warm saltwater rinses (8 oz water with 1 tsp salt) and utility wax (to cover the offending surface of the appliance) provide comfort until the situation can be resolved.

Evaluation

- The patient has demonstrated acceptable plaque biofilm control abilities; soft tissues are free of trauma; the patient is choosing a variety of foods based on *MyPlate*.

NUTRITIONAL DIRECTIONS

- Although a mechanically altered diet allows for ease of chewing and is less painful, it consists of soft, sticky, and retentive foods that can adhere around the brackets, contributing to plaque biofilm formation. Consequently, this diet can result in gingival inflammation and increased caries risk. Encourage and educate the patient regarding an optimal oral self-care regimen.
- Commonly chosen soft foods include mashed potatoes, rice, pasta, bananas, soups, cheese, and boiled vegetables.[1]
- Liquids such as milkshakes or smoothies may also be well tolerated. Since these drinks are fermentable carbohydrates, highlight the need for optimal oral self-care.
- Foods such as carrots and apples should not be avoided but rather cut into small pieces.
- Corn on the cob, meat dishes, nuts, chewing gum, chewy candy, and crackers are foods commonly identified as difficult to consume with orthodontic bands.[1]
- Soft drinks, energy drinks, specialized coffee drinks, and sports drinks often contain fermentable carbohydrates along with citric or phosphoric acid and should be avoided to minimize enamel decalcification and erosion.
- Adequate nutritional intake is indispensable for maintenance and repair of hard and soft tissue and to withstand the stresses of tooth movement.
- Foods with a low nutrient value and fermentable carbohydrates minimize success of orthodontic treatment and increase the risk of oral complications.

Xerostomia

Good oral health depends on adequate salivary flow. Common factors contributing to xerostomia are listed in Box 20.1. Because xerostomia is most commonly characterized by diminished or absent salivary flow or a change in the viscosity of saliva, xerostomia has a negative impact on oral tissues and dietary intake (Fig. 20.1). Chapter 3 provides some basic information about the functions of saliva and xerostomia.

The dental professional should determine from the medical history the patient's risk for xerostomia. Salivary flow does not significantly decrease as a result of aging. Adults most frequently experience xerostomia in relation to taking multiple medications (see Box 20.1). Xerostomia can also be a result of one or more chronic diseases, such as Sjögren syndrome (Fig. 20.2). An estimated 5% to 39% of the general population and 17% to

• BOX 20.1 Factors Contributing to Xerostomia

Medications

- Analgesics
- Antianxiety agents
- Anticholinergics
- Anticonvulsants
- Antidepressants
- Antihistamines
- Antihypertensives
- Antiinflammatories
- Antiobesity agents
- Antiparkinson agents
- Antipsychotics
- Bronchodilators
- Decongestants
- Diuretics
- Gastrointestinal agents
- Narcotics

Other Considerations

- Antineoplastic therapy (chemotherapy and radiation)
- Systemic diseases (diabetes, Sjögren syndrome)
- Stress and depression
- Significant nutrient deficiency (e.g., vitamins A and C, protein)
- Liquid diets, due to lack of mastication
- Dehydration
- Females—smaller salivary glands and produce less saliva[2]

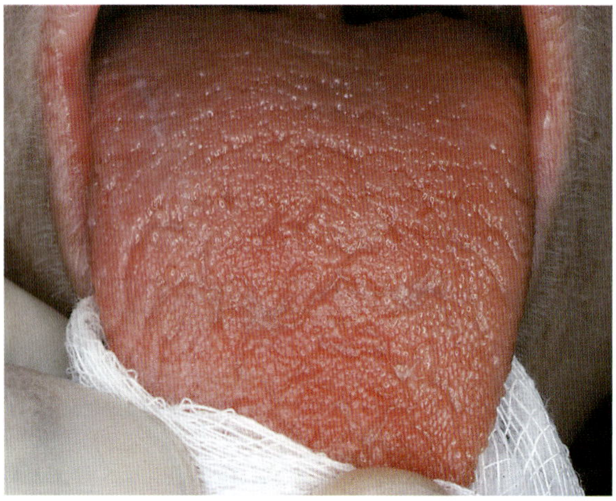

• **Figure 20.1** Appearance of mouth of patient with xerostomia. (Reproduced with permission from Ibsen OAC, Phelan JA. *Oral Pathology for the Dental Hygienist*. 6th ed. St Louis, MO: Saunders Elsevier; 2014.)

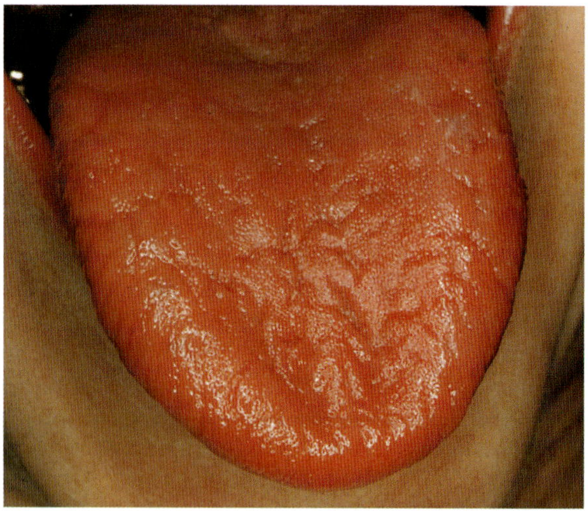

• **Figure 20.2** Appearance of mouth of patient with Sjögren syndrome causing xerostomia. Note the absence of filiform papilla. (Reproduced with permission from Ibsen OAC, Phelan JA. *Oral Pathology for the Dental Hygienist*. 6th ed. St. Louis, MO: Saunders Elsevier; 2014.)

40% of older adults experience some level of xerostomia. This jumps to as high as 72% in older adults residing in nursing home care.[2] Xerostomia results in various oral complications compromising a patient's nutrient intake (Box 20.2). Overall, the goals for a patient with xerostomia are to protect the oral cavity from the destructive effects of xerostomia, treat existing conditions, and provide relief from the dryness to improve the quality of the diet and quality of life. The dental professional should be able to recognize and provide suggestions for patients experiencing xerostomia.

DENTAL CONSIDERATIONS

Assessment

- *Physical:* Dry mouth; dysgeusia; burning sensation of the tongue or oral mucous membranes; dry and crusty mucosa; difficulty in swallowing and speaking (see Box 20.2); medications (see Box 20.1); antineoplastic therapy (chemotherapy and radiation); systemic diseases (diabetes, Sjögren syndrome, acquired immune deficiency syndrome); stress and depression; dehydration; and weight loss.
- *Dietary:* Inadequate intake of vitamins A and C, fluid, fiber, potassium, vitamin B_6, iron, calcium, zinc, and protein; taste changes; lack of interest in eating; and poor appetite.

Interventions

- If the patient complains of oral dryness, the dental hygienist can place a mouth mirror or tongue blade on the oral mucosa and watch for stickiness on removal. Milking the major salivary glands (submandibular, sublingual, and parotid) to observe the amount of saliva produced is another assessment option.
- After a thorough oral examination of the patient with oral dryness, a sialometric test can be performed. Saliva flow tests take approximately 10 to 15 minutes and provide fast results of not only the flow but also consistency, pH, and quantity of saliva. A low salivary rate with this type of test may raise suspicion and indicate systemic disease. A more invasive procedure, scintigraphy, is a diagnostic test performed in the hospital to observe salivary function. Examples include tumors, cysts, salivary stones, duct blockage, and trauma.
- Because burning mouth syndrome cannot be identified clinically, listen to the patient's symptoms. Patients may compare the burning sensation to consumption of hot peppers, typically complaining of having an intense burning sensation on the anterior two-thirds of the tongue or oral mucous membranes. This is commonly associated with taste changes and xerostomia.
- Discomfort with a removable appliance may occur because of the tongue sticking to the prosthesis, an inability to retain the appliance properly, and gingival lesions created by an improperly fitting denture.
- A complete assessment, as described in Chapter 21, allows the dental professional to formulate appropriate intervention strategies for xerostomia.
- Each patient's situation is unique; thus, oral therapy must be individualized.
- Educate the patient about techniques and procedures to relieve symptoms of xerostomia effective in minimizing oral discomfort and related conditions, especially increased dental caries.
- More than 400 over-the-counter and prescription medications indicate xerostomia to be a possible side effect. Because drugs are a common cause of xerostomia, review the patient's medications to identify any drugs associated with xerostomia (see Box 20.1). The patient may want to discuss an alternative medication or a reduction in dosage with the health care provider. If the medication cannot be changed or the dosage cannot be reduced, provide alternative options for maintaining oral health.
- Schedule frequent recare appointments to monitor the oral cavity.
- Discuss the importance of excellent daily oral hygiene.
- Fluoride therapy to reduce the risk of caries.
- Pilocarpine or cevimeline may be prescribed by the health care provider for relief of xerostomia.[3]
- After assessing food intake, note any changes in appetite affecting overall dietary adequacy resulting in weight changes.
- Malic acid may counteract the harmful effects of drug-induced xerostomia on enamel.[3]

Evaluation

- The patient uses oral hygiene and dietary interventions to relieve xerostomia.

NUTRITIONAL DIRECTIONS

- Use products formulated to relieve xerostomia (e.g., sprays or oral rinses).
- Use unflavored or mildly flavored oral hygiene products that have a neutral pH.
- Use lip balm to help keep lips moist.
- Consume fluids with meals and between meals; frequent sips of fluids between bites facilitate chewing and swallowing.
- Use a humidifier to maintain the humidity in the air.
- Choose nutrient-dense, soft, moist foods (e.g., macaroni and cheese, cottage cheese, or applesauce).
- Use gravies and sauces to moisten dry foods (e.g., roast beef).
- Choose foods principally made with a nonnutritive sweetener or sugar alcohols (e.g., gum, hard candy, lozenges, or popsicles), especially between meals.
- Avoid or limit foods that are dry (e.g., saltines), crumbly (e.g., whole-wheat muffins), sticky (e.g., peanut butter), and spicy (e.g., salsa or chili peppers); alcohol; commercial mouthwashes containing alcohol; tobacco; and caffeine.
- Suck on ice chips between meals.
- Carry a water bottle during the day.
- Tart, sour, and citrus foods and drinks may help stimulate saliva flow (e.g., sugar-free lemonade, sour candy, and dill pickles).
- Enhance appetite by presenting foods in interesting, appealing, and appetizing ways. Suggestions to improve the appearance and appeal of food can involve colorful combinations of foods. Imagine the lack of appeal of a plate with cauliflower, mashed potatoes, and baked white fish compared with a colorful plate of baked salmon, steamed broccoli, and a baked yam.

Root Caries and Dentin Hypersensitivity

Because the population of older adults who have retained their teeth is increasing, root caries are increasingly common. New carious lesions in adults are typically located on the root, below the cementoenamel junction, in areas of gingival recession. The area around the cementoenamel junction is particularly susceptible because it often has an anatomically thin layer of enamel. The cementum, which is thinner and contains fewer minerals than enamel, is also more susceptible. Demineralization of cementum can occur at a pH of 6.7 or less. Adequate removal of plaque biofilm from exposed root surfaces is very difficult because of root morphology allowing bacteria and cariogenic material to accumulate, thus increasing caries risk. Xerostomia frequently compounds the risk for root caries because of limited buffering and dilution capacity of decreased amounts of saliva along with poor oral clearance. Also, prevalence of root caries is increased when carbohydrates are consumed frequently.

In addition to root caries, other problems often associated with gingival recession are abrasion and erosion of enamel and cementum.

• BOX 20.2 Consequences of Xerostomia Influencing Nutrient Intake

- Increased rate of root caries and oral infections
- Inability to keep mouth moist
- Sticky or tacky saliva
- Absence of salivary pooling
- Difficulty in chewing and swallowing
- Burning or sensitive oral mucosa
- Dry, crusty, smooth, or shiny mucosa
- Low tolerance to spicy and acidic foods
- Ulcerations
- Food sticks to hard palate or tongue
- Painful tongue—atrophied, fissured, inflamed, edematous, burning sensation
- Angular cheilosis—cracking or burning at the corners of the mouth
- Altered or lack of taste—lack of interest in eating, possible unintentional weight loss
- Difficulty wearing dentures
- Dentin hypersensitivity—hot, cold, sweet, touch
- Dry nose—impairment of sense of smell
- Dry throat—difficulty with swallowing

Erosion is the permanent depletion of tooth surfaces due to the action of an external or internal chemical substance (Fig. 20.3). Erosion is the major cause of hypersensitivity and often occurs as a consequence of exposure to acids such as those found in food and beverages (extrinsic) and acid from gastroesophageal reflux or excessive vomiting (intrinsic). **Abrasion** is the permanent depletion of tooth surfaces as a result of pathologic tooth wear, such as toothbrush abrasion (Fig. 20.4). Erosion and abrasion produce dentin exposure, which can lead to dentin hypersensitivity. **Dentin hypersensitivity** is an extremely painful feeling resulting from a stimulus to the exposed dentin.

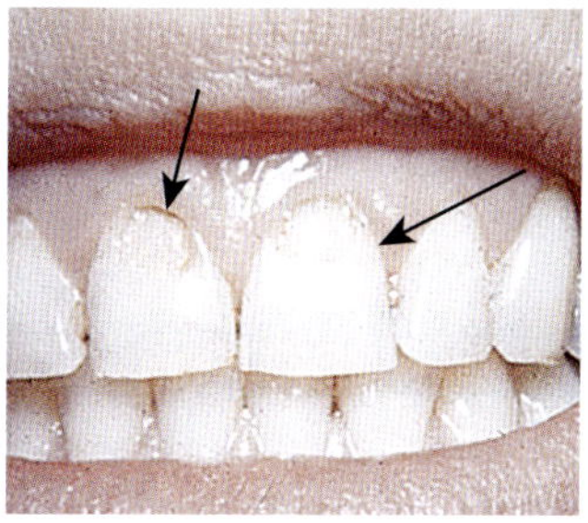

• **Figure 20.3** Erosion (*arrows*) caused by frequently sucking on lemons. (Reproduced with permission from Darby ML, Walsh MM. *Dental Hygiene: Theory and Practice*. 4th ed. St. Louis, MO: Saunders Elsevier; 2015.)

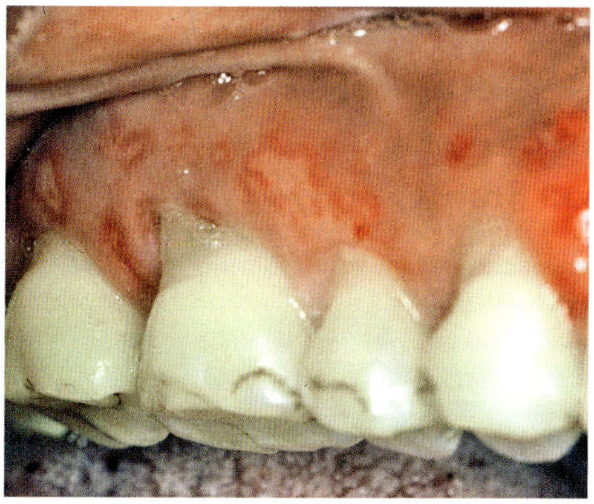

• **Figure 20.4** Toothbrush abrasion. (Reproduced with permission from Newman MG, Takei HH, Klokkevold PR, Carranza FA: *Carranza's Clinical Periodontology*. 12th ed. St. Louis, MO: Saunders Elsevier; 2014.)

DENTAL CONSIDERATIONS

Assessment

- *Physical:* Gingival recession, oral infections, a narrow region of attached gingiva, toothbrush abrasion, use of fluoridated water, oral hygiene status, and xerostomia.
- *Dietary:* Diet history and carbohydrate analysis, frequency of eating, use of sugar-sweetened medications (cough syrup or lozenges), or intake of hard candy.

Interventions

- Patients who complain of a sudden, sharp pain in areas where dentin is exposed and recession exists may be experiencing dentin hypersensitivity.
- Onset of dentin hypersensitivity is often related to temperature, primarily cold, or touch.
- Recommend 3-month recare visits, meticulous oral hygiene, topical fluoride treatments at home, and fluoridated water. Self-applied fluoride gels reduce enamel solubility and oral bacteria. Desensitizing toothpastes and mouthrinses may also be beneficial.[4]
- For patients with areas of hypersensitivity, recommend the following: (a) brushing before consuming acidic foods to neutralize the pH of saliva; (b) using a straw for acidic drinks; (c) decreasing frequency of intake or following with a chewing gum containing xylitol or a noncariogenic food (e.g., cheese or milk); or (d) avoiding foods causing discomfort (e.g., hot coffee or iced beverages).
- Brushing immediately after consuming acidic foods can hasten the erosion process. Wait at least 40 minutes to brush.
- Recommend using soft-bristled toothbrushes.
- Saliva is one of the best protective measures for the demineralizing effects of erosion by neutralizing the acid. Tips to increase saliva flow should be recommended.

Evaluation

- The patient is free of pain, can eat comfortably, has avoided controllable risk factors, and has incorporated appropriate oral hygiene procedures into a home care regimen.

NUTRITIONAL DIRECTIONS

- Minimize the acidic attacks on teeth. Consumption of carbonated beverages (regular and diet), sports drinks, energy drinks, pickled products, wine, citrus products (e.g., grapefruit and orange juice), and ciders are acidic and should be minimized because they can contribute to erosion.
- Because dairy products, especially cheddar cheese, are cariostatic, their consumption with or without cariogenic foods can decrease the risk of caries. A reduced-fat cheese (5 g of fat per oz or less) or smaller portion size is appropriate for many patients.

Dentition Status

Over the decades, a steady reduction in tooth loss has occurred. However, 18% of individuals older than age 65 years still incur loss of all natural teeth.[5] Although many mistakenly believe that tooth loss is a normal element of aging, education level and race/ethnicity of the patient are the strongest determinants of tooth loss.[6] Smoking status has also been identified as a variable. Although complete dentition is not required for adequate nutrient intake, loss of teeth or supporting periodontium and/or an improperly fitting prosthesis are frequently associated with poor food selection and limited chewing ability. Compromised nutritional intake may be a result of tooth loss, tooth mobility, edentulous status, and discomfort from removable appliances. Malnutrition or inability to comply with nutritional recommendations may result from declining dentition status.

A patient with complete dentures, less than 20 functioning teeth, or few pairs of opposing teeth has lower nutrient intakes than a patient with adequate dentition.[7] The patient's masticatory efficiency and biting force increasingly decline with each tooth lost. The number of teeth and presence of advanced mobility determine food choices. Well-fitting dentures and/or implants may improve quality of the diet; with loss of chewing ability, however, the patient may choose predominantly soft foods with less variety.[8] Because of the number of variables that can have an impact on nutrient intake, it is imperative for the dental professional to provide personalized nutrition education for patients who are edentulous, wear a dental prosthesis, or have missing or compromised teeth. It is also essential for dental professionals to work collaboratively with and educate registered dietitian nutritionists (RDNs) and physicians to assess patients at risk of malnutrition due to their dentate status.

DENTAL CONSIDERATIONS

Assessment

- *Physical:* Masticatory efficiency, biting force, number of teeth and location, and fit of dentures.
- *Dietary:* Adequacy of calories and nutrients, especially protein; fiber; vitamins A, B_{12}, and C, folic acid; iron, magnesium, zinc; and fluids; interest in foods.

Interventions

- Most tooth loss is a result of caries or periodontal disease. Tooth loss can be prevented with education, early diagnosis, and regular care. As a dental health educator, it is important to educate the patient, community, and other health care providers regarding prevention and recognition of signs and symptoms of oral disease.
- Nutrient deficiencies frequently interfere with maintenance and repair of oral soft and hard tissues.
- During the appointment preceding placement of a new denture, educate the patient about the initial days of adaptation so that appropriate foods can be available for the adjustment period.
- Swallowing foods may initially present a challenge to a new denture wearer because a full upper denture interferes with the ability to determine the location of food in the mouth. Days 1 and 2 of placement may necessitate a full liquid diet (see Chapter 19, Box 19.2) to allow the patient to master swallowing with the new prosthesis before having to deal with chewing or biting firmer textured foods.
- A high-protein liquid nutrition supplement may be necessary to meet caloric and nutrient needs to promote healing from extractions or sore spots or both.
- Encourage intake of dairy products fortified with vitamin D to slow the rate of bone loss.
- During the next 2 to 3 days, the patient should advance as tolerated to a mechanically altered diet (see Chapter 19, Box 19.3), which slowly introduces foods that require limited mastication.
- Discuss the possible decline in taste, a limited ability to identify texture and temperature of foods, and challenges in forming a bolus with food (mass of food) to be swallowed (Chapter 3) for patients with a complete set of dentures.
- As sore spots heal, the patient should add firmer-textured foods. This process is essential for masticatory efficiency and stability of the denture and to enhance the patient's nutritional status and increase fiber intake.
- Examine the denture for fit. An appointment to reline or make new dentures may be needed. Explain the significance of a properly fitting denture to the patient, including its relationship to a poor-quality diet.
- Patients with a compromised dentition status frequently have inadequate intake of whole grains, fruits, vegetables, and proteins.

DENTAL CONSIDERATIONS—cont'd

- Chewy, hard, or fibrous foods are often avoided because of low masticatory performance.
- Ensure adequate nutrient intake by encouraging a variety of food and beverages based on *MyPlate* and *Dietary Guidelines.*

Evaluation

- The patient is choosing a variety of foods from each of the *MyPlate* groups and understands the importance of a complete and functioning dentition to overall general health.

NUTRITIONAL DIRECTIONS

- Fortified foods may improve nutrient intake.
- Cut food into small pieces.
- Peel and chop fruits and vegetables; cooked fruits and vegetables may be better tolerated.
- Chew food well and longer.
- Evenly distribute food on both sides of the mouth.
- Chew in a straight up-and-down motion rather than a rotary motion and avoid biting with anterior teeth.
- Avoid foods such as chewing gum, sticky foods (e.g., caramels), berries with seeds, and nuts.

Oral and Maxillofacial Surgery

Oral and maxillofacial surgeries include extractions, orthognathic surgery (to correct conditions of the jaw and face), dental implants, and maxillomandibular fixation. The dental hygienist is a vital part of the dental team providing comprehensive treatment to a patient for optimal outcomes.

The role of the dental hygienist includes obtaining an assessment of the nutritional needs for patients before a surgical procedure to cope better with the postsurgical demands and to minimize complications. The patient must have an adequate nutrient and fluid intake to meet the stress of surgery (e.g., blood loss and catabolism), provide for optimal healing, and increase resistance to infection, which shortens the recovery period. Patients who are malnourished as a result of various chronic diseases and conditions—such as anorexia nervosa, chemotherapy, or alcohol abuse—are at increased risk because they are likely to be immunosuppressed. A compromised immune response may compound the severity of complications. These patients should be referred to an RDN for medical nutrition therapy before the procedure. Based on a nutrition assessment and consideration of the procedure, recommendations can be developed to help the patient plan and purchase appropriate food for the recovery period. Postoperative recommendations should also be addressed by the dental professional.

DENTAL CONSIDERATIONS

Assessment

- *Physical:* Oral dysfunction that affects speech, mastication, or swallowing; medical history.
- *Dietary:* Dietary intake, including decaffeinated fluids.

Interventions

- When general anesthesia is used for the surgical procedure, the stomach should be empty at the time of the operation to avoid aspirating vomitus.
- If the patient loses weight unintentionally, healing seems delayed, history of bisphosphonate use exists, or overall health declines, the patient should be referred to a health care provider or RDN.
- Provide written instructions to reinforce nutrition education. Tailor the information to meet the patient's needs, attitudes, and behaviors.
- For successful nutrition intervention, it is important to obtain information before discussing dietary interventions, including food preferences, eating patterns, living conditions, economic status, lifestyle, and physical capabilities.
- Recommendations for oral surgery such as extractions include reminding the patient to avoid alcohol and smoking, avoid sipping through a straw, drink adequate decaffeinated fluids, and refrain from brushing during the first 24 hours to avoid a dry socket.
- Emphasize meeting the recommendations of *MyPlate.* The key factor for optimal healing during the recovery process is adequate intake of calories, carbohydrates, protein, fat, vitamins, minerals, and fluids.
- Depending on severity of the operative procedure, the patient may tolerate solid foods after surgery. If not, the dental hygienist can suggest a full liquid diet (see Chapter 19, Box 19.2) for 1 to 2 days with progression to a mechanically altered diet (see Chapter 19, Box 19.3) and then to a regular diet when tolerated.
- Suggest nutrient-dense, enriched and fortified foods and fluids that the patient enjoys.
- Because nutrient requirements increase after surgery, patients may find it difficult to consume adequate amounts of food. To increase protein and calories, suggest a high-protein liquid nutritional supplement or add milk powder to milk, milkshakes, soups, yogurt, or pudding. A multivitamin with minerals may be necessary.

Evaluation

- The patient is able to verbalize the problem and discuss ways to continue maintaining a healthy oral cavity and an adequate nutrient intake.

NUTRITIONAL DIRECTIONS

- Cold foods may be soothing to the oral cavity postoperatively.
- Frequent small meals with nutrient-dense foods help meet nutrient needs.

Loss of Alveolar Bone

Several factors, including poor calcium intake over a lifetime, create a physiologic negative calcium balance. To maintain a normal serum calcium level, the body obtains calcium from other internal sources. The calcium from spongy cancellous bone, the primary component of the alveolar process, can readily be absorbed. The status of the alveolus, which may undergo resorption before other bones, may be an early indicator of osteoporosis. When osteoporotic change in the alveolus is detected, the dental professional should refer the patient to a health care provider for further evaluation. Progressive loss of the alveolar ridge leads to tooth loss.

After tooth extractions, accelerated atrophy of alveolar bone occurs (within months). A reduction in masticatory efficiency, as occurs in individuals with dentures, also increases resorption, loss of bone mass, or alveolar osteoporosis. The mandible has greater resorption than the maxilla. As the alveolar ridge reduces in height and volume, it becomes increasingly difficult to fit dentures properly, and relined or new dentures are necessary. Management of osteoporosis is discussed in *Health Application 9* in Chapter 9.

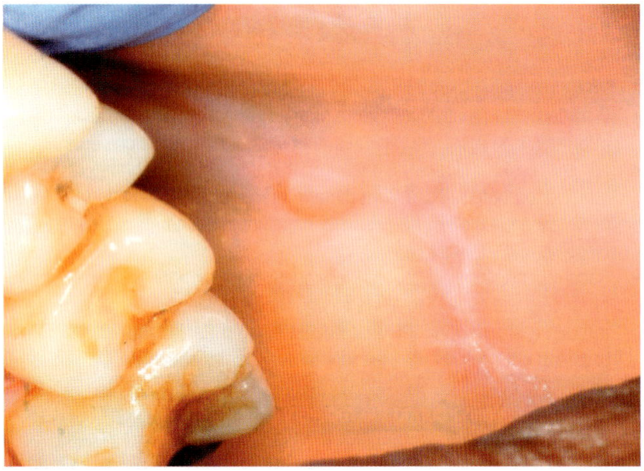

• **Figure 20.5** Mild lichen planus on the buccal mucosa. The patient was prescribed a mouthwash and pain subsided within 24 hours. (Courtesy of Amy L. Sullivan, University of Mississippi Medical Center, Jackson, MS.)

Glossitis

A chronic inflammation of the tongue, or glossitis, is very painful. Glossitis may be caused by bacteria, fungus, virus, or disease, and unknown causes. Nutrient deficiency (e.g., B vitamins) or an allergic reaction to food or drugs can result in glossitis. Additionally, psychological stress can be related to psychogenic glossitis. There are many forms of glossitis. One of the most common forms of glossitis is "geographic tongue" or **benign migratory glossitis**. Clinically, benign migratory glossitis appears as multiple reddish flat areas with a loss of filiform papillae on the dorsum of the tongue. The dental hygienist may also identify and document a grooved or fissured tongue as part of the intraoral examination.[9] Although usually asymptomatic, having a patient avoid dietary triggers such as hot, spicy, or acidic foods is recommended. Dental professionals should also closely examine the oral cavity for any signs of lichen planus, considering a potential link.[9]

Lichen planus is a chronic inflammatory disease with an itchy rash found most often in the mouth. It is associated with various systemic diseases, such as hypertension and diabetes.[10] A mouthwash consisting of Maalox, Benadryl, and dexamethasone (Decadron)—or similar variations—is another commonly prescribed treatment for pain and irritation for patients with glossitis, lichen planus, and benign migratory glossitis (Fig. 20.5). Ultimately, more options for pain control provide a better quality of life for the patient. Once pain is controlled, patients can continue with normal eating, consuming the balanced diet based on the *Dietary Guidelines*.

Glossitis typically appears reddish with a slight to total atrophy of the filiform and fungiform papillae on the dorsum of the tongue. Depending on the degree of atrophy, the tongue inevitably appears shiny, smooth, and red (see Chapter 11, Fig. 11.4). The atrophy can be localized or generalized. The tongue size can shrink because of dehydration or become enlarged (macroglossia) as a result of edema. A thorough assessment determines the extent and cause of glossitis.

With benign migratory glossitis, an assessment of the tongue might reveal erythematous or atrophic patches surrounded by a yellow-white border, often changing pattern or appearance. These erythematous patches may extend onto the buccal mucosa (Fig. 20.6). When patients engage in the previously mentioned triggers (spicy foods), antihistamine or corticosteroid rinses may be suggested.[11] In those cases in which lichen planus is also observed, an assessment might reveal whitish plaques on the dorsal part of the tongue and even the buccal mucosa.

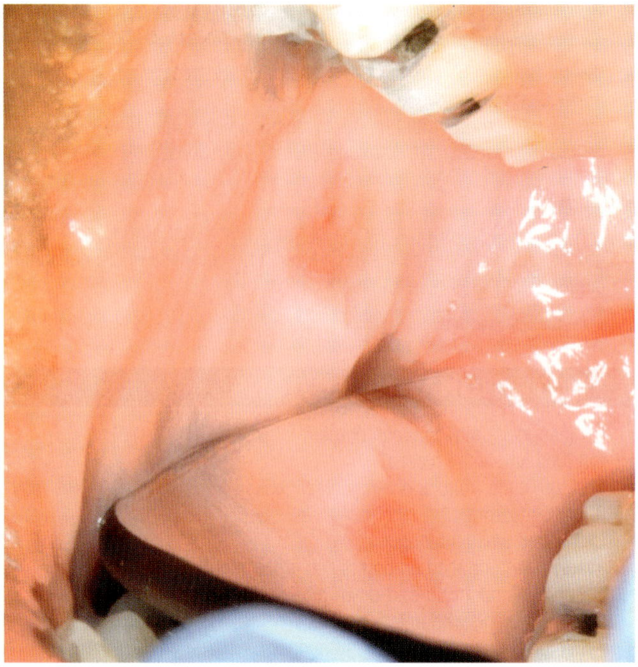

• **Figure 20.6** The irritation on the buccal mucosa appeared after eating acidic and spicy foods. (Courtesy of Amy L. Sullivan, University of Mississippi Medical Center, Jackson, MS.)

DENTAL CONSIDERATIONS

Assessment

- *Physical:* Burning sensation, pain, or tenderness of the tongue; atrophy of papillae on the dorsum of the tongue; tongue size (microglossia or macroglossia); appearance of the tongue (e.g., shiny, smooth, red); diminished, altered, or lost taste sensation; change in the alveolus.
- *Dietary:* Nutritional status.

Intervention

- Macroglossia is commonly observed in individuals who are edentulous.
- Individualize dietary instructions with the goal of improving nutritional quality of the diet.
- Suggest enhancing the taste and appearance of foods on the plate.

Evaluation

- The patient is developing or maintaining healthful eating and exercise patterns and behaviors and has met with the health care provider for further evaluation.

NUTRITIONAL DIRECTIONS

- Choose soft, nutrient-dense, enriched, and fortified foods (e.g., tuna salad, cream soups, cottage cheese).
- Liquid nutrition supplements, such as instant breakfast, may help provide adequate nutrients.

Temporomandibular Disorder

When a patient complains of orofacial pain, frequent headaches, impaired mandibular movement, or **tinnitus** (ringing in the ears), and the extraoral examination reveals clicking, **crepitus** (crackling or crunching sound), and popping of the temporomandibular joint, the diagnosis can be **temporomandibular disorder**. Clenching, grinding, stress, malocclusion, injury, and bone abnormalities are common conditions that result in temporomandibular disorder. Limited jaw opening and associated discomfort can inhibit intake. Recommendations may include avoiding gum chewing and foods that require significant chewing, such as caramels, taffy, and bagels. A mechanically altered diet (see Chapter 19, Box 19.3) may also be warranted.

HEALTH APPLICATION 20

Functional Nutrition

"Functional" implies that the food has value in providing some type of health benefits beyond basic nutrition and may function to optimize health by reducing or minimizing the risk of certain diseases and other health conditions. **Functional foods** are found in virtually all food categories and can include conventional foods and fortified, enriched, or enhanced foods with potentially beneficial effects on health when consumed as a part of a varied diet. The term functional foods has no legal meaning in the United States. In fact, the Academy of Nutrition and Dietetics, the International Food Information Council, Institute of Food Technologists, the European Commission, Health Canada, European Commission, and the Japanese Ministry of Health, Labour, and Welfare all define functional foods slightly differently.

Foods have always been known to provide therapeutic benefits. Thus, all foods, because they provide nutritive value, are functional to some extent. After determining the role for essential elements (e.g., protein, carbohydrates, vitamins) of foods in deficiency diseases, scientists began to recognize physiologically active components in plant and animal products that can reduce risk for various chronic diseases or otherwise provide desirable physiologic effects. Implying that some foods are "good" and others are "bad" leads to misinformed food choices. Dietary supplements are not foods. Some food components—not the traditional nutrients of carbohydrate, protein, fat, vitamins, and minerals—may provide positive health benefits. Foods containing these components are defined by the Academy of Nutrition and Dietetics as functional foods.[12]

The scientifically sound approach to labeling and marketing a functional food is through the use of U.S. Food and Drug Administration (FDA)–approved health claims as outlined by the Nutrition Labeling and Education Act (1990) discussed in Chapter 1. Under the Nutrition Labeling and Education Act, a health claim can be authorized by the FDA with the consensus of qualified experts acknowledging that scientific studies support the validity of the relationship described in that claim. Scientific agreement requires consistent findings from well-designed clinical and epidemiologic studies and expert opinions from independent scientists. Strong evidence supports some of the claims, but there is only weak evidence for others. When research confirms links between food components and health, the FDA permits additional health claims (see Box 1.5).

Health-related statements or claims allowed on labels include[13]:

- nutrient content claims that indicate a specific nutrient at a certain level
- structure and function claims that describe the effect of dietary components on the normal structure or function of the body
- dietary guidance claims in reference to health benefits of broad categories of foods or diets, not a disease or health-related condition
- qualified health claims that convey a relationship between components in the diet and reduced risk of disease

Examples of functional foods include natural components of fruits and vegetables, milk, fortified or enhanced foods, and even some foods previously thought of as unhealthy, such as chocolate and red wine. More than a dozen classes of biologically active plant chemicals are known as phytochemicals and antioxidants (Table 20.1). These natural components found in vegetables such as cabbage, carrots, broccoli, and tomatoes may reduce the risk of cancer. Foods that have been fortified to enhance the level of a specific food component include products such as calcium-fortified orange juice, fiber-supplemented snack bars, or folate-enriched cereals. Oat products reduce serum cholesterol, reducing risk of coronary heart disease. Food products are constantly being developed with beneficial components, such as cholesterol-lowering margarine and products with soy protein.

Frequently, the press reports about a perfectly legitimate scientific study or a firm will begin marketing a functional food on the basis of "emerging evidence." (For more information, see Chapter 16.) Conversely, consumers worry that new technological developments may influence the safety of the food. For instance, many prefer natural additives as opposed to synthetics. Lack of nutritional knowledge may limit the acceptance of functional foods. However, people should not automatically assume that consuming functional foods will necessarily improve their health. Adding a food containing a particular nutrient does not mean that the nutrient will always have the desired effect.

Research regarding how foods or food components and dietary supplements may promote health and reduce chronic disease is providing a steady stream of new information. Dietary recommendations from established scientific authorities are slow in coming because of the need for a strong, consensus-based body of evidence before changing dietary advice for the public. Increasing intake of selected foods may not be wise without considering potential negative consequences and whether or not these specific elements are needed. Factors such as overall nutritional value and calorie intake of an individual's diet and whether sound scientific evidence backs the claims on package labels should be considered before routinely encouraging or choosing these foods. When evaluating functional foods, safe levels of intake must be considered. In many cases, optimal levels of nutrients and other physiologically active components in the foods have yet to be determined.

A person who does not have cardiovascular disease (CVD) or an elevated cholesterol level would not benefit from using sterol-enhanced products. The vitamins in vitamin-enhanced drinks are probably well absorbed, but the vitamins may not be the ones deficient in the diet and most of these products have more sugar than a regular soda. Many of these products indicate improvement of athletic performance, conditioning, recovery from fatigue after exercise, and avoidance of injury. Some of these claims may be valid. However, these foods should be used only when scientific evidence clearly supports the claim and when the physiologic changes caused by the functional ingredient are understood. The best way a consumer can evaluate the effectiveness of a food product is by trying it for several weeks to observe for benefits.

Functional foods are an important part of wellness because they offer great potential for consumers to optimize their health through diet, but they are not "magic bullets" or a universal panacea for poor health habits. Functional foods are not a substitute for a well-balanced diet and regular physical activity within the framework of a healthy lifestyle. Consumers will probably continue to choose functional foods they enjoy eating, with which they are familiar, and which are readily accessible. When referring to functional foods, the important thing is that what *is* eaten may be more important to health than what is *not* eaten. The best advice is to discuss appropriate intake of functional foods and strategies for achieving dietary intake goals in the context of a healthful diet based on the *Dietary Guidelines* and *MyPlate* to optimize health and potentially decrease the risk of chronic diseases.

TABLE 20.1 Examples of Functional Components

Class/Component	Source[a]	Potential Benefit
Carotenoids		
Beta carotene	Carrots, pumpkin, sweet potato, cantaloupe, spinach, tomatoes	Neutralizes free radicals that may damage cells; bolsters cellular antioxidant defenses; can be made into vitamin A in the body
Lutein, zeaxanthin	Kale, collard, spinach, corn, eggs, citrus fruits, asparagus, carrots, broccoli	Supports maintenance of eye health
Lycopene	Tomatoes and processed tomato products (more effective after heating), watermelon, red/pink grapefruit	Supports maintenance of prostate health
Dietary (Functional and Total) Fiber		
Insoluble fiber	Wheat bran, corn bran, fruit skins	Supports maintenance of digestive health; may reduce risk of some types of cancer
Beta glucan[b]	Oat bran, oatmeal, oat flour, barley, rye	May reduce risk of cardiovascular disease (CVD)
Soluble fiber[b]	Psyllium seed husk, peas, beans, apples, citrus fruit	May reduce risk of CVD and some types of cancer
Whole grains[b]	Cereal grains, whole-wheat bread, oatmeal, brown rice	May reduce risk of CVD and some types of cancer; may contribute to maintenance of healthy blood glucose levels
Fatty Acids		
Monounsaturated fatty acids (MUFAs)[b]	Tree nuts, olive oil, canola oil	May reduce risk of CVD
Polyunsaturated fatty acids (PUFAs)-Omega-3 fatty acids—delta-aminolevulinic acid (ALA)	Walnuts, flaxseeds, flaxseed oil	Support maintenance of heart and eye health; supports maintenance of mental function
PUFAs—Omega-3 fatty acids—docosahexaenoic acid (DHA)/eicosapentaenoic acid (EPA)	Salmon, tuna, marine, other fish oils	May reduce risk of CVD; contributes to maintenance of eye health and mental function
Conjugated linoleic acid (CLA)	Beef and lamb; some cheese	Supports maintenance of desirable body composition and immune health
Flavonoids		
Anthocyanins—cyanidin, delphinidin, malvidin	Berries, cherries, red grapes	Bolster cellular antioxidant defenses; supports maintenance of healthy brain function
Flavonols—catechins, epicatechins, epigallocatechin	Tea, cocoa, chocolate, apples, grapes	Support maintenance of heart health
Procyanidins and proanthocyanidins	Cranberries, cocoa, apples, strawberries, grapes, red wine, peanuts, cinnamon, tea, chocolate	Support maintenance of urinary tract health and heart health
Flavanones—hesperetin, naringin	Citrus fruits	Neutralize free radicals that may damage cells; bolster cellular antioxidant defenses
Flavonols—quercetin, kaempferol, isorhamnetin, myricetin	Onions, apples, tea, broccoli	Neutralize free radicals that may damage cells; bolster cellular antioxidant defenses
Isothiocyanates		
Sulforaphane	Cauliflower, broccoli, brussels sprouts, cabbage, kale, horseradish	May enhance detoxification of undesirable compounds; bolster cellular antioxidant defenses
Minerals		
Calcium[b]	Sardines, spinach, yogurt, low-fat dairy products, fortified foods and beverages	May reduce the risk of osteoporosis
Magnesium	Spinach, pumpkin seeds, whole-grain breads and cereals, halibut, almonds, brazil nuts, beans	Supports maintenance of normal muscle and nerve function, immune health, and bone health
Potassium[b]	Potatoes, low-fat dairy products, whole-grain breads and cereals, citrus juices, beans, banana, leafy greens	May reduce risk of high blood pressure and stroke in combination with a low sodium diet

TABLE 20.1 **Examples of Functional Components—cont'd**

Class/Component	Source[a]	Potential Benefit
Selenium	Fish, red meat, whole grains, garlic, liver, eggs	Neutralizes free radicals that may damage cells; supports maintenance of immune and prostate health
Phenolic Acids		
Caffeic acid, ferulic acid	Apples, pears, citrus fruits, some vegetables, whole grains, coffee	Bolster cellular antioxidant defenses; support maintenance of eye and heart health
Plant Stanols/Sterols		
Free stanols/sterols[b]	Corn, soy, wheat, fortified foods and beverages	May reduce risk of CVD
Stanol/sterol esters[b]	Stanol ester dietary supplements, fortified foods and beverages, including table spreads	May reduce risk of CVD
Polyols		
Sugar alcohols[b]—xylitol, sorbitol, mannitol, lactitol	Some chewing gums and other food applications	May reduce risk of dental caries
Prebiotics		
Inulin, fructo-oligosaccharides (FOS), polydextrose	Whole grains, onions, some fruits, garlic, honey, leeks, fortified foods and beverages	Supports maintenance of digestive health; supports calcium absorption
Probiotics		
Yeast, *Lactobacilli*, *Bifidobacteria*, other specific strains of beneficial bacteria	Certain yogurts and other cultured dairy and nondairy products	Support maintenance of digestive and immune health; benefits are strain specific
Phytoestrogens		
Isoflavones—daidzein, genistein	Soybeans and soy-based foods	Support maintenance of bone and immune health, and healthy brain function; for women, support menopausal health
Lignans	Flax seeds, rye, some vegetables, seeds and nuts, lentils, triticale, broccoli, cauliflower, carrots	Support maintenance of heart and immune health
Soy Protein		
Soy protein	Soybeans and soy-based foods like milk, yogurt, cheese and tofu	May reduce risk of CVD
Sulfides/Thiols		
Diallyl sulfide, allyl methyl trisulfide	Garlic, onions, leeks, scallions	May enhance detoxification of undesirable compounds; support maintenance of heart, immune and digestive health
Dithiolthiones	Cruciferous vegetables	May enhance detoxification of undesirable compounds; support maintenance of healthy immune function
Vitamins		
A[c]	Organ meats, milk, eggs, carrots, sweet potato, spinach	Supports maintenance of eye, immune and bone health; contributes to cell integrity
Thiamin (vitamin B_1)	Lentils, peas, brown or enriched white rice, pistachios, certain fortified breakfast cereals	Supports maintenance of mental function; helps regulate metabolism
Riboflavin (vitamin B_2)	Lean meats, eggs, green leafy vegetables, dairy products, certain fortified breakfast cereals	Supports cell growth; helps regulate metabolism
Niacin (vitamin B_3)	Dairy products, poultry, fish, nuts, eggs, certain fortified breakfast cereals	Supports cell growth; helps regulate metabolism
Pantothenic acid (vitamin B_5)	Sweet potato, organ meats, lobster, soybeans, lentils, certain fortified breakfast cereals	Helps regulate metabolism and hormone synthesis

[a]Examples are not an all-inclusive list.
[b]U.S. Food and Drug Administration–approved health claim for component.
[c]Preformed vitamin A is found in foods that come from animals. Provitamin A carotenoids are found in many darkly colored fruits and vegetables and are a major source of vitamin A for vegetarians.
Data from International Food Information Council Foundation. Functional Foods, July 2011. http://www.foodinsight.org/Content/3842/Final%20Functional%20Foods%20Backgrounder.pdf. Accessed May 23, 2017.

CASE APPLICATION FOR THE DENTAL HYGIENIST

Mrs. Owen is a 73-year-old patient with complete dentition in the maxillary arch and a removable mandibular partial denture. The mandibular canines and incisors are present, all of which have periodontal involvement with 3 to 5 mm of gingival recession. Root caries are present on the mandibular right and left canine. Examination reveals dry, cracked lips; a lack of salivary pool; and an ill-fitting mandibular prosthesis. The medical history reveals high blood pressure and a 10-year history of antihypertensive drug use. Mrs. Owen complains of difficulty in swallowing dry food, xerostomia, and taste alterations.

While obtaining a 24-hour food recall, the dental hygienist realizes that Mrs. Owen has lost interest in food. She states: "I just don't feel like eating. Food doesn't taste good, and I don't like cooking for myself." If she eats breakfast, she typically has orange juice and a doughnut; for lunch, she has canned soup; and before bedtime, part of a frozen dinner. A jar of hard candy sits in her living room from which she periodically takes a piece throughout the day, and she is constantly drinking soda for relief of xerostomia.

Nutritional Assessment

- Food intake for possible nutrient deficiencies
- Oral factors affecting motivation to eat
- Social and medical factors affecting nutrient intake
- Knowledge and motivation level
- Financial status

Nutritional Diagnosis

Several factors are involved with Mrs. Owen's poor nutrient intake: xerostomia; root caries; an ill-fitting prosthesis; frequent intake of hard candy; lack of variety in food; choice of soft, low nutrient-dense foods; and social isolation.

Nutritional Goals

Mrs. Owen has agreed to improve her overall nutritional status gradually by replacing soft, low nutrient-dense foods with high-fiber foods and using sugar-free candies and soda to prevent root caries.

Nutritional Implementation

Intervention: Increase intake of calcium-rich foods, such as low-fat milk, yogurt, and cheese.

Rationale: Adequate calcium and vitamin D intakes help to protect the alveolar bone from resorption.

Intervention: Provide education on xerostomia and its effects on the oral cavity and dietary process.

Rationale: An understanding of the cause and effect of xerostomia can help Mrs. Owen make necessary changes.

Intervention: Limit the intake of commercial frozen prepared meals and other processed foods high in sodium. Suggest that she could prepare several meals and freeze them in individual portion sizes when she feels like cooking.

Rationale: An occasional frozen meal is quick and effortless and a better choice than not eating. However, they are expensive and generally need to be supplemented with other foods for adequate nutrients. Because many are high in sodium, an important factor because of Mrs. Owen's hypertension, remind her to read labels and to purchase ones that contain less than 500 mg of sodium per serving.

Intervention: Suggest (a) frequent sips of a nutritious beverage (e.g., milk or juices) or a noncariogenic fluid (e.g., water) throughout the day; (b) use of products designed for patients with xerostomia, such as Bioténe or Oral Balance; (c) foods containing nonnutritive sweeteners or sugar alcohols (e.g., products containing xylitol); and (d) foods that stimulate saliva flow, such as citrus, tart, or sour foods (e.g., sugar-free lemon drops). Remind the patient of gastrointestinal distress associated with excessive consumption of products containing sugar alcohols.

Rationale: High-nutrient or noncariogenic fluids keep the mouth moist to relieve xerostomia. Products containing xylitol consumed after a meal can deter demineralization and promote remineralization. Citrus, tart, or sour foods and chewing gum stimulate saliva flow.

Intervention: Emphasize the importance of practicing proper oral hygiene techniques and explain the caries and periodontal disease process.

Rationale: Because dentition status is related to nutritional status, Mrs. Owen would benefit from retaining each natural tooth as long as possible. Xerostomia is also a contributing factor to root caries; however, plaque biofilm must be present for xerostomia to play a role in caries development. Proper daily oral hygiene care would improve her oral status and prevent further complications.

Intervention: Apply topical fluoride in the office, and instruct the patient on self-applied home fluoride treatments.

Rationale: Topical fluoride application reduces caries risk by disrupting destructive bacteria from metabolizing fermentable carbohydrates. Application of fluoride is based on caries risk, not age.

Intervention: Instruct the patient to use a daily antimicrobial rinse for 2 weeks after each treatment.

Rationale: Antimicrobial agents are used as an adjunct to other strategies for caries reduction. Antimicrobial agents effectively control plaque biofilm formation and maturation.

Intervention: Avoid dry, spicy, and some acidic foods. Avoid alcohol, caffeine, and tobacco as well.

Rationale: These choices can worsen xerostomia or irritate the mucosa.

Intervention: Encourage involvement with a local senior group and provide information for food assistance programs for older adults, such as Meals on Wheels.

Rationale: An older adult who lives alone may experience a decreased appetite and lack motivation to prepare appropriate meals. Socializing with others during meals enhances the enjoyment of eating.

Evaluation

Mrs. Owen's mandibular partial denture has been adjusted. The nutrition goals established with the dental hygienist are gradually being met. She has substituted a few pieces of sugar-free candy for hard sugar-containing candy, prepares more meals, and has joined the community senior citizen center. She recently began using home fluoride treatments, completed the antimicrobial rinse, and remains caries free. She appears to be a much happier individual.

Student Readiness

1. To understand what a patient with xerostomia experiences, eat several saltine crackers with no fluid, and note the dryness of the oral cavity. Imagine this situation indefinitely and its impact on a patient's food intake. Now, try a product designed to relieve xerostomia to understand its effect before recommending it to a patient.
2. Discuss at least two changes in the oral cavity that can change a patient's taste sensation. What recommendations can a dental hygienist provide?
3. Prepare an educational program for interdisciplinary health care professionals on recognizing changes in the oral cavity affecting nutrient intake and, ultimately, general health. List at least three health care professionals who would benefit from this knowledge.

References

1. Al Jawad FA, Cunningham SJ, Croft N, et al. A qualitative study of the early effects of fixed orthodontic treatment on dietary intake and behavior in adolescent patients. *Eur J Orthod.* 2011;34:432–436.
2. Liu B, Dion MR, Jurasic M, et al. Xerostomia and salivary hypofunction in vulnerable elders: prevalence and etiology. *Oral Surg Oral Med Oral Pathol Oral Radiol Endod.* 2012;114(1):52–60.
3. Gil-Montoya JA, Silvestre FJ, Barrios R, et al. Treatment of xerostomia and hyposalivation in the elderly: a systematic review. *Med Oral Patol Oral Cir Bucal.* 2016;21(3):355–366.
4. Molina A, Garcia-Gargallo M, Montero E, et al. Clinical efficacy of desensitizing mouthwashes for the control of dentin hypersensitivity and root sensitivity: as systematic review and meta-analysis. *Int J Dent Hyg.* 2017;15:84–94.
5. Centers for Disease Control and Prevention, Oral Health Resources. Complete tooth loss. https://www.cdc.gov/mmwr/preview/mmwrhtml/mm5632a6.htm. Accessed May 24, 2017.
6. Kim JK, Baker LA, Seirawan H, et al. Prevalence of oral health problems in US adults, NHANES 1999-2004: exploring differences by age, education, and race/ethnicity. *Spec Care Dentist.* 2012;32(6):234–241.
7. Cousson PY, Bessadet M, Nicolas E, et al. Nutritional status, dietary intake and oral quality of life in elderly complete denture wearers. *Gerodontology.* 2012;29:e685–e692.
8. Saarela RKT, Lindroos E, Soini H, et al. Dentition, nutritional status and adequacy of dietary intake among older residents in assisted living facilities. *Gerodontology.* 2016;33:225–232.
9. Scariot R, Bastista TBD, Olandoski M, et al. Host and clinical aspects in patients with benign migratory glossitis. *Arch Oral Biol.* 2017;73:259–268.
10. Mozaffari HR, Sharifi R, Sadeghi M. Prevalence of oral lichen planus in diabetes mellitus: a meta-analysis study. *Acta Inform Med.* 2016;24(6):390–393.
11. Huber MA. White oral lesions, actinic cheilitis, and leukoplakia: confusions in terminology and definition: facts and controversies. *Clin Dermatol.* 2010;28(3):262–268.
12. Crowe KM, Francis C. Position of the Academy of Nutrition and Dietetics: functional foods. *J Acad Nutr Diet.* 2013;113(8):1096–1103.
13. International Food Information Council Foundation. Functional foods. July 2011. http://www.foodinsight.org/Content/3842/Final%20Functional%20Foods%20Backgrounder.pdf. Accessed May 23, 2017.

e EVOLVE RESOURCES

Please visit http://evolve.elsevier.com/Stegeman/nutritional for additional practice and study support tools.

21 Nutritional Assessment and Education for Dental Patients

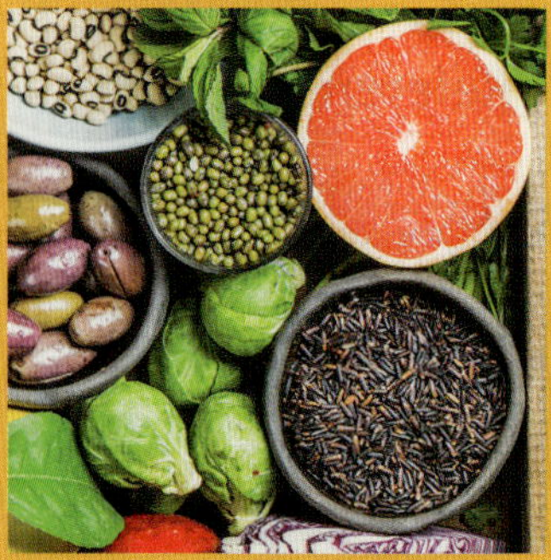

STUDENT LEARNING OUTCOMES

Upon completion of this chapter, the student will be able to achieve the following student learning outcomes:

1. Discuss the importance of a thorough health, social, and dental history in relation to assessment of nutritional status.
2. Describe the components needed to assess the nutritional status of a patient.
3. Explain the types of diet histories and determine situations in which each may be used effectively.
4. Discuss the following related to dietary treatment plans and nutrition education sessions:
   - Formulate a dietary treatment plan for a dental problem influenced by nutrition.
   - Identify steps and considerations in implementing a dietary treatment plan.
   - Assimilate the steps of a nutrition education session.
   - Integrate EXPLORE-GUIDE-CHOOSE techniques of motivational interviewing into a clinical setting.
5. Practice several communication skills that the dental professional should employ when educating a patient.

KEY TERMS

Anthropometry
Diet history
Explore
Food frequency questionnaire
Goal
Guide
Motivational interviewing
24-Hour recall

TEST YOUR NQ

1. **T/F** When health and dental histories have been reviewed, the dental professional has adequate information to begin nutrition education with the patient.
2. **T/F** A clinical oral examination is a very sensitive tool for identifying nutritional deficiencies.
3. **T/F** Using food models helps the patient to learn how to determine portion sizes quickly and accurately.
4. **T/F** When providing nutrition education, the dental professional should suggest minimal changes to the patient's usual intake and reinforce positive practices.
5. **T/F** Results of dietary discussion sessions do not need to be documented or communicated with other dental staff members.
6. **T/F** Providing a standardized low-carbohydrate menu is sufficient for most patients with a high caries rate.
7. **T/F** The dental professional should highlight all foods on the food diary that may contribute to increasing the risk for caries.
8. **T/F** After the nutrition education session, the patient should have enough information and motivation to make the necessary changes.
9. **T/F** "What type of snacks do you eat?" is an example of an open-ended question.
10. **T/F** Listening involves interpreting the words spoken, the manner in which they are said, and nonverbal actions directly observed.
11. **T/F** In motivational interviewing, inappropriate behaviors are discussed and a course of treatment is presented.
12. **T/F** It is better to elicit a patient's motivation and thoughts than to present the dental professional's opinions.

Health is a multidimensional and interprofessional concept, encompassing the interaction of many elements. Dissemination of information to a patient does not guarantee that the patient will establish healthier patterns. For example, millions of people start or continue smoking despite innumerable documented health risks. To facilitate positive changes toward a desired health behavior, the health care educator must tailor the message to meet the patient's needs, practices, habits, attitudes, beliefs, and values.

The relationship between nutrition and the oral cavity has already been established in this book. As you have learned, signs of a nutrient deficiency, excess, or imbalance are detectable in the mouth. Conversely, integrity of the oral cavity is a factor in nutrient intake. Nutrition education should be patient centered, should emphasize prevention, and provide evidence-based information. Through the dental hygiene process of care (assessment, diagnosis, planning, implementation, and evaluation), the dental hygienist is ideally situated to address nutritional status as it relates to oral health.[1] The position of the Academy of Nutrition and Dietetics states, "The Academy supports the integration of oral health with nutrition services, education, and research. Collaboration between dietetics and oral healthcare professionals is recommended for oral health promotion and disease prevention and intervention."[2] Nutrition is essential for general health and dental health. The American Dental Hygienists' Association *Standards for Clinical Dental Hygiene Practice*[1] state that one of the dental hygienist's responsibilities is assessment of nutrition history and dietary practices with integration of nutrition counseling into comprehensive dental hygiene care. Poor eating habits are widespread among Americans; nutrition education as it relates to oral care is justifiable for most patients. When the instruction requires more than general nutrition information, involves complex medical nutrition therapy, or the consumption of unfamiliar foods, a referral to the health care provider or registered dietitian nutritionist (RDN) is necessary.

A nutrition assessment involves compiling and comparing data about the patient from various resources to provide meaningful evaluation and effective education. Providing nutritional information without a complete assessment is inappropriate. All steps in the assessment require critical thinking by the dental professional. The evaluation tools to be discussed in this chapter include health, social, and dental histories; clinical evaluations; dietary intake evaluation; and biochemical analysis.

Evaluation of the Patient

For effective education, a comprehensive picture of the patient is essential. If information gathered is incomplete, the treatment plan is distorted and may be ineffective or even detrimental to the patient's overall health. Consider this scenario: a patient with rampant caries is told to substitute sugar-free candy for mints. The patient agrees to try this until she discovers that sugar-free mints cost more money and are unrealistic with her limited income. The patient is unaware of other acceptable alternatives and continues with the mints. Thus, information essential for making appropriate recommendations for the patient was overlooked. Another example: a dental hygienist recommends a fluoride supplement to a young patient who drinks only bottled water containing fluoride, without assessing all fluoride sources being consumed. This could potentially lead to fluorosis.

Health History

The health history is designed to identify health-related considerations and side effects from medications putting a patient at nutritional risk. The presence of some medical conditions could affect nutritional status by interfering with a patient's ability to chew, digest, absorb, metabolize, or excrete nutrients. Medications (over the counter and prescription), herbs, and supplements have numerous side effects and interactions altering eating behaviors or affecting nutritional status or both. A patient taking an antihypertensive medication may experience drug-induced xerostomia and its consequent dental complications. Changes in taste and appetite, increased risk of dental problems, gastrointestinal distress, nausea or vomiting, and xerostomia are just a few drug-induced side effects. Many medications also have drug–nutrient interactions (e.g., prednisone), which may influence nutrient needs.

By reviewing the health history and clarifying statements with the patient, the clinician can discover additional health-related information. Patients may not report valuable information because they (a) perceive it as irrelevant for dental professionals, (b) have forgotten it, (c) are confused by the question, or (d) are apprehensive about their visit to the dental office. Patients frequently neglect to disclose the use of oral contraceptives, antiobesity drugs, or dietary supplements, which can have several dental and nutrition implications. A few minutes of further questioning by the dental professional can save hours of time and effort spent trying to treat the complications. A thorough health history provides the dental professional with a strong foundation for developing a plan for dietary education. In addition, a blood pressure measurement for all patients and a blood glucose level of patients with diabetes can be obtained to augment the assessment.

Screening tools, such as a nutrition assessment questionnaire (see Evolve), are helpful. When a nutritional screening is obtained during the initial steps of the assessment, the dental professional can detect warning signs to investigate further.

Psychosocial History

A social history identifies factors influencing food intake. Personal, environmental, or economic influences can imply nutritional problems (Box 21.1). The dental professional obtains much of this information through conversation and further questioning. In addition, by asking a patient to describe a "typical day," the dental professional can determine routine activities reflective of the patient's

• BOX 21.1 Social Influences of Food Intake

Examples of factors collected by the dental professional to understand further the basis of the patient's eating practices.

- Economic resources
- Food preparation and storage facilities
- Cultural, ethnic, or religious background
- Living or eating alone
- Frequency of dining out
- Responsibility of grocery shopping and food preparation
- Motivation level
- Education level
- Transportation issues
- Physical or mental challenges of an individual
- Occupation
- Work or school status
- Physical activity level
- Emotional experiences
- Peer and media movements

lifestyle. Understanding reasons for food choices and considering emotional patterns provide directions for suggesting dietary modifications. Considerations in choosing foods or establishing eating patterns can be found in Chapter 16.

Dental History

A knowledge of how patients perceive or value their oral health assists the dental professional in developing strategies for education. Such information is part of a dental history. Explanations of past and current dental practices, past dental treatment, and behaviors that impact oral care (e.g., clenching teeth, biting fingernails, sinus trouble) should also be collected. Tobacco and alcohol use, fluoride history, and snacking patterns are also important components.

The most effective technique for gathering a medical, social, and dental history is for the dental professional to interview the patient.

Assessment of Nutritional Status

A thorough assessment provides the dental professional with enough information to determine the nutritional status of the patient. An assessment of a healthy patient may identify nutritional aspects that can be improved or "fine-tuned" for optimal health. When patients are experiencing medical or dental complications, the assessment provides information alerting the dental professional to nutritional factors that can impede responses to dental treatment or recovery (e.g., a patient with anorexia nervosa, whose fragile nutritional status would delay recovery after periodontal surgery). During the assessment, the dental professional can also identify the level of patient readiness for change to provide appropriate guidelines directed toward modifying behavior. Overall, assessment provides the basis for the dental professional's well-informed recommendations or referrals.

Clinical Observation

Clinical observation begins as soon as the patient walks through the door. General appraisal should include posture, gait, mobility, skin tone and color, general weight status, significant weight loss or gain since previous visit, emotional state, personal hygiene, and physical limitations. Unintentional weight loss can be indicative of numerous disease states or even oral problems.

Extraoral and Intraoral Assessments

Visual inspection during an extraoral and intraoral examination identifies abnormal clinical signs. Table 21.1 lists physical signs and symptoms that may indicate an alteration in nutrition. These findings are not sensitive tools for determining nutrient deficiencies or excesses because they can mirror nonnutritional complications

TABLE 21.1 Nutrition-Related Complications of the Oral Cavity

Nutrient	Deficiency Symptoms
Thiamin (B_1)	Increased sensitivity and burning sensation of oral mucosa; burning tongue; loss of taste and appetite
Riboflavin (B_2)	Angular cheilosis; blue to purple mucosa; glossitis, magenta tongue, enlarged fungiform papillae, atrophy and inflammation of filiform papillae, burning tongue
Niacin (B_3)	Glossitis, ulcerations of tongue, atrophy of papillae; cheilosis; thin epithelium; burning of oral mucosa, stomatitis, erythematous marginal and attached gingiva; loss of appetite
Pyridoxine (B_6)	Cheilosis; glossitis, atrophy and burning of tongue; stomatitis
Cobalamin (B_{12})	Stomatitis; hemorrhaging; pale to yellow mucosa; glossitis, atrophy and burning of tongue; altered taste; loss of appetite
Folic acid	Glossitis with enlargement of fungiform papillae, ulcerations along edge of tongue; gingivitis; erosion and ulcerations on buccal mucosa, pale mucosa
Biotin	Glossitis; gray mucosa; atrophy of lingual papillae
Vitamin C	Odontoblast atrophy; porotic dentin formation; alterations in pulp; gingival inflammation with easy bleeding, deep red to purple gingiva; ulceration and necrosis; slow wound healing; muscle and joint pain; defects in collagen formation
Vitamin A	Ameloblast atrophy; faulty bone and tooth formation; accelerated periodontal destruction; hypoplasia; xerostomia; cleft lip; keratinization of epithelium; drying and hardening of salivary glands *Toxicity symptoms:* Hypertrophy of bone; cracking and bleeding lips; thinning of epithelium; erythematous gingiva; cheilosis
Vitamin D, calcium, and phosphorus	Failure of bones to heal; mild calcification to enamel hypoplasia; loss of alveolar bone; delayed dentition; increased caries rate; loss of lamina dura around roots of tooth; reduced plasma calcium levels
Vitamin K	Gingival hemorrhaging
Iron	Painful oral cavity; stomatitis; thinned buccal mucosa with ulcerations; pale to gray mucosa, lips, and tongue; angular cheilosis; burning tongue; reddening at lip and margins of tongue; salivary gland dysfunction
Zinc	Thickening of epithelium; thickening of tongue with underlying muscle atrophy; impaired taste
Protein	Smooth, edematous tongue; angular cheilosis; fissures on lower lip; smaller teeth; delayed eruption; salivary gland dysfunction

or the possibility of several nutritional difficulties. For example, cheilosis can be the result of a vitamin B complex, iron, or protein deficiency; uncontrolled diabetes, excess or lack of saliva; constantly licking lips; allergies; yeast or fungal infections; or environmental exposure. Observations are used as an adjunct to supplement other assessment techniques.

Examples of extraoral signs and symptoms for the dental professional to document are multiple skin bruises or pallor, excessively dry or easily plucked hair, dry eyes, and cracked or spoon-shaped fingernails. Intraoral inspection of the integrity of soft tissues, status of the periodontium, and presence of plaque biofilm and calculus are examples of valuable indicators of the need for nutrition intervention. Data obtained during an extraoral and intraoral examination can supply valuable evidence of a nutrition problem that can be confirmed with other assessment procedures.

Other health professionals, such as RDNs, provide a physical assessment that includes the performance of a basic oral screening. A dental professional is capable of sharing expertise related to oral health concepts. Educating other health professionals to recognize normal and nonnormal oral conditions that interfere with dietary intake and encouraging performance of oral screenings can lead to identifying potential problems with oral issues and an increase in referrals to dental professionals.[2,3] Ultimately, the patient benefits from the strategies formulated by an interdisciplinary team.

Anthropometric Evaluation

Anthropometry involves measurements of physical characteristics such as height, weight, and change in weight. Indirectly, an anthropometric evaluation provides an image of body composition and helps to monitor progress of pregnant women and growth of infants, children, and adolescents. This assessment alone is not sensitive enough to determine nutritional status; however, anthropometric measures may be useful in diagnosis.

It is appropriate in most dental environments to request a patient's height and weight, as this information may be needed to determine appropriate dosage for medications and local anesthesia used during dental care. It may also be needed for a basic screening for obesity that may be a factor in periodontal disease. The height and weight information can easily be put into a body mass index (BMI) calculator (available on the Evolve website). The BMI, as described in the *Dietary Guidelines* (see Chapter 1 or http://www.usda.gov/cnpp), provides the general weight category and associated health risk, and is a guide for measuring nutritional status. However, BMI does not consider variables such as body composition and should not be the only anthropometric measure assessed. BMI is not used for pregnant or lactating women, older adults, or athletes. Visual inspection also assists in detecting unusual leanness, indicating undernutrition, or notable obesity.

Concern arises when weight loss is unintentional. A reduction of 10% of usual weight over 6 months is significant, and a loss of 20% of body weight or greater may indicate depletion of body mass, which may affect the immune response and the patient's ability to heal after invasive dental treatment.

Laboratory Information

When available, laboratory tests provide another piece of the puzzle in determining nutritional status. Generally, blood and urine samples supply the most sensitive data. As with other assessment techniques, a laboratory test alone should not be used to diagnose malnutrition because nonnutritional factors also can influence these data. A health care provider or RDN usually interprets nutrition-related laboratory tests. Dental professionals generally do not have access to this information, and it is not commonly used in a dental nutrition assessment.

In a dental environment, laboratory evaluations can include measuring salivary flow, plaque indices, caries risk assessment, determining the number of destructive bacterial cells, testing the pH of saliva, or monitoring blood glucose. Each of these tests provides valuable information to be included in the assessment.

DENTAL CONSIDERATIONS

Assessment

- *Physical:* Deviations from normal anatomy, particularly of the head and neck areas; diseases or conditions; emotional state; activity level; abnormal anthropometric measurements; blood pressure, respiration, and pulse; if accessible or practical, laboratory tests, such as blood glucose or HbA_{1c}values for individuals with diabetes.
- *Dietary:* Medications responsible for difficulties in eating; conditions that interfere with obtaining adequate nutrients (e.g., financial status, ability to shop for or prepare food); oral health issues interfering with food intake.

Interventions

- To be an effective nutrition educator, the dental professional must understand eating habits of local cultural, ethnic, or religious groups (see Chapter 16). If a patient presents with unfamiliar foods and/or food behaviors, refer to an RDN.
- Encourage patients who are challenged by remembering their list of medications and supplements to bring all the containers to the appointment.
- Questioning the patient about mode of transportation and mobility in the community may reveal difficulties in food procurement related to immobility or isolation.
- Ask the patient to describe past dental experiences to gauge knowledge level and perception and attitude toward dentistry.
- Information about previous fluoride exposure provides valuable indicators for the assessment. Additional questions include the following: "Were you raised in an area with fluoridated water?" "Did you take fluoride supplements growing up?" "How often did the dentist provide fluoride treatments?" "Were fluoride treatments given at school?" "Have you used fluoridated rinses or gels at home?"
- Observations of the patient's attentiveness, anxiety level, motivation, previous dental treatment, and present oral conditions provide direction when initiating a nutrition assessment as part of the dental hygiene care plan.
- A simple method to determine a patient's readiness for behavior change is to ask, "On a scale from 1 to 10, how ready are you to substitute 12 oz of milk for 12 oz of soda?" (1 being not ready to change and 10 being ready to change).[4]
- Questions and comments made by the patient reflect existing knowledge and understanding of information presented as well as their needs and desires. A dental professional should practice active listening skills to gain valuable information needed in the assessment.
- While interviewing, maintain verbal and nonverbal neutrality in response to the patient's statements.

Evaluation

- When histories and other information about the patient have been obtained and the clinical examination has been performed, the dental professional should have some understanding of the patient's preferences and needs. For greater compliance, tailor the message to meet the patient's preferences, based on the needs.

NUTRITIONAL DIRECTIONS

- Take the time to gather as much nutrition information about the patient as possible to provide individualized suggestions for greater patient compliance. Generic and vague health messages and meal plans are ineffective.

Determining Diet History

To assess the patient's nutritional status further, the evaluation process should include a screening of the **diet history** or a review of usual patterns of food intake and various factors that determine food selection. The overall goal is to determine usual dietary habits to individualize recommendations and suggest minor changes while improving dietary quality. Reviewing intake of the parent, guardian, or caregiver is necessary to understand food choices of a child or adolescent. Questioning may be necessary to clarify information provided. Explain the need for a nutrition assessment before asking the patient to complete the diet history form. Additional questioning may be necessary to clarify the information provided. Inquire about food preparation, whether foods chosen are nonfat or dietetic, and use of beverages or condiments. Also, use of food models, pictures of foods in measured portions, and measuring devices are helpful to easily and precisely identify usual serving sizes.

The diet history can be evaluated based on *MyPlate* (see Fig. 21.1) and the *Dietary Guidelines* for adequacy and variety of nutrients. Use of the U.S. Department of Agriculture government-operated websites is free. Other nutrition software programs are available, including on the Evolve website. An analysis of daily carbohydrate exposures identifies cariogenic potential of the diet. Practical tools used to collect data on dietary intake include the 24-hour recall, food frequency questionnaire, and 3- to 7-day food diary.

Twenty-Four-Hour Recall

The **24-hour recall** (see Figs. 18.7 and 21.2) allows the dental professional to collect data on food consumed during a single day. It is easy, quick, and presents a representative sample of the patient's dietary intake. The information is most accurate when interviewing the patient or the parent, guardian, or caregiver of a child and requesting intake from the previous day. This requires little time and is easy to obtain. The patient is generally able to recreate the dietary intake from the preceding day with minimal effort. Obtaining as much detail as possible elicits an accurate view of usual food and beverage intake (Box 21.2). The use of

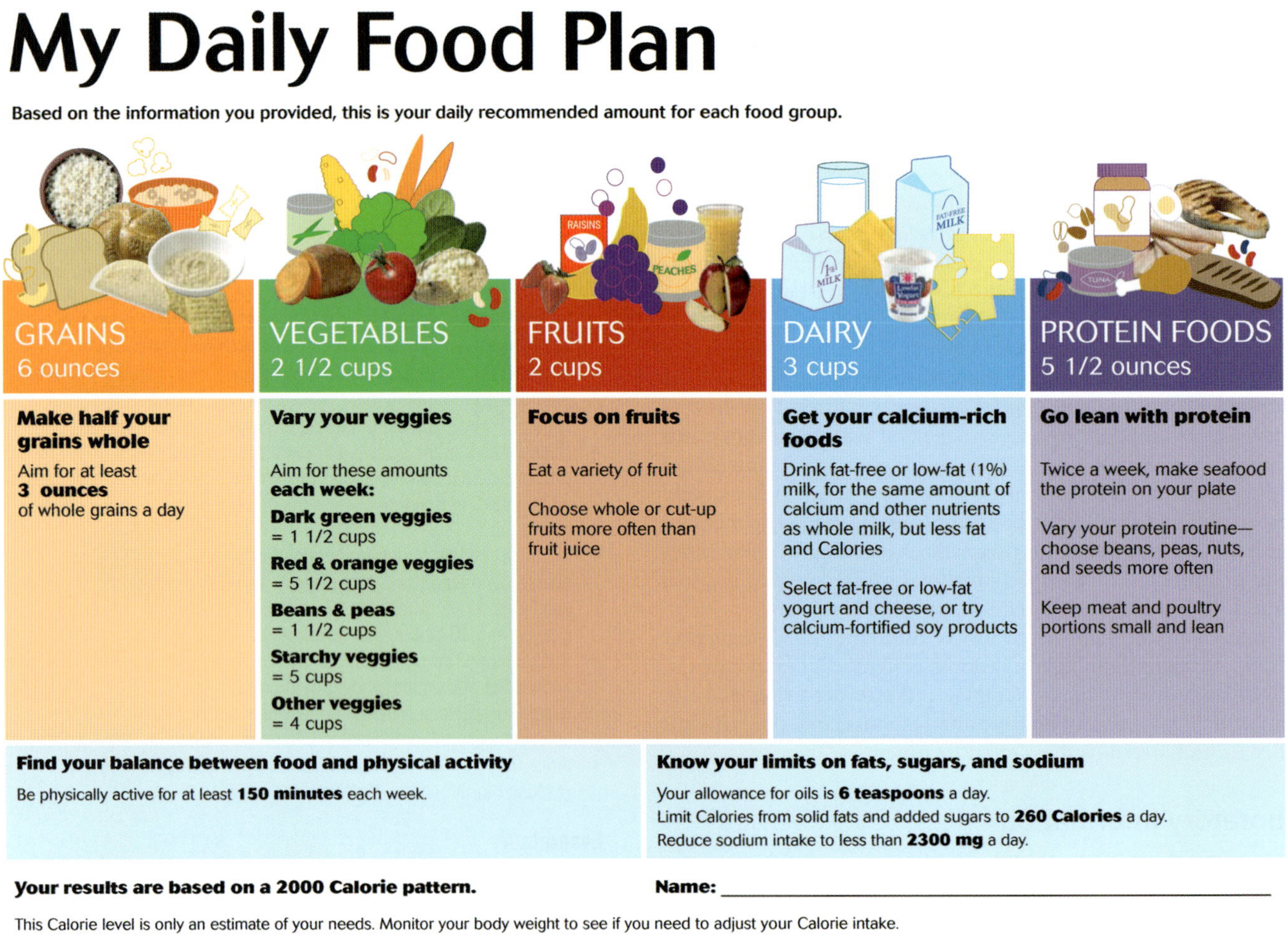

My Daily Food Plan

Based on the information you provided, this is your daily recommended amount for each food group.

GRAINS 6 ounces	VEGETABLES 2 1/2 cups	FRUITS 2 cups	DAIRY 3 cups	PROTEIN FOODS 5 1/2 ounces
Make half your grains whole Aim for at least **3 ounces** of whole grains a day	**Vary your veggies** Aim for these amounts **each week:** **Dark green veggies** = 1 1/2 cups **Red & orange veggies** = 5 1/2 cups **Beans & peas** = 1 1/2 cups **Starchy veggies** = 5 cups **Other veggies** = 4 cups	**Focus on fruits** Eat a variety of fruit Choose whole or cut-up fruits more often than fruit juice	**Get your calcium-rich foods** Drink fat-free or low-fat (1%) milk, for the same amount of calcium and other nutrients as whole milk, but less fat and Calories Select fat-free or low-fat yogurt and cheese, or try calcium-fortified soy products	**Go lean with protein** Twice a week, make seafood the protein on your plate Vary your protein routine—choose beans, peas, nuts, and seeds more often Keep meat and poultry portions small and lean

Find your balance between food and physical activity
Be physically active for at least **150 minutes** each week.

Know your limits on fats, sugars, and sodium
Your allowance for oils is **6 teaspoons** a day.
Limit Calories from solid fats and added sugars to **260 Calories** a day.
Reduce sodium intake to less than **2300 mg** a day.

Your results are based on a 2000 Calorie pattern. **Name:** ____________________

This Calorie level is only an estimate of your needs. Monitor your body weight to see if you need to adjust your Calorie intake.

• **Figure 21.1** *MyPlate* food record worksheet for a 2000-calorie intake goal. (From U.S. Department of Agriculture (USDA) Center for Nutrition Policy and Promotion. http://www.choosemyplate.gov. Accessed August 23, 2017.)

My Food Diary **Day** ____________________

Meal/Snack (Indicate time of day)	What You Ate and Drank	Where and With Whom	Notes (Feelings, hunger, etc.)
Breakfast			
Snack			
Lunch			
Snack			
Dinner			

• **Figure 21.2** Food record worksheet. (From the Centers for Disease Control and Prevention. http://www.cdc.gov/healthyweight/pdf/food_diary_cdc.pdf. Accessed August 23, 2017.)

• BOX 21.2 How to Keep Your Food Record

- Record foods and beverages as soon after eating as possible.
- Record on days when *not* sick or fasting.
- Record all meals and snacks for each day, including one weekend day.
- Estimate portion sizes (e.g., 3 oz fish, 1 cup of cereal, ½ cup of milk, 1 tsp of vegetable oil) as closely as possible.
- Document the food preparation method (e.g., baked, broiled, fried, or grilled).
- Include amounts of added sugar, creamer, sauces, gravies, and condiments (e.g., mayonnaise or mustard).
- For combination dishes—such as casseroles, soups, chili, or pasta—record all the ingredients and the amounts accurately and the portion eaten.
- Record brand names (e.g., Cheerios or Promise Margarine).
- Enter the time of consumption.
- Include miscellaneous items, such as mints, gum, and cough drops.

food models or visuals of common serving sizes helps the patient provide a more accurate estimation of portion size. Snacking patterns and spacing of meals may also be revealed in a 24-hour recall. Another advantage is that it allows a general analysis of basic nutrient adequacy, variety, and cariogenicity.

An account of the previous day may not be optimal, however, if it was not a typical day. For example, the patient may have been extremely busy the day before and ate only one meal instead of the usual three meals and two snacks. In addition, it does not capture long-term behaviors and may miss foods that could have an impact on the assessment. Or, the patient may consume raw carrots as snacks on most days except the day of the 24-hour recall. The interviewer would miss the carotenes and other valuable nutrients that are part of this patient's dietary intake. Requesting recall of a typical day also may result in unreliable estimates because the patient is more likely to supply information about a "fictitious" day with optimal nutrient intake. It is an option, however, for obtaining a typical day's intake when the past 24 hours were atypical. Another problem may be that a patient has difficulty recollecting the previous day's food intake. Take a minute to write down what you ate yesterday to understand how arduous this task can be and how easy it is to omit snacks, gum, condiments, beverages, and other foods of lesser importance but could reveal important in the dental assessment.

Food Frequency Questionnaire

Another dietary evaluation tool is the **food frequency questionnaire**. The purpose of this questionnaire is to determine how often a patient consumes foods from groupings containing similar nutrient content. A list of commonly eaten foods is provided with instructions for the patient to circle the number of times per day, week, or month the food is chosen (Table 21.2). It requires limited explanation and little time; the questionnaire can be completed in the waiting room. The data gained allow for an analysis of food group consumption and carbohydrate intake. It is specifically relevant in determining caries risk.

TABLE 21.2 Food Frequency Questionnaire

Directions: THE FOLLOWING QUESTIONS WILL HELP SHOW YOUR (OR YOUR CHILD'S) NORMAL EATING BEHAVIOR. THIS INFORMATION WILL ALLOW THE DENTAL HEALTH TEAM TO THOROUGHLY EVALUATE YOUR (OR YOUR CHILD'S) DENTAL STATUS. PLEASE MARK HOW OFTEN YOU (OR YOUR CHILD) ATE OR DRANK EACH OF THESE ITEMS IN THE PAST WEEK.

Food Item	Never	1 to 3 Times per Month	1 to 3 Times per Week	5 or More Times per Week	1 to 2 Times per Day	3 to 4 Times per Day	5 or More Times per Day
Fruit and juices							
Vegetables, other than starchy choices							
Potatoes and other starchy choices							
Milk and yogurt							
Meat, fish, poultry, eggs							
Cheese							
Cereals (cold and hot)							
Cookies, cake, pies, pastries							
Candy							
Regular soda							
Diet soda							
Gum							
Sugar-free gum							
Alcohol							

Reprinted with permission from Thompson FE, Byers TB. Dietary Assessment Resource Manual. *J Nutr.* 1994;124(II Suppl):2297S.

Because of the lack of a comprehensive food list, the food frequency questionnaire is not specific and does not garner enough data to evaluate nutrient content. Nutrient intakes derived from food frequency questionnaires are often under- or overestimated. Dietary intake also relies on the patient's memory, and the patient can easily improve the choices by documenting only healthy foods. A food frequency questionnaire can be used to supplement the 24-hour recall to increase reliability of the information collected. For instance, a patient may have had a glass of milk yesterday; however, the food frequency questionnaire indicates this is unusual. The dental professional may not have concentrated on dairy products with only the 24-hour recall, but in combination with the food frequency questionnaire, it becomes a component of the nutrition education session.

Food Diary

The patient (or parent or guardian) may also be asked to record food and drink consumption for 3 to 7 days, including a weekend day, to evaluate intake. Fig. 21.2 is an example of 1 day of a food diary (see Fig. 18.7 for another example). Verbal and written instructions for using the food diary can be provided at the prophylaxis appointment (see Box 21.2). For accuracy, important points to stress include recording the intake when it is consumed, as well as weighing and measuring foods and beverages. The patient can return the diary at the recare or follow-up appointment. Overall, this is the most effective method of obtaining dietary information because the data are more likely to be representative of actual intake, and the analysis of nutrient and fermentable carbohydrate intake is more accurate. In addition, the patient becomes actively involved when recording the information and may see obscure eating patterns emerge.

Patient compliance is a deterring factor. Requesting records for too many days may decrease cooperation. The validity of the food diary is threatened when the patient underestimates food intake and neglects to record all foods or accurate portion sizes. The patient also may adjust the food diary to reflect healthier eating patterns. By emphasizing that this is not a test but rather an instrument to evaluate actual food patterns and to identify areas for potential modifications to improve overall health and oral health, the dental professional can concentrate on applying the data or may be able to dispel myths and misinformation that surface from the food diary. Finally, the food diary represents food consumed only for the time period documented, which does not always reflect usual intake.

The dental hygienist and other members of the dental team can cooperatively establish the most practical and realistic approach for determining food intake in their setting. Along with other components of assessment, the dental professional can generally evaluate the nutritional status of the patient and be knowledgeable about the effect of food habits on oral status.

DENTAL CONSIDERATIONS

Assessment

- *Physical:* Age or status of patient may require a caregiver to provide information.
- *Dietary:* Current dietary practices and requirements, adequacy of diet, fermentable carbohydrate intake, frequency of eating.

Interventions

- When interviewing a patient for a 24-hour recall, you may want to begin with, "What was the first thing you ate or drank after you got up?" or "What was the first thing you ate or drank yesterday morning?" Do not assume that breakfast was eaten. Other questions commonly used are the following: "Do you use gum, mints, antacids, or cough drops?" "Do you eat snacks?" "Tell me what you do to clean your mouth." "What do you usually drink?"
- If the operatory has a computer or netbook with Internet access, the practitioner can put the patient's 24-hour recall directly into the *Choose MyPlate* computer program for quick analysis.
- Use of standardized food models and food pictures, measuring cups, and/or actual foods may guide the patient toward actual portion size consumed.
- Allow as much participation by patients as possible, encouraging them to make their own decisions and to prescribe their own dietary modifications. Active involvement in problem solving is more effective in changing patients' habits and making them more accountable for their actions.

Evaluation

- The patient participates in the nutrition assessment process, asking appropriate questions and making statements that reflect understanding.

NUTRITIONAL DIRECTIONS

- Nutrition analysis of food intake, even if it is computer generated, cannot be used exclusively for diagnosing a deficiency and cannot replace nutrition education. Many software programs do not have complete or current data, and they do not consider other factors such as overcooking or caries risk. Nutrient intakes may not be accurately estimated. Nutritional analysis provides only an approximation of nutrient content and should be used only as an assessment tool and a guide in educating patients.

Identification of Nutritional Status

When all of the information is collected, the dental professional can begin to identify nutritional status and cariogenicity of the dietary intake and help the patient establish goals. (Chapter 18 describes the cariogenic potential of the diet.) A thorough understanding of the nutrients in each group of *MyPlate* helps to identify nutrients that may be deficient or excessive. For example, a commonly omitted food group is the dairy group, which, if evaluated, would alert the dental professional to possible inadequate intake of calcium, vitamin D, protein, and riboflavin. If such inadequacies are found, the dental hygienist could concentrate on helping the patient identify suitable food choices that are appetizing, accessible, and affordable. Preferably, choices providing these nutrients would be from foods, rather than supplements.

Several methods are available to evaluate a dietary intake. Fig. 21.3 provides an example to use as an assessment and/or education tool. The foods from the 24-hour recall or 3-day food record (Table 21.3) are transferred to the appropriate food categories with assistance from the patient. It is helpful to have the parent or guardian present when educating a child or adolescent, encouraging the child or adolescent to participate as much as possible. The patient easily determines adequacy of intake, and ideas for modifications or substitutions can follow. The number of servings consumed from each group is totaled. Average intakes are determined by dividing the totals by the number of days in the diary, and the averages are compared with *MyPlate*. As described in Chapter 18, the patient should be encouraged to circle or highlight each carbohydrate exposure and identify form, frequency, and time eaten (i.e., with a meal or as a snack) to evaluate the cariogenic potential of the diet.

Combination foods can be problematic for the patient because of numerous ingredients and difficulties of assigning different components into appropriate food groups. Each ingredient is considered separately and placed in the appropriate food group with servings. A 1-cup serving of spaghetti and meatballs generally is categorized as two grain servings (spaghetti), one protein serving (meatballs), one oil serving (if oil is present in spaghetti sauce or meatballs are fried), and one vegetable serving (tomato sauce).

Computer dietary analysis software packages, online programs, websites, and phone applications are available to assess dietary intake. Patients should be advised to investigate these tools before relying on them completely. Because anyone can publish on the Internet, professionals and patients should examine accuracy, authority, credibility, currency, objectivity, and coverage when using these tools (see "Relevant Websites" on Evolve). Several packages are specifically designed for the dental office. Nutrients usually available include calories, vitamins, minerals, protein, fiber, fat, and cholesterol. Programs vary in complexity, visuals, efficiency, number of food items, and accuracy. A printout of the comparison with the recommended dietary allowances, dietary goals, and exchanges provides a useful and "eye-opening" adjunct to the nutrition education session.

Use of a computer software program is limited by the cost of the hardware and software and the time factor. Not all software is reliable and accurate. Before relying on the data, randomly compare the nutrient content of several foods to U.S. Department of Agriculture nutrient data (https://ndb.nal.usda.gov/ndb/) or the manufacturer's information. Most important, use computer feedback to supplement nutrition education sessions but not to replace them.

These approaches to determining dietary intake are adequate and practical for most dental patients. The primary goal of a dietary assessment in dentistry is to identify patients with oral concerns related to eating and to improve these habits to prevent dental disease. If a more thorough assessment is required, the patient should be referred to an RDN.

Formation of Nutrition Treatment Plan

After evaluation of data, the results can be shared with the patient and parent or guardian, if appropriate. The dental professional and patient can begin to establish an individualized dietary plan and course of action. The patient should be involved in as many processes as possible to improve compliance. When assisting the patient in preparing an altered meal pattern, several strategies need to be considered. As discussed earlier, accommodating factors affecting food intake, whenever possible, are advantageous. The

DIETARY ANALYSIS

NAME ______________________
AGE ______________________
ACTIVITY LEVEL *SEDENTARY* *MODERATE* *ACTIVE*
CALORIE LEVEL ______________________

Food Groups	Day 1	Day 2	Day 3	Daily Average	Recommended Daily Amounts (Based on appropriate calorie level)	Comparison		
						Adequate	Low	High
Milk					______ cups			
Protein Foods					______ oz. equivalents			
Vegetables					______ cups			
Fruits					______ cups			
Grains					______ oz. equivalents			

• **Figure 21.3** Assessment of dietary intake form. This tool can also be used as an educational tool for patient understanding. (A customizable version is available on Evolve.)

TABLE 21.3 Checklist for Food Records*

Type of Food	Did You Specify
All	Amount eaten? By cup, tablespoon, or teaspoon? By size, giving dimensions (length, width, thickness, or diameter)? By number, for standard-size items? By weight?
Cereals	Size of servings? Brand name? Additions, such as milk, sugar, or fruit? Instant or ready-to-eat type?
Baked goods	Homemade or commercial? From scratch or mix? Topping or frosting? Portion size? Number eaten? Low fat? Low carbohydrate?
Fruits and juices	Cooked, raw, or dried? Peeled? Fresh, frozen, or canned? Sweetened? Size of serving? 100% fruit juice?
Vegetables	Cooked or raw? Fresh, frozen, or canned? Sauces, other additions? Serving size?
Milk products	Percent fat? Made with sweetener? Regular, low fat, or nonfat? Powder or liquid?
Meat, fish, poultry	Type of cut? Oil or water packed? Fat, skin removed? Preparation method? Additions? Cooked weight or dimensions of amount eaten?
Eggs	Added fat? Egg substitutes? Quantity? Preparation method?
Mixed dishes	Homemade or commercial? From scratch or mix? Brand? Major ingredients and proportions? Cooking method?
Soups	Homemade or commercial? Brand? Broth or milk base? Type of milk? Principal ingredients?
Fats and oils	Stick, tub, diet, whipped, liquid, or nonfat margarine? Brand? Major oil? Type of shortening? Homemade or commercial salad dressing? Low calorie or nonfat? Creamy?
Beverages	Brand? Sweetened? Diet? Decaffeinated? Alcohol content? Additions? Amount?
Snacks	Brand? Size, weight, or number eaten?
Restaurant meals	Type? Fast food, ethnic, seafood, steak? How often?
Vitamin-mineral supplements	Type? Reasons? Amount?

Note: Use this list to help clarify and increase accuracy of a food diary.
Reprinted with permission from Aronson V. Checklist for food records. In: Virginia Aronson, Barbara Fitzgerald, and Lynn Vincent Hewes, *Guidebook for Nutrition Counselors.* 2nd ed. Englewood Cliffs, NJ: Prentice Hall; 1990: 16-17.

goal is patient adherence so that oral health is improved. Other important considerations are food preferences, habits and behaviors, allergies, and prescribed diets. Compliance is more likely if changes are minimal or deviate as little as possible from the patient's normal pattern of eating. The patient should verify other results indicated by the assessment. For instance, if a patient's intake seems deficient in fruits, further questioning may reveal that no fruit was available during the days of recording because of the patient's inability to go to the grocery store. The dental professional would interpret this deficiency as atypical or that the situation may occur frequently because of lack of transportation.

Integration and Implementation

The purpose of nutrition education is to provide practical, accurate, evidence-based information; motivate and encourage positive changes in behavior; and continue healthful practices (Fig. 21.4). Obtaining knowledge and changing a personal habit requires a patient to internalize and accept that modifying a specific behavior is beneficial for overall health. A large gap exists between gaining information and applying the information because of difficulties in changing eating patterns. The patient and dental hygienist work together to bridge the gap. Knowledge alone does not determine desired behavior. Providing a sheet with a textbook diet or a list of nutrition "dos and don'ts" is unlikely to effect change. These written guidelines are not meaningful because they do not account for each patient's individuality and unique nutrition needs and for the difficulty in changing established eating patterns. Consider a patient who accurately describes *MyPlate* but continues to omit vegetables. This patient is knowledgeable but is not motivated enough to change behavior; learning is ineffective.

Effective nutrition education involves the patient and dental professional working together to define the diet/dental problem and formulate solutions. An education session in which the dental professional points out each negative behavior is not conducive to learning. The dental professional's responsibility is to supply accurate information and guide the patient in making healthful decisions toward improving the diet/dental situation. The dental professional can offer some suggestions and encouragement; however, it is the patient's responsibility to make changes in food patterns.

Motivational Interviewing

As far back as the early 1980s and early 1990s in medical settings, motivational interviewing was initiated as an education tool for changing health-related behaviors.[5,6] **Motivational interviewing** is a patient-centered, respectful, collaborative conversation in which the dental professional concentrates on strengthening and supporting a patient's motivation for a positive change in behavior. A three-component model is proposed to help dental professionals educate patients using motivational interviewing.[7] The first step is to **explore** the patient's behavior (Fig. 21.5). Professionals do this by building rapport and trust, asking open-ended questions, attentive listening (Fig. 21.6), affirming the patient's thoughts and feelings (with respect and nonjudgment), and summarizing what the patient is saying. It is ideal to find out what is important to patients, their concerns and values, and their health and nutrition history.

The second step after this enlightening conversation is to **guide** (Fig. 21.7). Professionals should inquire about the patient's own motivation and commitment rather than imposing ideas and suggestions. Dental professionals could easily ask, "On a scale from 1 to 10, how interested are you in changing your eating behavior?" The power for change resides solely in the hands of the patient, not the dental professional. When patients recognize a difference between where they are and where they want to be, they become more motivated. If the patient expresses some interest in a commitment to change, then the final step in the model is to

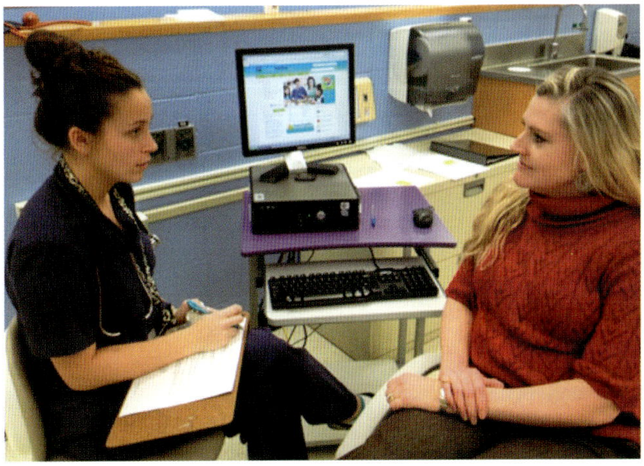

• **Figure 21.5** Motivational interviewing: exploring, establishing good rapport, and listening. (Courtesy of Amy L. Sullivan, University of Mississippi Medical Center, Jackson, MS.)

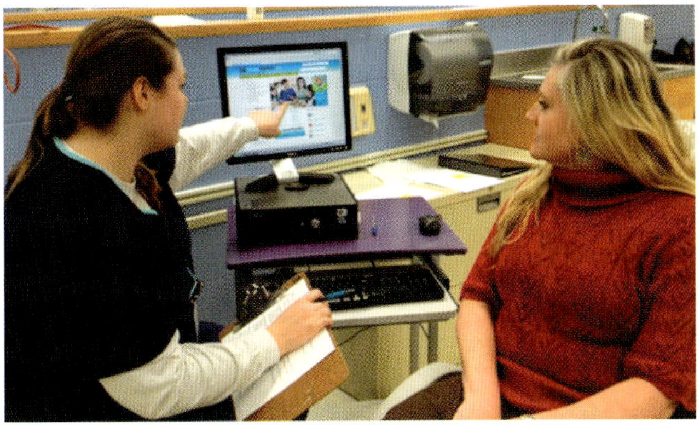

• **Figure 21.4** Educating the patient. (Courtesy of Amy L. Sullivan, University of Mississippi Medical Center, Jackson, MS.)

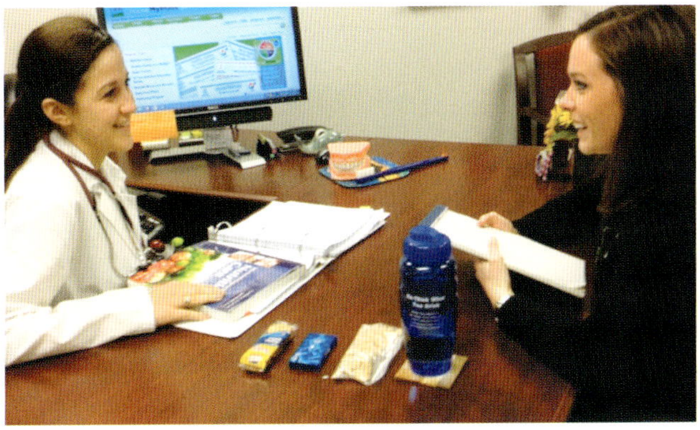

• **Figure 21.6** Listening to the patient. (Courtesy of Amy L. Sullivan, University of Mississippi Medical Center, Jackson, MS.)

choose. Dental professionals assist the patient by identifying specific, patient-oriented goals to build an action plan. Multiple options should be offered to avoid patient rejection (Fig. 21.8). Acknowledging resistance may help the patient not feel judged or pressured. Professionals can reflect back on things the patient has previously mentioned and use that information to move forward, focusing on reasons for the importance of changing. Professionals can also help foresee potential barriers that the patient may encounter and monitor the patient's follow through (Box 21.3).

Setting Goals

Resistance to change, despite knowledge, is a natural response of an individual. Consider the dental health professional who does not floss regularly yet encourages patients to floss. Box 21.4 presents an exercise to facilitate further understanding. Establishing a **goal** is an important aspect of changing behaviors because it sets a concrete standard for change. A meaningful and realistic goal should be something achievable by the patient. The goal chosen should be difficult enough to be challenging but not so difficult as to seem impossible. Occasionally, behaviors may need to be prioritized; a behavior with the most significant impact on oral health is addressed first. Perhaps frequent use of cough drops has led to an increased caries rate. The dental professional should emphasize the reason that this behavior is detrimental and guide the patient in establishing goals to decrease use of or eliminate cough drops. This guidance may include referring the patient to a health care provider to determine what is causing the sore throat or cough or explaining why the mouth is so dry.

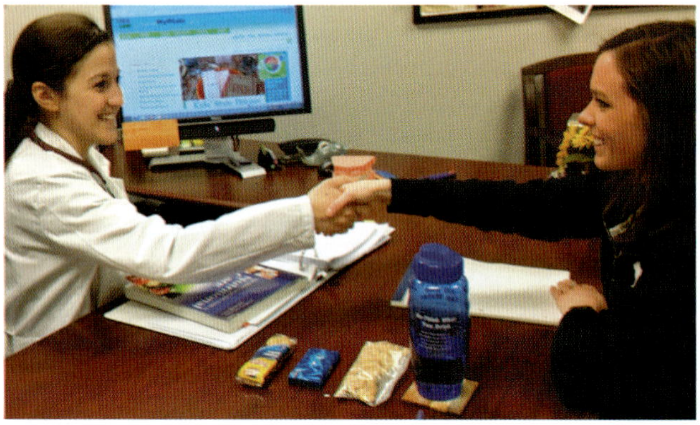

• **Figure 21.7** Motivational interviewing: guiding—getting a commitment. (Courtesy of Amy L. Sullivan, University of Mississippi Medical Center, Jackson, MS.)

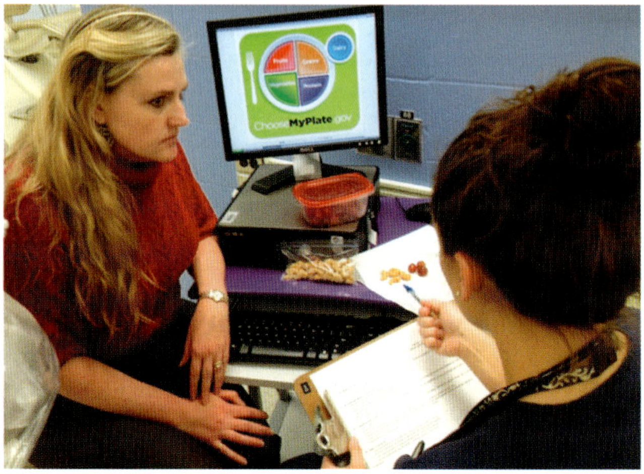

• **Figure 21.8** Motivational interviewing: choosing—offering multiple options. (Courtesy of Amy L. Sullivan, University of Mississippi Medical Center, Jackson, MS.)

• BOX 21.3 Motivational Interviewing: Three-Component Model

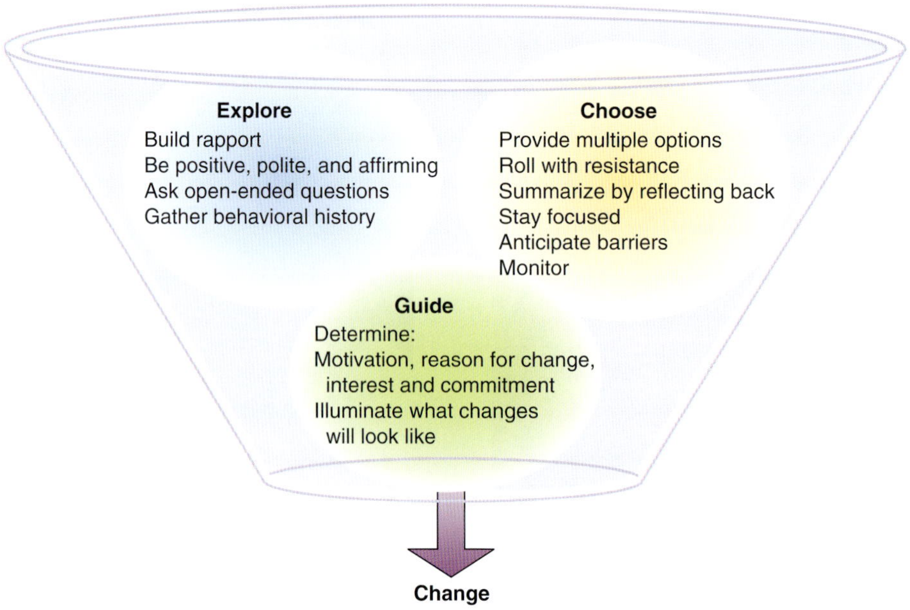

• BOX 21.4 Exercise to Understand Resistance to Change

Fold your arms in front of you. Do not glance down to identify which arm rests on top. Quickly unfold your arms and refold them the opposite way. For example, if the right arm was initially on top, it should be under the left arm after the switch.

Note the awkwardness. Does this reflect a change in an established behavior? If even this slight physical change leads to some resistance, think of the implications for more substantial behavioral changes asked of a patient.

Adapted from Newstrom JW, Scannell EE. Games Trainers Play. New York: McGraw-Hill; 1980.

A goal needs to be measurable or observable. "Eat one vegetable each day" is a very specific goal that can readily be measured. However, "improve oral health" is vague and difficult to observe; this goal should be more specific. Creating goals for multiple behavior changes at one time could be overwhelming. Gradual changes in behavior are more successful and can be accomplished by breaking goals into small steps. The dental professional can work with the patient to select and develop a realistic goal. When established, the goal should be modified as needs change. For example, "Eat one vegetable every other day" may be more appropriate for someone eating no vegetables at all than "Eat three to five servings of vegetables each day as recommended." The latter example may prove to be too difficult, and the patient may give up. Successful achievement of smaller steps motivates the patient toward larger changes. When smaller steps are accomplished, the patient can modify the goal to eating one vegetable every day and eventually work toward eating three to five vegetables per day.

Menu Creation

When the patient has a grasp of the dietary need and has direction as to how to accomplish it, the patient should create a realistic menu for a day or possibly make modifications on the dietary intake sheet previously recorded. The dental professional assists the patient in documenting a menu that follows the principles discussed, including nutritionally adequate and noncariogenic situations (Fig. 21.9). It should vary as little as possible from the original intake and include foods the patient likes. Often, the patient may suggest an ideal intake, modeling *MyPlate*. The dental professional can intervene and suggest individualized or personalized options to improve long-term compliance. For instance, most individuals know that it is unwise to eat frequently at fast food restaurants, but it is unrealistic to instruct patients never to eat there. The dental professional can help the patient determine the best food selections available if fast food establishments are necessary several times each week.

The feedback given by the patient to formulate a menu is one indicator for determining whether learning has occurred. An ideal menu reflects knowledge-based skills, but the patient may need to be redirected toward more realistic modifications.

Follow-up

A follow-up appointment to monitor progress and to evaluate the care provided can be scheduled separately or in conjunction with another dental appointment. Primary approaches for the dental professional include supporting continued change, establishing challenging goals or revising existing goals, and clarifying information. Reviewing a new food record with the patient promotes feedback of progress, particularly when compared with the original. Rather than expressing disappointment over failure to achieve a goal, the dental professional praises any positive behaviors, no matter how small. Praise and encouragement are more motivating. Perhaps the initial interventions established did not meet the patient's needs. Follow-up appointments can be used to listen, reassess the plan, identify new needs, and formulate new goals.

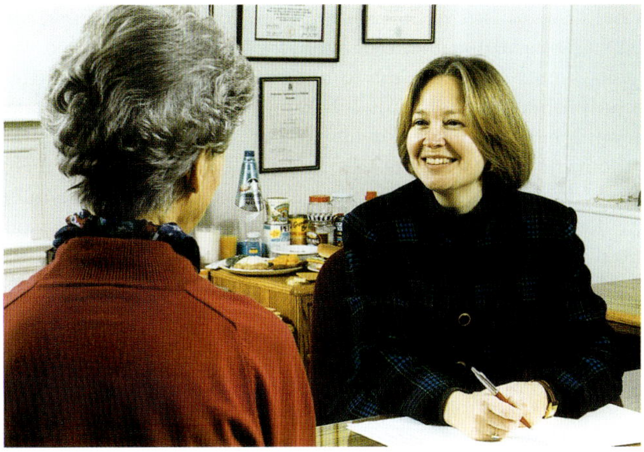

• Figure 21.9 Menu planning. (A customizable version is available on Evolve.)

Review

The dental professional concludes the session by summarizing the pertinent points and giving the patient a sense of accomplishment and direction after leaving the appointment. A firm commitment toward change may not always occur, but an agreement to think about it can be a successful conclusion. Providing a work phone number, email address or other social media forum, and encouraging contact with you with questions also helps the patient recognize your concern.

Evaluation

Evaluation is an ongoing process that occurs in all stages of assessment and education. The dental hygienist needs to revise the nutrition assessment and educate continuously, making appropriate changes as needed.

Documentation

The nutrition assessment process must be documented in the treatment record. Because this is a permanent legal document, if it is not recorded, presumably the intervention did not occur. Also, the treatment record serves as a tool to communicate with other members of the dental team and health care professionals. At a restorative appointment, another dental team member can reinforce the nutrition message already initiated from the information provided on the treatment record. Documentation should include the dental issues, assessment, plan, and outcomes.

Facilitative Communication Skills

Intertwined with implementing an effective nutrition care plan is the interpersonal communication skills of the dental professional. An atmosphere of sincerity, trust, and empathy should be established to help the patient relax and feel more comfortable in revealing accurate information and to be more cooperative in working toward a goal. Good rapport is the foundation; without it, very little is accomplished. Using nonjudgmental and noncritical responses encourages a patient to provide accurate accounts of food intake without the threat of being reprimanded. If a patient's food record reveals donuts and soda for breakfast, it would be judgmental to say, "I can't believe you eat that for breakfast!" Instead, a noncommittal verbal and nonverbal acknowledgment of the food, such as, "Is this usual?" would elicit a more accurate reply. Phrases discounting a patient's feelings do not promote the warm and caring atmosphere essential for good rapport. Phrases such as, "You're making a mountain out of a molehill," "Don't be ridiculous," or "It is good, but…," are guaranteed to inhibit the patient's participation.

Listening

Listening to the patient is an important and distinguishing feature of effective communication that the dental professional must practice. Listening involves more than hearing. It includes interpreting what is said, how it is said, and nonverbal actions observed. Attentive listening is difficult, requiring the full attention of the dental hygienist. Attentive listening can actually save time, however, because it gains a better understanding of a situation and results in better communication (see Fig. 21.6).

Impediments to attentive listening include interrupting, preparing a response while the other person is speaking, distracting mannerisms, daydreaming, multitasking with devices such as phones or computers, and finishing the speaker's sentences. Awareness of personal barriers to listening allows the dental professional to focus on establishing appropriate alternatives for more effective communication.

To improve listening skills, the dental professional can practice being attentive by shutting out external distractions or not interrupting (e.g., decreasing the number of questions asked, not taking the subject in another direction). Patients feel more comfortable and important when they are being heard.

Nonverbal Communication

Facial expressions (Fig. 21.10), eye contact, body movements, personal distance, head nodding, and vocal cues (e.g., tone of voice, rate of speaking) are nonverbal behaviors that enhance or substitute for verbal messages. Positive nonverbal communications increase the effectiveness of the message and create a comfortable atmosphere for the patient. Eye contact is a significant interaction between the dental professional and patient. Good eye contact communicates interest, understanding, and warmth, whereas a lack of eye contact or staring can be interpreted as indifference or preoccupation. Eye contact and other nonverbal signals can communicate what cannot be verbalized.

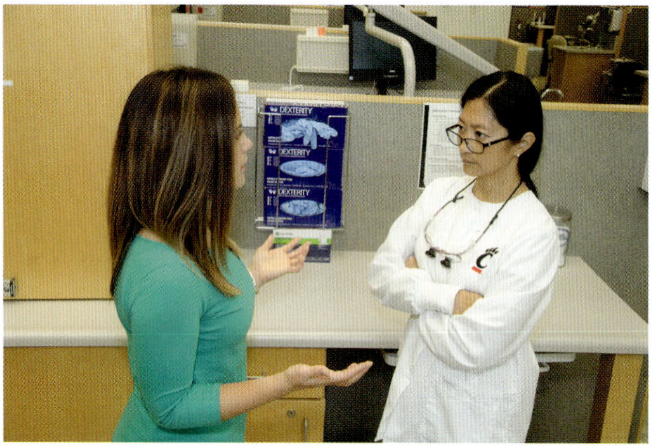

• Figure 21.10 Nonverbal facial expressions can show emotion. (Photo courtesy of Peter Bender, Cincinnati, OH.)

Verbal Communication

Asking open-ended questions encourages the patient to expand on the answers, which can include much more information about food choices than anticipated. "What is your evening routine?" would evoke a more detailed response than a question with a yes or no reply, such as, "Do you snack in the evening?"

Dental hygienists can also demonstrate effective communication by reflecting back on what a patient has previously mentioned. This demonstrates that the professional heard what the patient stated and offers a sense of understanding to the patient. An example might be, "If I heard you correctly, you said that snacking in the evenings is your biggest downfall."

DENTAL CONSIDERATIONS

Assessment

- *Physical:* Attitude and interest of patient toward behavior change; nonverbal signs from patient.
- *Dietary:* Completed and analyzed dietary intake.

Interventions

- Avoid scheduling nutrition education sessions after a long or difficult dental appointment.
- The operatory causes anxiety for many patients; when possible, choose a quiet and private location for nutrition education so that the patient feels more relaxed and less apprehensive.
- When possible, designate a room for nutrition education that is equipped with a computer with Internet access and educational material—such as pertinent literature, posters, flannel boards, food packages, food models, and measuring utensils—to enhance the learning experience.
- Standing with arms folded is often viewed as negative nonverbal behavior for indifference, unfriendliness, and aloofness.
- Explain to the patient that you will be taking notes of the discussion so you will not forget important information.
- Resist the temptation to create an ideal diet prescription and solve all nutrition problems. Help patients to adapt and develop a less-than-perfect menu plan that is more likely to be followed routinely.
- When appropriate, request that a family member or friend participate with the patient in the education session, especially an individual who is responsible for the cooking and food shopping. Assistance is also warranted when a physical or mental impairment interferes with the patient's understanding.
- Treat all patients without judgement and with respect and dignity.

Evaluation

- The patient is an active participant, making a change toward food choices and behaviors agreed to in the nutrition education session. At the follow-up visit or next recare appointment, there is successful achievement of the first set of goals and advancement to implement other, more difficult suggestions. Many questions are asked and comments are made that verify interest and understanding.

NUTRITIONAL DIRECTIONS

- Establishing good eating habits is a wise investment toward lifelong positive health and dental status. Prevention, alleviation, or postponing the onset of a disease is possible with good nutrition.

HEALTH APPLICATION 21

Health Literacy

Snrettap reihtlaeh hsilbatse lliw tneitap eht that eetnaraug ton seod tneitap a ot noitamrofni fo noitanimessid. Stnemele ynam fo noitcaretni eht gnissapmocne, tpecnoc lanoisnemiditlum a si htlaeh.

While reading this passage, how did you feel? Are you confused, frustrated, uncertain, too embarrassed to ask what it means, feeling a sense of shame, or did you stop trying to understand the two sentences? These are examples of feelings that people with low-proficiency health literacy skills may experience during our discussions with them. *Fermentable carbohydrates*, *gingiva*, *suppuration*, *xerostomia*, *periodontal disease*, and *calculus* may be unfamiliar, complex, and technical terms that we frequently use with our patients. The above passage simulates what a patient may view on a printed page or the gibberish they may hear in conversation. (*Note:* It is the first two sentences of this chapter written backwards.) Miscommunication is recognized for failure to follow health instructions.

Healthy People 2020 defines health literacy as the "degree to which individuals have the capacity to obtain, process and understand basic health information and services needed to make appropriate health decisions." An objective of *Healthy People 2020* is to improve health literacy of the population by (a) increasing the number of people receiving easy-to-understand instructions about what to do to take care of their health, (b) being asked to repeat health care instructions, and (c) being offered help in filling out the health history or other dental forms.[8] It is the responsibility of all dental health professionals to recognize misunderstanding of patients and to work toward presenting information to match their needs and abilities.

Thirteen percent of English-speaking adults in the United States have proficient health literacy skills, while 44% have basic or below-basic literacy skills (Box 21.5).[9] Low health literacy has been linked to poor health outcomes, such as less frequent use of preventive services. However, the dental hygienist should appreciate that any patient can have difficulty understanding the health information provided. A well-educated individual in a discipline not related to health care, for example, may not fully understand complex dental information. Situations in which comprehension of health information may be a challenge include those individuals with limited English proficiency, obvious cultural differences, a lack of knowledge and experience, and communication or developmental disorders. Populations at risk of low health literacy include older adults, racial and ethnic groups, people with less than a high school education, people with low income levels, and nonnative English speakers. The dental hygienist should tailor the dental health information to meet the learning needs of the patient (Box 21.6).

Look at the description below provided by the dental hygienist. The information is at a college level. Box 21.7 provides a list of terms that can be used in place of complex terms. What are examples of simple words that you have used in place of complex words?

Hyperglycemia can cause many complications including nephropathy, retinopathy, neuropathy, and periodontal disease.

Below is an example of how you can you get this message across to a patient with basic or below basic levels of health literacy.

High blood sugar can be dangerous to your health. It can cause problems with your kidneys, your eyes, your ability to walk, and your gums.

• BOX 21.5 Levels of Health Literacy

Below Basic

- Able to sign name
- Do simple addition
- Find a country in an article
- Read or complete a brief and uncomplicated document

Basic

- Able to do one-step arithmetic problems
- Locate information in a newspaper article
- Make low-level inferences from a text
- Integrate easily identifiable pieces of information

Intermediate

- Can apply information from a moderately dense text and make simple inferences
- Determine appropriate arithmetic operations
- Identify quantities needed to perform the arithmetic operation

Proficient

- Demonstrate proficiencies associated with long and complex documents and text

From National Assessment of Adult Literacy. Health literacy of America's adults: results of the National Assessment of Adult Literacy (NAAL) 2003. http://nces.ed.gov/naal/multimedia.asp. Accessed June 12, 2017.

• BOX 21.6 Strategies the Dental Professional Can Utilize to Minimize or Avoid Misunderstanding

- Simple, short, common, and plain terms
- Communicate in short sentences.
- Employ jargon-free language.
- Break complex information into understandable chunks.
- Supplement the discussion with relevant and simple pictures and other visual cues.
- Use concrete examples rather than abstract principles.
- Avoid numbers and statistics.
- Present essential information first.
- Communicate using clear messages.
- Limit the number of messages at one time.
- Repeat key messages.
- Have the patient repeat instructions.
- Modify the explanation until it is clear to the patient.
- Ask open-ended questions.
- Provide the information in multiple ways.
- Provide forms in multiple languages.
- Provide written instructions.
- Offer assistance to the patient in completing the paperwork.
- Arrange for a medically trained interpreter.

• BOX 21.7 Substituting Simple Words for Complex Words

Complex	Simple	Complex	Simple
Administer	Give	Periodontal disease	Gum disease
Anesthetic	Numbing medicine	Plaque	Germs
Bacteria	Germs	Physician	Doctor
Calculus	Tartar, germs that are hard	Procedure	Test
Diagnosis	Problem, condition	Prone	Lying down
Discontinue	Stop	Purulent, suppuration	Pus
Facial, buccal	Cheek side	Remain	Stay
Fermentable carbohydrates	Foods that can cause cavities	Requirement	Need
Gingiva	Gums	Substantial	Large, much
Identify	Find, name, show	Supine	Lay back
Lesion	Cut, injury	Suture	Stitch
Lingual	Tongue side	Validate	Confirm
Minimum	Least, smallest	Xerostomia	Dry mouth

Adapted from Improving Communication from the Federal Government to the Public. http://www.plainlanguage.gov/howto/wordsuggestions/simplewords.cfm. *Accessed June 12, 2017.*

◆ CASE APPLICATION FOR THE DENTAL HYGIENIST

As 70-year-old Mr. B walks into the operatory, it is noted that he continues to lose weight and has less energy than at his previous 4-month recare visit. His health history reveals no significant findings except one daily medication to control hypertension. The social history reveals that his wife has been deceased for 2 years and his limited income makes it difficult to purchase the foods he needs. He complains of a loose-fitting maxillary denture and xerostomia.

Nutritional Assessment

- Medical, dental, and social history
- Nutrition assessment questionnaire (see Evolve)
- Extraoral and intraoral examination
- Periodontal evaluation
- Anthropometric evaluation for weight changes
- Three-day food record

Nutritional Diagnosis

Social and oral factors are affecting the desire and ability to obtain adequate nutrition.

Nutritional Goals

The patient will seek support from suggested referrals and begin to improve his caloric intake and variety of food.

Nutritional Implementation

Intervention: Ask open-ended questions pertaining to his late wife.

Rationale: Weight change can stem from lack of transportation and education. Mr. B's late wife may have done all the shopping (primary driver) and cooking previously. Educating Mr. B on finding transportation or educating him on what foods should be included in a meal may be appropriate.

Intervention: Examine the oral cavity for any deviation from normal and the fit of the maxillary denture.

Rationale: Ill-fitting dentures can be a result of weight loss, which can be responsible for creating sore spots. The presence of oral infections can decrease the ability and desire to eat, ultimately affecting nutritional status. Identifying such areas can allow for treatment and education on prevention.

Intervention: Provide instruction for completing a 3-day food record.

Rationale: This component completes the assessment process. Determining typical eating habits and patterns and the variety of foods gives direction to the nutrition education. Look for the predominant use of soft foods, highly salted foods, convenience foods, and fermentable carbohydrates; variety; low calories; and number of meals daily.

Intervention: Educate Mr. B regarding basic information about nutrient needs and the relationship between diet and health status.

Rationale: Depression over a spouse's death and dining alone are two factors decreasing an older individual's desire to eat. Referral to a community-based senior citizen program may provide support and companionship needed to improve his desire to eat.

Intervention: Explain to Mr. B that frequent consumption of acid-containing beverages (e.g., sodas, citrus juices) can put him at high risk for caries. Due to his xerostomia, the lack of protection by saliva may even allow sugar alcohols to create a cariogenic environment, especially if his remaining teeth have gingival recession.

Rationale: Patients with xerostomia have limited cleansing and buffering capabilities because of reduced quantities of saliva. Even foods generally noncariogenic when saliva flow is adequate can be detrimental when saliva flow is diminished. Suggest rinsing with water to dilute the effects of citrus juices or to remove carbohydrates (e.g., rinsing away remnants of crackers or pretzels).

Intervention: Provide positive feedback on any changes, even small ones, that Mr. B makes.

Rationale: An older adult may be more resistant to modifications in well-established habits. Small goals are more realistic. Allow him to make the goals based on the information presented to him. Recognize any change is a sign of effort. A follow-up on his progress is important to establish new goals or modify goals as necessary.

Evaluation

At a return visit, Mr. B's new 24-hour recall reveals adequate caloric intake and improvement in variety of food choices. He has slowly begun to gain back some of his weight. He has sought the support of various local senior citizen groups. His denture has been repaired, and he presents a healthy oral cavity.

Student Readiness

1. Examine your own health, social, and dental histories, and identify health-related factors that a dental professional would find useful in developing a dietary plan.
2. Interview a partner to obtain health, social, and dental histories. What questions were effective in clarifying or obtaining additional pertinent information?
3. Establish a nutrition goal you can realistically apply this week, and have a partner evaluate. Review progress with the partner at the conclusion of the week. Would you do anything differently to increase the likelihood of accomplishing the goal?
4. Select and explain at least two reasons why a dental professional should conduct a nutrition assessment for patients.
5. Describe the components needed for an assessment of a patient's nutritional status, and explain the rationale of each.
6. The following 24-hour recall was obtained by a dental hygienist. What questions need to be asked to get a more accurate estimate of the patient's intake?
   Breakfast: Bagel and cream cheese, coffee
   Lunch: Hamburger, french fries, soda
   Snack: Candy bar
   Dinner: Roast beef, potatoes, salad, corn
7. Explain why the following question asked during a nutrition education session is undesirable: "Do you realize omitting fruits and vegetables from your day could lead to a deficiency in vitamins A and C?" Reword the question to enhance effectiveness.

CASE STUDY

The dental hygienist has reviewed Jim S's medical, dental, and social histories at the prophylaxis appointment, indicating no significant changes. Jim presents with observable weight gain since the last 6-month recare appointment and three new areas of dental caries. He has no idea why the areas of decay occurred. A 3-day food diary is explained, and a nutrition education session is established following his restorative treatment. At the restorative appointment, the patient forgot to bring his completed food diary. The dental hygienist attributed this to a lack of interest. A 24-hour recall is obtained, and the session is conducted in the operatory.

1. Prioritize the diet and dental information that Jim S needs.
2. Explain why and how a nutrition education session could be beneficial to Jim.
3. What questions should be asked before and during the session to gain additional information?
4. State several reasons why the education session may not be effective to motivate behavior change. How could these situations be modified to enhance motivation?

References

1. American Dental Hygienists' Association (ADHA). Standards for Clinical Dental Hygiene Practice. Chicago, ADHA. 2016. https://www.adha.org/resources-docs/2016-Revised-Standards-for-Clinical-Dental-Hygiene-Practice.pdf. Accessed June 10, 2017.
2. Touger-Decker R, Mobley C. Position of the Academy of Nutrition and Dietetics: Oral health and nutrition. *J Acad Nutr Diet*. 2013;113(5):693–701.
3. Mallonee LF, Boyd LD, Stegeman CA. Practice Paper of the Academy of Nutrition and Dietetics: Oral health and nutrition. *J Acad Nutr Diet*. 2014;114(6):958.
4. Chapman-Novakofski K. Education and counseling: behavioral change. In: Mahan LK, Raymond JL, eds. *Krause's Food and the Nutrition Care Process*. 14th ed. St. Louis, MO: Saunders Elsevier; 2017.
5. Miller WR. Motivational interviewing with problem drinkers. *Behav Psychother*. 1983;11:147–172.
6. Rollnick S, Heather N, Bell A. Negotiating behaviour change in medical settings: the development of brief motivational interviewing. *J Ment Health*. 1992;1(1):25–37.
7. Arnett M, Gwozdek A. Motivational interviewing for dental hygienists. *Dimens Dent Hyg*. 2017;54–57.
8. U.S. Department of Health and Human Services: *Healthy People 2020*. Health communication and health information technology. http://www.healthypeople.gov/2020/topicsobjectives2020/objectiveslist.aspx?topicId=18. Accessed June 12, 2017.
9. National Assessment of Adult Literacy. Demographics. http://nces.ed.gov/naal/kf_demographics.asp#3. Accessed June 12, 2017.

EVOLVE RESOURCES

Please visit http://evolve.elsevier.com/Stegeman/nutritional for additional practice and study support tools.

Glossary

abrasion permanent depletion of tooth surfaces as a result of pathologic tooth wear, such as toothbrush abrasion.

Acceptable Macronutrient Distribution Ranges (AMDRs) a part of the latest dietary reference intakes (DRIs); established for the macronutrients (fat, carbohydrate, protein, and two polyunsaturated fats) to ensure sufficient intakes of essential nutrients while reducing risk of chronic diseases.

accessory organs organs, such as salivary glands, liver, gallbladder, and pancreas, that provide secretions essential for the digestive process.

achlorhydria absence of hydrochloric acid in the stomach, a condition that occurs primarily in older patients.

acidogenic foods and beverages that cause a reduction of salivary pH to less than 5.5.

active site the region of an enzyme that selectively binds a substrate and contains the amino acids that directly participate in the chemical transformation converting a substrate into a product.

active transport absorption within the gastrointestinal tract from a region of lower concentration to one of a higher concentration; requires a carrier and cellular energy.

ad libitum as desired, at will.

added sugars sugars added to foods during processing or at the table.

adenosine triphosphate (ATP) main form of energy used by the cells.

adequate intake (AI) average amount of a nutrient that seems to maintain a defined nutritional state; derived from mean nutrient intakes by groups of healthy people.

adipose tissue body fat.

aerobic lives and grows in the presence of oxygen.

age-related macular degeneration (AMD) deterioration in the central area of the retina (back of the eye) in which lesions lead to loss of central vision.

aldosterone hormone secreted by the adrenal cortex that signals the kidney to retain sodium and water, and excrete potassium and hydrogen ions; ultimately causes edema and high blood pressure.

alimentary canal all the body parts through which food passes, extending from the mouth to the anus.

alopecia hair loss.

α-linolenic acid organic compound found in many vegetable oils.

alternative medicine use of medical and health care systems that are not considered part of conventional Western medicine.

alveolar bone the bone of the maxillae and mandible that contains the sockets for the teeth.

alveolar process crest of the maxilla and mandible.

ameloblasts tall columnar epithelial cells in the inner layer of the enamel; enamel-forming cells.

amenorrhea absence of menses.

amino acids basic building blocks or monomer units for proteins.

amorphous having no definite form.

amphiphilic compound with molecules with a water-soluble group attached to a water-insoluble grouping.

amylase an enzyme that begins the process of digesting dietary carbohydrates.

anabolism use of absorbed nutrients to build or synthesize more complex compounds.

anencephaly absence of a major portion of the brain and skull.

aneurysm bulge or ballooning in the wall of an artery. When an aneurysm becomes too large, it may burst and cause dangerous bleeding or death.

anhydrous contains no water, a hydrophobic or "water-fearing" substance

anion ion carrying a negative charge as a result of an accumulation of electrons.

anorexia lack or loss of appetite.

anosmia loss of smell.

anthropometric measurements of physical characteristics, such as height, weight, and change in weight.

anticariogenic foods and beverages that may reduce the risk of caries by preventing plaque from recognizing a cariogenic food.

anticholinergic medication used to block parasympathetic nerve impulses.

anticoagulant drug or substance that delays or prevents the clotting of blood (e.g., heparin).

antidiuretic hormone (ADH) hormone released by the pituitary gland to act on the kidneys that control urine output.

antigenic having the properties of an antigen (substance that comes in contact with target cells, inducing an immune response or sensitivity).

antioxidant synthetic or natural substance that prevents or delays the damaging effects of a reactive substance seeking an electron.

apatite calcium phosphate complex that forms crystalline salts within the matrix of bone and teeth.

appetite external factors that influence people to seek and eat food even when not hungry.

ariboflavinosis symptoms associated with riboflavin deficiency (angular cheilitis, glossitis, dermatitis, and anemia).

ataxia gait disorder characterized by uncoordinated muscle movements.

atherosclerosis degenerative disease caused by progressive accumulation of fatty materials on smooth inner walls of the arteries of the heart, narrowing the arteries and disrupting blood flow.

atrophic gastritis chronic stomach inflammation with atrophy of the mucous membrane and glands, resulting in diminished hydrochloric acid production.

atrophic gingivitis condition characterized by redness, pain, and wasting of the gingival tissue owing to local and systemic causes.

atrophic glossitis atrophy of the filiform and fungiform papillae beginning at the tip and lateral borders of the tongue and gradually spreading to the entire dorsum of the tongue.

avoidant/restrictive food intake disorder (ARFID) children who have difficulty eating; body image is not a characteristic of this eating disorder classification.

autoimmune disorder condition in which the body produces antibodies against one's own tissues (e.g., celiac disease).

avidin biotin-binding glycoprotein substance present in raw egg white.

baby bottle tooth decay (BBTD) see early childhood caries.

bariatric surgery surgical procedure that promotes weight loss by restricting food intake or interrupting the digestive process to prevent absorption of some kilocalories and nutrients.

basal energy expenditure person's total caloric requirement.

basal metabolic rate energy required for involuntary physiological functions to maintain life, including respiration, circulation, and maintenance of muscle tone and body temperature.

benign migratory glossitis "geographic tongue"; multiple reddish flat areas with a loss of filiform papillae on the dorsum of the tongue, which may also be grooved or fissured.

beriberi dietary deficiency of thiamin characterized by neuropathy, diarrhea, weight loss, fatigue, and poor memory.

bile emulsifier that helps in digestion of fats.

binges periods of overeating.

bioactive a substance that has an effect on a living organism; in nutrition, bioactive substances are nonessential, since the body can function properly without them.

bioavailability amount of nutrient available to the body based on its absorption.

bioinformation the language of communication of biological information in an organism, including the transfer of biological information from deoxyribonucleic acid (DNA) to ribonucleic acid (RNA) to protein.

biological value measure of protein quality, with a higher score for proteins of higher quality.

biomolecule any molecule that is produced by a living cell or organism and other organic compounds found in living organisms.

bisphosphonates medications primarily prescribed for osteoporosis, multiple myeloma, and used intravenously during cancer chemotherapy; they decrease bone turnover and inhibit the bone's reparative ability.

body mass index (BMI) mathematical calculation using a person's height and weight to determine weight status and to predict health risks that increase at higher levels of overweight and obesity (see p. v).

bolus mass of food that is swallowed and passed into the stomach.

botanical plant or plant part valued for its medicinal or therapeutic properties, flavor, and/or scent.
bradycardia low or slow heart rate.
bradykinesia slowness of movement.
brown tumors giant cell tumor replacement of bone evidenced radiologically.
bruxism clenching and grinding of teeth that erodes and diminishes the height of dental crowns.
calcitonin polypeptide hormone regulating the balance of calcium and phosphate in the blood by direct action on bone and kidney; secreted by the parathyroid, thyroid, and thymus tissue.
calorie amount of heat needed to increase the temperature of 1 kg of water 1° C; measurement of the potential energy value of foods and energy within the body, equivalent to 1000 calories; more accurately called kilocalorie.
calorie-dense foods term used for food usually high in fats (or fat and sugar) and low in vitamins and minerals and other nutrients. A characteristic of calorie-dense foods is that less volume of food is needed to furnish energy requirements.
calorimeter device used to measure kilocalories.
cancellous bone internal bone that appears spongy.
Candida invasive fungal microorganism.
carbohydrate a biomolecule containing carbon, hydrogen, and oxygen with twice as much hydrogen as oxygen; 1 g yields 4 cal; produced by plants through photosynthesis.
cardiovascular disease (CVD) condition involving the heart and blood vessels and producing various pathologic effects; also referred to as coronary heart disease (CHD) or coronary artery disease (CAD).
Caries Management by Risk Assessment (CaMBRA) used by dental professionals to identify risk of caries and to determine preventive and therapeutic goals for both children and adult patients.
cariogenic fermentable carbohydrate that causes a reduction of salivary pH to less than 5.5, resulting in demineralization of enamel and dental caries.
cariostatic (also see noncariogenic) carbohydrates that are caries inhibiting; not metabolized by microorganisms in plaque biofilm; do not cause a reduction of salivary pH to less than 5.5.
casein principal protein in cow's milk and chief constituent of cheese.
catabolism breakdown of complex into simpler substances.
catecholamine an organic compound that consists of a single amine and a catechol; obtained from dietary tyrosine and/or phenylalanine.
cation ion carrying a positive charge as a result of a deficiency of electrons.
celiac disease malabsorption syndrome in which individuals are hypersensitive to gluten, a protein inherent to wheat, rye, barley, and triticale.
cheilosis unilateral or bilateral presence of cracks and dry scaling around the vermilion border of lips and corners of the mouth; the skin is scaly with red fissures.
chelation therapy use of specific chemicals to bind and eliminate heavy metals from the body.
chemical bonds hold together atoms in a compound.
chemotherapy treatment of disease by chemical agents.
cholesterol waxy lipid found in all body cells; found only in animal products.
cholinergic parasympathetic (autonomic) nerves stimulated by acetylcholine.
chyme bolus entering the stomach, a semifluid material produced by gastric juices on ingested food.
circumvallate lingual papillae 8 to 10 large and distinctive structures forming a V shape on the posterior end of the anterior two-thirds of the dorsum of the tongue.
***cis* isomer** the geometric arrangement of hydrogen atoms on the same side of the plane of a C=C double bond.
cleft lip/palate split where parts of the upper lip or palate fail to grow together.
clinical attachment loss (CAL) loss of periodontal attachment.
coenzyme molecule needed to activate an enzyme.
cofactor element similar to an enzyme necessary to activate reactions, but the molecule required is a mineral or electrolyte.
Coliforms a bacterial indicator of sanitation, universally present in the feces of animals.
collagen basic protein substance of connective tissue helping support body structures such as skin, bones, teeth, and tendons.
colonics a method to cleanse the lower intestines is based on the assumption that years of bad diet causes the colon to become caked with layers of accumulated toxins.
complementary feeding period first introduction of solid foods to an infant occurring between 4 months of age when neither breast milk nor formula adequately meets all the nutrient requirements to promote growth and development.
complementary medicine use of untraditional medical and health care systems and products along with conventional medical treatments.
complex carbohydrates see *polysaccharides*.
compound lipids triglycerides with at least one of the fatty acids replaced with carbohydrate, phosphate, or nitrogenous compounds.
compressional forces actions in which the pressure attempts to diminish a structure's volume, which usually increases density.
condensation reaction biochemical reaction in which two molecules combine, eliminating water or some other simple molecule.
conditionally essential amino acids amino acids that are essential in the diet during certain stages of development or in certain nutritional or disease states.
conditionally indispensable amino acids amino acids normally not required by the body, but in certain physiological conditions become indispensable.
conjugated linoleic acid (CLA) family of at least 13 isomers (or forms) of linoleic acid, found especially in meats and dairy products.
constipation having a bowel movement fewer than three times per week with hard, dry, small, and difficult-to-pass stools.
covalent bond bond formed when electrons are equally shared between two nonmetals.
crepitus crackling or grating sound made by a joint, such as the temporomandibular joint.
cretinism stunting of growth often characterized by mental deficits and deaf mutism; a result of inadequate iodine intake during pregnancy.
Daily Value (DV) term used on food labels indicating the percentage of the DV provided by a serving to show the amount of nutrients provided as a percentage of established standards; based on a 2000-cal diet.
demineralization removal or loss of calcium, phosphate, and other minerals from tooth enamel, causing tooth enamel to dissolve.
dental erosion chemical removal of minerals from the tooth structure that occurs when an acidic environment causes the enamel to dissolve gradually; occurs with frequent exposure to foods with a pH below 4.2.
dental stomatitis traumatization and chronic inflammation of mucus membranes supporting a removable denture.
dentin hypersensitivity extremely painful feeling of exposed dentin resulting from a stimulus, such as temperature or tactile.
detoxification ("detox") the biochemical process that transforms non-water-soluble toxins and metabolites into water-soluble compounds that can be excreted in urine, sweat, bile, or stool.
dextrins intermediate products of the digestive enzymes on starch molecules; they are long glucose chains split into shorter ones.
dialysate material that passes through the membrane during dialysis.
diaphoresis excessive sweating.
diet history detailed dietary record; may include 24-hour recall; food frequency questionnaire; and other information such as weight history, previous diet changes, use of supplements, and food intolerances.
dietary acculturation dietary changes that occur as a result of adapting to food resources of a new location.
dietary fiber several different types of nondigestible carbohydrates and lignin intrinsic and intact in plants.
Dietary Reference Intakes (DRIs) set of nutrient-based reference values that identify amounts of required nutrients for various stages of life.
dipeptide two amino acids together.
diplopia perception of two images of a single object; also known as double vision.
disaccharides double sugars (two simple sugars joined together) containing 12 carbon atoms.
disease a condition of a living animal or plant body or of one of its parts that impairs normal functioning and is typically manifested by distinguishing signs and symptoms.
dispensable amino acids amino acids essential for the body, but they can be produced from indispensable amino acids so are not required in normal conditions.
docosahexaenoic acid (DHA) omega-3 fatty acid with 22 carbons and 6 double bonds synthesized by the body from linolenic acid; present in fish oils.
dysesthesia condition in which a burning sensation is produced by ordinary stimuli.
dysgeusia persistent, abnormal distortion of taste, including sweet, sour, bitter, salty, or metallic.
dysphagia difficulty in swallowing.
early childhood caries (ECC) early rampant tooth decay associated with inappropriate feeding practices.
edentulous without teeth or lacking some or all teeth.
eicosapentaenoic acid (EPA) omega-3 fatty acid with 20 carbon atoms and 5 double bonds synthesized by the body from linolenic acid; present in fish oils.
emulsification the breakdown of fats into smaller particles by lowering the surface tension.
enamel hypoplasia developmental disturbance of the teeth characterized by defective formation of the enamel matrix.
energy ability or power to do work.
enrichment process of restoring nutrients removed from food during processing.
enteral feedings feeding that delivers liquid food through a tube; may be used for infants and children with a functioning gastrointestinal tract unable to ingest nutrients orally to meet their metabolic needs.
enteric general term for the intestines.
enzymes complex proteins enabling metabolic reactions to proceed at a faster rate without being exhausted themselves.
epigenetics the scientific study of how nutrition and environmental factors regulate gene activity without changing the underlying DNA sequence.
epilepsy transient disturbance of brain function that results in episodic impairment or loss of consciousness.

epinephrine the "fight or flight" hormone secreted in time of immediate energy need; activates glycogen degradation for energy.
epiphyses growing points at ends of long bones.
epithelialization natural healing process in which the area is covered with or converted to epithelium.
ergogenic enhanced physical performance, stamina, or recovery.
erosion permanent depletion of tooth surfaces due to the action of an external or internal chemical substance.
erythema marginated redness of mucous membranes caused by inflammation.
erythropoiesis formation of red blood cells.
esophagitis inflammation of the lower esophagus.
essential amino acids (EAAs) amino acids that must be supplied by the diet. Also known as indispensable amino acids.
essential fatty acids (EFAs) fatty acids (linoleic acid and linolenic acid) that must be supplied by the diet.
essential hypertension elevated blood pressure of unknown cause.
Estimated Average Requirement (EAR) amount of a nutrient estimated to meet the needs of half of the healthy individuals in a specific age and gender group.
Estimated Energy Requirement (EER) dietary energy intake predicted to maintain energy balance in healthy normal-weight individuals of a defined age, gender, weight, height, and physical activity level consistent with good health.
Evidence Analysis Library (EAL) a process in which an expert work group identifies practice-related questions, performs a systematic literature review, and develops and rates a conclusive statement for each question; such a library was developed by the Academy of Nutrition and Dietetics (AND).
evidence-based medical practices that have been thoroughly evaluated using scientific methods.
explore the first step of motivational interviewing, the patient's behavior is to be looked into.
extracellular fluid (ECF) fluid outside the cells.
fatty acids structural component of fats.
fermentable carbohydrate carbohydrates that can be metabolized by bacteria in plaque biofilm to decrease the pH to a level causing demineralization; this includes all sugars and cooked or processed starches.
fibroblasts collagen-forming cells.
fibrotic formation of fibrous tissue of the gingiva and other mucous membranes because of chronic inflammation; tissue may clinically appear to be healthy, concealing the disease.
filiform papillae smooth, threadlike structures that are covered by a nonkeratinized epithelium, on the anterior two-thirds of the dorsum of the tongue.
flavin adenine nucleotide (FAD/FADH$_2$) a redox coenzyme derived from riboflavin.
flexitarian person who primarily follows a plant-based diet, but occasionally eats small amounts of meat, poultry or fish; also known as a *semivegetarian*.
fluid volume deficit (FVD) relatively equal losses of sodium and water in relation to their gains.
fluid volume excess (FVE) relatively equal gains of water and sodium in relation to their losses.
fluorapatite fluoride-containing crystalline substance produced during bone and tooth development; resistant to acid.
fluorosis hypomineralization of enamel, caused by excessive fluoride intake during the formation of enamel.
foliate papillae vertical ridges or grooves scattered along the lateral borders of the tongue.
follicular hyperkeratosis condition characterized by the appearance of cone-shaped, horny, hyperkeratinized, scaly eruptions resulting from blocked pores as a result of vitamin A deficiency.
food deserts located in lower-income, inner-city, and rural areas, with few supermarkets but numerous small stores that stock limited nutritious food items, particularly produce, at affordable prices.
food fad catch-all term covering all aspects of nutritional nonsense, characterized by exaggerated beliefs about the value of nutrition in health and disease.
food frequency questionnaire checklist of many foods used to determine how often specific foods are consumed.
food insecurity lack of access to enough food to fully meet basic needs at all times.
food jags refusing to eat anything except one food for several days.
food pattern customary way of eating, reflecting a person's ethnic or cultural, social, religious, geographical, economic, and psychological components and family lifestyle.
food quackery promotion of nutrition-related products or services having questionable safety or effectiveness, or both, for the claims made.
fortification process of adding nutrients not present in the natural product or to increase the amount above that in the original product.
full liquid diet nutrients provided in a liquid form when solid food is not tolerated; a transition between a clear liquid and soft diet.
functional fiber isolated, nondigestible carbohydrates with beneficial physiological effects in humans.
functional foods foods that contain potentially healthful products, including any modified food or food ingredients providing a health benefit beyond its traditional nutrients.
functional group a group of atoms that gives a family of molecules its characteristic chemical and physical properties.
fungating producing fungus-like growth.
fungiform papillae red, knoblike structures on the tongue scattered throughout the filiform papillae.
gastroesophageal reflux disease (GERD) return of gastric contents into the esophagus, causing a severe burning sensation under the sternum.
gastrostomy establishment of a new opening into the stomach to insert a tube for nutrition, foods, or medications directly into the stomach, bypassing the mouth and esophagus.
gene region of DNA sequence that contains the instructions to produce a specific protein required for life.
genome all of the DNA contained in an organism or cell, which includes chromosomes in the nucleus and DNA in the mitochondria.
genomics scientific discipline of mapping, sequencing, and analyzing the genome.
ghrelin peptide hormone secreted in the gastrointestinal tract by exocrine cells.
gingivitis inflammation of the gingival tissue.
ginseng fleshy root of a plant; stimulant used in energy drinks that may improve concentration and thinking, physical stamina, and athletic endurance, but may cause abdominal pain and headaches.
glossitis chronic inflammation of the tongue, characterized by the loss of filiform papillae on the dorsum of the tongue.
glossodynia pain in the tongue.
glossopyrosis pain, burning, itching, and stinging of the tongue with no apparent lesions.
glucagon a signal of the "starved" state; secreted when blood glucose levels are low.
glucogenic amino acids can be converted into glucose as a fuel for the body.
gluconeogenesis synthesis of glucose from noncarbohydrate sources.
gluten protein found mainly in wheat and to a lesser degree in rye, oat, and barley.
gluten sensitivity a condition in which individuals are unable to tolerate gluten; not an allergic or autoimmune response.
glycemic index a measure of the effect of different carbohydrate foods on blood glucose levels.
glycogen carbohydrate storage form of energy in humans.
glycogenesis process by which sugars, including fructose, galactose, sorbitol, and xylitol, are stored as glycogen.
glycolysis anaerobic conversion of glucose to produce energy in the form of adenosine triphosphate (ATP).
glycosidic bond a bond that combines two monosaccharides into a disaccharide.
goal achievable aim or target that would be meaningful in changing behaviors by setting a concrete standard for change.
goiter chronic enlargement of the thyroid gland occurring most frequently in areas with low iodine in the soil.
goitrogens naturally occurring substances in foods that interfere with the synthesis of thyroid hormone production; may cause goiter if consumed in large amounts.
gravida pregnant woman; gravida followed by a Roman numeral or preceded by a Latin prefix (e.g., "primi-," "secundi-") designates the number of pregnancies for the woman (e.g., gravida I or primigravida is a woman in her first pregnancy).
guarana a seed containing four times as much caffeine as coffee beans.
guide the second step of motivational interviewing in which the patient's motivation and commitment is identified.
gustatory sense of taste.
health claim claim that describes a health relationship between a food, food component, or dietary supplement ingredient and reduced risk of a disease or a health-related condition.
Healthy U.S.-Style Eating Pattern (U.S.-Pattern) an eating pattern introduced in the *2015-2020 Dietary Guidelines for Americans* indicating the number of food equivalents from each food group and subgroups for 12 caloric levels to be consumed each week for an adequate healthful diet.
hematopoiesis formation of red blood cells.
heme iron iron provided from animal sources.
hemochromatosis an uncommon disorder in which iron is absorbed at a high rate despite elevated iron stores in the liver.
hemosiderin storage form of iron in the liver when the amount of iron in the body exceeds storage capacity.
herbs leafy green parts of a plant.
herpetic related to the herpes virus; ulceration on the tongue or esophagus or both.
hiatal hernia partial protrusion (herniation) of the stomach through the diaphragm.
high-energy phosphate compounds instant source of energy for cells; also called *ATP*.
high-quality proteins foods that contain adequate amounts of the nine essential amino acids to maintain nitrogen balance and permit growth.
hirsutism excessive hair growth.
homeopathy treatment of diseases and conditions with minute doses of drugs that cause symptoms of a disease in healthy people to cure similar symptoms in sick people.
homeostatic mechanisms body's ability to correct nutritional imbalances, for instance, decreased nutrient intake accompanied by an increase in absorption or efficiency or use.

hormone compound produced and secreted by cells of the body, transported in the blood to another site where it has a specific regulatory function.
hormone replacement therapy (HRT) therapy using medication that contains one or more female hormones, usually estrogen and progestin.
hunger physiological drive to eat or an uneasy or painful sensation caused by lack of food.
hydrocarbon the hydrophobic chain "tail" of a fatty acid that contains only carbon and hydrogen atoms.
hydrogenation process in which polyunsaturated vegetable oil is converted to a solid by a commercial process whereby hydrogen is added to the oil; increases the proportion of saturated fatty acids, alters the shape of the fatty acid, and creates *trans* fatty acids.
hydrolysis splitting of a large molecule into smaller water-soluble ones that can be used by cells; the reaction requires water.
hydrolysis reactions cleavage of a compound with the addition of water.
hydrolyzed protein proteins broken down into amino acids.
hydrophilic "water-loving" biomolecules.
hydrophobic "water-fearing" compounds that do not readily combine with water.
hydroxyapatite inorganic component of bones and teeth.
hypercalcemia excessive levels of calcium in the blood.
hypercalciuria high levels of calcium in the urine.
hypercarotenemia excessive levels of carotene in the blood, characterized by yellowing of the palms of the hands and soles of the feet.
hypergeusia heightened taste acuity.
hyperglycemia elevated blood sugar.
hyperkalemia elevated potassium concentrations in the blood.
hyperlipidemia elevated concentrations of any or all of the serum lipids, especially triglycerides or cholesterol or both.
hypernatremia elevated serum sodium level.
hypertension persistent high arterial blood pressure; considered a risk factor for heart and kidney disease, and stroke.
hypervitaminosis A condition resulting from the ingestion of excessive amounts of vitamin A.
hypocalcemia deficient levels of calcium in the blood.
hypodipsia diminished thirst.
hypogeusia loss of taste.
hypoglycemia low blood sugar (less than 70 mg/dL).
hypokalemia low potassium concentrations in the blood.
hyponatremia low 0 sodium levels in the blood.
hypotonic solution having less osmotic pressure than another solution.
iatrogenic adverse condition resulting from treatment (e.g., medications, irradiation, or surgery) by a health care provider.
immune response body's ability to protect itself from destructive bacteria and infection present in the body.
immunocompromised immune response weakened by a disease or pharmacologic agent.
immunoglobulins antibodies, the body's main protection from disease.
incontinence inability to control urinary or fecal excretion.
indispensable amino acids nine amino acids required in the diet.
indirect calorimetry method to estimate metabolic energy by measuring oxygen consumption, carbon dioxide production, respiratory quotient, and resting energy expenditure as a means to assess and manage a patient's nutrition.
innate inborn.
insulin hormone that lowers blood sugar levels.
interesterified fats a new type of customized fat suitable for commercial preparation produced to replace *trans* fats; they affect blood lipids, but not as much as *trans* fats.
interstitial spaces between cells within a tissue or organ.
interstitial fluid fluid located between cells and in body cavities, including joints, pleura, and gastrointestinal tract.
intracellular fluid (ICF) liquid within cells.
intrinsic factor glycoprotein synthesized by parietal cells in the stomach; required for vitamin B_{12} absorption.
ionic bond bond formed between a positively charged metal ion and a negatively charged nonmetal ion.
irradiated foods process of treating food with controlled amounts of ionized radiation to kill the spoilage-causing and disease-causing bacteria and molds in food.
ischemia inadequate blood flow and lack of oxygen because of constriction or obstruction of arteries.
Kaposi sarcoma malignant tumor of blood vessel origin that occurs on skin and oral mucosa.
Kayser-Fleischer ring greenish-yellow pigmented ring encircling the cornea; consists of copper deposits in the Descemet membrane.
keratinized epithelium a protein, main component of epidermis and horny tissues on the skin.
Keshan disease cardiomyopathy (disease of the heart muscle) resulting from deficiency of selenium found in women and children, primarily in Keshan, China.
ketoacidosis accumulation of ketone bodies in the blood.
ketogenic formation of ketone bodies.
ketogenic amino acids certain amino acids degrade into acetyl CoA and are converted into ketone bodies.
ketone bodies soluble forms of lipids that can be used as fuel for the body.
ketones normal products of lipid metabolism in the liver; can be used by muscles for energy if adequate amounts of glucose are available.
ketonuria ketones excreted in the urine as a result of high levels in the blood.
ketosis accumulation of ketone bodies in the blood.
kilocalorie see calorie.
kwashiorkor nutritional deficiency disease due to inadequate protein but adequate calories.
lactovegetarian person who consumes only products from plants and dairy products.
large intestine cecum, colon, and rectum.
leukemia generalized malignant disease characterized by distorted proliferation and development of white blood cells.
leukoplakia white, yellow, or gray thickened patches on mucous membranes of the oral mucosa that cannot be wiped away; appearance may be wrinkled, fissured, nodular, or smooth.
lichen planus a chronic inflammatory disease presenting as an itchy rash, mostly in the oral cavity.
linoleic acid essential fatty acid with 18 carbon atoms and 2 double bonds; also called omega-6 fatty acid.
lipase an enzyme that begins the process of digesting dietary lipids.
lipids compounds that contain carbon, hydrogen, and oxygen, with less oxygen in proportion to hydrogen and carbon than carbohydrates; provide 9 cal/g; a biomolecule that is produced by a living cell or organism.
lipoatrophy loss of fat from specific areas of the body, especially the face, arms, legs, and buttocks.
lipodystrophy rearrangement of fat cells in the face.
lipogenesis process of converting glucose to fats.
lipohypertrophy accumulation of fat on the back or the neck between the shoulders.
lipolysis fat breakdown.
lipoprotein compound lipids composed of triglycerides, phospholipids, and cholesterol combined with protein; produced by the body.
Listeriosis serious infection caused by food contaminated with the bacterium *Listeria monocytogenes*, which principally affects infants and adults with weakened immune systems.
long-chain fatty acids fatty acid that contains 12 or more carbon atoms.
longitudinal fissure slits or wrinkles that extend lengthwise on the tongue.
low birth weight (LBW) weighing less than 5½ lb (2500 g) at birth.
lower esophageal sphincter (LES) group of very strong circular muscle fibers located just above the stomach.
low nutrient density foods having a high fat, alcohol, or sugar content with nominal amounts of vitamins and minerals.
low-quality proteins plant proteins that lack one or more essential amino acids or may lack a proper balance of amino acids; also called incomplete proteins.
lymphatic system comprised of lymph (plasma-like tissue fluid), the lymph nodes, and lymph vessels that are not connected to the blood system; carries fat-soluble nutrients through the thoracic duct and into venous blood at the left subclavian vein.
lysosomes intracellular bodies containing hydrolytic enzymes that promote breakdown of materials taken into the cells.
macrodontia larger than normal teeth.
macroglossia large, protruding tongue.
macronutrients nutrients needed in large amounts by the body to provide energy—carbohydrates, protein, and fats.
macules flat lesions of abnormal color.
manganese madness severe psychotic and neuromuscular symptoms that resemble symptoms of parkinsonism.
marasmus nutritional deficiency caused by inadequate protein and caloric intake.
mastication process in which teeth crush and grind food into smaller pieces to initiate digestion.
masticatory efficiency how well a person prepares the food for swallowing.
materia alba soft-white deposit around the necks of teeth.
mechanically altered diet regular diet altered in consistency during periods when chewing is difficult; a transition between a full liquid diet and a regular diet.
medium-chain fatty acids fatty acid with 6 to 10 carbon atoms.
megaloblastic anemia condition in which red blood cells are extra large in size but fewer in number.
melting point temperature at which a product becomes a liquid.
menopausal gingivostomatitis changes in the oral mucosa resulting in a dry, shiny gingiva that bleeds easily; color ranges from an abnormally pale pink to a deep red may be alleviated with estrogen hormone replacement.
menopause cessation of the menses; occurs when production of the hormones estrogen and progesterone ceases.
meta-analysis systematic analysis that is applied to separate experiments on a related topic involving pooling the data to provide larger study samples that generate information about statistically significant results from the cumulative research on a topic.

metabolism continuous processes whereby living organisms and cells convert nutrients into energy, body structure, and waste.

microflora microorganisms living in the large intestine.

microbiome all microbial cells in the human body, including bacterial, fungal, protozoal, and other single-cell microorganisms.

micrognathia abnormally small jaw.

micronutrients nutrients needed by the body in small amounts (e.g., vitamins and minerals).

microvilli minute cylindrical processes located on the surface of intestinal cells, greatly increasing their absorptive surface area.

mineralization deposition of inorganic minerals on an organic matrix.

mitochondria power source of the cell.

modified barium swallow assessment to measure physiological and anatomical abnormalities associated with swallowing.

molecule the smallest particle of a substance that retains all the properties of the substance.

monomer the smallest repeating unit present in a polymer.

monosaccharides simple sugars containing two to six carbon atoms.

monounsaturated fatty acid (MUFA) fatty acid containing one double bond; found in olive, peanut, and canola oil.

motivational interviewing an educational tool for changing behaviors involving a respectful, collaborative conversation.

mucositis ulcerations and sores of the mucous membrane in the mouth or throat, usually caused by chemotherapy or radiation.

myelin lipid substance that insulates nerve fibers and affects transmission of nerve impulses.

myxedema severe hypothyroidism.

nanotechnology the ability to measure and detect molecular structures nanometers or smaller, allowing determination and manipulation of minute amounts of substances in the food supply.

naturopathy support of the body's inherent ability to maintain and restore health, using noninvasive treatments with minimal use of surgery and drugs.

necrosis degeneration and death of cells.

necrotizing enterocolitis (NEC) condition in neonates with development of cellular dead patches in the intestines interfering with digestion and absorption.

necrotizing ulcerative gingivitis (NUG) oral condition caused by nutritional deficiencies, stress, infection, and depressed immune responses; characterized by erythema and necrosis of the interdental papillae.

neoplasia an abnormal mass of tissue, more frequently referred to as a tumor.

neural tube defects (NTD) birth defects of the skull, brain, and spinal cord.

neutropenia diminished number of neutrophils in the blood; also called leukopenia or agranulocytosis.

nicotinamide adenine dinucleotide (NAD+/NADH) a redox coenzyme derived from niacin

night blindness inability to adapt to bright lights when the eyes are adapted to darkness.

nitrogen balance balance of reactions in which protein substances are broken down and rebuilt.

nocturia excessive urination at night.

noma severe gangrenous process usually manifesting as a small ulcer on the gingiva that becomes necrotic and spreads to the lips, cheek, and tissues covering the jaw; caused by inadequate amounts of protein.

noncariogenic (also see cariostatic) foods and beverages that do not decrease salivary pH below 5.5 and are not a factor in demineralization.

non-celiac gluten sensitivity (NCGS) intestinal and other symptoms related to ingesting gluten-containing foods but without celiac disease or wheat allergy.

nondigestible enzymes in the gastrointestinal tract cannot digest and absorb the substance; plant cells that remain largely intact through the digestive process.

nonessential amino acids (NEAAs) amino acids essential to the body, but not required in the diet. Also known as dispensable amino acids.

nonheme iron iron provided primarily from plant sources and supplements; less efficiently absorbed than heme iron.

nonnutritive sucking sucking on objects that do not provide nutrition (i.e., pacifier, fingers).

normoglycemia normal blood glucose range.

nucleic acid a biomolecule that is produced by a living cell or organism forms the genetic material in the cell; synthesizes cellular protein.

nucleotide building blocks for nucleic acids.

nutrient content claim characterizes the level of a nutrient in a food; terms used are "free," "low," "high," and "reduced."

nutrient-dense containing a high percentage of nutrients in relation to the number of calories provided.

nutrient density amount of nutrients in a food relative to its calories.

nutrients biochemical substances that can be supplied in adequate amounts only from an outside source, normally from food.

nutrigenomics/nutritional genomics scientific study of how foods or their components interact with genes and how individual genetic differences affect prevention or treatment of disease with regard to nutrients (and other naturally occurring compounds).

nutrition study of foods and nutrients and their effect on health, growth, and development.

nutrition and dietetic technician, registered (NDTR) nutritional professional having completed a 2-year degree in a Dietetic Technician Program or a 4-year degree from an approved (Accreditation Council for Education in Nutrition and Dietetics) program.

Nutrition Facts panel label on food products providing nutrient content of food and the number of servings in the package.

nutritional deficiency inadequate amounts of a nutrient available to sustain biochemical functions.

nutritional insult deficiency or excessive amounts of specific nutrients.

nutritionist person who may have a 4-year degree in foods and nutrition and usually works in a public health setting; may be legally defined in some states denoting licensure or certification.

nystagmus involuntary rapid movement of the eyeball.

obesity excess weight for height, with a BMI above 30.0.

observational studies epidemiologic research studies with no type of intervention or experiment.

odontoblasts tissue cells that deposit dentin and form the outer surface of dental pulp adjacent to the dentin; dentin-forming cells.

odynophagia pain associated with swallowing.

oils fats liquid at room temperature.

olfactory nerves receptors for smell.

omega-3 fatty acid unsaturated fatty acid with its first double bond at the third carbon atom from the methyl end; includes eicosapentaenoic acid and docosahexaenoic acid.

omega-6 fatty acid unsaturated fatty acid with its first double bond at the sixth carbon atom from the methyl end; includes linoleic acid and linolenic acid.

organic foods that meet U.S. Department of Agriculture (USDA) standards and do not contain parts of other slaughtered animals, were not given growth hormones or antibiotics, and allowed outdoors; not genetically engineered or irradiated; grown on land that has not been fertilized with sewage sludge or chemical fertilizers or treated with pesticides.

osmoreceptors neurons in the hypothalamus stimulated by increased osmolality, enhancing the release of ADH.

osmosis movement of water from an area of lower solute concentration to a higher solute concentration. When solute concentrations in the body are different, water moves across the membrane.

osteoblasts assists in production of collagen; helps in building and reformation of new bone.

osteocalcin vitamin K–dependent, bone-specific protein that is released into blood from resorbed bone matrix and originating osteoblasts.

osteoclasts resorbed bone in microscopic cavities.

osteodystrophy abnormal bone development, similar to osteomalacia.

osteoid young bone that has not undergone calcification.

osteomalacia softening of bones.

osteonecrosis a condition in which bone dies or undergoes necrosis.

osteoporosis age-related disorder characterized by decreased bone mass, causing bones to be more susceptible to fracture.

osteosclerosis increased bone formation resulting in reduced marrow spaces and increased radiopacity.

overjet horizontal projection of upper teeth beyond the lower teeth.

overweight excess accumulation of body fat or a BMI between 25.0 and 29.9.

ovolactovegetarian vegetarian diet supplemented with milk, eggs, and cheese.

ovovegetarian type of vegetarian whose diet consists of foods from plants with the addition of eggs (no meat, poultry, fish, or dairy products).

oxidation process of hydrolyzing triglycerides into two-carbon entities to enter the TCA (Krebs) cycle for energy production.

oxidation-reduction reaction a chemical reaction that can convert functional groups into other functional groups.

oxidative phosphorylation a metabolic process that synthesizes phosphoric bonds from the energy released by the oxidation of various substrates.

pancreatic enzymes enzymes that hydrolyze carbohydrates, protein, and fats.

papillae epithelium surrounding taste buds; papillae appear on the tongue as little red dots, or raised bumps, and are most prevalent on the dorsal epithelium.

parasympathetic nerves division of autonomic nervous system.

Parkinson disease progressive neurologic condition characterized by involuntary muscle tremors, muscular weakness, rigidity, stooped posture, and peculiar gait.

parotitis inflammation of the parotid gland.

passive diffusion passage of a permeable substance from a more concentrated solution to an area of lower concentration.

pathogenic harmful.

pedometer instrument used by a walker; measures approximate distance walked by recording steps.

pellagra deficiency resulting from inadequate intake of niacin, which results in the four Ds (diarrhea, dermatitis, dementia, and death).

peptide bond a strong covalent bond that forms polypeptides.

periapical area around the root apex.

perimenopause time leading up to menopause, in which the ovaries begin to shut down, making less amounts of certain hormones, such as estrogen and progesterone.
periodontal disease infections and lesions affecting tissues that form the attachment apparatus of a tooth or teeth.
periodontitis inflammatory process involving interproximal and marginal areas of two or more adjacent teeth.
periodontium hard and soft tissues that surround and support teeth: gingiva, alveolar mucosa, cementum, periodontal ligament, and alveolar bone.
peripheral edema in the extremities, such as the legs and feet.
peristalsis involuntary rhythmic waves of contraction traveling the length of the alimentary tract.
pernicious anemia megaloblastic anemia with a decrease in red blood cells; occurs when the body cannot properly absorb vitamin B_{12} in the gastrointestinal tract.
petechia (*pl.* petechiae) small, pinpoint, round red spot caused by submucous hemorrhage.
phantom taste dysgeusia without identifiable taste stimuli.
phenylketonuria genetic disorder characterized by inability to metabolize the amino acid phenylalanine.
phospholipid fat-related substances that contain phosphorus, fatty acids, and a nitrogen-containing base; constituent of every cell.
photosynthesis compounding or building up of chemical substances under the influence of light; green plants use chlorophyll and energy from sunlight to produce carbohydrates from water and carbon dioxide and to liberate oxygen.
physical activity any body movement produced by skeletal muscles resulting in energy expenditure.
physical fitness ability to perform physical activity.
phytochemical biologically active substances found in plants.
pica abnormal consumption of specific food and nonfood substances, such as dirt, clay, starch, or ice; occurs more frequently during pregnancy.
plant sterols essential components of plant membranes resembling the chemical structure of cholesterol that perform similar cellular functions in plants; naturally present in small quantities in fruits, vegetables, nuts, seeds, legumes, and oils.
plaque biofilm well-organized community of bacteria embedded in a slime layer that adheres tenaciously to tooth surfaces, restorations, and prosthetic appliances.
plethora red appearance resulting from an excess of blood.
pocketed foods foods retained in the mouth, especially in the vestibule.
polycythemia sustained increase in number of red blood cells; may result in iron-deficiency anemia.
polymer a large molecule containing numerous repeating units.
polyols sugar alcohols formed from or converted to sugar; sorbitol, xylitol, and mannitol are present in the body or added to foods.
polypeptide several amino acids joined together.
polypharmacy use of at least 5 or more prescription medications.
polysaccharides (complex carbohydrates) sugars containing more than 12 carbon atoms.
polyunsaturated fatty acid (PUFA) fatty acid containing two or more double bonds.
portal circulation passage of nutrients from the gastrointestinal tract and spleen through the portal vein to the liver.
postabsorptive state time when digestive and absorptive processes are minimal, not affecting the basal metabolic rate.
ppb parts per billion.
prebiotics nondigestible food ingredients having beneficial effects on the host by stimulating growth or activity of probiotics in the colon.
precursor substance from which another biologically active substance is formed.
preeclampsia development of hypertension as a result of pregnancy or the influence of recent pregnancy; usually occurs after the 20th week of pregnancy.
premature born before the state of maturity, occurring with a gestational age (length of pregnancy) of less than 37 weeks.
primigravida woman in her first pregnancy.
probiotics products containing live bacteria that aid in restoring and maintaining an intestinal balance of healthful bacteria.
prognathism overgrowth of the mandible.
prostaglandins hormone-like compounds derived from unsaturated fatty acids.
protease an enzyme that begins the process of digesting dietary proteins.
protein a biomolecule that is produced by a living cell or organism; chains of amino acids joined by peptide linkage; essential for physiological structure and function; contains nitrogen.
protein-energy malnutrition (PEM) nutritional deficiency condition caused by consistently consuming inadequate amounts of energy and protein.
protein-sparing energy source that allows protein to be used for building and repairing (i.e., fats and carbohydrates).
proteolytic enzymes enzymes that hydrolyze proteins.
prothrombin first stage in forming an insoluble clot; a deficiency results in impaired blood coagulation.
purging use of laxatives, enemas, emetics, diuretics, or exercise to negate effects of overindulgence.
purpura condition characterized by hemorrhaging into tissues, under the skin, and through the mucous membranes; the three types are petechiae, ecchymoses, and hematomas.
purulent exudates consisting of or containing pus; generally the result of inflammation.
pyogenic producing pus.
qualified health claims statements on food labels that are supported by some evidence but do not meet the scientific standard; must be accompanied by a disclaimer specified by the U.S. Food and Drug Administration (FDA).
quality of life an individual's perception of one's position in life in the context of the culture and value systems and in relation to the person's goals, expectations, standards, and concerns.
quercetin bioflavonoid reported to energize muscles (unsubstantiated claim).
radical group of atoms forming a fundamental constituent of a molecule.
R-binder protein produced by salivary glands necessary for absorption of vitamin B_{12}.
Recommended Dietary Allowances (RDAs) specific amounts of essential nutrients that adequately meet the known nutrient needs of 97% to 98% of healthy Americans.
redox coenzymes coenzymes that capture and transfer electrons.
reduction a gain of electrons, a decrease in charge, a loss of oxygen atoms, or a gain of hydrogen atoms.
registered dietitian-nutritionist (RDN) person who has completed a bachelor's degree in foods and nutrition with training in normal and clinical nutrition, food science, and food service management, and advanced training in medical nutrition therapy.
remineralization restoration or return of calcium, phosphates, and other minerals into areas that have been damaged, as by incipient caries, abrasion, or erosion.
remodeling resorption and reformation of bone.
renal failure inability of the kidneys to maintain normal function of excreting toxic waste materials.
renal osteodystrophy changes in bones associated with renal failure.
renin enzyme synthesized in the kidney; released in response to low blood pressure.
residue total amount of fecal solids, including undigested or unabsorbed food, and metabolic (bile pigments) and bacterial products.
respiration a process in which animals hydrolyze glucose into carbon dioxide and water, and plants use these products for photosynthesis.
retinoic acid form of vitamin A that can be produced by the body and can be made in the laboratory; used in combination with other drugs to treat leukemia and acne.
retrognathic mandible posterior to its normal relationship with other facial positions.
rhodopsin light-sensitive pigment that allows the eye to adjust to changes in light.
rickets condition resulting from vitamin D deficiency, especially in infancy and childhood; causes disturbance of normal bone formation.
sarcopenia progressive loss of muscle mass, strength, and function due to the aging process.
satiety feeling of fullness.
saturated fatty acid fatty acid that does not contain any double bonds.
scorbutic similar to scurvy.
sealants clear or shaded plastic material applied to the occlusal surfaces of permanent teeth.
secretory immunoglobulin antibody present in oral, nasal, intestinal, and other mucosal secretions; provides the first line of defense in the oral cavity.
sensory neuropathy impairment of the ability to feel.
severe early childhood caries (SECC) see early childhood caries (ECC).
severe sensory neuropathy impairment of the ability to sense touch, vibration, temperature, and pinprick.
short-chain fatty acid fatty acid that contains fewer than six carbon atoms.
side chain (R group) the part of the amino acid that varies to form 22 different amino acids that varies from one amino acid to another.
signs objective evidence of disease perceptible to the clinician.
silver diamine fluoride (SDF) colorless ammonia solution containing silver and fluoride ions. The silver ion acts as an antibacterial agent. SDF is showing to be effective in inhibiting demineralization.
small intestinal bacterial overgrowth (SIBO) impaired gastric and intestinal emptying due to overuse of probiotics, causing excessive bacteria in the gastrointestinal tract, resulting in nausea, vomiting, bloating, flatulence, and diarrhea.
small intestine duodenum, jejunum, and ileum.
soluble dietary fiber dietary fibers that become viscous (sticky, thick) in solution (oats, legumes, psyllium seeds).
solutes dissolved substances in fluid.
solvent fluid in which substances are dissolved.
sphincter muscles any of the ringlike muscles encircling an opening that is able to contract to close the opening, such as the sphincter pylori between the stomach and small intestine.
spices botanical seasonings from seeds, berries, fruit, bark, or roots.

squamous metaplasia change in oral cavity cell structures with keratin production in the duct cells of salivary glands, caused by vitamin A deficiency.
stable nutrients nutrients of which more than 85% is retained during processing and storage.
stannous containing tin.
stomatitis inflammation of the oral mucosa.
Streptococcus mutans bacteria found in dental plaque biofilm.
structural lipids fats that are a component of cell membranes, tooth enamel, and dentin (e.g., phospholipids).
structural polysaccharides see dietary fiber.
substrate the substance acted upon and changed by an enzyme.
suckling process the infant uses to extract breastmilk by moving the jaws back and forth and squeezing with the gingiva; this encourages mandibular development by strengthening the jaw muscle.
sugar alcohols formed from or converted to sugar; also called polyols.
suppuration discharge or formation of pus.
symbiotic intimate relationship of two dissimilar organisms in a mutually beneficial relationship; for example, prebiotics stimulate growth or activity of beneficial bacteria from probiotics in the gut.
sympathetic nerves exhibiting a mutual relationship between two organ systems or parts of the body.
symptoms subjective evidence of abnormality as perceived by the patient.
synergistic effect for example, combined sweeteners yield a sweeter taste than each sweetener alone.
syrup of ipecac cardiotoxic drug induces vomiting after accidental ingestion of a chemical or poison.
systematic reviews reliable information based on all relevant published and unpublished evidence, selecting studies for inclusion, assessing the quality of each study, then compiling the findings and interpreting them to present a balanced and impartial summary while defining limitations of the evidence.
systemic condition disease or disorder that affects the whole body.
tachycardia rapid heartbeat.
taste buds receptors for sense of taste.
taurine an amino acid with antioxidant properties.
temporomandibular disorder (TMD) group of symptoms that cause pain and dysfunction in the head, face, and temporomandibular region.
tensional forces actions in which pressure stretches or strains the structure.
tetany neuromuscular disorder of uncontrollable muscular cramps and tremors.
thermic effect increase in metabolism that occurs during digestion, absorption, and metabolism of energy-yielding nutrients.
thermogenesis process of heat production in warm-blooded organisms; occurs when the metabolic rate increases above normal, influenced by many factors, including digestion of food and activity.
thiaminase active enzyme found naturally in foods (e.g., raw fish) inactivating thiamin.
thromboembolism plug or clot in a blood vessel formed by coagulation of blood.
thrombus blood clot.
tinnitus noise in the ears, which sometimes may be heard by others.
tocopherols name given to vitamin E and compounds chemically related to it.
tocotrienols component of vitamin E.
Tolerable Upper Intake level (UL) maximum daily level of nutrient intake that probably would not cause adverse health effects or toxic effects for most individuals.
total fiber sum of dietary fiber and added fiber.
total parenteral nutrition (TPN) nutrition provided to a patient with impaired digestive tract; special liquid food mixture administered into the blood through a vein.
toxoplasmosis infection caused by a parasite; gravida may be symptom-free because the immune system prevents the parasite from causing illness, but the infection is passed on to the fetus.
trabecular bone internal bone.
***trans* fatty acid** unsaturated fatty acid that is usually monounsaturated; may be formed during hydrogenation, in which the hydrogen ions rotate so that the hydrogens stick out on opposite sides of the bond.
***trans* isomer** the geometric arrangement of hydrogen atoms on opposite sides of the plane of a C=C double bond
transferrin serum protein transports iron in the blood.
tricarboxylic acid cycle (TCA cycle) the central metabolic pathway that produces energy, also known as the citric acid cycle or Krebs cycle.
triglycerides major form of lipid in the body and food composed of three fatty acids bonded to glycerol, an alcohol.
24-hour recall a method of assessing everything a person has consumed (foods, supplements, and beverages) in a 24-hour period; may or may not reflect a typical day.
umami flavorful, pleasant taste detected in foods containing L-glutamine present in amino acids and proteins.
unqualified health claims statements allowed on food labels by FDA; must be supported by qualified experts agreeing that scientific evidence is available determining a relationship between a nutrient and a specific disease.
unsaturated fatty acid (UFA) of or related to an organic compound, especially fatty acids, containing one or more double or triple bonds between carbons.
Upper Level (UL) see tolerable upper intake level.
uremic condition in which too much urea and other nitrous waste products are present in the blood.
valves/sphincter muscles circular muscles regulating the flow of bolus between different segments of the gastrointestinal tract.
variants different forms of genes.
varicose veins unnaturally and permanently distended veins.
vegan person who eats only plant foods.
vegetarian person who purposefully does not eat meat (beef, pork, poultry, seafood, and the flesh of any animal, and sometimes animal by-products).
very low food security at times food intake of household members is reduced and normal eating patterns disrupted because of insufficient funds or other resources to obtain food.
vitamins general term for numerous related organic, noncaloric substances present in foods in small amounts.
wheat allergy adverse immunologic reaction to wheat proteins.
whole grains grains and grain products made from the entire grain seed, usually called the kernel (consisting of bran, germ, and endosperm); a cracked, crushed, or flaked kernel must retain nearly the same relative proportions of bran, germ, and endosperm as the original grain to be called whole grain.
xeroderma dry, rough, scaly skin.
xerophthalmia abnormally dry and thickened surface of the conjunctiva and cornea of the eye.
xerostomia dryness of the mouth resulting from inadequate salivary secretion.
xylitol sugar alcohol used as a sugar substitute; considered a nutritive sweetener; provides four calories per gram.

Answers to Nutritional Quotient Questions

Chapter 1: Overview of Healthy Eating Habits

1. False. No single food contains all the essential nutrients in amounts needed for optimal health.
2. False. Only consumption of added sugars should be reduced. Naturally occurring sugars, especially from milk and fruits, are desirable.
3. True.
4. False. DRIs are a set of nutrient-based reference values that include the Estimated Average Requirements, Recommended Dietary Allowances, Adequate Intakes, and Tolerable Upper Intake Levels intended to be used for planning and assessing diets of healthy Americans and Canadians.
5. True.
6. False. Three to five servings are recommended for vegetables and two to four servings are recommended for fruit.
7. True.
8. False. Sugar is implicated as a cause of dental caries but not in other major diseases, such as hypertension, cardiovascular disease, or diabetes mellitus.
9. True.
10. False. The nutrients that provide energy are fats, carbohydrates, and proteins.

Chapter 2: Concepts in Biochemistry

1. False. A hydrolysis reaction requires H_2O as a reactant to degrade molecules. A condensation reaction produces H_2O as a product.
2. False. Amino acids are the building blocks of proteins. Nucleotides are the building blocks of nucleic acids.
3. True.
4. False. Sucrose is a disaccharide containing glucose and fructose.
5. True.
6. True.
7. True.
8. False. Catabolism involves the oxidation of carbohydrates into CO_2 and H_2O. Oxidation is the loss of electrons. The electrons released in catabolism are captured by NADH and $FADH_2$ and used to synthesize ATP in oxidative phosphorylation.
9. False. Insulin is a signal of the "fed" state and is secreted when blood glucose levels are high. It activates metabolic pathways that will lower blood glucose levels, like glycolysis and glycogen biosynthesis, not glycogen degradation.
10. True.

Chapter 3: the Alimentary Canal: Digestion and Absorption

1. True.
2. False. Gurgling sounds, caused by air and fluid in the normal abdomen, indicate peristalsis is occurring.
3. False. Absorption occurs primarily in the small intestine.
4. False. Long-chain triglycerides enter the lymphatic system; short-chain and medium-chain triglycerides enter the portal circulation.
5. True.
6. False. Door-like mechanisms between the digestive segments are called valves or sphincter muscles.
7. True.
8. False. Villi are located in the small intestine.
9. True.
10. True.

Chapter 4: Carbohydrate: the Efficient Fuel

1. False. The FDA has labeled raw sugar as unfit for direct use as a food or a food ingredient because of the impurities it contains.
2. True.
3. False. Oral bacteria are unable to metabolize xylitol, which is a calorie-containing sugar alcohol.
4. False. The desire for sweetness is not considered an acquired taste because newborn infants exhibit a preference for it.
5. True.
6. True.
7. False. Excessive caloric intake leads to obesity, whether from carbohydrates, proteins, fats, or alcohol.
8. False. Sucrose is table sugar.
9. False. Many other factors, including consumption of other fermentable carbohydrates, contribute to development of caries.
10. True.

Chapter 5: Protein: the Cellular Foundation

1. True.
2. False. Malnourished children are highly susceptible to dental caries possibly related to alterations in the structure of tooth crowns and diminished salivary flow, or changes in saliva composition.
3. False. Gelatin does not contain all the indispensable amino acids.
4. False. The protein requirement for an older adult is at least equal to that of a young adult and may be increased.

5. False. Adequate amounts of protein are needed for development of healthy teeth, but increasing protein beyond the RDA would not have any effect on tooth enamel.
6. False. Excessive amounts of protein without decreasing intake of other energy-containing nutrients may lead to an increase in fat stores and possibly leading to obesity.
7. True.
8. False. Marasmus is caused because of protein and calorie deficiency.
9. True.
10. True.

Chapter 6: Lipids: the Condensed Energy

1. False. The overall average of fat intake is important with respect to total energy intake; but foods such as margarine and oils, which are 100% fat, can be used safely in the diet.
2. False. As an antioxidant, vitamin E protects the oil to which it is added to some degree; however, in doing so, vitamin E may be inactivated, so it cannot be used by the body.
3. True.
4. False. The AMDR for fat is estimated to be 20% to 35% of energy intake for adults.
5. False. Bananas contain a trace of fat; avocados are 88% fat. However, they are both plant products, so they do not contain any cholesterol.
6. False. All fats produce 9 kcal/g.
7. True.
8. False. Even though they are nutritious foods, for most Americans, their use may need to be limited because of their high concentration of calories.
9. True.
10. True.

Chapter 7: Use of the Energy Nutrients: Metabolism and Balance

1. True.
2. True.
3. False. BMR stands for basal metabolic rate, which is the amount of energy needed to maintain involuntary physiologic functions.
4. True.
5. True.
6. False. Hunger is the physiologic drive to eat, whereas appetite implies a desire for specific types of food.
7. False. Fats are stored by the body for energy, but they must first be converted into a form that the body can use. Glycogen stores, which depend on carbohydrate intake, are readily available for energy.
8. True.
9. True.
10. False. Only fats, carbohydrates, proteins, and alcohol provide energy (cals).

Chapter 8: Vitamins Required for Calcified Structures

1. True.
2. True.
3. True.
4. True.
5. False. Retinol is obtained from animal foods; beta carotene is found in fruits and vegetables.
6. True.
7. True.
8. False. A deficiency of vitamin D causes rickets.
9. False. Vitamin K is essential for blood clotting; vitamin D functions to regulate blood calcium and phosphorus levels.
10. True.

Chapter 9: Minerals Essential for Calcified Structures

1. True.
2. False. Many nutrients work together in building strong healthy bones, including protein, calcium, phosphorus, magnesium, fluoride, and vitamins C and D.
3. True.
4. True.
5. False. Based on the DRIs, teenagers need 1300 mg of calcium. If milk is the only calcium source, a teen would need to consume 4 1/2 cups.
6. False. Fluoridation of community water supplies is the most effective method of preventing dental caries.
7. False. Although many women take calcium supplements to prevent osteoporosis, they are not essential for all women. Excessive calcium intake may increase the risk of CHD and symptoms including dizziness, kidney stone formation, and irregular heartbeat.
8. True.
9. False. Caffeine decreases calcium absorption.
10. False. Bottled waters vary in fluoride content.

Chapter 10: Nutrients Present in Calcified Structures

1. False. The National Academy of Medicine has established ULs for copper, manganese, and molybdenum, but not for chromium.
2. True.
3. True.
4. False. Although the evidence is not conclusive, some research studies suggest a possible association between aluminum toxicity and Alzheimer disease.
5. True.
6. False. Unrefined foods generally provide more trace minerals.
7. False. Aluminum is cariostatic, especially in combination with fluoride.
8. True.
9. False. Sugar is not a good source of any nutrients except calories. Good sources of chromium include meats, whole-grain cereals, mushrooms, green beans, and broccoli.
10. False. Selenium supplements are not recommended because selenium can be toxic.

Chapter 11: Vitamins Required for Oral Soft Tissues and Salivary Glands

1. True.
2. False. Vitamin D is called the sunshine vitamin because sun facilitates the body's production of vitamin D; vitamin B_6 is also called pyridoxine, pyridoxal, and pyridoxamine.
3. False. Beriberi is caused by a thiamin deficiency; niacin deficiency causes pellagra.
4. True.
5. False. Flushing and intestinal disturbances are symptoms of niacin toxicity. No toxicity symptoms have been observed for thiamin.
6. True.
7. True.
8. False. Liver, leafy vegetables, legumes, grapefruit, and oranges are rich sources of folate.
9. True.
10. True.

Chapter 12: Water and Minerals Required for Oral Soft Tissues and Salivary Glands

1. True.
2. True.
3. True.
4. True.
5. False. The National Academy of Medicine has established an AI for total fluid (beverages, water, and food) requirements to be 15 to 16 cups per day for men and 11 to 12 cups per day for women.
6. False. The minimum requirement for sodium is 500 mg per day for adults, but no RDA has been established for sodium. The *Dietary Guidelines* recommend less than 2300 mg sodium daily.
7. True.
8. False. Potassium is principally within the cells (intracellular).
9. True.
10. False. Oral pallor is a sign of iron-deficiency anemia.

Chapter 13: Nutritional Requirements Affecting Oral Health in Women

1. False. These cravings do not reflect natural instincts for required nutrients.
2. True.
3. False. If the diet is deficient in calcium, the fetal calcium requirements would be met first, but some of the calcium may come from her bones, not from her teeth.
4. False. Although she is "eating for two," normal energy requirements are not doubled. Depending on the prepregnancy weight, approximately 300 cal more than her usual caloric requirement are needed during the second and third trimesters.
5. True.
6. False. Iron and folate are usually the nutrients needing supplementation.
7. True.
8. False. Breast milk is normally thin and is nutritionally adequate.
9. False. The more often an infant nurses, the more milk is produced. Milk production is most active during infant sucking.
10. True.

Chapter 14: Nutritional Requirements During Growth and Development and Eating Habits Affecting Oral Health

1. True.
2. False. Fluoride supplements are not recommended for infants before age 6 months even though breast milk and artificial breast milk are low in fluoride.
3. False. Solid foods are introduced between 4 and 6 months of age, not at 6 weeks.
4. False. The previous recommendation to withhold foods that most commonly cause allergies until after 12 months of age has been replaced with new recommendations to introduce high allergenic foods (including peanuts) between 4 and 6 months of age along with introduction of other solid foods. However, they are a choking hazard; thus, small nuts should be withheld or closely monitored until the molars erupt.
5. True.
6. True.
7. False. Breastfed infants need a supplement of 200 IU vitamin D beginning during the first 2 months to prevent rickets.
8. False. Suckling, as occurs when extracting milk from the breast, encourages maximum development of the genetically defined jaw and chin; breastfed infants are less likely to develop malocclusion.
9. False. Milk and dairy products are essential components of children's and adolescent's diets because of the high calcium requirement to increase bone mineral density and other important components of these products.
10. False. Toddlers and children need snacks because of their high energy needs; however, wholesome snacks (e.g., cheese cubes, fresh fruit, raw vegetable sticks, milk, or yogurt) that do not promote tooth decay are recommended.

Chapter 15: Nutritional Requirements for Older Adults and Eating Habits Affecting Oral Health

1. False. Because of changes in nutrient requirements secondary to physiologic changes, the National Academy of Medicine has developed DRIs for individuals 51 to 70 years old and older than 70 years.
2. True.
3. True.
4. False. The texture for edentulous patients is determined by their own preferences.
5. False. Dehydration is a frequent occurrence in elderly individuals for many reasons—impaired homeostatic mechanisms, decreased thirst sensation, inability of the kidney to concentrate urine, changes in functional status, side effects of medications, and mobility disorders.
6. True.
7. False. Iron intake requirement is lower after menopause.
8. True.
9. False. Although it is highly likely that an elderly individual may benefit from taking a dietary supplement, toxicity or nutrient imbalances may occur. An older individual should consult a health care provider before deciding to take a vitamin supplement.

10. False. Physical activity can help ameliorate some chronic health problems, improve physiological well-being, and relieve symptoms of depression and anxiety.

Chapter 16: Food Factors Affecting Health

1. True.
2. False. Patterns and attitudes internalized during childhood promote a sense of stability and security for older patients.
3. False. No culture has ever been known to make food choices solely on the basis of nutritional values of food. The factors that seem to predominate in food choices are cultural and economic.
4. False. Only about 10% of the American food dollar is spent on food.
5. False. Fad diets may be physically harmless, but they are usually not based on sound nutritional principles.
6. False. Scientific research to date has not shown any nutritional benefits from the use of organically grown foods.
7. False. Although some food processing is detrimental to the nutritive value of foods, the goal of food processing is to maintain optimum qualities of color, flavor, texture, and nutritive value.
8. True.
9. True.
10. True.

Chapter 17: Effects of Systemic Disease on Nutritional Status and Oral Health

1. True.
2. True.
3. False. Supplements for anemia should not be prescribed without the results of blood testing to determine the type of anemia. High intakes of iron could possibly complicate the situation.
4. False. Because of the various considerations involved in constructing a meal plan and lifestyle changes for a patient with diabetes, the patient must be referred to a certified diabetes educator.
5. True.
6. True.
7. False. Kaposi sarcoma is a tumor that occurs frequently in immunocompromised patients.
8. True.
9. False. Although a patient with an eating disorder should be referred to a physician or an eating disorder program, it is the dental hygienist's responsibility to approach the patient with the objective findings.
10. False. Patients with bulimia are generally of normal weight or sometimes above recommended body weight.

Chapter 18: Nutritional Aspects of Dental Caries: Causes, Prevention, and Treatment

1. False. A combination of diet, host, environment, and saliva are necessary for initiation of dental decay.
2. True.
3. True.
4. True.
5. False. Sugar alcohols are fermented slowly by oral bacteria, and they are noncariogenic. Xylitol is cariostatic because of its ability to inhibit production of *Streptococcus mutans*.
6. False. An acid environment is required to demineralize a tooth; a cariogenic food causes the plaque pH to decrease to less than 5.5.
7. False. It is the least important factor to consider. Identifying frequency of intake, physical form, and spacing of food within a day or meal would provide a more accurate assessment.
8. True.
9. False. Although the RDAs provide a lot of factual information, they are too overwhelming for most patients. *MyPlate* and *Dietary Guidelines for Americans* provide practical and general nutrition information relevant to preventing dental decay and improving overall health.
10. False. Information alone does not guarantee a behavioral change.

Chapter 19: Nutritional Aspects of Gingivitis and Periodontal Disease

1. True.
2. False. Indirectly, firm, fibrous foods reduce the amount of bacterial plaque biofilm by stimulating salivary flow, which promotes oral clearance of food and lessens food retention.
3. False. A nutrient deficiency can be a contributing factor to gingivitis, but local irritants (plaque biofilm and calculus) must be present. The inflammation can be exaggerated by a nutrient deficiency and by reduced resistance and recovery time.
4. True.
5. False. A patient may interpret this advice as condoning ice cream, gelatin, and chicken noodle soup, which would not provide enough nutrients or calories for quick recovery. The dental hygienist should provide a specific list of nutrient-dense foods for the patient to purchase before the periodontal surgery.
6. True.
7. True.
8. True.
9. True.
10. False. If surgery is indicated for a periodontal patient, optimally, the nutritional assessment and counseling should be completed before the procedure to increase nutrient reserves that would expedite the recovery period.

Chapter 20: Nutritional Aspects of Alterations in the Oral Cavity

1. False. Although root surface caries can be a complication of xerostomia, other causes are possible, such as frequent intake of hard candy. Also, a complete and thorough assessment of the patient is essential. No single factor is adequate to diagnose the presence, extent, or cause of root caries. An inaccurate evaluation can lead to inappropriate recommendations.
2. False. Although xerostomia is a common complaint in an older adult, the changes in saliva in a healthy older individual are minimal. Xerostomia has been strongly associated with multiple factors, such as use of medications, one or more systemic diseases, and radiation, all of which are common to this population.
3. True.

4. False. Root caries appear on the root surface, in areas of gingival recession. This condition is seen more often in older adults who have experienced periodontal disease or toothbrush trauma.
5. False. Spongy cancellous bone is the major component of alveolar bone.
6. True.
7. True.
8. True.
9. False. It is important to have nutrient dense foods available, but in different consistencies. A full liquid diet progressing to a mechanically altered diet and on to a regular diet would allow the patient to adjust to swallowing, chewing and biting with the new appliance.
10. True.

Chapter 21: Nutritional Assessment and Education for Dental Patients

1. False. Although the health and dental histories provide valuable information, they are not enough to determine the patient's nutritional status. Other evaluation tools include clinical assessment and dietary intake.
2. False. Clinical oral examinations detect physical signs and symptoms of many nutrient deficiencies. However, deficiencies generally do not appear until an advanced state exists. An oral examination, and dental histories could be used as an adjunct in identifying potential nutritional deficiencies.
3. True.
4. True.
5. False. Dietary counseling must be documented and other staff members informed about the nutritional counseling for consistency and reinforcement of the information at future appointments.
6. False. Changing a dietary habit is difficult and requires a meal plan and lifestyle behavior changes tailored to meet the patient's needs. A thorough assessment identifies many factors that should be considered. Active involvement of the patient in establishing a meal pattern enhances compliance.
7. False. The dental hygienist is responsible for providing information and guiding the patient to make healthier decisions. Active participation, problem solving, and decision making allow for greater compliance. The patient should highlight the fermentable carbohydrates.
8. False. Changing food habits is very difficult. The first attempt established by the dental hygienist and patient may not have been successful, and other alternatives may need to be established. Follow-up is an essential component of the nutritional counseling process.
9. True.
10. True.
11. False. The patient's behavior is "explored" by building rapport and not being confronted; the patent is then "guided" by the dental professional and the patient "chooses" the course of treatment.
12. True.

Index

Page numbers followed by "*f*" indicate figures, "*t*" indicate tables, and "*b*" indicate boxes.

E

F